Anatomical Directions

DIRECTIONAL TERMS	DEFINITION	EXAMPLE OF USAGE
Left	To the left of body (not *your* left, the subject's)	The stomach is to the *left* of the liver.
Right	To the right of the body or structure being studied	The *right* kidney is damaged.
Lateral	Toward the side; away from the midsagittal plane	The eyes are *lateral* to the nose.
Medial	Toward the midsagittal plane; away from the side	The eyes are *medial* to the ears.
Anterior	Toward the front of the body	The nose is on the *anterior* of the head.
Posterior	Toward the back (rear)	The heel is *posterior* to the head.
Superior	Toward the top of the body	The shoulders are *superior* to the hips.
Inferior	Toward the bottom of the body	The stomach is *inferior* to the heart.
Dorsal	Along (or toward) the vertebral surface of the body	Her scar is along the *dorsal* surface.
Ventral	Along (toward) the belly surface of the body	The navel is on the *ventral* surface.
Caudad (caudal)	Toward the tail	The neck is *caudad* to the skull.
Cephalad	Toward the head	The neck is *cephalad* to the tail.
Proximal	Toward the trunk (describes relative position in a limb or other appendage)	The joint is *proximal* to the toenail.
Distal	Away from the trunk or point of attachment	The hand is *distal* to the elbow.
Visceral	Toward an internal organ; away from the outer wall (describes positions inside a body cavity)	This organ is covered with the *visceral* layer of the membrane.
Parietal	Toward the wall; away from the internal structures	The abdominal cavity is lined with the *parietal* peritoneal membrane.
Deep	Toward the inside of a part; away from the surface	The thigh muscles are *deep* to the skin.
Superficial	Toward the surface of a part; away from the inside	The skin is a *superficial* organ.
Medullary	Refers to an inner region, or medulla	The *medullary* portion contains nerve tissue.
Cortical	Refers to an outer region, or cortex	The *cortical* area produces hormones.

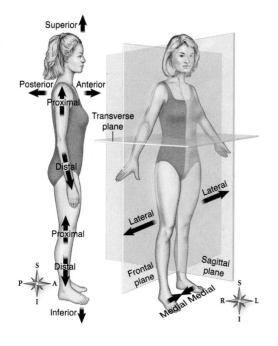

To make the reading of anatomical figures a little easier, an anatomical compass is used throughout this book. On many figures, you will notice a small compass rosette similar to those on geographical maps. Rather than being labeled N, S, E, and W, the anatomical rosette is labeled with abbreviated anatomical directions.

A = Anterior	**P** (opposite A) = Posterior
D = Distal	**P** (opposite D) = Proximal
I = Inferior	**S** = Superior
L (opposite M) = Lateral	**M** = Medial
L (opposite R) = Left	**R** = Right

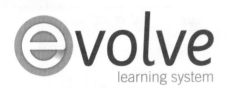

evolve
learning system

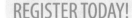

To access your Student Resources, visit the web address below:

http://evolve.elsevier.com/ThibodeauPatton/humanbody/

Register today and gain access to:

- **Appendixes**
  Supplemental information helps you become more familiar with pathological conditions, medical terminology and abbreviations, and clinical laboratory values.

- **Audio Chapter Summaries**
  Downloadable MP3s allow you to listen to chapter summaries anywhere, making your A&P studies completely portable!

- **Audio Glossary**
  Definitions and audio pronunciations of more than 1000 terms from the *Anatomy & Physiology* glossary improve your vocabulary comprehension.

- **Body Spectrum Electronic Coloring Book**
  With more than 80 illustrations that you can color online or offline, this provides a fun and effective way to reinforce elements from the textbook.

- **Frequently Asked Questions**
  Common questions related to the material covered in the textbook with answers from the authors guide you through difficult A&P topics.

- **Matching Exercises**
  Matching exercises with answers provided help you review the important terms covered in the text.

- **Online Tutoring**
  Online help from expert mentors gives you support with any questions you may have regarding anatomy and physiology.

- **Panorama of Anatomy and Physiology**
  Software program filled with interactive exercises, quizzes, and activities that reinforce key anatomy and physiology concepts.

- **Student Post-Test Questions**
  Multiple-choice questions with instant scoring help you review important content and gauge your comprehension of topics.

- **WebLinks**
  A carefully selected set of websites, organized by chapter, supplement the content of the book.

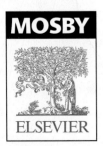

MOSBY

ELSEVIER

THE HUMAN BODY
IN HEALTH & DISEASE

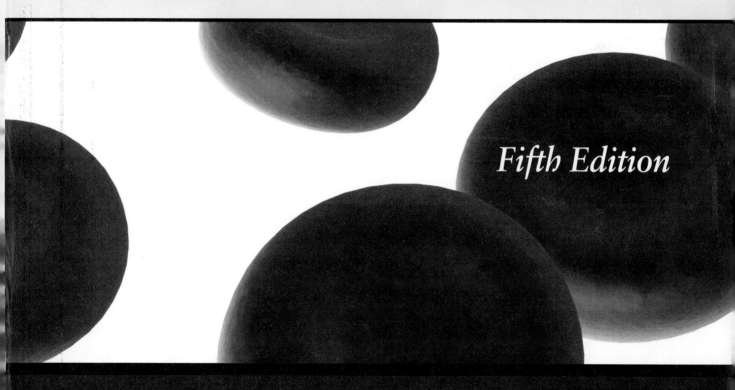

Fifth Edition

GARY A. THIBODEAU, PhD
Chancellor Emeritus and Professor Emeritus of Biology
University of Wisconsin–River Falls
River Falls, Wisconsin

MOSBY

ELSEVIER

KEVIN T. PATTON, PhD
Professor of Life Sciences
St. Charles Community College
Cottleville, Missouri

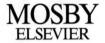
MOSBY
ELSEVIER

11830 Westline Industrial Drive
St. Louis, Missouri 63146

THE HUMAN BODY IN HEALTH & DISEASE   ISBN: 978-0-323-05492-8

Library of Congress Cataloging in Publication Data
Thibodeau, Gary A., 1938-
  The human body in health & disease / Gary A. Thibodeau, Kevin T. Patton. -- 5th ed.
     p. ; cm.
  Includes index.
  ISBN 978-0-323-05491-1 (hardcover : alk. paper) -- ISBN 978-0-323-05492-8 (pbk. : alk. paper) 1.
Human physiology. 2. Human anatomy. 3. Physiology, Pathological. I. Patton, Kevin T. II. Title. III.
Title: Human body in health and disease.
  [DNLM: 1. Physiology. 2. Anatomy. 3. Pathology. QT 104 T427h 2010]
  QP34.5.T495 2010
  612--dc22
                          2009000728

Executive Publisher: Tom Wilhelm
Acquisitions Editor: Jeff Downing
Developmental Editor: Karen C. Turner
Editorial Assistant: Jennifer Shropshire
Publishing Services Manager: Deborah L. Vogel
Senior Project Manager: Ann E. Rogers
Design Direction and Cover Design: Kim Denando

Printed in the United States of America

Last digit is the print number: 9 8 7 6 5 4 3 2

Contributors

Ed Calcaterra, BS, MEd
Instructor
DeSmet Jesuit High School
Creve Coeur, Missouri

Rhonda J. Gamble, PhD
Professor of Physiology and Life Sciences
Mineral Area College
Park Hills, Missouri

Jeff Kingsbury, MD
Professor, Life Sciences
Mohave Community College;
Associate Professor, Department of Biological Sciences
Northern Arizona University
Flagstaff, Arizona

Amy L. Way, PhD
Associate Professor of Health Science
Lock Haven University of Pennsylvania
Clearfield, Pennsylvania

Scientific Review Panel

Bert Atsma
Union County College
Cranford, New Jersey

Janis Baker
Instructor, School of Vocational Nursing
Valley Baptist Medical Center
Harlingen, Texas

Rachel Beecham
Assistant Professor, Natural Science and Environmental Health
Mississippi Valley State University
Itta Bena, Mississippi

Christi A. Blair
Holmes Community College
Kosciusko Practical Nursing Program
Kosciusko, Mississippi

Andrew Case
Academic Transfer Program
Southeast Community College
Lincoln, Nebraska

Erin Clason
Health Sciences Faculty
Spokane Community College
Spokane, Washington

Virginia Clevenger
Mercer County Vocational School
Trenton, New Jersey

Mentor David
Barton County Community College
Great Bend, Kansas

Leslie Day
Lecturer, Biology
Northeastern University
Boston, Massachusetts

Judith Diehl
Reid State Technical Campus
Atmore, Alabama

Paul Ellis
Professor, Health Studies
St. Louis College of Health Careers
Saint Louis, Missouri

Judy Fair
Sandusky School of Practical Nursing
Sandusky, Ohio

Beth Forshee
Assistant Professor of Physiology
Lake Erie College of Osteopathic Medicine
Erie, Pennsylvania

Linda Fulton
North Hills School of Health Occupations
Pittsburgh, Pennsylvania

Christy Gee
Medical Assisting Department Chair
South College
Asheville, North Carolina

Sharon Harris-Pelliccia
Division Chair, Medical Studies
Mildred Elley College
Latham, New York

Beulah Hoffman
Indiana Vocational Technical College
Terre Haute, Indiana

Rita Hoots
Yuba College
Woodland, California

Marilyn Hunter
Daytona Beach Community College
Daytona Beach, Florida

Jon-Phillippe Hyatt
Assistant Professor, Human Science
Georgetown University
Washington, DC

Pablo Irusta
Assistant Professor, Human Science
Georgetown University
Washington, DC

Tanys Gene James
Instructor/Professor of Nursing
North Central Texas College
Gainesville, Texas

Michelle Kennedy
Morgan County High School
Madison, Georgia

Brian Kipp
Assistant Professor, Biomedical Sciences
Grand Valley State University
Allendale, Michigan

Kathy Korona
Community College of Allegheny County
West Mifflin, Pennsylvania

Anne Lilly
Santa Rosa Junior College
Santa Rosa, California

Caleb Makukutu
Kingwood Junior College
Kingwood, Texas

Susan Caley Opsal
Instructor, Natural Sciences Department
Illinois Valley Community College
Oglesby, Illinois

Darrell Pietarila
Flint Hills Technical School
Emporia, Kansas

Henry M. Seidel
Professor Emeritus of Pediatrics
The Johns Hopkins University School of Medicine
Baltimore, Maryland

Donna Silsbee
SUNY Institute of Technology
Utica, New York

Gerry Silverstein
Emeritus Lecturer in Health Sciences
University of Vermont
Burlington, Vermont

Greg K. Sitorius
Minden High School
Minden, Nebraska

Sharon Spalding
Professor of Physical Education and Director of
    Athletics and Wellness
Mary Baldwin College
Staunton, Virginia

William Sproat
Associate Professor of Biology
Walters State Community College
Morristown, Tennessee

Karen Tvedten
School of Radiologic Technology
Madison, Wisconsin

Rebecca S. Wiggins
Health Science Education Instructor
West Florida High School of Advanced Technology
Pensacola, Florida

Shirley Yeargin
Rend Lake College
Ina, Illinois

Nina Zanetti
Associate Professor
Siena College
Loudonville, New York

Preface

THIS BOOK ABOUT the human body represents the latest and best information available. *The Human Body in Health & Disease* is a guide for future health professionals who are just beginning their exploration of the complex human organism. It not only presents introductory material on the elegance and efficiency of the healthy human body but also shows what happens when things go wrong. To truly understand the human body, one must appreciate both normal and abnormal structure and function.

In this time of rapid scientific advances, our understanding of the human body is increasing at an explosive rate. Almost daily, new discoveries cause scientists to overturn old, established hypotheses and replace them with new concepts. Recent advances in medicine, biotechnology, biochemistry, immunology, neuroendocrinology, molecular biology, and other fields are truly overwhelming. New fields, such as genomics and proteomics, have burst upon the scene and assumed a major role in uncovering new information about human structure, function, and disease. This explosion of new understanding presents instructors with the challenge of selecting that which will be the most appropriate information for presentation in introductory but nonetheless rigorous courses. *The Human Body in Health & Disease* has been carefully designed to do just that and succeeds in presenting up-to-date information that is both accurate and easy to comprehend.

As we prepared this newest edition, each decision regarding how concepts were to be presented in our book was evaluated by teachers actually working in the field—teachers currently helping students learn about human structure, function, and disease for the first time. We also consulted closely with working health professionals and medical writers to ensure that our references to disease processes and related topics are current, accurate, and clearly summarized. The result is a text that students will read with enthusiasm—one designed to help the teacher teach and the student learn. It is particularly suited to introductory courses about the human body in relation to various health professions. *The Human Body in Health & Disease* emphasizes concepts that are required knowledge for entry into more advanced courses, completion of professional licensing examinations, and success in a practical, work-related environment.

SPECIAL FEATURES

Unifying Themes

Anatomy, physiology, and introductory pathology encompass a body of knowledge that, because of its sheer magnitude, can easily discourage and overwhelm the new student. There is no question, however, that competency in these fields is essential for student success in almost every clinical or advanced course in a health-related or science curriculum. If a textbook is to be successful as a teaching tool in such a complex and important learning environment, it must assist and complement the efforts of instructor and student. It must help unify information, stimulate critical thinking, and motivate students to master a new vocabulary as they learn about the beauty and "connectedness" of human structure and function and the "disjointedness" of human disease.

The Human Body in Health & Disease is dominated by two major unifying themes: the *complementarity of normal structure and function* and *homeostasis*. In every chapter of the book the student is shown how organized anatomical structures of a particular size, shape, form, or placement serve unique and specialized functions. Repeated emphasis of this principle encourages students to integrate otherwise isolated factual information into a cohesive and understandable whole. This integration of knowledge is further developed in each chapter as the breakdown of normal integration of form and function is identified as the basis for many disease processes. As a result, anatomy, physiology, and pathology emerge as vital, dynamic topics of personal interest and importance to the student. The integrating principle of homeostasis is used to show how the "normal" interaction of structure and function is achieved and maintained by dynamic counterbalancing of forces within the body. Failures of homeostasis are shown as basic mechanisms of disease—a concept that reinforces understanding of the regulatory systems of the human body.

Organization and Content

The 24 chapters of *The Human Body in Health & Disease* present the core material of anatomy, physiology, and pathology *most important* for introductory students. The selection of appropriate information in these disciplines was designed to eliminate the confusing mix of nonessential and overly specialized material that unfortunately accompanies basic information in many introductory textbooks. Information is presented in a way that lets students know and understand what is *important*.

An equally important goal for us in designing this text was to present information using a conceptual framework on which the student can build an understanding of the human body. Rather than simply listing a set of facts, each chapter outlines the broad concepts that allow students to relate the facts to one another in a meaningful way. This approach is especially apparent in the passages that deal with human disease and related topics. Most anatomy and physiology books present diseases as a disjointed list of definitions or descriptions at the end of each chapter—almost as an afterthought. Our book, however, presents disease conditions within a framework that facilitates a more complete understanding of the *process* of disease and allows the student to compare and contrast related disorders easily.

The sequence of chapters in the book follows that most commonly used in courses taught at the undergraduate level. Basic concepts of human biology—anatomy, physiology, biochemistry, cytology, histology, and pathology—are presented in Chapters 1 through 5. Chapters 6 through 24 present material on more specialized topics, such as individual organs or systems, the senses (Chapter 10), immunity (Chapter 15), and genetics and genetic diseases (Chapter 24). Because each chapter is self-contained, instructors are given the flexibility to alter the sequence of material to fit personal teaching preferences or the special content or time constraints of their courses.

Instructors who teach courses with less emphasis on concepts of pathology may wish to examine

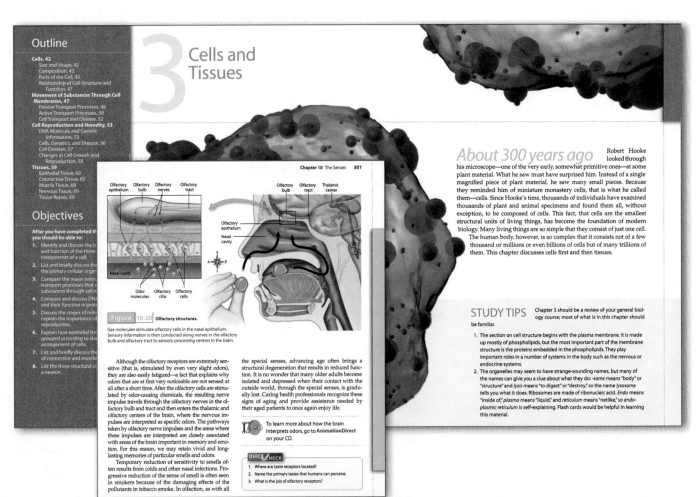

an alternate text with a similar instructional design: *Structure & Function of the Body*, also available from Elsevier. Students who are entering the health professions or any field related to the human body may wish to acquire a copy of *Mosby's Handbook of Anatomy & Physiology*. This compact book acts as a ready reference and patient-teaching aid to be used during your workday to help you remember essential facts or to help you guide patients in understanding how their bodies work. Students may also wish to get a copy of the *Survival Guide for Anatomy & Physiology*, written by Kevin Patton, which is an easy-to-read handbook that helps students achieve success in anatomy and physiology. Survival skills, hints for developing effective study habits, and guidelines for how best to prepare for tests and quizzes all help students learn to read with greater comprehension, and a Quick Reference filled with illustrations, tables, and diagrams conveys all of the important facts and concepts students need to know to succeed.

Pedagogical Features

The Human Body in Health & Disease is a student-oriented text. Written in a very readable style, it has numerous learning aids that maintain interest and motivation. Every chapter contains the following elements, each of which facilitates teaching and learning.

Chapter Outline: An overview outline introduces each chapter and enables the student to preview the content and direction of the chapter at the major concept level before embarking on the detailed reading.

Chapter Objectives: Each chapter opening page contains five to ten measurable objectives for the student to work toward. Each objective clearly identifies for the student, before he or she reads the chapter, what the key goals should be and what information should be mastered.

Study Tips: Each chapter opens with an updated list of approximately five specific tips and hints on how to most effectively study the concepts presented in the chapter. Prepared by veteran teacher Ed Calcaterra, in consultation with Kevin Patton, these tips are a unique and useful feature that make this text even more "student friendly."

Key Terms and Pronunciation Guide: Key terms, when introduced and defined in the text

body, are identified in boldface to highlight their importance. A simplified pronunciation guide follows each new term that students may find difficult to pronounce correctly.

Boxed Inserts and Essays: Brief boxed inserts or sometimes longer essays appear in every chapter. These boxes include information ranging from clinical applications of the information to sidelights on recent research or related topics to relevant discussions of exercise and fitness. Pathological conditions are sometimes explained in essay format to help students better understand the relationship between normal structure and function. All boxed materials are highlighted with an easily recognized symbol so that students can see at a glance whether the box contains wellness, clinical, research, or science application information. In this edition, the featured boxes cover four categories:

- The *Health & Well-Being* boxes contain information about wellness, fitness and exercise, athletics, public health, and related issues and problems.

- The *Clinical Application* boxes emphasize interesting facts and trends related to disease processes and therapies.

- The *Research, Issues, & Trends* sidebars illustrate the dynamic nature of human science today as well as the importance of ethical and legal issues in applying new research information.

- The *Science Applications* boxes summarize a few of the professions that make use of the concepts in the chapter to improve our quality of life. These essays also feature significant individuals who have contributed to human science and medicine. Thus they help place the study of the human body in a historical and social context.

AnimationDirect icons: For the first time, each chapter has boxes identified with a special icon that point the reader to animations of important principles. These are available in AnimationDirect, which is included on the Companion CD. The brief animated sequences are designed to demonstrate concepts that are not easily illustrated in static diagrams. In effect they help put a student's understanding in motion and thus help solidify learning.

Outline Summaries: Extensive and detailed end-of-chapter summaries in outline format provide excellent guides for students as they review the text materials when preparing for examinations. Many students also find these detailed guides to be useful as a chapter preview in conjunction with the chapter outline.

Audio Chapter Summary icons: New to this edition are audio chapter summaries for each chapter in the book. Called out with an icon at the start of each chapter outline summary, these MP3s, which can be downloaded onto a portable media player, provide students with an easy way to review chapter content while on the go. These can be found on the Companion CD and the Evolve website.

Word Lists: A comprehensive word list appears at the end of each chapter. The first part is a list of new terms related to basic, normal anatomy and physiology. The second is a brief list of new terms related to diseases and other clinical topics. These lists organize essential terminology so that students can study it more easily.

Chapter Tests: Objective-type Chapter Test questions are included at the end of each chapter. They serve as quick checks for the recall and mastery of important subject matter. They are also designed as aids to increase the retention of information. Answers to all Chapter Test questions are provided at the end of the text.

Review Questions: Subjective review questions at the end of each chapter allow students to use a narrative format to discuss concepts and also serve to synthesize important chapter information that can then be reviewed by the instructor to assess comprehension of the material. The answers to these review questions are available in the *TEACH Instructor Resource Manual* that accompanies the text.

Critical Thinking Questions: Review questions that encourage students to use critical thinking skills are highlighted at the end of the Review Questions section. Answers to these questions are found in the *TEACH Instructor Resource Manual* along with the answers to the other Review Questions.

Case Studies: Each chapter ends with a few case studies or other application questions that ask students to apply their knowledge of the human body to specific, practical problems. The questions range from simple applications to moderately complex problem-solving items. Complete narrative answers to each application question appear in the back of the book so that students can verify their answers or find the answer to a question that stumps them.

Glossary: An extensive listing of key terms, pronunciations, and definitions serves as a handy reference for students as they progress through the course.

Index: A comprehensive index aids in locating information anywhere in the book quickly and easily.

Companion CD

Resources that are called out in the text and additional learning and study aids that may be useful to students are available on the Companion CD bound into the back of this book.

AnimationDirect

New to this edition is a resource called AnimationDirect, a set of more than 75 animations that further demonstrate difficult concepts presented in the book. Throughout the text, boxes with a special icon alert the reader to particular animations, all of which can be accessed on the Companion CD. They help visualize important processes and thus promote deeper understanding of key concepts.

APPENDIXES

Appendix A: Examples of Pathological Conditions: Also appearing at the end of the text, a series of tables in this appendix summarizes specific pathological conditions by characteristic. The tables serve as a mini-reference tool to supplement material presented in the chapters of the text. Summary tables include:

Leading health problems

Viral conditions

Bacterial conditions

Mycotic (fungal) conditions

Conditions caused by protozoa

Conditions caused by pathogenic animals

Conditions caused by physical agents

Endocrine conditions

Autoimmune conditions

Deficiency diseases

Genetic conditions

Appendix B: Medical Terminology: A list of word parts commonly used in terms related to medicine and pathology is given along with tips on dissecting complex terms to determine their meanings. Many of these word parts are also used within chapters to emphasize how knowledge of medical terminology can help in learning basic concepts.

Appendix C: Clinical and Laboratory Values: Commonly observed ranges of values for various human body components and the physiological conditions related to them are listed along with the tests used to determine the values in a given individual. Normal and pathological indicators of blood, urine, and other values are summarized. This information supplements related information presented in appropriate chapters.

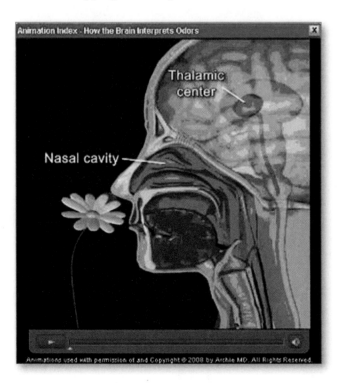

Animation Index - How the Brain Interprets Odors

Thalamic center

Nasal cavity

Animations used with permission of and Copyright © 2008 by Archie MD. All Rights Reserved.

Appendix D: Common Medical Abbreviations and Symbols: A brief list of abbreviations, acronyms, and symbols commonly used by nurses, medical specialists, pharmacists, and other health care professionals is presented to assist in mastering relevant terminology.

AUDIO CHAPTER SUMMARIES

New to this edition are audio chapter summaries for each chapter in the book. These concise, narrated overviews are called out at the start of each chapter outline summary and can be accessed on the Companion CD. Students can listen to the audio files on their computers or download them to their iPod, smart phone, or other portable media player so they can either preview or review chapter content while on the go. Some students find that these audio summaries improve their retention of chapter concepts when used immediately after reading the chapter. All of the audio summaries can also be found on the Evolve website.

BODY SPECTRUM: MOSBY'S ELECTRONIC COLORING BOOK

This feature is one of our most popular interactive programs. It simplifies the way students learn anatomy and medical terminology by offering 80 detailed anatomy illustrations that can be colored online or printed out to color and study offline.

Illustrations and Design

A major strength of *The Human Body in Health & Disease* is the exceptional quality, accuracy, and beauty of the illustration program. The illustration program in this edition has been heavily revised to provide the best available illustrations that both engage the reader and assist in learning important concepts. Plus, new to this edition is a more intuitive internal design that integrates the illustrations and other pedagogy more closely with the text.

The truest test of any illustration is how effectively it can complement and strengthen written information found in the text and how successfully it can be used by the student as a learning tool. In this edition, we have been very careful to position illustrations where they will best fit into the flow of reading, in most cases on the same page where they are called out. This helps students easily

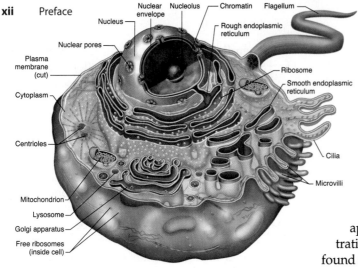

out the text. Photos and charts proven pedagogically effective in the previous edition of *The Human Body in Health & Disease* have been retained or updated to provide accurate information and visual appeal. New diagrams and illustrations have been added where appropriate to demonstrate important concepts. New photographs of pathological conditions have been added to the text as well.

As in previous editions, directional rosettes appear inconspicuously in all anatomical illustrations. These rosettes, like the compass rosettes found on all modern maps, orient the user, pointing which way is left and which way is right—directions that in anatomy may appear "backwards" to the beginning student. The rosettes also point to "superior" and "inferior" and "lateral" and "medial" directions in a manner that orients the user to the exact

understand concepts visually, without forcing them to flip back and forth through pages. Extensive use has been made of full-color illustrations, micrographs, and dissection photographs through-

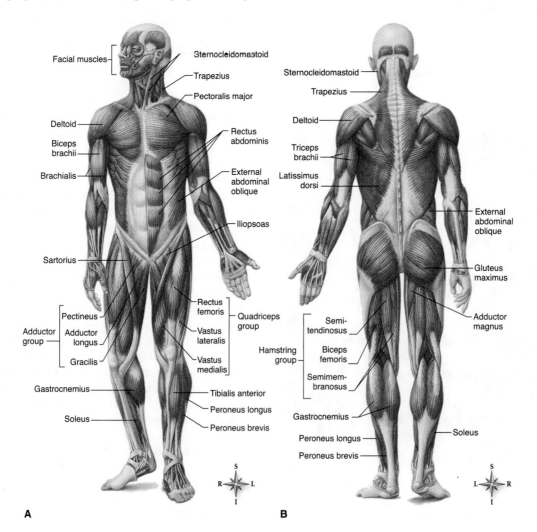

A

B

positioning of the body or organ in the illustration. As happens with map users, the user of this book will become more and more familiar with the "territory" of the human body and, by the end of this text, will no longer need to rely on these anatomical rosettes for orientation.

Color has been used extensively in this edition of *The Human Body in Health & Disease*. It not only makes the book more attractive but also makes the subject matter less intimidating to students. The use of color has been updated in illustrations to unify the art program throughout the book. Having consistent color for cellular and chemical structures, certain body processes, and other related concepts helps emphasize the student-friendly and "big picture" approach this book takes.

Clear View of the Human Body

We are particularly excited to present a full-color, semitransparent model of the body called the Clear View of the Human Body. Located between Chapters 3 and 4 in the textbook, this feature permits the virtual dissection of male and female human bod-

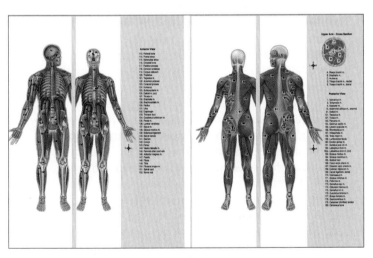

ies along several different planes. Developed by Kevin Patton and Paul Krieger, this tool helps learners assimilate their knowledge of the complex structure of the human body. It also helps students visualize human anatomy in the manner of today's clinical and athletic body-imaging technology.

SUPPLEMENTS

The supplements package has been carefully planned and developed to assist instructors and to enhance their use of the text. Each supplement, including the test items and study guide, has been thoroughly reviewed by many of the same instructors who reviewed the text.

TEACH Instructor Resource Manual

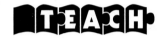 The TEACH Instructor Resource Manual, prepared by Sally Flesch, provides text adopters with substantial support in teaching from the text. The following features are included in every chapter:

- Chapter synopsis of major components and principles covered in the chapter
- Learning objectives with rationales for review of chapter objectives
- Lecture outline that parallels the textbook summary
- Lesson plan grid that follows the learning objectives and refers instructors to the entire suite of ancillaries
- Suggestions for student activities and assignments
- Sources of audiovisual and computer software support
- Health-related sources on the World Wide Web
- Information resources for distribution to students
- Answers to the text Review Questions and Case Studies Questions
- Additional exercises including labeling, matching, and critical thinking questions

Electronic Test Bank

An electronic test bank of more than 3400 questions with answers gives instructors an easy way to test students' comprehension of text material and create comprehensive exams for students. The test bank questions are available on the *Instructor's Electronic Resource DVD* and on the Evolve website.

Electronic Image Collection

The image collection includes nearly 300 anatomy and physiology images from the text—available in jpeg and PowerPoint form—to enhance your lectures. The image collection is available on the *Instructor's Electronic Resource DVD* and on the Evolve website.

Study Guide

The *Study Guide*, written by Linda Swisher, provides students with additional self-study aids, including chapter overviews, topic reviews, and application and labeling exercises (such as matching, crossword puzzles, fill in the blank, and multiple choice), as well as answers to the questions in the *Study Guide*. These learning aids have been specially designed to help prepare students for class discussion and exams.

Anatomy and Physiology Online

Anatomy and Physiology Online is a 24-module online course that brings A&P to life and helps you understand the most important concepts presented in *The Human Body in Health & Disease*. This online

ANATOMY AND PHYSIOLOGY ONLINE *to accompany*

THE **HUMAN BODY** IN **HEALTH & DISEASE** *Fifth Edition*

course includes instructionally sound learning modules with over 150 animations, 300 interactive exercises, and quizzes and exams to assess student comprehension. To learn more, visit the Evolve website (see below).

Evolve

The Evolve interactive website provides students with access to online tutoring from A&P experts, WebLinks created especially for this text, the A&P AudioGlossary, online study activities, the audio chapter summaries, and student-generated frequently asked questions with answers from the authors. Instructors will have access to an electronic version of the *TEACH Instructor Resource Manual,* an image collection, PowerPoint presentations with integrated figures, the electronic test bank, and audience response questions. To learn more, point your browser to: http://evolve.elsevier.com/ThibodeauPatton/humanbody/.

A WORD OF THANKS

Many people have contributed to the development and success of *The Human Body in Health & Disease*. We extend our thanks and deep appreciation to the various students and classroom instructors who have provided us with helpful suggestions following their use of the earlier editions of this text. For this edition, we would like to thank the following experts for their contributions: Sally Flesch for the *TEACH Instructor Resource Manual,* Linda Swisher for the *Study Guide* and A&P Online, Ed Calcaterra for the Test Bank and contributions to the text pedagogy, and David Hill for the audio chapter summaries. We are grateful for the contributions of Rhonda Gamble, Jeff Kingsbury, and Amy Way, who helped us to revise some of the chapters in this edition.

At Elsevier, thanks are due to all on the talented and creative team that produced this fifth edition. We wish especially to acknowledge the support and effort of Sally Schrefer, executive vice president; Tom Wilhelm, executive publisher; Jeff Downing, editor; Karen Turner, developmental editor; Debbie Vogel, publishing services manager; Ann Rogers, senior project manager; Gail Brower, copy editor; and Kim Denando, senior book designer, all of whom were instrumental in bringing this edition to successful completion.

Gary A. Thibodeau
Kevin T. Patton

Contents

23
Growth and Development, 638

24
Genetics and Genetic Diseases, 664

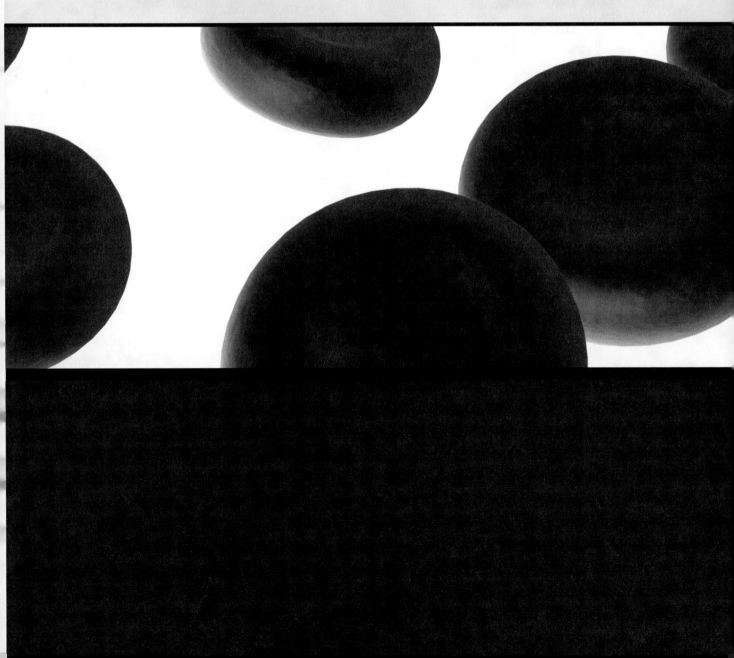

THE HUMAN BODY
IN HEALTH & DISEASE

1

An Introduction to the Structure and Function of the Body

Outline

Objectives

After you have completed this chapter, you should be able to:

1. Define the following terms: *anatomy,* *physiology,* and *pathology.*

2. List and discuss in order of increasing complexity the levels of organization of the body.

3. Define the term *anatomical position.*

4. List and define the principal directional terms and sections (planes) used in describing the body and the relationship of body parts to one another.

5. List the nine abdominopelvic regions and the abdominopelvic quadrants.

6. List the major cavities of the body and the subdivisions of each.

7. Discuss and contrast the axial and the appendicular subdivisions of the body. Identify a number of specific anatomical regions in each area.

8. Explain the meaning of the term *homeostasis* and give an example of a typical homeostatic mechanism.

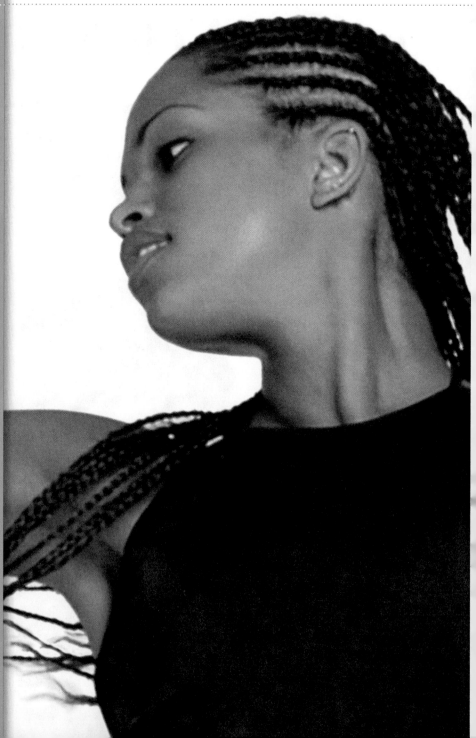

There are many wonders in our world, but none is more wondrous than the human body. This is a textbook about that incomparable structure. It deals with two very distinct and yet interrelated sciences: **anatomy** and **physiology.**

As a science, anatomy is often defined as the study of the structure of an organism and the relationships of its parts. The word *anatomy* is derived from two Greek words that mean "a cutting up." Anatomists learn about the structure of the human body by cutting it apart. This process, called **dissection,** is still the principal technique used to isolate and study the structural components or parts of the human body.

Physiology, on the other hand, is the study of the functions of living organisms and their parts. It is a dynamic science that requires active experimentation. In the chapters that follow, you will see again and again that anatomical structures are exactly suited to perform specific functions. Each has a particular size, shape, form, or position in the body related directly to its ability to perform a unique and specialized activity.

STUDY TIPS

A number of topics are introduced in this chapter that will be important throughout the rest of the course.

1. The most important one is probably homeostasis. The word itself tells you what it means: *homeo* means "the same," *stasis* means "staying." Homeostasis is the balance the body tries to maintain by making sure its internal environment "stays the same." Make sure you understand this concept.
2. Another important topic introduced in this chapter is the structural levels of organization. The lower levels are the building blocks on which the upper levels depend. As various disease processes are explained in later chapters, notice how many of these processes cause failure at the chemical or cellular level and how this failure affects organs, systems, and even the body as a whole.
3. Become familiar with the directional terms; you will see them in almost every diagram in the text. The terms are also used in naming several body structures (for example, superior vena cava, distal convoluted tubule). The

continued on page 21

Although an understanding of the normal structure and function of the body is important, it is also important to know the mechanisms of **disease.** Disease conditions result from abnormalities of body structure or function that prevent the body from maintaining the internal stability that keeps us alive and healthy. **Pathology,** the scientific study of disease, uses principles of anatomy and physiology to determine the nature of particular diseases. The term *pathology* comes from *pathos,* the Greek word for "disease." Chapter 5 provides an overview of the basic mechanisms of disease, such as infection and cancer. Throughout the rest of this textbook, explanations of normal structure and function are supplemented by discussions of related disease processes. By knowing the structure and function of the healthy body, you will be better prepared to understand what can go wrong to cause disease. At the same time, a knowledge of disease states will enhance your understanding of normal structure and function.

Structural Levels of Organization

Before you begin the study of the structure and function of the human body and its many parts, it is important to think about how those parts are organized and how they might logically fit together into a functioning whole. Examine Figure 1-1. It illustrates the differing levels of organization that influence body structure and function. Note that the levels of organization progress from the least complex (chemical level) to the most complex (organism level).

Organization is one of the most important characteristics of body structure. Even the word *organism,* used to denote a living thing, implies organization.

Although the body itself is considered a single structure, it is made up of trillions of smaller structures. Atoms and molecules are often referred to as the **chemical level** of organization. The existence of life depends on the proper levels and proportions of many chemical substances in the cells of the body.

Many of the physical and chemical phenomena that play important roles in the life process are reviewed in Chapter 2. Such information provides an understanding of the physical basis for life and for the study of the next levels of organization that are so important in the study of anatomy and physiology—cells, tissues, organs, and systems.

SCIENCE APPLICATIONS

MODERN ANATOMY

Anatomists study the structure of the human body. Modern anatomy started during the Renaissance in Europe with the

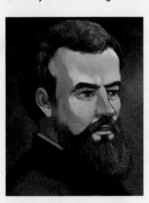

Andreas Vesalius (1514–1564)

Flemish scientist Andreas Vesalius *(shown at left)* and his contemporaries. Vesalius was the first to apply a scientific method (see the box on p. 16) to the study of the human body. Most anatomists still dissect *cadavers* (preserved human remains). However, today many anatomists also use imaging technologies such as x-rays, computerized scans, and even digitized photographs of thin slices of the body as you can see *in the figure at right* from the National Library of Medicine's Visible Human Project. Such digitized images can be reconstructed into dissectible, three-dimensional body views by computers.

Applications of modern anatomy are also found in the fields of forensic science, anthropology, medicine and allied health professions, sports and athletics, dance, and even art and computerized animation.

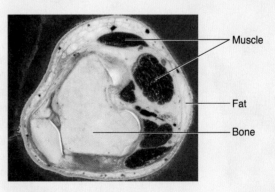

Horizontal section of the human arm

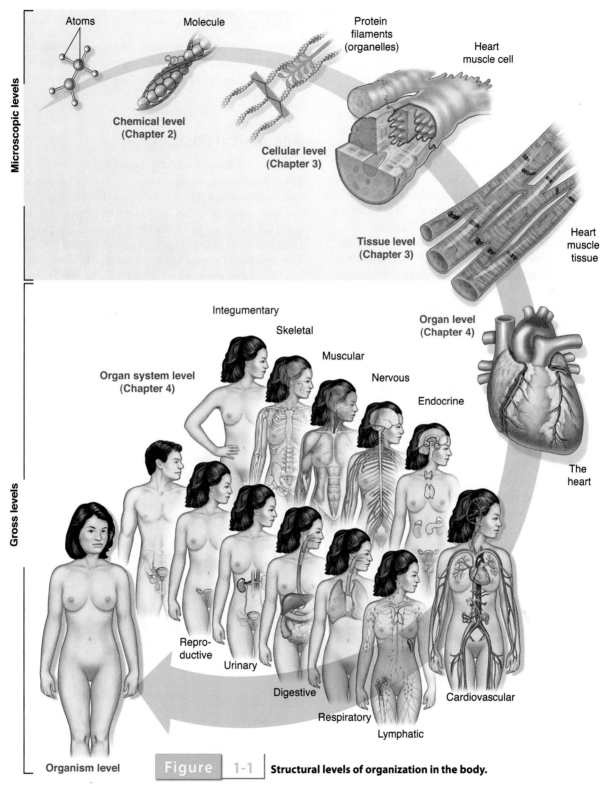

Microscopic levels

Atoms

Molecule

Chemical level (Chapter 2)

Protein filaments (organelles)

Cellular level (Chapter 3)

Heart muscle cell

Tissue level (Chapter 3)

Heart muscle tissue

Gross levels

Integumentary

Skeletal

Muscular

Nervous

Endocrine

Organ system level (Chapter 4)

Organ level (Chapter 4)

The heart

Reproductive

Urinary

Digestive

Respiratory

Lymphatic

Cardiovascular

Organism level

> Figure 1-1 **Structural levels of organization in the body.**
>
> Atoms, molecules, and cells ordinarily can be seen only with a microscope, but the gross (large) structures of tissues, organs, systems, and the whole organism can be seen easily with the unaided eye.

Cells are considered to be the smallest "living" units of structure and function in our bodies. Although long recognized as the simplest units of living matter, cells are far from simple. They are extremely complex, a fact you will discover in Chapter 3.

Tissues are somewhat more complex than cells. By definition a tissue is an organization of many cells that act together to perform a common function. The cells of a tissue may be of several types but all are working together in some way to produce the structural and functional qualities of the tissue. Cells of a tissue are often held together and surrounded by varying amounts and varieties of gluelike, nonliving intercellular substances.

Organs are larger and even more complex than tissues. An organ is a group of several different kinds of tissues arranged so that they can act together as a unit to perform a special function. For instance, the heart shown in Figure 1-1 is an example of organization at the organ level. Unlike microscopic molecules and cells, some tissues and most organs are gross (large) structures that can be seen easily without a microscope.

Systems are the most complex units that make up the body. A system is an organization of varying numbers and kinds of organs arranged so that they can together perform complex functions for the body. The organs of the cardiovascular system shown in Figure 1-1 allow blood to carry nutrients, oxygen, and wastes to and from the tissues of the body. The heart and each of the blood vessels are the organs that pump blood and carry it throughout the body as it performs its functions.

The *body as a whole*—the human organism—is all the atoms, molecules, cells, tissues, organs, and systems that you will study in subsequent chapters of this text. Although capable of being dissected or broken down into many parts, the body is a unified and complex assembly of structurally and functionally interactive components, each working together to ensure healthy survival.

 For a brief 3-D tour of each of the body's organ systems, go to **AnimationDirect** on your CD.

QUICK CHECK

1. What is *anatomy?* What is *physiology?* What is *pathology?*
2. What are the major levels of organization in the body?
3. How is a *tissue* different from an *organ?*

Anatomical Position

Discussions about the body, the way it moves, its posture, or the relationship of one area to another assume that the body as a whole is in a specific position called the **anatomical position.** In this reference position (Figure 1-2) the body is in an erect or standing posture with the arms at the sides and palms turned forward. The head also points forward, as do the feet, which are aligned at the toe and set slightly apart. The anatomical position is a reference position that gives

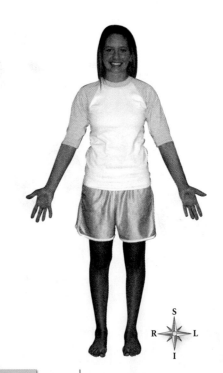

Figure 1-2   **Anatomical position.**

The body is in an erect or standing posture with the arms at the sides and the palms forward. The head and feet also point forward. The anatomical compass rosette is explained on pp. 7-8.

meaning to the directional terms used to describe the body parts and regions. In other words, you need to know the anatomical position so that you know how to apply **directional terms** correctly no matter what position the body being described is in.

Supine and prone are terms used to describe the position of the body when it is not in the anatomical position. In the supine position the body is lying face upward, and in the prone position the body is lying face downward.

Anatomical Directions

When studying the body, it is often helpful to know where an organ is in relation to other structures. The following directional terms are used in describing relative positions of body parts. To help you understand them better, they are listed here in sets of opposite pairs:

1. **Superior** and **inferior** (Figure 1-3)—*superior* means "toward the head," and *inferior* means "toward the feet." *Superior* also means "upper" or "above," and *inferior* means "lower" or "below." For example, the lungs are located superior to the diaphragm, whereas the stomach is located inferior to the diaphragm (refer to Figure 1-7 if you are not sure where these organs are located).

2. **Anterior** and **posterior** (Figure 1-3)—*anterior* means "front" or "in front of"; *posterior* means "back" or "in back of." In humans, who walk in an upright position, *ventral* (toward the belly) can be used in place of anterior, and *dorsal* (toward the back) can be used for posterior. For example, the nose is on the anterior surface of the body, and the shoulder blades are on its posterior surface.

3. **Medial** and **lateral** (Figure 1-3)—*medial* means "toward the midline of the body"; *lateral* means "toward the side of the body or away from its midline." For example, the great toe is at the medial side of the foot, and the little toe is at its lateral side. The heart lies medial to the lungs, and the lungs lie lateral to the heart.

4. **Proximal** and **distal** (Figure 1-3)—*proximal* means "toward or nearest the trunk of the body, or nearest the point of origin of one of its parts";

distal means "away from or farthest from the trunk or the point of origin of a body part." For example, the elbow lies at the proximal end of the lower arm, whereas the hand lies at its distal end.

5. **Superficial** and **deep**—*superficial* means nearer the surface; *deep* means farther away from the body surface. For example, the skin of the arm is superficial to the muscles below it, and the bone of the upper arm is deep to the muscles that surround and cover it.

To make the reading of anatomical figures a little easier for you, we have used an anatomical compass rosette throughout this book. On many figures, you will see a small compass rosette like you might see on a geographical map. Instead of being labeled **N,** **S, E,** or **W,** the anatomical rosette is labeled with abbreviated anatomical directions. For example, in Figure 1-2 (p. 6), the rosette is labeled S (for *superior*) on top and I (for *inferior*) on the bottom. Notice that in

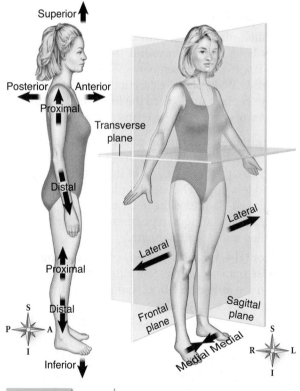

Figure   1-3   **Directions and planes of the body.**

Figure 1-2 the rosette shows R *(right)* on the subject's right—not your right. Here are the directional abbreviations used with the rosettes in this book:

A	Anterior
D	Distal
I	Inferior
L (opposite R)	Left
L (opposite M)	Lateral
M	Medial
P (opposite A)	Posterior
P (opposite D)	Proximal
R	Right
S	Superior

QUICK CHECK

1. What is the anatomical position?
2. Why are the anatomical directions listed in pairs?

Planes or Body Sections

To facilitate the study of individual organs or the body as a whole, it is often useful to first subdivide or "cut" it into smaller segments. To aid in doing this uniformly, body **planes** or sections have been identified by special names. Read the following definitions and identify each of these terms in Figure 1-3.

1. **Sagittal**—a sagittal cut or section is a lengthwise plane running from front to back. It divides the body or any of its parts into right and left sides. The sagittal plane shown in Figure 1-3 divides the body into two *equal halves.* This unique type of sagittal plane is called a midsagittal plane.

2. **Frontal**—a frontal *(coronal)* plane is a lengthwise plane running from side to side. As you can see in Figure 1-3, a frontal plane divides the body or any of its parts into anterior and posterior (front and back) portions.

3. **Transverse**—a transverse plane is a horizontal or crosswise plane. Such a plane (see Figure 1-3) divides the body or any of its parts into upper and lower portions.

Body Cavities

Contrary to its external appearance, the body is not a solid structure. It is made up of open spaces or cavities that in turn contain compact, well-ordered arrangements of internal organs. The two major body cavities are called the **ventral** and **dorsal body cavities.** The location and outlines of the body cavities are illustrated in Figure 1-4. The upper part of the ventral cavity includes the thoracic cavity, a space that you may think of as your chest cavity. Its midportion is a subdivision of the thoracic cavity called the **mediastinum;** its other subdivisions are called the right and left **pleural cavities.** The lower part of the ventral cavity in Figure 1-4 includes an **abdominal cavity** and a **pelvic cavity.** Actually, these two form only one cavity, the **abdominopelvic cavity,** because no physical partition separates them. In Figure 1-4 a dotted line shows the approximate point of separation between the abdominal and pelvic subdivisions. Notice, however, that an actual physical partition separates the thoracic cavity from the abdominal cavity. This muscular sheet is the **diaphragm.** It is dome-shaped and is the most important muscle for breathing.

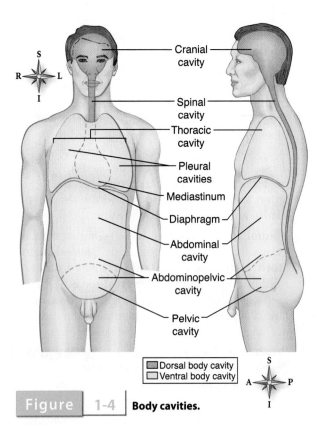

Cranial cavity
Spinal cavity
Thoracic cavity
Pleural cavities
Mediastinum
Diaphragm
Abdominal cavity
Abdominopelvic cavity
Pelvic cavity

Dorsal body cavity
Ventral body cavity

Figure 1-4 **Body cavities.**

Location and subdivisions of the dorsal and ventral body cavities as viewed from the front (anterior) and from the side (lateral).

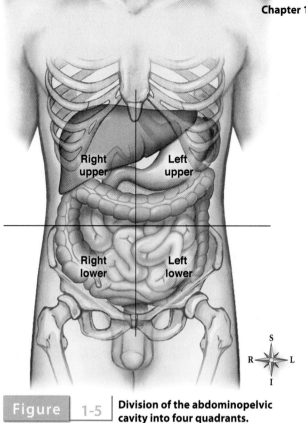

Right
upper

Left
upper

Right
lower

Left
lower

| Figure | 1-5 | **Division of the abdominopelvic cavity into four quadrants.** |

Diagram showing relationship of internal organs to the four abdominal quadrants.

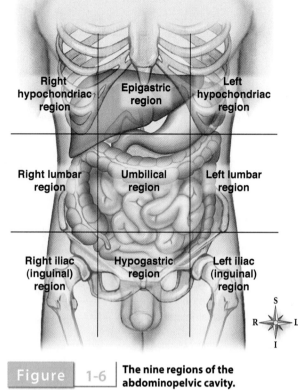

Right
hypochondriac
region

Epigastric
region

Left
hypochondriac
region

Right lumbar
region

Umbilical
region

Left lumbar
region

Right iliac
(inguinal)
region

Hypogastric
region

Left iliac
(inguinal)
region

| Figure | 1-6 | **The nine regions of the abdominopelvic cavity.** |

The most superficial organs are shown. Look at Figure 1-7 (p. 10); can you identify the deeper structures in each region?

To make it easier to locate organs in the large abdominopelvic cavity, anatomists have divided the abdominopelvic cavity into **four quadrants:** right upper or superior, right lower or inferior, left upper or superior, and left lower or inferior. As you can see in Figure 1-5, the midsagittal and transverse planes, which were described in the previous section, pass through the navel (umbilicus) and divide the abdominopelvic region into the four quadrants. This method of subdividing the abdominopelvic cavity is frequently used by health professionals and is useful for locating the origin of pain or describing the location of a tumor or other abnormality.

Another and perhaps more precise way to divide the abdominopelvic cavity is shown in Figure 1-6. Here, the abdominopelvic cavity is subdivided into nine regions defined as follows:

1. **Upper abdominopelvic regions**—the **right** and **left hypochondriac regions** and the **epigastric region** lie above an imaginary line across the abdomen at the level of the ninth rib cartilages.

2. **Middle regions**—the **right** and **left lumbar regions** and the **umbilical region** lie below an imaginary line across the abdomen at the level of the ninth rib cartilages and above an imaginary line across the abdomen at the top of the hip bones.

3. **Lower regions**—the **right** and **left iliac** (or *inguinal*) **regions** and the **hypogastric region** lie below an imaginary line across the abdomen at the level of the top of the hip bones.

The dorsal cavity shown in Figure 1-4 includes the space inside the skull that contains the brain; it is called the **cranial cavity.** The space inside the spinal column is called the **spinal cavity;** it contains the spinal cord. The cranial and spinal cavities are **dorsal cavities,** whereas the thoracic and abdominopelvic cavities are **ventral cavities.**

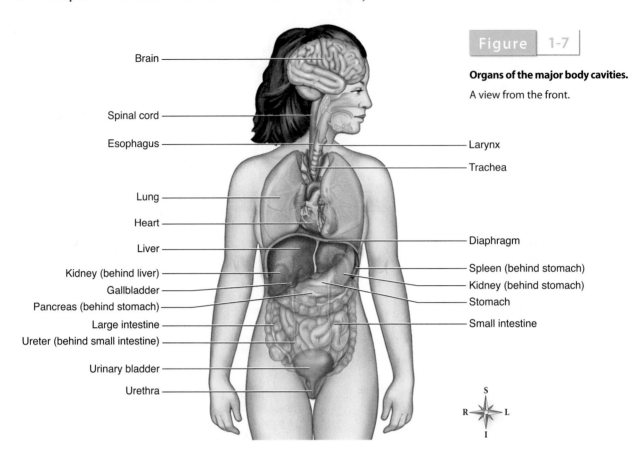

Figure **1-7**

Organs of the major body cavities.

A view from the front.

Brain

Spinal cord

Esophagus

Lung

Heart

Liver

Kidney (behind liver)

Gallbladder

Pancreas (behind stomach)

Large intestine

Ureter (behind small intestine)

Urinary bladder

Urethra

Larynx

Trachea

Diaphragm

Spleen (behind stomach)

Kidney (behind stomach)

Stomach

Small intestine

Knowledge of the body cavities has important clinical applications. For example, one can locate specific organs by knowing in which cavity they are found. Some of the organs in the largest body cavities are visible in Figure 1-7 and are listed in Table 1-1. Find each body cavity in a model of the human body if you have access to one. Try to identify the organs in each cavity, and try to visualize their locations in your own body. Study Figures 1-4 and 1-7.

Table **1-1** | **Body Cavities**

BODY CAVITY	ORGAN(S)
VENTRAL BODY CAVITY	
Thoracic cavity	
Mediastinum	Heart, trachea, esophagus, thymus, blood vessels
Pleural cavities	Lungs
Abdominopelvic cavity	
Abdominal cavity	Liver, gallbladder, stomach, spleen, pancreas, small intestine, parts of large intestine
Pelvic cavity	Lower (sigmoid) colon, rectum, urinary bladder, reproductive organs
DORSAL BODY CAVITY	
Cranial cavity	Brain
Spinal cavity	Spinal cord

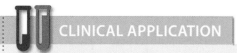

AUTOPSY

Knowledge of human anatomy is important in conducting an autopsy (AW-top-see) or postmortem examination. The term *autopsy* comes from the Greek words *auto* (meaning "self") and *opsis* (meaning "view"). Autopsies are procedures in which a human body is examined after death to accurately determine the cause of death, to confirm the accuracy of diagnostic tests, to discover previously undetected problems, and to assess the effectiveness of surgeries or other treatments. Medical and allied health students often attend autopsies to improve their knowledge of human anatomy and pathology.

Autopsies are usually performed in three stages. In the first stage, the exterior of the body is examined for abnormalities such as wounds or scars from injuries or surgeries. In the second stage, the ventral body cavity is opened by a deep, Y-shaped incision. The arms of the Y start at the anterior surface of the shoulders and join at the inferior point of the breastbone (sternum) to form a single cut that extends to the pubic area. After the rib cage is sawn through, the walls of the thoracic and abdominopelvic cavities can be opened like hinged doors to expose the internal organs. The second stage of the autopsy includes careful dissection of many or all of the internal organs. If the brain is to be examined, a portion of the skull must be removed. The face, arms, and legs are usually not dissected unless there is a specific reason for doing so. After the organs are returned to their respective body cavities, and the body is sewn up, the third phase of the autopsy begins. It is a microscopic examination of tissues collected during the first two phases. Tests to analyze the chemical content of body fluids or to determine the presence of infectious organisms also may be performed.

QUICK CHECK

1. What is meant by a *section* of the body?
2. What are the two major cavities of the body?
3. What is the difference between the *abdominal cavity* and the *abdominopelvic cavity*?

Body Regions

To recognize an object, you usually first notice its overall structure and form. For example, a car is recognized as a car before the specific details of its tires, grill, or wheel covers are noted. Recognition of the human form also occurs as you first identify overall shape and basic outline. However, for more specific identification to occur, details of size, shape, and appearance of individual body areas must be described. Individuals differ in overall appearance because specific body areas such as the face or torso have unique identifying characteristics. Detailed descriptions of the human form require that specific regions be identified and appropriate terms be used to describe them.

The ability to identify and correctly describe specific body areas is particularly important in the health sciences. For a patient to complain of pain in the head is not as specific and therefore not as useful to a health professional as a more specific and localized description would be. Saying that the pain is facial provides additional information and helps to more specifically identify the area of pain. By using correct anatomical terms such as forehead, cheek, or chin to describe the area of pain, attention can be focused even more quickly on the specific anatomical area that may need attention. Familiarize yourself with the more common terms used to describe specific body regions identified in Figure 1-8 and listed in Table 1-2.

The body as a whole can be subdivided into two major portions or components: **axial** and **appendicular.** The axial portion of the body consists of the head, neck, and torso or trunk; the appendicular portion consists of the upper and lower extremities. Each major area is subdivided as shown in Figure 1-8. Note, for example, that the torso is composed of thoracic, abdominal, and pelvic areas, and the upper extremity is divided into arm, forearm, wrist, and hand components. Although most terms used to describe gross body regions are well understood, misuse is common. The word *leg* is a good example: it refers to the area of the lower extremity between the knee and ankle and not to the entire lower extremity.

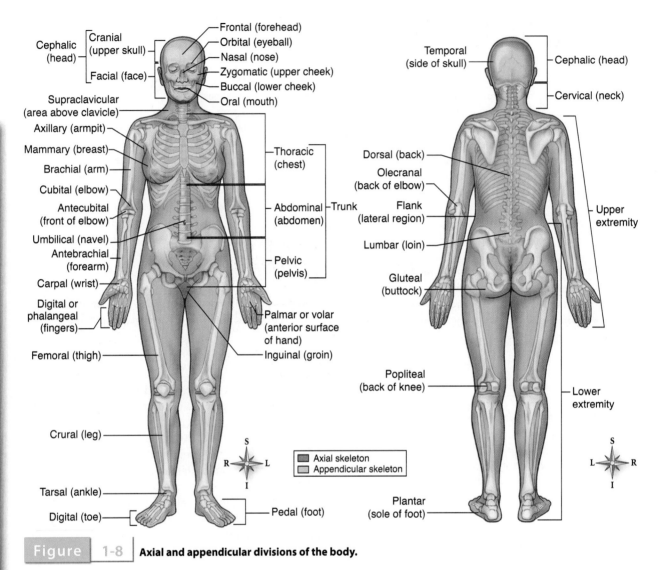

Cephalic (head) — Cranial (upper skull), Facial (face)
Frontal (forehead)
Orbital (eyeball)
Nasal (nose)
Zygomatic (upper cheek)
Buccal (lower cheek)
Oral (mouth)
Supraclavicular (area above clavicle)
Axillary (armpit)
Mammary (breast)
Brachial (arm)
Cubital (elbow)
Antecubital (front of elbow)
Umbilical (navel)
Antebrachial (forearm)
Carpal (wrist)
Digital or phalangeal (fingers)
Femoral (thigh)
Crural (leg)
Tarsal (ankle)
Digital (toe)
Thoracic (chest)
Abdominal (abdomen) — Trunk
Pelvic (pelvis)
Palmar or volar (anterior surface of hand)
Inguinal (groin)
Pedal (foot)

Temporal (side of skull)
Cephalic (head)
Cervical (neck)
Dorsal (back)
Olecranal (back of elbow)
Flank (lateral region)
Lumbar (loin)
Gluteal (buttock)
Popliteal (back of knee)
Plantar (sole of foot)
Upper extremity
Lower extremity

Axial skeleton
Appendicular skeleton

Figure 1-8 Axial and appendicular divisions of the body.

Specific body regions are labeled.

The structure of the body changes in many ways and at varying rates during a lifetime. Before young adulthood, the body develops and grows; after young adulthood, it gradually undergoes degenerative changes. With the reduced activity of the body as one advances through older adulthood, a generalized decrease in size or a wasting away of many body organs and tissues occurs that affects the structure and function of many body areas. This degenerative process, which results from disuse, is called **atrophy.** In many cases, atrophy can be reversed with therapy. Some tissues simply lose their elasticity or ability to regenerate as we get older. Nearly every chapter of this book refers to a few of those changes.

QUICK CHECK

1. What is the difference between the *axial* portion of the body and the *appendicular* portion of the body?
2. What are some of the regions of the upper extremity and lower extremity?
3. What is meant by the term *atrophy?*

Table 1-2	Descriptive Terms for Body Regions		
BODY REGION	**AREA OR EXAMPLE**	**BODY REGION**	**AREA OR EXAMPLE**
Abdominal (ab-DOM-i-nal)	Anterior torso below diaphragm	**Femoral** (FEM-or-al)	Thigh
Antebrachial (an-tee-BRAY-kee-al)	Forearm	**Gluteal** (GLOO-tee-al)	Buttock
Antecubital (an-tee-KYOO-bi-tal)	Depressed area just in front of elbow	**Inguinal** (ING-gwi-nal)	Groin
Axillary (AK-si-lair-ee)	Armpit	**Lumbar** (LUM-bar)	Lower back between ribs and pelvis
Brachial (BRAY-kee-all)	Arm	**Mammary** (MAM-ar-ee)	Breast
Buccal (BUK-all)	Cheek	**Occipital** (ock-SIP-it-al)	Back of lower skull
Carpal (KAR-pul)	Wrist	**Olecranal** (oh-LEK-rah-nal)	Back of elbow
Cephalic (seh-FAL-ik)	Head	**Palmar** (PAHL-mar)	Palm of hand
Cervical (SER-vi-kal)	Neck	**Pedal** (PEED-al)	Foot
Cranial (KRAY-nee-all)	Skull	**Pelvic** (PEL-vik)	Lower portion of torso
Crural (KROOR-all)	Leg	**Perineal** (per-i-NEE-al)	Area (perineum) between anus and genitals
Cubital (KYOO-bi-tall)	Elbow	**Plantar** (PLAN-tar)	Sole of foot
Cutaneous (kyoo-TAYN-ee-us)	Skin (or body surface)	**Popliteal** (pop-li-TEE-all)	Area behind knee
Digital (DIJ-i-tal)	Fingers or toes	**Supraclavicular** (soo-prah-klah-VIK-yoo-lar)	Area above clavicle
Dorsal (DOHR-sal)	Back	**Tarsal** (TAR-sal)	Ankle
Facial (FAY-shal)	Face	**Temporal** (TEM-poh-ral)	Side of skull
Frontal (FRUN-tal)	Forehead	**Thoracic** (tho-RASS-ik)	Chest
Nasal (NAY-zal)	Nose	**Umbilical** (um-BIL-i-kul)	Area around navel or umbilicus
Oral (OR-al)	Mouth		
Orbital *or* **ophthalmic** (OR-bi-tal *or* off-THAL-mik)	Eyes	**Volar** (VOH-lar)	Palm or sole
Zygomatic (zye-go-MAT-ik)	Upper cheek		

The Balance of Body Functions

Although they may have very different structures, all living organisms maintain mechanisms that ensure survival of the body and success in propagating its genes through its offspring.

Survival depends on the body maintaining relatively constant conditions within the body. **Homeostasis** is what physiologists call the *relative constancy* of the internal environment. The cells of the body live in an internal environment made up mostly of water combined with salts and other dissolved substances.

Like fish in a fishbowl, the cells are able to survive only if the conditions of their watery environment remain relatively stable—that is, only if conditions stay within a narrow range. The temperature, salt content, acid level (pH), fluid volume and pressure, oxygen concentration, and other vital conditions must remain within acceptable limits. To maintain a narrow range of water conditions in a fishbowl, one may add a heater, an air pump, and filters. Likewise, the body has mechanisms that act as heaters, air pumps, and the like to maintain the relatively stable conditions of its internal fluid environment.

Because the activities of cells and external disturbances are always shifting the conditions inside the body, fluctuations occur frequently. Therefore, the body must constantly work to maintain or restore stability, or homeostasis. For example, the heat generated by muscle activity during exercise may cause the body's temperature to rise above normal. The body must then release sweat, which evaporates and cools the body back to a normal temperature. To accomplish such self-regulation, a highly complex and integrated communication control system is required. The basic type of control system in the body is called a **feedback loop.**

The idea of a feedback loop is borrowed from engineering. Figure 1-9, *A,* shows how an engineer would describe the feedback loop that maintains

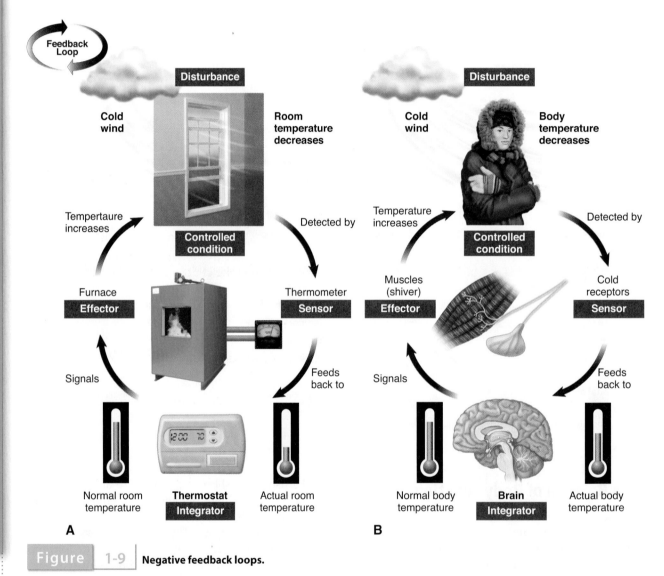

Figure 1-9 | **Negative feedback loops.**

A, An engineer's diagram showing how relatively constant room temperature (controlled condition) can be maintained. A thermostat (control center) receives feedback information from a thermometer (sensor) and responds by counteracting change from normal by activating a furnace (effector). **B,** A physiologist's diagram showing how a relatively constant body temperature (controlled condition) can be maintained. The brain (control center) receives feedback information from nerve endings called *cold receptors* (sensors) and responds by counteracting a change from normal by activating shivering by muscles (effectors).

stability of temperature in a building. Cold winds outside a building may cause a decrease in building temperature below normal. A **sensor,** in this case a thermometer, detects the change in temperature. Information from the sensor *feeds back* to a **control center**—a thermostat in this example—that compares the actual temperature to the normal temperature and responds by activating the building's furnace. The furnace is called an **effector** because it has an effect on the controlled condition (temperature). Because the sensor continually feeds information back to the control center, the furnace will be automatically shut off when the temperature has returned to normal.

As you can see in Figure 1-9, *B,* the body uses a similar feedback loop in restoring body temperature when we become chilled. Nerve endings that act as temperature sensors feed information to a control center in the brain that compares actual body temperature to normal body temperature. In response to a chill, the brain sends nerve signals to muscles that shiver. Shivering produces heat that increases our body temperature. We stop shivering when feedback information tells the brain that body temperature has increased to normal.

Feedback loops such as those shown in Figure 1-9 are called **negative feedback** loops because they oppose, or negate, a change in a controlled condition. Most homeostatic control loops in the body involve negative feedback because reversing changes back toward a normal value tends to stabilize conditions—exactly what homeostasis is all about. An example of a negative feedback loop occurs when decreasing blood oxygen concentration caused by muscles using oxygen during exercise is counteracted by an increase in breathing to bring the blood oxygen level back up to normal. Another example is the excretion of larger than usual volumes of urine when the volume of fluid in the body is greater than the normal, ideal amount.

Although not common, **positive feedback** loops do exist in the body and are also involved in normal function. Positive feedback control loops are stimulatory. Instead of opposing a change in the internal environment and causing a "return to normal," positive feedback loops temporarily amplify or reinforce the change that is occurring. This type of feedback loop causes an ever-increasing rate of events to occur until something stops the process. An example of a positive feedback loop includes the events that cause rapid increases in uterine contractions before the birth of a baby. Another example is the increasingly rapid sticking together of blood cells called *platelets* to form a plug that begins formation of a blood clot.

In each of these cases, the process increases rapidly until the positive feedback loop is stopped suddenly by the birth of a baby or the formation of a clot. In the long run, such normal positive feedback events also help maintain constancy of the internal environment.

It is important to realize that homeostatic control mechanisms can maintain only a *relative* constancy. All homeostatically controlled conditions in the body do not remain absolutely constant. Rather, conditions normally fluctuate near a normal, ideal value. Thus body temperature, for example, rarely remains exactly the same for very long; it usually fluctuates up and down near a person's normal body temperature.

Because all organs function to help maintain homeostatic balance, we will be discussing negative and positive feedback mechanisms often throughout the remaining chapters of this book.

Before leaving this brief introduction to physiology, we must pause to state an important principle: the ability to maintain the balance of body functions is related to age. During childhood, homeostatic functions gradually become more and more efficient and effective. They operate with maximum efficiency and effectiveness during young adulthood. During late adulthood and old age, they gradually become less and less efficient and effective. Changes and functions occurring during the early years are called *developmental processes;* those occurring after young adulthood are called *aging processes.* In general, developmental processes improve efficiency of functions; aging processes usually diminish it.

QUICK CHECK

1. Why is *homeostasis* also called "balance" of body function?
2. What is a *feedback loop* and how does it work?
3. How does *negative feedback* differ from *positive feedback?*

RESEARCH, ISSUES, AND TRENDS

THE SCIENTIFIC METHOD

What we call the **scientific method** is merely a systematic approach to discovery. Although there is no single method for scientific discovery, many scientists follow the steps outlined here (see figure at right) to discover the concepts of human biology discussed in this textbook.

First, one makes a tentative explanation, called a **hypothesis.** A hypothesis is a reasonable guess based on previous informal observations or on previously tested explanations.

After a hypothesis has been proposed, it must be tested—a process called **experimentation.** Scientific experiments are designed to be as simple as possible, to avoid the possibility of errors. Often, **experimental controls** are used to ensure that the test situation itself is not affecting the results. For example, if a new cancer drug is being tested, half the test subjects will get the drug and half the subjects will be given a harmless substitute. The group getting the drug is called the *test group,* and the group getting the substitute is called the *control group.* If both groups improve, or if only the control group improves, the drug's effectiveness hasn't been demonstrated. If the test group improves, but the control group doesn't, the hypothesis that the drug works is tentatively accepted as true. Experimentation requires accurate measurement and recording of data.

If the results of experimentation support the original hypothesis, it is tentatively accepted as true, and the researcher moves on to the next step. If the data do not support the hypothesis, the researcher tentatively rejects the hypothesis. Knowing which hypotheses are untrue is as valuable as knowing which hypotheses are true.

Initial experimental results are published in scientific journals so that other researchers can benefit from them and verify them. If experimental results cannot be reproduced by other scientists, then the hypothesis is not widely accepted. If a hypothesis withstands this rigorous retesting, the level of confidence in the hypothesis increases. A hypothesis that has gained a high level of confidence is called a **theory** or **law.**

The facts presented in this textbook are among the latest theories of how the body is built and how it functions. As methods of imaging the body and measuring functional processes improve, we find new data that cause us to replace old theories with newer ones.

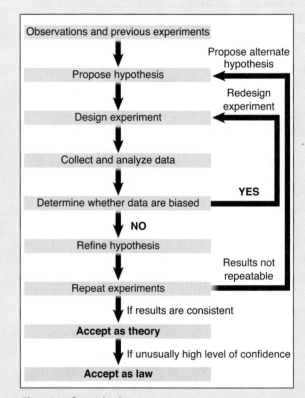

The scientific method.

In this classic example, initial observations or results from other experiments may lead to formation of a new hypothesis. As more testing is done, eliminating outside influences or biases and ensuring consistent results, scientists begin to have more confidence in the tested principle and then call it a theory or law

HEALTH & WELL-BEING

EXERCISE PHYSIOLOGY

Exercise physiologists study the effects of exercise on the body's organ systems. For example, many are interested in the complex control mechanisms that preserve or restore homeostasis during or immediately after periods of strenuous physical activity. Exercise, defined as any significant use of skeletal muscles, is a normal activity with beneficial results. However, exercise disrupts homeostasis. For example, when muscles are worked, the core body temperature rises and blood CO_2 levels increase. These and many other body functions quickly deviate from "normal ranges" that exist at rest. Complex control mechanisms must then "kick in" to restore homeostasis.

As a scientific discipline, exercise physiology often attempts to explain many body processes in terms of how they maintain homeostasis. Exercise physiology has many practical applications in therapy and rehabilitation, athletics, occupational health, and general wellness. This specialty concerns itself with the function of the whole body, not just one or two body systems.

Outline Summary

To download an MP3 version of the chapter summary for use with your iPod or portable media player, access the **Audio Chapter Summaries** on your CD.

Structural Levels of Organization (Figure 1-1)

A. Organization is the most important characteristic of body structure
B. The body as a whole (organism) is a unit constructed of the following smaller units:
  1. Atoms and molecules—chemical level
  2. Cells—the smallest structural units; organizations of various chemicals
  3. Tissues—organizations of similar cells
  4. Organs—organizations of different kinds of tissues
  5. Systems—organizations of many different kinds of organs

Anatomical Position (Figure 1-2)

A. Reference position in which the body is standing erect with the feet slightly apart and arms at the sides with palms turned forward
B. Anatomical position gives meaning to directional terms

Anatomical Directions

A. Superior—toward the head, upper, above; inferior—toward the feet, lower, below
B. Anterior—front, in front of (same as ventral in humans); posterior—back, in back of (same as dorsal in humans)
C. Medial—toward the midline of a structure; lateral—away from the midline or toward the side of a structure
D. Proximal—toward or nearest the trunk, or nearest the point of origin of a structure; distal—away from or farthest from the trunk, or farthest from a structure's point of origin
E. Superficial—nearer the body surface; deep—farther away from the body surface

Planes or Body Sections (Figure 1-3)

A. Sagittal plane—lengthwise plane that divides a structure into right and left sections
B. Midsagittal—sagittal plane that divides the body into two equal halves

C. Frontal (coronal) plane—lengthwise plane that divides a structure into anterior and posterior sections

D. Transverse plane—horizontal plane that divides a structure into upper and lower sections

Body Cavities (Figure 1-4)

A. Ventral cavity
1. Thoracic cavity
   a. Mediastinum—midportion of thoracic cavity; heart and trachea located in mediastinum
   b. Pleural cavities—right lung located in right pleural cavity, left lung in left pleural cavity
2. Abdominopelvic cavity
   a. Abdominal cavity contains stomach, intestines, liver, gallbladder, pancreas, and spleen
   b. Pelvic cavity contains reproductive organs, urinary bladder, and lowest part of intestine
   c. Abdominopelvic regions (Figures 1-5 and 1-6)
      (1) Four quadrants
      (2) Nine regions

B. Dorsal cavity
1. Cranial cavity contains brain
2. Spinal cavity contains spinal cord

Body Regions (Figure 1-8)

A. Axial region—head, neck, and torso or trunk
B. Appendicular region—upper and lower extremities

The Balance of Body Functions

A. Survival of the individual and of the genes that make up the body is of the utmost importance
B. Survival depends on the maintenance or restoration of homeostasis (relative constancy of the internal environment; Figure 1-9)
1. The body uses negative feedback loops and, less often, positive feedback loops to maintain or restore homeostasis
2. Feedback loops involve a sensor, a control center, and an effector
C. All organs function to maintain homeostasis
D. Ability to maintain balance of body functions is related to age; peak efficiency occurs during young adulthood, diminishing efficiency occurs after young adulthood

New Words

abdominal	anatomical position	axial	control center
abdominopelvic quadrants (4)	anatomy	cavities	cranial
	anterior	cell	deep
abdominopelvic regions (9)	appendicular	chemical level	diaphragm

directional terms	hypothesis	physiology	superior
disease	iliac (region)	planes (of body)	supine
dissection	inferior	pleural	system
distal	lateral	positive feedback	theory
dorsal	lumbar (region)	posterior	thoracic
effector	medial	prone	tissue
epigastric (region)	mediastinum	proximal	transverse
experimentation	midsagittal plane	sagittal	ventral
feedback loop	negative feedback	scientific method	
frontal	organ	sections (of body)	**Diseases and Other**
homeostasis	organization (structural	sensor	**Clinical Terms**
hypochondriac (region)	levels)	spinal	atrophy
hypogastric (region)	pelvic	superficial	pathology

Review Questions

1. Define *anatomy, physiology,* and *pathology.*
2. Disease results from what general conditions in the body?
3. List and explain the levels of organization in the human body.
4. Describe the anatomical position.
5. Name and explain the three planes or sections of the body.
6. List two organs of the mediastinum, two organs of the abdominal cavity, and two organs of the pelvic cavity.
7. From the upper left to lower right, list the nine regions of the abdominopelvic cavity.
8. Name the two subdivisions of the dorsal cavity. What structure does each contain?
9. Explain the difference between the terms *lower extremity, thigh,* and *leg.*
10. List four conditions in the cell that must be kept in homeostatic balance.

11. List the three parts of a negative feedback loop and give the function of each.

Critical Thinking

12. Name a structure that is inferior to the heart; superior to the heart; anterior to the heart; posterior to the heart; and lateral to the heart.
13. The maintenance of body temperature and the birth of a baby are two body functions that are regulated by feedback loops. Explain the different feedback loops that regulate each process.
14. If a person complained of pain in the epigastric region, what organs could be involved?

Chapter Test

1. _Cutting up_ is a term derived from two Greek words meaning "cutting up."
2. _Physiology_ means the study of the function of living organisms and their parts.
3. _Pathology_ is the scientific study of disease.
4. _cells_, _tissues_, _organs_, _systems_, and _body as a whole_ are the five levels of organization in a living thing.
5. _supine_ and _prone_ are terms used to describe the body position when it is not in anatomical position.
6. A _superior_ section cuts the body or any of its parts into upper and lower portions.
7. A _anterior_ section cuts the body or any of its parts into front and back portions.
8. A _medial_ section cuts the body or any of its parts into left and right portions.
9. If the body is cut into equal right and left sides, the cut is called a _Sagittal_ section or plane.
10. The body portion that consists of the head, neck, and torso is called the _axial region_ portion.
11. The body portion that consists of the upper and lower extremities is called the _appendicular region_ portion.
12. The two major cavities of the body are the:
    a. thoracic and abdominal
    b. abdominal and pelvic
    c. dorsal and ventral
    d. anterior and posterior

13. The structure that divides the thoracic cavity from the abdominal cavity is the:
    a. mediastinum
    b. diaphragm
    c. lungs
    d. stomach
14. The epigastric region of the abdominopelvic cavity is:
    a. inferior to the umbilical region
    b. lateral to the umbilical region
    c. medial to the umbilical region
    d. none of the above
15. The hypogastric region of the abdominopelvic cavity is:
    a. inferior to the umbilical region
    b. lateral to the left iliac region
    c. medial to the right iliac region
    d. both a and c
16. Which of the following is an example of a positive feedback loop?
    a. Maintaining a constant body temperature
    b. Contractions of the uterus during childbirth
    c. Maintaining a constant volume of water in the body
    d. Both a and c
17. Which of the following is an example of a negative feedback loop?
    a. Maintaining a constant body temperature
    b. Contractions of the uterus during childbirth
    c. Maintaining a constant volume of water in the body
    d. Both a and c

Match each directional term in column B with its opposite term in column A.

Column A		Column B
18. _inferior_ superior		a. posterior
19. _proximal_ distal		b. superficial
20. _posterior_ anterior		c. medial
21. _medial_ lateral		d. proximal
22. _superficial_ deep		e. inferior

Study Tips

continued from page 3

terms are fairly easy to learn because they are presented in opposite pairs, so if you learn one term, you almost always automatically know its opposite. Flash cards will help you learn them. Table 1-2 and Appendix B on the CD that accompanies your book are helpful resources to keep in mind when you see an unfamiliar term.

4. In your study group, try to come up with examples of negative feedback loops that help maintain a balance. Be creative; don't just use the furnace example. Go over your directional flash cards or photocopy Figure 1-3 and then blacken out the terms so you and your fellow students can use the illustration to quiz each other. Go over the questions at the end of the chapter and discuss possible test questions.

Case Studies

1. Mrs. Miller was referred to the clinic by her regular physician to have a mole on her skin examined. The referral form states that the mole is on the left upper quadrant of her abdomen. Give a more detailed description of its location. In preparing Mrs. Miller for the examination, how would you position her? Should you ask her to assume a supine or prone position? During the examination, the physician notices that the referral form states that Mrs. Miller has a similar mole in the occipital region. What position should she assume so that the physician can examine that mole?

2. Mr. Sanchez has just severed the distal tip of the fourth digit on his upper extremity. Describe in layman's terms which body part he has injured. As blood poured out of the injured tissue, his blood pressure dropped. His heart then pumped faster to restore normal pressure. What effect would this response have on Mr. Sanchez's homeostasis? Would such a response be an example of negative or positive feedback?

Outline

Objectives

After you have completed this chapter, you should be able to:

1. Define the terms *atom*, *element*, *molecule*, and *compound*.

2. Describe the structure of an atom.

3. Compare and contrast ionic and covalent types of chemical bonding.

4. Distinguish between *organic* and *inorganic* chemical compounds.

5. Discuss the chemical characteristics of water.

6. Explain the concept of pH.

7. Discuss the structure and function of the following types of organic molecules: *carbohydrate, lipid, protein,* and *nucleic acid*.

2 Chemistry of Life

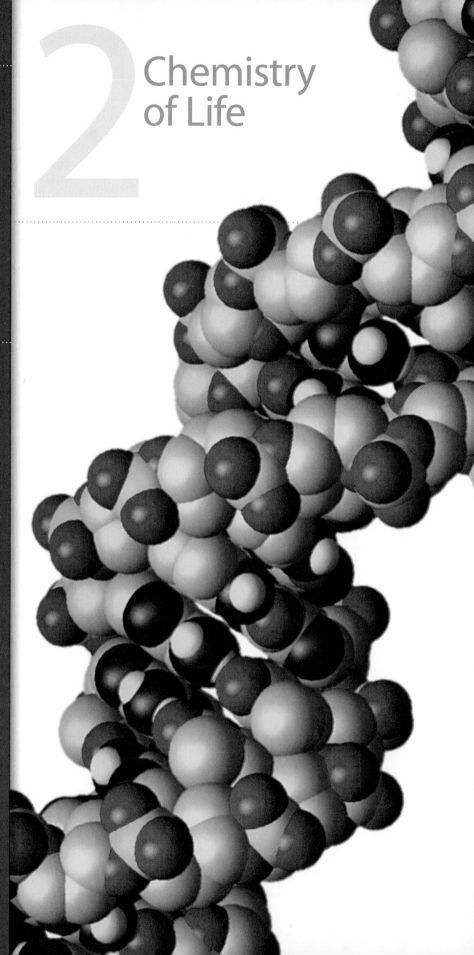

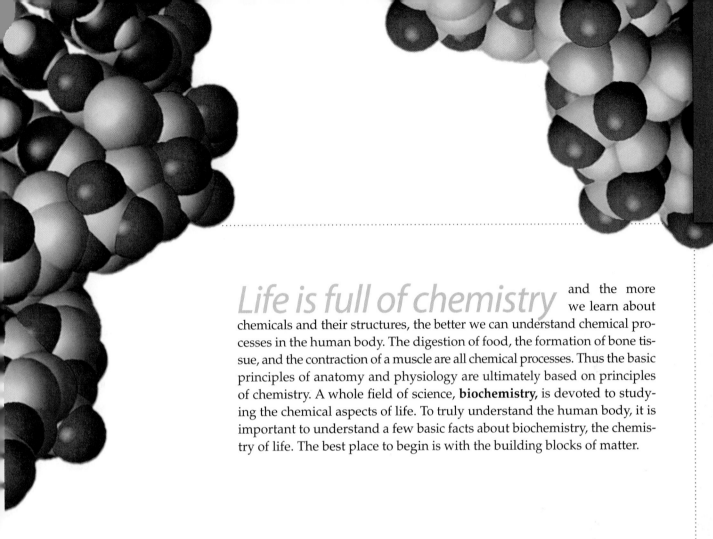

Life is full of chemistry and the more we learn about chemicals and their structures, the better we can understand chemical processes in the human body. The digestion of food, the formation of bone tissue, and the contraction of a muscle are all chemical processes. Thus the basic principles of anatomy and physiology are ultimately based on principles of chemistry. A whole field of science, **biochemistry,** is devoted to studying the chemical aspects of life. To truly understand the human body, it is important to understand a few basic facts about biochemistry, the chemistry of life. The best place to begin is with the building blocks of matter.

STUDY TIPS

This chapter introduces you to some basic chemical concepts that are used later in other chapters to describe structures and functions of the body. First of all, it's important that you can read and understand a handful of important chemical symbols and equations.

1. Practice by putting the chemical symbols found in Tables 2-1 and 2-2 on flash cards and then pair up with a classmate and quiz each other on what the symbols stand for. Also learn to identify whether each one *is* or *is not* an ion.

2. If your instructor requires you to know the parts of the atom, make your own labeled diagram of an atom or make a three-dimensional model out of household items such as marshmallows, toothpicks, and string. Using multiple senses will help you learn and remember the information.

3. It is important that you learn the concept of pH value, which will be an integral part of later discussions. Practice identifying whether particular pH values are neutral, acid, or base by making a simple "wheel of fortune" out

continued on page 39

Levels of Chemical Organization

Matter is anything that occupies space and has mass. Biochemists classify matter into several levels of organization for easier study. The smallest unit of matter is the **atom.** Atoms are used to build more complicated substances in the body. In the body, most chemicals are in the form of molecules. **Molecules** are particles of matter that are composed of one or more atoms.

Atoms

Atoms are units that are so small they can be observed only with very sophisticated techniques. Atoms are composed of several kinds of *subatomic particles:* **protons, electrons,** and **neutrons.** At the core of each atom is a nucleus composed of positively charged protons and uncharged neutrons. The number of protons in the nucleus is an atom's **atomic number.** The number of protons and neutrons combined is the atom's **atomic mass.**

Negatively charged electrons surround the nucleus at a distance. If an atom is neutral (carries no electrical charge), there is one electron for every proton. Electrons don't stay still. Instead, they move about within certain limits called *orbitals.* Imagine the electrons orbiting the nucleus like planets orbit the sun. Orbitals are arranged into **energy levels** (shells), depending on their distance from the nucleus. The farther an orbital extends from the nucleus, the higher its energy level. The energy level closest to the nucleus has one orbital, so it can hold two electrons. The next energy level has up to four orbitals, so it can hold eight electrons. Figure 2-1 shows a carbon (C) atom. Notice that the first energy level (the innermost shell) contains two electrons and the outer energy level contains four electrons. The outer energy level of a carbon atom could hold up to four more electrons (for a total of eight). The number of electrons in the outer energy level of an atom determines how it behaves chemically (that is, how it may unite with other atoms). This behavior, called *chemical bonding,* will be discussed later.

Elements, Molecules, and Compounds

Substances can be classified as **elements** or **compounds.** Elements are pure substances, composed of only one of more than a hundred types of atoms that exist in nature. Only four kinds of atoms (**oxygen, carbon, hydrogen,** and **nitrogen**) make up about 96% of the human body. There are traces of about

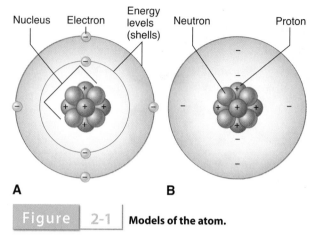

Figure 2-1 | **Models of the atom.**

The nucleus—protons (+) and uncharged neutrons—is at the core. Electrons inhabit outer regions called *energy levels* **(A),** which look more like a cloud because the electrons do not stay in one place **(B).** This is a carbon atom, a fact that is determined by the number of its protons. All carbon atoms (and only carbon atoms) have six protons. (One proton in the nucleus is not visible in this illustration.)

20 other elements in the body. Table 2-1 lists some of the elements in the body and also gives their universal chemical *symbols*—the abbreviations used by chemists worldwide.

Atoms usually unite with each other to form larger chemical units called *molecules.* Some molecules are made of several atoms of the same element. *Compounds* are substances whose molecules have more than one element in them. In order to describe which atoms are present in a compound, a chemical *formula* is used. The formula for a compound contains symbols that represent each element in the molecule. The number of atoms of each element in the molecule is expressed as a subscript after the elemental symbol. For example, each molecule of the compound **carbon dioxide** has one carbon (C) atom and two oxygen (O) atoms; thus its molecular formula is CO_2.

 To learn more about molecule formation, go to **AnimationDirect** on your CD.

QUICK CHECK

1. What kinds of particles make up matter?
2. What is a *compound?* An *element?*
3. Can you describe an *energy level?*

Table	2-1	**Important Elements in the Human Body**		
		NAME	**SYMBOL**	**NUMBER OF ELECTRONS IN OUTER SHELL***
Major elements (more than 96% of body weight)		Oxygen	O	6
		Carbon	C	4
		Hydrogen	H	1
		Nitrogen	N	5
Trace elements (examples of some of the more than 20 trace elements found in the body)		Calcium	Ca	2
		Phosphorus	P	5
		Sodium (Latin *natrium*)	Na	1
		Potassium (Latin *kalium*)	K	1
		Chlorine	Cl	7
		Iodine	I	7

*Maximum is eight, except for hydrogen. The maximum for that element is two.

Chemical Bonding

Chemical bonds form to make atoms more stable. An atom is said to be chemically stable when its outer energy level is "full" (that is, when its energy shells have the maximum number of electrons they can hold). All but a handful of atoms have room for more electrons in their outermost energy level. A basic chemical principle states that atoms react with one another in ways that make their outermost energy level full. To create this full energy level, atoms can share, donate, or borrow electrons.

CLINICAL APPLICATION

RADIOACTIVE ISOTOPES

Each element is unique because of the number of protons it has. In short, each element has its own *atomic number*. However, atoms of the same element can have different numbers of neutrons. Two atoms that have the same atomic number but different atomic masses are **isotopes** of the same element. An example is hydrogen. Hydrogen has three isotopes: ^{1}H (the most common isotope), ^{2}H, and ^{3}H. The accompanying figure shows that each different isotope has only one proton but different numbers of neutrons.

Some isotopes have unstable nuclei that radiate (give off) particles. Radiation particles include protons, neutrons, electrons, and altered versions of these normal subatomic particles. An isotope that emits radiation is called a **radioactive isotope.**

Radioactive isotopes of common elements are sometimes used to evaluate the function of body parts. Radioactive iodine (^{125}I) that is put into the body and then taken up by the thyroid gland gives off radiation that can be easily measured. Thus the rate of thyroid activity can be determined us-

ing this method. Images of internal organs can be formed by radiation scanners that plot out the location of injected or ingested radioactive isotopes. For example, radioactive technetium (^{99}Tc) is commonly used to image the liver and spleen. The radioactive isotopes ^{13}N, ^{15}O, and ^{11}C are often used to study the brain by way of a technique called the *PET scan*.

Radiation can damage cells. Exposure to high levels of radiation may cause cells to develop into cancer cells. Higher levels of radiation completely destroy tissues, causing *radiation sickness*. Low doses of radioactive substances are sometimes given to cancer patients to destroy cancer cells. The side effects of these treatments result from the unavoidable destruction of normal cells along with the cancer cells.

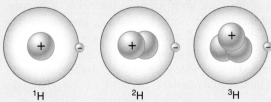

^{1}H ^{2}H ^{3}H

For example, a hydrogen atom has one electron and one proton. Its single energy shell has one electron but *can* hold two—so it's not full. If two hydrogen atoms "share" their single electrons with each other, then both will have full energy shells, making them more stable *as a molecule* than either would be as an atom. This is one example of how atoms **bond** to form molecules. Other atoms may donate or borrow electrons until the outermost energy level is full.

Ionic Bonds

One common way in which atoms make their outermost energy level full is to form **ionic bonds** with other atoms. Such a bond forms between an atom that has only one or two electrons in the outermost level (which would normally hold eight) and an atom that needs only one or two electrons to fill its outer level. The atom with one or two electrons simply "donates" its outer shell electrons to the one that needs one or two.

For example, as you can see in Table 2-1, the sodium (Na) atom has one electron in its outer level and the chlorine (Cl) atom has seven. Both need to have eight electrons to fill their outer shell. Figure 2-2 shows how sodium and chlorine form an ionic bond when sodium "donates" the electron in its outer shell to chlorine. Now both atoms have full outer shells (although sodium's outer shell is now one energy level lower). Because the sodium atom lost an electron, it now has one more proton than it has electrons. This makes it a positive **ion,** an electrically charged atom. Chlorine has "borrowed" an electron to become a negative ion called the *chloride ion.* Because oppositely charged particles attract one another, the sodium and chloride ions are drawn together to form a sodium chloride (NaCl) molecule—common table salt. The molecule is held together by an *ionic bond.*

Ionic molecules usually dissolve easily in water because water molecules wedge between the ions and force them apart. When this happens, we say the molecules **dissociate** (dis-SOH-see-ayt) to form free ions. Molecules that form ions when dissolved in water are called **electrolytes** (ee-LEK-troh-lytes). Chapter 20 describes mechanisms that maintain the homeostasis of electrolytes in the body. Table 2-2 lists some of the more important ions present in body fluids. Ions are used by the body for muscle contraction, to generate nerve impulses, and for numerous other processes that will be described throughout your study of the human body.

The formula of an ion always shows its charge by a "+" or "−" superscript after the chemical symbol.

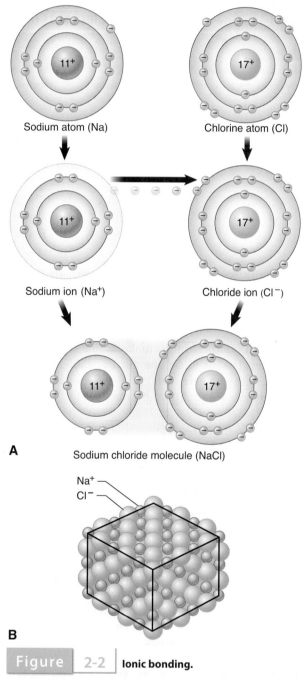

A, The sodium atom donates the single electron in its outer energy level to a chlorine atom having seven electrons in its outer level. Then both have eight electrons in their outer shells. Because the electron/proton ratio changes, the sodium atom becomes a positive sodium ion. The chlorine atom becomes a negative chloride ion. The positive-negative attraction between these oppositely charged ions is called an *ionic bond.* **B,** A cube-shaped crystal of sodium chloride (table salt).

Sodium atom (Na) Chlorine atom (Cl)

Sodium ion (Na$^+$) Chloride ion (Cl$^-$)

A Sodium chloride molecule (NaCl)

Na$^+$
Cl$^-$

B

Figure 2-2 | Ionic bonding.

Table 2-2	Important Ions in Body Fluids
NAME	**SYMBOL**
Sodium (Latin *natrium*)	Na^+
Chloride	Cl^-
Potassium (Latin *kalium*)	K^+
Calcium	Ca^{++}
Hydrogen	H^+
Magnesium	Mg^{++}
Hydroxide	$OH-$
Phosphate	$PO_4^=$
Bicarbonate	HCO_3^-

Thus the sodium ion is Na^+, and the chloride ion is Cl^-. Calcium (Ca) atoms lose two electrons when they form ions, so the calcium ion is written as Ca^{++}.

Covalent Bonds

Atoms may also fill their energy levels by sharing electrons rather than donating or receiving them. When atoms share electrons, a **covalent** (koh-VAY-lent) **bond** forms. Figure 2-3 shows how two hydrogen atoms may move together closely so that their energy levels overlap. Each energy level contributes its one electron to the sharing relationship. That way, both outer levels have access to both electrons. Because atoms involved in a covalent bond must stay close to each other, it is not surprising that covalent bonds are not easily broken. Covalent bonds normally do not break apart in water. Carbon, nitrogen, oxygen, and hydrogen almost always share electrons to form covalent bonds, making this type of bonding important in the human body. Covalent bonding is used to form all of the major organic compounds found in the body.

Hydrogen Bonds

Another type of bonding that is important in the human body but that does *not* result in the formation of a new molecule is hydrogen bonding. **Hydrogen bonds** do not create molecules, but rather, weakly bond neighboring molecules. This type of bonding is present in **water, DNA,** and **proteins,** among others. It is responsible for some of the unique characteristics of water and helps to stabilize DNA and large proteins. Figure 2-11 depicts the hydrogen bonding that occurs between two strands of DNA.

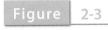

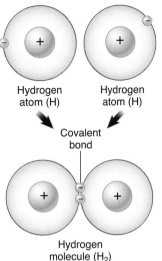

Hydrogen atom (H)   Hydrogen atom (H)

Covalent bond

Hydrogen molecule (H₂)

Covalent bonding.

Two hydrogen atoms move together, overlapping their energy levels. Although neither gains nor loses an electron, the atoms share the electrons, thereby forming a covalent bond.

QUICK CHECK

1. How is an *ion* formed?
2. What is meant by an electrolyte *dissociating* in water?
3. How does hydrogen bonding differ from ionic and covalent bonding?

Inorganic Chemistry

In living organisms, there are two kinds of compounds: **organic** and **inorganic.** Organic compounds are composed of molecules that contain carbon-carbon (C—C) covalent bonds or carbon-hydrogen (C—H) covalent bonds—or both kinds of bonds. Few inorganic compounds have carbon atoms in them and none have C—C or C—H bonds. Organic molecules are generally larger and more complex than inorganic molecules. The human body has both kinds of compounds because both are equally important to the chemistry of life. We will discuss the chemistry of inorganic compounds first, then move on to some of the important types of organic compounds.

Water

Although it is an inorganic compound, water is essential to life. Water is the most abundant compound in the body, found in and around each cell. It is the **solvent** in which most other compounds or **solutes** are dissolved. When water is the solvent for a *mixture* (a blend of two or more kinds of molecules), the mixture is called an **aqueous solution.**

An aqueous solution containing common salt (NaCl) and other molecules forms the "internal sea" of the body. Water molecules not only compose the basic internal environment of the body but also participate in many important *chemical reactions*. Chemical reactions are interactions among molecules in which atoms regroup into new combinations. Interestingly, all four of the major organic compounds in the body are formed by the same type of chemical reaction, and all involve water.

Dehydration synthesis reactions are a common type of chemical reaction in the body. In any kind of synthesis reaction, the **reactants** combine to form a larger **product.** In dehydration synthesis, reactants combine only after hydrogen (H) and oxygen (O) atoms are removed. These leftover H and O atoms come together, forming H_2O, or water. As Figure 2-4 shows, the result is both the large product molecule and a water molecule. Just as dehydration of a cell is a loss of water from the cell and dehydration of the body is loss of fluid from the entire internal environment, dehydration synthesis is a reaction in which water is lost from the reactants.

Another common reaction in the body, **hydrolysis** (hye-DROL-i-sis), also involves water. In this reaction, water (*hydro-*) disrupts the bonds in large molecules, causing them to be broken down into smaller molecules (*lysis*). Hydrolysis is virtually the reverse of dehydration synthesis, as Figure 2-4 shows.

Chemical reactions always involve energy transfers. Energy is required to build the molecules. Some of that energy is stored as potential energy in the chemical bonds. The stored energy can then be released when the chemical bonds in the molecule are later broken apart. For example, a molecule called **adenosine triphosphate (ATP)** breaks apart in the muscle cells to yield the energy needed for muscle contraction (see Figure 18-2 on p. 527).

Chemists often use a *chemical equation* to represent a chemical reaction. In a chemical equation, the reactants are separated from the products by an arrow ($\rightarrow$) showing the "direction" of the reaction. Reactants are separated from each other, and products are separated from each other by addition, or plus, signs (+). Thus the reaction *potassium and chloride combined to form potassium chloride* can be expressed as the following equation:

$$K^+ + Cl^- \rightarrow KCl$$

The single arrow $\rightarrow$ is used for equations that occur in only one direction. For example, when hydrochloric acid (HCl) is dissolved in water, all of it dissociates to form H^+ and Cl^-.

$$HCl \rightarrow H^+ + Cl^-$$

The double arrow $\leftrightarrow$ is used for reactions that happen in "both directions" at the same time. When carbonic acid (H_2CO_3) dissolves in water, some of it dissociates into H^+ (hydrogen ion) and HCO_3^- (bicarbonate), but not all of it. As additional ions dissociate, previously dissociated ions bond together again, forming H_2CO_3.

$$H_2CO_3 \leftrightarrow H^+ HCO_3^-$$

In short, the double arrow indicates that at any instant in time both reactants and products are present in the solution at the same time.

Acids, Bases, and Salts

Besides water, many other inorganic compounds are important in the chemistry of life. For example, acids and bases are compounds that profoundly affect chemical reactions in the body, and as such are closely regulated. As explained in more detail at the beginning of Chapter 19, a few water molecules dissociate to form the H^+ ion and the OH^- (hydroxide) ion:

$$H_2O \leftrightarrow H^+ + OH^-$$

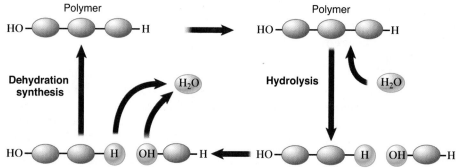

Dehydration synthesis

Hydrolysis

Figure 2-4

Water-based chemistry.

Dehydration synthesis (*on the left*) is a reaction in which small molecules are assembled into large molecules by removing water (H and O atoms). Hydrolysis (*on the right*) operates in the reverse direction; H and O from water are added as large molecules are broken down into small molecules.

RESEARCH, ISSUES, AND TRENDS

BOTTLED OR TAP?

As the demand for bottled water has increased over recent years, have you ever asked yourself, "Which source of water really is better for my body, bottled or tap?" It may be of interest to you that 40% to 60% of the bottled water sold worldwide is actually nothing more than packaged tap water that *may* have been reprocessed in some way. Overall, both sources of water in the United States are safe to drink. Some believe that bottled water is healthier than tap, but EPA regulations for tap water are stricter than FDA regulations for bottled water. Taste preference seems to be a major factor in which is chosen, and it may be this reason most

of all that could impact health and homeostasis. If you don't like the way your water tastes, you won't drink as much of it, so taste and hydration are related, and this could affect your health. However, many of us can't tell the difference between bottled water and tap water in a taste test. Additionally, fluoride, an important mineral that is widely accepted as being beneficial in reducing the incidence of cavities, is often missing from bottled water but generally added to tap water. So, the next time you consider whether to pay extra for bottled water or simply turn on the faucet, you may want to do a little research before you decide, "bottled or tap?"

In pure water, the balance between these two ions is equal. However, when an acid such as hydrochloric acid (HCl) dissociates into H^+ and Cl^-, it shifts this balance in favor of excess H^+ ions. In the blood, carbon dioxide (CO_2) forms carbonic acid (H_2CO_3) when it dissolves in water. Some of the carbonic acid then dissociates to form H^+ ions and HCO_3^- (bicarbonate) ions, producing an excess of H^+ ions in the blood. Thus high CO_2 levels in the blood make the blood more acidic.

Bases, or **alkaline** compounds, on the other hand, shift the balance in the opposite direction. For example, sodium hydroxide (NaOH) is a base that forms OH^- ions but no H^+ ions. In short, **acids** are compounds that produce an excess of H^+ ions, and **bases** are compounds that produce an excess of OH^- ions (or a decrease in H^+).

The relative H^+ concentration is a measure of how acidic or basic a solution is. The H^+ concentration is usually expressed in units of **pH.** The formula used to calculate pH units gives a value of 7 to pure water. A higher pH value indicates a low relative concentration of H^+—a base. A lower pH value indicates a higher H^+ concentration—an acid. Figure 2-5 shows a scale of pH from 0 to 14. Notice that when the pH of a solution is less than 7, the scale "tips" toward the side marked "high H^+." When the pH is more than 7, the scale "tips" toward the side marked "low H^+." pH units increase or decrease by factors of 10. Thus a pH 5 solution has 10 times the H^+ concentration of a pH 6 solution. A pH 4 solution has 100 times the H^+ concentration of a pH 6 solution.

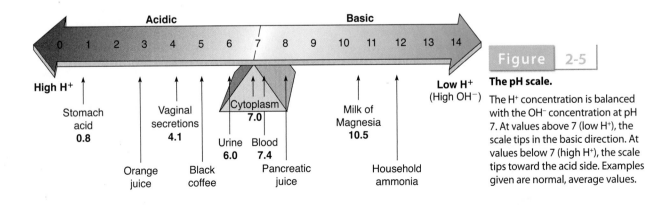

Figure 2-5

The pH scale.

The H^+ concentration is balanced with the OH^- concentration at pH 7. At values above 7 (low H^+), the scale tips in the basic direction. At values below 7 (high H^+), the scale tips toward the acid side. Examples given are normal, average values.

A *strong acid* is an acid that completely, or almost completely, dissociates to form H^+ ions. A *weak acid,* on the other hand, dissociates very little and therefore produces few excess H^+ ions in solution.

When a strong acid and a strong base mix, excess H^+ ions may combine with the excess OH^- ions to form water. That is, they may *neutralize* each other. The remaining ions usually form neutral ionic compounds called **salts.** For example:

$$HCl + NaOH \rightarrow H^+ + Cl^- + Na^+ + OH^- \rightarrow H_2O + NaCl$$

acid   base   water   salt

The pH of body fluids affects body chemistry so greatly that normal body function can be maintained only within a narrow range of pH. Acidosis (low blood pH) and alkalosis (high blood pH) are equally dangerous and thankfully rarely occurs because of the homeostatic mechanisms of the body. The body can remove excess H^+ ions by excreting them in the urine (see Chapter 19). Another way to remove acid is by increasing the loss of CO_2 (an acid) by way of the respiratory system (see Chapter 16). A third way to adjust the body's pH is by using **buffers**—chemicals in the blood that maintain pH. Buffers maintain pH balance by preventing sudden changes in the H^+ ion concentration. Buffers do this by forming a chemical system that neutralizes acids and bases as they are added to a solution. The mechanisms by which the body maintains pH homeostasis, or acid-base balance, are discussed further in Chapter 21.

> **QUICK CHECK**
>
> 1. Define an organic compound.
> 2. What is the difference between dehydration synthesis and hydrolysis?
> 3. Does an acid have a low pH or a high pH? A base?

Organic Chemistry

Organic compounds are much more complex than inorganic compounds. In this section, we describe the basic structure and function of each major type of organic compound found in the body: **carbohydrates, lipids** (fats), **proteins,** and **nucleic acids.** Table 2-3 summarizes the structure and the function of each type. Refer to this table as you read through the descriptions that follow. All four of these organic compounds are formed by dehydration synthesis reactions. Conversely, their bonds can be broken by hydrolysis.

Table 2-3 | Major Types of Organic Compounds

EXAMPLE	COMPONENTS	FUNCTIONS
CARBOHYDRATE		
Monosaccharide (glucose, galactose, fructose)	Single monosaccharide unit	Unit as source of energy; used to build other carbohydrates
Disaccharide (sucrose, lactose, maltose)	Two monosaccharide units	Can be broken into monosaccharides
Polysaccharide (glycogen, starch)	Many monosaccharide units	Used to store monosaccharides (thus to store energy)
LIPID		
Triglyceride	One glycerol, three fatty acids	Stores energy
Phospholipid	Phosphorus-containing unit, two fatty acids	Forms cell membranes
Cholesterol	Four carbon rings at core	Stabilizes cell membranes; is basis of steroid hormones
PROTEIN		
Structural proteins (fibers)	Amino acids	Form structures of the body
Functional proteins (enzymes, hormones)	Amino acids	Facilitate chemical reactions; send signals; regulate functions
NUCLEIC ACID		
Deoxyribonucleic acid (DNA)	Nucleotides (contain deoxyribose)	Contains information (genetic code) for making proteins
Ribonucleic acid (RNA)	Nucleotides (contain ribose)	Serves as a copy of a portion of the genetic code

BIOCHEMISTRY

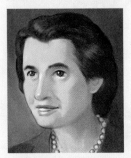

Rosalind Franklin
(1920–1958)

British scientist Rosalind Franklin was one of the leading biochemists of the modern age. Franklin used x-rays to cast shadows through DNA to analyze its structure. When she was only 32 years old, she discovered the unusual helical (spiral) structure of the DNA molecule and how the sugars and phosphates form an outer backbone for the molecule (see Figure 2-11). Her breakthrough helped James Watson, Francis Crick, and Maurice Wilkins to finally work out the structure and function of DNA in 1953 and thus crack the "code of life." The three men received a Nobel Prize for their achievement in 1962, but Franklin's early death from cancer in 1958 prevented her from sharing in the credit for one of the greatest discoveries of all time.

Biochemists continue to make important discoveries that increase our understanding of human structure and function. Aided by laboratory technicians and assistants, biochemists also find ways to help other professionals apply biochemistry to solve everyday problems. For example, clinical laboratory professionals analyze samples from the bodies of patients for signs of health or disease. Others who use biochemistry as a basis for their work include pharmacists and pharmacy technicians, dietitians, forensic investigators, genetic counselors, and even science journalists.

Carbohydrates

The name *carbohydrate* literally means "carbon (C) and water (H_2O)," signifying the types of atoms that form carbohydrate molecules. The basic unit of carbohydrate molecules is called a *monosaccharide* (mon-oh-SAK-ah-ryde) (Figure 2-6). Glucose (dextrose) is an important monosaccharide in the body; cells use it as their primary source of energy (see Chapter 18). A molecule made of two saccharide units is a double sugar, or *disaccharide.* The disaccharides sucrose (table sugar) and lactose (milk sugar) are important dietary carbohydrates. After they are eaten, the body breaks them down, or digests them, to form monosaccharides that can be used as cellular fuel. Many saccharide units joined together form *polysaccharides.* Examples of polysaccharides are **glycogen** (GLYE-koh-jen) and *starch.* Glycogen is the polysaccharide of glucose that the human body stores. Plants store glucose as starch. Each glycogen molecule is a chain of glucose molecules joined together. Liver cells and muscle cells form glycogen when there is an excess of glucose in the blood, thus putting them into "storage" for later use.

Carbohydrates have potential energy stored in their bonds. When the bonds are broken in cells, the energy is released and then trapped by the cell's chemistry to do work. Chapter 18 explains more about the process by which the body extracts energy from carbohydrates and other food molecules.

Carbohydrates

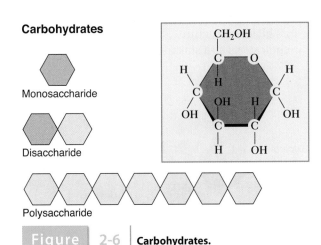

Monosaccharide

Disaccharide

Polysaccharide

Figure 2-6 **Carbohydrates.**

Monosaccharides are single carbohydrate units joined by dehydration synthesis to form disaccharides and polysaccharides. The detailed chemical structure of the monosaccharide *glucose* is shown in the inset.

Lipids

Lipids are fats and oils. Fats are lipids that are solid at room temperature, such as the fat in butter and lard. Oils, such as corn oil and olive oil, are liquid at room temperature. There are several important types of lipids in the body:

1. **Triglycerides** (try-GLISS-er-ydes) are lipid molecules formed by a *glycerol* unit joined to three *fatty acids* (Figure 2-7). Like carbohydrates, their bonds can be broken apart to yield energy (see Chapter 18). Thus triglycerides are useful in storing energy in cells for later use.

2. **Phospholipids** are similar to triglycerides but have phosphorus-containing units in them, as their name implies. The phosphorus-containing unit in each molecule forms a "head" that attracts water. Two fatty acid "tails" repel water. Figure 2-8, *A*, shows the head and tail of the phospholipid molecule. This structure allows them to form a stable *bilayer* in water that forms the foundation for the cell membrane. In Figure 2-8, *B*, the water-attracting heads face the water and the water-repelling tails face away from the water (and toward each other).

3. **Cholesterol** is a *steroid* lipid (a multiple-ring structure) that performs several important functions in the body. It combines with phospholipids in the cell membrane to help stabilize its bilayer structure. The body also uses cholesterol as a starting point in making steroid

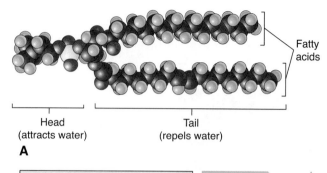

Head (attracts water)   Tail (repels water)

A

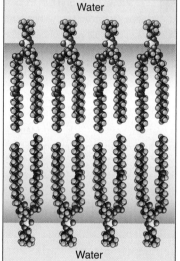

Water

Water

B

Figure 2-8

Phospholipids.

A, Each phospholipid molecule has a phosphorus-containing "head" that attracts water and a lipid "tail" that repels water. **B,** Because the tails repel water, phospholipid molecules often arrange themselves so that their tails face away from water. The stable structure that results is a bilayer sheet forming a small bubble.

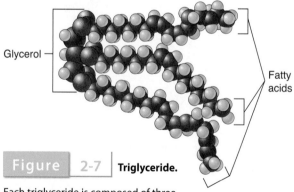

Glycerol

Fatty acids

Figure 2-7   **Triglyceride.**

Each triglyceride is composed of three fatty acid units attached to a glycerol unit.

hormones such as estrogen, testosterone, and cortisone (see Chapter 11).

Proteins

Proteins are very large molecules composed of basic units called **amino acids.** In addition to carbon, hydrogen, and oxygen, amino acids contain nitrogen (N). By means of a process described fully in Chapter 3, a particular sequence of amino acids is strung together and held by **peptide bonds.** Positive-negative attractions between different atoms in the long amino acid strand cause it to coil on itself and maintain its shape. The complex, three-dimensional molecule that results is a protein molecule (Figure 2-9).

The shape of a protein molecule determines its role in body chemistry. **Structural proteins** are shaped in ways that allow them to form essential structures

BLOOD LIPOPROTEINS

A lipid such as cholesterol can travel in the blood only after it has attached to a protein molecule—forming a lipoprotein. Some of these molecules are called *high-density lipoproteins (HDLs)* because they have a high density of protein (more protein than lipid). Another type of molecule contains less protein (and more lipid), so it is called *low-density lipoprotein (LDL)*.

The cholesterol in LDLs is often called "bad" cholesterol because high blood levels of LDL are associated with **atherosclerosis,** a life-threatening blockage of arteries. LDLs carry cholesterol *to cells,* including the cells that line blood vessels. HDLs, on the other hand, carry "good" cholesterol *away from cells* and toward the liver for elimination from the body. A high proportion of HDL in the blood is associated with a low risk of developing atherosclerosis. Factors such as cigarette smoking decrease HDL levels and thus contribute to the risk of atherosclerosis. Factors such as exercise increase HDL levels and thus decrease the risk of atherosclerosis.

---

of the body. Collagen, a protein with a fiber shape, holds most of the body tissues together. Keratin, another structural protein, forms a network of waterproof fibers in the outer layer of the skin. **Functional proteins** participate in chemical processes of the body. Functional proteins include some of the hormones, growth factors, cell membrane channels and receptors, and enzymes.

Enzymes are chemical catalysts. This means that they help a chemical reaction occur but are not reactants or products themselves. They participate in chemical reactions but are not changed by the reactions. Enzymes are vital to body chemistry. No reaction in the body occurs fast enough unless the specific enzymes needed for that reaction are present.

Primary (first level)
Protein structure is a sequence of amino acids in a chain.

— One amino acid

Amino acid chain

Secondary (second level)
Protein structure is formed by folding and twisting of amino acid chain.

Folded sheet   Twisted helix

Figure 2-9 | **Protein.**

Protein molecules are large, complex molecules formed by one or more strands of amino acids. Each amino acid is connected to the next by a type of covalent bond called a *peptide bond*. Additional weak forces between atoms of the larger molecule then cause the strand to twist or fold into a *secondary* (second-level) protein structure. New relationships among the atoms then cause the molecule to fold again on itself to form a three-dimensional *tertiary* (third-level) protein structure. Several tertiary proteins may join to form a *quaternary* (fourth-level) protein structure.

Tertiary (third level)
Protein structure is formed when the twists and folds of the secondary structure fold again to form a larger three-dimensional structure.

Quaternary (fourth level)
Protein structure is a protein consisting of more than one folded amino acid chain.

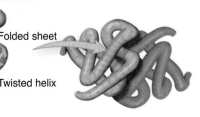

— Folded sheet

— Twisted helix

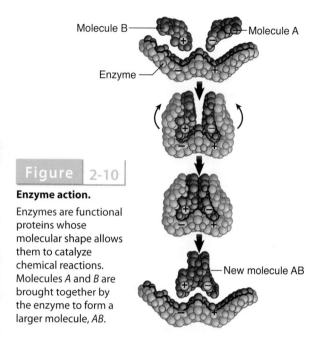

Molecule B — Molecule A

Enzyme

Figure 2-10

Enzyme action.

Enzymes are functional proteins whose molecular shape allows them to catalyze chemical reactions. Molecules *A* and *B* are brought together by the enzyme to form a larger molecule, *AB*.

New molecule AB

Table 2-4	**Components of Nucleotides**	
NUCLEOTIDE	**DNA**	**RNA**
Sugar	Deoxyribose	Ribose
Phosphate	Phosphate	Phosphate
Nitrogen base	Cytosine	Cytosine
	Guanine	Guanine
	Adenine	Adenine
	Thymine	Uracil

Figure 2-10 illustrates how shape is important to the function of enzyme molecules. Each enzyme has a shape that "fits" the specific molecules it works on, much as a key fits specific locks. This explanation of enzyme action is sometimes called the **lock-and-key model.**

Proteins can bond with other organic compounds and form "mixed" molecules. For example, *glycoproteins* (described in Chapter 3) are proteins with sugars attached and are found embedded in cell membranes. *Lipoproteins* (described on p. 33, Clinical Application box) are lipid-protein combinations.

Nucleic Acids

The two forms of nucleic acid are **deoxyribonucleic acid (DNA)** and **ribonucleic acid (RNA).** As outlined in Chapter 3, the basic building blocks of nucleic acids are called **nucleotides.** Each nucleotide consists of a *phosphate unit,* a sugar *(ribose or deoxyribose),* and a *nitrogen base.* DNA nucleotide bases include **adenine, thymine, guanine,** and **cytosine.** RNA uses the same set of bases, except for the substitution of **uracil** for thymine (Table 2-4).

Nucleotides bind to one another to form strands or other structures. In the DNA molecule, nucleotides are arranged in a twisted, double strand called a **double helix** (Figure 2-11).

The sequence of different nucleotides along the DNA double helix is the "master code" for assem-bling proteins and other nucleic acids. *Messenger RNA (mRNA)* molecules have a sequence that forms a temporary "working copy" of a portion of the DNA code called a gene. The code in nucleic acids ultimately directs the entire "symphony" of living chemistry.

QUICK CHECK

1. Which category of organic chemical is made up of *monosaccharides?* Of *fatty acids?* Of *amino acids?* Of *nucleotides?*
2. Why is the structure of a protein molecule important?
3. What is the role of DNA in the body?

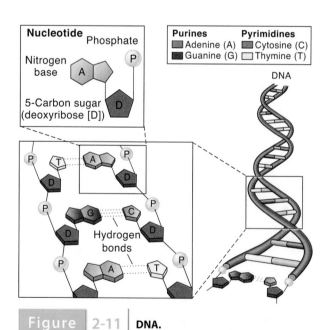

Nucleotide

Phosphate

Nitrogen base

5-Carbon sugar (deoxyribose [D])

Purines **Pyrimidines**
Adenine (A) Cytosine (C)
Guanine (G) Thymine (T)

DNA

Hydrogen bonds

Figure 2-11 DNA.

Deoxyribonucleic acid (DNA), like all nucleic acids, is composed of units called *nucleotides.* Each nucleotide has a phosphate, a sugar, and a nitrogen base. In DNA, the nucleotides are arranged in a double helix formation.

Outline Summary

 To download an MP3 version of the chapter summary for use with your iPod or portable media player, access the **Audio Chapter Summaries** on your CD.

Levels of Chemical Organization

A. Atoms
   1. Nucleus—central core of atom
      a. Proton—positively charged particle in nucleus
      b. Neutron—uncharged particle in nucleus
      c. Atomic number—number of protons in nucleus
      d. Atomic mass—number of protons and neutrons combined
   2. Energy levels—orbital regions surrounding atomic nucleus that contain electrons
      a. Electron—negatively charged particle
      b. May contain up to eight electrons in each level
      c. Energy level increases the farther it is from the nucleus
B. Elements, molecules, and compounds
   1. Element—a pure substance; made up of only one kind of atom
   2. Molecule—a group of atoms bound together in a group
   3. Compound—substances whose molecules have more than one kind of atom

Chemical Bonding

A. Chemical bonds form to make atoms more stable
   1. Atoms react with one another in ways that make their outermost energy level full
   2. Atoms may share electrons or donate or borrow them to become stable
B. Ionic bonds
   1. Ions form when an atom gains or loses electrons in its outer energy level to become stable
      a. Positive ion—has lost electrons; indicated by superscript positive sign(s), as in Na^+ or Ca^{++}
      b. Negative ion—has gained electrons; indicated by superscript negative sign(s), as in Cl^-
   2. Ionic bonds form when positive and negative (oppositely charged) ions attract each other

   3. Electrolyte—molecule that dissociates (breaks apart) in water to form individual ions; an ionic compound
C. Covalent bonds
   1. Covalent bonds form when atoms share their outer energy to fill up and thus become stable
   2. Covalent bonds do not ordinarily easily dissociate in water
   3. Covalent bonding is used to form all of the major organic compounds found in the body.
D. Hydrogen bonds
   1. Hydrogen bonds do not create new molecules
   2. Hydrogen bonds weakly bond neighboring molecules
   3. Hydrogen bonds are present in water, DNA, and proteins

Inorganic Chemistry

A. *Organic* molecules contain carbon-carbon covalent bonds and/or carbon-hydrogen covalent bonds; *inorganic* molecules do not
B. Organic molecules are generally larger and more complex than inorganic molecules
C. Water
   1. Water is an inorganic compound essential to life
   2. Water is a solvent (liquid in which solutes are dissolved), forming aqueous solutions in the body
   3. Water is involved in chemical reactions
      a. Dehydration synthesis—chemical reaction in which water is removed from small molecules so they can be strung together to form a larger molecule
      b. Hydrolysis—chemical reaction in which water is added to the subunits of a large molecule to break it apart into smaller molecules
      c. Chemical reactions always involve energy transfers, as when energy is used to build ATP molecules

  d. Chemical equations show how reactants interact to form products; arrows separate the reactants from the products

D. Acids, bases, and salts
  1. Water molecules dissociate to form equal amounts of H^+ (hydrogen ion) and OH^- (hydroxide ion)
  2. Acid—substance that shifts the H^+/OH^- balance in favor of H^+; opposite of base
  3. Base—substance that shifts the H^+/OH^- balance against H^+; also known as an *alkaline;* opposite of acid
  4. pH—mathematical expression of relative H^+ concentration in an aqueous solution
     a. 7 is neutral (neither acid nor base)
     b. pH values above 7 are basic; pH values below 7 are acidic
  5. Neutralization occurs when acids and bases mix and form salts
  6. Buffers form chemical systems that absorb excess acids or bases and thus maintain a relatively stable pH

Organic Chemistry

A. Carbohydrates—sugars and complex carbohydrates
  1. Contain carbon (C), hydrogen (H), oxygen (O)
  2. Monosaccharide—basic unit of carbohydrate molecules (e.g., glucose)
  3. Disaccharide—double sugar made up of two monosaccharide units (e.g., sucrose, lactose)
  4. Polysaccharide—complex carbohydrate made up of many monosaccharide units (e.g., glycogen; stored by the body)
  5. Function of carbohydrates is to store energy for later use

B. Lipids—fats and oils
  1. Triglycerides
     a. Formed by a glycerol unit joined to three fatty acids
     b. Store energy for later use
  2. Phospholipids
     a. Similar to triglyceride structure, but have phosphorus-containing units— each with a head and two tails
     b. The head attracts water and the double tail does not, thus forming stable double layers (bilayers) in water
     c. Form membranes of cells

  3. Cholesterol
     a. Molecules have a steroid structure made up of multiple rings
     b. Cholesterol stabilizes the phospholipid tails in cellular membranes and is also converted into steroid hormones by the body

C. Proteins
  1. Very large molecules made up of amino acids held together in long, folded chains by peptide bonds
  2. Structural proteins
     a. Form essential structures of the body
        (1) Collagen is a fibrous protein that holds many tissues together
        (2) Keratin forms tough, waterproof fibers in the outer layer of the skin
  3. Functional proteins
     a. Participate in chemical processes of the body
     b. Examples include hormones, cell membrane channels and receptors, and enzymes
  4. Enzymes—chemical catalysts
     a. Help chemical reactions occur
     b. Enzyme action sometimes called lock-and-key model
  5. Proteins can combine with other organic molecules to form "mixed" molecules such as glycoproteins or lipoproteins

D. Nucleic acids
  1. Made up of nucleotides that include:
     a. A phosphate unite
     b. A sugar (ribose or deoxyribose)
     c. A nitrogen base (adenine, thymine or uracil, guanine, cytosine)
  2. DNA (deoxyribonucleic acid)
     a. Used as the cell's "master code" for assembling proteins
     b. Uses deoxyribose as the sugar and A, T (not U), C, and G as bases
     c. Forms a double helix shape
  3. RNA (ribonucleic acid)
     a. Used as a temporary "working copy" of a gene (portion of the DNA code)
     b. Uses ribose as the sugar and A, U (not T), C, and G as bases
  4. By directing the formation of structural and functional proteins, nucleic acids ultimately direct overall body structure and function

New Words

acid	covalent bond	inorganic compound	protein (*structural* and *functional*)
adenine	cytosine	ion	
adenosine triphosphate (ATP)	dehydration synthesis	ionic bond	proton
	deoxyribonucleic acid (DNA)	isotope	radioactive isotope
alkaline		lipid	reactant
amino acid	dissociate	lock-and-key model	ribonucleic acid (RNA)
aqueous solution	double helix	matter	salt
atom	electrolyte	molecule	solute
atomic mass	electron	neutron	solvent
atomic number	element	nucleic acid	structural protein
base	energy level	nucleotide	thymine
biochemistry	enzyme	nucleus	uracil
bond	functional protein	organic compound	
buffer	glycogen	peptide bond	**Diseases and Other Clinical Terms**
carbohydrate	guanine	pH	
carbon dioxide	hydrogen bond	product	atherosclerosis
compound	hydrolysis		

Review Questions

1. Define the terms *element, compound, atom,* and *molecule.*
2. Name and define three kinds of particles within an atom.
3. What is an energy level?
4. What is a chemical bond?
5. What is an electrolyte? An ion?
6. Define the terms *organic compound* and *inorganic compound.*
7. What is a solvent? A solute?
8. Explain the concept of pH.
9. What is an acid? A base?
10. Briefly describe the structure of each of the following: protein, lipid, carbohydrate, nucleic acid.
11. Briefly state the principal functions of each of the following: carbohydrate, protein, lipid, nucleic acid.

Critical Thinking

12. Compare and contrast how ionic bonds and covalent bonds solve the problem of achieving stability in atoms.
13. A particular protein molecule is hydrolyzed by an enzyme. How would you explain that process to someone unfamiliar with chemical terminology?
14. Your blood normally has a pH of around 7.4—is your blood alkaline, acid, or neutral?
15. If a newly discovered protein was found to regulate how hormones influence the functions of cells in the body, would the protein be a structural protein or a functional protein?
16. What mechanism does DNA use to regulate all of the body's structures and function?
17. How would you explain the difference between ^1H, ^2H, and ^3H?

Chapter Test

1. _matter_ is anything that occupies space and has mass.
2. Molecules are made up of particles called _atoms_.
3. Positively charged particles within the nucleus of an atom are called _protons_.
4. Electrons inhabit regions of the atoms called _energy_ levels.
5. Substances with molecules having more than one kind of atom are called _compounds_.
6. A(n) _hydrogen atom_ chemical bond occurs when atoms share electrons.
7. The symbol K⁺ represents the potassium _Kalium ion_.

8. A compound that dissociates in water to form ions is called a(n) _covalent bonds_.
9. Molecules that have a carbon-carbon bond in them are classified as _organic_ compounds.
10. In salt water, salt is the solute and water is the _____.
11. When water is used to build up small molecules into larger molecules, the process is called _____.
12. _H⁺ ions_ are solutions that have an excess of hydrogen ions.
13. The blood contains chemicals called _buffer_ that maintain a stable pH.

Match each directional term in column B with its opposite term in column A.

Column A
14. _____ glycogen
15. _____ collagen
16. _____ RNA
17. _____ cholesterol
18. _____ NaCl
19. _____ NaOH
20. _____ HCl

Column B
a. salt
b. acid
c. base
d. carbohydrate
e. lipid
f. protein
g. nucleic acid

21. An ion is formed when:
    a. electrons are shared
    b. electrons remain in place
    c. electrons are gained or lost
    d. neutrons are added to the nucleus
22. In the equation $H_2O + CO_2 \rightarrow H^+ + HCO_3^-$, which of the compounds is a reactant?
    a. CO_2
    b. HCO_3^-
    c. O_2
    d. $\rightarrow$
23. Which of these chemical subunits is found in DNA?
    a. uracil
    b. ribose
    c. amino acid
    d. deoxyribose

24. Which of these values represents an acid?
    a. pH 7.5
    b. pH 6.1
    c. pH 9.0
    d. pH 7.0
25. Steroid hormones are:
    a. carbohydrates
    b. proteins
    c. lipids
    d. nucleic acids

Study Tips

continued from page 23
of a small square of poster board and a paper clip. On the various spokes of the wheel, print different pH values. Spin the paperclip and identify whether the value it lands on is acid, base, or neutral.

4. Table 2-3 summarizes some important concepts of the structure and function of the major organic compounds that you will be using later in the course.

Make your own version of the table on a poster-sized piece of paper and add simple pictures of the different molecules. Then make flash cards and practice identifying which category different molecules belong to: protein, carbohydrate, lipid, or nucleic acid. Then practice identifying which function each performs.

Case Studies

1. Grania knows that the pH of blood is normally 7.35 to 7.45. She sees that her blood test results show 7.57 as her blood plasma pH. Is Grania's blood too acid or too alkaline—or is her blood pH just what it should be?

2. Baraka has adopted a "high carb" dieting strategy to help him prepare for an upcoming athletic event. What category of organic compound will Baraka be eating in higher proportions than usual? What are some examples of this type of compound that might be found in Baraka's food? What role does this type of organic compound play in Baraka's body? Why might this be an advantage in an athletic event?

3. Sinead's husband Shane O'Shaunessey just received the results from his annual physical examination. Shane sheepishly reported to Sinead that his HDL cholesterol levels have increased significantly. Sinead smiled and told Shane not to worry. Why would Sinead not be troubled by this increase in Shane's cholesterol level?

Outline

Objectives

**After you have completed this chapter,
you should be able to:**

1. Identify and discuss the basic structure
   and function of the three major
   components of a cell.

2. List and briefly discuss the functions of
   the primary cellular organelles.

3. Compare the major passive and active
   transport processes that act to move
   substances through cell membranes.

4. Compare and discuss DNA and RNA
   and their function in protein synthesis.

5. Discuss the stages of mitosis and
   explain the importance of cellular
   reproduction.

6. Explain how epithelial tissue is
   grouped according to shape and
   arrangement of cells.

7. List and briefly discuss the major types
   of connective and muscle tissue.

8. List the three structural components of
   a neuron.

3 Cells and Tissues

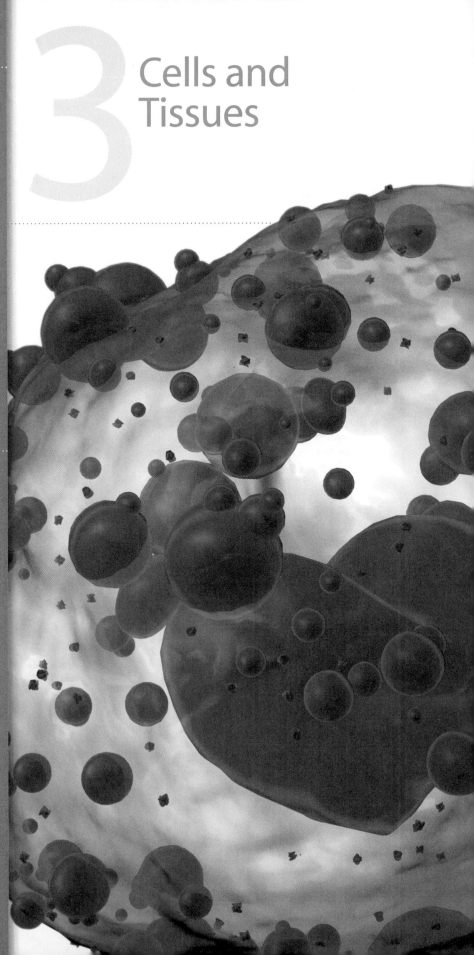

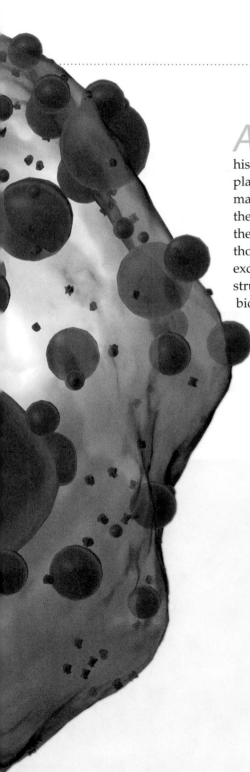

About 300 years ago Robert Hooke looked through his microscope—one of the very early, somewhat primitive ones—at some plant material. What he saw must have surprised him. Instead of a single magnified piece of plant material, he saw many small pieces. Because they reminded him of miniature monastery cells, that is what he called them—cells. Since Hooke's time, thousands of individuals have examined thousands of plant and animal specimens and found them all, without exception, to be composed of cells. This fact, that cells are the smallest structural units of living things, has become the foundation of modern biology. Many living things are so simple that they consist of just one cell. The human body, however, is so complex that it consists not of a few thousand or millions or even billions of cells but of many trillions of them. This chapter discusses cells first and then tissues.

STUDY TIPS

Chapter 3 should be a review of your general biology course; most of what is in this chapter should be familiar.

1. The section on cell structure begins with the plasma membrane. It is made up mostly of phospholipids, but the most important part of the membrane structure is the proteins embedded in the phospholipids. They play important roles in a number of systems in the body such as the nervous or endocrine systems.

2. The organelles may seem to have strange-sounding names, but many of the names can give you a clue about what they do: *-some* means "body" or "structure" and *lysis* means "to digest" or "destroy," so the name *lysosome* tells you what it does. Ribosomes are made of ribonucleic acid. *Endo* means "inside of," *plasma* means "liquid," and *reticulum* means "netlike," so *endoplasmic reticulum* is self-explaining. Flash cards would be helpful in learning this material.

continued on page 77

Cells

Size and Shape

Human cells are microscopic in size; that is, they can be seen only when magnified by a microscope. However, the different types of human cells vary considerably in size. An ovum (female sex cell), for example, has a diameter of about 150 micrometers, whereas red blood cells have a diameter of only 7.5 micrometers. Cells differ even more notably in shape than in size. Some are flat, some are brick shaped, some are thread-like, and some have irregular shapes.

Composition

Cells contain **cytoplasm** (SYE-toh-plaz-em), or "living matter," a substance that exists only in cells. The term *cyto-* is a Greek combining form and denotes a relationship to a cell. Each cell in the body is surrounded by a thin membrane, the **plasma membrane.** This membrane separates the cell contents from the dilute saltwater solution called **interstitial** (in-ter-STISH-all) **fluid,** or simply **tissue fluid,** that bathes every cell in the body. Numerous specialized structures called **organelles** (or-gah-NELLZ), which will be described in subsequent sections, are contained within the cytoplasm of each cell. A small, circular

body called the **nucleus** (NOO-klee-us) is also inside the cell.

Important information related to body composition is included in Chapter 2. You are encouraged to review this material, which includes a discussion of the chemical elements and compounds important to body structure and function.

Parts of the Cell

The three main parts of a cell are:

1. Plasma membrane
2. Cytoplasm
3. Nucleus

The plasma membrane surrounds the entire cell, forming its outer boundary. The cytoplasm is all the living material inside the cell (except the nucleus). The nucleus is a large, membrane-bound structure in most cells that contains the genetic code.

PLASMA MEMBRANE

As the name suggests, the **plasma membrane** is the membrane that encloses the cytoplasm and forms the outer boundary of the cell. It is an incredibly delicate structure—only about 7 nm (nanometers) or 3/10,000,000 of an inch thick! Yet it has a precise, or-

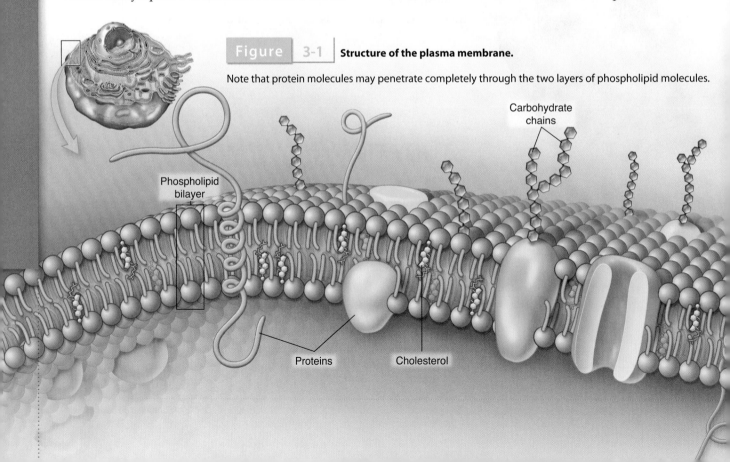

Figure **3-1** **Structure of the plasma membrane.**

Note that protein molecules may penetrate completely through the two layers of phospholipid molecules.

Carbohydrate chains

Phospholipid bilayer

Proteins

Cholesterol

derly structure (Figure 3-1). Two layers of phosphate-containing fat molecules called **phospholipids** form a fluid framework for the plasma membrane. Another kind of fat molecule called *cholesterol* is also a component of the plasma membrane. Cholesterol helps stabilize the phospholipid molecules to prevent breakage of the plasma membrane. Note in Figure 3-1 that protein molecules dot the surfaces of the membrane and extend all the way through the phospholipid framework.

Despite its seeming fragility, the plasma membrane is strong enough to keep the cell whole and intact and also performs other life-preserving functions for the cell. It serves as a well-guarded gateway between the fluid inside the cell and the fluid around it. Certain substances can move through the membrane, but others are barred from entry. The plasma membrane even functions as a communication device. In what way, you may wonder? Some proteins on the membrane's outer surface serve as receptors for certain other molecules when these other molecules contact the proteins. In other words, certain molecules bind to certain receptor proteins. For example, some hormones (chemicals secreted into blood from ductless glands) bind to membrane receptors, and a change in cell functions follows. We might therefore think of such hormones as chemical messages that are communicated to cells by way of binding to their cytoplasmic membrane receptors.

The plasma membrane also identifies a cell as being part of one particular individual. Its surface proteins serve as positive identification tags because they occur only in the cells of that individual. A practical application of this fact is made in *tissue typing*, a procedure performed before an organ from one individual is transplanted into another. Carbohydrate chains attached to the surface of cells often play a role in the identification of cell types.

CYTOPLASM

Cytoplasm is the internal living material of cells. It fills the space between the plasma membrane and the nucleus, which can be seen in Figure 3-2 as a round or

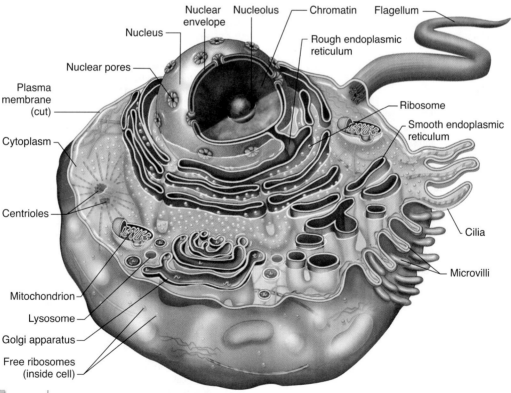

Nuclear envelope
Nucleus
Nuclear pores
Plasma membrane (cut)
Cytoplasm
Centrioles
Mitochondrion
Lysosome
Golgi apparatus
Free ribosomes (inside cell)
Nucleolus
Chromatin
Flagellum
Rough endoplasmic reticulum
Ribosome
Smooth endoplasmic reticulum
Cilia
Microvilli

Figure 3-2 | **General characteristics of the cell.**

Artist's interpretation of cell structure. Some of these structures, such as a flagellum or groups of cilia, are present only in certain types of cells.

spherical structure in the center of the cell. Numerous small structures are part of the cytoplasm, along with the fluid that serves as the interior environment of each cell. As a group, the small structures that make up much of the cytoplasm are called **organelles.** This name means "little organs," an appropriate name because they function for the cell like organs function for the body.

Look again at Figure 3-2. Notice how many different kinds of structures you can see in the cytoplasm of this cell. A little more than a generation ago, almost all of these organelles were unknown. They are so small that they are still invisible even when magnified 1000 times by a light microscope. The advent of electron microscopes finally brought them into view by magnifying them many thousands of times. Next we briefly discuss the following organelles, all of which are found in cytoplasm (Table 3-1):

1. Ribosomes
2. Endoplasmic reticulum
3. Golgi apparatus
4. Mitochondria
5. Lysosomes
6. Centrioles
7. Cilia
8. Flagella

Ribosomes

Organelles called **ribosomes** (RYE-boh-sohms), shown as dots in Figure 3-2, are very tiny particles found throughout the cell. They are each made up of two tiny subunits constructed mostly of a special kind of RNA called *ribosomal RNA (rRNA)*. Some ribosomes are found temporarily attached to a network of membranous canals called *endoplasmic reticulum (ER)*. Ribosomes also may be free-floating in the cytoplasm. Ribosomes perform a very complex function: they make enzymes and other protein compounds. Thus they are aptly nicknamed "protein factories."

Table 3-1	Structures and Function of Some Major Cell Parts	
CELL PART	**STRUCTURE**	**FUNCTION(S)**
Plasma membrane	Phospholipid bilayer studded with proteins	Serves as the boundary of the cell; protein and carbohydrate molecules on outer surface of plasma membrane perform various functions; for example, they serve as markers that identify cells as being from a particular individual or as receptor molecules for certain hormones
Ribosomes	Tiny particles, each made up of rRNA subunits	Synthesize proteins; a cell's "protein factories"
Endoplasmic reticulum (ER)	Membranous network of interconnected canals and sacs, some with ribosomes attached (rough ER) and some without attachments (smooth ER)	Rough ER receives and transports synthesized proteins (from ribosomes); smooth ER synthesizes lipids and certain carbohydrates
Golgi apparatus	Stack of flattened, membranous sacs	Chemically processes, then packages substances from the ER
Mitochondria	Membranous capsule containing a large, folded membrane encrusted with enzymes; contains its own DNA molecule	Adenosine triphosphate (ATP) synthesis; a cell's "powerhouses"
Lysosomes	"Bubble" of enzymes encased by membrane	A cell's "digestive system"
Centrioles	Pair of hollow cylinders, each made up of tiny tubules	Function in cell reproduction
Cilia	Short, hairlike extensions on surface of some cells	Move substances along surface of the cell
Flagella	Single and much longer projection of some cells	The only example in humans is the "tail" of a sperm cell, propelling the sperm through fluids
Nucleus	Double-membraned, spherical envelope containing DNA strands	Dictates protein synthesis, thereby playing an essential role in other cell activities, namely active transport, metabolism, growth, and heredity
Nucleolus	Dense region of the nucleus	Plays an essential role in the formation of ribosomes

Endoplasmic Reticulum

An **endoplasmic reticulum** (en-doh-PLAZ-mik reh-TIK-yoo-lum) **(ER)** is a system of membranes forming a network of connecting sacs and canals that wind back and forth through a cell's cytoplasm, from the nucleus almost to the plasma membrane. The tubular passageways or canals in the ER carry proteins and other substances through the fluid cytoplasm of the cell from one area to another. There are two types of ER: *rough* and *smooth*. Rough ER is named such because many ribosomes are attached to its outer surface, giving it a rough texture similar to sandpaper. As ribosomes make their proteins, they may attach to the rough ER and drop the protein into the interior of the ER. The ER then begins folding the new proteins and transports them to areas in which chemical processing takes place. These areas of the ER are so full of molecules that ribosomes have no room into which they can pass their proteins and so they do not attach. The absence of attached ribosomes gives this type of ER a smooth texture. Fats, carbohydrates, and proteins that make up cellular membrane material are manufactured in smooth ER. Thus the smooth ER makes new membrane for the cell. To sum up: rough ER receives, folds, and transports newly made proteins and smooth ER manufactures new membrane.

Golgi Apparatus

The **Golgi** (GOL-jee) **apparatus** consists of tiny, flattened sacs stacked on one another near the nucleus. Little bubbles, or sacs, break off the smooth ER and carry new proteins and other compounds to the sacs of the Golgi apparatus. These little sacs, also called **vesicles,** fuse with the Golgi sacs and allow the contents of both to mingle. The Golgi apparatus chemically processes the molecules from the ER by continuing the folding of proteins begun in the ER and combining them with other molecules to form quaternary proteins or combinations such as glycoproteins (carbohydrate/protein combinations). The Golgi apparatus then packages the processed molecules into new little vesicles that break away from the Golgi apparatus and move slowly outward to the plasma membrane. Each vesicle fuses with the plasma membrane, opens to the outside of the cell, and releases its contents. An example of a Golgi apparatus product is the slippery substance called *mucus*. If we wanted to nickname the Golgi apparatus, we might call it the cell's "chemical processing and packaging center."

Mitochondria

Mitochondria (my-toh-KON-dree-ah) are another kind of organelle found in all cells. Mitochondria are so tiny that a lineup of 15,000 or more of them would fill a space only about 2.5 cm (1 inch) long. Two membranous sacs, one inside the other, compose a single mitochondrion. The inner membrane forms folds that look like miniature incomplete partitions. Within a mitochondrion's fragile walls, complex, energy-releasing chemical reactions occur continuously. Because these reactions supply most of the power for cellular work, mitochondria have been nicknamed the cell's "power plants." The survival of cells and therefore of the body depends on mitochondrial chemical reactions. Enzymes (molecules that promote specific chemical reactions), which are found in mitochondrial walls and the mitochondrial fluids, use oxygen to break down glucose and other nutrients to release energy required for cellular work. The process is called *aerobic* or *cellular respiration*. Each mitochondrion has its own DNA molecule, sometimes called a *mitochondrial chromosome*, that contains information for building and running the mitochondrion.

Lysosomes

The **lysosomes** (LYE-soh-sohms) are membranous-walled organelles that in their active stage look like small sacs, often with tiny particles in them (see Figure 3-2). Because lysosomes contain enzymes that can digest food compounds, they have the nickname "digestive bags." Lysosomal enzymes also can digest substances other than foods. For example, they can digest and thereby destroy microbes that invade the cell. Thus lysosomes can protect cells against destruction by microbes. Formerly, scientists thought lysosomes were involved in programmed cell death. Now, however, we know a different set of mechanisms is responsible for "cell suicide," or **apoptosis** (ap-op-TOH-sis), which makes space for newer cells.

Centrioles

The **centrioles** (SEN-tree-ohlz) are paired organelles. Two of these rod-shaped structures exist in every cell. They are arranged so that they lie at right angles to each other (see Figure 3-2). Each centriole is composed of fine tubules that play an important role during cell division.

Microvilli

Microvilli (my-kroh-VILL-eye) are small fingerlike projections of the plasma membrane of some cells

(Figure 3-3, *A*). These projections increase the surface area of the cell and thus increase its ability to absorb substances. For example, cells that line the small intestine are covered with microvilli that increase the absorption rate of nutrients into the blood.

Cilia

Cilia (SIL-ee-ah) are extremely fine, almost hairlike extensions on the exposed or free surfaces of some cells (Figure 3-3, *A*). Cilia are organelles capable of movement. One cell may have a hundred or more cilia capable of moving together in a wavelike fashion over the surface of a cell. They often have highly specialized functions. For example, by moving as a group in one direction, they propel mucus upward over the cells that line the respiratory tract. Single, nonmoving cilia have a sensory function and are present in some sensory cells of the eye, ear, nose, and other sensory organs.

Flagella

A **flagellum** (flah-JEL-um) is a single projection extending from the cell surface. Flagella are much larger than cilia. In the human, the only example of a flagellum is the "tail" of the male sperm cell. Propulsive movements of the flagellum make it possible for sperm to "swim" or move toward the ovum after they are deposited in the female reproductive tract (Figure 3-3, *B*).

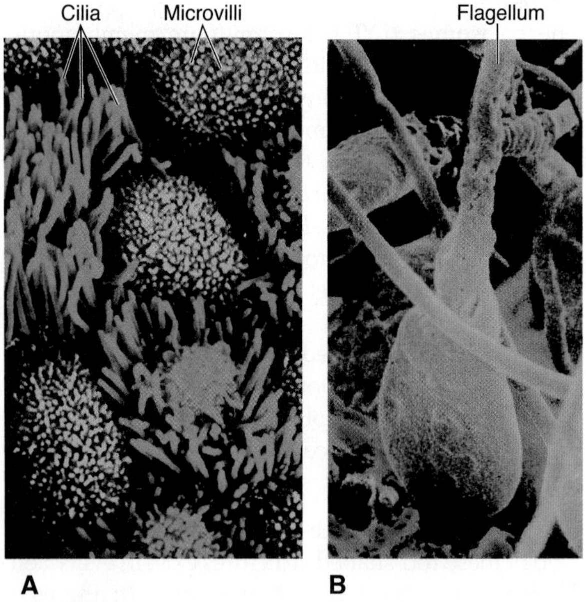

NUCLEUS

Viewed under a light microscope, the **nucleus** of a cell looks like a very simple structure—just a small sphere in the central portion of the cell. However, its simple appearance belies the complex and critical role it plays in cell function. The nucleus ultimately controls every organelle in the cytoplasm. It also controls the complex process of cell reproduction. In other words, the nucleus must function properly for a cell to accomplish its normal activities and be able to duplicate itself.

Note that the cell nucleus in Figure 3-2 is surrounded by a **nuclear envelope,** made up of two separate membranes. The nuclear envelope has many tiny openings called *nuclear pores* that permit large molecules to move into and out of the nucleus. The nuclear envelope encloses a special type of cell material within the nucleus called **nucleoplasm.** Nucleoplasm contains a number of specialized structures; two of the most important are shown in Figure 3-2. They are the **nucleolus** (noo-KLEE-oh-lus) and the **chromatin** (KROH-mah-tin) **granules.**

Nucleolus

The nucleolus is a dense region of the nuclear material that is critical in protein formation because it "programs" the formation of ribosomes in the nucleus. The ribosomes then migrate through the nuclear envelope into the cytoplasm of the cell and produce proteins.

Chromatin and Chromosomes

Chromatin granules in the nucleus are threadlike structures made of proteins and hereditary molecules called **DNA,** or **deoxyribonucleic** (dee-OK-see-rye-boh-noo-KLAY ik) **acid.** DNA is the genetic material often described as the chemical "cookbook" of the body. Because it contains the code for building both structural proteins and functional proteins, DNA determines everything from gender and metabolism rate to body build and hair color in every human being. During cell division, DNA molecules become tightly coiled. They then look like short, rodlike structures and are called **chromosomes.** Each cell of the body contains a total of 46 different DNA molecules in its nucleus and one copy of a 47th DNA molecule in each of its mitochondria. The importance and function of DNA are explained in greater detail in the section on cell reproduction later in this chapter.

Cilia   Microvilli   Flagellum

A   **B**

Figure 3-3 | **Cell extensions.**

A, Microvilli *(light blue)* are small, fingerlike extensions of the plasma membrane that increase the surface area for absorption. Cilia *(darker blue)* are longer than microvilli and move back and forth, pushing fluids along the surface. **B,** The tail-like flagellum that propels each sperm cell is so long that it does not fit into the photograph at this magnification.

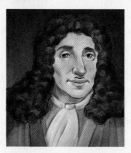

Antoni van Leeuwenhoek
(1632–1723)

MICROSCOPY

Until the very hour of his death in 1723, the Dutch drapery merchant Antoni van Leeuwenhoek *(left)* spent most of his 91 years pursuing adventures with the hundreds of microscopes he had built or collected. Using what were, even then, very simple lenses or combinations of lenses, van Leeuwenhoek discovered a whole world of tiny structures he called "animalcules" in body fluids. Although scientists a century later would declare that all living organisms are made up of cells, van Leeuwenhoek was the first to see and describe human blood cells (see Figure 3-22), human sperm cells (see Figure 3-3, *B*), and many other cells and tissues of the body. He was also the first to observe many microscopic organisms that live on or in the human body—many of which are capable of producing disease.

Scientists today use light microscopes that are much more advanced than those of van Leeuwenhoek's time. Some of the most modern microscopes, called *electron microscopes,* use electron beams instead of light to produce images of very high magnification (see Figure 3-3). Both cell biologists and *histologists* (tissue biologists) use microscopes to research the fine structure and function of the human body. A wide variety of professions have found practical applications for microscopy. Most health professionals use microscopes, or the images produced with microscopes, to perform routine duties. For example, clinical laboratory technicians and pathologists use microscopes to assess the health of human cells and tissues. Outside of the health sciences, professionals such as law enforcement investigators, archaeologists, anthropologists, and paleontologists often use microscopes to further their study of human and animal tissues.

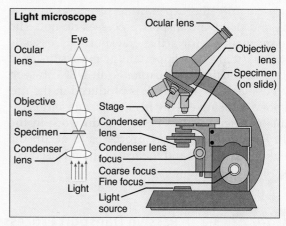

Modern compound light microscope

Relationship of Cell Structure and Function

Every human cell performs certain functions; some maintain the cell's survival, and others help maintain the body's survival. In many instances, the number and type of organelles within cells cause cells to differ dramatically in terms of their specialized functions. For example, cells that contain large numbers of mitochondria, such as heart muscle cells, are capable of sustained work. Why? Because the numerous mitochondria found in these cells supply the necessary energy required for rhythmic and ongoing contractions of the heart. Movement of the flagellum of a sperm cell is another example of the way a specialized organelle has a specialized function. The sperm's flagellum propels it through the reproductive tract of the female, thus increasing the chances of successful fertilization. This is how and why organizational structure at the cellular level is so important for function in living organisms. Examples in every chapter of the text illustrate how structure and function are intimately related at every level of body organization.

QUICK CHECK

1. What is the molecular structure of the *plasma membrane* of the cell?
2. What is *cytoplasm*? What does it contain?
3. List five major structures of the cell and briefly describe their function.
4. Which two kinds of cell structures contain DNA?

Movement of Substances Through Cell Membranes

The plasma membrane in every healthy cell separates the contents of the cell from the tissue fluid that surrounds it. At the same time the membrane must permit certain substances to enter the cell and allow others to leave. Heavy traffic moves continuously in both directions through cell membranes. Molecules of water, foods, gases, wastes, and many other substances stream in and out of all cells in endless procession. A number of processes allow this mass movement of substances into and out of cells. These **transport processes** are classified under two general headings:

1. Passive transport processes
2. Active transport processes

As implied by their names, active transport processes require the expenditure of energy by the cell, and passive transport processes do not. The energy required for active transport processes is obtained from a very important chemical substance called **adenosine triphosphate** (ah-DEN-oh-seen try-FOS-fayt), or **ATP.** ATP is produced in the mitochondria using energy from nutrients and is capable of releasing that energy to do work in the cell. For active transport processes to occur, the breakdown of ATP and the use of the released energy are required.

The details of active and passive transport of substances across cell membranes are much easier to understand if you keep in mind the following two key facts: (1) in passive transport processes, no cellular energy is required to move substances from a high concentration to a low concentration; and (2) in active transport processes, cellular energy is required to move substances from a low concentration to a high concentration.

Passive Transport Processes

The primary **passive transport** processes that move substances through the cell membranes include the following:

1. Diffusion
   a. Osmosis
   b. Dialysis
2. Filtration

Scientists describe the movement of substances in passive systems as going "down a concentration gradient." This means that substances in passive systems move from a region of high concentration to a region of low concentration until they reach equal

Table 3-2	**Passive Transport Processes**		
PROCESS	**DESCRIPTION**		**EXAMPLES**
Diffusion	Movement of particles through a membrane from an area of high concentration to an area of low concentration—that is, down the concentration gradient		Movement of carbon dioxide out of all cells; movement of sodium ions into nerve cells as they conduct an impulse
Osmosis	Diffusion of water through a selectively permeable membrane in the presence of at least one impermeant solute		Diffusion of water molecules into and out of cells to correct imbalances in water concentration
Filtration	Movement of water and small solute particles, but not larger particles, through a filtration membrane; movement occurs from area of high pressure to area of low pressure	High pressure Low pressure	In the kidney, water and small solutes move from blood vessels but blood proteins and blood cells do not, thus beginning the formation of urine

proportions on both sides of the membrane. As you read the next few paragraphs, refer to Table 3-2, which summarizes important information about passive transport processes.

DIFFUSION

Diffusion, a good example of a passive transport process, is the process by which substances scatter themselves evenly throughout an available space. The system does not require additional energy for this movement. To demonstrate diffusion of particles throughout a fluid, perform this simple experiment the next time you pour yourself a cup of coffee or tea. Place a cube of sugar on a teaspoon and lower it gently to the bottom of the cup. Let it stand for 2 or 3 minutes, and then, holding the cup steady, take a sip off the top. It will taste sweet. Why? Because some of the sugar molecules will have diffused from the area of high concentration near the sugar cube at the bottom of the cup to the area of low concentration at the top of the cup.

The process of diffusion is shown in Figure 3-4. Note that both substances diffuse rapidly through the membrane in both directions. However, as indicated by the green arrows, more of the solute (dissolved substance) moves out of the 20% solution, where the concentration is higher, into the 10% solution, where the concentration is lower, than in the opposite direction. This is an example of movement down a concentration gradient. Simultaneously, more water moves from the 10% solution, where there are more water molecules, into the 20% solution, where there are fewer water molecules. This is also an example of movement down a concentration gradient. Water moves from high to low concentration. The result? Equilibration (balancing) of the concentrations of the two solutions after an interval of time. From then on, equal amounts of solute will diffuse in both directions, as will equal amounts of water.

Osmosis and Dialysis

Osmosis (os-MOH-sis) and **dialysis** (dye-AL-i-sis) are specialized examples of diffusion. In both cases, diffusion occurs across a selectively permeable membrane. The plasma membrane of a cell is said to be selectively permeable because it permits the passage of certain substances but not others; that is, this necessary property permits some substances, such as nutrients, to gain entrance to the cell while excluding others. Osmosis is the diffusion of water, but not **solutes** (substances dissolved in the water), across a selectively permeable membrane.

FILTRATION

Filtration is the movement of water and solutes through a membrane as a result of a pushing force that is greater on one side of the membrane than on the other side. The force is called *hydrostatic pressure,* which is simply the force or weight of a fluid pushing against some surface (an example is blood pressure, in which blood pushes against vessel walls). A principle concerning filtration that is of great physiological importance is that it always occurs *down* a hydrostatic pressure gradient. This means that when two fluids have unequal hydrostatic pressures and are separated by a membrane, water and diffusible solutes or particles (those to which the membrane is permeable) will filter out of the solution that has the higher hydrostatic pressure into the solution that has the lower hydrostatic pressure. Filtration is the process responsible for urine formation in the kidney; wastes are filtered out of the blood into the kidney tubules because of a difference in hydrostatic pressure.

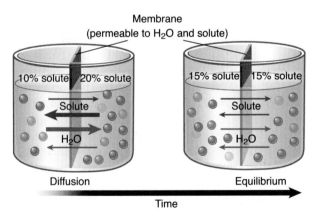

Membrane
(permeable to H₂O and solute)

| 10% solute | 20% solute |
Solute
H₂O

| 15% solute | 15% solute |
Solute
H₂O

Diffusion   Equilibrium

Time

Figure 3-4 | **Diffusion.**

Note that the membrane is permeable to solute and water and that it separates a 10% solution of solute particles from a 20% solution. The container on the left shows the two solutions separated by the membrane at the start of diffusion. The container on the right shows the result of diffusion after some time has passed.

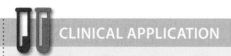

CLINICAL APPLICATION

TONICITY

A salt (NaCl) solution is said to be **isotonic** (*iso* = equal) if it contains the same concentration of salt normally found in a living red blood cell, which measures 0.9% NaCl. Salt particles (Na^+ and Cl^- ions) do not cross the plasma membrane easily, so salt solutions that differ in concentration from the cell's fluid will promote the osmosis of water one way or the other. A solution that contains a higher level of salt than the cell (above 0.9%) is said to be **hypertonic** (*hyper* = above) to the cell and one containing less (below 0.9%) is **hypotonic** (*hypo* = below) to the cell. With what you now know about filtration, diffusion, and osmosis, can you predict what would occur if red blood cells were placed in isotonic, hypotonic, and hypertonic solutions?

Examine the figures. Note that red blood cells placed in isotonic solution remain unchanged because there is no effective difference in salt or water concentrations. The movement of water into and out of the cells is about equal. This is not the case with red cells placed in hypertonic salt solution; they immediately lose water from their cytoplasm into the surrounding salty solution, and they shrink. This process is called **crenation.**

The opposite occurs if red cells are placed in a hypotonic solution; they swell as water enters the cell from the surrounding dilute solution. Eventually the cells break, or **lyse,** and the hemoglobin they contain is released into the surrounding solution.

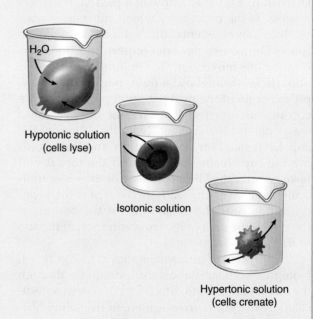

Hypotonic solution
(cells lyse)

Isotonic solution

Hypertonic solution
(cells crenate)

To learn more about passive transport, go to **AnimationDirect** on your CD.

Active Transport Processes

Active transport is the uphill movement of a substance through a living cell membrane. *Uphill* means "up a concentration gradient" (that is, from a lower to a higher concentration). The energy required for this movement is obtained from ATP. Because the formation and breakdown of ATP require complex cellular activity, active transport mechanisms can take place only through living membranes. Table 3-3 summarizes active transport processes.

ION PUMPS

A specialized cellular component called the *ion pump* makes possible a number of active transport mechanisms. An ion pump is a protein structure in the cell membrane called a *carrier*. The ion pump uses energy from ATP to actively move ions across cell membranes *against* their concentration gradients. "Pump" is an appropriate term because it suggests that active transport moves a substance in an uphill direction just as a water pump does, that is, moves water uphill.

An ion pump is specific to one particular ion; different ion pumps are required to move different types of ions. For example, sodium pumps move sodium ions only. Likewise, calcium pumps move calcium ions and potassium pumps move potassium ions.

Table	3-3	**Active Transport Processes**

PROCESS	DESCRIPTION		EXAMPLES
Ion pump	Movement of solute particles from an area of low concentration to an area of high concentration (up the concentration gradient) by means of a carrier protein structure		In muscle cells, pumping of nearly all calcium ions to special compartments—or out of the cell
Phagocytosis	Movement of cells or other large particles into cell by trapping it in a section of plasma membrane that pinches off inside the cell		Trapping of bacterial cells by phagocytic white blood cells
Pinocytosis	Movement of fluid and dissolved molecules into a cell by trapping them in a section of plasma membrane that pinches off inside the cell		Trapping of large protein molecules by some body cells

Some ion pumps are "coupled" to one another so that two or more different substances may be moved through the cell membrane at one time. For example, the **sodium-potassium pump** shown in Figure 3-5 pumps sodium ions out of a cell while it pumps potassium ions into the cell. Because both ions are moved against their concentration gradients, this pump creates a high sodium concentration outside the cell and a high potassium concentration inside the cell. Such a pump is required to remove sodium from the inside of a nerve cell after it has rushed in as a result of the passage of a nerve impulse. Some ion pumps are coupled with other specific carriers that transport glucose, amino acids, and other substances. However, there are no transporter pumps for moving water—it can move only passively by osmosis.

PHAGOCYTOSIS AND PINOCYTOSIS

Phagocytosis (fag-oh-sye-TOH-sis) is another example of how a cell can actively move an object or substance through the plasma membrane and into the cytoplasm. The term *phagocytosis* comes from a Greek word meaning "to eat." The word is appropriate because this process permits a cell to engulf and literally

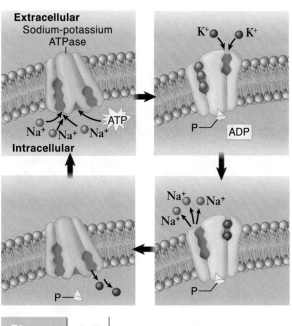

Figure	3-5	**Sodium-potassium pump.**

Three sodium ions (Na$^+$) are pumped out of the cell and two potassium ions (K$^+$) are pumped into the cell during one pumping cycle of this carrier molecule. ATP is broken down in the process so that the energy freed from ATP can be used to pump the ions.

"eat" foreign material (Figure 3-6). Certain white blood cells destroy bacteria in the body by phagocytosis. During this process the cell membrane forms a pocket around the bacterium, by expenditure of energy from ATP; then it is moved to the interior of the cell. Once inside the cytoplasm, the bacterium fuses with a lysosome and is destroyed.

Pinocytosis (pin-oh-sye-TOH-sis) is an active transport mechanism used to incorporate fluids or dissolved substances into cells by trapping them in a pocket of plasma membrane that pinches off inside the cell. Again, the term is appropriate because the word part *pino-* comes from the Greek word meaning "drink."

Cell Transport and Disease

Considering the importance of active and passive transport processes to cell survival, you can imagine the problems that arise when one of these processes fails. Several very severe diseases result from damage to cell transport processes. **Cystic fibrosis (CF),** for example, is an inherited condition in which chloride ion

(Cl^-) pumps in the plasma membrane are missing. Because chloride ion transport is altered, cells that rely heavily on chloride transporters may die and their remains then thicken the secretions of many exocrine glands. Such is the case when abnormally thick mucus in the lungs impairs normal breathing; frequently this leads to recurring lung infections. Figure 3-7 shows a child with CF next to a normal child of the same age. Because of the difficulty with breathing and digestion and other problems caused by the disease, the affected child has not developed normally. Digestion is compromised by thick pancreatic secretions that may plug the duct leading from the pancreas and thereby prevent important digestive juices from flowing into the intestines. Advances in treatment of CF, including gene therapy (see Chapter 23), have recently improved survivability and quality of life in many CF patients. There is real hope for even more improvements in the near future as our understanding of CF's cellular mechanisms increases.

Cholera (KAHL-er-ah) is a bacterial infection that causes cells lining the intestines to leak chlo-

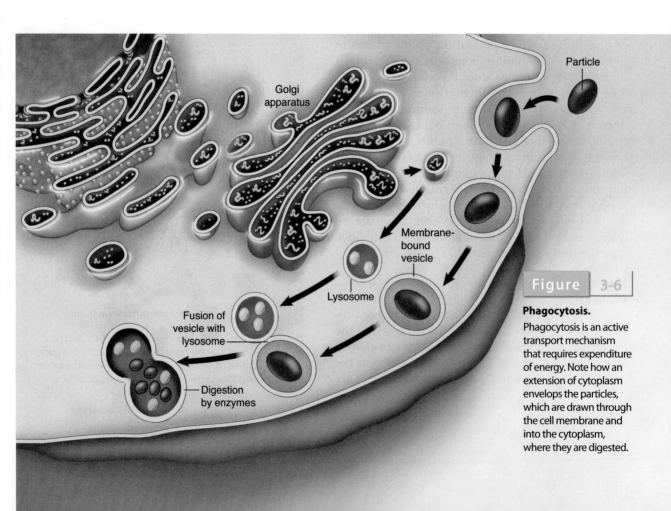

Golgi apparatus

Particle

Membrane-bound vesicle

Lysosome

Fusion of vesicle with lysosome

Digestion by enzymes

Figure 3-6

Phagocytosis.

Phagocytosis is an active transport mechanism that requires expenditure of energy. Note how an extension of cytoplasm envelops the particles, which are drawn through the cell membrane and into the cytoplasm, where they are digested.

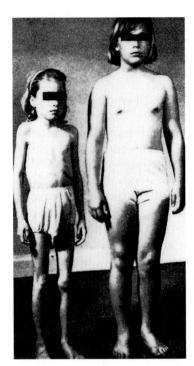

Figure 3-7

Cystic fibrosis. Even though both children in the photo are the same age, the child with cystic fibrosis (*left*) is smaller and thinner than the normal child (*right*). In cystic fibrosis, the absence of chloride ion pumps causes thickening of some glandular secretions. Because thickened secretions block airways and digestive ducts, children born with this disease become weakened, often dying before adulthood.

ride ions (Cl⁻). Water follows Cl⁻ out of the cells by osmosis, causing severe diarrhea and the resulting loss of water by the body. Death can occur in a few hours if treatment is not received.

 To learn more about active transport, go to **AnimationDirect** on your CD.

QUICK CHECK

1. What are the differences between *passive* and *active* transport processes?
2. What is *osmosis?*
3. How does an *ion pump* work? How do faulty ion pumps cause disease?
4. Describe the process of *phagocytosis.*

Cell Reproduction and Heredity

All human cells that reproduce do so by a process called **mitosis** (my-TOH-sis). During this process a cell divides to multiply; that is, one cell divides to form two cells. Cell reproduction and ultimately the transfer of heritable traits is closely tied to the production of proteins. Two *nucleic acids,* **ribonu-** **cleic acid,** or **RNA,** in the cytoplasm and **deoxyribonucleic acid,** or **DNA,** in the nucleus play crucial roles in protein synthesis.

DNA Molecule and Genetic Information

Chromosomes, which are composed largely of DNA, make heredity possible. The "genetic information" contained in segments of the DNA molecules that are called *genes* ultimately determines the transmission and expression of heritable traits such as skin color and blood group from each generation of parents to their children (Figure 3-8).

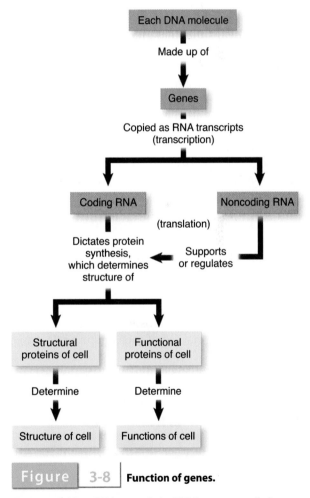

Figure 3-8 | **Function of genes.**

Genes copied from DNA are copied to RNA in a process called *transcription.* The RNA transcripts are then used in a process called *translation,* in which a code that determines the sequence of amino acids is translated to form a protein. The structure of the resulting protein determines the role of the protein in body structure and function—and ultimately, the structure and function of the body.

Structurally, the DNA molecule resembles a long, narrow ladder made of a pliable material. It is twisted round and round its axis, taking on the shape of a double helix. Each DNA molecule is made of many smaller units, namely, a sugar, bases, and phosphate units (Table 3-4). The bases are adenine, thymine, guanine, and cytosine. These nitrogen-containing chemicals are called *bases* because by themselves they have a high pH and chemicals with a high pH are called "bases" (see pp. 28-30 for a discussion of acids and bases). As you can see in Figure 3-9 (also Figure 2-11, p. 34), each step in the DNA ladder consists of a pair of bases. Only two combinations of bases occur, and the same two bases invariably pair off with each other in a DNA molecule. Adenine always binds to thymine, and cytosine always binds to guanine. This characteristic of DNA structure is called **complementary base pairing.**

A **gene** is a specific segment of base pairs in a chromosome. Although the types of base pairs in all chromosomes are the same, the order or *sequence* of base pairs is not the same. This fact has tremendous functional importance because it is the sequence of base pairs in each gene of each chromosome that determines heredity. Each gene directs the synthesis of one kind of protein molecule that may function, for example, as an enzyme, a structural component of a cell, or a specific hormone. In humans, having 46 chromosomes in each body cell, the nuclear DNA has a content of genetic information totaling more than 3 *billion* base pairs in 80,000 or so genes. This means that each parent contributes about one and a half billion bits of genetic information in the 23 chromosomes each parent provides for the original cell of each offspring. Is it any wonder, then, with all of this genetic information packed into each of our cells, that no two of us inherit exactly the same traits?

GENETIC CODE

How do genes bring about heredity? There is, of course, no short and easy answer to that question. We know that the genetic information contained in each gene is capable of "directing" the synthesis of a specific protein. The unique sequence of a thousand or so base pairs in a gene determines the sequence of specific building blocks required to form a particular protein. This store of information in each gene is called the *genetic code.* In summary, the coded information in genes controls protein and enzyme production, enzymes facilitate cellular chemical reactions, and cellular chemical reactions determine cell structure and function and therefore heredity.

RNA MOLECULES AND PROTEIN SYNTHESIS

DNA, with its genetic code that dictates directions for protein synthesis, is contained in the nucleus of the cell. The actual process of protein synthesis, however, occurs in ribosomes and on ER. Another specialized nucleic acid, ribonucleic acid (RNA), transfers this genetic information from the nucleus to the cytoplasm.

Both RNA and DNA are composed of four bases, a sugar, and phosphate. RNA, however, is a single rather than a double-stranded molecule, and it contains a different sugar and base component. The base uracil replaces thymine.

The process of transferring genetic information from the nucleus into the cytoplasm where proteins are actually produced requires completion of two specialized steps called *transcription* and *translation.*

Transcription

During **transcription** the double-stranded DNA molecule separates or unwinds, and a special type of RNA called **messenger RNA** or **mRNA** is formed (Figure 3-9, *step 1*). Each strand of mRNA is a duplicate or copy of a particular gene sequence along one of the newly separated DNA spirals. The messenger RNA is said to have been "transcribed" or copied from its DNA mold or template. The mRNA molecules pass from the nucleus to the cytoplasm to direct protein synthesis in the ribosomes and ER (Figure 3-9, *step 2*).

Table 3-4	Components of Nucleotides	
NUCLEOTIDE	**DNA**	**RNA**
Sugar	Deoxyribose	Ribose
Phosphate	Phosphate	Phosphate
Nitrogen base	Cytosine	Cytosine
	Guanine	Guanine
	Adenine	Adenine
	Thymine	Uracil

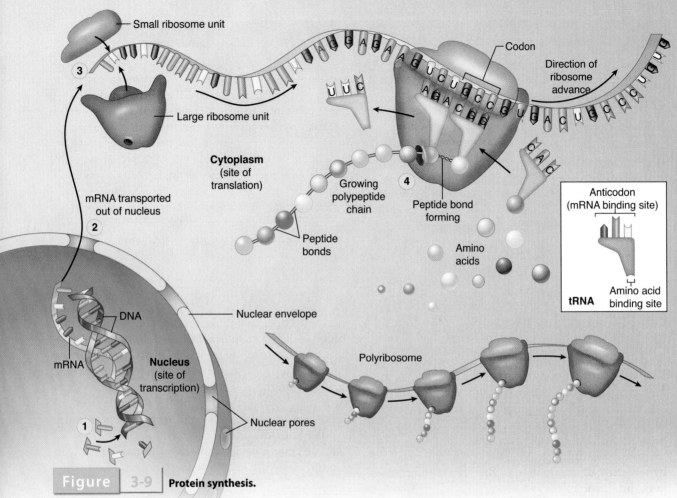

Small ribosome unit

Large ribosome unit

Codon

Direction of ribosome advance

Cytoplasm (site of translation)

mRNA transported out of nucleus

Growing polypeptide chain

Peptide bond forming

Peptide bonds

Amino acids

Anticodon (mRNA binding site)

Amino acid binding site

tRNA

DNA

Nuclear envelope

mRNA

Nucleus (site of transcription)

Polyribosome

Nuclear pores

Figure 3-9 | **Protein synthesis.**

1, Protein synthesis begins with transcription, a process in which an mRNA molecule forms along one gene sequence of a DNA molecule within the cell's nucleus. As it is formed, the mRNA molecule separates from the DNA molecule. *2,* The mRNA transcript then leaves the nucleus through the large nuclear pores. *3,* Outside the nucleus, ribosome subunits attach to the beginning of the mRNA molecule and begin the process of translation. *4,* In translation, transfer RNA (tRNA) molecules bring specific amino acids—encoded by each mRNA codon—into place at the ribosome site. As the amino acids are brought into the proper sequence, they are joined together by peptide bonds to form long strands called *polypeptides.* Several polypeptide chains may be needed to make a complete protein molecule.

TRANSLATION

Translation is the synthesis of a protein by ribosomes, which use the information contained in an mRNA molecule to direct the choice and sequencing of the appropriate chemical building blocks called *amino acids.* First, the two subunits of a ribosome attach at the beginning of the mRNA molecule (Figure 3-9, *step 3*). The ribosome then moves down the mRNA strand and amino acids are assembled into their proper sequence (Figure 3-9, *step 4*). **Transfer RNA (tRNA)** molecules assist the process by bringing specific amino acids in to "dock" at each **codon** along the mRNA strand. A codon is a series of three nucleotide bases that act as a code representing a specific amino acid. Each gene is made up of a series of codons that tell the cell the sequence of amino acids to string together to form a protein strand. This strand then folds on itself and perhaps even combines with another strand to form a complete protein molecule (see Figure 2-9, p. 33). The specific, complex shape of each type of protein molecule allows the molecule to perform specific functions in the cell. It is clear that because DNA directs the shape of each protein, DNA also directs the function of each protein in a cell.

RESEARCH, ISSUES, AND TRENDS

HUMAN GENOME

The sum total of all of the DNA in each cell of the body is called the **genome** (JEE-nohm). With intense, coordinated effort, a team of scientists recently mapped all of the gene locations in the human genome. Efforts at reading the different genetic codes possible at each location are still underway. Much of the work of mapping the human genome was done as part of the Human Genome Project (HGP), which was started in 1990. Besides producing a human genetic map and developing tools of genetic mapping, a new field called *genomics*, the HGP also addresses the ethical, legal, and social issues that may arise—a notable first for such a massive scientific research effort. The HGP is sponsored by the Department of Energy (DOE) and the National Institutes of Health (NIH), and its first director was James Watson, one of the scientists credited with originally discovering the structure of the DNA molecule in 1953. With the human genome already mapped, many scientists are working now to fill in the details concerning the many genes and gene variants found in the human genome. Many are also working in the emerging field of *proteomics*—the study of all the proteins encoded by each of the genes of the human genome.

Cells, Genetics, and Disease

Many diseases have a cellular basis; that is, they are basically cell problems even though they may affect the entire body. Because individual cells are members of an interacting "community" of cells, it is no wonder that a problem in just a few cells can have a "ripple effect" that influences the entire body. Most of these cell problems can be traced to abnormalities in the DNA itself or in the process by which DNA information is transcribed and translated into proteins.

In individuals with inherited diseases, abnormal DNA from one or both parents may cause production of dysfunctional proteins in certain cells or prevent a vital protein from being synthesized. For example, DNA may contain a mistake in its genetic code that prevents production of normal blood-clotting proteins. Deficiency of these essential proteins results in excessive, uncontrollable bleeding—a condition called *hemophilia* (see Chapters 12 and 24). Chemical or mechanical irritants, radiation, bacteria, viruses, and other factors can directly damage DNA molecules and thus disrupt a cell's normal function. For example, the virus that causes *acquired immunodeficiency syndrome (AIDS)* eventually inserts its own genetic codes into the DNA of certain cells. The viral codes trigger synthesis of viral molecules, detouring raw materials intended for use in building normal human products. This does two things: it prevents human white blood cells from performing their normal functions and it provides a mechanism by which the virus can reproduce itself and spread to other cells. When enough cells of the human immune system are affected, they can no longer protect us from infections and cancer—a condition that eventually leads to death.

The genetic basis for disease discussed briefly in Chapter 5 is fully explained in Chapter 24.

Table	3-5	**Stages of Cell Division**

STAGE	CHARACTERISTICS
Prophase	The chromatin condenses into visible chromosomes Chromatids become attached at the centromere Spindle fibers appear The nucleolus and nuclear envelope disappear
Metaphase	Spindle fibers attach to each chromatid Chromosomes align across the center of the cell
Anaphase	Centromeres break apart Chromosomes move away from the center of the cell The cleavage furrow appears
Telophase	The nuclear envelope and both nuclei appear The cytoplasm and organelles divide equally The process of cell division is completed

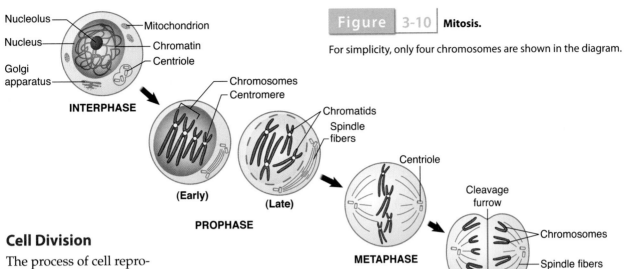

Figure 3-10 **Mitosis.**

For simplicity, only four chromosomes are shown in the diagram.

Cell Division

The process of cell reproduction involves the division of the nucleus (mitosis) and the cytoplasm. After the process is complete, two daughter cells result; both have the same genetic material as the cell that preceded them. When a cell is not dividing—but instead going about its usual functions—it is in a period called **interphase** (IN-ter-fayz). Interphase includes the initial growing stages of a newly formed cell, followed by a period during which the cell prepares for possible cell division. During this preparatory part of interphase, the DNA of each chromosome replicates itself. The cell then enters another growth period of interphase before it begins to actively divide.

The stages of mitosis are listed in Table 3-5, along with a brief description of the changes that occur during each stage.

DNA REPLICATION

DNA molecules possess a unique ability that no other molecules in the world have. They can make copies of themselves, a process called **DNA replication.** Before a cell divides to form two new cells, each DNA molecule in its nucleus forms another DNA molecule just like itself. When a DNA molecule is not replicating, it has the shape of a tightly coiled double helix. As it begins replication, short segments of the DNA molecule uncoil and the two strands of the molecule pull apart between their base pairs. The separated strands therefore contain unpaired bases. Each unpaired base in each of the two separated strands attracts its complementary base (in the nucleoplasm) and binds to it. Specifically, each adenine attracts and binds to a thymine, and each cytosine attracts and binds to a guanine. These steps are repeated over and over throughout the length of the DNA molecule. Thus each half of a DNA molecule becomes a whole DNA molecule identical to the original DNA molecule. After DNA replication is complete, the cell continues to grow until it is ready for the first phase of mitosis.

PROPHASE

Look at Figure 3-10 and note the changes that identify the first stage of mitosis, **prophase** (PRO-fayz). The chromatin becomes "organized." Chromosomes in the nucleus have formed two strands called **chromatids** (KROH-mah-tids). Note that the two chromatids are held together by a beadlike structure called the **centromere** (SEN-troh-meer). In the cytoplasm the centrioles are moving away from each other as a network of tubules called **spindle fibers** forms between them. These spindle fibers serve as "guidewires" and assist the chromosomes to move toward opposite ends of the cell later in mitosis.

METAPHASE

By the time **metaphase** (MET-ah-fayz) begins, the nuclear envelope and nucleolus have disappeared. Note in Figure 3-10 that the chromosomes have aligned themselves across the center of the cell. Also, the centrioles have migrated to opposite ends of the cell, and spindle fibers are attached to each chromatid.

ANAPHASE

As **anaphase** (AN-ah-fayz) begins, the beadlike centromeres, which were holding the paired chromatids together, break apart. As a result, the individual chromatids, identified once again as chromosomes, move away from the center of the cell. Movement of chromosomes occurs along spindle fibers toward the centrioles. Note in Figure 3-10 that chromosomes are being pulled to opposite ends of the cell. A **cleavage furrow** that begins to divide the cell into two daughter cells can be seen for the first time at the end of anaphase.

TELOPHASE

During **telophase** (TEL-oh-fayz) cell division is completed. Two nuclei appear, and chromosomes become less distinct and appear to break up. As the nuclear envelope forms around the chromatin, the cleavage furrow completely divides the cell into two parts. Before division is complete, each nucleus is surrounded by cytoplasm in which organelles

have been equally distributed. By the end of telophase, two separate daughter cells, each having identical genetic characteristics, are formed. Each cell is fully functional and will perhaps itself undergo mitosis in the future.

RESULTS OF CELL DIVISION

Mitosis results in the production of identical new cells. In the adult, mitosis replaces cells that have become less functional with age or have been damaged or destroyed by illness or injury. During periods of body growth, mitosis allows groups of similar cells to *differentiate*, or develop into different **tissues.**

Changes in Cell Growth and Reproduction

Cells have the ability to adapt to changing conditions. Cells may alter their size, reproductive rate, or other characteristics to adapt to changes in the internal environment. Such adaptations usually allow cells to work more efficiently. However, sometimes cells alter their characteristics abnormally—decreasing their efficiency and threatening the health of the body. Common types of changes in cell growth and reproduction are summarized below and in Table 3-6.

Cells may respond to changes in function, hormone signals, or availability of nutrients by increasing or decreasing in size. The term **hypertrophy** (hye-PER-troh-fee) refers to an increase in cell size, and the term **atrophy** (AT-roh-fee) refers to a decrease in cell size. Either type of adaptive change can occur easily in muscle tissue. When a person continually uses muscle cells to pull against heavy resistance, as in weight training, the cells respond by increasing

| Table | 3-6 | **Alterations in Cell Growth and Reproduction** |

TERM	DEFINITION	EXAMPLE
CHANGES IN GROWTH OF INDIVIDUAL CELLS		
Hypertrophy	Increase in size of individual cells	Strength training stimulates increase in size of skeletal muscle fibers
Atrophy	Decrease in size of individual cells	Immobility of limbs causes skeletal muscles that move limbs to decrease in size
CHANGES IN CELL REPRODUCTION		
Hyperplasia	Increase in cell reproduction	Skin tumor causes thickening of skin by overproduction of skin cells
Anaplasia	Production of abnormal, undifferentiated cells	Lung cancer causes production of abnormal cells that do not function properly

in size. Bodybuilders thus increase the size of their muscles by hypertrophy—increasing the size of muscle cells. Atrophy often occurs in underused muscle cells. For example, when a broken arm is immobilized in a cast for a long period, muscles that move the arm often atrophy. Because the muscles are temporarily out of use, muscle cells decrease in size. Atrophy also may occur in tissues whose nutrient or oxygen supply is diminished.

Sometimes cells respond to changes in the internal environment by increasing their rate of reproduction—a process called **hyperplasia** (hye-per-PLAY-zha). The word part *-plasia* comes from a Greek word that means "formation"—referring to formation of new cells. Because *hyper-* means "excessive," *hyperplasia* means excessive cell reproduction. Like hypertrophy, hyperplasia causes an increase in the size of a tissue or organ. However, hyperplasia is an increase in the *number of cells* rather than an increase in the size of each cell. A common example of hyperplasia occurs in the milk-producing glands of the female breast during pregnancy. In response to hormone signals, the glandular cells reproduce rapidly, preparing the breast for nursing.

If the body loses its ability to control mitosis, abnormal hyperplasia may occur. The new mass of cells thus formed is a tumor or **neoplasm** (NEE-oh-plaz-em). Many neoplasms also exhibit a characteristic called **anaplasia** (an-ah-PLAY-zha). Anaplasia is a condition in which cells change in orientation to each other and fail to mature normally; that is, they fail to differentiate into a specialized cell type. Neoplasms may be relatively harmless growths called *benign* (be-NYNE) tumors. If tumor cells can break away and travel through the blood or lymphatic vessels to other parts of the body (Figure 3-11), the neoplasm is a *malignant* (mah-LIG-nant) *tumor* or **cancer.** Neoplasms are discussed further in Chapter 4.

QUICK CHECK

1. How do *genes* determine the structure and function of the body?
2. What are the main steps in making proteins in the cell?
3. What are the four phases of *mitotic cell division*?
4. What is the relationship between *cell division* and *cancer*?

Tissues

The four main kinds of tissues that compose the body's many organs include:

1. Epithelial tissue
2. Connective tissue
3. Muscle tissue
4. Nervous tissue

Tissues differ from each other in the size and shape of their cells, in the amount and kind of material between the cells, and in the special functions they

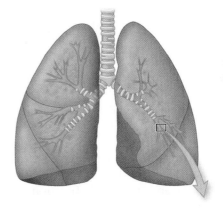
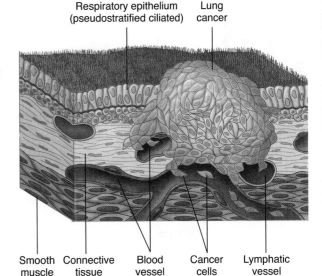

Respiratory epithelium (pseudostratified ciliated) — Lung cancer — Smooth muscle — Connective tissue — Blood vessel — Cancer cells — Lymphatic vessel

Figure 3-11 Cancer.

This depiction of an abnormal mass of proliferating cells in the lining of lung airways is a malignant tumor—lung cancer. Notice how some cancer cells are leaving the tumor and entering the blood and lymph vessels.

| Table | 3-7 | **Epithelial Tissues** |

TISSUE	STRUCTURE	LOCATION(S)	FUNCTION(S)
Simple squamous	Single layer of flattened cells	Alveoli of lungs	Diffusion of respiratory gases between alveolar air and blood
		Lining of blood and lymphatic vessels	Diffusion, filtration, and osmosis
Stratified squamous	Many layers; outermost layer(s) is flattened cells	Surface of lining of mouth and esophagus	Protection
		Surface of skin (epidermis)	Protection
Simple columnar	Single layer of tall, narrow cells	Surface layer of lining of stomach, intestines, parts of respiratory tract	Protection; secretion; transport (absorption)
Stratified transitional	Many layers of varying shapes, capable of stretching	Urinary bladder	Protection, ability to stretch
Pseudostratified	Single layer of tall cells that wedge together to appear as if there are two or more layers	Surface of lining of trachea	Protection
Simple cuboidal	Single layer of cells that are as tall as they are wide	Glands; kidney tubules	Secretion, absorption

perform to help maintain the body's health and survival. In Tables 3-7 through 3-9, you will find a listing of the four major tissues and the various subtypes of each. The tables also include the structure of each subtype along with examples of the location of the tissues and a primary function of each tissue type.

Epithelial Tissue

Epithelial (ep-i-THEE-lee-all) tissue covers the body and many of its parts. It also lines various parts of the body. Because epithelial cells are packed close together with little or no intercellular material between them, they form continuous sheets that contain no blood vessels. Examine Figure 3-12. It illus-

| Table | 3-8 | **Connective Tissues** |

TISSUE	STRUCTURE	LOCATION(S)	FUNCTION(S)
Areolar	Loose arrangement of fibers and cells	Area between other tissues and organs	Connection
Adipose (fat)	Cells contain large fat compartments	Area under skin	Protection
		Padding at various points	Insulation; support; nutrient reserve
Dense fibrous	Dense arrangement of collagen fiber bundles	Tendons; ligaments; fascia; scar tissue	Flexible but strong connection
Bone	Hard, calcified matrix arranged in osteons	Skeleton	Support; protection
Cartilage	Hard but flexible matrix with embedded chondrocytes	Part of nasal septum; area covering articular surfaces of bones; larynx; rings in trachea and bronchi	Firm but flexible support
		Disks between vertebrae	Withstand pressure
		External ear	Flexible support
Blood	Liquid matrix with flowing red and white cells	Blood vessels	Transportation, immunity
Hematopoietic	Liquid matrix with dense arrangement of blood cell–producing cells	Red bone marrow	Blood cell formation

Table 3-9	Muscle and Nervous Tissue		
TISSUE	**STRUCTURE**	**LOCATION(S)**	**FUNCTION(S)**
MUSCLE			
Skeletal (striated voluntary)	Long, threadlike cells with multiple nuclei and striations	Muscles that attach to bones	Maintenance of posture; movement of bones
		Eyeball muscles	Eye movements
		Upper third of esophagus	Involved in first part of swallowing
Cardiac (striated involuntary)	Branching, interconnected cylinders with faint striations	Wall of heart	Contraction of heart
Smooth (nonstriated involuntary or visceral)	Threadlike cells with single nuclei and no striations	Walls of tubular viscera of digestive, respiratory, and genitourinary tracts	Movement of substances along respective tracts
		Walls of blood vessels and large lymphatic vessels	Changing of diameter of vessels
		Ducts of glands	Movement of substances along ducts
		Intrinsic eye muscles (iris and ciliary body)	Changing of diameter of pupils and shape of lens
		Arrector muscles of hairs	Erection of hairs (goose pimples)
NERVOUS			
	Nerve cells with large cell bodies and thin fiberlike extensions; supportive glial cells also present	Brain; spinal cord; nerves	Irritability; conduction

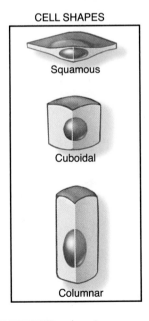

CELL SHAPES

Squamous

Cuboidal

Columnar

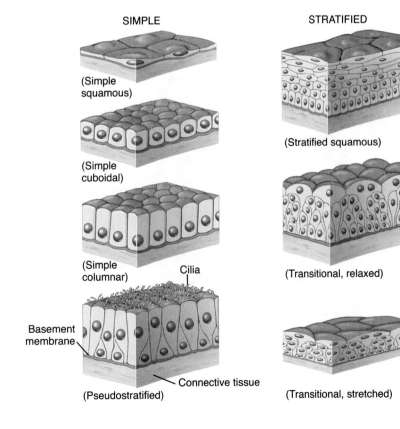

SIMPLE

(Simple squamous)

(Simple cuboidal)

(Simple columnar)

Cilia

Basement membrane

Connective tissue

(Pseudostratified)

STRATIFIED

(Stratified squamous)

(Transitional, relaxed)

(Transitional, stretched)

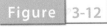

Figure 3-12

Classification of epithelial tissues.
The tissues are classified according to the shape and arrangement of cells.

trates how this large group of tissues can be subdivided according to the *shape* and *arrangement* of the cells found in each type.

SHAPE OF CELLS

If classified according to *shape,* epithelial cells are:

1. Squamous (flat and scalelike)
2. Cuboidal (cube shaped)
3. Columnar (more tall than wide)
4. Transitional (varying shapes that can stretch)

ARRANGEMENT OF CELLS

If classified according to *arrangement* of cells, epithelial tissue can be labeled as one of the following:

1. Simple (a single layer of cells of the same shape)
2. Stratified (many layers of cells; named for the shape of cells in the outer layer)

Several types of epithelium are described in the paragraphs that follow and are illustrated in Figures 3-12 to 3-16.

SIMPLE SQUAMOUS EPITHELIUM

Simple squamous (SKWAY-muss) **epithelium** consists of a single layer of very thin and irregularly shaped cells. Because of its structure, substances can readily pass through simple squamous epithelial tissue, making transport its special function. Absorption of oxygen into the blood, for example, takes place through the simple squamous epithelium that forms the tiny air sacs in the lungs (Figure 3-13).

STRATIFIED SQUAMOUS EPITHELIUM

Stratified squamous epithelium (Figure 3-14) consists of several layers of closely packed cells, an arrangement that makes this tissue especially adept at protection. For instance, stratified squamous epithelial tissue protects the body against invasion by microorganisms. Most microbes cannot work their way through a barrier of stratified squamous tissue such as that which composes the surface of skin and of mucous membranes.

One way of preventing infections, therefore, is to take good care of your skin. Don't let it become cracked from chapping, and guard against cuts and scratches.

SIMPLE COLUMNAR EPITHELIUM

Simple columnar epithelium can be found lining the inner surface of the stomach, intestines, and some areas of the respiratory and reproductive tracts. In Figure 3-15 the simple columnar cells are arranged

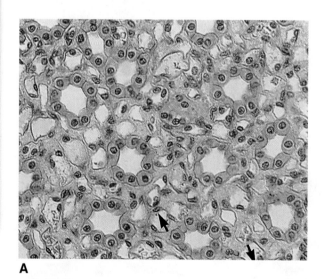

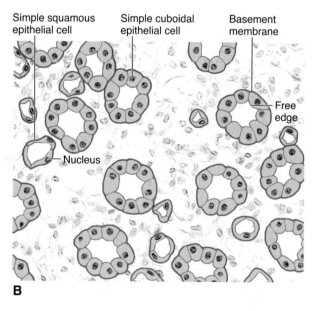

A   **B**

Figure | 3-13 | **Simple squamous and simple cuboidal epithelium.**

A, Photomicrograph shows thin simple squamous epithelium forming some tubules *(arrows)* and simple cuboidal epithelium forming the walls of other tubules. **B,** Sketch of photomicrograph.

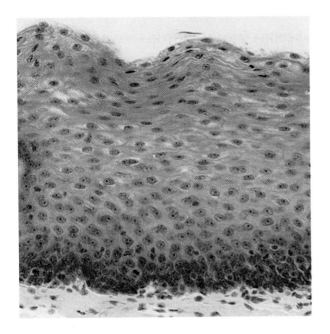

A

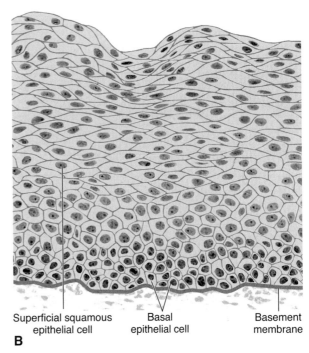

Superficial squamous   Basal   Basement
epithelial cell   epithelial cell   membrane

B

Figure 3-14   **Stratified squamous epithelium.**

A, Photomicrograph. Note the many layers of cells and flattened (squamous) nucleated cells in the outer layer. **B,** Sketch of the photomicrograph.

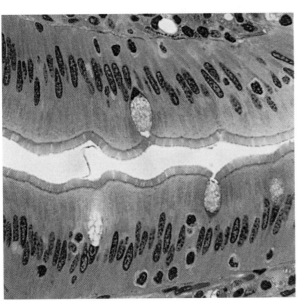

A

Goblet cell   Columnar
epithelial cells

B

Figure 3-15   **Simple columnar epithelium.**

A, Photomicrograph. Note the oblong nuclei and the striated border. **B,** Sketch of the photomicrograph. Note the goblet or mucus-producing cells that are present.

in a single layer lining the inner surface of the colon or large intestine. These epithelial cells are taller than they are wide, and the nuclei are located toward the bottom of each cell. The "open spaces" among the cells are specialized **goblet cells** that produce mucus. The regular columnar-shaped cells specialize in absorption.

STRATIFIED TRANSITIONAL EPITHELIUM

Stratified transitional epithelium is typically found in body areas subjected to stress and must be able to stretch; an example would be the wall of the urinary bladder. In many instances, up to 10 layers of differently shaped cells of varying sizes are present in the absence of stretching. When stretching occurs, the epithelial sheet expands, the number of cell layers decreases, and cell shape changes from roughly cuboidal to nearly squamous (flat) in appearance. This ability of transitional epithelium keeps the bladder wall from tearing under the pressures of stretching. Stratified transitional epithelium is shown in Figures 3-12 and 3-16.

PSEUDOSTRATIFIED EPITHELIUM

Pseudostratified epithelium, illustrated in Figure 3-11, is typical of that which lines the trachea or windpipe. Look carefully at the illustration. Note that each cell actually touches the gluelike **basement membrane** that lies under all epithelial tissues. Although the epithelium in Figure 3-12 (pseudostratified) appears to be two cell layers thick, it is not. This is the reason it is called *pseudo* (or false) stratified epithelium. The cilia that extend from the cells are capable of moving in unison. In doing so, they move mucus along the lining surface of the trachea, thus affording protection against entry of dust or other foreign particles into the lungs.

CUBOIDAL EPITHELIUM

Simple cuboidal epithelium does not form protective coverings but instead forms tubules or other groupings specialized for secretory activity (Figures 3-13 and 3-17). These secretory cuboidal cells usually function in clusters or tubes of secretory cells commonly called **glands.** Glands of the body

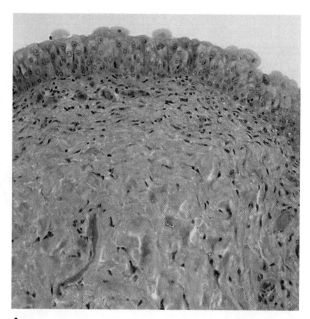

A

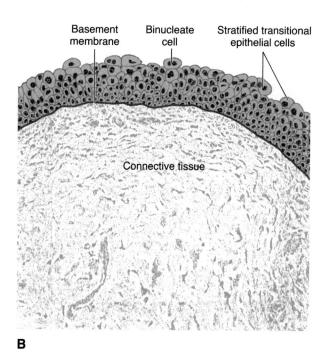

B

Figure 3-16 | **Stratified transitional epithelium.**

A, Photomicrograph of tissue lining the urinary bladder wall. **B,** Sketch of the photomicrograph. Note the many layers of epithelial cells of various shapes.

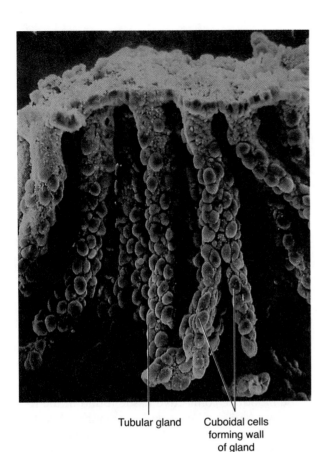

Tubular gland   Cuboidal cells
forming wall
of gland

Figure 3-17 **Simple cuboidal epithelium.**

This scanning electron micrograph shows how a single layer of cuboidal cells can form glands. The secreting cells arrange themselves into single or branched tubules that open onto a surface—the lining of the stomach in this case.

may be classified as **exocrine** if they release their secretion through a duct or as **endocrine** if they release their secretion directly into the bloodstream. Examples of glandular secretions include saliva produced by the salivary glands, digestive juices, sweat or perspiration, and hormones such as those secreted by the pituitary or thyroid glands. Simple cuboidal epithelium also forms the tubules that form urine in the kidneys.

Connective Tissue

Connective tissue is the most abundant and widely distributed tissue in the body. It also exists in more varied forms than any of the other tissue types. It is found in skin, membranes, muscles, bones, nerves, and all internal organs. Connective tissue exists as delicate, paper-thin webs that hold internal organs together and give them shape. It also exists as strong and tough cords, rigid bones, and even in the form of a fluid—blood.

The functions of connective tissue are as varied as its structure and appearance. It connects tissues to each other and forms a supporting framework for the body as a whole and for its individual organs. As blood, it transports substances throughout the body. Several other kinds of connective tissue function to defend us against microbes and other invaders.

Connective tissue differs from epithelial tissue in the arrangement and variety of its cells and in the amount and kinds of intercellular material, called **matrix,** found between its cells. In addition to the relatively few cells embedded in the matrix of most types of connective tissue, varying numbers and kinds of fibers are also present. The structural quality and appearance of the matrix and fibers determine the qualities of each type of connective tissue. The matrix of blood, for example, is a liquid, but other types of connective tissue, such as cartilage, have the consistency of firm rubber. The matrix of bone is hard and rigid, although the matrix of connective tissues such as tendons and ligaments is strong and flexible.

The following list identifies a number of the major types of connective tissue in the body. Photomicrographs of several are also shown.

1. Areolar connective tissue
2. Adipose, or fat tissue
3. Fibrous connective tissue
4. Bone
5. Cartilage
6. Blood
7. Hematopoietic tissue

AREOLAR AND ADIPOSE CONNECTIVE TISSUE

Areolar (ah-REE-oh-lar) **connective tissue** is the most widely distributed of all connective tissue types. It is the "glue" that gives form to the internal organs. It consists of delicate webs of fibers and of a variety of cells embedded in a loose matrix of soft, sticky gel.

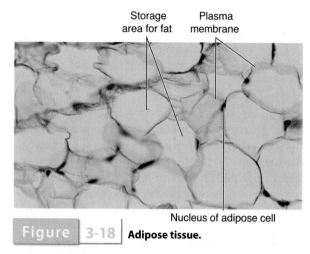

Storage area for fat | Plasma membrane

Nucleus of adipose cell

Figure 3-18 | **Adipose tissue.**

Photomicrograph showing the large storage spaces for fat inside the adipose tissue cells.

Adipose (AD-i-pohs), or **fat tissue,** is specialized to store lipids. In Figure 3-18, numerous spaces have formed in the tissue so that large quantities of fat can accumulate inside cells.

FIBROUS CONNECTIVE TISSUE

Fibrous connective tissue (Figure 3-19) consists mainly of bundles of strong, white **collagen** fibers arranged in parallel rows. This type of connective tissue composes tendons. It provides great strength and flexibility, but it does not stretch. Such characteristics are ideal for these structures that anchor our muscles to our bones.

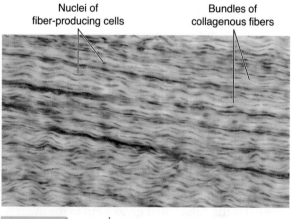

Nuclei of fiber-producing cells | Bundles of collagenous fibers

Figure 3-19 | **Dense fibrous connective tissue.**

Photomicrograph of tissue. Note the multiple bundles of collagenous fibers in parallel and wave-form arrangements. Collagen is white in living tissue but is stained pink here to make it visible.

BONE AND CARTILAGE

Bone is one of the most highly specialized forms of connective tissue. The matrix of bone is hard and calcified. It forms numerous structural building blocks called **osteons** (AHS-tee-onz), or *Haversian* (hah-VER-shun) *systems.* When bone is viewed under a microscope, we can see these circular arrangements of calcified matrix and cells that give bone its characteristic appearance (Figure 3-20). Bones are a storage area for calcium and provide support and protection for the body.

Cartilage differs from bone in that its matrix is the consistency of a firm plastic or a gristle-like gel. Cartilage cells, which are called **chondrocytes** (KON-droh-sytes), are located in many tiny spaces distributed throughout the matrix (Figure 3-21).

BLOOD AND HEMATOPOIETIC TISSUE

Because its matrix is liquid, **blood** is perhaps the most unusual form of connective tissue. It has transportation and protective functions in the body. Red and white blood cells are the cell types common to blood (Figure 3-22).

Hematopoietic (hee-mat-oh-poy-ET-ik) **tissue** is the bloodlike connective tissue found in the red marrow cavities of bones and in organs such as the spleen, tonsils, and lymph nodes. This type of tissue is responsible for the formation of blood cells and lymphatic system cells important in our defense against disease (Table 3-8).

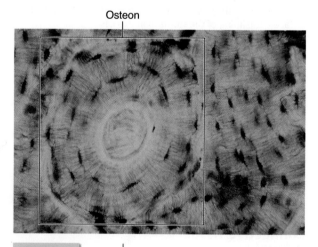

Osteon

Figure 3-20 | **Bone tissue.**

Photomicrograph of dried, ground bone. A wheel-like structural unit of bone, known as an osteon (Haversian system), is apparent in this section.

Matrix   Chondrocyte
in lacuna

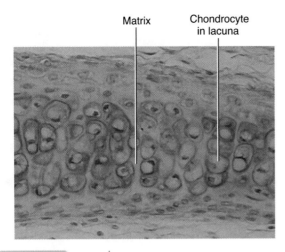

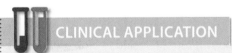

Cartilage.

Photomicrograph showing the chondrocytes distributed throughout the gel-like matrix.

Matrix   White   Red
(liquid)   blood cell blood cells

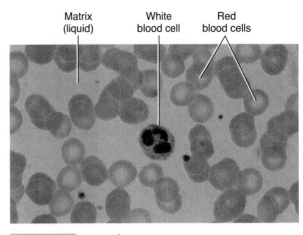

Figure 3-22 **Blood.**

Photomicrograph of a human blood smear. This smear shows a white blood cell surrounded by a number of smaller red blood cells. The liquid matrix of this tissue is also called *plasma.*

CLINICAL APPLICATION

SCREENING DONATED ORGANS AND TISSUES

Tissue typing is a screening process in which cell markers in a donated organ or tissue are identified so that they can be matched to recipients with similar cell markers. Cell markers are specific protein molecules (called **antigens** [see Chapter 15]) on the surface of plasma membranes. If the cell markers in donated tissue are different than those in the recipient's normal tissue, the recipient's immune system will recognize the tissue as foreign. When the immune system mounts a significant attack against the donated tissue, a **rejection reaction** occurs. The inflammation and tissue destruction that occurs in a rejection reaction not only destroys or "rejects" the donated tissue but may also threaten the life of the recipient. Although drugs such as cyclosporine can be used to inhibit the immune system's attack against donated tissue, crossmatching of tissues by their cell markers is the primary method of preventing rejection reactions.

If you know your blood type, you already know some of your tissue markers. In the ABO system (see Chapter 12), type A blood has the A marker, type B blood has the B marker, type AB blood has both A and B markers, and type O blood has neither A nor B markers. It is important to type and crossmatch blood before a blood transfusion takes place to prevent a rejection reaction that could kill the recipient. The American Red Cross and other agencies that

coordinate procurement of organs and tissues for transplantation are developing computer networks to monitor availability of organs with specific cell markers. Such high-speed computer networks allow physicians to immediately locate organs or tissues for emergency transplants or transfusions.

Another procedure used to screen potential donor organs and tissues involves checking for the presence of infectious agents, especially viruses. Because viruses are difficult to find, most screening tests screen for the presence of specific antibodies. Antibodies are protein molecules produced by some white blood cells upon exposure to a virus or other infectious agent. Each type of virus triggers production of a specific kind of antibody, so the presence of a specific antibody type means that the tissue may have the corresponding virus. For example, a test called *ELISA (enzyme-linked immunosorbent assay)* is used to test for the presence of antibodies produced in response to HIV (human immunodeficiency virus). HIV causes *acquired immunodeficiency syndrome (AIDS),* a fatal disease that can be transmitted through HIV-contaminated tissues or body fluids. Routine screening for hepatitis-B antigen and other viral antibodies is also done by most tissue and blood banks. Because there is some lag time between infection by a virus and the resulting production of antibodies, such screening tests may fail to identify a virus-contaminated tissue from a recently infected donor.

Muscle Tissue

Muscle cells are the movement specialists of the body. They have a higher degree of contractility (ability to shorten or contract) than any other tissue cells. There are three kinds of muscle tissue: **skeletal, cardiac,** and **smooth.**

SKELETAL MUSCLE TISSUE

Skeletal, or striated, muscle is called **voluntary** because willed or voluntary control of skeletal muscle contractions is possible. Note in Figure 3-23 that when viewed under a microscope, skeletal muscle is characterized by many cross striations and many nuclei per cell. Individual cells are long and threadlike and are often called *fibers*. Skeletal muscles are attached to bones and when contracted, produce voluntary and controlled body movements.

CARDIAC MUSCLE TISSUE

Cardiac muscle forms the walls of the heart, and the regular but involuntary contractions of cardiac muscle produce the heartbeat. Under the light microscope (Figure 3-24), cardiac muscle fibers have faint cross striations (like skeletal muscle) and thicker dark bands called *intercalated disks*. Cardiac muscle fibers branch and reform to produce an interlocking mass of contractile tissue.

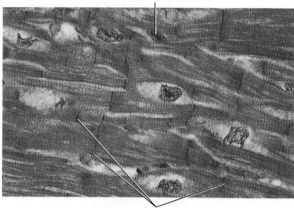

Nucleus of muscle cell

Intercalated disks

Figure 3-24 | **Cardiac muscle.**

Photomicrograph showing the branched, lightly striated fibers. The darker bands, called intercalated disks, which are characteristic of cardiac muscle, are easily identified in this tissue section.

SMOOTH MUSCLE TISSUE

Smooth (visceral) muscle is said to be *involuntary* because it is not under conscious or willful control. Under a microscope (Figure 3-25), smooth muscle cells are seen as long, narrow fibers but not nearly as long as skeletal or striated fibers. Individual smooth muscle cells appear smooth (that is, without cross striations) and have only one nucleus per fiber. Smooth

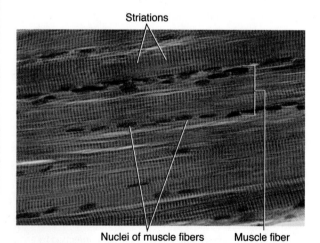

Striations

Nuclei of muscle fibers   Muscle fiber

Figure 3-23 | **Skeletal muscle.**

Photomicrograph showing the striations of the muscle cell fibers in longitudinal section.

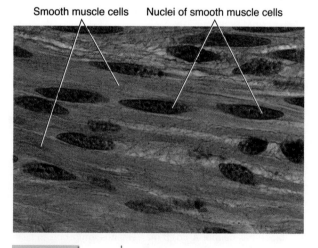

Smooth muscle cells   Nuclei of smooth muscle cells

Figure 3-25 | **Smooth muscle.**

Photomicrograph, longitudinal section. Note the central placement of nuclei in the spindle-shaped smooth muscle fibers.

muscle helps form the walls of blood vessels and hollow organs such as the intestines and other tube-shaped structures in the body. Contractions of smooth (visceral) muscle propel food material through the digestive tract and help regulate the diameter of blood vessels. Contraction of smooth muscle in the tubes of the respiratory system, such as the bronchioles in the lungs, can impair breathing and result in asthma attacks and labored respiration.

Nervous Tissue

The function of **nervous tissue** is rapid communication between body structures and control of body functions (Table 3-9). Nervous tissue consists of two kinds of cells: nerve cells, or **neurons** (NOO-rons), which are the functional or conducting units of the system, and special connecting and supporting cells called **glia** (GLEE-ah), or *neuroglia.*

All neurons are characterized by a **cell body** and two types of processes: one **axon,** which transmits a nerve impulse away from the cell body, and one or more **dendrites** (DEN-drytes), which carry impulses toward the cell body. The neurons in Figure 3-26 have many dendrites extending from the cell body.

Tissue Repair

When damaged by mechanical or other injuries, tissues have a varying capacity to repair themselves.

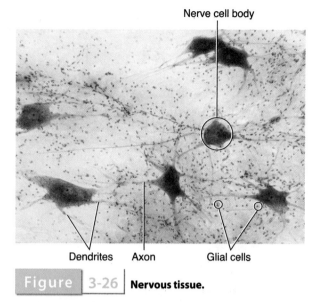

Figure 3-26 **Nervous tissue.**

Light micrograph of neurons in a smear of the spinal cord. The neurons in this slide show characteristic cell bodies and multiple cell processes.

Damaged tissue will regenerate or be replaced by tissue we know as scars. Tissues usually repair themselves by allowing the phagocytic cells to remove dead or injured cells, then filling in the gaps that are left. This growth of new tissue is called **regeneration.**

 HEALTH & WELL-BEING

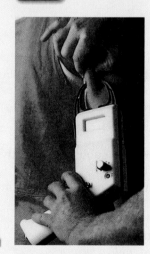

TISSUES AND FITNESS

Achieving and maintaining an ideal body weight is a health-conscious goal. However, a better indicator of health and fitness is **body composition.** Exercise physiologists assess body composition to identify the percentage of the body made of lean tissue and the percentage made of fat. Body-fat percentage is often determined by using calipers to measure the thickness of skin folds at certain places on the body (see figure). A person with low body weight may still have a high ratio of fat to muscle, an unhealthy condition. In this case the individual is "underweight" but "over fat." In other words, fitness depends more on the percentage and ratio of specific tissue types than the overall amount of tissue present.

Therefore one goal of a good fitness program is a desirable body-fat percentage. For men, the ideal is 15% to 18%, and for women, the ideal is 20% to 22%. Because fat contains stored energy (measured in calories), a low fat percentage means a low energy reserve. High body-fat percentages are associated with several life-threatening conditions, including diabetes and cardiovascular disease. A balanced diet and an exercise program can ensure that the ratio of fat to muscle tissue stays at a level appropriate for maintaining homeostasis.

Epithelial and connective tissues have the greatest capacity to regenerate. When a break in an epithelial membrane occurs, as in a cut, cells quickly divide to form daughter cells that fill the wound. In connective tissues, cells that form collagen fibers become active after an injury and fill in a gap with an unusually dense mass of fibrous connective tissue. If this dense mass of fibrous tissue is small, it may be replaced by normal tissue later. If the mass is deep or large, or if cell damage was extensive, it may remain a dense fibrous mass called a **scar.** An unusually thick scar that develops in the lower layer of the skin, such as that shown in Figure 3-27, is called a **keloid** (KEE-loyd).

Skeletal muscle tissue often regenerates itself when injured. Cardiac and smooth muscle seems to have less ability to regenerate—especially when the damage is severe.

Nerve tissue has been viewed as having a limited capacity to regenerate, but new evidence shows that these limitations are not as great as once thought. Neurons outside the brain and spinal cord can sometimes regenerate on their own, but very slowly and only if certain neuroglia are present to "pave the way." In the normal adult brain and spinal cord, neurons may not always grow back when injured. Thus brain and spinal cord injuries often result in permanent damage. Fortunately, the discovery of *nerve growth factors* produced by neuroglia offers the promise of treating brain damage by stimulating release of these factors.

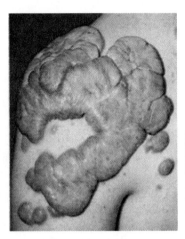

Figure 3-27

Keloid.

Keloids are thick scars that form in the lower layer of the skin in predisposed individuals.

QUICK CHECK

1. What is the difference between *simple* and *stratified* epithelial tissue?
2. What are the three main types of *muscle tissue?*
3. What are the two main cell types found in *nervous tissue?*
4. What is meant by the term *regeneration* of tissue?

Outline Summary

 To download an MP3 version of the chapter summary for use with your iPod or portable media player, access the **Audio Chapter Summaries** on your CD.

Cells

A. Size and shape
  1. Human cells vary considerably in size
  2. All are microscopic
  3. Cells differ notably in shape
B. Composition
  1. Cells contain cytoplasm—substance found only in cells
  2. Organelles are specialized structures within the cytoplasm
  3. Cell interior is surrounded by a plasma membrane
C. Parts of the cell
  1. Plasma membrane (Figure 3-1)
    a. Forms outer boundary of cell
    b. Composed of a thin, two-layered membrane of phospholipids containing proteins
    c. Is selectively permeable
  2. Cytoplasm (Figure 3-2)—internal cell fluid and numerous organelles
    a. Ribosomes
      (1) Made of two tiny subunits of mostly ribosomal RNA
      (2) May attach to rough ER or lie free in cytoplasm
      (3) Manufacture enzymes and other protein compounds
      (4) Often called *protein factories*
    b. Endoplasmic reticulum (ER)

(1) Network of connecting sacs and canals
(2) Carry substances through fluid cytoplasm
(3) Two types—rough and smooth
(4) Rough ER collects, folds, and transports proteins made by ribosomes
(5) Smooth ER synthesizes chemicals; makes new membrane

c. Golgi apparatus
(1) Group of flattened sacs near nucleus
(2) Collect chemicals into vesicles that move from the smooth ER outward to plasma membrane
(3) Called the *chemical processing and packaging center*

d. Mitochondria
(1) Composed of inner and outer membranous sacs
(2) Involved with energy-releasing chemical reactions
(3) Often called *power plants* of the cell
(4) Contains one DNA molecule

e. Lysosomes
(1) Membranous-walled organelles
(2) Contain digestive enzymes
(3) Have protective function (eat microbes)
(4) Formerly thought to be responsible for apoptosis (programmed cell death)

f. Centrioles
(1) Paired organelles that lie at right angles to each other near the nucleus
(2) Function in cell reproduction

g. Microvilli
(1) Small, fingerlike extensions of the plasma membrane
(2) Increase absorptive surface area of the cell

h. Cilia
(1) Fine, hairlike extensions found on free or exposed surfaces of some cells
(2) Some are found in groups and capable of moving in unison in a wavelike fashion
(3) Single, nonmoving cilia in some cells serve sensory functions

i. Flagella
(1) Single projections extending from cell surfaces
(2) Much larger than cilia
(3) "Tails" of sperm cells only example of flagella in humans

3. Nucleus
   a. Controls cell because it contains DNA, the genetic code—instructions for making proteins, which in turn determine cell structure and function
   b. Component structures include nuclear envelope, nucleoplasm, nucleolus, and chromatin granules
   c. DNA molecules become tightly coiled chromosomes during cell division
   d. Each cell has 46 chromosomes in the nucleus

D. Relationship of cell structure and function
   1. Every human cell has a designated function—some help maintain the cell; others regulate life processes of the body itself
   2. Specialized functions of a cell differ depending on number and type of organelles

Movements of Substances Through Cell Membranes

A. Passive transport processes do not require added energy and result in movement "down a concentration gradient"
   1. Diffusion (Figure 3-4)
      a. Substances scatter themselves evenly throughout an available space
      b. It is unnecessary to add energy to the system
      c. Movement is from high to low concentration
      d. Osmosis and dialysis are specialized examples of diffusion across a selectively permeable membrane
      e. Osmosis is diffusion of water (when some solutes cannot cross the membrane)
      f. Dialysis is diffusion of solutes
   2. Filtration
      a. Movement of water and solutes caused by hydrostatic pressure on one side of membrane
      b. Responsible for urine formation

B. Active transport processes occur only in living cells; movement of substances is "up the concentration gradient"; requires energy from ATP

1. Ion pumps
   a. An ion pump is protein complex in cell membrane
   b. Ion pumps use energy from ATP to move substances across cell membranes against their concentration gradients
   c. Examples: sodium-potassium pump (Figure 3-5), calcium pump
   d. Some ion pumps work with other carriers so that glucose or amino acids are transported along with ions
2. Phagocytosis and pinocytosis
   a. Both are active transport mechanisms because they require cell energy
   b. Phagocytosis is a protective mechanism often used to destroy bacteria (Figure 3-6)
   c. Pinocytosis is used to incorporate fluids or dissolved substances into cells

C. Cell transport and disease
   1. Cystic fibrosis, characterized by abnormally thick secretions in the airways and digestive ducts, results from failed Cl⁻ transport (Figure 3-7)
   2. Cholera is a bacterial infection that causes Cl⁻ and water to leak from cells lining the intestines, resulting in severe diarrhea and water loss

Cell Reproduction and Heredity

A. DNA molecule and genetic information (Figure 3-8)
   1. DNA molecule resembles a long, narrow ladder twisted round and round its axis; shaped in a double helix
   2. Each molecule made of a sugar (deoxyribose), bases, and phosphate units
   3. Bases are nitrogen-containing chemicals: adenine, thymine, guanine, and cytosine
   4. Complementary base pairing—each step of DNA ladder contains a base pair; adenine-thymine or cytosine-guanine
   5. A gene is a specific segment of base pairs in a chromosome
   6. Genetic code—sequence of base pairs determines heredity

   a. Coded information in genes controls protein and enzyme production
   b. Enzymes facilitate chemical reactions
   c. Cellular chemical reactions determine cell structure and function
7. RNA molecules and protein synthesis
   a. DNA contained in cell nucleus
   b. Protein synthesis—occurs in cytoplasm, thus genetic information must pass from the nucleus to the cytoplasm
   c. Process of transferring genetic information from nucleus to cytoplasm where proteins are produced requires completion of *transcription* and *translation* (Figure 3-9)
8. Transcription
   a. Double-stranded DNA separates to form messenger RNA (mRNA)
   b. Each strand of mRNA duplicates a particular gene (base-pair sequence) from a segment of DNA
   c. mRNA molecules pass from the nucleus to the cytoplasm, where they direct protein synthesis in ribosomes and ER
9. Translation
   a. Involves synthesis of proteins in cytoplasm by ribosomes
   b. Requires use of information contained in mRNA
   c. Codon—a series of three nucleotide bases that act as a code for a specific amino acid

B. Cells, genetics, and disease
   1. Abnormal DNA that is inherited or that results from damage is often the basis of disease
   2. Factors that cause damage to DNA molecules include chemical or mechanical irritants, radiation, bacteria, and viruses
C. Cell division—reproduction of cell involving division of the nucleus (mitosis) and the cytoplasm
   1. Two daughter cells result from the division
   2. Period when the cell is not actively dividing is called *interphase*
   3. DNA replication—process by which each half of a DNA molecule becomes a whole

molecule identical to the original DNA molecule; precedes mitosis
4. Mitosis—process in cell division that distributes identical chromosomes (DNA molecules) to each new cell formed when the original cell divides; enables cells to reproduce their own kind; makes heredity possible (Figure 3-10)
 a. Prophase—first stage
  (1) Chromatin granules become organized
  (2) Chromosomes (pairs of linked chromatids) appear
  (3) Centrioles move away from nucleus
  (4) Nuclear envelope disappears, freeing genetic material
  (5) Spindle fibers appear
 b. Metaphase—second stage
  (1) Chromosomes align across center of cell
  (2) Spindle fibers attach themselves to each chromatid
 c. Anaphase—third stage
  (1) Centromeres break apart
  (2) Separated chromatids now called *chromosomes*
  (3) Chromosomes are pulled to opposite ends of cell
  (4) Cleavage furrow develops at end of anaphase
 d. Telophase—fourth stage
  (1) Cell division is completed
  (2) Nuclei appear in daughter cells
  (3) Nuclear envelope and nucleoli appear
  (4) Cytoplasm is divided (cytokinesis)
  (5) Daughter cells become fully functional
D. Changes in cell growth and reproduction
 1. Hypertrophy—increase in size of individual cells; increasing size of tissue
 2. Atrophy—decrease in size of individual cells; decreasing size of tissue
 3. Hyperplasia—increase in cell reproduction, increasing size of tissue
 4. Anaplasia—production of abnormal, undifferentiated cells
 5. Uncontrolled cell reproduction results in formation of a benign or malignant neoplasm (tumor) (Figure 3-11)

Tissues (Tables 3-7 through 3-9)

A. Epithelial tissue
 1. Covers body and lines body cavities
 2. Cells packed closely together with little matrix
 3. Classified by shape of cells (Figure 3-12)
  a. Squamous
  b. Cuboidal
  c. Columnar
  d. Transitional
 4. Classified by arrangement of cells
  a. Simple
  b. Stratified
 5. Simple squamous epithelium (Figure 3-13)
  a. Single layer of scalelike cells
  b. Transport (e.g., absorption) is function
 6. Stratified squamous epithelium (Figure 3-14)
  a. Several layers of closely packed cells
  b. Protection is primary function
 7. Simple columnar epithelium (Figure 2-15)
  a. Columnar cells arranged in a single layer
  b. Line stomach and intestines
  c. Contain mucus-producing goblet cells
  d. Specialized for absorption
 8. Stratified transitional epithelium (Figure 3-16)
  a. Found in body areas, such as urinary bladder, that stretch
  b. Up to 10 layers of roughly cuboidal-shaped cells that distort to squamous shape when stretched
 9. Pseudostratified epithelium
  a. Each cell touches basement membrane
  b. Lines the trachea
 10. Simple cuboidal epithelium (Figure 3-17)
  a. Often specialized for secretory activity
  b. Cuboidal cells may be grouped into glands
  c. May secrete into ducts, directly into blood, and on body surface
  d. Examples of secretions include saliva, digestive juice, and hormones
  e. Cuboidal epithelium also forms the urine-producing tubules of the kidney
B. Connective tissue
 1. Most abundant tissue in body
 2. Most widely distributed tissue in body
 3. Multiple types, appearances, and functions
 4. Relatively few cells in intercellular matrix
 5. Types
  a. Areolar—glue that holds organs together

b. Adipose (fat)—lipid storage is primary function (Figure 3-18)
c. Fibrous—bundles of strong collagen fibers; example is tendon (Figure 3-19)
d. Bone—matrix is calcified; function is support and protection (Figure 3-20)
e. Cartilage—matrix is consistency of gristle-like gel; chondrocyte is cell type (Figure 3-21)
f. Blood—matrix is fluid; functions are transportation and protection (Figure 3-22)

C. Muscle tissue (Figures 3-23 to 3-25)
1. Skeletal muscle tissue—attaches to bones; also called *striated* or *voluntary;* control is voluntary; striations apparent when viewed under a microscope (Figure 3-23)
2. Cardiac muscle tissue—also called *striated involuntary;* composes heart wall; ordinarily cannot control contractions (Figure 3-24)
3. Smooth muscle tissue—also called *nonstriated (visceral)* or *involuntary;* no cross striations; found in blood vessels and other tube-shaped organs (Figure 3-25)

D. Nervous tissue (Figure 3-26)
1. Function—rapid communication between body structures and control of body functions
2. Neurons—conduction cells
   a. All neurons have a cell body and two types of processes: axon and dendrite
      (1) Axon (one) carries nerve impulse away from cell body
      (2) Dendrites (one or more) carry nerve impulse toward the cell body
3. Glia (neuroglia)—supportive and connecting cells

E. Tissue repair—usually accomplished by means of regeneration of tissue

New Words

adipose	endocrine	nuclear envelope	spindle fiber
anaplasia	epithelial tissue	nucleoplasm	squamous
antigen	exocrine	organelles	transcription
apoptosis	genome	cilia	transfer RNA (tRNA)
areolar connective tissue	gland	endoplasmic reticulum (ER)	translation
atrophy	glia	flagellum (*pl.,* flagella)	transport processes
axon	goblet cell	Golgi apparatus	dialysis
centriole	hematopoietic tissue	lysosome	diffusion
centromere	hyperplasia	microvillus (*pl.,* microvilli)	filtration
chondrocyte	hypertonic	mitochondrion	osmosis
chromatid	hypertrophy	(*pl.,* mitochondria)	phagocytosis
chromatin granule	hypotonic	nucleolus	pinocytosis
cleavage furrow	interphase	nucleus	
codon	interstitial	plasma membrane	**Diseases and Other**
collagen	isotonic	ribosome	**Clinical Terms**
complementary base	lyse	vesicle	
pairing	matrix	osteon	cancer
connective tissue	messenger RNA (mRNA)	passive transport	cholera
crenation	mitosis	phospholipid	cystic fibrosis (CF)
cytoplasm	anaphase	pseudostratified	keloid
dendrite	metaphase	epithelium	neoplasm
deoxyribonucleic acid	prophase	ribonucleic acid (RNA)	regeneration
(DNA)	telophase	solute	rejection reaction
DNA replication	neuron	sodium-potassium pump	scar
			tissue typing

Review Questions

1. Describe the structure of the plasma membrane.
2. List three functions of the plasma membrane.
3. Give the function of each of the following organelles: ribosome, Golgi apparatus, mitochondria, lysosome, and centrioles.
4. Give the function of the nucleus and nucleolus.
5. Explain the difference between chromatin and chromosomes.
6. Describe the processes of diffusion and filtration.
7. Describe the functioning of the ion pump and explain the process of phagocytosis.
8. What cell transport mechanism failure results in the disease cystic fibrosis?
9. Describe the process of transcription.
10. Describe the process of translation.
11. List the four stages in active cell division (mitosis) and briefly describe what occurs in each stage.
12. What important event in mitosis occurs during interphase?
13. Name and describe three epithelial tissues.
14. Name and describe three connective tissues.
15. Name and describe two muscle tissues.
16. Name the two types of nervous tissue. Which is functional nerve tissue and which is support tissue?

Critical Thinking

17. Explain what is meant by tissue typing. Why has this become so important in recent years?
18. Explain what would happen if a cell containing 97% water were placed in a 10% salt solution.
19. If one side of a DNA molecule had the following base sequence: adenine-adenine-guanine cytosine-thymine-cytosine-thymine, what would the sequence of bases on the opposite side of the molecule be?
20. If a molecule of mRNA was made from the DNA base sequence in question 19, what would the sequence of bases be in the RNA?
21. Compare and contrast tissue repair in epithelial, connective, muscle, and nervous tissue.

Chapter Test

1. _____ and _____ are two fat-based molecules that make up part of the structure of the plasma membrane.
2. _____ is a term that refers to small structures inside the cell, it means "little organs."
3. _____ is the movement of substances across a cell membrane using cell energy, whereas _____ is the movement of substances across a cell membrane without using cell energy.
4. _____ refers to the movement of fluids or dissolved molecules into the cell by trapping them in the plasma membrane.
5. _____ is a disease caused by the inability of cells to transport Cl^- ions.
6. _____ is the process in protein synthesis that uses the information in mRNA to build a protein molecule.
7. _____ is the process in protein synthesis that forms the mRNA molecule.
8. _____ is a segment of base pairs in a chromosome.
9. _____ is the total genetic information packaged in a cell.
10. _____, _____, _____, and _____ are the four main tissues in the body.
11. Which of the following is not a form of diffusion?
    a. Filtration
    b. Dialysis
    c. Osmosis
    d. All of the above are examples of diffusion
12. The disease caused by the muscle cell's inability to control chloride ion movement is:
    a. cystic fibrosis
    b. hemophilia
    c. Duchenne muscular dystrophy
    d. AIDS
13. The disease caused by an inherited mistake in the genetic code that prevents production of normal blood clotting proteins is:

a. cystic fibrosis
b. hemophilia
c. Duchenne muscular dystrophy
d. AIDS

14. During what stage of mitosis do the chromosomes move away from the center of the cell?
    a. Interphase
    b. Metaphase
    c. Anaphase
    d. Telophase

15. During what stage of mitosis does the DNA replicate?
    a. Interphase
    b. Metaphase
    c. Prophase
    d. Telophase

16. During what stage of mitosis do the chromosomes align in the center of the cell?
    a. Interphase
    b. Metaphase
    c. Prophase
    d. Telophase

17. During what stage of mitosis does the chromatin condense into chromosomes?
    a. Interphase
    b. Metaphase

c. Prophase
d. Telophase

18. During what stage of mitosis do the nuclear envelope and nuclei reappear?
    a. Interphase
    b. Prophase
    c. Anaphase
    d. Telophase

19. Which of the following terms refers to an increase in cell size?
    a. Hyperplasia
    b. Hypertrophy
    c. Anaplasia
    d. Atrophy

20. Which of the following terms refers to the production of abnormal, undifferentiated cells?
    a. Hyperplasia
    b. Hypertrophy
    c. Anaplasia
    d. Atrophy

21. Which tissue is least likely to regenerate itself?
    a. Simple squamous epithelium
    b. Striated muscle tissue
    c. Dense fibrous connective tissue
    d. Stratified squamous epithelium

Match the cell structure in column A with its corresponding description in column B.

Column A
22. _____ ribosome
23. _____ endoplasmic reticulum
24. _____ Golgi apparatus
25. _____ mitochondria
26. _____ lysosomes
27. _____ flagella
28. _____ cilia
29. _____ nucleus
30. _____ nucleolus

Column B
a. along cell projection used to propel sperm cells
b. bags of digestive enzymes in the cell
c. tubelike passages that carry substances throughout the cell
d. short hairlike structures on the free surfaces of some cells
e. chemically processes and packages substances from the endoplasmic reticulum
f. directs protein synthesis, contains DNA; the "brain" of the cell
g. "protein factories" in the cell, made of RNA
h. small structure in the nucleus that helps in the formation of ribosomes
i. "powerhouse" of the cell; where most of the cell's ATP is formed

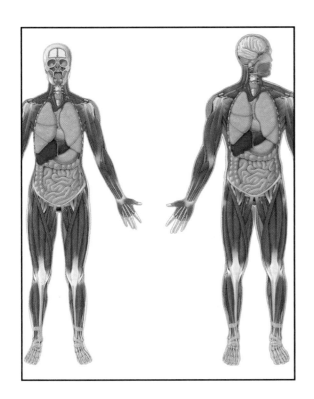

Clear View of the Human Body

Developed by: **KEVIN PATTON and PAUL KRIEGER**

Illustrated by: **Dragonfly Media Group**

INTRODUCTION

A complete understanding of human anatomy and physiology requires an appreciation for how structures within the body relate to one another. Such appreciation for anatomical structure has become especially important in the 21st century with the explosion in the use of diverse methods of medical imaging that rely on the ability to interpret sectional views of the human body.

The best way to develop your understanding of overall anatomical structure is to carefully dissect a large number of male and female human cadavers—then have those dissected specimens handy while reading and learning about each system of the body. Obviously, such multiple dissections and constant access to specimens are impractical for nearly everyone. However, the experience of a simple dissection can be approximated by layering several partially transparent, two-dimensional anatomical diagrams in a way that allows a student to "virtually" dissect the human body simply by paging through the layers.

This **Clear View of the Human Body** provides a handy tool for dissecting simulated male and female bodies. It also provides views of several different parts of the human body in a variety of cross sections. The many different anterior and posterior views also give you a perspective on body structure that is not available with ordinary anatomical diagrams. This Clear View is an always-available tool to help you learn the three-dimensional structure of the body in a way that allows you to see how they relate to each other in a complete body. It will always be right here in your textbook, so place a bookmark here and refer to the Clear View frequently as you study each of the systems of the human body.

HINTS FOR USING THE CLEAR VIEW OF THE BODY

1. Starting at the first page of the Clear View, slowly lift the page as you look at the anterior view of the male and female bodies. You will see deeper structures appear, as if you had dissected the body. As you lift each successive layer of images, you will be looking at deeper and deeper body structures. A key to the labels is found in the gray sidebar.
2. Starting with the second section of the Clear View, notice that you are looking at the posterior aspect of the male and female body. Lift each layer from the left edge to reveal body structures in successive layers from the back to the front. This very unique view will help you understand structural relationships even better.
3. On each page of the Clear View, look at the horizontal section represented in the sidebar. The section you are looking at on any one page is from the location shown in the larger diagram as a red line. In other words, if you cut the body at the red line and tilted the upper part of the body toward you, you would see what is shown in the section diagram. Notice that each section has its own labeling system that is separate from the labels used in the larger images.

KEY

1. Epicranius m.
2. Temporalis m.
3. Orbicularis oculi m.
4. Masseter m.
5. Orbicularis oris m.
6. Pectoralis major m.
7. Serratus anterior m.
8. Basilic vein
9. Brachial fascia
10. Cephalic vein
11. Rectus sheath
12. Linea alba
13. Rectus abdominis m.
14. Umbilicus
15. Abdominal oblique m., external
16. Abdominal oblique m., internal
17. Transverse abdominis m.
18. Inguinal ring, external
19. Fossa ovalis
20. Fascia of the thigh
21. Great saphenous vein
22. Parietal bone
23. Frontal bone
24. Temporal bone
25. Zygomatic bone
26. Maxilla
27. Mandible
28. Sternocleidomastoid m.
29. Sternohyoid muscle
30. Omohyoid muscle
31. Deltoid m.
32. Pectoralis minor m.
33. Sternum
34. Rib (costal) cartilage
35. Rib
36. Greater omentum
37. Frontal lobe
38. Parietal lobe
39. Temporal lobe
40. Cerebellum
41. Nasal septum
42. Brachiocephalic vein
43. Superior vena cava
44. Thymus gland
45. Right lung
46. Left lung
47. Pericardium
48. Liver
49. Gall bladder
50. Stomach
51. Transverse colon
52. Small intestines
53. Biceps brachii m.
54. Brachioradialis m.
55. Adductor longus m.
56. Sartorius m.
57. Quadriceps femoris m.
58. Patellar ligament
59. Tibialis anterior m.
60. Sup. extensor retinaculum
61. Inf. extensor retinaculum
62. Cerebrum of brain
63. Cerebellum
64. Brain stem
65. Maxillary sinus
66. Nasal cavity
67. Tongue
68. Thyroid gland
69. Heart
70. Hepatic veins
71. Esophagus
72. Spleen
73. Celiac artery
74. Portal vein
75. Duodenum
76. Pancreas
77. Mesenteric artery
78. Ascending colon
79. Transverse colon
80. Descending colon
81. Sigmoid colon
82. Mesentery
83. Appendix
84. Inguinal ligament
85. Pubic symphysis
86. Extensor carpi radialis m.
87. Pronator teres m.
88. Flexor carpi radialis m.
89. Flexor digitorum profundus m.
90. Quadraceps femoris m.
91. Extensor digitorum longus m.
92. Thyroid cartilage
93. Trachea
94. Aortic arch
95. Right lung
96. Left lung
97. Pulmonary artery
98. Right atrium
99. Right ventricle
100. Left atrium
101. Left ventricle
102. Coracobrachialis m.
103. Inferior vena cava
104. Descending aorta
105. Right kidney
106. Left kidney
107. Right ureter
108. Rectum
109. Urinary bladder
110. Prostate gland
111. Iliac artery and vein
112. Uterus
113. Parietal bone
114. Frontal sinus
115. Sphenoidal sinus
116. Occipital bone
117. Palatine process
118. Cervical vertebrae
119. Corpus callosum
120. Thalamus
121. Trapezius m.
122. Acromion process
123. Coracoid process
124. Humerus
125. Subscapularis m.
126. Deltoid m. (cut)
127. Triceps m.
128. Brachialis m.
129. Brachioradialis m.
130. Radius
131. Ulna
132. Diaphragm
133. Thoracic duct
134. Quadratus lumborum m.
135. Psoas m.
136. Lumbar vertebrae
137. Iliacus m.
138. Gluteus medius m.
139. Iliofemoral ligament
140. Sacral nerves
141. Sacrum
142. Coccyx
143. Femur
144. Vastus lateralis m.
145. Femoral artery and vein
146. Adductor magnus m.
147. Patella
148. Fibula
149. Tibia
150. Fibularis longus m.
151. Spinal cord
152. Nerve root
153. Platysma m.
154. Splenius capitis m.
155. Levator scapulae m.
156. Rhomboideus m.
157. Infraspinatis m.
158. Teres major m.
159. Lumbodorsal fascia
160. Erector spinae m.
161. Serratus post. inf. m.
162. Latissimus dorsi m.
163. Gluteus medius m.
164. Gluteus maximus m.
165. Iliotibial tract
166. Flexor carpi ulnaris m.
167. Extensor carpi ulnaris m.
168. Extensor digitorum m.
169. Carpal ligament, dorsal
170. Interosseus m.
171. Gluteus minimus m.
172. Piriformis m.
173. Gemellus sup. m.
174. Obturator internus m.
175. Gemellus inf. m.
176. Quadratus femoris m.
177. Biceps femoris m.
178. Gastrocnemius m.
179. Calcaneal (Achilles) tendon
180. Calcaneus bone
181. Subcutaneous fat
182. Corpus spongiosum
183. Corpora cavernosa
184. Umbilical ligaments
185. Epigastric artery and vein
186. Right testis
187. Transverse thoracic m.
188. Parietal pleura
189. Common bile duct
190. Lesser omentum
191. Flexor digitorum profundus
192. Epiglottis

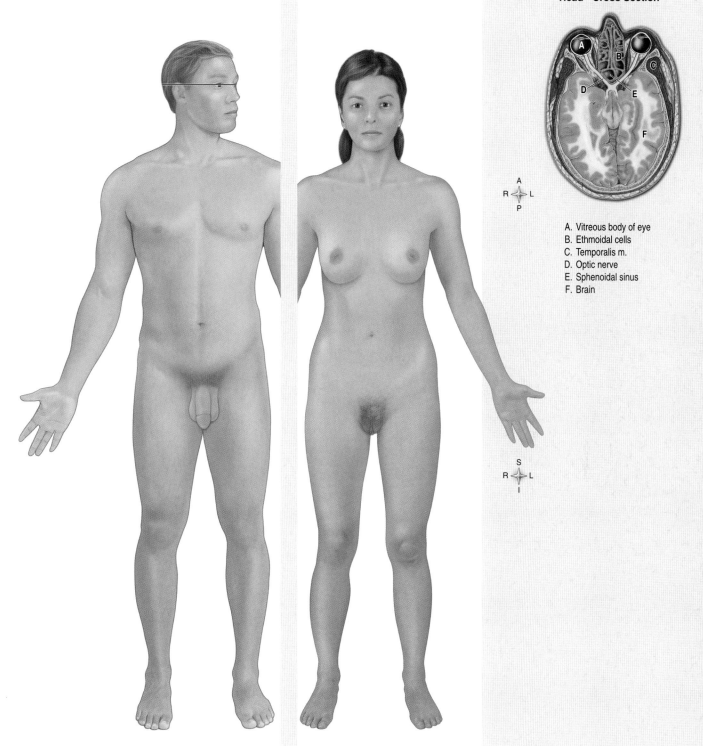

Head - Cross Section

A. Vitreous body of eye
B. Ethmoidal cells
C. Temporalis m.
D. Optic nerve
E. Sphenoidal sinus
F. Brain

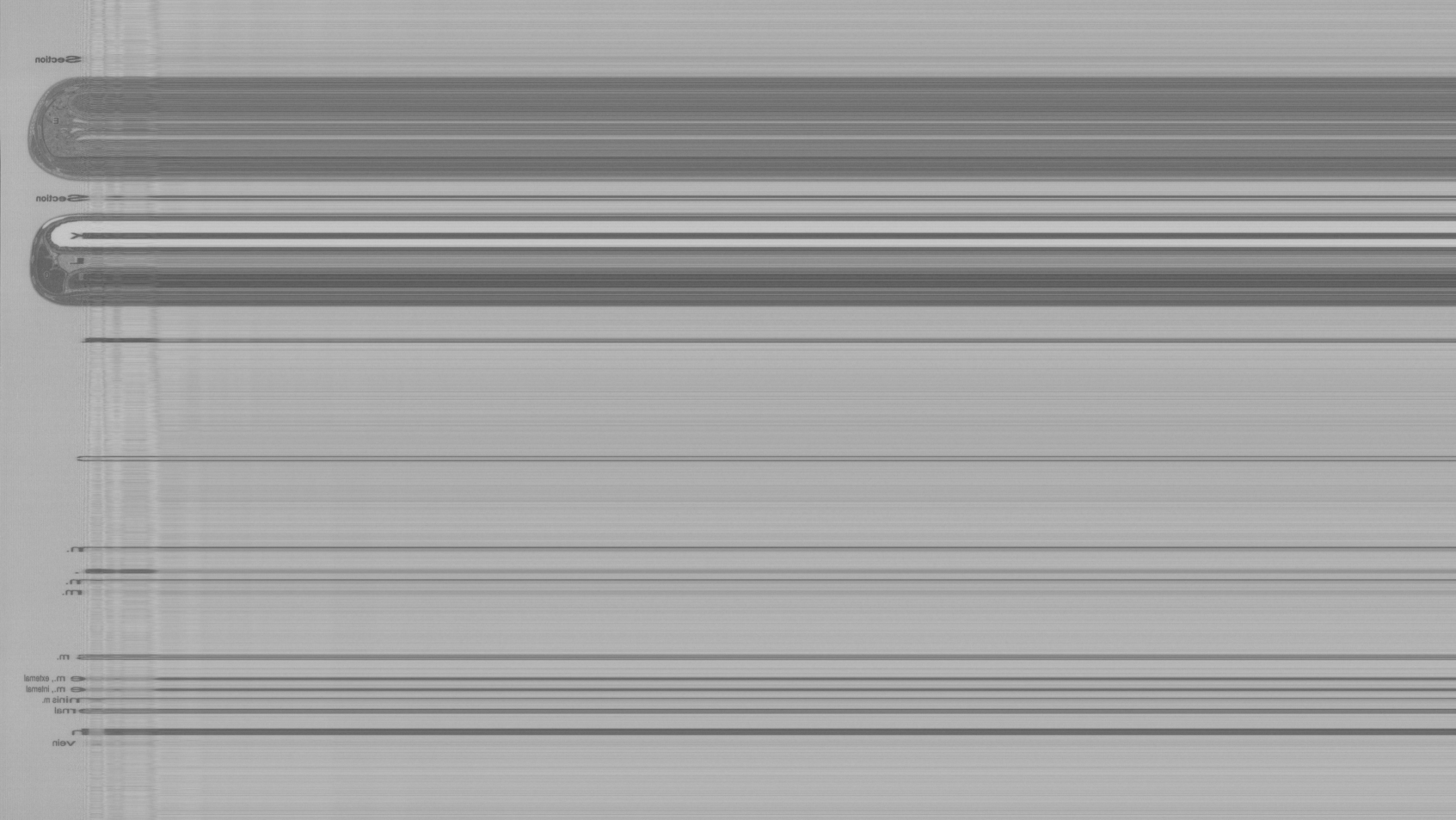

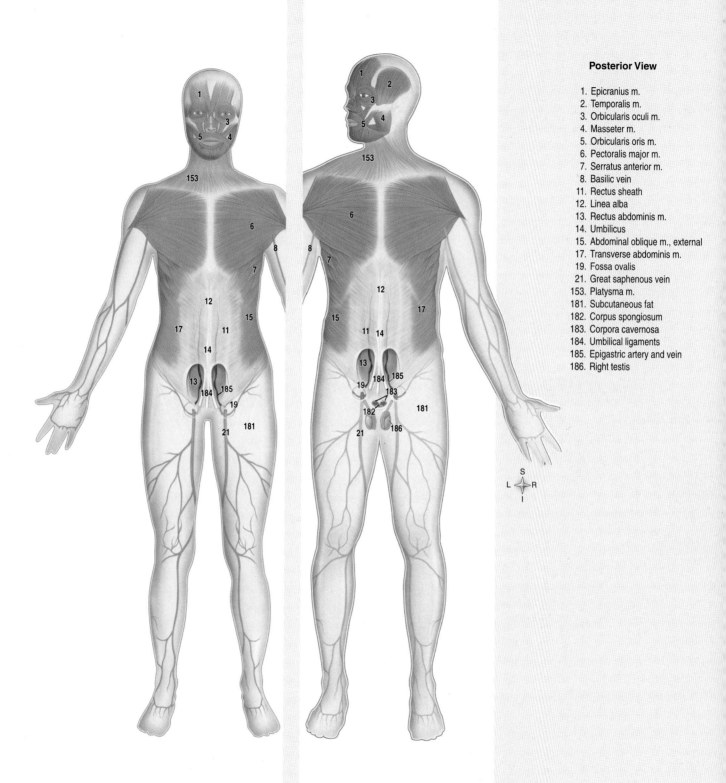

Study Tips

continued from page 41

3. The transport processes of osmosis and dialysis are special cases of diffusion—osmosis with water and dialysis with solutes. Filtration uses a pressure rather than a concentration difference to move substances.

4. *Phago* means "to eat," *pino* means "to drink," *cyto* means "cell," and *-sis* means "condition." *Phagocytosis* and *pinocytosis* are descriptions of what the cell is doing.

5. When studying protein synthesis, keep the goal of the process in mind. The cell wants a protein made, the DNA has the plans, but the ribosome is the factory. The DNA needs to tell the ribosome what to build (transcription), and the factory needs to put the protein together in the correct order (translation).

6. Use flash cards to study the phases of mitosis; remember that the phases are based on what is happening to the chromosomes.

7. Make and use flash cards to learn the terms used to describe changes in cell growth and reproduction.

8. Tissue types are additional topics that could be learned using flash cards. It may be helpful to remember that epithelial tissues are covering and protective tissues, and the important thing about connective tissue is the matrix surrounding the cells.

9. Link the diseases or conditions described in the chapter with the cell structure or function that is abnormal. Cystic fibrosis is caused by abnormal cell transport function; hemophilia and AIDS are caused by abnormal DNA structure.

10. In your study group, review the flash cards for the organelles, mitosis, changes in cell growth and reproduction, and tissues. Be sure to discuss steps in protein synthesis and the cell transport processes. Go over the questions at the end of the chapter and discuss possible test questions.

Case Studies

1. One form of the inherited condition *glycogen storage disease*—a form called *Pompe's disease*—results in accumulation of excessive glycogen in cells of the heart, liver, and other organs. The accumulation of glycogen can disrupt cell function, causing heart and other problems that can progress to death. Glycogen is a large carbohydrate molecule formed by linking numerous glucose molecules into a branched chain (see Chapter 2). Glycogen formation is normal in the affected cells. The accumulation of excessive glycogen results from the failure of enzymes that are supposed to break apart the glycogen so that the cell can use the glucose subunits. In what organelle would you expect to find these glycogen-digesting enzymes? Explain how the presence of nonfunctional enzymes could have been inherited.

2. Malignant tumors are sometimes treated with drugs that halt mitosis, and thus stop the production of new cancer cells. Two such drugs, vincristine sulfate and vinblastine sulfate, interfere with the formation of spindle fibers. How could this action halt mitosis? Antibiotics such as mitomycin C and inorganic compounds such as *cis*-platinum can also be used to stop the growth of tumors. These drugs interfere with DNA synthesis in treated cells. How could this action halt mitosis?

3. Lauren is a 2-year-old girl with cystic fibrosis (CF). Because Lauren has this condition, her mother frequently turns her over, cups her hand, and quickly but firmly pats her sharply on the back between the shoulder blades. How could this help Lauren's condition?

Outline

Objectives

After you have completed this chapter, you should be able to:

1. Define and contrast the terms organ and *organ system*.

2. List the 11 major organ systems of the body.

3. Identify and locate the major organs of each major organ system.

4. Briefly describe the major functions of each major organ system.

5. Identify and discuss the major subdivisions of the reproductive system.

6. Describe current approaches to organ replacement.

4 Organ Systems of the Body

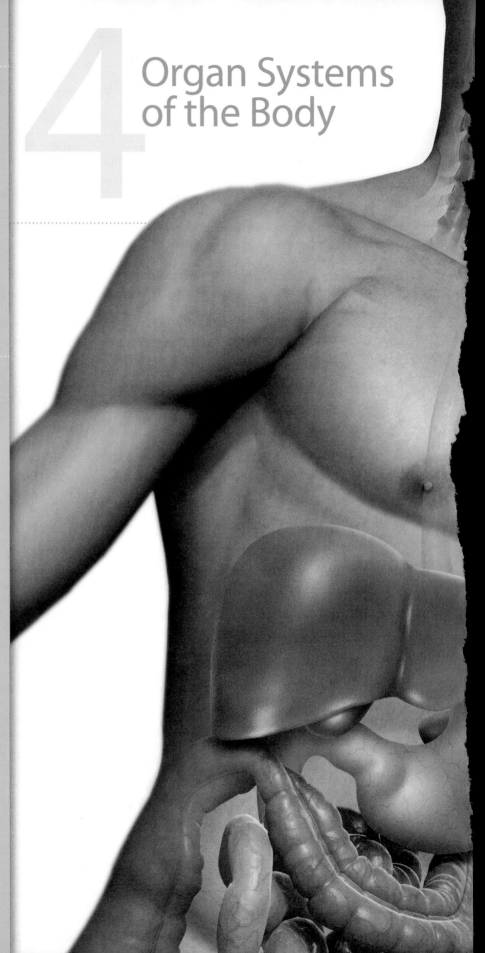

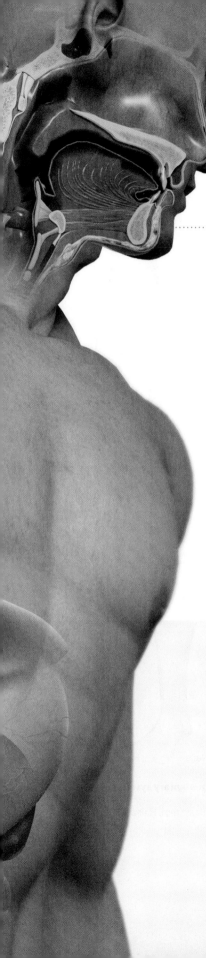

The words organ and *system*, discussed in Chapter 1, have special meanings when applied to the body. An **organ** is a structure made up of two or more kinds of tissue and is organized to perform a more complex function than just one tissue. A **system** is a group of organs that together perform a more complex function than does one organ. This chapter gives an overview of the major organ systems of the body.

In the chapters that follow, the presentation of information on individual organs and an explanation of how they work together to accomplish complex body functions will form the basis for the discussion of each organ system. For example, we cover the skin as the primary organ of the integumentary system in Chapter 6 and information on the bones as organs of the skeletal system in Chapter 7. Knowledge of individual organs and how they are organized into groups makes much more meaningful the understanding of how a particular organ system functions as a unit in the body.

STUDY TIPS

Chapter 4 is the "big picture" chapter. It is a preview of the systems discussed in the remaining chapters.

1. Put the names of the systems on one side of a flash card and the functions of the systems and their organs on the other side. Notice how each organ contributes to the functioning of the system.
2. Review the various types of artificial organs, transplants, and some of the problems in transplantation.
3. Before you begin the chapter dealing with a particular system, it would be helpful to get an overview of that system by reviewing the synopsis of that system in this chapter. That will give you a quick look at its major functions and the organs in that system.
4. In your study group, review the body system flash cards you have made. Discuss how several systems need to be involved in accomplishing one function in the body, such as getting food or oxygen to the cells. Go over the questions at the back of the chapter and discuss possible test questions.

When you have completed your study of the major organ systems in the chapters that follow, it will be possible to view the body not as an assembly of individual parts but as an integrated and functioning whole. This chapter names the systems of the body and the major organs that compose them, and it briefly describes the functions of each system. It provides a basic "road map" to help you anticipate and prepare for the more detailed information that follows in the remainder of the text.

Organ Systems of the Body

In contrast to cells, which are the smallest structural units of the body, organ systems are its largest and most complex structural units. Table 4-1 lists the 11 major organ systems that compose the human body. Figures throughout this chapter represent each system visually as well.

Notice that Table 4-1 also groups the 11 major organ systems into larger systems or divides some of them into smaller systems. We group or split the major organ systems when it makes a particular situation easier to understand. For example, physical therapists sometimes find it most useful to use the concept of a "skeletomuscular system" rather than thinking of the skeletal and muscular systems separately. The nervous system is so complex that often it is easier to understand if it is split into central and peripheral nervous systems. Notice also that some organs belong to more than one system. For example, the hypothalamus is part of the brain and therefore is in the nervous system, but it also secretes hormones, so it is in the endocrine system as well.

 For a brief 3-D tour of each of the body's organ systems, go to **AnimationDirect** on your CD.

Integumentary System

The **integumentary** (in-teg-yoo-MEN-tar-ee) **system** includes only one organ: the skin (Figure 4-1). In most adults, the skin alone weighs 20 pounds or more, accounting for about 16% of total body weight and making it the body's heaviest organ.

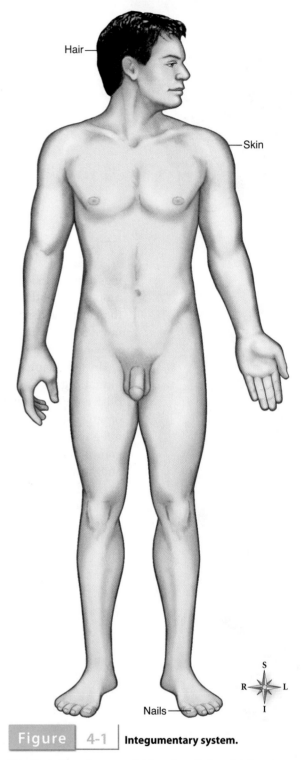

Figure 4-1 **Integumentary system.**

The skin is the only organ of this system. Hair and nails are appendages of this organ.

Table 4-1 | Organ Systems of the Body

GROUPED SYSTEM*	MAJOR BODY SYSTEMS	SPLIT SYSTEM*	PRINCIPAL ORGANS	
Skeletomuscular	Integumentary		Skin (includes hair, nails, glands)	
	Skeletal		Bones (many)	Ligaments (many)
	Muscular		Muscles (many)	
Neuroendocrine	Nervous	Central	Brain	Spinal cord
		Peripheral†	Cranial nerves (and branches) Peripheral nerves (and branches)	Sense organs (many)
	Endocrine		Pituitary gland Pineal gland Hypothalamus Thyroid gland Adrenal glands	Pancreatic islets Ovaries Testes Other glands
	Cardiovascular (also known as *circulatory*)		Heart Arteries (many)	Veins (many) Capillaries (many)
	Lymphatic/immune	Lymphatic‡	Lymph nodes Lymph vessels Thymus	Spleen Tonsils
		Immune	Lymph nodes	All other lymphoid organs
	Respiratory		Nose Pharynx Larynx	Trachea Bronchi Lungs
	Digestive		PRIMARY ORGANS Mouth Pharynx Esophagus Stomach Small intestine Large intestine Rectum Anal canal	ACCESSORY ORGANS Teeth Salivary glands Tongue Liver Gallbladder Pancreas Appendix
Urogenital	Urinary		Kidneys Ureters	Urinary bladder Urethra
	Reproductive	Male	Testes (gonads) Vas deferens Urethra	Prostate Penis Scrotum
		Female	Ovaries (gonads) Uterus Uterine (fallopian) tubes	Vagina Vulva Mammary glands (breasts)

*Some systems are grouped or split into other systems when needed; a few examples are given here.

†The nervous system often is split in other ways, such as sensory/motor or somatic/autonomic.

‡The lymphatic system includes both lymphoid organs and an extensive network of lymph vessels, whereas the immune system includes only lymphoid organs with defensive functions.

Although the integumentary system has only one organ, that one organ, the skin, has many millions of *appendages* (structures attached to a main part) and glands. These skin structures include the hair, nails, and sweat- and oil-producing glands. The skin includes many microscopic sense receptors, making it the largest sensory organ of the body. Skin sense receptors permit the body to respond to pain, pressure, touch, texture, vibration, and changes in temperature.

The integumentary system is crucial to survival. Its primary function is *protection.* The skin protects underlying tissue against invasion by harmful bacteria, bars entry of most chemicals, and minimizes the chances of mechanical injury to underlying structures. In addition, the skin regulates body temperature by sweating, synthesizes important chemicals, and functions as a sophisticated sense organ.

Skeletal System

Bones are the primary organs of the skeletal system. Figure 4-2 shows examples of the 206 individually named bones found in the **skeletal system.** Each individual also has some variable bones that differ from person to person and do not have specific names.

The skeletal system includes not only bones but also related tissues such as cartilage and ligaments. Cartilage can cushion bones that are linked together and can act as the connection between one bone and another. **Ligaments** are bands of fibrous connective tissue that help hold bones together. Connections between two or more bones are called **joints.** The moveable joints between bones makes various movements of individual body parts possible. Without joints, our bodies would be rigid, immobile hulks.

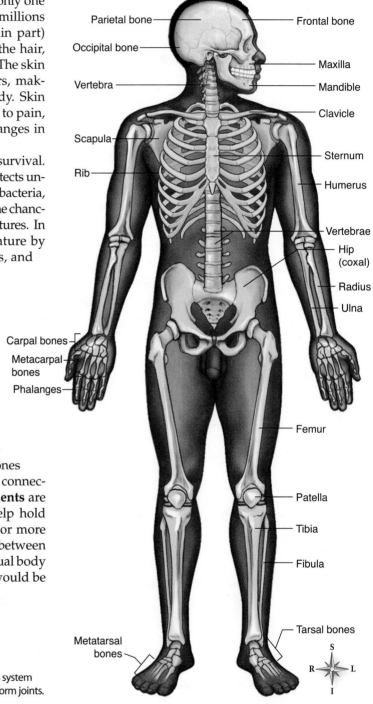

Figure 4-2 | **Skeletal system.**

Only a few of the 206 named bones that are organs of this system are labeled here. Ligaments help hold bones together to form joints.

The skeleton provides protection and a supporting framework for the brain and other internal organs. Bones also serve as storage areas for important minerals such as calcium and phosphorus. The formation of blood cells in the red marrow of certain bones is another crucial function of the skeletal system.

Muscular System

Individual skeletal muscles are the organs of the **muscular system.** Muscles are made up of mostly **skeletal muscle** tissue. Also called **voluntary muscle,** this tissue has the ability to contract when stimulated by conscious nerve regulation. Although movement of the body is the primary function of the muscular system, it also maintains our posture (body position) and provides heat to maintain our body temperature.

A **tendon** is the part of a muscle organ that attaches the muscle to a bone (or another muscle). The patellar tendon of the leg labeled in Figure 4-3 shows how tendons attach muscles to bones. When stimulated by a nervous impulse, muscle tissue shortens or contracts. Voluntary movement occurs when skeletal muscles shorten—a function of the way muscles are attached to bones and the way bones articulate (join) with one another in joints. Sometimes it is useful to think of this cooperative functioning of the bones and muscles as the *skeletomuscular system*.

In addition to skeletal muscle organs, the body contains **smooth muscle** tissue in the walls of hollow organs such as the stomach and small intestine. A third type of muscle tissue is the **cardiac muscle** in the wall of the heart. These muscle tissue types are **involuntary** because they are stimulated by subconscious regulation.

| Figure | 4-3 | **Muscular system.** |

A few of the major muscle organs are labeled here. A tendon is the part of a muscle that attaches to a bone (or another muscle).

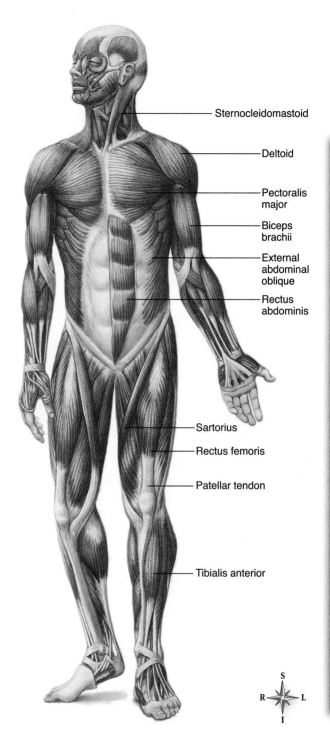

Sternocleidomastoid

Deltoid

Pectoralis major

Biceps brachii

External abdominal oblique

Rectus abdominis

Sartorius

Rectus femoris

Patellar tendon

Tibialis anterior

Nervous System

The brain, spinal cord, and nerves are the organs of the **nervous system** (Figure 4-4). The brain and spinal cord make up the *central nervous system (CNS)*. These two organs provide the central control of the whole nervous system. The *cranial nerves* extend from the brain and the *spinal nerves* extend from the spinal cord. The cranial and spinal nerves, and all their branches, make up the *peripheral nervous system (PNS)*. The word peripheral (per-IF-er-al) means "around the boundary," an apt term for the nerve branches that extend all the way to the farthest boundaries of the body.

The extensive networking of the components of the nervous system makes it possible for this complex system to perform its primary functions. These include the following:

1. Communication between body organs
2. Integration of body functions
3. Control of body functions
4. Recognition of sensory stimuli

These functions are performed by signals called **nerve impulses.** In general, the functions of the nervous system result in rapid activity that lasts usually for a short duration. For example, we can chew our food normally, walk, and perform coordinated muscular movements only if our nervous system functions properly. The nerve impulses permit the rapid and precise control of diverse body functions. Other types of nerve impulses cause glands to secrete fluids.

In addition, elements of the peripheral nervous system can recognize certain **stimuli** (STIM-yoo-lye), such as heat, light, sound, pressure, or temperature,

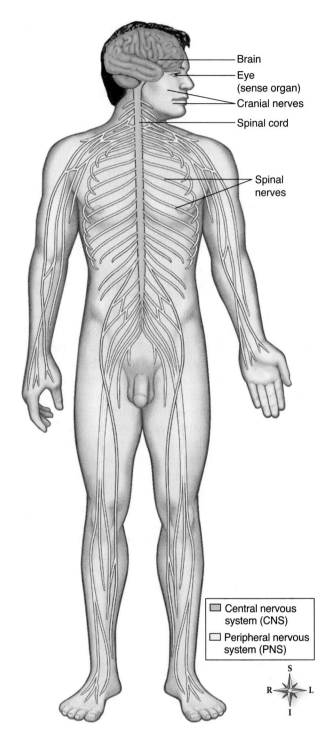

Brain

Eye
(sense organ)

Cranial nerves

Spinal cord

Spinal nerves

Central nervous system (CNS)

Peripheral nervous system (PNS)

Figure   4-4   Nervous system.

The brain and spinal cord make up the central nervous system. Cranial and spinal nerves, as well as all their branches and sensory organs, make up the peripheral nervous system.

that affect the body. When stimulated, these **sense organs** (discussed in Chapter 10) generate nerve impulses that travel to the brain or spinal cord where analysis or relay occurs and, if needed, appropriate action is initiated.

Endocrine System

The **endocrine system** is composed of glands that secrete chemicals known as **hormones** directly into the blood. Sometimes called *ductless glands,* the organs of the endocrine system perform the same general functions as the nervous system: communication, integration, and control. The nervous system provides rapid, brief control by fast-traveling nerve impulses. The endocrine system provides slower but longer-lasting control by hormone secretion; for example, secretion of growth hormone controls the rate of development over long periods of gradual growth. It is no wonder that the nervous and endocrine systems are sometimes thought of as one large regulatory system—the *neuroendocrine system.*

In addition to controlling growth, hormones are the main regulators of metabolism, reproduction, and other body activities. They play important roles in fluid and electrolyte balance and acid-base balance. The various roles of major hormones are integrated into discussions throughout the rest of this book.

As you can see in Figure 4-5, endocrine glands are widely distributed throughout the body. But this is not the complete picture—endocrine glands are far more numerous and widespread than is shown here. We look at just a few of the major endocrine glands.

The **pituitary** (pi-TOO-i-tair-ee) **gland, pineal** (PIN-ee-al) **gland,** and **hypothalamus** (hye-poh-THAL-ah-muss) are located in the skull. The **thyroid** (THY-royd) and **parathyroid** (PAIR-ah-THY-

royd) **glands** are in the neck, and the **thymus** (THY-muss) **gland** is in the thoracic cavity, specifically in the mediastinum (see Figure 1-4, p. 8). The **adrenal** (ah-DREE-nal) **glands** and **pancreas** (PAN-kree-ass) are found in the abdominal cavity. Note in Figure 4-5 that some reproductive glands (ovaries in the female and the testes in the male) also function as endocrine glands.

Cardiovascular System

The **cardiovascular system** consists of the heart and a closed system of vessels made up of **arteries, veins,**

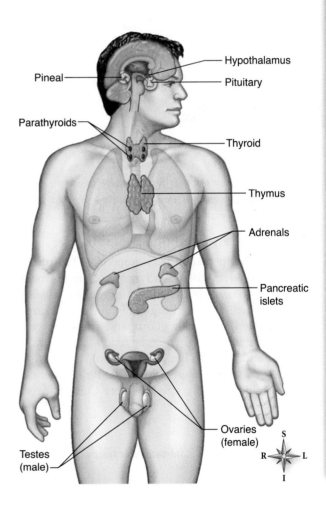

| Figure | 4-5 | **Endocrine system.** |

Some of the major endocrine glands are shown here.

and **capillaries** (Figure 4-6). As the name implies, blood contained in this system is pumped by the heart around a closed circle, or circuit, of vessels as it passes through the body. The cardiovascular system is sometimes called the **circulatory system.**

The primary function of the cardiovascular or circulatory system is *transportation.* The need for an efficient transportation system in the body is critical. Transportation needs include continuous movement of oxygen and carbon dioxide, nutrients, hormones, and other important substances. Wastes produced by the cells are released into the bloodstream on an ongoing basis and are transported by the blood to the excretory organs. The cardiovascular system also helps regulate body temperature by distributing heat throughout the body and by assisting in retaining or releasing heat from the body by regulating blood flow near the body surface. Some cells of the cardiovascular system also function in defense of the body by way of immunity.

> **QUICK CHECK**
>
> 1. What is the *integument?*
> 2. Give examples of organs of the skeletal system.
> 3. What are the major functions of the nervous system?
> 4. What organs make up the cardiovascular system?

Lymphatic and Immune Systems

The **lymphatic system** is composed of **lymphatic vessels** together with other lymphatic organs made up of masses of defensive cells often called *lymphoid tissue.* These lymphoid organs include the **lymph nodes, tonsils, thymus gland,** and **spleen** (Figure 4-7). Note that the thymus functions as an endocrine gland and as a lymphatic organ.

Instead of containing blood, the lymphatic vessels are filled with **lymph,** a watery fluid that con-

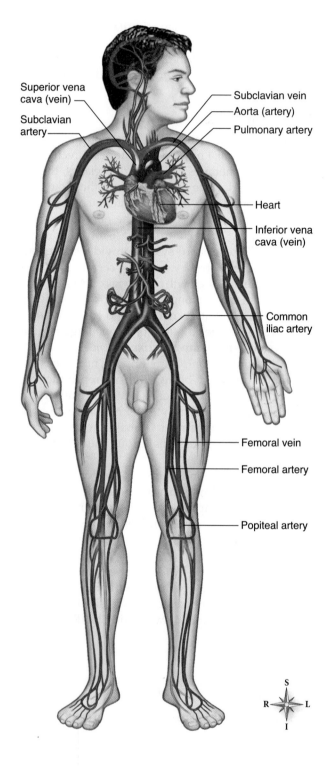

Figure 4-6 | **Cardiovascular system.**

The heart and a few of the major arteries and veins are shown. Capillaries are too small to be visible in this sketch.

Superior vena cava (vein)

Subclavian artery

Subclavian vein

Aorta (artery)

Pulmonary artery

Heart

Inferior vena cava (vein)

Common iliac artery

Femoral vein

Femoral artery

Popliteal artery

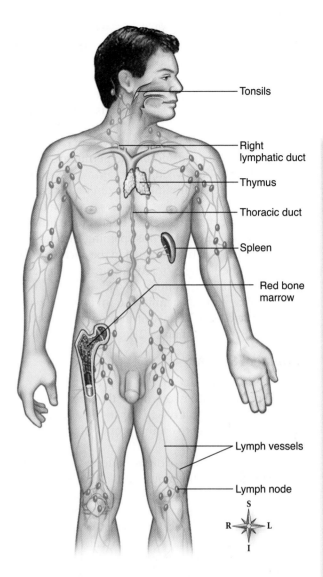

Figure 4-7 | **Lymphatic and immune systems.**

Besides lymphatic organs, the red marrow of the bone is included in this system because it produces many of the immune cells of the body.

Labels on figure:
- Tonsils
- Right lymphatic duct
- Thymus
- Thoracic duct
- Spleen
- Red bone marrow
- Lymph vessels
- Lymph node

tains lymphocytes, proteins, and some fatty molecules, but no red blood cells. The lymph is formed from the fluid around the body cells and diffuses into the lymph vessels. However, unlike blood, lymph does not circulate repeatedly through a closed circuit, or loop, of vessels. Instead, lymph flowing through lymphatic vessels eventually enters the cardiovascular, or circulatory, system by passing through large ducts, such as the **thoracic duct**, which in turn connect with veins in the upper thoracic cavity. Many biologists consider the lymphatic system to be part of the cardiovascular system.

The functions of the lymphatic system include movement of fluids and small particles from the tissue spaces around the cells and movement of fats absorbed from the digestive tract back to the blood.

Lymph nodes and other lymphoid structures act as small filters that trap and destroy bacterial cells, cancerous cells, and other debris that are carried by the lymph fluid as it flows through the tissues. As such, the organs of the lymphatic system play a role in immunity. Figure 4-7 shows groupings of lymph nodes in the axillary (armpit) and in the inguinal (groin) areas of the body.

All of the body's defense systems together make up the **immune system.** It protects us from disease-causing microorganisms, harmful toxins, transplanted tissue cells, and any of our own cells that have turned malignant or cancerous. The immune system is composed of protective cells (such as phagocytes) and various types of defensive protein molecules (produced by secretory immune cells). Some immune system cells have the ability to attack, engulf, and destroy harmful bacteria directly by phagocytosis. Other more numerous immune system cells secrete protein compounds called **antibodies** (AN-ti-bod-ees) and **complements** (KOM-pleh-ments). These substances produce chemical reactions that

help protect the body from many harmful agents. The lymphatic and immune systems, which are linked to each other and to the cardiovascular system, are discussed in Chapter 15.

Respiratory System

The major organs of the **respiratory system** include the **nose, pharynx** (FAIR-inks), **larynx** (LAIR-inks), **trachea** (TRAY-kee-ah), **bronchi** (BRONG-kye), and **lungs** (Figure 4-8). Together these organs facilitate the movement of air into the tiny, thin-walled sacs of the lungs called **alveoli** (al-VEE-oh-lye), where the oxygen from the air is exchanged for carbon dioxide, a waste product. The carbon dioxide is carried to the lungs by the blood so it can be eliminated from the body. Figure 4-8 also shows the *diaphragm*, which is a sheet of muscle that plays a major role in inflating the lungs during breathing.

The organs of the respiratory system perform a number of functions in addition to permitting movement of air into the alveoli. For example, if you live in a cold or dry environment, incoming air can be warmed and humidified as it passes over the lining of the respiratory air passages. In addition, inhaled irritants such as pollen or dust passing through the respiratory tubes can be trapped in the sticky mucus that covers the lining of many respiratory passages and then eliminated from the body.

The respiratory system is also involved in regulating the acid-base balance of the body—a function that is discussed in Chapter 21.

Digestive System

The organs of the **digestive system** (Figure 4-9) are often separated into two groups: the *primary organs* and the *secondary* or *accessory organs* (see Table 4-1). They work together to ensure proper digestion and absorption of nutrients.

The primary organs of digestion form the digestive tract. They include the mouth, pharynx, esophagus, stomach, small intestine, large intestine, rectum, and anal canal. The accessory organs of digestion may attach to the digestive tract (or be inside it). Accessory digestive organs include the teeth, salivary glands, tongue, liver, gallbladder, pancreas, and appendix.

The digestive tract is a tube, open at both ends. It is also called the **alimentary** (al-ih-MEN-tah-ree) **canal** or **gastrointestinal** (GAS-troh-in-TESS-ti-nal) **(GI) tract.** Food that enters the tract is digested, its nutrients are absorbed, and the undigested residue is eliminated from the body as waste material called **feces** (FEE-seez).

Urinary System

The organs of the **urinary system** include the **kidneys, ureters** (yoo-REE-ters), **bladder,** and **urethra** (yoo-REE-thrah).

The kidneys (Figure 4-10) "clear," or clean, the blood of the waste products continually produced by the metabolism of foodstuff in the body cells. The kidneys also play an important role in maintaining the electrolyte, water, and acid-base balances in the body.

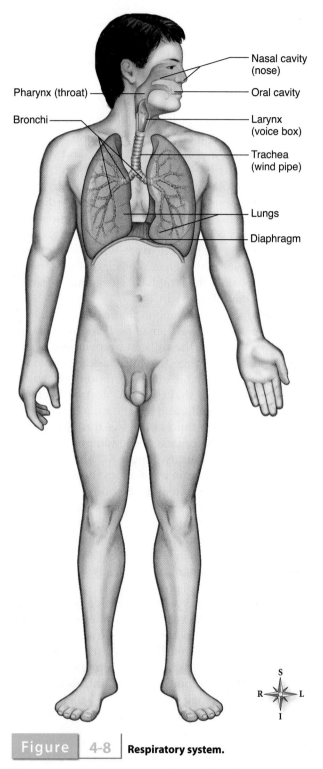

Figure 4-8 | **Respiratory system.**

The lungs are the primary organs of respiration. The nasal cavity, pharynx, larynx, trachea, and bronchi move air to and from the lungs.

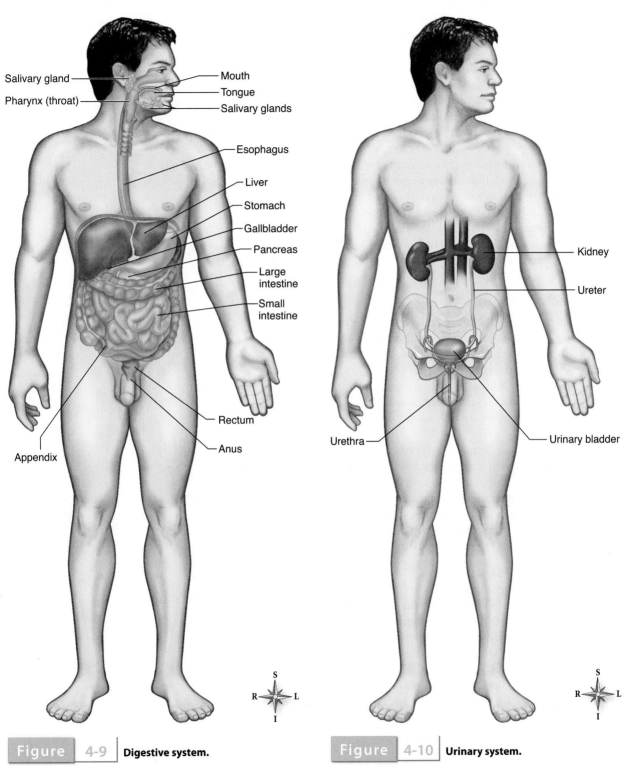

Figure 4-9 | **Digestive system.**

The primary organs (digestive tract) and major accessory organs are shown.

Figure 4-10 | **Urinary system.**

The kidneys are the primary urinary organs. Accessory structures help conduct urine out of the body.

The waste product produced by the kidneys is called **urine** (YOOR-in). After it is produced by the kidneys, it flows out of the kidneys through the ureters into the urinary bladder, where it is temporarily stored. Urine passes from the bladder to the outside of the body through the urethra. In the male the urethra passes through the penis and has a double function; it transports urine and semen (seminal fluid). Therefore it has urinary and reproductive purposes. In the female the urinary and reproductive passages are completely separate, so the urethra performs only a urinary function.

Other organs, in addition to the organs of the urinary system, also are involved in the elimination of body wastes. Undigested food residues and metabolic wastes are eliminated from the intestinal tract as feces, and the lungs rid the body of carbon dioxide. The skin also serves an excretory function by eliminating water and some salts in sweat.

Reproductive Systems

The normal function of the **reproductive system** is different from the normal function of other organ systems of the body. The proper functioning of the reproductive systems ensures survival, not of the individual but of the genes. In addition, production of the hormones that permit the development of sexual characteristics also affects other structures and functions of the body.

Humans reproduce sexually (two-parent reproduction) and therefore we have two systems: the male reproductive system and the female reproductive system. An individual has either the male or the female system. Both systems have **gonads** (GOH-nads) that both produce sex cells for forming the offspring and produce hormones that regulate reproductive functions.

MALE REPRODUCTIVE SYSTEM

The male reproductive structures shown in Figure 4-11 include the **testes** (TES-teez), which produce the sex cells and thus serve as the male gonads. The testes produce **sperm** as well as the male hormone *testosterone*. A tube called the **vas deferens** (vas DEF-er-enz) extends from each testis and leads to the urethra. Surrounding the upper urethra is the **prostate** (PROSS-tayt), which is an exocrine gland.

The **penis** (PEE-nis) and **scrotum** (SKROH-tum) are external structures and together are known as the external **genitalia** (jen-i-TAIL-yah). The urethra, which is identified in Figure 4-10 as part of the urinary system, passes through the penis. It carries sperm to the exterior and acts as a passageway for the elimination of urine.

Functioning together, the male reproductive structures produce sperm and introduce them into the female reproductive tract, where fertilization can occur. Sperm produced by the testes travel through a

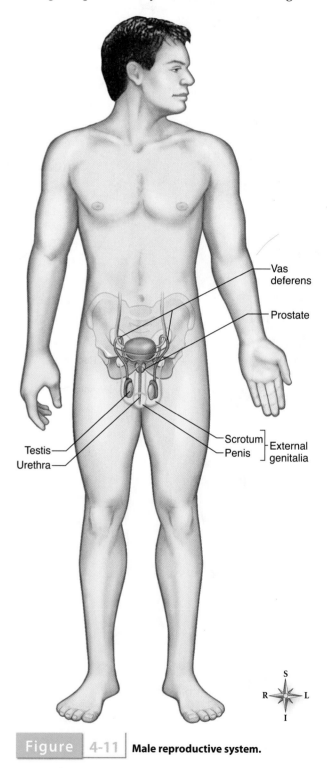

Figure **4-11** **Male reproductive system.**

number of ducts, including the vas deferens, to exit the body. The prostate and other accessory organs, which add fluid and nutrients to the sex cells as they pass through the ducts and the supporting structures (especially the penis), facilitate transfer of sex cells into the female reproductive tract.

FEMALE REPRODUCTIVE SYSTEM

The female gonads are the **ovaries.** Other reproductive organs shown in Figure 4-12 include the **uterus** (YOO-ter-us); **uterine** (YOO-ter-in), or **fallopian, tubes;** and the **vagina** (vah-JYE-nah). In the female the term **vulva** (VUL-vah) is used to describe the external genitalia.

Eggs, or **ova,** are sex cells produced by the ovaries. Ova travel through the uterine tubes, where they may be fertilized by sperm. As the offspring formed by the union of sperm and ovum matures, it moves down the uterine tube to the uterus, where it implants and forms a connection with the mother's blood vessels. After about 9 months, the offspring is delivered through the *cervix* (neck) of the uterus and through the vagina.

The breasts are fatty extensions of the skin that house the **mammary glands**, which produce milk to nurture offspring. They are present in both males and females, but normally only produce milk in females. Because of their role in supporting development of offspring, mammary glands usually are classified as accessory sex organs, rather than as skin glands.

The reproductive organs in the female produce the ova; receive the male sex cells (sperm); permit fertilization and transfer of the sex cells to the uterus; and facilitate the development, birth, and nourishment of offspring.

> **QUICK CHECK**
>
> 1. What are the functions of the lymphatic system?
> 2. What functions besides gas exchange are performed by the respiratory system?
> 3. What are some of the accessory organs of the digestive system?
> 4. What organ in males is shared by both the urinary system and the reproductive system?

Integration of Body Organ System Functions

As you study the details of structure and function of the various organ systems in the chapters that follow, it is important that you focus on how each system and its component organs relate to other systems and to the body as a whole. Look at Figure 4-13. It depicts the body as a bag of fluid separated from the external environment. The concept of homeostasis, introduced in Chapter 1, explains how the body maintains or is able

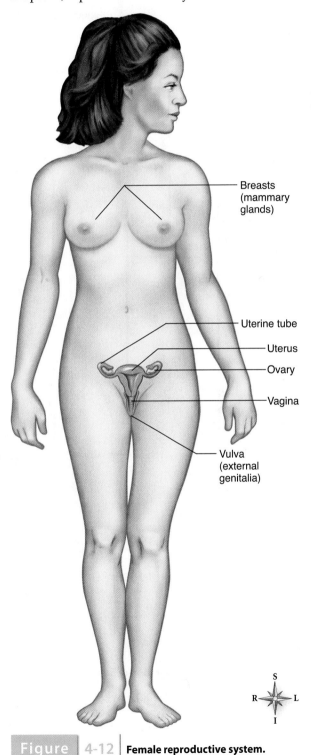

Breasts (mammary glands)

Uterine tube

Uterus

Ovary

Vagina

Vulva (external genitalia)

Figure 4-12 **Female reproductive system.**

Integumentary system

Separates internal environment from external environment.

Nervous system

Major regulatory system of the internal environment: senses changes, integrates, and sends signals to effectors (muscular organs, glands).

Digestive system

Breaks down nutrients from the external environment and absorbs them into the internal environment.

Respiratory system

Exchanges O_2 and CO_2 between the internal and external environment.

Endocrine system

Regulates internal environment by secreting hormones that travel through the bloodstream to target areas.

Circulatory system

Transports nutrients, water, oxygen, hormones, wastes, and other materials within the internal environment.

Skeletal system

Supports, protects, and moves body. Also stores minerals.

Muscular system

Powers and directs skeletal movement.

Reproductive system

Produces sex cells that form offspring, ensuring survival of genes. Female system is also site of fertilization and early development.

Urinary system

Adjusts internal environment by excreting excess water, salt, and other substances.

Immune system

Defends internal environment against injury from foreign cells and other irritants.

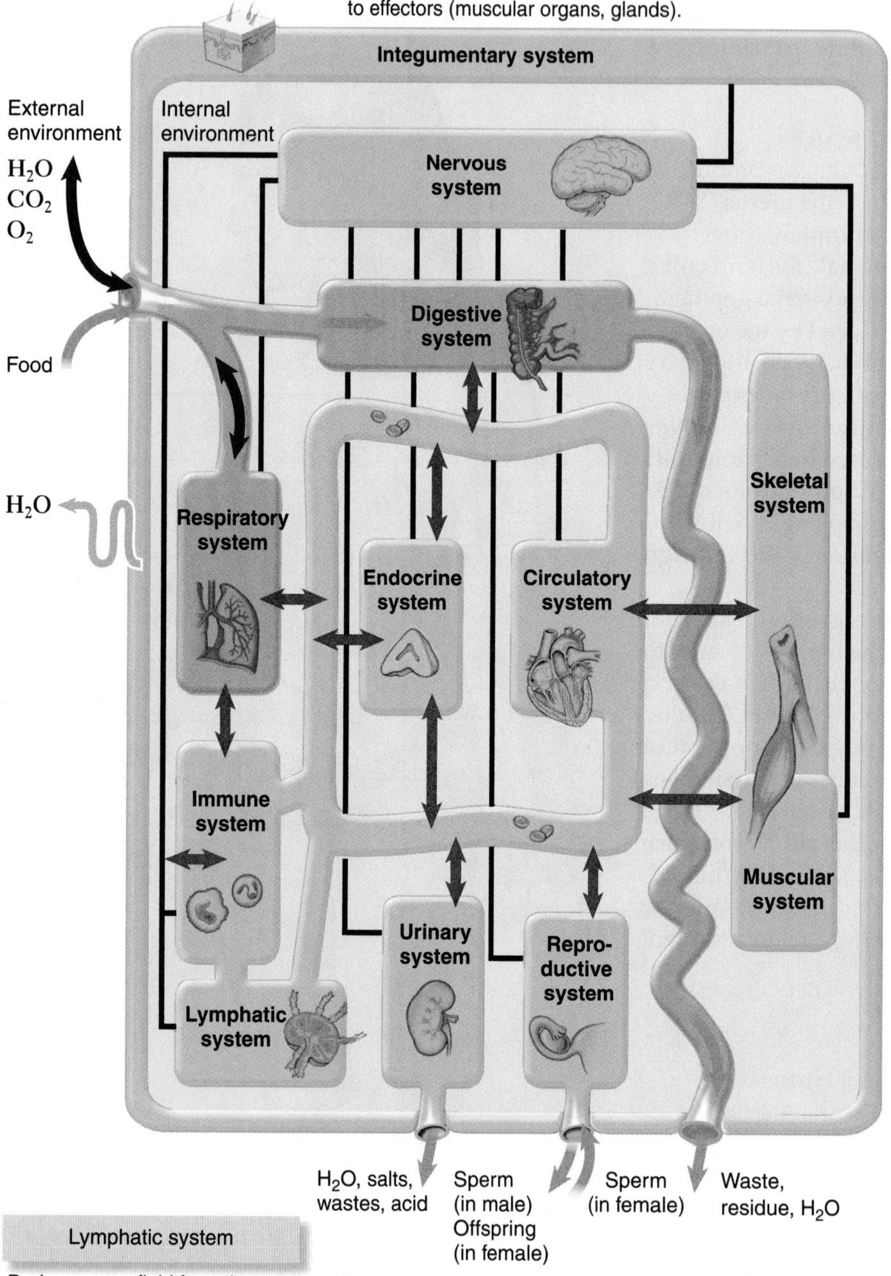

Lymphatic system

Drains excess fluid from tissues, cleans it, and returns it to the blood.

Figure 4-13 | **Integration of body organ systems.**

In this illustration, the human body is compared to a bag of fluid separated from the external environment. Note how the digestive and respiratory systems are represented as tubes that bring the external environment to deeper parts of the bag where substances transported by the cardiovascular (circulatory) system may be absorbed into the internal fluid environment or excreted into the external environment. It is the interrelated functioning of the body organ systems that makes homeostasis possible.

to restore relative constancy to its internal environment even when faced with changing external surroundings or internal needs.

For example, contraction of a muscle can produce a specific body movement only if it is attached appropriately to a bone in the skeletal system. In order for contraction to begin, muscles must first be stimulated by nervous impulses generated in the nervous system. Then, in order to continue contracting, they must receive both oxygen from the respiratory system and nutrients absorbed from the digestive system. Numerous waste products produced by contracting muscles must be eliminated by the urinary and respiratory systems. The cardiovascular system provides transportation for the respiratory gases, nutrients, and waste products of metabolism. No one body system functions entirely independently of other systems. Instead, you will find that they are structurally and functionally interrelated and interdependent. Homeostasis can be maintained only by the coordinated and carefully regulated functioning of all body organ systems.

Organ Replacement

As we all know, disease and injury are sometimes unavoidable. It is common therefore to suffer damage that renders an organ incapable of proper function. By def-

inition, a nonvital organ is not required for life to continue—a vital organ is. If a *nonvital organ* is damaged, a person's health may be in some peril, but even permanent loss of that organ will not result in death. For example, we can survive easily without the use of our spleen, appendix, and tonsils. We can also survive, although less easily, without the use of our eyes, arms, and legs. However, if the functions of a *vital organ* are lost, we are in immediate danger of dying. For example, when the heart or brain ceases to function, death will result.

Over the past few decades, health science professionals have made great advances in the ability to replace or repair lost or damaged organs. In the case of nonvital organs, these techniques have improved the quality of life for many patients. In the case of vital organs, these techniques have extended life.

Artificial Organs

A nonvital organ, especially, is often successfully replaced or enhanced by an artificial organ or **prosthesis** (pros-THEE-sis). Figure 4-14 shows examples of many types of prostheses now in use or in development. Crude artificial limbs have been used for centuries, but the availability of new materials and advanced engineering has made more efficient types possible. For example, new computer-

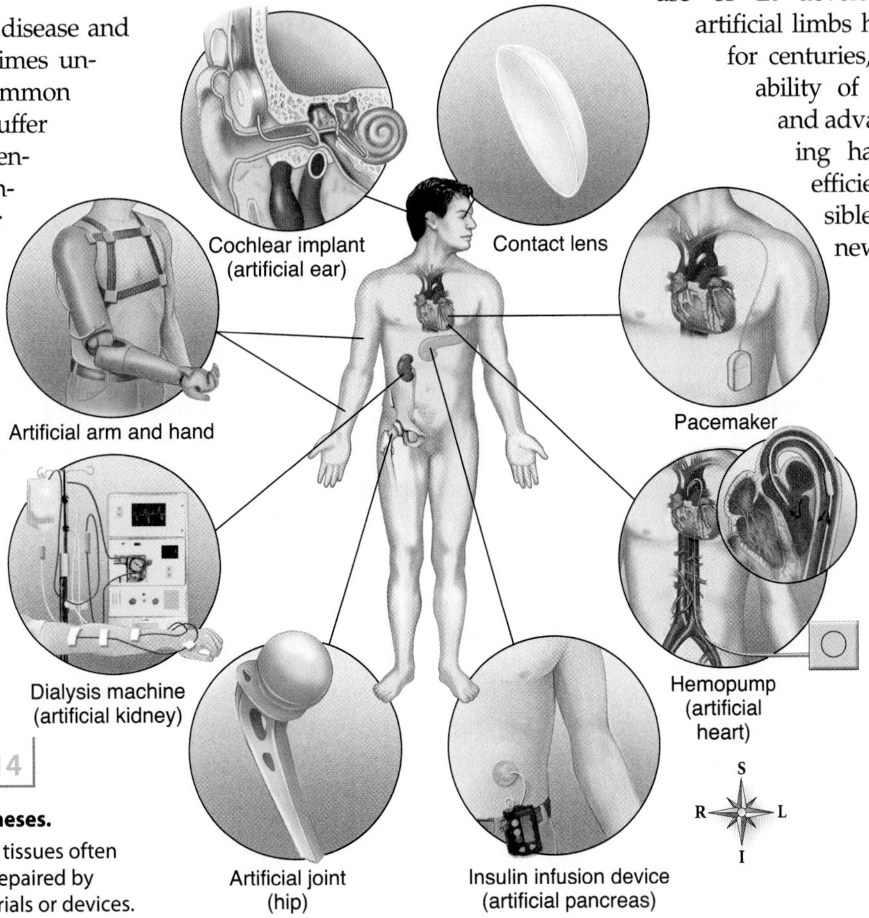

Figure 4-14

Examples of prostheses.
Damaged organs or tissues often can be replaced or repaired by using artificial materials or devices.

Cochlear implant (artificial ear) · Contact lens · Artificial arm and hand · Pacemaker · Dialysis machine (artificial kidney) · Hemopump (artificial heart) · Artificial joint (hip) · Insulin infusion device (artificial pancreas)

assisted arm and hand replacements can manipulate small objects with amazing dexterity. Artificial sense organs have even been able to restore sight to the blind and hearing to the deaf. For example, many people suffering from deafness have had their hearing partially restored by "artificial ears" called **cochlear** (KOH-klee-er) **implants**. In cochlear implants, a miniature microphone is surgically implanted under the skin near the outer ear and wired to an electrode in the inner ear, or *cochlea*. Sound picked up by the microphone is converted to electrical signals that are relayed directly to the auditory nerve in the cochlea.

The use of artificial materials—transplanted animal or human tissues or mechanical devices—to partially or completely replace vital organs or to augment their functions, is occurring more and more frequently in modern medical practice. One of the earliest devices to augment vital functions was the "artificial kidney," or *dialysis machine* (see Chapter 19). **Dialysis** machines pump blood through permeable tubes in an external apparatus, allowing waste products to diffuse out of the blood and into a saltwater type of electrolyte fluid that surrounds the permeable dialysis tubes. Patients with kidney failure must be "hooked up" to the machine, generally for 2- to 4-hour periods two or three times each week. Although ongoing machine-based dialysis treatments can extend the lives of kidney failure victims for long periods, this process is generally considered an interim solution while awaiting kidney transplantation.

The first permanent artificial heart (called the *Jarvik-7*) was implanted in a human in 1982. Since that time, great progress has been made in the development of smaller and much more efficient electromechanical devices that help keep blood pumping in patients suffering from end-stage heart disease. A number of these devices, called *left ventricular assist systems (LVAS)*, are implanted in the abdomen and connected to the heart. They are regulated and controlled by an external battery pack. One of the most successful LVAS devices, called the *Novacor,* has been used by growing numbers of patients worldwide for extended periods until a heart transplant becomes possible. Another more short-term option is the **Hemopump**, which is inserted through a tiny incision in the artery in the left leg and controlled by a small external motor.

Unfortunately, because of the critical shortage of donor organs, only about 2500 heart transplants occur in the United States each year, although the need is much greater. In addition to LVAS devices, cardiovascular surgeons now have a wide array of heart valve replacement and repair products available. Some replacement valves are totally mechanical, whereas others are fabricated from porcine (pig), bovine (cow), or human tissues. Although new materials and bioengineering advances are encouraging, total artificial replacement for vital organs, if possible at all, is generally employed only to ensure survival until a more permanent solution (most often organ transplantation) can occur.

Organ Transplantation

One approach that offers the hope of a permanent solution to loss of vital organ function is *organ transplantation.* In this technique, a normal living organ from a donor is surgically transplanted into the recipient. Kidney, liver, pancreas, lung, small intestine, and heart transplants are now done at many hospitals throughout the world. When a new organ is transplanted into the body, the old organ may or may not be removed. For example, failed kidneys are of-

HEALTH & WELL-BEING

PAIRED ORGANS

Have you ever wondered what advantage there might be in having two kidneys, two lungs, two eyes, and two of many other organs? Although the body could function well with only one of each, most of us are born with a pair of these organs. For paired organs that are vital to survival, such as the kidneys, this arrangement allows for the accidental loss of one organ without immediate threat to the survival of the individual. Athletes who have lost one vital organ through injury or disease are often counseled against participating in contact sports that carry the risk of damaging the remaining organ. If the second organ is damaged, total loss of a vital function, such as sight, or even death may result.

ten left in place at the back of the ventral body cavity. As Figure 4-15 shows, the "new" kidney is nestled far below it in the curve of the pelvic bone, where it is attached to major blood vessels and to the bladder. Using this strategy, the trauma of removing the damaged kidneys is avoided and the transplanted kidney can still process blood efficiently.

Despite its many successes, organ transplantation still has some problems. One is that a recipient's immune system often rejects a transplanted organ. Some **immunosuppressive drugs** that suppress the immune system and inhibit rejection reactions also pose the risk of severe infection. Cyclosporine is an immunosuppressive drug that solves this problem to some degree by suppressing rejection reactions without severely inhibiting infection control. In addition, better tissue-typing procedures, continued development of new and more effective antirejection drugs, selective use of certain steroids, and new uses for other established drugs such as rapamycin and azathioprine also offer the hope of reducing organ-rejection problems.

Another way to solve the rejection problem is to build "new" organs from a patient's own tissues. For example, in a method called *free-flap surgery,* pieces of tissue from one part of the body are surgically remodeled and then grafted to a new part of the body.

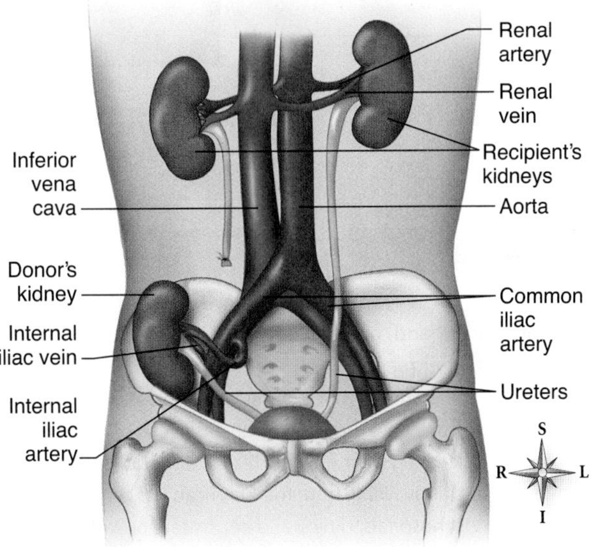

Inferior vena cava

Donor's kidney

Internal iliac vein

Internal iliac artery

Renal artery

Renal vein

Recipient's kidneys

Aorta

Common iliac artery

Ureters

Figure 4-15 | **Kidney transplantation.**

In kidney transplantations, the diseased organs are left in place, and the donated organ is nestled in another part of the body.

After cancerous breasts are removed, "new" breasts can be formed from skin and muscle tissue taken from the thighs, buttocks, or abdomen. Parts of the intestine can be used to repair the urinary bladder. Toes can even be transplanted to the hand to replace missing fingers. The advantage of using a patient's own tissues is that the possibility of rejection is greatly reduced.

Another major problem with organ transplants is the limited availability of donor organs. One solution is to eliminate or reduce the need for human donors. Researchers are now working on a variety of methods by which new organs or tissues can be "grown" in a tissue culture or in a patient's body. For example, it is hoped that one day normal liver cells can be safely removed from a healthy donor and implanted in a plastic sponge that will be placed in the recipient's body. The transplanted cells may then reproduce and form a mass capable of producing some liver function. Researchers are also culturing colonies of healthy nervous tissue in laboratory dishes in the hope that it can someday be used to repair damaged sections of the brain or spinal cord.

Recent discoveries that have allowed scientists to culture adult or embryonic **"stem cells"** in the laboratory and then control the differentiation of these primitive cells into specific cell and tissue types, such as blood cells, muscle, or nerve, are exciting and complex advances in biology that will have a profound impact on human health. Stem cells can be taken from early embryonic tissue, adult donors, or from the umbilical cord blood of newborn infants (see "Freezing Umbilical Cord Blood" box in Chapter 23). Although many scientific and ethical questions remain unanswered, the potential now exists for cell, tissue, and organ "engineering" that may well permit repair or total replacement of diseased or damaged organs in a functioning organ system. Many scientists believe that information obtained from stem cell research may become the basis for some of the most important advances in clinical medicine in the decade ahead, including treatment of such diverse conditions as Parkinson disease and other types of neurologic disease, diabetes, spinal cord injury, and stroke. In the case of Parkinson disease, transplantation of stem cells into specific areas of the brain in selected patients has proved effective in reducing symptoms such as tremor, muscle rigidity, and a slow shuffling gait.

SCIENCE APPLICATIONS

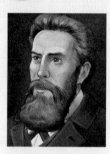

Wilhelm Röntgen
(1845–1923)

RADIOGRAPHY

In 1895, the German physicist Wilhelm Röntgen (*at left*) made one of the most important medical discoveries of the modern age—radiographic imaging of the body. **Radiography**, or x-ray photography, is the oldest and still the most widely used method of noninvasive imaging of internal body structures; it earned Röntgen a Nobel Prize. While studying the effects of electricity passing through gas under low pressures, Röntgen accidentally discovered x-rays when they caused a plate coated with special chemicals to glow. Not long after that, he showed that they could produce shadows of internal structures such as bones on photographic film. His first, and most famous, radiograph was of his wife Bertha's hand. Although a little fuzzy, it clearly showed Bertha's finger bones and the outline of her ring. When this radiograph was published by a Vienna newspaper, the entire world became instantly aware of his breakthrough discovery.

The figure at right shows how radiography works. A source of waves in the x band of the radiation spectrum beams the x-rays through a body and onto a piece of photographic film or phosphorescent screen. The resulting image shows the outlines of bones and other dense structures that absorb the x-rays. As the figure shows, one way to make soft, hollow structures such as digestive organs more visible is to use radiopaque contrast material. For example, barium sulfate (which absorbs x-rays) can be injected into the colon to make it more visible in a radiograph.

Today, many variations of Röntgen's invention are used to study internal organs without having to cut into the body. For example, computed tomography (CT) scanning is a modern, computerized type of x-ray photography. Radiographic technicians are health professionals whose chief responsibility is to make radiographs, and radiologists are responsible for interpreting these images. Many medical, veterinary, and dental professionals rely on these images and interpretations of them in their diagnosis, assessment, and treatment of patients. In addition, radiography is used in many industrial and investigative settings—and even by archaeologists studying mummies.

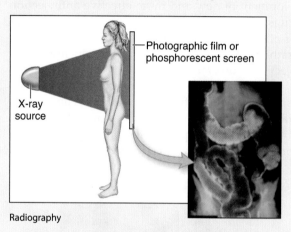

Photographic film or phosphorescent screen

X-ray source

Radiography

HEALTH & WELL-BEING

CANCER SCREENING TESTS

A knowledge of the structure and function of the body organ systems is a critically important "first step" in understanding and using information that empowers us to become more sophisticated guardians of our own health and well-being. For example, a better understanding of the reproductive system helps individuals participate in a more direct and personal way in cancer-prevention screening techniques.

Breast and testicular self-examinations to detect cancer are two important ways that women and men can participate directly in protecting their own health. Information on these screening tests is available from the American Cancer Society and from most hospitals, clinics, and health care providers.

Outline Summary

 To download an MP3 version of the chapter summary for use with your iPod or portable media player, access the **Audio Chapter Summaries** on your CD.

A. Organ—a structure made up of two or more kinds of tissues that can together perform a more complex function than a single tissue
B. Organ system—a group of organs that perform a more complex function than can any organ alone
C. A knowledge of individual organs and how they are organized into groups makes more meaningful the understanding of how a particular organ system functions as a whole

Organ Systems of the Body

A. Integumentary system (Figure 4-1)
  1. Structure
    a. Only one organ, the skin, but has many appendages (attached structures)
    b. Skin appendages
      (1) Hair
      (2) Nails
      (3) Microscopic sense receptors
      (4) Sweat glands
      (5) Oil glands
  2. Functions
    a. Protection—primary function
    b. Regulation of body temperature
    c. Synthesis of chemicals
    d. Sense organ
B. Skeletal system (Figure 4-2)
  1. Structure
    a. Bones—organs of the skeletal system
      (1) 206 named bones in the skeleton
      (2) Additional variable bones occur in each individual
    b. Cartilage connects and cushions joined bones
    c. Ligaments—bands of fibrous tissue that hold bones together
    d. Joints—connections between bones that make movement possible
  2. Functions
    a. Supporting framework for entire body

    b. Protection of brain and internal organs
    c. Movement (with joints and muscles)
    d. Storage of minerals
    e. Formation of blood cells
C. Muscular system (Figure 4-3)
  1. Structure
    a. Muscles are the primary organs
      (1) Voluntary or striated skeletal muscle
      (2) Involuntary or smooth muscle tissue in walls of some organs
      (3) Cardiac muscle in wall of the heart
  2. Functions
    a. Movement
    b. Maintenance of body posture
    c. Production of heat
  3. Skeletomuscular system—combination of the skeletal and muscular systems
D. Nervous system (Figure 4-4)
  1. Structure
    a. Central nervous system (CNS)
      (1) Brain
      (2) Spinal cord
    b. Peripheral nervous system (PNS)
      (1) Cranial nerves and their branches
      (2) Spinal nerves and their branches
      (3) Sense organs
  2. Functions
    a. Communication between body organs
    b. Integration of body functions
    c. Control of body functions
    d. Recognition of sensory stimuli
E. Endocrine system (Figure 4-5)
  1. Structure—ductless glands that secrete signaling hormones directly into the blood
  2. Functions
    a. Same as nervous system—communication, integration, control
    b. Control is slow and of long duration
    c. Neuroendocrine system—combination of nervous and endocrine systems

  d. Examples of functions regulated by hormones:
  (1) Growth
  (2) Metabolism
  (3) Reproduction
  (4) Fluid and electrolyte balance
F. Cardiovascular system (also called *circulatory system*) (Figure 4-6)
  1. Structure
    a. Heart
    b. Blood vessels
  2. Functions
    a. Transportation of substances throughout the body
    b. Regulation of body temperature
    c. Immunity (body defense)
G. Lymphatic and immune systems (Figure 4-7)
  1. Lymphatic system
    a. Structure
      (1) Lymphatic vessels
      (2) Lymph nodes and tonsils
      (3) Thymus
      (4) Spleen
    b. Functions
      (1) Transportation of lymph
      (2) Immunity
  2. Immune system
    a. Structure
      (1) Unique cells
        (a) Phagocytes
        (b) Secretory cells
      (2) Defensive protein compounds
        (a) Antibodies
        (b) Complements
    b. Functions
      (1) Phagocytosis of bacteria
      (2) Chemical reactions that provide protection from harmful agents
H. Respiratory system (Figure 4-8)
  1. Structure
    a. Nose
    b. Pharynx
    c. Larynx
    d. Trachea
    e. Bronchi
    f. Lungs
  2. Functions

    a. Exchange of waste gas (carbon dioxide) for oxygen in the alveoli of the lungs
    b. Filtration of irritants from inspired air
    c. Regulation of acid-base balance
I. Digestive system (Figure 4-9)
  1. Structure
    a. Primary organs—form alimentary canal, or GI tract
      (1) Mouth
      (2) Pharynx
      (3) Esophagus
      (4) Stomach
      (5) Small intestine
      (6) Large intestine
      (7) Rectum
      (8) Anal canal
    b. Accessory organs—assist the digestive process
      (1) Teeth
      (2) Salivary glands
      (3) Tongue
      (4) Liver
      (5) Gallbladder
      (6) Pancreas
      (7) Appendix
  2. Functions
    a. Mechanical and chemical breakdown (digestion) of food
    b. Absorption of nutrients
    c. Elimination of undigested waste product—referred to as *feces*
    d. Appendix holds bacteria that assist digestion
J. Urinary system (Figure 4-10)
  1. Structure
    a. Kidneys
    b. Ureters
    c. Urinary bladder
    d. Urethra (part of both urinary and reproductive systems in males)
  2. Functions
    a. "Clearing," or cleaning, blood of waste products—excreted from the body as *urine*
    b. Electrolyte balance
    c. Water balance
    d. Acid-base balance

K. Reproductive systems
    1. Structure
        a. Male (Figure 4-11)
            (1) Gonads—testes
            (2) Other structures—vas deferens, urethra, prostate, external genitalia (penis and scrotum)
        b. Female (Figure 4-12)
            (1) Gonads—ovaries
            (2) Other structures—uterus, uterine (fallopian) tubes, vagina, external genitalia (vulva), mammary glands (breasts)
    2. Functions
        a. Survival of genes
        b. Production of sex cells (male: sperm; female: ova)
        c. Transfer and fertilization of sex cells
        d. Development and birth of offspring
        e. Nourishment of offspring
        f. Production of sex hormones

Integration of Body Organ System Functions (Figure 4-13)

A. No one body system functions entirely independently of other systems
B. All body systems are structurally and functionally interrelated and interdependent

Organ Replacement

A. Loss of function in nonvital organs is not immediately life-threatening; loss of function in vital organs *is* immediately life-threatening
B. Loss of function in organs can be treated by organ replacement
    1. Artificial organs (prostheses) (Figure 4-14)
    2. Organ transplantation
    3. Free-flap surgery
    4. Stem cell treatment

New Words

Review the names of organ systems and individual organs in Figures 4-1 through 4-12.	complement feces fimbriae gastrointestinal (GI) tract genitalia	lymph nerve impulse ovum (*pl.,* ova) sense organ sperm	**Diseases and Other Clinical Terms** cochlear implant dialysis

alimentary canal
alveolus (*pl.,* alveoli)
antibody (*pl.,* antibodies)
cardiac muscle
	hormone
	involuntary (smooth)
	   muscle
	ligament
		stimulus (*pl.,* stimuli)
		tendon
		voluntary (skeletal)
		   muscle
			Hemopump
			immunosuppressive drug
			prosthesis
			radiography

Review Questions

1. Define organ and organ system.
2. Give examples of the stimuli to which skin organs can respond.
3. How is the skin able to assist in the body's ability to regulate temperature?
4. What is the function of tendons?
5. What are some of the differences between the lymphatic and cardiovascular systems?
6. Name the organs that help rid the body of waste. What type of waste does each organ remove?
7. Besides bone, what other types of tissue are included in the skeletal system?

8. List the eleven organ systems discussed in this chapter.
9. Most of the organ systems have more than one function. List two functions for the following systems: integumentary, skeletal, muscular, lymphatic, respiratory, and urinary.
10. What is unique about the reproductive system?
11. Name three artificial organs or prostheses. What organs do they replace or assist?
12. What is the role of drugs such as cyclosporine in organ transplantation?

Critical Thinking

13. Explain the difference between the nervous and endocrine systems. Include what types of functions are regulated and the "message carriers" for each system.
14. The term *balance* is used in this chapter. This is another term for *homeostasis*. Review the functions of the body systems and list the homeostatic functions of each.

Chapter Test

1. The primary organs of the digestive system make up a long tube called the _____.
2. _____ is another name for voluntary muscle.
3. _____ is another name for involuntary muscle.
4. The nervous system can generate special electrochemical signals called _____.
5. The _____, _____, and _____ are called appendages of the skin.
6. The _____ is part of both the lymphatic and endocrine systems.

7. The _____ is part of both the male reproductive system and urinary system.
8. The gonads for the male reproductive system are the _____; the gonads for the female reproductive system are the _____.
9. The skeletal system is composed of bone and what two related tissues: _____ and _____.
10. _____ is an "artificial ear" used to improve hearing.
11. _____ are undifferentiated cells taken from embryonic tissue or cord blood and can be used in "organ engineering."

Match each system in column A with its corresponding function in column B.

Column A
12. _____ integumentary
13. _____ skeletal
14. _____ muscular
15. _____ nervous
16. _____ endocrine
17. _____ cardiovascular
18. _____ lymphatic
19. _____ respiratory
20. _____ digestive
21. _____ urinary
22. _____ reproductive

Column B
a. Provides movement, body posture, and heat
b. Uses hormones to regulate body function
c. Transports fatty nutrients from the digestive system into the blood
d. Causes physical and chemical changes in nutrients so they can be absorbed into the blood
e. Cleans the blood of metabolic waste and regulates water and electrolyte balance
f. Protects underlying structures, has sensory receptors, and regulates body temperature
g. Responsible for the transport of substances from one part of the body to another
h. Ensures the survival of the species rather than the individual
i. Uses electrochemical signals to integrate and control body functions
j. Exchanges oxygen and carbon dioxide and helps regulate acid-base balance
k. Provides a rigid framework for the body and stores minerals

Case Studies

1. Tommy has been diagnosed as having irreversible kidney failure. Which system of the body is involved in this condition? What functions has Tommy lost? What options do his physicians have in treating Tommy's condition?

2. Mr. Davidson was referred to a urologist for diagnosis and treatment of an obstruction in his urethra. What bodily functions may be affected by Mr. Davidson's conditions?

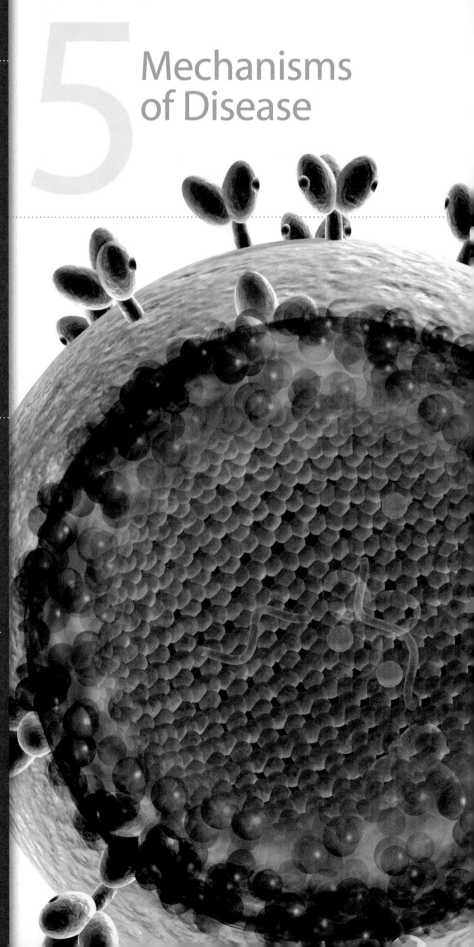

Outline

Objectives

**After you have completed this chapter,
you should be able to:**

1. Define the terms *health* and *disease*.

2. List and describe the basic
mechanisms of disease and risk factors
associated with disease.

3. List and describe five categories of
pathogenic organisms and explain
how they cause disease.

4. Distinguish between the terms *benign*
and *malignant* as they apply to tumors.

5. Describe the pathogenesis of cancer.

6. Outline the events of the inflammatory
response and explain its role in disease.

5 Mechanisms of Disease

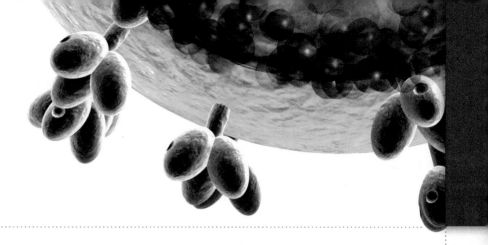

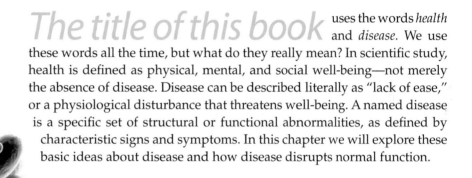

The title of this book

uses the words *health* and *disease*. We use these words all the time, but what do they really mean? In scientific study, health is defined as physical, mental, and social well-being—not merely the absence of disease. Disease can be described literally as "lack of ease," or a physiological disturbance that threatens well-being. A named disease is a specific set of structural or functional abnormalities, as defined by characteristic signs and symptoms. In this chapter we will explore these basic ideas about disease and how disease disrupts normal function.

STUDY TIPS

This is a very challenging chapter. It presents a great deal of information, much of which may be new to you.

1. Divide the chapter into parts: disease terminology, mechanisms and risk factors, pathogenic organisms, tumors and cancer, and inflammation. In each of these sections, go over the terms in bold print. You may be surprised at how many you already know. Put the ones you don't know on flash cards.

2. Use flash cards to learn the mechanisms of disease; most of them are self-explanatory. Divide the pathogenic organisms into viruses, bacteria, fungi, protozoa, and pathogenic animals. Use flash cards for each group. Write a brief description of each type of organism.

3. Methods of disease spread are fairly self-explanatory. Make sure you know the distinction between prevention (e.g., vaccination) and treatment (e.g., antibiotic). In the cancer section, be sure you understand the difference between a carcinoma and a sarcoma.

4. The causes of cancer are also self-explanatory, as are the methods of detection and types of treatment. When studying the types of treatment, don't forget about surgery; it is not in bold type and therefore could be missed.

5. As you study inflammation, make flash cards for the four primary signs and their causes. Be sure you understand what chemotaxis is. Learn the positive effects of fever and the different effects fever has on the young and the elderly.

continued on page 131

Studying Disease

Disease Terminology

Pathology is the study of disease. Researchers want to know the scientific basis of abnormal conditions. Health practitioners want to know how to prevent and treat a wide variety of diseases. When we suffer from the inevitable "cold" or something more serious, we all want to know what is going on and how best to deal with it. Pathology has its own terminology, as in any specialized field. Most of these terms are derived from Latin and Greek word parts. For example, *patho-* comes from the Greek word for "disease" *(pathos)* and is used to form many terms, including *pathology* itself. If you are unfamiliar with word parts commonly used in medical science, refer to Appendix B on the CD that accompanies your book.

Disease conditions are usually *diagnosed* or identified by signs and symptoms. **Signs** are objective abnormalities that can be seen or measured by someone other than the patient, whereas **symptoms** are the subjective abnormalities felt only by the patient.

Although *sign* and *symptom* are distinct terms, we often use them interchangeably. A **syndrome** (SIN-drohm) is a collection of different signs and symptoms, usually with a common cause, that presents a distinct picture of a pathological condition. The condition or syndrome, as defined by a characteristic set of signs and symptoms, is what we commonly refer to as a **disease.** When signs and symptoms appear suddenly, persist for a short time, then disappear, we say that the disease is **acute.** On the other hand, diseases that develop slowly and last for a long time (perhaps for life) are labeled **chronic** diseases. The term *subacute* refers to diseases with characteristics somewhere between acute and chronic.

The study of all factors involved in causing a disease is referred to as **etiology** (ee-tee-OHL-oh-jee). The etiology (causes or origin) of a skin infection often involves a cut or abrasion and subsequent invasion and growth of a bacterial population. Diseases with undetermined causes are said to be **idiopathic** (id-ee-oh-PATH-ik). **Communicable,** or **infectious** diseases can be transmitted from one individual to another.

The term *etiology* refers to the theory of a disease's cause, but the actual pattern of a disease's development is called its **pathogenesis** (path-oh-JEN-eh-sis). The common cold, for example, begins with a *latent,* or "hidden," stage during which the cold virus establishes itself in the patient. No signs of the cold are yet evident at that stage. In infectious diseases, the latent stage is also called **incubation.** After incubating, the cold may then manifest itself as a mild nasal drip, triggering a few sneezes. It then progresses to its full fury and continues for a few days. After the cold has run its course, *convalescence,* or recovery, occurs. During this stage, body functions return to normal. Those who develop a chronic disease such as cancer may exhibit a temporary reversal of symptoms that seems to be a recovery. Such reversal of a chronic disease is called a **remission.** If a remission is permanent, we say that the person is "cured."

Patterns of Disease

Epidemiology (EP-i-dee-mee-OHL-oh-jee) is the study of the occurrence, distribution, and transmission of diseases in humans. Epidemiologists are physicians or medical scientists who study patterns of disease occurrence in specific groups of people. For example, a hospital may employ a staff epidemiologist who is responsible for infection-control programs within the hospital. Many governments and other agencies employ epidemiologists who track the spread of disease through a local community or even the world at large.

A disease that is native to a local region is called an **endemic** disease. If the disease spreads to many individuals at the same time within a defined geographic region the situation is called an **epidemic. Pandemics** are epidemics that spread throughout the world. HIV (human immunodeficiency virus) is now considered a pandemic because it is found worldwide. Because of the speed and availability of modern air travel, pandemics are more common than they once were. Almost every flu season, we see a new strain of influenza virus quickly spreading from continent to continent.

Tracking the cause of a disease and its pattern of spread through a population can be very difficult. One reason is that there are so many different factors involved in the spread of disease. Nutrition, age, gender, sanitation practices, and socioeconomic conditions may play a role in the spread of disease. Infectious agents, for example, can spread quickly and easily through an unsanitary water supply. Likewise, accumulation of untreated sewage or garbage can harbor disease-causing organisms or chemicals. Infectious agents or other contaminants in food also may spread disease to a large number of people. Crowded conditions may often play a role in spreading disease because more people come in close contact with one another. In crowded regions with poor sanitation and food-handling practices, disease may spread quickly.

The pattern of a disease's spread may be difficult to explain because of the different kinds of agents that can cause disease. For example, imagine that the majority of students in your class became ill with headaches and nausea (upset stomach) at about the same time. One would have to investigate many possible causes and modes of transmission before an explanation could be offered. Is it food poisoning? Is it an outbreak of the "flu" or another virus? Is the water supply for the drinking fountain contaminated? Is there a leak of toxic fumes in the building? Is there radioactive material nearby? Because any of these can cause the situation that is described, a thorough investigation is needed to distinguish the *causal* relationships from the *coincidental* relationships.

Causal relationships establish the cause of a disease outbreak (any of the possibilities listed in the previous paragraph are potentially causal). Coincidental relationships are events that coincide by chance. Using the example above, the professor may have worn a particularly unattractive sweater on the day the students became ill. However, it is much more likely that is a coincidental relationship, than a causal one. Only when all possible causal factors have been investigated can a reasonable answer be proposed that would explain the etiology of the disease outbreak.

Epidemiologists study the spread of disease so that ways of stopping it can be found. The two most obvious strategies for combating disease are *prevention* and *therapy.*

Therapy or treatment of diseases was perhaps the first strategy used by humans to fight disease. The continued search for therapeutic treatments for almost all known diseases is evidence that we still value this strategy. However, we have always known that an even more effective disease-fighting strategy is prevention. Only recently have we understood many diseases well enough to know how to prevent them. Although the war on human disease will probably never end, we have had some dramatic successes. The often fatal viral infection *smallpox* once caused catastrophic epidemics, but natural outbreaks have been eliminated at this point in history because of successful prevention strategies such as worldwide *vaccination* and education (Figure 5-1).

Unfortunately, smallpox and other pathogens that rarely if ever now produce natural outbreaks of disease may nonetheless become available for use as weapons. Such biological weapons could produce epidemics in local regions and would thus not

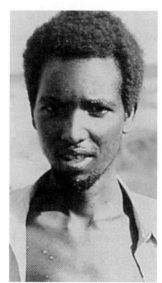

Figure 5-1

The last smallpox victim.

Ali Maow Maalin of Somalia contracted the last known naturally occurring case of smallpox in 1977. Successful disease prevention techniques completely eradicated natural outbreaks of this disease that once killed millions worldwide. The World Health Organization (WHO) considers naturally occurring cases to be eradicated; thus the vaccine for smallpox is no longer required in the United States. Unfortunately, the potential of smallpox being used as a biological weapon remains a threat.

only generate alarm but would also severely burden public health resources. See the Research, Issues, and Trends box on p. 117.

See the Research, Issues, and Trends box on p. 117.

> **QUICK CHECK**
>
> 1. What is the difference between a *sign* and a *symptom?*
> 2. What is *pathogenesis?* Give an example.
> 3. What is the difference between an *epidemic* and a *pandemic?*
> 4. What does an *epidemiologist* do?

Pathophysiology

Mechanisms of Disease

Pathophysiology is the study of the underlying physiological processes associated with disease. Pathophysiology is a branch of pathology, the general study of disease. Pathophysiologists attempt to understand the mechanisms of a disease and its pathogenesis. Although pathophysiologists uncover information that leads to the discovery of strategies of prevention and treatment, developing and applying these strategies is left to other professionals.

Many diseases are best understood as disturbances of homeostasis, the relative constancy of the body's internal environment. Under normal physiologic conditions, if homeostasis is disturbed, a variety of negative-feedback mechanisms returns the body to normal. Negative feedback, or feedback loops, were introduced in Chapter 1. When a disturbance of homeostasis goes beyond normal fluctuations, a disease condition exists. In acute conditions, the body recovers its homeostatic balance quickly. In chronic diseases, a normal state of balance may never be restored. If the disturbance keeps the body's internal environment too far from normal for too long, death may result (Figure 5-2).

Disturbance of homeostasis and the body's responses to that disturbance are the basic mechanisms of disease. Because of the variety of disease mechanisms, they are easier to study if categorized as follows:

1. **Genetic mechanism**—altered or *mutated* genes that can cause production of abnormal proteins. These abnormal proteins often simply do not perform their originally intended function, resulting in the absence of an essential function. On the other hand, such proteins may perform an abnormal, disruptive function instead. Either case may be a threat to the constancy of the body's internal environment. The basis for genetic diseases is discussed in Chapter 24, and important genetic conditions are summarized in Appendix A on page A-1 of your book.

2. **Infectious mechanism**—*pathogenic* (disease-causing) organisms or particles that damage the body in some way. An organism that lives in or on another organism to obtain its nutrients is called a **parasite.** The presence of microscopic-size or larger parasites may interfere with normal body functions of the *host* and thereby cause disease. Organisms other than parasites can poison or otherwise damage the human body to cause disease. Some of the major pathogenic organisms are listed later in this chapter and in Appendix A on page A-1 of your book.

3. **Neoplastic mechanism**—abnormal tissue growths or *neoplasms* (tumors [benign or

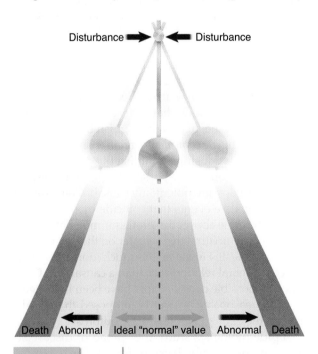

Disturbance ➡ ⬅ Disturbance

Death | Abnormal | Ideal "normal" value | Abnormal | Death

Figure 5-2 | **Model of homeostatic balance.**

Movement of the parameter in question, away from the ideal normal value, is depicted as normal fluctuations. Sometimes a physiological disturbance pushes the body beyond its capacity to maintain homeostasis and into the abnormal range for a given physiological parameter. Disturbances in the extreme may result in death.

malignant] and cancers) that can cause a variety of physiological disturbances. Many such mechanisms are described later in this chapter.

4. **Traumatic mechanism**—physical and chemical agents such as toxic or destructive chemicals, extreme heat or cold, mechanical injury (trauma), and radiation that can affect the normal homeostasis of the body. Examples of pathological conditions caused by physical agents are summarized in Appendix A on page A-1 of your book. These conditions include injuries such as fractures and lacerations caused by physical trauma or poisoning caused by chemical agents.

5. **Metabolic mechanism**—endocrine imbalances or malnutrition that cause insufficient or imbalanced intake of nutrients. A variety of diseases caused by this mechanism are outlined in Chapter 18 and Appendix A on page A-1 of your book.

6. **Inflammatory mechanism**
   a. **Autoimmunity**—faulty response or overreaction of the immune system that causes it to attack the body. Autoimmunity, literally "self-immunity," is discussed in Chapter 15 along with other immune system disturbances. Examples of autoimmune conditions are listed in Appendix A on page A-1 of your book.
   b. **Inflammation**—common response of the body to disturbances. The *inflammatory response* is a normal mechanism that usually speeds recovery from an infection or injury. However, when the inflammatory response occurs at inappropriate times or is abnormally prolonged or severe, normal tissues may be damaged. Thus some disease symptoms are *caused by* the inflammatory response.

7. **Degeneration**—breaking apart, or *degeneration,* of tissues by means of many still unknown processes. Although a normal consequence of aging, degeneration of one or more tissues resulting from disease can occur at any time. The degeneration of tissues associated with aging is discussed in Chapter 23.

Risk Factors

Other than direct causes or disease mechanisms, certain *predisposing conditions* may make the development of a disease more likely to occur. Usually called **risk factors,** they often do not actually cause a dis-

ease but may put one "at risk" for developing it. Some of the major categories of risk factors follow:

1. **Genetic factors**—There are several types of genetic risk factors. Sometimes, an inherited trait puts a person at a greater than normal risk for developing a specific disease. For example, light-skinned people are more at risk for developing certain forms of skin cancer than are dark-skinned people. This occurs because light-skinned people have less pigment in their skin to protect them from cancer-causing ultraviolet radiation (see Chapter 6). Membership in a certain ethnic group or *gene pool* involves the "risk" of inheriting a disease-causing gene that is common in that gene pool. For example, certain Africans and their descendants are at a greater-than-average risk of inheriting *sickle cell anemia*—a deadly blood disorder.

2. **Age**—Biological and behavioral variations inherent during different phases of the human life cycle put us at greater risk for developing certain diseases at certain times in life. For example, middle ear infections are more common in infants than in adults because of the difference in ear structure at different ages.

3. **Lifestyle**—The way we live and work can put us at risk for some diseases. People whose work or personal activity puts them in direct sunlight for long periods have a greater chance of developing skin cancer because they are in more frequent contact with ultraviolet radiation from the sun. Research has shown that the high-fat, low-fiber diet common among people in the developed nations increases their risk of developing certain cancers such as colon cancer.

4. **Stress**—Physical, psychological, or emotional stress can put one at risk of developing problems such as headaches, chronic high blood pressure (hypertension), depression, heart disease, and cancer. Conditions caused by psychological factors are sometimes called **psychogenic** (mind-caused) disorders.

5. **Environmental factors**—Although environmental factors such as climate and pollution can cause injury or disease, some environmental situations simply put us at greater risk for getting certain diseases. For example, because some parasites survive only in tropical environments, we are at risk for diseases caused by

those particular organisms only if we live in or travel to that climate.

6. **Preexisting conditions**—A preexisting disease, such as an infection, can adversely affect our capacity to defend ourselves against further attack. Thus a *primary* (preexisting) condition can put a person at risk of developing a *secondary* condition. For example, blisters from a preexisting burn may break open and thus increase the risk of a bacterial infection of the skin.

Combined risk factors can increase a person's chances of developing a specific disease even more. For example, a light-skinned person can add to the genetic risk of developing skin cancer by spending a long time in the sun without skin protection—a lifestyle risk added to a genetic risk. As you may have guessed, many of these categories of risk factors overlap. For example, stress can be a component of lifestyle, or it could be considered a preexisting condition. Sometimes a high-risk group is identified by epidemiologists, but the exact mechanism that puts them at high risk may be uncertain. For example, a high incidence of heart disease in a small ethnic group may point to a genetic risk factor but could also result from some aspect of a shared lifestyle.

Risk factors for many deadly diseases can be avoided. Risk of heart disease, diabetes, cancer, infections, and other types of disease can be decreased by making informed choices about lifestyle that influence diet and exercise, stress management, the environment, and treatment of preexisting conditions.

QUICK CHECK

1. How is *pathophysiology* different from *pathology?*
2. List eight general mechanisms that may cause disease.
3. List six factors that may cause risk of developing a disease.
4. How is a *primary* condition different from a *secondary* condition?

Pathogenic Organisms and Particles

Many kinds of organisms and particles can cause disease in humans. Even humans can cause human disease through accidental or intentional injury to themselves or others. In pathophysiology, the pathogenic organisms most often studied are microscopic or just barely visible to the unaided eye. Microscopic organisms, also called **microbes,** include *bacteria, fungi,* and *protozoa.* Larger organisms, the pathogenic *animals,* are

also medically important. The smallest of all pathogens, microscopic nonliving particles called *viruses* and *prions,* lead our list of important disease-causing agents.

Viruses

Viruses are intracellular parasites that consist of a nucleic acid (DNA or RNA) core surrounded by a protein coat and sometimes a lipoprotein envelope. Although they are not technically living organisms, viruses have a genetic code (genome) and, like living organisms, they multiply. They are particles that invade cells and insert their own genetic code into the host cell's genetic processes, causing the host cell to produce viral DNA or RNA and protein coats. They thus pirate the host cell's nutrients and organelles to produce more virus particles. These newly formed viruses may leave the cell to infect other cells by exocytosis or by bursting the cell membrane (Figure 5-3).

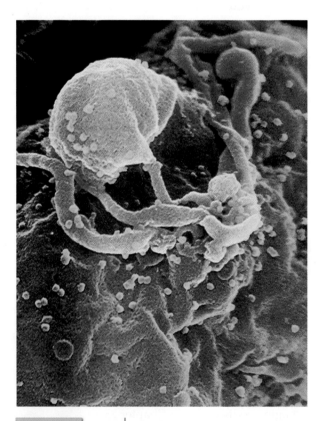

Figure 5-3 ┃ **HIV.**

The human immunodeficiency virus, or HIV (*blue* in this electron micrograph), which is released from infected white blood cells, soon spreads over neighboring cells, infecting them in turn. The individual viruses are very small; more than 200 million would fit on the period at the end of this sentence.

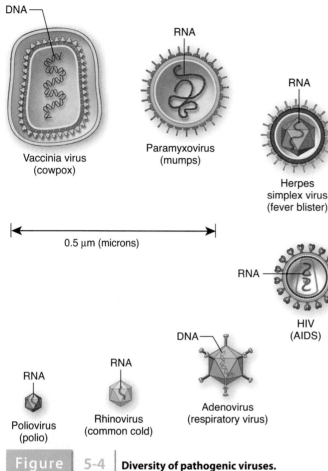

Figure 5-4 **Diversity of pathogenic viruses.**

Some viruses are relatively large; others are extremely tiny. A human hair would be 8 meters thick if drawn at the same scale as the particles depicted here.

The symptoms of viral infections may not appear right away. The viral genetic code may not become active for some time, or viral multiplication may not immediately cause significant cellular damage. In any case, the effects of the intracellular viral parasite may eventually take their toll and thus produce symptoms of disease.

Viruses are a very diverse group, as illustrated in Figure 5-4. They are usually classified according to their shape, DNA or RNA content, and their method of multiplying. Some examples of medically important viruses are listed in Table 5-1. Many of these and some other viral diseases are discussed in detail in later chapters.

HIV

The most discussed virus in recent history is HIV (human immunodeficiency virus). If untreated, this virus causes AIDS (acquired immunodeficiency syndrome). HIV attacks the immune system, thus rendering the host organism susceptible to a variety of infections. The immune system gives our bodies the ability to fight infections. HIV finds and destroys a type of white blood cell (T cells called CD4 cells) that the immune system must have to fight disease.

HIV was first identified in the United States in 1981 after a number of homosexual men started getting sick with a rare type of cancer. It took several years for scientists to develop a test for the virus, to understand how HIV was transmitted between humans, and to determine what people could do to

Table 5-1 Examples of Pathogenic Viruses

VIRAL TYPE	VIRUS	DISEASES CAUSED
DNA	Human papillomavirus (HPV)	Warts
	Hepatitis B	Hepatitis B (viral liver infection)
	Herpes simplex 1 and 2	Fever blisters and genital herpes
	Epstein-Barr virus (EBV)	Mononucleosis
RNA	Influenza A, B, and C	Various influenza infections
	Human immunodeficiency virus (HIV)	Acquired immunodeficiency syndrome (AIDS)
	Flavivirus	West Nile virus (WNV), yellow fever, dengue, St. Louis encephalitis
	Paramyxovirus	Measles, mumps, and parainfluenza
	Rhinovirus	Common cold and upper respiratory infections
	Coronavirus (CoV)	Respiratory infections, including severe acute respiratory syndrome (SARS)
	Hepatitis A and C	Hepatitis A and C (viral liver infections)

See Table 2 in Appendix A on page A-1 of your book for a list of viral diseases and their descriptions.

protect themselves against being infected. During the early 1980s, as many as 150,000 people became infected with HIV each year in the United States. By the early 1990s, this rate had dropped to about 40,000 each year, where it remains today.

The spread of HIV in regions of the world that are economically disadvantaged remains a major global health concern. This persists as a consequence of lack of education about disease prevention and lack of resources needed to treat the infected individuals with antiviral therapy.

It is also important to note that antiviral therapy prevents the immune system collapse characteristic of AIDS, but does not eliminate HIV from the infected individual, who thus remains contagious. HIV is a fragile virus, and cannot live for very long outside the body. The virus is not transmitted through day-to-day activities such as shaking hands, hugging, or a casual kiss. HIV is not spread from a toilet seat, drinking fountain, doorknob, dishes, drinking glasses, food, or pets. Unlike other infections discussed later, HIV infection is not an arthropod-borne disease and cannot be spread by mosquitoes or other biting arthropods.

HIV is primarily found in the blood, semen, or vaginal fluid of an infected person. HIV is transmitted in three main ways:

- Sexual contact (anal, vaginal, or oral) with someone infected with HIV

- Sharing needles and syringes with someone infected with HIV

- Being exposed (fetus or infant) to HIV before or during birth or through breastfeeding

SARS-CoV AND FLAVIVIRUS

Viruses such as the *SARS-associated coronavirus (SARS-CoV)*, the cause of **severe acute respiratory syndrome (SARS)**, are spread when virus particles are shed by an infected body by way of respiratory fluids or other body fluids, and these particles then come in contact with another person's body fluids. A person is most likely to pick up shed viruses in the moist mucous membranes of the mouth, nose, eyes, or genitals. On the other hand, viruses such as the *flaviviruses* that cause **West Nile virus (WNV)** infection, yellow fever, and other potentially serious infections, must be transmitted less directly. Flaviviruses move from an infected bird or other animal to a mosquito or other biting insect and then finally to the human host. Such viruses cannot move directly from an infected

bird to a human—they require the insect to carry the virus to humans. This role of animals, including biting insects, in disease transmission is discussed later in this chapter.

 To learn more about virus replication, go to **AnimationDirect** on your CD.

Prions

The word **prion** is a shortened form of the phrase "PROteinaceous INfectious particle." Prions are pathogenic protein molecules that convert normal proteins of the body into abnormal proteins, causing abnormalities of function (Figure 5-5). The abnormal form of the protein also may be inherited by offspring of an affected person. Being a newly discovered type of pathogen, not much is known yet about how the prion works.

We do know that prions can affect proteins in the nervous system and cause diseases such as *bovine*

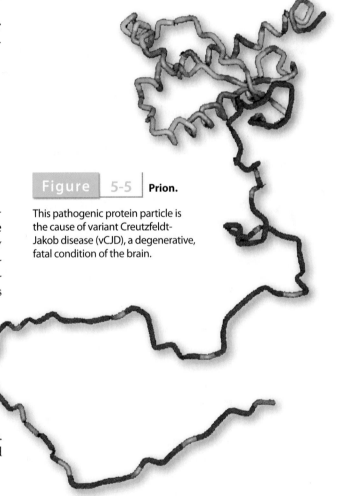

Figure 5-5 | **Prion.**

This pathogenic protein particle is the cause of variant Creutzfeldt-Jakob disease (vCJD), a degenerative, fatal condition of the brain.

spongiform encephalopathy (BSE; "mad cow disease") and *variant Creutzfeldt-Jakob disease* (vCJD). Both of these diseases are very rare, fatal conditions characterized by degeneration of brain tissue and progressive loss of nervous system function. Many scientists believe that prions from infected cattle were consumed as beef by humans with these diseases, but there are many unanswered questions about the exact mechanisms of transmission of prion diseases.

Bacteria

A **bacterium** (*pl.*, bacteria) is a tiny, primitive cell without a nucleus. Bacteria produce disease in a variety of ways. They can secrete toxic substances that damage human tissues, they may become parasites inside human cells, or they may form populations in the host body that disrupt normal human function. Like viruses, bacteria also are a diverse group of *pathogens* ("disease-producers"). There are several ways to classify bacteria:

1. **Growth requirements**—Bacteria can be categorized according to whether they need oxygen to grow. For example, they can be categorized as *aerobic* (requiring oxygen for their metabolism) or *anaerobic* (requiring an absence of oxygen).

2. **Staining properties**—Bacteria stain differently, depending on the compounds in their walls. For example, *gram-positive* bacteria are stained purple by the Gram staining technique, whereas *gram-negative* bacteria are not (see Clinical Application box on p. 113).

3. **Shape and size**—Bacteria are most commonly classified by their varied shapes (Table 5-2). Medically significant bacteria range in size from less than 0.5 μm to more than 5 μm, making size a useful characteristic for classification. The abbreviation μm represents *micrometers* or *microns,* one millionth of a meter. Some major groupings based on shape and size follow:

Table 5-2	Examples of Pathogenic Bacteria		
STRUCTURAL CLASSIFICATION	**GRAM STAIN CLASSIFICATION**	**BACTERIUM**	**DISEASES CAUSED**
Bacilli (rods)	Gram-positive	*Bacillus* organisms	Anthrax and gastroenteritis
	Gram-positive	*Clostridium* organisms	Botulism, tetanus, and soft tissue infections
	Gram-negative	*Enterobacteria* organisms	*Salmonella* diseases and gastroenteritis
	Gram-negative	*Pseudomonas* organisms	External otitis (swimmer's ear), endocarditis, and pulmonary infections
Cocci (spheres)	Gram-positive	*Staphylococcus* organisms	Staphylococci infections, food poisoning, urinary tract infections, and toxic shock syndrome
	Gram-positive	*Streptococcus* organisms	Throat infections, pneumonia, sinusitis, otitis media, rheumatic fever, and dental caries
	Gram-negative	*Neisseria* organisms	Meningitis, gonorrhea, and pelvic inflammatory disease
Curved or spiral rod	Gram-negative	*Vibrio* organisms	Cholera, gastroenteritis, and wound infections
	Gram-negative	*Campylobacter* organisms	Diarrhea
	Gram-negative	Spirochetes	Syphilis and Lyme disease
Small bacterium	Gram-negative	*Rickettsia* organisms	Rocky Mountain spotted fever and Q fever
	Gram-negative	*Chlamydia* organisms	Genital infections, lymphogranuloma venereum, pelvic inflammatory disease, conjunctivitis, and parrot fever

See Table 3 in Appendix A on page A-1 of your book for a list of bacterial diseases and their descriptions.

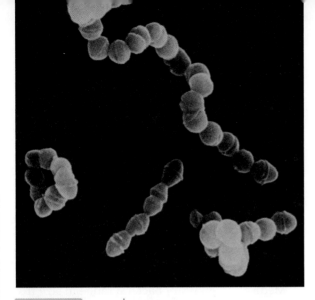

Figure 5-6 **Streptococci bacteria.**

As this scanning electron micrograph shows, individual spherical bacteria (cocci) may adhere to each other to form chains.

a. **Bacilli** (bah-SILL-eye)—large, rod-shaped cells found singly or in groups.
b. **Cocci** (KOK-sye)—large, round bacteria found singly, in pairs *(diplococci)*, in strings *(streptococci)* as shown in Figure 5-6, or in clusters *(staphylococci)*.
c. **Curved or spiral rods**—curved rods arranged singly or in strands, or large curved or spiral cells arranged singly or in cell colonies.
d. **Small bacteria**—round or oval bacteria that are so small that some of them were once thought to be viruses. They can reproduce only inside other living cells, so they are sometimes called *obligate intracellular parasites*. **Rickettsia** (ri-KET-see-ah) and *chlamydia* (klah-MID-ee-ah) are two types of small bacteria.

Table 5-2 summarizes bacterial types and some of the diseases each group causes.

Some bacteria can develop into resistant dormant forms called **spores** when subjected to adverse environmental conditions. Spores are resistant to chemicals, heat, and dry, arid conditions. When environmental conditions become more suitable for life processes such as reproduction, the spores revert back to the active form of bacterium. Although advantageous for the bacterium, this transformation ability often makes it difficult for humans to destroy pathogenic bacteria.

Another type of microbe that is similar to bacteria is the **archaea** (ark-EE-ah). They differ from bacteria in their chemical makeup and metabolism. Also, unlike bacteria, many archaea thrive in extremely harsh environments that are very hot, very acid, or very salty. Although archaea have been found in the human body, in the mouth for example, none have yet been proven to cause disease.

Fungi

Fungi (FUN-jye; *sing.,* fungus) are a group of simple organisms similar to plants but without chlorophyll (green pigment). Without chlorophyll, pathogenic fungi cannot produce their own food, so they must consume or parasitize other organisms. Most pathogenic fungi parasitize tissue on or near the skin or mucous membranes, as in athlete's foot and vaginal yeast infections. A few systemic (body-wide) fungal infections, such as San Joaquin fever, can disrupt the entire body. Figure 5-7 shows that *yeasts* are small, single-celled fungi and *molds* are large, multicellular fungi. Fungal, or **mycotic** (my-KOT-ik), **infections** often resist treatment, so they can become a quite serious health problem. Table 5-3 lists some of the important pathogenic fungi and the diseases that they cause.

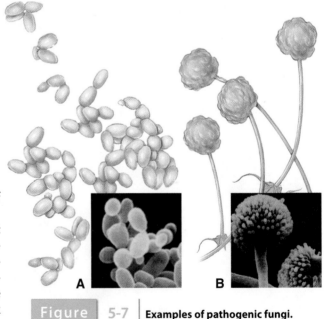

Figure 5-7 **Examples of pathogenic fungi.**

Electron micrographs and drawings. **A,** Scanning electron micrograph of yeast cells. Yeasts commonly infect the urinary and reproductive tracts. **B,** This electron micrograph shows *Aspergillus* organisms, a mold that can infect different parts of the body where it forms characteristic "fungus balls."

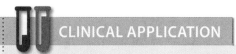

CLINICAL APPLICATION

LABORATORY IDENTIFICATION OF PATHOGENS

Often the evident signs or symptoms of a disease caused by bacteria or other pathogens provide enough information for a health professional to make a diagnosis. To be sure that the correct course of treatment is given, laboratory tests are often required to positively identify a pathogen.

Sometimes pathogens can be observed in specimens of blood, feces (stool), cerebrospinal fluid (CSF), mucus, urine, or other substances from the body. To view a microscopic pathogen, a portion of the collected specimen is smeared on a microscope slide and then stained to enhance visibility. Certain stains color only certain types of cells. For example, only gram-positive bacteria retain the violet stain used in the Gram staining technique (Figure **A**). Gram-negative bacteria do not retain the violet stain; they retain only a red counterstain (Figure **B**). Thus gram-positive (violet) bacteria can be distinguished from gram-negative (red) bacteria using the Gram method. The staining properties, shape, and size of a pathogen are a few of the characteristics sometimes used to identify pathogens in specimen samples.

Pathogens are sometimes identified by **cultures** (propagation of microorganisms in special media conducive to their growth) that originate from specimens taken from a patient. These populations of bacteria can be grown only on certain *media* (liquid or *agar* gel–containing nutrients). Thus pathogenic bacteria are often identified by the type of medium in which they grow best. For example, mucus swabbed from a sore throat and placed in a medium that contains blood may produce pinpoint-sized colonies of pathogenic streptococci bacteria. The streptococci bacteria that cause "strep throat" typically have a distinct, transparent ring around each colony. The rings result from hemolysis—bursting of red blood cells in the surrounding medium. A few viruses also can be cultivated but only within living cells.

Some infections can be diagnosed on the basis of immunological tests that check for antibodies against a particular pathogen. If antibodies are found, it is assumed that the patient has been exposed to a pathogen; a large number of antibodies usually indicates an active infection. An example is the test for anti-HIV antibodies used to identify HIV infections. Recall from Chapter 4 that such tests are often used to screen donated tissues and organs for pathogenic organisms. Even newer tests use rapid biological sensors that borrow the recognition mechanisms from immune cells sensitive to particular pathogens and link them to special proteins from jellyfish that cause the sensor to glow when the pathogen is present. A wide variety of different immunological tests are now available for bacterial and viral infections and other new technologies are on the horizon.

The recent explosion of knowledge in genetics and genomics (see Chapter 24) has led to many newer methods of rapidly and accurately identifying a variety of pathogens. For example, patterns of DNA or RNA code that are unique to a particular virus, bacterium, or other pathogen can be detected by special sensors or laboratory tests.

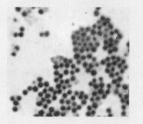 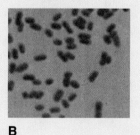

A   **B**

Table 5-3	**Examples of Pathogenic Fungi**
FUNGUS	**DISEASES CAUSED**
Candida organisms	Thrush and mucous membrane infections (including vaginal yeast infections)
Epidermophyton and *Microsporum* organisms	Tinea infections: ringworm, jock itch, and athlete's foot
Histoplasma organisms	Histoplasmosis
Aspergillus organisms	Aspergillosis and pneumonia
Coccidioides organisms	Coccidioidomycosis (San Joaquin fever)

See Table 4 in Appendix A on page A-1 of your book for a list of mycotic diseases and their descriptions.

Protozoa

Protozoa (proh-toh-ZOH-ah) are *protists,* one-celled organisms that are larger than bacteria and whose DNA is organized in a nucleus. Table 5-4 illustrates some of the pathogenic protozoa. Protozoa can infect human fluids and cause disease by parasitizing cells or directly destroying them (Figure 5-8). Some major groups of pathogenic protozoa include the following:

1. **Amoebas** (ah-MEE-bahs)—large cells of changing shape; amoebas extend their membranes to form *pseudopodia* ("false feet") that pull themselves along.
2. **Flagellates** (FLAJ-eh-layts)—protozoa that are similar to amoebas but move by wiggling long, whiplike extensions called **flagella**.
3. **Ciliates** (SILL-ee-ayts)—protozoa that move by means of many short, hairlike projections called cilia.
4. **Sporozoa** (spor-oh-ZOH-ah)—protozoa with unusual organelles at their tips that allow them to

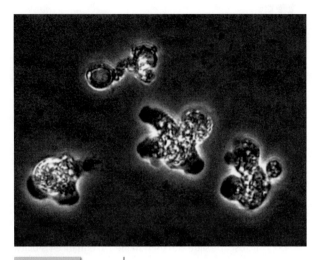

Figure 5-8 | *Naegleria fowlerii.*

N. fowlerii is an emerging pathogen in the southern United States. It is found in warm, fresh-water ponds, lakes, streams, and warm springs. The organism enters the body by swimming up the nose and invading the brain through the thin ethmoid bone. It causes a fatal central nervous system infection.

Table 5-4 | **Examples of Pathogenic Protozoa**

CLASSIFICATION	PROTOZOAN	DISEASES CAUSED
Amoeba	*Entamoeba* organisms	Diarrhea, amebic dysentery, and liver and lung infections
Flagellate	*Giardia* organisms	Giardiasis, diarrhea, and malabsorption syndrome
	Trichomonas organisms	Trichomoniasis, vaginitis, and urinary tract infections
Ciliate	*Balantidium* organisms	Gastrointestinal disturbances, including pain, nausea, and anorexia
Sporozoan (coccidium)	*Isospora* organisms	Isosporiasis infection of gastrointestinal tract, diarrhea, and malabsorption syndrome
	Plasmodium organisms	Malaria
	Toxoplasma organisms	Toxoplasmosis and congenital damage to fetus

See Table 5 in Appendix A on page A-1 of your book for a list of diseases caused by protozoa.

enter host cells; also called *coccidia*. They often oscillate between two different hosts, having two different stages in their life cycle. The sporozoa that cause malaria exhibit this pattern.

Table 5-4 lists some of the major disease-causing protozoa.

Pathogenic Animals

Pathogenic animals sometimes called *metazoa* (met-ah-ZOH-ah) are large, multicellular organisms. Animals can cause disease by parasitizing humans or causing injury in some other way. Table 5-5 illustrates some animals that cause disease. The major groups of pathogenic animals include the following:

1. **Nematodes** (nem-ah-TOHDS)—large parasites, also called *roundworms*, that infest a variety of different human tissues. They are often transmitted by food or by flies that bite.

2. **Platyhelminths** (plaht-ih-HEL-minths)—large parasites, otherwise known as *flatworms* and *flukes*, that can infest several different human organs. The *Schistosoma* flukes shown in Figure 5-9 cause "snail fever," or *schistosomiasis*.

3. **Arthropods** (AR-throh-pods)—group of parasites that include *mites*, *ticks*, *lice*, and *fleas*. Also included are biting or stinging *wasps*, *bees*,

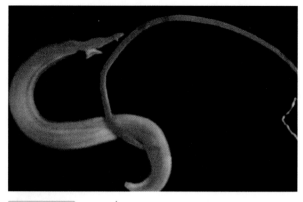

Figure 5-9 **Platyhelminths.**

This light micrograph shows both male and female *Schistosoma* flukes mating in the human bloodstream (the male is the larger of the two).

mosquitoes, and *spiders*. All are capable of causing injury or infestation themselves but also can carry other pathogenic organisms. An organism that spreads disease to other organisms is called a **vector** of the disease.

Table 5-5 summarizes some of the major health problems associated with selected pathogenic animals.

Table 5-5 | Examples of Pathogenic Animals

CLASSIFICATION	ANIMAL	DISEASES CAUSED
Nematode	*Ascaris* organisms	Intestinal roundworm infestation, gastrointestinal obstruction, and bronchial damage
	Enterobius organisms	Pinworm infestation of the lower gastrointestinal tract, itching around the anus, and insomnia
	Trichinella organisms	Trichinosis, fever, and muscle pain
Platyhelminth	*Schistosoma* organisms	Schistosomiasis (snail fever)
	Fasciola organisms	Liver fluke infestation
	Taenia organisms	Pork and beef tapeworm infestation
Arthropod	*Arachnida* organisms	Infestation by mites and ticks; toxic bites by spiders, scorpions; and transmission of other pathogens
	Insecta	Infestation by fleas and lice; toxic bites by wasps, mosquitoes, and bees; and transmission of other pathogens; ticks (Lyme disease)

See Table 6 in Appendix A on page A-1 of your book for a list of diseases caused by pathogenic animals.

Prevention and Control

The key to preventing many diseases caused by pathogenic organisms is stopping them from entering the human body. This sounds simple enough but is often very difficult to accomplish. The following is a partial list of the ways in which pathogens can spread:

1. **Person-to-person contact**—Small pathogens often can be carried in the air from one person to another. Also, direct contact with an infected person or with contaminated materials handled by the infected person is a common mode of transmission. The *rhinovirus* that causes the common cold is often transmitted in these ways. Some viruses, such as those that cause *hepatitis B, hepatitis C,* and *AIDS* are transmitted when infected blood, semen, or another body fluid enters a person's bloodstream. Preventing the spread of these diseases often involves educating people about avoiding certain types of contact with individuals known or suspected of carrying the disease. Another strategy, called **aseptic** (ay-SEP-tik) **technique,** involves killing or disabling pathogens on surfaces before they can spread to other people. Table 5-6 summarizes the major approaches taken when using aseptic technique.

2. **Environmental contact**—Many pathogens are found throughout the local environment—in food, water, soil, and on assorted surfaces. Under normal conditions, these pathogens infect only individuals who happen to come across them or who are already weakened by some other condition. If improper sanitation practices create an environment that promotes increased growth and spread of pathogens, an epidemic could result. Disease caused by environmental pathogens can often be prevented by avoiding contact with certain materials and by maintaining safe sanitation practices.

3. **Opportunistic invasion**—Some potentially pathogenic organisms are found on the skin and mucous membranes of nearly everyone. However, they do not cause disease until they have the opportunity. That is, they do not create a problem until and unless conditions change or they enter the body's internal environment. For example, the fungi that cause athlete's foot are often present on the skin of people who do not have symptoms of this infection. Only when the skin is kept warm and moist for prolonged periods can the fungus reproduce and create an infection. Preventing opportunistic infection involves avoiding conditions that could promote infections. Changes in the pH (acidity), moisture, temperature, or other characteristics of skin and mucous membranes often promote opportunistic infections. Cleansing and aseptic treatment of accidental or surgical wounds also can prevent these infections.

4. **Transmission by a vector**—As stated previously, a vector such as an arthropod acts as a carrier of a pathogenic organism. For example, the spirochete bacterium that causes *Lyme disease* is not usually

Table	5-6	Common Aseptic Methods that Prevent the Spread of Pathogens*
METHOD	**ACTION**	**EXAMPLES**
Sterilization	Destruction of all living organisms	Pressurized steam bath, extreme temperature, or radiation used to sterilize surgical instruments and garments or other surfaces
Disinfection	Destruction of most or all pathogens on inanimate objects but not necessarily all harmless microbes	Chemicals such as iodine, chlorine, alcohol, phenol, and soaps
Antisepsis	Inhibition or inactivation of pathogens	Chemicals such as alcohol, iodine, quaternary ammonium compounds (quats), and dyes
Isolation	Separation of potentially infectious people or materials from noninfected people	Quarantine of affected patients; protective apparel worn while giving treatments; and sanitary transport, storage, and disposal of body fluids, tissues, and other materials

*Spores (special bacterial forms) may resist methods that would ordinarily kill active bacterial cells.

transmitted directly from human to human. Instead, a vector such as the deer tick carries it from one person to another or between animals and humans. The most effective way to stop such diseases from spreading is a combination of reducing the population of vectors and reducing the number of contacts with vectors. *Malaria,* still a major killer in some parts of the world, was virtually eliminated from North America in this way. Many mosquitoes that transmit the malaria organism were destroyed with pesticides, and at the same time, people were educated about ways to prevent mosquito bites. Consistent use of both strategies resulted in the collapse of the pathogen population in the vector and host. The fact that sporadic cases of malaria still occur in North America demonstrate the need for ongoing monitoring of vector populations, as well as incidence of the disease.

A prevention strategy that has worked with some bacterial and viral pathogens has been the **vaccine.** A vaccine is a killed or attenuated (weakened) pathogen or part of a pathogen that is given to a person to stimulate immunity. Vaccination is a preventive method that stimulates a person's own immune system in a way that promotes development of resistance to a particular pathogen. More discussion of vaccination and other immune system strategies of disease prevention is found in Chapter 15.

After an infection has begun, there are several ways to treat the patient and attempt to gain control of the disease. One common approach is the use of chemicals to destroy pathogens or inhibit their growth. **Antibiotics,** for example, are compounds produced by certain living organisms or in a laboratory that kill or inhibit pathogens. *Penicillin—*

RESEARCH, ISSUES, AND TRENDS

DISEASE AS A WEAPON

World events have shown us that the intentional transmission of disease can be used as a weapon of terror. **Anthrax,** a bacterial infection caused by *Bacillus anthracis*, is an example of a pathogen that has been intentionally distributed to otherwise healthy victims in acts of **bioterrorism**. This particular bacterium ordinarily affects mainly plant-eating animals such as sheep, cattle, and goats, often resulting in their death.

The anthrax bacterium can assume the form of a **spore** that is resistant to heat, drying, and chemicals and then later becomes active to cause infection. Rarely, humans inhale some anthrax spores or get the spores in an open cut when handling infected animals or their hides. The inhaled form may be fatal if not treated quickly with antibiotics. The cutaneous (skin) form is less serious, characterized by a reddish brown patch on the skin that ulcerates and then forms a dark, nearly black scab (see figure), followed by muscle pain, internal hemorrhage (bleeding), headache, fever, nausea, and vomiting. Anthrax causes disease by releasing a toxin that latches onto receptors on the cells of the host, then punching a hole in the cell's membrane, and inserting a portion of the toxin called "lethal factor" that destroys proteins in the cell and kills it.

If the infection is discovered before the anthrax bacteria have time to make large amounts of toxin, antibiotics such as doxycycline and ciprofloxacin can cure anthrax. Scientists are also working to perfect drugs that imitate the cell's re-

ceptors and would thus "gum up" the toxin on fake receptors before it can attack cells. Vaccines are available, but these must be given long before possible exposure to the spores.

Anthrax spores have been refined for military purposes, even though this is outlawed by various global treaties, and have been used by terrorists to attempt to intimidate or disrupt civilian populations. Such a situation occurred in the United States when anthrax-contaminated packages were sent through the mail in the fall of 2001. Other bacteria such as *Yersinia pestis* (plague), viruses such as smallpox, and a variety of genetically engineered forms of known pathogens continue to be added to the potential arsenal of terrorists.

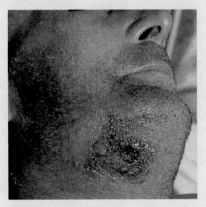

Cutaneous anthrax

produced by a fungus—and *streptomycin*—produced by a bacterium—are well-known antibiotics. A few synthetic chemicals are now used to treat bacterial and viral infections. Among the growing list of synthetic antiviral agents are *acyclovir (ACV)* for treating herpes infections and *efavirenz,* used to treat AIDS. These antiviral agents, especially when used in carefully formulated combinations (often called "drug cocktails"), do not stop infections but merely inhibit viral reproduction and thus slow down the progression of viral diseases.

Antibiotic resistance is an important consideration in the treatment of infectious diseases today. As we continue to use antibiotics to treat bacterial disease, bacteria develop resistance to antibiotic drugs. Some of this occurs as a natural consequence of bacterial adaptation. However, we accelerate this process by prescribing antibiotics for diseases that are not of bacterial etiology, or by using the medications inappropriately after they are prescribed.

QUICK CHECK

1. What are four ways that a disease can be spread?
2. What is *aseptic technique?*
3. How is an *antibiotic* drug different from an *antiviral* drug?

Tumors and Cancer

Neoplasms

The term *neoplasm* literally means "new matter" and refers to an abnormal growth of cells. Neoplasms, also called **tumors,** can take the form of distinct lumps of abnormal cells or, in blood tissue, can be diffuse. Neoplasms are often classified as **benign** or **malignant** (Table 5-7). Benign tumors remain localized within the tissue from which they arose. Malignant tumors

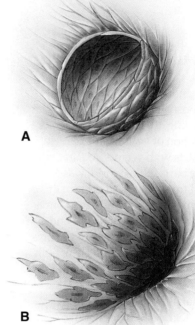

Figure 5-10

Types of neoplasms.
A, Benign neoplasms (tumors) are usually encapsulated and grow slowly. **B,** Malignant neoplasms or cancers are not encapsulated. They grow rapidly, extending into surrounding tissues. Some cells metastasize, that is, they fall away from the original tumor and form tumors in other parts of the body.

tend to spread to other regions of the body. **Cancer** is another term for a malignant tumor.

Benign tumors are called such because they do not spread to other tissues and they usually grow very slowly. Their cells are often well differentiated, unlike the undifferentiated cells typical of malignant tumors. Cells in a benign tumor tend to stay together, and they are often surrounded by a capsule of dense tissue. Benign tumors are usually not life threatening but can be if they disrupt the normal function of a vital organ (Figure 5-10).

Malignant tumors, on the other hand, are not encapsulated and do not stay in one place. Their cells tend to fall away from the original neoplasm and may start new tumors in other parts of the body. For example, cells from malignant breast tumors usually form new (secondary) tumors in bone, brain, and lung tissues. The cells migrate by way of lymphatic or blood vessels. This manner of spread-

Table 5-7 | Comparison of Benign and Malignant Tumors

CHARACTERISTIC	BENIGN TUMOR	MALIGNANT TUMOR
Rate of growth	Slow	Rapid
Structure	Encapsulated	Nonencapsulated (infiltrates surrounding tissue)
Pattern of growth	Expanding but not spreading to other tissues	Metastasizing (spreading) to other tissues
Cell type	Well differentiated (similar to normal tissue cells)	Undifferentiated (abnormal in structure and function)
Mortality rate	Low	High if condition remains untreated

ing is called **metastasis** (meh-TASS-tah-sis). Cells that do not metastasize still can spread, but in another way: they grow rapidly and extend the tumor into nearby tissues. Malignant tumors may replace part of a vital organ with abnormal, undifferentiated tissue—a life-threatening situation (Figures 5-10 and 5-11).

Benign and malignant neoplasms are classified into subgroups depending on appearance and the location where they originate. Benign and malignant tumors can be divided into three types—epithelial tissue, connective tissue, and miscellaneous tumors. Some examples of each follow:

1. Benign tumors that arise from epithelial tissues
   a. **Papilloma** (pap-i-LOH-mah)—a type of tumor that forms a fingerlike projection, as in a wart.
   b. **Adenoma** (ad-eh-NO-mah)—a general term for benign tumors of glandular epithelium.
   c. **Nevus** (NEE-vus)—a variety of small, pigmented tumors of the skin, such as moles.

2. Benign tumors that arise from connective tissues
   a. **Lipoma** (lip-OH-mah)—a tumor arising from adipose (fat) tissue.
   b. **Osteoma** (os-tee-OH-mah)—a tumor that involves bone tissues.
   c. **Chondroma** (kon-DROH-mah)—tumors of cartilage tissue.

3. Malignant tumors that arise from epithelial tissues, generally called **carcinomas** (kar-sih-NO-mahs)
   a. **Melanoma** (mel-ah-NO-mah)—a type of cancer that involves melanocytes, the pigment-producing cells of the skin.
   b. **Adenocarcinoma** (ad-en-oh-kar-sih-NO-mah)—the general term for malignant tumors of glandular epithelium.

4. Malignant tumors that arise from connective tissues, generally called **sarcomas** (sar-KOH-mahs)
   a. **Lymphoma** (lim-FOH-mah)—a term used to describe a cancer of lymphatic tissue.
   b. **Osteosarcoma** (os-tee-oh-sar-KOH-mah)—term that refers to a malignant tumor of bone tissue.
   c. **Myeloma** (my-eh-LOH-mah)—a type of malignant bone marrow tumor.
   d. **Fibrosarcoma** (fye-broh-sar-KOH-mah)—a general term used to describe cancers involving fibrous connective tissues.

Miscellaneous tumors do not fit either of the other categories. For example, an *adenofibroma* (ad-en-oh-fye-BROH-mah) is a benign neoplasm formed by epithelial and connective tissues. Another example is *neuroblastoma* (noo-roh-blas-TOH-mah), a malignant tumor that arises from nerve tissue.

Cancers can be further classified by their location. For example, malignant tumors may be labeled *skin cancer*, *stomach cancer*, or *lung cancer* according to the location of the affected tissues. The more common

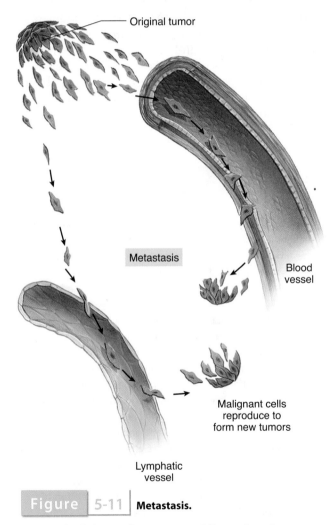

Original tumor

Metastasis

Blood vessel

Malignant cells reproduce to form new tumors

Lymphatic vessel

Figure 5-11 **Metastasis.**

Abnormal cells from malignant tumors fall away from the original neoplasm and travel along lymphatic vessels, through which they can enter and exit easily. Malignant cells also can travel through the bloodstream and burrow through a blood vessel wall to invade other tissues.

BOX 5-1

MAJOR FORMS OF CANCER*

Lung cancer

Colorectal cancer

Breast cancer

Prostate cancer

Uterine cancer (including cervical cancer)

Urinary (bladder and kidney) cancer

Oral (lip, mouth, and throat) cancer

Pancreatic cancer

Leukemia (cancer of blood tissue)

Lymphoma (cancer of lymphatic tissue)

Ovarian cancer

Skin cancer

*By location.

forms of cancer in the United States are listed in Box 5-1 and are described in later chapters.

Causes of Cancer

The etiologies of various forms of cancer puzzle researchers no less today than they did 100 years ago. The more we know about how cancer develops, the more questions we have. Currently, the best answer to the question "What causes cancer?" is "Many different things." We know that cancer is a type of neoplasm, which means that it involves uncontrolled cell division. A process called **hyperplasia** (hye-per-PLAY-zha) produces too many cells. Also, abnormal, undifferentiated tumor cells are often produced by a process called **anaplasia** (an-ah-PLAY-zha). Thus the mechanism of all cancers is a mistake or problem in cell division. We are uncertain of all the triggers of the abnormal cell division. Currently, the following factors are known to play a role:

SCIENCE APPLICATIONS

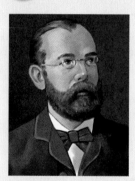

Robert Koch (1843–1910)

PUBLIC HEALTH

Robert Koch astounded his parents when, at the age of five (in 1848), he showed his parents that he had taught himself to read. His determination and his methodical use of newspapers in his home not only helped young Robert teach himself to read, it also foreshadowed a brilliant career as an investigative scientist. Koch became a physician, and while still a young man, he proved that the anthrax bacillus (bacterium) causes the anthrax infection (see box, p. 117). Thus he was the first to prove that specific bacteria cause specific diseases. He later went on to do similar ground-breaking work with wound infections, tuberculosis, cholera, and many other infections. Perhaps more importantly, he laid the groundwork for the laboratory study of bacteria and the control of individual infections as well as epidemics. In so doing, Robert Koch laid the groundwork for modern *public health*, the field that strives to prevent and control disease and promote good health in the human population.

Public health is a field that includes many different endeavors, all aimed at promoting the health and wellness of us all. For example, medical and allied health workers treat disease and work to prevent and control epidemics. Pathologists and laboratory technicians help us better understand diseases that affect the human population, and researchers help develop effective prevention and treatment. Many public health advisors, environmental health scientists, and activists work to help us understand and resolve issues related to exposure to pollutants, the affects of our lifestyle, technological advances, and social choices that effect our health. Public health administrators and staff, including volunteers, help organize and support the worldwide effort to promote public health.

1. **Genetic factors**—More than a dozen forms of cancer are known to be directly inherited, perhaps involving abnormal "cancer genes" called **oncogenes** (ON-koh-jeens). The way in which every known oncogene works is not yet clearly understood and is likely to involve a number of different mechanisms. Other cancers may develop primarily in those people with genetic predispositions to specific forms of cancer. Cancers with known genetic risk factors include basal cell carcinoma (a type of skin cancer), breast cancer, and neuroblastoma (a cancer of nerve tissue). These cancers probably require a combination of the "at risk" version of a gene plus one or more environmental factors.

2. **Carcinogens** (kar-SIN-oh-jens)—Carcinogens ("cancer makers") are chemicals that affect genetic activity in some way, causing abnormal cell reproduction. Some carcinogens are **mutagens** (MYOO-tah-jens) ("mutation makers"). Mutagens cause changes in a cell's DNA structure. Although many industrial products such as benzene are known to be carcinogens, a wide variety of natural vegetable and animal materials are also carcinogenic.

3. **Age**—Certain cancers are found primarily in young people (for example, leukemia) and others primarily in older adults (for example, colon cancer). The age factor may result from changes in the genetic activity of cells over time or from accumulated effects of cell damage.

4. **Environment**—Exposure to damaging types of radiation or chronic mechanical injury can cause cancer. For example, sunlight can cause skin cancer, and breathing asbestos fibers can cause lung cancer. Also, exposure to high concentrations of certain metals such as nickel or chromium can cause tumors to develop.

5. **Viruses**—Several cancers have now been identified as having a viral origin. This makes sense because we know that viruses often change the genetic machinery of infected cells. For example, human papillomaviruses have been found to have a causal relationship in some cases of cervical cancer in women and penile cancer in men.

BOX 5-2

THE WARNING SIGNS OF CANCER

Sores that do not heal
Unusual bleeding
A change in a wart or mole
A lump or thickening in any tissue
Persistent hoarseness or cough
Chronic indigestion
A change in bowel or bladder function
Bone pain that wakes one at night and is located on only one side

---

Pathogenesis of Cancer

Signs of cancer include those a person would expect of a malignant neoplasm—the appearance of abnormal, rapidly growing tissue. Cancer specialists, or *oncologists*, have summarized some major signs of early stages of cancer. These signs are listed in Box 5-2.

Early detection of cancer is important because in the early stages of development of primary tumors, before metastasis and the development of secondary tumors has begun, cancer is most treatable. Some methods currently used to detect the presence of cancer include the following:

1. **Self-examination**—Examining the self for the early signs of cancer is one method of detection. For example, women are encouraged to perform a monthly breast self-examination. Likewise, men are encouraged to perform a monthly testicular self-examination. If an abnormality is found, it can be further investigated with one of the methods described later. Self-examination of the skin and other accessible organs or tissues is also recommended by cancer specialists.

2. **Diagnostic imaging**—A variety of methods are available for forming images of internal body organs to detect tumors without exploratory surgery. **Radiography** is the oldest and still the most widely used method of noninvasive imag-

ing of internal body structures. Radiography is the use of *x-rays* to form a still or moving picture of some of the internal tissues of the body. A *mammogram*, for example, is an x-ray photograph of a breast. Potentially cancerous lumps show up as small, white areas on the mammogram (Figure 5-12, *A*). **Computed tomography (CT)** scanning is a type of radiography in which x-rays produce a cross-sectional image of body regions (Figure 5-12, *B*). **Magnetic resonance imaging (MRI)** is a type of scanning that uses a magnetic field to induce tissues to emit radio waves. Different tissues can be distinguished because each emits different signals. With MRI, tumors can then be visualized on a computer screen in cross sections similar to

those produced in CT scanning (Figure 5-12, *C*). MRI is also sometimes called *nuclear magnetic resonance (NMR)* imaging. In **ultrasonography,** high-frequency sound waves can be reflected off internal tissues to produce images, or *sonograms,* of tumors (Figure 5-12, *D*). For more detailed information regarding medical imaging, refer to the box below and on p. 123.

3. **Biopsy**—After a neoplasm has been identified with one of the previously mentioned techniques, a biopsy of the tumor may be done. Biopsy of an accessible tumor may precede or even eliminate the need for extensive medical imaging. A biopsy is the removal and examination of living tissue. Microscopic examination of tumor tissue re-

CLINICAL APPLICATION

MEDICAL IMAGING OF THE BODY

Cadavers (preserved human bodies used for scientific study) can be cut into sagittal, frontal, or transverse sections for easy viewing of internal structures, but living bodies, of course, cannot. This limitation has hampered medical professionals who strive to determine whether internal organs are injured or diseased. In some cases the only sure way to detect a *lesion* or variation from normal is by performing extensive *exploratory surgery*. Fortunately, recent advances in medical imaging allow physicians to visualize internal structures of the body without risking the trauma or other complications associated with extensive surgery. Some of the more widely used techniques are briefly described here.

Radiography

Radiography, or x-ray photography, is the oldest and still most widely used method of noninvasive imaging of internal body structures. The boxed essay on p. 96 discusses the origins of radiography. With this method, energy in the x band of the radiation spectrum is beamed through the body and onto photographic film (Figure **A**). The x-ray photograph shows the outlines of the bones and other dense structures that partially absorb the x-rays. In *fluoroscopy,* a phosphorescent screen sensitive to x-rays is used instead of photographic film. A visible image is formed on the screen as x-rays passing through the subject cause the screen to glow. Fluoroscopy allows a medical professional to view the internal structures of the subject's body in present time as it moves. Without enhancement aids, radiography works best as a tool to view solid objects such as bones. One way to make soft, hollow structures such as blood vessels or digestive organs more visible is to use

radiopaque contrast media. Substances such as barium sulfate that absorb x-rays are injected into or swallowed by the patient to fill the hollow organ of interest. As the screen in Figure **A** shows, the hollow organ then shows up as distinctly as a dense bone.

Computed Tomography

A newer variation of traditional x-ray photography is **computed tomography (CT)** or computed axial tomography (CAT) scanning. In this method, a device with an x-ray source on one side of the body and an x-ray detector on the other side is rotated around a central axis of the subject's body (Figure **B**). Information from the x-ray detectors is interpreted by a computer, which generates a video image of the body as if it were cut into anatomical sections. The term *computed tomography* literally means "picturing a cut using a computer." Because CT scanning and other recent advances in diagnostic imaging produce images of the body as if it were actually cut into sections, it has become especially important for students of the health sciences to become familiar with *sectional anatomy,* which is the study of the structural relationships visible in anatomical sections.

Magnetic Resonance Imaging

Magnetic resonance imaging (MRI) is a type of scanning that uses a magnetic field to induce tissues to emit radiofrequency (RF) waves. An RF detector coil senses the waves and sends the information to a computer that constructs sectional images similar to those produced in CT scanning (Figure **C**). Different tissues can be distinguished from each other because each emits different radio signals. MRI, also called *nuclear magnetic resonance (NMR)* imaging, avoids the use of potentially harmful x radiation and often produces sharper images of soft tissues than other imaging methods.

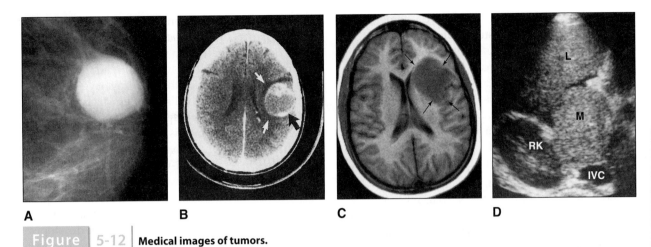

Figure 5-12 | **Medical images of tumors.**

A, A mammogram showing carcinoma of a breast duct. **B,** CT scan of the brain showing a tumor in the left hemisphere. **C,** MR image of the brain showing a tumor in the left hemisphere. **D,** Sonogram showing a transverse view of an abdominal tumor. *IVC,* inferior vena cava; *L,* liver; *M,* mass; *RK,* right kidney.

Ultrasonography

During **ultrasonography,** high-frequency (ultrasonic) waves are reflected off internal tissues to produce an image called a *sonogram* (Figure **D**). Because it does not involve x radiation, and because it is relatively inexpensive and easy to use, ultrasonography has been used extensively—especially in studying maternal or fetal structures in pregnant women. However, the image produced is not nearly as clear or sharp as those produced by MRI, CT scanning, or traditional radiography.

Variations of these and other technological advances that have improved the ability to study the structure and functions of the human body are discussed more in later chapters.

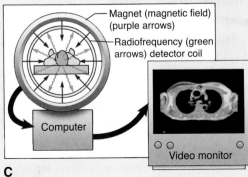

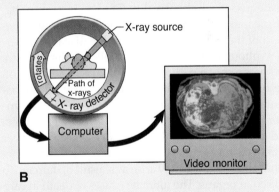

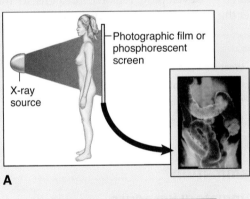

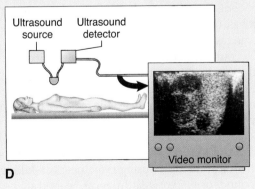

moved surgically or through a needle sometimes reveals whether the tissue is malignant or benign. A very simple, noninvasive type of biopsy used to detect some types of cancer involves simply scraping cells from an exposed surface and smearing them on a glass microscope slide. For example, the *Papanicolaou* (pah-pah-NI-kah-lah-oo) *test* or "Pap smear" is a common screening procedure in which cells from the neck of the uterus (cervix) are examined (see Chapter 22).

4. **Blood test**—Changes in the concentration of normal blood components, such as ions or enzymes, sometimes can indicate cancer. Cancer cells also may produce or trigger production of abnormal substances—substances often referred to as *tumor markers*. For example, bone cancer and some other malignancies can elevate the blood concentration of calcium ions (Ca^{++}) above normal levels. Blood tests to help detect tumor markers of prostate and other cancers are being developed and introduced.

The information gained from these and other techniques can be used to *stage* and *grade* malignant tumors. Staging involves classifying a tumor based on its size and the extent of its spread. Grading is an assessment of what the tumor is likely to do based on the degree of cell abnormality. Grading is a useful basis for making a **prognosis** (prog-NO-sis), or statement of the probable outcome of the disease.

Without treatment, cancer usually results in death. The progress of a particular type of cancer depends on the type of cancer and its location. Many cancer patients suffer from **cachexia** (kah-KEK-see-ah), a syndrome involving loss of appetite, severe weight loss, and general weakness. The cause of cachexia in cancer patients is uncertain. A variety of anatomical or functional abnormalities may arise as a result of damage to particular organs. The ultimate causes of death in cancer patients include secondary infection by pathogenic microbes, organ failure, hemorrhage (blood loss), and in some cases, undetermined factors.

Of course, after cancer has been identified, every effort is made to treat it and thus prevent or delay its development. Surgical removal of cancerous tumors is preferable; although for anatomic reasons, that is not always possible. Even with surgical removal, the possibility that malignant cells have been left behind must be addressed. **Chemotherapy** (kee-moh-THAYR-ah-pee), or "chemical therapy," using *cytotoxic* ("cell-killing") compounds or *antineoplastic* drugs can be used after sur-

gery to destroy any remaining malignant cells. **Radiation therapy,** also called *radiotherapy,* using destructive x-ray or gamma radiation may be used alone or with chemotherapy to destroy remaining cancer cells. Chemotherapy and radiation therapy may have severe side effects because normal cells are often killed along with the cancer cells. **Laser therapy,** in which an intense beam of light destroys a tumor, is also sometimes performed in addition to chemotherapy or radiation therapy.

Immunotherapy (im-yoo-no-THAYR-ah-pee), a newer type of cancer treatment, bolsters the body's own defenses against cancer cells. Because viruses cause some types of cancer, oncologists hope that vaccines against certain forms of cancer will be developed. Another newer approach is the use of *rational drugs* in chemotherapy. Rational drugs are those that target only specific molecules, enzymes, or receptors unique to cancer cells or tumor growth, thereby affecting only the cancer and sparing the normal cells. Rational drugs thus increase the efficiency of chemotherapy and reduce its side effects.

Although new and different approaches to cancer treatment are being investigated, many researchers are concentrating on improving existing methods and promoting cancer prevention. Despite progress in reducing cancers in developed countries, the steep rise in smoking in developing regions threatens to make cancer the major killer worldwide.

QUICK CHECK

1. What is metastasis?
2. Give examples of the four major types of tumors.
3. Name five general causes of cancer.
4. How is cancer treated?

Inflammation

Inflammatory Response

The **inflammatory response** is a combination of processes that attempt to minimize injury to tissues, thus maintaining homeostasis. Inflammation may occur as a response to any tissue injury, including mechanical injuries such as cuts and burns or damage caused by many other irritants such as chemicals, radiation, or toxins released by bacteria. The processes of inflammation eventually eliminate the irritant, after which tissue repair can begin.

As you learned in Chapter 3, tissue repair is the replacement of dead cells with living cells. In a type of tissue repair called *regeneration*, the new cells are similar to those that they replace. Another type of tissue repair is *replacement*. In replacement, the new cells are different from those that they replace, resulting in a scar. Often, *fibrous* tissue replaces the old tissue, a condition called *fibrosis*. Most tissue repairs are a combination of regeneration and replacement.

Inflammation also may accompany specific immune system reactions (which are discussed in Chapter 15). First described by a Roman physician almost 2000 years ago, the inflammatory response has four primary signs—redness, heat, swelling, and pain. These signs are indicators of a complex process that is summarized in the following paragraphs and in Figures 5-13 and 5-14.

As tissue cells are damaged, they release **inflammation mediators** such as *histamine, prostaglandins,* and compounds called *kinins*. Some inflammation mediators cause blood vessels to dilate (widen), increasing blood volume in the tissue. Increased blood volume produces the redness and heat of inflammation. This response is important because it allows

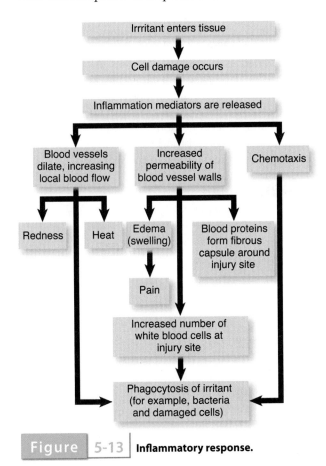

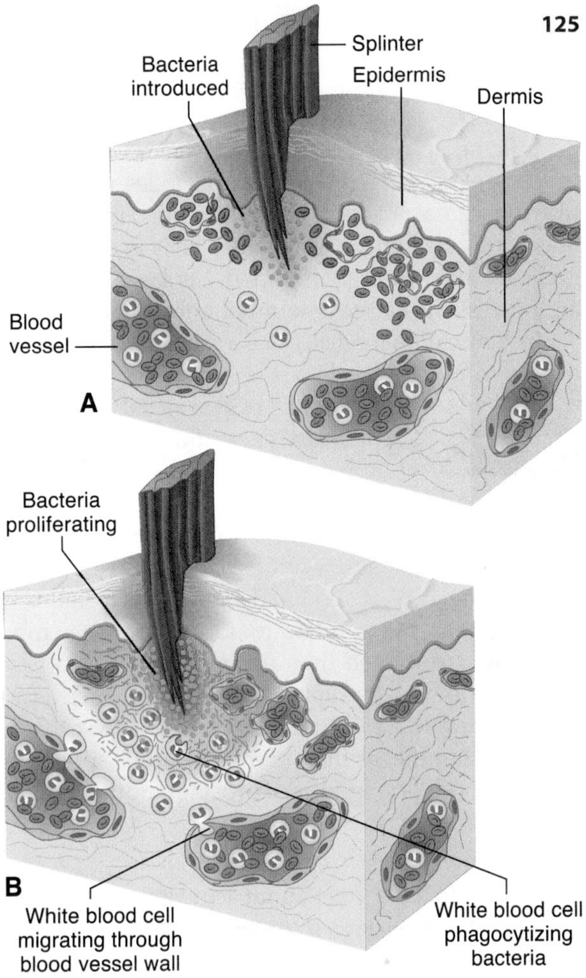

Figure 5-14 **Typical inflammatory response to a mechanical injury.**

A, A splinter damages tissue and carries bacteria into the body. Blood vessels dilate and begin leaking fluids, causing swelling and redness. **B,** White blood cells are attracted to the injury site and begin to consume bacteria and damaged tissue cells. A fibrous capsule separates the injury site from surrounding tissue.

immune system cells (white blood cells) in the blood to travel quickly and easily to the site of injury.

Some inflammation mediators increase the permeability of blood vessel walls. This allows immune system cells and other blood components to move out of the blood vessels easily where they can deal directly with injured tissue. As water leaks out of the vessel, tissue swelling, or **edema** (ed-EE-mah), results. The pressure caused by edema triggers pain receptors, consciously alerting an individual of the damage. The excess fluid often has the beneficial effect of diluting the irritant. The fluid that accumulates in inflamed tissue is called **inflammatory exudate** (EKS-oo-dayt). Blood proteins that leak into tissue spaces begin to clot within a few minutes. The clot forms a fibrous capsule

Figure 5-13 | **Inflammatory response.**

around the injury site, preventing the irritant from spreading to nearby tissues.

Inflammatory exudate is slowly removed by lymphatic vessels and is carried to lymph nodes, which act as filters. Bacteria and damaged cells trapped in the lymph nodes are acted on by white blood cells in each lymph node. In some cases, lymph nodes enlarge when they are processing a large amount of infectious material.

Inflammation mediators also can act as signals that attract white blood cells to the injury site. The movement of white blood cells in response to chemical attractants is called **chemotaxis** (kee-moh-TAK-sis). Once in the tissue, white blood cells often consume damaged cells and pathogenic bacteria by means of *phagocytosis*. When the inflammatory exudate becomes thick with the accumulation of white blood cells, dead tissue and bacterial cells, and other debris, **pus** is formed.

Occasionally, the inflammatory response is more intense or prolonged than desirable. In such a case, inflammation can be suppressed by drugs such as antihistamines or aspirin. Antihistamines block the action of histamine, as their name implies. Aspirin disrupts the body's synthesis of prostaglandins, a group of inflammation mediators.

 To learn more about acute inflammatory response, go to **AnimationDirect** on your CD.

Inflammatory Disease

Although many inflammation events are *local*, some affect the entire body, producing *systemic* inflammation. Local inflammation occurs when damage caused by an irritant remains isolated in a limited area, as in a small cut that becomes infected. Systemic inflammation occurs when the irritant spreads widely throughout the body or when inflammation mediators cause changes throughout the body.

One example of a systemic (body-wide) manifestation of the inflammatory response is a **fever.** The irritant or inflammation mediators can cause the "thermostat" of the brain to reset at a higher temperature. Instead of the normal body temperature, the body achieves and maintains a new, higher temperature. Increased temperature often kills or inhibits pathogenic microbes. Some pathophysiologists also believe that the higher temperature enhances the activity of the immune system. Fevers usually subside or "break" after the irritant has been eliminated. Fevers also can be reduced by drugs that block the fever-producing agents.

The fever response in children and in the elderly often differs from that in the normal adult. Young children often develop very high temperatures in response to mild infections as compared with adults, sometimes causing *seizures* (abnormal brain activity). Elderly people often have reduced or absent fever responses during infections, which may reduce their ability to resist the infectious agent.

Acute inflammation is an immediate, protective response that promotes elimination of an irritant and subsequent tissue repair. Occasionally, chronic inflammatory conditions occur. Chronic inflammation, whether local or systemic, is always damaging to affected tissues. Thus conditions involving chronic inflammation are classified as *inflammatory diseases.* Although some inflammatory diseases are caused by known pathogens or by an abnormal immune response (allergy or autoimmunity), the causes of many of them are uncertain. Inflammatory conditions such as arthritis, asthma, eczema, and chronic bronchitis are among the most common chronic diseases in the world.

QUICK CHECK

1. What are the four principal signs of inflammation?
2. What is the role of an *inflammation mediator*?
3. What happens in the body to cause a *fever*?

Outline Summary

 To download an MP3 version of the chapter summary for use with your iPod or portable media player, access the **Audio Chapter Summaries** on your CD.

Studying Disease

A. Disease terminology
   1. Health—physical, mental, and social well-being—not merely the absence of disease
   2. Disease—an abnormality in body function that threatens health
   3. Etiology—the study of the factors that cause a disease
   4. Idiopathic—refers to a disease with an unknown cause
   5. Signs and symptoms—the objective and subjective abnormalities associated with a disease

6. Pathogenesis—the pattern of a disease's development
B. Patterns of disease
1. Epidemiology is the study of occurrence, distribution, and transmission of diseases in human populations
2. Endemic diseases are native to a local region
3. Epidemics occur when a disease affects many people at the same time
4. Pandemics are widespread, perhaps global, epidemics
5. Discovering the cause of a disease is difficult because many factors affect disease transmission
6. Disease can be fought through prevention and therapy (treatment)

Pathophysiology

A. Mechanisms of disease
1. Pathophysiology—the study of underlying physiological aspects of disease
2. Genetic mechanism
3. Infectious mechanism (pathogenic organisms and particles)
4. Neoplastic mechanism (tumors and cancer)
5. Traumatic mechanism (physical and chemical agents)
6. Metabolic mechanism (endocrine imbalances or malnutrition)
7. Inflammatory mechanism
   a. Autoimmunity
   b. Inflammation
8. Degeneration
B. Risk factors (predisposing conditions)
1. Genetic factors
2. Age
3. Lifestyle
4. Stress
5. Environmental factors
6. Preexisting conditions

Pathogenic Organisms and Particles

A. Viruses (Table 5-1 and Figure 5-4)
1. Microscopic, intracellular parasites that consist of a nucleic acid core with a protein coat
2. Invade host cells and pirate organelles and raw materials
3. May be transmitted directly from human to human, or may be transmitted indirectly through a biting insect
4. Classified by shape, nucleic acid type, and method of reproduction

B. Prions (Figure 5-5)
1. Pathogenic protein molecules
2. Convert normal proteins to abnormal proteins, causing abnormal functions that produce disease; may be passed on to offspring
3. Cause rare, degenerative disorders of the nervous system such as BSE (bovine spongiform encephalopathy) and vCJD (variant Creutzfeldt-Jakob disease)
C. Bacteria (Table 5-2 and Figure 5-6)
1. Tiny cells without nuclei
2. Secrete toxins, parasitize host cells, or form colonies
3. Classification
   a. By growth requirements
      (1) Aerobic—require oxygen
      (2) Anaerobic—require no oxygen
   b. By staining properties (depend on composition of cell wall)
      (1) Gram-positive
      (2) Gram-negative
   c. By shape and size
      (1) Bacilli—rod-shaped cells
      (2) Cocci—round cells
      (3) Curved or spiral rods
      (4) Small bacteria—obligate parasites
   d. Spores—nonreproducing forms of bacteria that resist unfavorable environmental conditions
   e. Archaea are similar to bacteria but have a different chemical makeup and different metabolism (allowing them to survive harsh conditions); none found that infect humans
D. Fungi (Table 5-3 and Figure 5-7)
1. Simple organisms similar to plants but lacking chlorophyll
2. Yeasts—small, single-celled fungi
3. Molds—large, multicellular fungi
4. Mycotic infections—often resist treatment
E. Protozoa (Table 5-4 and Figure 5-8)
1. Large, one-celled organisms having organized nuclei
2. May infest human fluids and parasitize or destroy cells
3. Major groups
   a. Amoebas—possess pseudopodia
   b. Flagellates—possess flagella
   c. Ciliates—possess cilia
   d. Sporozoa (coccidia)—enter cells during one phase of a two-part life cycle; borne by vectors (transmitters) during the other phase

F. Pathogenic animals (Table 5-5)
  1. Large, complex multicellular organisms
  2. Parasitize or otherwise damage human tissues or organs
  3. Major groups
    a. Nematodes—roundworms
    b. Platyhelminths—flatworms and flukes
    c. Arthropods
      (1) Parasitic mites, ticks, lice, fleas
      (2) Biting or stinging wasps, bees, mosquitoes, spiders
      (3) Are often vectors of disease

Prevention and Control

A. Mechanisms of transmission
  1. Person-to-person contact
    a. Can be prevented by education
    b. Can be prevented by using aseptic technique (Table 5-6)
  2. Environmental contact
    a. Can be prevented by avoiding contact
    b. Can be prevented by safe sanitation practices
  3. Opportunistic invasion
    a. Can be prevented by avoiding changes in skin and mucous membranes
    b. Can be prevented by cleansing of wounds
  4. Transmission by a vector
    a. Can be prevented by reducing the population of vectors and reducing contact with vectors
B. Other prevention and treatment strategies
  1. Vaccination—stimulates immunity
  2. Chemicals—destroy or inhibit pathogens
    a. Antibiotics—natural compounds derived from living organisms
    b. Synthetic compounds (for example, ACV and efavirenz)

Tumors and Cancer

A. Neoplasms (tumors)—abnormal growths of cells
  1. Benign tumors remain localized
  2. Malignant tumors spread, forming secondary tumors
  3. Metastasis—cells leave a primary tumor and start a secondary tumor at a new location (Figure 5-11)
  4. Classification of tumors

    a. Benign, epithelial tumors
      (1) Papilloma—fingerlike projection
      (2) Adenoma—glandular tumor
      (3) Nevus—small, pigmented tumor
    b. Benign, connective tissue tumors
      (1) Lipoma—adipose (fat) tumor
      (2) Osteoma—bone tumor
      (3) Chondroma—cartilage tumor
    c. Carcinomas (malignant epithelial tumors)
      (1) Melanoma—involves melanocytes
      (2) Adenocarcinoma—glandular cancer
    d. Sarcomas (connective tissue cancers)
      (1) Lymphoma—lymphatic cancer
      (2) Osteosarcoma—bone cancer
      (3) Myeloma—bone marrow tumor
      (4) Fibrosarcoma—cancer of fibrous tissue
B. Causes of cancer—varied and still not clearly understood
  1. Cancer involves hyperplasia (growth of too many cells) and anaplasia (development of undifferentiated cells)
  2. Factors known to play a role in causing cancer
    a. Genetic factors (for example, oncogenes—cancer genes)
    b. Carcinogens—chemicals that alter genetic activity
    c. Age—changes in cell activity over time or accumulated effects of cell damage
    d. Environment—chronic exposure to damaging substances
    e. Viruses—cause change in genetic "machinery"
C. Pathogenesis of cancer
  1. Signs of cancer
  2. Methods of detecting cancers (Figure 5-12)
    a. Self-examination
    b. Diagnostic imaging—radiography (for example, mammogram and CT scan), magnetic resonance imaging (MRI), ultrasonography
    c. Biopsy (for example, Pap smear)
    d. Blood tests
  3. Staging—classifying tumors by size and extent of spread
  4. Grading—assessing the likely pattern of a tumor's development
  5. Cachexia—syndrome including appetite loss, weight loss, and general weakness

6. Causes of death by cancer—secondary infections, organ failure, hemorrhage, and undetermined factors
7. Treatments
   a. Surgery
   b. Chemotherapy (chemical therapy)
   c. Radiation therapy (radiotherapy)
   d. Laser therapy
   e. Immunotherapy
   f. New strategies (for example, rational drugs that target specific molecules, enzymes, or receptors)

Inflammation

A. Inflammatory response—reduces injury to tissues, thus maintaining homeostasis (Figures 5-13 and 5-14)
   1. Signs—redness, heat, swelling, and pain

2. Inflammation mediators (histamine, prostaglandins, and kinins)
   a. Some cause blood vessels to dilate, increasing blood volume (redness and heat)—white blood cells travel quickly to injury site
   b. Some increase blood vessel permeability (causing swelling, or edema, and pain)—white blood cells move easily out of vessels, irritant is diluted, and exudate accumulates
   c. Some attract white blood cells to injury site (chemotaxis)
B. Inflammatory diseases
   1. Inflammation can be local or systemic (body-wide)
   2. Fever—high body temperature caused by a resetting of the body's "thermostat"—destroys pathogens and enhances immunity
   3. Chronic inflammation can constitute a disease itself because it causes damage to tissues

New Words

Review the names of organ systems and individual organs in Figures 4-1 through 4-12.

amoeba
archaea
arthropod
autoimmunity
bacillus (*pl.*, bacilli)
bacterium (*pl.*, bacteria)
bioterrorism
chemotaxis
ciliate
coccus (*pl.*, cocci)
edema
epidemiology
flagellate
flagellum (*pl.*, flagella)
fungus (*pl.*, fungi)
inflammation
inflammation mediators
inflammatory exudate
inflammatory response
microbe
mycotic infection
nematode
oncogene

parasite
pathogenesis
pathophysiology
platyhelminth
prion
protozoa
psychogenic
pus
risk factor
spore
sporozoa
vector
virus

Diseases and Other Clinical Terms

acute
adenocarcinoma
adenoma
anaplasia
anthrax
antibiotic
aseptic technique
benign
biopsy
cachexia
carcinogen
carcinoma

chemotherapy
chlamydia
chondroma
chronic
communicable
computed tomography (CT)
culture
endemic
epidemic
etiology
fever
fibrosarcoma
Gram-staining technique
hyperplasia
idiopathic
immunotherapy
incubation
infectious
laser therapy
lipoma
lymphoma
magnetic resonance imaging (MRI)
malignant
melanoma
metastasis
morbidity
mortality

mutagen
myeloma
neoplasm
nevus
osteoma
osteosarcoma
pandemic
papilloma
prognosis
radiation therapy
remission
rickettsia
sarcoma
severe acute respiratory syndrome (SARS)
sign
spongiform encephalopathy (MSE; "mad cow disease")
symptom
syndrome
tumor
ultrasonography
vaccine
variant Creutzfeldt-Jakob disease (vCJD)
West Nile virus (WNV)

Review Questions

1. Define or explain the following terms: etiology, idiopathic, communicable, latent or incubation period.
2. What is the difference between an *epidemic* and a *pandemic*. What factor makes pandemics increasingly common in modern times?
3. List four factors involved in the spread of disease.
4. List the eight mechanisms of disease.
5. What is a risk factor?
6. List the six risk factors discussed in the chapter.
7. Describe a virus. How does a virus damage a cell?
8. Briefly describe a bacterium. List the ways in which bacteria produce disease.
9. Distinguish between anaerobic and aerobic bacteria.
10. Name the shapes and sizes used to classify bacteria. Which of these include the obligate parasites?
11. Describe fungi. Distinguish between yeasts and molds.
12. Describe protozoa. List the four major groups of protozoa.
13. Name and give an example of each of the pathogenic animals. Which of the arthropods are parasitic? What is a vector?
14. List the four ways disease can be spread.
15. Distinguish between *malignant* and *benign* tumors.
16. List the three benign tumors that arise from epithelial tissue.
17. List the three benign tumors that arise from connective tissue.
18. What are sarcomas? List the four sarcomas discussed in the chapter.
19. List the five factors that are known to play a role in the development of cancer. What is a mutagen?
20. List the four methods used to detect the presence of cancer.
21. List four methods of cancer treatment.
22. What are the four primary signs of inflammation? What causes each of them?
23. What is chemotaxis?
24. What are two positive effects of fever?

Critical Thinking

25. The doctor noticed a rash on a boy's arm. The boy complained that the rash itched. Which of these was a sign? Which was a symptom? What is the difference between the two?
26. Of the risk factors listed in the text, which can you change, and which can't you change?
27. Why do bacteria that form spores present a greater health risk than those that do not form spores?
28. Explain the difference in function between an antibiotic and a vaccine.

Chapter Test

1. _____ are objective abnormalities that can be seen or measured.
2. _____ are subjective abnormalities felt only by the patient.
3. A disease with an undetermined cause is said to be _____.
4. A _____ affects a larger geographical region than does an epidemic.
5. _____ is an attenuated pathogen given to a person to stimulate immunity.
6. A _____ tumor tends to spread to other regions of the body.
7. _____ is a process by which cancer cells are spread by lymphatic or blood vessels.
8. _____ are malignant tumors that arise from connective tissue.
9. _____ are malignant tumors that arise from epithelial tissue.
10. _____ a cause of cancer that damages or changes DNA structure.
11. The four primary signs of inflammation are _____, _____, _____, and _____.
12. Which of the following is not a risk factor for disease?
    a. Stress
    b. Genetic factors
    c. Age
    d. Autoimmunity
13. Which of the following is not a means by which pathogens can spread?
    a. Environmental contact

b. Vectors
c. Person-to-person contact
d. All of the above can spread pathogens
14. Treatment for cancer includes everything but:
a. biopsy
b. surgery
c. chemotherapy
d. all of the above are treatments for cancer

15. Which of the following is not an inflammation mediator?
a. Prostaglandins
b. Edema
c. Histamine
d. Kinins

Match the descriptions in Column A with the corresponding pathogenic organism in Column B.

Column A
16. _____ intracellular parasites made up of DNA or RNA and surrounded by a protein coat
17. _____ causes mycotic infections
18. _____ roundworms
19. _____ can be gram-positive or gram-negative
20. _____ causes malaria
21. _____ vector for Lyme disease
22. _____ insert their genetic code into the host's genetic code
23. _____ one-celled organism with a nucleus; can be a ciliate
24. _____ similar to plants but with no chlorophyll
25. _____ mites, lice, and fleas
26. _____ tiny primitive cells without nuclei; can be rod shaped
27. _____ flatworms and flukes
28. _____ can be bacilli or cocci shaped

Column B
a. virus
b. bacteria
c. fungus
d. protozoa
e. nematodes
f. platyhelminths
g. arthropods

Study Tips

continued from page 103
6. Meet with your study group early and often. This is not material you can master in one night. You may want to go over only one or two parts of the chapter per session.

Review definitions, flash cards, major concepts, questions at the end of the chapter, and possible test questions. Keep your study material for this chapter handy; you may wish to refer to it as you study future chapters.

Case Studies

1. Without warning, Mr. Lee begins to feel sick. His most obvious symptom is a high fever. Within 24 hours, everyone in the Lee household also feels sick and has a high temperature. Before long, nearby households have the same experience—many people in the community are now sick. The local health department would probably call on what type of health professional to investigate this situation? Would the health professional label this situation an epidemic or a pandemic? If the symptoms are caused by a bacterial infection, list some ways the pathogen could have been transmitted to so many people within a short span of time.
2. Sandy is a nurse at the local university hospital. One of her patients has a severe staphylococcal infection.

What would the pathogen responsible for this infection look like under a microscope? Sandy's patient is taking a newly developed antibiotic in the hope that it will cure the infection. Do you think that this drug is natural or synthetic?
3. Fred is a first-year medical student. He received a minor scrape during a basketball game on the parking lot outside his dorm. He has cleansed the wound and applied an antibiotic as a preventive measure. The affected area is red, swollen, and mildly painful. How do you explain these symptoms? Fred's roommate suggested applying an antiinflammatory drug to the wound, but Fred refuses. What advantage might Fred see in avoiding such treatment?

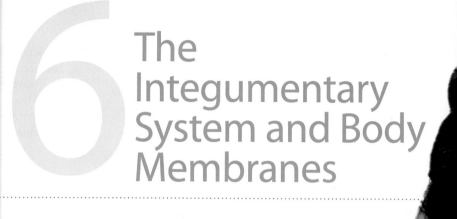

6

The Integumentary System and Body Membranes

Objectives

After you have completed this chapter, you should be able to:

1. Classify, compare the structure of, and give examples of each type of body membrane.

2. Describe the structure and function of the epidermis and dermis.

3. List and briefly describe each accessory organ of the skin.

4. List and discuss the three primary functions of the integumentary system.

5. List and describe major skin disorders and infections.

6. Classify burns and describe how to estimate the extent of a burn injury.

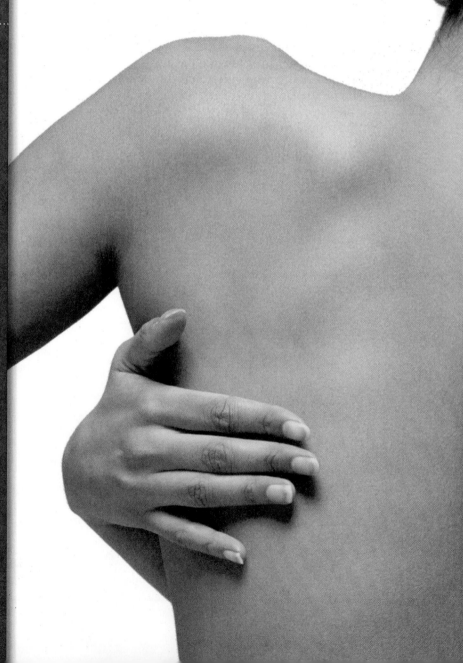

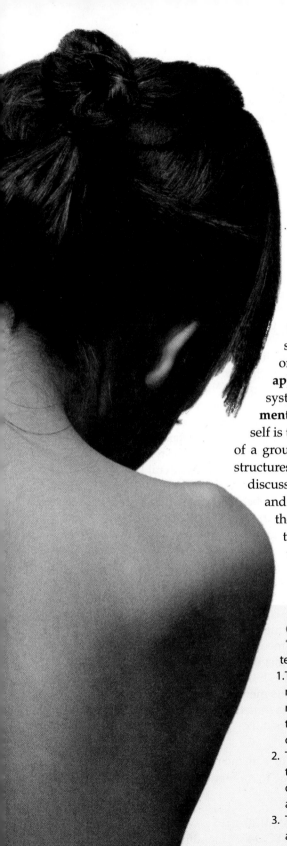

In Chapter 1 the concept of progressive organization of body structures from simple to complex was established. Complexity in body structure and function progresses from cells to tissues and then to organs and organ systems. This chapter discusses the skin and its **appendages**—the hair, the nails, and the skin glands—as an organ system. This system is called the **integumentary system. Integument** (in-TEG-yoo-ment) is another name for the skin, and the skin itself is the principal organ of the integumentary system. The skin is one of a group of anatomically simple but functionally important sheetlike structures called **membranes.** This chapter begins with classification and discussion of the important body membranes. Study of the structure and function of the integument follows. Ideally, you should study the skin and its appendages before proceeding to the more traditional organ systems in the chapters that follow to improve your understanding of how structure is related to function.

STUDY TIPS

Before starting your study of Chapter 6, go back to Chapter 4 and review the synopsis of the integumentary system.

1. The body membranes are either epithelial or connective. The epithelial membranes cover or protect. The difference between mucous and serous membranes is their location in the body. If the membrane is exposed to the environment, it is mucous membrane. Connective tissue membranes cover joints.

2. The skin is divided into two parts: epidermis and dermis. *Epi-* means "on," so the epidermis is *on* the dermis. The job of the epidermis is protection. The dermis contains most of the skin appendages: nails, sense receptors, hair, and glands.

3. The functions of the skin are related to its location: protection, sensation, and heat regulation.

4. Burns are classified by how much damage has been done and how deep the damage goes.

continued on page 161

Classification of Body Membranes

The term *membrane* refers to a thin, sheetlike structure that may have many important functions in the body. Membranes cover and protect the body surface, line body cavities, and cover the inner surfaces of the hollow organs such as the digestive, reproductive, and respiratory passageways. Some membranes anchor organs to each other or to bones, and others cover the internal organs. In certain areas of the body, membranes secrete lubricating fluids that reduce friction during organ movements such as the beating of the heart or lung expansion and contraction. Membrane lubricants also decrease friction between bones in joints. There are two major categories or types of body membranes:

1. **Epithelial membranes**, composed of epithelial tissue and an underlying layer of specialized connective tissue

2. **Connective tissue membranes**, composed exclusively of various types of connective tissue; no epithelial cells are present in this type of membrane

Epithelial Membranes

There are three types of epithelial tissue membranes in the body:

1. Cutaneous membrane

2. Serous membranes

3. Mucous membranes

CUTANEOUS MEMBRANE

The **cutaneous** (kyoo-TAY-nee-us) **membrane,** or **skin,** is the primary organ of the integumentary system. It is one of the most important and certainly one of the largest and most visible organs of the body. In most individuals the skin composes some 16% of the body weight. It fulfills the requirements necessary for an epithelial tissue membrane in that it has a superficial layer of epithelial cells and an underlying layer of supportive connective tissue. Its structure is uniquely suited to its many functions. The skin is discussed in depth later in the chapter.

SEROUS MEMBRANES

Serous (SEER-us) **membranes** are found only on surfaces within closed cavities. Like all epithelial membranes, a serous membrane is composed of two distinct layers of tissue. The epithelial sheet is a thin layer of simple squamous epithelium. The connective tissue layer forms a very thin, gluelike **basement membrane** that holds and supports the epithelial cells.

The serous membrane that lines body cavities and covers the surfaces of organs in those cavities is in reality a single, continuous sheet of tissue covering two different surfaces. The name of the serous membrane is determined by its location. Using this criterion results in two types of serous membranes; the first type lines body cavities, and the second type covers the organs within those cavities. The serous membrane, which lines the walls of a body cavity much like wallpaper covers the walls of a room, is called the **parietal** (pah-RYE-i-tal) **portion.** The other type of serous membrane, which covers the surface of organs found in body cavities, is called the **visceral** (VISS-er-al) **portion.**

The serous membranes of the thoracic and abdominal cavities are identified in Figure 6-1. In the thoracic cavity the serous membranes are called **pleura** (PLOOR-ah), and in the abdominal cavity, they are called **peritoneum** (pair-i-toh-NEE-um). Look again at Figure 6-1 to note the placement of the **parietal** and **visceral pleura** and the **parietal** and **visceral peritoneum.** In both cases the parietal layer forms the lining of the body cavity, and the visceral layer covers the organs found in that cavity.

Serous membranes secrete a thin, watery fluid that helps reduce friction and serves as a lubricant when organs rub against one another and against the walls of the cavities that contain them. **Pleurisy** (PLOOR-i-see) is a very painful pathological condition characterized by inflammation of the serous membranes (pleura) that line the chest cavity and cover the lungs. Pain is caused by irritation and friction as the lungs rub against the walls of the chest cavity. In severe cases the inflamed surfaces of the pleura fuse, and permanent damage may develop. The term **peritonitis** (pair-i-toh-NYE-tis) is used to describe inflammation of the serous membranes in the abdominal cavity. Peritonitis is sometimes a serious complication of an infected appendix.

 To learn more about serous membranes, go to **AnimationDirect** on your CD.

MUCOUS MEMBRANES

Mucous (MYOO-kus) **membranes** are epithelial membranes that line body surfaces opening directly to the exterior. Examples of mucous membranes include

Epithelial membranes

☐ Mucous membranes

☐ Cutaneous membrane (skin)

■ Serous membranes

  ■ *Parietal layer*

  ☐ *Visceral layer*

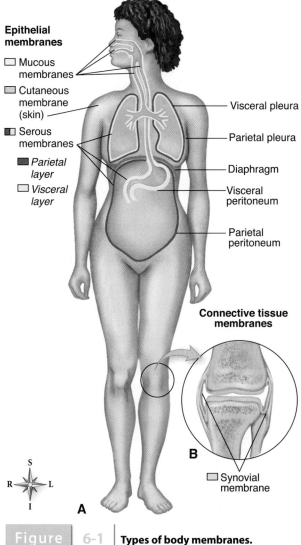

— Visceral pleura

— Parietal pleura

— Diaphragm

— Visceral peritoneum

— Parietal peritoneum

Connective tissue membranes

B

☐ Synovial membrane

A

Figure 6-1 **Types of body membranes.**

A, Epithelial membranes, including cutaneous membrane (skin), serous membranes (parietal and visceral pleura and peritoneum), and mucous membranes. **B,** Connective tissue membranes, including synovial membranes.

those lining the respiratory, digestive, urinary, and reproductive tracts. The epithelial component of a mucous membrane varies, depending on its location and function. In the esophagus, for example, a tough, abrasion-resistant stratified squamous epithelium is found. A thin layer of simple columnar epithelium covers the walls of the lower segments of the digestive tract.

The epithelial cells of most mucous membranes secrete a thick, slimy material called **mucus** that keeps the membranes moist and soft.

The term **mucocutaneous** (myoo-koh-kyoo-TAY-nee-us) **junction** is used to describe the transitional

area that serves as a point of "fusion" where skin and mucous membranes meet. Such junctions lack accessory organs such as hair or sweat glands that characterize the skin. These transitional areas are generally moistened by mucous glands within the body orifices, or openings, where these junctions are located. The eyelids, nasal openings, vulva, and anus have mucocutaneous junctions that may become sites of infection or irritation.

To learn more about mucous membranes, go to **AnimationDirect** on your CD.

Connective Tissue Membranes

Unlike cutaneous, serous, and mucous membranes, connective tissue membranes do not contain epithelial components. The **synovial** (si-NO-vee-all) **membranes** lining the spaces between bones and joints that move are classified as connective tissue membranes (Figure 6-1, *B*). These membranes are smooth and slick and secrete a thick and colorless lubricating fluid called **synovial fluid.** The membrane itself, with its specialized fluid, helps reduce friction between the opposing surfaces of bones in movable joints. Synovial membranes also line the small, cushionlike sacs called **bursae** (BER-see) found between moving body parts.

To learn more about connective tissue and synovial membrane, go to **AnimationDirect** on your CD.

QUICK CHECK

1. What are the four main types of membranes in the body?
2. Which of the body's membranes are types of epithelial membranes?
3. What fluid(s) is/are produced by each of the four main membrane types? What is the function of each fluid?

The Skin

The brief description of the skin in Chapter 4 (see pp. 81-82) identified it as not only the primary organ of the integumentary system but also as the largest and one of the most important organs of the body. Architecturally the skin is a marvel. Consider the incredible number of structures fitting into 1 square inch of skin: 500 sweat glands; more than 1000 nerve endings; yards of tiny blood vessels; nearly 100 oil or **sebaceous** (seh-BAY-shus) **glands**; 150 sensors for pressure, 75 for heat, 10 for cold; and millions of cells.

Structure of the Skin

The skin, or cutaneous membrane, is a sheetlike organ that covers the body and acts as a barrier between the internal and external environment. The skin is composed of two main layers (Figure 6-2):

1. The **epidermis** is the outermost layer of the skin. It is a relatively thin sheet of stratified squamous epithelium.
2. The **dermis** is the deeper of the two layers. It is thicker than the epidermis and is made up largely of connective tissue.

As you can see in Figure 6-2, the layers of the skin are supported by a thick layer of loose connective tissue and fat called **subcutane-**

ous (sub-kyoo-TAY-nee-us) **tissue,** or the **hypodermis** (hye-poh-DER-mis). Fat in the subcutaneous layer insulates the body from extremes of heat and cold. It also serves as a stored source of energy for the body and can be used as a food source if required. In addition, the subcutaneous tissue acts as a shock-absorbing pad and helps protect underlying tissues from injury caused by bumps and blows to the body surface.

EPIDERMIS

The tightly packed epithelial cells of the epidermis are arranged in many distinct layers. The cells of the innermost layer, called the **stratum germinativum** (STRA-tum jer-mi-nah-TYE-vum), undergo mitosis and reproduce themselves (see Figure 6-2). As they move toward the surface of the skin, these new cells "specialize" in ways that increase their ability to provide protection for the body tissues that lie below them. This ability is of critical clinical significance. It enables the skin to repair itself if it is injured. The self-repair-

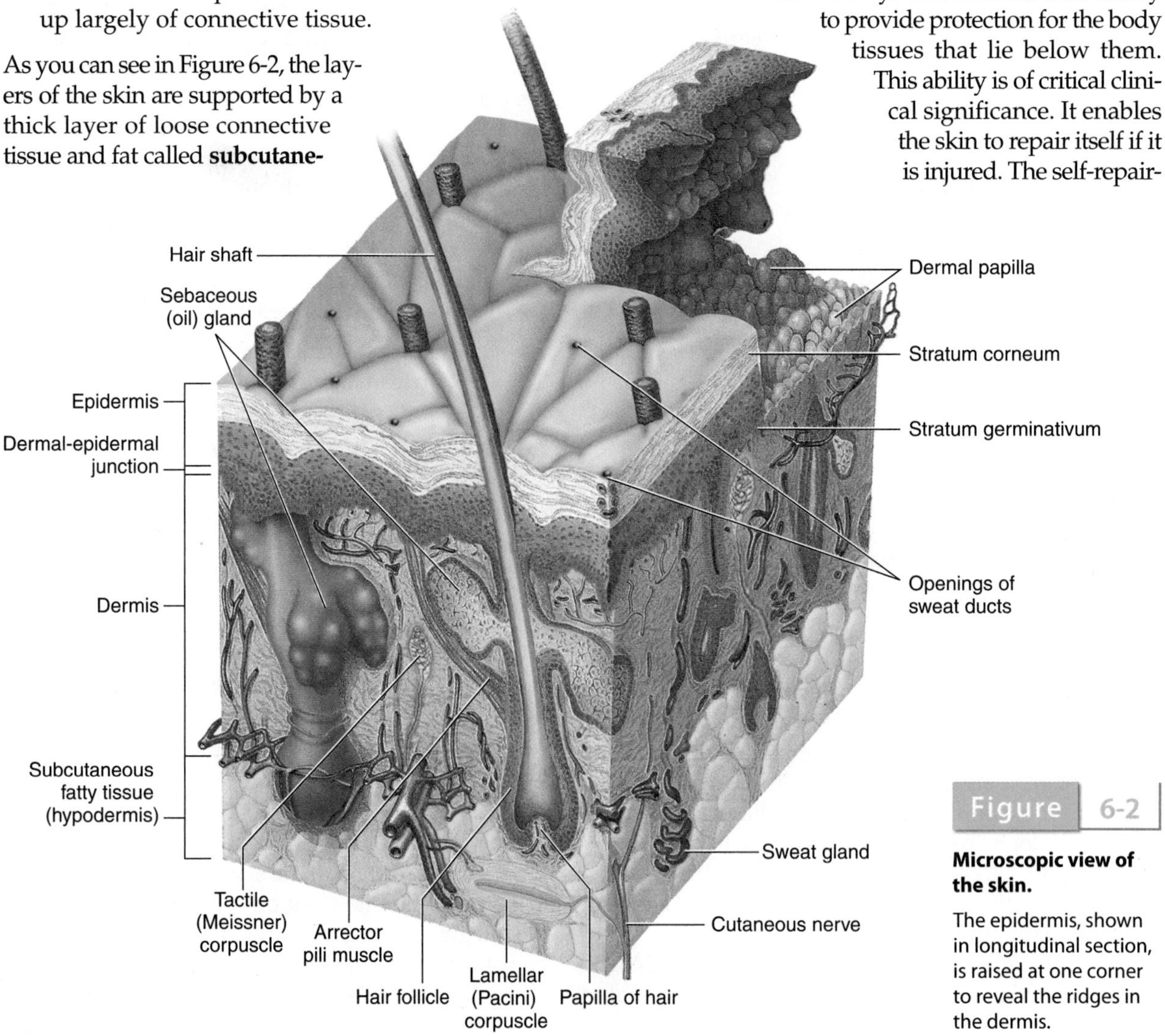

Hair shaft
Sebaceous (oil) gland
Epidermis
Dermal-epidermal junction
Dermis
Subcutaneous fatty tissue (hypodermis)
Tactile (Meissner) corpuscle
Arrector pili muscle
Hair follicle
Lamellar (Pacini) corpuscle
Papilla of hair
Sweat gland
Cutaneous nerve
Dermal papilla
Stratum corneum
Stratum germinativum
Openings of sweat ducts

Figure 6-2

Microscopic view of the skin.

The epidermis, shown in longitudinal section, is raised at one corner to reveal the ridges in the dermis.

CLINICAL APPLICATION

SUBCUTANEOUS INJECTION

Although the subcutaneous layer is not part of the skin, it carries the major blood vessels and nerves that supply the skin above it. The rich blood supply and loose, spongy texture of the subcutaneous layer make it an ideal site for the rapid and relatively pain-free absorption of injected material. Liquid medicines such as insulin and pelleted implant materials such as synthetic hormones are often administered by **subcutaneous injection** into this spongy and porous layer beneath the skin.

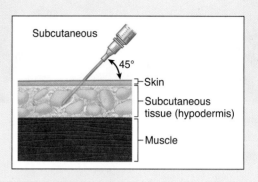

ing characteristic of normal skin makes it possible for the body to maintain an effective barrier against infection, even when it is subjected to injury and normal wear and tear. As new cells are produced in the deep layer of the epidermis, they move upward through additional layers, or "strata" of cells. As they approach the surface, the cytoplasm is replaced by one of nature's most unique proteins, a substance called **keratin** (KAIR-ah-tin). Keratin is a tough, waterproof material that provides cells in the outer layer of the skin with a horny, abrasion-resistant, and protective quality. The tough outer layer of the epidermis is called the **stratum corneum** (KOR-nee-um). Cells filled with keratin are continually pushed to the surface of the epidermis. In the photomicrograph of the skin shown in Figure 6-3, many of the outermost cells of the stratum corneum have been dislodged. These dry, dead cells filled with keratin "flake off" by the thousands onto our clothes and bedding, into our bathwater, and onto things we handle. Millions of epithelial cells reproduce daily to replace the millions shed—just one example of the work our bodies do without our knowledge, even when we seem to be resting.

The deepest cell layer of the epidermis identified in Figure 6-2 is the stratum germinativum. It is sometimes called the **pigment layer** because it is responsible for the production of a pigment called **melanin** (MEL-ah-nin) that gives color to the skin. The term *pigment* comes from a Latin word meaning "paint." The pigment-producing cells in this layer are called **melanocytes** (MEL-ah-no-sytes). The amount and type of melanin produced by these cells will determine skin color, which may vary from almost white to yellow, brown, reddish brown, or deep brown. Your skin color depends first on the skin color genes you have inherited. That is, hered-

ity determines your basic skin color and how dark or light it is. However, other factors such as sunlight exposure can modify this hereditary effect. Prolonged exposure to sunlight in light-skinned people darkens the exposed area because the exposure leads to increased melanin deposits in the epidermis.

If the skin contains little melanin, as under the nails where there is often no melanin at all, a change in color can occur if the volume of blood in the skin changes significantly or if the amount of oxygen in the blood is increased or decreased. In light-skinned individuals, increased blood flow to the skin or increased blood oxygen levels can cause a pink flush to appear. However, if blood oxygen levels decrease

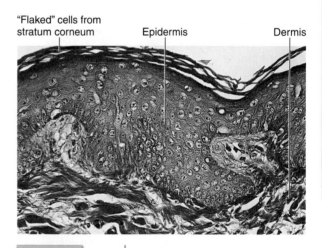

Figure 6-3 | **Photomicrograph of the skin.**

Many dead cells of the stratum corneum have flaked off from the surface of the epidermis. Note that the epidermis is very cellular. The dermis has fewer cells and more connective tissue.

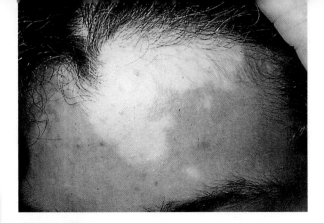

Figure 6-4 | **Vitiligo.**

Note the patchy loss of pigment on the face.

or if actual blood flow is reduced dramatically, the skin turns a bluish gray color—a condition called **cyanosis** (sye-ah-NO-sis). In general, the less abundant the melanin deposits in the skin, the more visible the changes in color caused by the change in skin blood volume or oxygen level. Conversely, the richer the skin's pigmentation, the less noticeable such changes will be.

The term **vitiligo** (vit-i-LYE-go) is used to describe a condition characterized by patchy looking areas of light skin resulting from the acquired loss of epidermal melanocytes. The term *vitiligo* is derived from the Greek word for calf. Early physicians compared the white spots caused by the loss of pigment to the patches often seen on calves. Although not as apparent in light-skinned individuals, the condition may be disfiguring in those with darker skin. About 50% of cases begin before age 20 and progress slowly over a period of years. The backs of the hands, face, genitalia, and body folds, including the axillae are often involved (see Figure 6-4 and Table 6-1). Most cases of vitiligo are apparently genetic in origin and occur in individuals who have no other associated findings. Occasionally, the condition is related to au-

Table 6-1 | **Common Skin Lesions**

LESION	DESCRIPTION	EXAMPLE
ELEVATED		
Papule	Firm, raised lesion (less than 1 cm in diameter)	Warts
Plaque	Large, raised lesion (greater than 1 cm in diameter)	Plaque caused by friction
Vesicle	Thin-walled blister filled with fluid that is smaller than 1 cm (a vesicle larger than 1 cm is a bulla)	Non-genital herpes vesicles
Pustule	Elevated lesion filled with pus	Acne

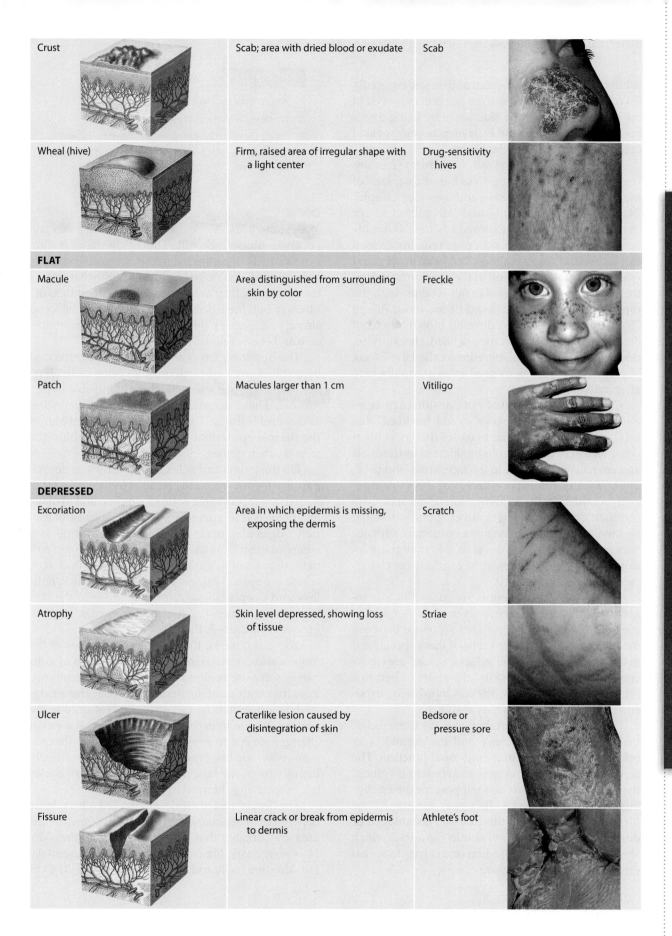

Crust		Scab; area with dried blood or exudate	Scab
Wheal (hive)		Firm, raised area of irregular shape with a light center	Drug-sensitivity hives

FLAT

Macule		Area distinguished from surrounding skin by color	Freckle
Patch		Macules larger than 1 cm	Vitiligo

DEPRESSED

Excoriation		Area in which epidermis is missing, exposing the dermis	Scratch
Atrophy		Skin level depressed, showing loss of tissue	Striae
Ulcer		Craterlike lesion caused by disintegration of skin	Bedsore or pressure sore
Fissure		Linear crack or break from epidermis to dermis	Athlete's foot

toimmune- or endocrine-related diseases, especially thyroid disorders. Some success has been achieved in darkening depigmented skin areas by using drugs and steroid hormones and by transplantation of skin epidermis containing melanocytes.

A hereditary condition called **albinism** (AL-bin-iz-em) is characterized by a partial or total lack of melanin pigment in the skin and eyes (see Chapter 24, p. 669). Affected individuals are subject to eye damage and sunburn if exposed to direct sunlight.

A normal increase in skin pigmentation caused by hormonal changes is almost universal in pregnant women. It is most common in the skin surrounding the nipples called the **areolae** (ah-REE-oh-lay), the nipples, and genital area. In addition, about 70% to 75% of pregnant women develop blotchy areas of brown pigmentation over the forehead, cheeks, nose, upper lip, and chin. It is sometimes called the "mask of pregnancy." The pigmented areas gradually fade after delivery.

One common variant of normal skin pigmentation is the small light brown or red **freckle** (Table 6-1). Freckles are small flat **macules** that most often occur as a genetic trait in light-skinned individuals and are usually confined to the face, arms, and back. In chronically sun-exposed areas of the skin, especially in older adults, brown-colored *"age spots"* are common. Incorrectly called "liver spots," these flat pigmented lesions become more numerous with advancing age. They may develop into malignant lesions and should be monitored carefully for changes in size and appearance.

The cells of the epidermis are packed tightly together. They are held firmly to one another and to the dermis below by specialized junctions between the membranes of adjacent cells. If these specialized links, sometimes described as "spot welds," are weakened or destroyed, the skin falls apart. When this occurs because of burns, friction injuries, or exposure to irritants, **blisters** may result.

The junction that exists between the thin epidermal layer of the skin above and the dermal layer below is called the **dermal-epidermal junction.** The area of contact between dermis and epidermis "glues" them together and provides support for the epidermis, which is attached to its upper surface. Blister formation also occurs if this junction is damaged or destroyed. The junction is visible in Figure 6-2, which shows the epidermis raised on one corner to reveal the underlying dermis more clearly.

QUICK CHECK

1. What are the two major layers of the skin?
2. Where in the skin would you find keratin?
3. How is the condition called *vitiligo* related to melanin?
4. Give two examples each of elevated, flat, and depressed skin lesions.

DERMIS

The dermis is the deeper of the two primary skin layers and is much thicker than the epidermis. It is composed largely of connective tissue. Instead of cells being crowded close together like the epithelial cells of the epidermis, they are scattered far apart, with many fibers in between. Some of the fibers are tough and strong (collagen or white fibers), and others are stretchable and elastic (elastic or yellow fibers).

The upper region of the dermis is characterized by parallel rows of peglike projections called **dermal papillae** (pah-PIL-ee), which are visible in Figure 6-2. These upward projections are interesting and useful features. They form an important part of the dermal-epidermal junction that helps bind the skin layers together.

On the palms and soles, distinct rows of dermal papillae form the roughly parallel *friction ridges* that help us to walk upright without slipping and to make and hold tools (Figure 6-5, *A*). The uniqueness of friction ridges also make possible fingerprinting as a means of identification. The palms and soles (and palmar surfaces of fingers and toes) possess *thick skin*, which is a special category of skin that is thick, hairless, and deeply ridged. However, most of the skin is *thin skin*, which has hair and irregular, shallow grooves (Figure 6-5, *B*).

You can observe these ridges on the tips of the fingers and on the skin covering the palms of your hands. Observe in Figure 6-2 how the epidermis follows the contours of the dermal papillae. These ridges develop sometime before birth. Not only is the pattern unique in each individual but also it never changes except to grow larger—two facts that explain why our fingerprints or footprints positively identify us. Many hospitals identify newborn babies by footprinting them soon after birth.

The deeper area of the dermis is filled with a dense network of interlacing fibers. Most of the fibers in this area are collagen that gives toughness to the skin. However, elastic fibers are also present. These make the skin stretchable and elastic (able to rebound). Dur-

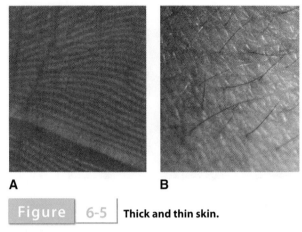

A   **B**

Figure   6-5 | **Thick and thin skin.**

A, Thick skin is hairless and has roughly parallel friction ridges.
B, Thin skin has hairs and shallow, irregular grooves.

ing pregnancy, the skin over a woman's abdomen may stretch beyond the ability of the elastic and connective tissue elements in the dermis to rebound. The result is creation of "stretch marks" called **striae** (STREYE-ay). Although they fade after delivery they never completely disappear (see Table 6-1). As we age, the number of elastic fibers in the dermis decreases, and the amount of fat stored in the subcutaneous tissue is reduced. Wrinkles develop as the skin loses elasticity, sags, and becomes less soft and pliant.

In addition to connective tissue elements, the dermis contains a specialized network of nerves and nerve endings to process sensory information such as pain, pressure, touch, and temperature. At various levels of the dermis, there are muscle fibers, hair follicles, sweat and sebaceous glands, and many blood vessels. Developmental malformation of dermal blood vessels can result in pigmented *birthmarks* in significant numbers of newborns. One of the most common (Figure 6-6) is a collection of dilated vessels that may initially appear as a bruise at birth and then grow rapidly during the first year into a bright red nodule called a **strawberry hemangioma** (hee-MAN-jee-OH-mah). A vast majority of these birthmarks shrink, fade, and disappear without treatment of any kind by age 7. Unfortunately, some pigmented vascular birthmarks, such as the **port-wine stain,** are permanent and do not fade with age. In these cases several types of laser-based therapy or use of specialized makeup can often provide effective cosmetic treatment. Dilation of dermal capillaries at the nape of the neck in a baby that occur during development

results in a birthmark called a **"stork bite"** in 50% to 70% of newborns. Although they often persist for life, these birthmarks generally are covered by hair and are inconspicuous.

Appendages of the Skin

HAIR
The human body is covered with millions of hairs. Indeed, at the time of birth most of the specialized structures called **follicles** (FOL-li-kuls) that are required for hair growth are already present. They develop early in fetal life and by birth are present in most parts of the skin. The hair of a newborn infant is extremely fine and soft; it is called **lanugo** (lah-NOO-go) from the Latin word meaning "down." In premature infants, lanugo may be noticeable over most of the body, but soon after birth the lanugo is lost and replaced by new hair that is stronger and more pigmented. Although only a few areas of the skin are hairless—notably the lips, the palms of the hands, and the soles of the feet—most body hair remains almost invisible. Hair is most visible on the scalp, eyelids, and eyebrows. The coarse hair that first appears in the pubic and axillary regions at the time of puberty develops in response to the secretion of hormones.

Hair growth begins when cells of the epidermal layer of the skin grow down into the dermis, forming a small tube called the **hair follicle.** The relationship of a hair follicle and its related structures to the

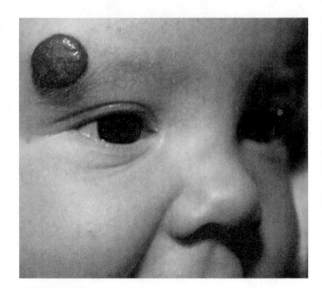

Figure   6-6 | **Strawberry hemangioma.**

epidermal and dermal layers of the skin is shown in Figure 6-2. Hair growth begins from a small, cap-shaped cluster of cells called the **hair papilla** (pah-PIL-ah), which is located in the larger hair bulb at the base of the follicle. The papilla is nourished by a dermal blood vessel. Note in Figure 6-2 that part of the hair, namely the *hair root,* lies hidden in the follicle. The visible part of a hair is called the *shaft.* Figure 6-7 shows shafts of hair extending from their follicles.

As long as cells in the papilla of the hair follicle remain alive, new hair will replace any that is cut or plucked. Contrary to popular belief, frequent cutting or shaving does not make hair grow faster or become coarser. Why? Because neither process affects the epithelial cells that form the hairs because the cells are embedded in the dermis.

Hair loss of any kind is called **alopecia** (al-oh-PEE-she-ah). Some forms of alopecia, such as *male pattern baldness* are not diseases but are simply inherited traits. Alopecia also may be a normal consequence of aging. Sudden loss of hair in round or oval "exclamation point" patches on the scalp, such as that seen in Figure 6-8, is called *alopecia areata.* It can occur without a known cause but is sometimes associated with certain metabolic or endocrine diseases. Scalp infections, che-

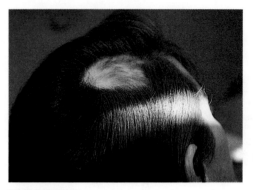

Figure 6-8 | **Alopecia areata.**

motherapy, radiation treatment, severe emotional or physical stress, and reactions to various types of drugs also can cause rapid hair loss. In most cases, regrowth of hair begins in 1 to 3 months, and the condition generally clears completely in 1 year without treatment. A significant number of women experience hair loss, especially on the front and sides of the scalp, 1 to 4 months after childbirth. The condition is called *postpartum* (*post*, after; + *partus*, birth) *alopecia.* As in alopecia areata, full regrowth of hair generally occurs in less than a year. Occasionally, and most often in young people, total loss of scalp hair occurs without apparent cause and in the absence of other findings. The condition, called *alopecia totalis* may be accompanied by cycles of partial hair regrowth and loss, but the chances for significant long-term regrowth are poor.

A tiny, smooth (involuntary) muscle can be seen in Figure 6-2. It is called an **arrector pili** (ah-REK-tor PYE-lye) muscle. It is attached to the base of a dermal papilla above and to the side of a hair follicle below. Generally, these muscles contract only when we are frightened or cold. When contraction occurs, each muscle simultaneously pulls on its two points of attachment (that is, up on a hair follicle but down on a part of the skin). This produces little raised places, called *goose pimples,* between the depressed points of the skin and at the same time pulls the hairs up until they are more or less straight.

Hair follicle   Shafts of hair   Stratum corneum cells

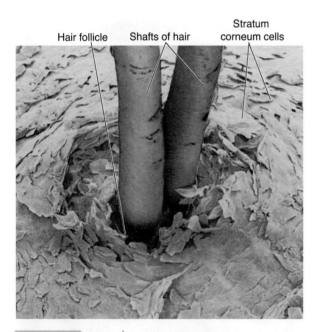

Figure 6-7 | **Hair shaft and follicle.**

Scanning electron micrograph showing shafts of hair extending from their follicles.

QUICK CHECK

1. What are dermal papillae? Why are they important?
2. What are birthmarks? List three types.
3. How is hair formed?
4. What is alopecia?

RECEPTORS

Receptors in the skin make it possible for the body surface to act as a sense organ, relaying messages to the brain concerning sensations such as touch, pain, temperature, and pressure. The receptors of the skin, which differ in structure from the highly complex to the very simple, are discussed in detail in Chapter 10. Two skin receptors are visible in Figure 6-2. One is a **lamellar (Pacini)** (pah-SIN-ee) **corpuscle**, which detects pressure deep in the dermis. The other is the more superficial **tactile (Meissner)** [MEYES-ner] **corpuscle**, which detects light touch. Burn injuries, which are discussed later in the chapter, destroy skin receptors. By doing so they also may destroy the ability of the burned skin to function as a sense organ.

NAILS

Nails are classified as accessory organs of the skin and are produced by cells in the epidermis. They form when epidermal cells over the terminal ends of the fingers and toes fill with keratin and become hard and platelike. The components of a typical fingernail and its associated structures are shown in Figure 6-9. In this illustration the fingernail of the index finger is viewed from above and in a sagittal section. (Recall that a sagittal section divides a body part into right and left portions.) Look first at the nail as seen from above. The visible part of the nail is called the *nail body.* The rest of the nail, namely, the *nail root,* lies in a groove and is hidden by a fold of skin called the **cuticle** (KYOO-ti-kul). In the sagittal section you can see the nail root from the side and note its relationship to the cuticle, which is folded back over its upper surface. The nail body nearest the root has a crescent-shaped white area known as the **lunula** (LOO-nyoo-lah), or "little moon." You should be able to identify this area easily on your own nails; it is most noticeable on the thumbnail. Under the nail lies a layer of epithelium called the *nail bed,* which is labeled on the sagittal section in Figure 6-9. Because it contains abundant blood vessels, it appears pink through the translucent nail bodies. If blood oxygen levels drop and cyanosis develops, the nail bed will turn blue.

Age and race can influence the normal shape and appearance of the nails. For example, longitudinal ridges are common in those with light skin of all ages and are especially prominent in the elderly, whereas pigmented bands are a normal finding in blacks (Figure 6-10). Pathologic changes in the appearance of the nails often occur as a result of certain diseases

Figure 6-9

Structure of nails.

A, Fingernail viewed from above. **B,** Sagittal section of fingernail and associated structures.

Free edge
Nail body
Lunula
Cuticle
Nail root

A

Cuticle Nail body
Nail bed
Nail root
Free edge
Bone

B

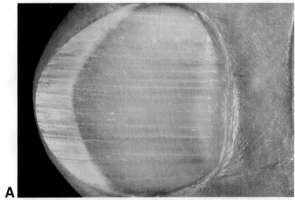

A

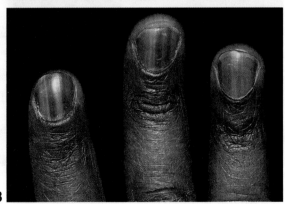

B

Figure 6-10 | **Normal variations in nail structure.**

A, Longitudinal ridges in light-skinned people are common. **B,** Pigmented bands are a normal finding in dark-skinned individuals.

and because of trauma. For example, even minor trauma to long fingernails can sometimes result in a loosening of the nail from the nail bed with a resulting separation that starts at the distal or free edge of the affected nail (Figure 6-11, *A*). The condition, called **onycholysis** (on-i-KOHL-i-sis), is common. Figure 6-11, *B*, shows pitting of the nail. Nail pitting often occurs in individuals with *psoriasis* (soh-RYE-ah-sis), a skin disorder described later in the chapter (see p. 152). Cyanosis and nail pitting are examples of how distinctive changes in the appearance of the skin or its appendages can point to disease in other areas of the body. Many of the pathologic conditions listed in Appendix A on page A-1 of your book and described throughout the text, including infectious and internal diseases, congenital syndromes, and tumors, have symptoms that appear as changes in appearance of the integumentary system and body membranes.

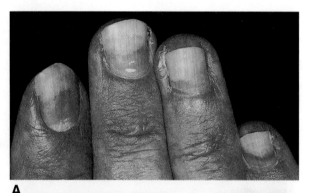

A

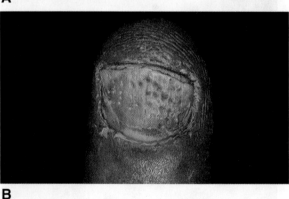

B

| Figure | 6-11 | **Abnormal nail structure.** |

A, Onycholysis. Separation of nail from the nail bed begins at the free edge. **B**, Nail pitting. A common finding in persons with psoriasis.

SKIN GLANDS

The skin glands include the two varieties of **sudoriferous** (soo-doh-RIF-er-us), or **sweat, glands** and the microscopic **sebaceous glands.**

Sweat (Sudoriferous) Glands

Sweat glands are the most numerous of the skin glands. They can be classified into two groups—**eccrine** (EK-rin) and **apocrine** (AP-oh-krin)—based on type of secretion and location. **Eccrine sweat glands** are by far the more numerous, important, and widespread sweat glands in the body. They are quite small and, with few exceptions, are distributed over the total body surface. Throughout life they produce a transparent, watery liquid called **perspiration,** or **sweat.** Sweat assists in the elimination of waste products such as ammonia and uric acid. In addition to elimination of waste, sweat plays a critical role in helping the body maintain a constant temperature. Anatomists estimate that a single square inch of skin on the palms of the hands contains about 3000 eccrine sweat glands. With a magnifying glass you can locate the pinpoint-size openings on the skin that you probably call **pores.** The pores are outlets of small ducts from the eccrine sweat glands.

Apocrine sweat glands are found primarily in the skin of the armpit (axilla) and in the pigmented skin areas around the genitals. They are larger than the eccrine glands, and instead of watery sweat, they secrete a thicker, milky secretion. The odor associated with apocrine gland secretion is not caused by the secretion itself. Instead, it is caused by the contamination and decomposition of the secretion by skin bacteria. Apocrine glands enlarge and begin to function at puberty.

Sebaceous Glands

Sebaceous glands secrete oil for the hair and skin. Oil, or sebaceous, glands grow where hairs grow. Their tiny ducts open into hair follicles (see Figure 6-2) so that their secretion, called **sebum** (SEE-bum), lubricates the hair and skin. Someone aptly described sebum as "nature's skin cream" because it prevents drying and cracking of the skin. Sebum secretion increases during adolescence, stimulated by the increased blood levels of the sex hormones. Frequently sebum accumulates in and enlarges some of the ducts of the sebaceous glands, forming white pimples. This sebum often darkens, forming a **blackhead.** Sebum secretion decreases in late adulthood,

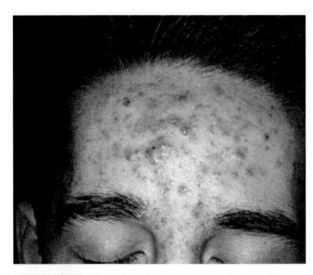

Figure 6-12 | **Acne.**

contributing to increased wrinkling and cracking of the skin.

Acne

The most common kind of acne, **acne vulgaris** (AK-nee vul-GAIR-is) (Figure 6-12), occurs most frequently during adolescence. This condition results from the more than fivefold increase in sebum secretion between the ages of 10 and 19. The oversecretion of sebum results in blockage of the sebaceous gland ducts with sebum, skin cells, and bacteria. The inflamed lesions that result are called **papules** (PAP-yools). Pus-filled pimples called **pustules** (PUS-tyools) often develop and then rupture, resulting in secondary infections in the surrounding skin. Formation of acne lesions can be minimized by careful cleansing of the skin to remove sebaceous plugs and to inhibit anaerobic skin bacteria.

Combinations of topical (external) medications are now used to effectively treat many types of acne. Topical use of vitamin A acid (Retin-A) is often combined with drying and peeling agents such as benzoyl peroxide and externally applied antibiotics in many treatment programs. In addition, physicians or other trained health professionals may use a specialized surgical instrument called an *extractor* to remove "blackheads" and the contents of acne pustules ("whiteheads") to hasten healing. More severe cases may require additional treatment with oral antibiotics and other drugs such as iso-tretinoin (Accutane). Surgical drainage and injection of large pustular legions with corticosteroids are sometimes necessary.

Functions of the Skin

The skin, or cutaneous membrane, serves three important functions that contribute to survival. The most important functions are as follows:

1. Protection
2. Temperature regulation
3. Sense organ activity

PROTECTION

The skin as a whole is often described as our "first line of defense" against a multitude of hazards. It protects us against the daily invasion of deadly microbes. The tough, keratin-filled cells of the stratum corneum also resist the entry of harmful chemicals and protect against physical tears and cuts. Because it is waterproof, keratin also protects the body from excessive fluid loss. Melanin in the pigment layer of the skin prevents the sun's harmful ultraviolet rays from penetrating the interior of the body.

Physical damage can cause bruising of the skin when blood vessels in the skin break open (Figure 6-13). Release of red blood cells initially produces a reddish color in the skin. It then begins to darken and produce bluish colors when hemoglobin loses oxygen. As the blood clots, it may begin to appear darker blue or even black. Cells break down the hemoglobin into iron-containing *hemosiderin* (a brownish pigment) and several iron-free *bile pigments* that are greenish and yellowish.

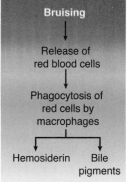

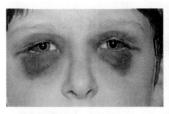

Figure 6-13 | **Bruising.** Color changes caused by the deoxygenation, clotting, and breakdown of blood are easily seen in light-skinned individuals.

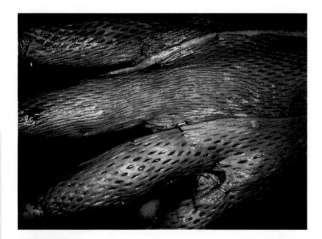

Figure 6-14 | **Skin graft.**

Illustration shows a skin graft covering a severe burn to the hand. Multiple slits allow the grafted piece of skin to stretch over a larger area than would otherwise be possible.

Skin grafts may be required to provide some degree of protection to areas of the body that are no longer covered by skin because of burns or to replace skin destroyed by disease or trauma. Figure 6-14 shows a skin graft covering a burned hand.

TEMPERATURE REGULATION

The skin plays a key role in regulating the body's temperature. Incredible as it seems, on a hot and humid day the skin can serve as a means for releasing almost 3000 calories of body heat—enough heat energy to boil more than 20 liters of water! It accomplishes this feat by regulating sweat secretion and by regulating the flow of blood close to the body surface. When sweat evaporates from the body surface, heat is also lost. The principle of heat loss through evaporation is basic to many cooling systems. When increased quantities of blood are allowed to fill the vessels close to the skin, heat is also lost by radiation. Blood supply to the skin far exceeds the amount needed by the skin. The overabundant blood supply primarily enables the regulation of body temperature.

SENSE ORGAN ACTIVITY

The skin functions as an enormous sense organ. Its millions of nerve endings serve as antennas or receivers for the body, keeping it informed of changes in its environment. The specialized receptors shown in Figure 6-2 make it possible for the body to detect sensations of light touch (tactile [Meissner] corpuscles) and pressures (lamellar [Pacini] corpuscles). Other receptors make it possible for us to respond to the sensations of pain, heat, and cold.

QUICK CHECK

1. Identify the structural components of a nail.
2. How do eccrine and apocrine sweat glands differ?
3. How is sebaceous gland function related to acne?
4. List the major functions of the skin.

Disorders of the Skin

Any disorder of the skin can be called a **dermatosis** (der-mah-TOH-sis), which simply means "skin condition." Many dermatoses involve inflamma-

HEALTH & WELL-BEING

EXERCISE AND THE SKIN

Excess heat produced by the skeletal muscles during exercise increases the core body temperature far beyond the normal range. Because blood in vessels near the skin's surface dissipates heat well, the body's control centers adjust blood flow so that more warm blood from the body's core is sent to the skin for cooling. During exercise, blood flow in the skin can be so high that the skin takes on a redder coloration.

To help dissipate even more heat, sweat production increases to as high as 3 L per hour during exercise. Each individual sweat gland produces very little sweat, but more than 3 million individual sweat glands are found throughout the skin, which account for the high total output. Sweat evaporation is essential to keeping body temperature in balance, but excessive sweating can lead to a dangerous loss of fluid. Because normal drinking may not replace the water lost through sweating, it is important to increase fluid consumption during and after any type of exercise to avoid **dehydration.**

tion of the skin, or **dermatitis** (der-mah-TYE-tis). Only a few of the many disorders of the skin are discussed here.

Skin Lesions

A **lesion** (LEE-zhun) is any measurable variation from the normal structure of a tissue. Lesions are not necessarily signs of disease; they may be benign variations that do not constitute a disorder. For example, freckles are considered lesions but are not signs of disease.

Almost all diseases affecting the skin are discovered and diagnosed after observing the nature of the lesions present. Lighting the skin from the side with a penlight is a method used to determine the category of a lesion: elevated, flat, or depressed. Elevated lesions cast shadows outside their edges; flat lesions do not cast shadows, and depressed lesions cast shadows inside their edges. Important examples of each type of lesion are summarized in Table 6-1 on pp. 138-139.

Lesions are often distinguished by abnormal density of tissue or abnormal coloration. Overgrowth or deficient growth of skin cells, calcification, and edema can cause changes in skin density. Discoloration can result from overproduction or underproduction of skin pigments such as the increase in melanin seen in a mole. A decrease in blood flow or oxygen content can give the skin a bluish cast (cyanosis), whereas an increased blood flow or oxygen content can give a red or darker hue to the skin. Discoloration of the affected area is associated with most skin lesions.

Some of the most common lesions result from scrapes and cuts that our skin often endures in its role of protection. Figure 6-15 shows the way in which such injuries typically repair themselves. First, clotting of blood stops blood loss. Then cells of stratum germinativum produce more epithelial cells to rebuild the epidermis as the clot dissolves. At the same time, fiber-producing cells of the dermis replace torn collagen fibers. Often, the replaced fibrous tissue is denser than the original tissue—providing extra strength in the case of further injury but also sometimes producing a scar.

Burns

Burns constitute one of the most serious and frequent problems that affect the skin. Typically, we think of a burn as an injury caused by fire or by contact of the skin with a hot surface. However, overexposure to ultraviolet light (sunburn) or contact of the skin with an electric current or a harmful chemical such as an acid also can cause burns.

CLASSIFICATION AND SEVERITY OF BURNS

The classification and seriousness of a burn injury as well as appropriate treatment and the possibility for recovery are determined by three major factors:

1. Depth and number of tissue layers involved
2. Total body surface area affected
3. Type of homeostatic mechanisms, such as respiratory or blood pressure control and fluid and electrolyte balance, that are damaged or destroyed

The age and general state of health of the individual at the time of injury are also important. A "moderately severe" burn in an otherwise healthy young adult may become a life-threatening "major" burn in an infant or an elderly individual with preexisting respiratory problems or heart disease.

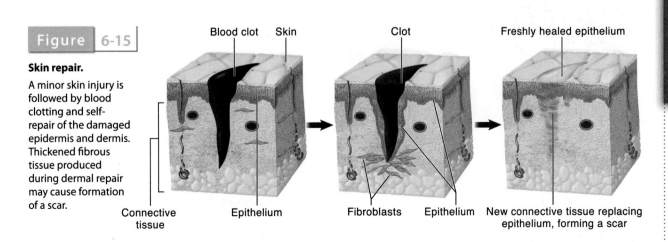

Figure 6-15

Skin repair.

A minor skin injury is followed by blood clotting and self-repair of the damaged epidermis and dermis. Thickened fibrous tissue produced during dermal repair may cause formation of a scar.

Blood clot   Skin

Connective tissue   Epithelium

Clot

Fibroblasts   Epithelium

Freshly healed epithelium

New connective tissue replacing epithelium, forming a scar

Depth Classification

Burns can be classified in a variety of ways, including how deeply the tissues are damaged (Figure 6-16).

First-degree burns. A **first-degree burn** (for example, a typical sunburn) causes minor discomfort and some reddening of the skin. Although the surface layers of the epidermis may peel in 1 to 3 days, no blistering occurs, and actual tissue destruction is minimal.

Second-degree burns. A **second-degree burn** (Figure 6-17, *A*) involves the deep epidermal layers and always causes injury to the upper layers of the dermis. Although deep second-degree burns damage sweat glands, hair follicles, and sebaceous glands, complete destruction of the dermis does not occur. Blisters, severe pain, generalized swelling, and fluid loss characterize this type of burn. Scarring is common. First- and second-degree burns are called **partial-thickness burns.**

Third-degree, or full-thickness, burns. A **third-degree burn** is characterized by complete destruction of the epidermis and dermis. In addition, tissue death extends below the primary skin layers into the subcutaneous tissue. The term **fourth-degree burn** (Figure 6-17, *B*) is used to describe a **full-thickness burn** that extends below the subcutaneous tissue to reach muscle or bone. Such injuries may occur as a result of high-voltage electrical burns or by exposure to very intense heat over time. Treatment may require extensive skin grafting, and even amputation of limbs. One distinction between partial-thickness and full-thickness burns is that full-thickness lesions are insensitive to pain immediately after injury because of the destruction of nerve endings; however, intense pain occurs soon thereafter. Serious burns result in more than 50,000 hospital admissions each year. Circulatory shock, fluid imbalances, respiratory injury, and infections are common complications. Although the number of deaths from severe burns continues to decline as a result of improvements in medical treatment, these injuries often result in long-term medical problems and lifelong disability.

Estimating Body Surface Area

When burns involve large areas of the skin, treatment and the possibility for recovery depend in large part on the *total area involved* and the

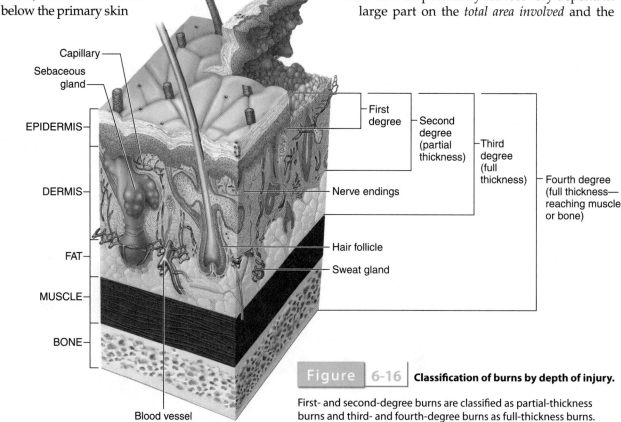

Figure 6-16 | **Classification of burns by depth of injury.** First- and second-degree burns are classified as partial-thickness burns and third- and fourth-degree burns as full-thickness burns.

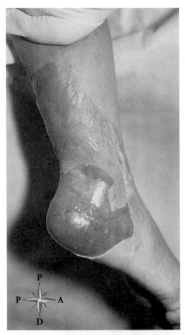

Partial- and full-thickness burns.

A, Second-degree (partial-thickness) burn showing a scald injury in a young child. **B**, Fourth-degree (full-thickness) high-voltage electrical burn resulting in underlying muscle and bone damage.

A

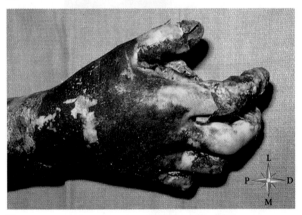

B

severity of the burn. The severity of a burn is determined by the depth of the injury, as well as by the amount of body surface area affected.

The **"rule of nines"** is one of the most frequently used methods of determining the extent of a burn injury. With this technique (Figure 6-18) the body is divided into 11 areas of 9% each, with the area around the genitals representing the additional 1% of body surface area. As you can see in Figure 6-18, in the adult 9% of the skin covers the head and each upper extremity, including front and back surfaces. Twice as much, or 18%, of the total skin area covers the front and back of the trunk and each lower extremity, including front and back surfaces.

To learn more about burns, go to **AnimationDirect** on your CD.

Skin Infections

The skin is the first line of defense against microbes that might otherwise invade the body's internal environment. So the skin is a common site of infection. Viruses, bacteria, fungi, or larger parasites cause skin conditions such as those listed here. Refer to Appendix B on the CD that accompanies your book for more information on these and other skin infections.

1. **Impetigo** (im-peh-TYE-go)—This highly contagious condition results from staphylococcal or streptococcal infection and occurs most often in young children. It starts as a reddish discoloration, or **erythema** (er-i-THEE-mah), but soon develops into vesicles and yellowish **crusts** (Figure 6-19, *A*). Occasionally, it becomes systemic (body-wide) and thus life threatening.

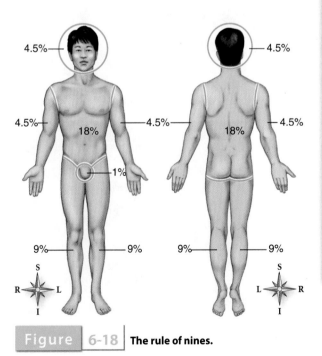

Figure 6-18 **The rule of nines.**

Dividing the body into 11 areas of 9% each helps in estimating the amount of skin surface burned in an adult.

2. **Tinea** (TIN-ee-ah)—Tinea is the general name for many different *mycoses* (fungal infections) of the skin. Ringworm, jock itch, and athlete's foot are classified as tinea. Signs of tinea include erythema, scaling, and crusting. Occasionally, **fissures**, or cracks, develop at creases in the epidermis. Figure 6-19, *B*, shows a case of ringworm, a tinea infection that typically forms a round rash that heals in the center to form a ring. Antifungal agents usually stop the acute infection. Recurrence can be avoided by keeping the skin dry because fungi require a moist environment to grow.

3. **Warts**—Caused by a papillomavirus, warts are a type of benign neoplasm of the skin. However, some warts do transform and become malignant. The nipplelike projections characteristic of this contagious condition are shown

in Table 6-1, pp. 138-139. Transmission of warts generally occurs through direct contact with lesions on the skin of an infected person. Warts can be removed by freezing, drying, laser therapy, or application of chemicals.

4. **Boils**—Also called **furuncles** (FUR-un-kulz), boils are most often local staphylococcal infections of hair follicles and are characterized by large, inflamed pustules (Figure 6-19, *C*). A group of untreated boils may fuse into even larger pus-filled lesions called **carbuncles** (KAR-bung-kulz).

5. **Scabies** (SKAY-beez)—Scabies is a contagious skin condition caused by the itch mite (*Sarcoptes scabiei*). Transmitted by skin-to-skin contact, as in sexual activity, the female mite digs under the hard stratum corneum and forms a short, winding burrow where she deposits her eggs

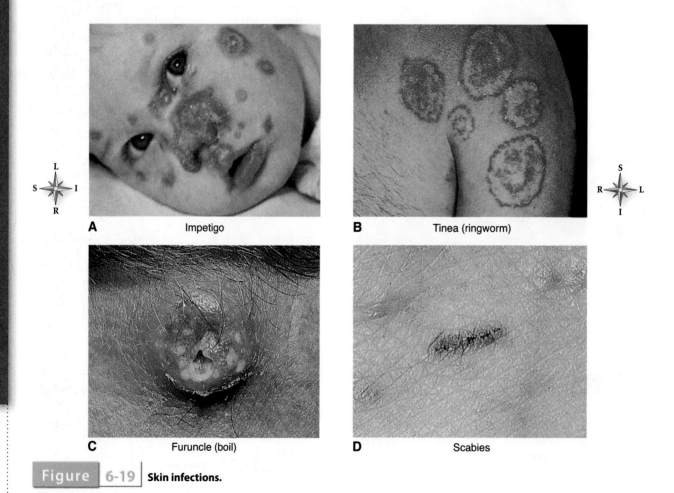

A   Impetigo

B   Tinea (ringworm)

C   Furuncle (boil)

D   Scabies

Figure 6-19 **Skin infections.**

(Figure 6-19, *D*). Young mites called *larvae* hatch, forming tiny, red papules. After a month or so, a hypersensitivity reaction (see Chapter 14) may cause a rash characterized by erythema and numerous papules. As the name of the culprit indicates, infestation of the skin by itch mites causes intense itching. **Excoriation** that results from scratching the itchy infested areas may lead to secondary bacterial infections.

Vascular and Inflammatory Skin Disorders

Every caregiver should be aware of the causes and nature of pressure sores or **decubitus** (deh-KYOO-bi-tus) **ulcers** (Figure 6-20, *A*). *Decubitus* means "lying down," a name that hints at a common cause of pressure sores: lying in one position for long periods. Also called *bedsores,* these lesions appear after blood flow to a local area of skin slows or is obstructed because of pressure on skin covering bony prominences such as the heel. Ulcers form and infections develop because lack of blood flow causes tissue damage or death. Frequent changes in body position and soft support cushions help prevent decubitus ulcers.

Hives, or **urticaria** (ur-ti-KAIR-ee-ah), is a common condition characterized by raised red lesions called **wheals** (Figure 6-20, *B*). Urticaria is often associated with severe itching. Hives are generally short lived, lasting from a few hours to a few weeks.

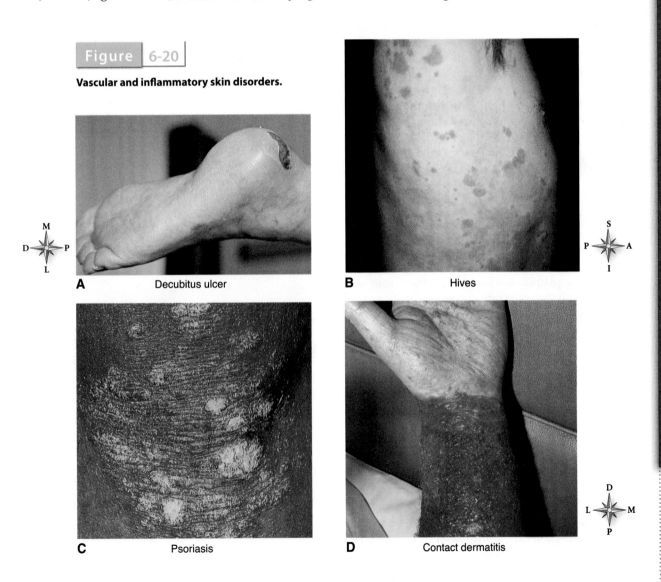

Figure 6-20

Vascular and inflammatory skin disorders.

A Decubitus ulcer

B Hives

C Psoriasis

D Contact dermatitis

The lesions are caused by leakage of fluid from the skin's blood vessels. They change in size and shape over time; new lesions erupt as old ones disappear when fluid in the raised wheals is reabsorbed by the body. Hypersensitivity or allergic reactions to drugs or food, physical irritants, and systemic diseases are common causes of urticaria.

Scleroderma (skleer-oh-DER-mah) is an autoimmune disease that affects the blood vessels and connective tissues of the skin. The name *scleroderma* comes from the word parts *sclera*, which means "hard," and *derma*, which means "skin." Hard skin is a good description of the lesions characteristic of scleroderma. Scleroderma begins as an area of mild inflammation that later develops into a patch of yellowish, hardened skin. Scleroderma most commonly remains a mild, localized condition. Very rarely, localized scleroderma progresses to a systemic form, affecting large areas of the skin and other organs. Persons with advanced systemic scleroderma seem to be wearing a mask because skin hardening prevents them from moving their mouths freely. Both forms of scleroderma occur more commonly in women than in men.

Psoriasis (soh-RYE-ah-sis) is a common, chronic, and often lifelong skin disease that affects 1% to 3% of the population. It is characterized by silvery white, scalelike **plaques** that may remain fixed on the skin for months (Figure 6-20, *C*). Psoriasis is thought to have a genetic basis and tends to affect skin on the elbows, knees, and scalp most often. Individuals with psoriasis often show pitting of the nails (Figure 6-11, *B*). The scales or plaques associated with the disease develop from an excessive rate of epithelial cell growth.

Eczema (EK-zeh-mah) is the most common inflammatory disorder of the skin. This condition is characterized by inflammation that is often accompanied by papules, vesicles, and crusts. Eczema is not a distinct disease but rather a sign or symptom of an underlying condition. For example, an allergic reaction called *contact dermatitis* can progress to become eczematous. The blisters and marked redness on the arm shown in Figure 6-20, *D* are the result of contact dermatitis caused by soap used in laundering a long-sleeved shirt.

Skin Cancer

Of the many types of skin cancer, the most common are **squamous cell carcinoma, basal cell carcinoma,** and malignant **melanoma:**

1. **Squamous cell carcinoma**—This slow-growing malignant tumor of the epidermis is the most common type of skin cancer. Lesions typical of this form of skin cancer are hard, raised nodules that are usually painless (Figure 6-21, *A*). If not treated, squamous cell carcinoma will metastasize, invading other organs.

2. **Basal cell carcinoma**—Usually occurring on the upper face, this type of skin cancer is much less likely to metastasize than other types. This malignancy begins in cells at the base of the epidermis (the basal layer of stratum germinativum). Basal cell carcinoma lesions typically begin as papules that erode in the center to form a bleeding, crusted crater (Figure 6-21, *B*).

3. **Melanoma**—Malignant melanoma is the most serious form of skin cancer. Unfortunately, the incidence of melanoma in the U.S. population is increasing. In the absence of early treatment, it causes death in about one in every four cases. This type of cancer sometimes develops from a pigmented **nevus (mole)** and transforms into a dark, spreading lesion (Figure 6-21, *C*). Benign moles should be checked regularly for warning signs of melanoma because early detection and removal are essential in treating this rapidly spreading cancer. The "ABCD" rule of self-examination of moles is summarized in Table 6-2.

Table 6-2	Warning Signs of Malignant Melanoma
ABCD	**RULE**
Asymmetry	Benign moles are usually symmetrical; their halves are mirror images of each other. Melanoma lesions are asymmetrical or lopsided
Border	Benign moles are outlined by a distinct border, but malignant melanoma lesions are often irregular or indistinct in shape
Color	Benign moles may be any shade of brown but are relatively evenly colored; melanoma lesions tend to be unevenly colored, exhibiting a mixture of shades or colors
Diameter	By the time a melanoma lesion exhibits characteristics A, B, and C, it also is probably larger than 6 mm (¼ inch)

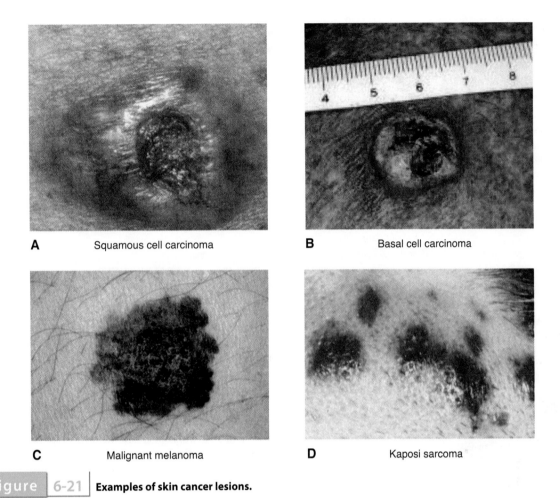

A   Squamous cell carcinoma   **B**   Basal cell carcinoma

C   Malignant melanoma   **D**   Kaposi sarcoma

Figure 6-21 | **Examples of skin cancer lesions.**

Although genetic predisposition also plays a role, many pathophysiologists believe that exposure to the sun's ultraviolet (UV) radiation is the most important causal factor in the common skin cancers. UV radiation damages the DNA in skin cells, causing the mistakes in mitosis that produce cancer. Skin cells have a natural ability to repair UV damage to the DNA, but in some people, this inherent mechanism may not be able to deal with a massive amount of damage. People with the rare, inherited condition *xeroderma* (zee-roh-DERM-ah) *pigmentosum* cannot repair UV damage at all and almost always develop skin cancer.

One of the rarer skin cancers, **Kaposi** (kah-POH-see) **sarcoma (KS),** has increased recently in some parts of the world. Once associated mainly with certain ethnic groups, a form of this cancer now appears in many cases of AIDS and other immune deficiencies. Kaposi sarcoma, first appearing as purple papules (Figure 6-21, *D*), quickly spreads to the lymph nodes and internal organs. Some pathophysiologists believe that a virus or other agent, perhaps transmitted along with HIV, is a possible cause of this cancer.

QUICK CHECK

1. How are burns classified?
2. How can the skin surface area damaged by a burn be estimated?
3. Identify five skin infections and four vascular and inflammatory skin disorders.
4. List the three major types of skin cancer.
5. What are the warning signs of malignant melanoma?

HEALTH & WELL-BEING

SUNBURN AND SKIN CANCER

Burns caused by exposure to harmful ultraviolet (UV) radiation in sunlight are commonly called *sunburns.* As with any burn, serious sunburns can cause tissue damage and lead to secondary infections and fluid loss. Cancer researchers have recently theorized that blistering (second-degree) sunburns during childhood may trigger the development of malignant melanoma later in life. Epidemiologic studies now show that adults who had more than two blistering sunburns before the age of 20 have a much greater risk of developing melanoma than someone who experienced no such burns. This theory helps explain the dramatic increase in skin cancer rates in the United States observed in recent years. Those who grew up sunbathing and experienced sunburns in the 1950s, 1960s, and 1970s are now, as older adults, exhibiting melanoma at a much higher rate than those in previous generations.

SCIENCE APPLICATIONS

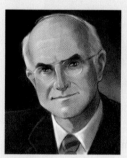

Dr. Joseph E. Murray (b. 1919)

SECRETS OF THE SKIN

The skin is our most visible organ, so it is no wonder that observing the structure and function of skin has generated sparks that have lit the fires of scientific discovery through the ages. The ancient Romans outlined the process of inflammation in detail after observing it first in the skin. In the twentieth century, Joseph Murray (see figure) noticed that skin he grafted onto burned soldiers he treated during World War II would eventually be rejected by the body. After the war, Murray tried to understand the body's immune reactions to transplanted tissues and his work led to the first successful kidney transplants. His breakthroughs in transplanting kidneys not only earned him a Nobel Prize in 1990, it also paved the way for all the different types of tissue and organ transplantation that we see today.

Many scientists continue to study the secrets of the skin and many physicians and other health care professionals are also pioneers in developing new methods of skin care and treatment in the fields of dermatology, allergy, burn medicine, and reconstructive and cosmetic surgery. Additional practical applications of some of this skin science are practiced by people working with cosmetics and other skin treatments, nail treatments, and hair treatments. For example, industrial researchers, product developers, cosmeticians, spa specialists, and hair stylists all require some knowledge of current skin science to do their jobs effectively.

Outline Summary

 To download an MP3 version of the chapter summary for use with your iPod or portable media player, access the **Audio Chapter Summaries** on your CD.

Classification of Body Membranes

A. Classification of body membranes (Figure 6-1)
   1. Epithelial membranes—composed of epithelial tissue and an underlying layer of connective tissue
   2. Connective tissue membranes—composed exclusively of various types of connective tissue
B. Epithelial membranes
   1. Cutaneous membrane—the skin
   2. Serous membranes—simple squamous epithelium on a connective tissue basement membrane
      a. Parietal—line walls of body cavities
      b. Visceral—cover organs found in body cavities
      c. Examples
         (1) Pleura—parietal and visceral layers line walls of thoracic cavity and cover the lungs
         (2) Peritoneum—parietal and visceral layers line walls of abdominal cavity and cover the organs in that cavity
      d. Diseases
         (1) Pleurisy—inflammation of the serous membranes that line the chest cavity and cover the lungs
         (2) Peritonitis—inflammation of the serous membranes in the abdominal cavity that line the walls and cover the abdominal organs
   3. Mucous membranes
      a. Line body surfaces that open directly to the exterior
      b. Produce mucus, a thick secretion that keeps the membranes soft and moist
C. Connective tissue membranes
   1. Do not contain epithelial components
   2. Produce a lubricant called synovial fluid
   3. Examples are the synovial membranes in the spaces between joints and in the lining of the bursal sacs

The Skin

A. Structure (Figure 6-2)—two primary layers called *epidermis* and *dermis*
   1. Epidermis
      a. Outermost and thinnest primary layer of skin
      b. Composed of several layers of stratified squamous epithelium
      c. Stratum germinativum—innermost (deepest) layer of cells that continually reproduce; the new cells move toward the surface
         (1) Sometimes called the pigment layer
         (2) Pigment cells called melanocytes that produce the brown pigment melanin
      d. As cells approach the surface, they are filled with a tough, waterproof protein called *keratin* and eventually flake off
      e. Stratum corneum—outermost layer of keratin-filled cells
      f. Skin color changes
         (1) Pink flush indicates increased blood volume or increased blood oxygen
         (2) Cyanosis—bluish gray color indicates decreased blood oxygen level
         (3) Vitiligo—patchy light skin areas resulting from acquired loss of epidermal melanocytes (Figure 6-4)
         (4) Increased skin pigmentation caused by hormonal changes in pregnant women
         (5) Freckles—small, flat macules' common normal skin pigment variation
      g. Dermal-epidermal junction—specialized area of contact between the epidermis and dermis
         (1) Provide support for epidermis
         (2) Weakened or destroyed junctions (sometimes described as "spot welds") can cause blisters

2. Dermis
   a. Deeper and thicker of the two primary skin layers; composed largely of connective tissue
   b. Upper area of dermis characterized by parallel rows of peglike dermal papillae
   c. Thick skin has parallel friction ridges in dermis and no hairs (Figure 6-5)
   d. Thin skin has irregular, shallow grooves and hair
   e. Deeper area of dermis is filled with network of tough collagenous and stretchable elastic fibers
   f. Number of elastic fibers decreases with age and contributes to wrinkle formation
      (1) Striae—"stretch marks"; elongated marks caused by overstretching of skin
   g. Dermis also contains nerve endings, muscle fibers, hair follicles, sweat and sebaceous glands, and many blood vessels
      (1) Birthmarks—malformation of dermal blood vessels
         (a) Strawberry hemangioma (Figure 6-6)
         (b) Port-wine stain
         (c) Stork bite

B. Appendages of the skin
   1. Hair (Figure 6-7)
      a. Soft hair of fetus and newborn called *lanugo*
      b. Hair growth requires epidermal tubelike structure called *hair follicle*
      c. Hair growth begins from hair papilla
      d. Hair root lies hidden in follicle; visible part of hair called *shaft*
      e. Alopecia (Figure 6-8)—hair loss
      f. Arrector pili—specialized smooth muscle that produces "goose pimples" and causes hair to stand up straight
   2. Receptors (Figure 6-2)
      a. Specialized nerve endings—make it possible for skin to act as a sense organ
      b. Tactile (Meissner) corpuscle—capable of detecting light touch
      c. Lamellar (Pacini) corpuscle—capable of detecting pressure

3. Nails (Figure 6-9)
   a. Produced by epidermal cells over terminal ends of fingers and toes
   b. Visible part called *nail body*
   c. Root lies in a groove and is hidden by cuticle
   d. Crescent-shaped area nearest root called *lunula*
   e. Nail bed may change color with change in blood flow
   f. Normal variations in nail structure (Figure 6-10)
      (1) Longitudinal ridges in light-skinned individuals
      (2) Pigmented bands in dark-skinned individuals
   g. Abnormal variations in nail structure (Figure 6-11)
      (1) Onycholysis—separation of nail from nail bed
      (2) Pitting—common in psoriasis

4. Skin glands—two main types: sweat, or sudoriferous, and sebaceous
   a. Sweat, or sudoriferous, glands
      (1) Eccrine sweat glands
         (a) Most numerous, important, and wide-spread of the sweat glands
         (b) Produce perspiration or sweat, which flows out through pores on skin surface
         (c) Function throughout life and assist in body heat regulation
      (2) Apocrine sweat glands
         (a) Found primarily in axilla and around genitalia
         (b) Secrete a thicker, milky secretion quite different from eccrine perspiration
         (c) Breakdown of secretion by skin bacteria produces odor
      (3) Sebaceous glands
         (a) Secrete oil, or sebum, for hair and skin
         (b) Level of secretion increases during adolescence
         (c) Amount of secretion regulated by sex hormones

(d) Sebum in sebaceous gland ducts may darken to form a blackhead

(e) Acne vulgaris (Figure 6-12)—inflammation of sebaceous gland ducts

C. Functions of the skin

1. Protection—first line of defense
   a. Against infection by microbes
   b. Against ultraviolet rays from sun
   c. Against harmful chemicals
   d. Against cuts and tears
   e. Bruising can cause discoloration of skin as blood release from damaged vessels breaks down (Figure 6-13)
   f. Skin grafts may be needed to replace skin destroyed by disease or trauma (Figure 6-14)

2. Temperature regulation
   a. Skin can release almost 3000 calories of body heat per day
   b. Mechanisms of temperature regulation
      (1) Regulation of sweat secretion
      (2) Regulation of flow of blood close to the body surface

3. Sense organ activity
   a. Receptors serve as receivers for the body, keeping it informed of changes in its environment
   b. Skin can detect sensations of light touch, pressure, pain, heat, and color

Disorders of the Skin

A. Skin lesions (Table 6-1)—any measurable variation from the normal structure

1. Elevated lesions—cast a shadow outside their edges
   a. Papule—small, firm raised lesion
   b. Plaque—large raised lesion
   c. Vesicle—blister
   d. Pustule—pus-filled lesion
   e. Crust—scab
   f. Wheal (hive)—raised, firm lesion with a light center

2. Flat lesions—do not cast a shadow
   a. Macule—flat, discolored region

3. Depressed lesions cast a shadow within their edges
   a. Excoriation—missing epidermis, as in a scratch wound

   b. Ulcer—craterlike lesion
   c. Fissure—deep crack or break

4. Some lesions are produced by scrapes and cuts—the skin can repair itself (Figure 6-15)

B. Burns

1. Treatment and recovery or survival depend on total area involved and severity or depth of the burn

2. Classification of burns (Figure 6-16)
   a. First-degree (partial-thickness) burns—only surface layers of epidermis involved
   b. Second-degree (partial-thickness) burns—involve the deep epidermal layers and always cause injury to the upper layers of the dermis
   c. Third-degree (full-thickness) burns (Figure 6-17)—characterized by complete destruction of the epidermis and dermis
      (1) May involve underlying muscle and bone (fourth degree)
      (2) Lesion is insensitive to pain because of destruction of nerve endings immediately after injury—intense pain is experienced soon thereafter

3. Estimating body surface area using the "rule of nines" (Figure 6-18) in adults
   a. Body divided into 11 areas of 9% each
   b. Additional 1% of body surface area around genitals

C. Skin infections (Figure 6-19)

1. Impetigo—highly contagious staphylococcal or streptococcal infection
2. Tinea—fungal infection (mycosis) of the skin; several forms occur
3. Warts—benign neoplasm caused by papillomavirus
4. Boils—furuncles; staphylococcal infection in hair follicles
5. Scabies—parasitic infection

D. Vascular and inflammatory skin disorders (Figure 6-20)

1. Decubitus ulcers (bedsores) develop when pressure slows down blood flow to local areas of the skin
2. Urticaria or hives—red lesions caused by fluid loss from blood vessels

3. Scleroderma—disorder of vessels and connective tissue characterized by hardening of the skin; two types: localized and systemic
4. Psoriasis—chronic inflammatory condition accompanied by scaly plaques
5. Eczema—common inflammatory condition characterized by papules, vesicles, and crusts; not a disease itself but a symptom of an underlying condition
E. Skin cancer (Figure 6-21)
   1. Three common types
      a. Squamous cell carcinoma—the most common type, characterized by hard, raised tumors
      b. Basal cell carcinoma—characterized by papules with a central crater; rarely spreads
      c. Melanoma—malignancy in a nevus (mole); the most serious type of skin cancer
   2. The most important causative factor in common skin cancers is exposure to sunlight
   3. Kaposi sarcoma, characterized by purple lesions, is associated with AIDS and other immune deficiencies

New Words

Review the names of organ systems and individual organs in Figures 4-1 through 4-12.

apocrine sweat gland
appendage
areola (*pl.,* areolae)
arrector pili
basement membrane
blister
bursa (*pl.,* bursae)
cutaneous membrane (skin)
cuticle
dermal-epidermal junction
dermal papilla (*pl.,* papillae)
dermis
eccrine sweat gland
epidermis
follicle
freckle
hair follicle
hair papilla
hypodermis
integument
integumentary system
keratin
lamellar (Pacini) corpuscle
lanugo

lunula
Meissner (tactile) corpuscle
melanin
melanocyte
membrane
mucocutaneous junction
mucous membrane
mucus
parietal
parietal peritoneum
parietal pleura
peritoneum
perspiration (sweat)
pigment layer
pleura
pore
sebaceous gland
sebum
serous membrane
stratum corneum
stratum germinativum
subcutaneous tissue
sudoriferous (sweat) gland
synovial fluid
synovial membrane
visceral
visceral peritoneum
visceral pleura

Diseases and Other Clinical Terms

acne vulgaris
albinism
alopecia
basal cell carcinoma
blackhead
blister
burn
carbuncle
crust
cyanosis
decubitus ulcer
dehydration
dermatitis
dermatosis
eczema
erythema
excoriation
first-degree burn
fissure
fourth-degree burn
full-thickness burn
furuncle (boil)
impetigo
Kaposi sarcoma (KS)
lesion
macule

melanoma
nevus (mole)
onycholysis
papule
partial-thickness burn
peritonitis
plaque
pleurisy
port-wine stain
psoriasis
pustule
rule of nines
scabies
scleroderma
second-degree burn
skin graft
squamous cell carcinoma
stork bite
strawberry hemangioma
striae (*sing.,* stria)
subcutaneous injection
tinea
urticaria (hives)
vitiligo
wart
wheal

Review Questions

1. Define *membrane*.
2. Explain the structure of a serous membrane, including the difference between the visceral and parietal membranes.
3. Explain the structure of a mucous membrane, including an explanation of the mucocutaneous junction.
4. Explain the structure of a synovial membrane. What is the function of synovial fluid?
5. Name and briefly describe the layers of the epidermis.
6. Explain the structure of the dermis.
7. Differentiate between the hair papilla, the hair root, and the hair shaft.
8. Explain what happens when the arrector pili contracts.
9. Name two receptors of the skin. To what stimuli does each respond?
10. Give the location of eccrine glands, their function, and what type of fluid they produce.
11. Give the location of apocrine glands, their function, and what type of fluid they produce.
12. Give the location of sebaceous glands, their function, and what type of fluid they produce.
13. Explain the difference between a second- and third-degree burn. Which is considered a full-thickness burn?
14. List the three most common forms of skin cancer and explain the factors involved in their development.
15. List the types of skin infections and list the cause as viral, bacterial, fungal, or arthropod.
16. What is the cause of a decubitus ulcer, and what are methods of prevention?

Critical Thinking

17. Explain the protective function of melanin.
18. Explain fully the role of the skin in temperature regulation.
19. If a person burned all of his back, the back of his right arm, and the back of his right thigh, approximately what percent of his body surface area would be involved? How did you determine this?

Chapter Test

1. _____, _____, and _____ are the three types of epithelial membranes.
2. Epithelial membranes are usually composed of two distinct layers: the epithelial layer and a supportive layer called the _____.
3. The membrane lining the interior of the chest wall is called the _____.
4. The membrane covering the organs of the abdomen is called the _____.
5. The connective tissue membrane that lines the space between bone and joint capsule is called _____.
6. The two main layers of the epidermis of the skin are the _____ and the _____.
7. As new skin cells approach the surface of the skin, their cytoplasm is replaced by a unique waterproof protein called _____.
8. The upper region of the dermis forms projections called _____ that form unique fingerprints.
9. The _____ are the sweat glands found in armpits; they produce a thicker secretion.
10. The _____ are the sweat glands found all over the body; they produce a transparent, watery liquid.
11. Sebaceous glands secrete an oil called _____.

12. _____, _____, and
_____ are the three functions of the
skin.

13. The "rule of nines" is used in the treatment
and prognosis of _____.

14. _____ are pressure sores caused by
reduced blood flow to local areas of the skin.

15. The most common type of skin cancer is
_____ carcinoma.

16. _____ results from a fivefold
increase in sebum secretions and usually
occurs during adolescence.

17. The receptors in the skin that respond to pain
are the:
a. Meissner corpuscles
b. lamellar corpuscles
c. free nerve endings
d. Krause end bulbs

18. The receptors in the skin that respond to
light touch are:
a. Meissner corpuscles
b lamellar corpuscles
c. free nerve endings
d. Krause end bulbs

Match each structure in column A with its description of the part of the hair in column B.

Column A
19. _____ hair follicle
20. _____ hair papilla
21. _____ hair root
22. _____ hair shaft

Column B
a. the part of the hair hidden in the follicle
b. the growth of the epidermal cells into the dermis forming a small tube
c. the part of the hair that is visible
d. a cuplike cluster of cells where hair growth begins

Match each skin condition in column A with its description in column B.

Column A
23. _____ furuncle
24. _____ urticaria
25. _____ excoriation
26. _____ melanoma
27. _____ scleroderma
28. _____ Kaposi
sarcoma

Column B
a. an autoimmune skin condition
b. skin cancer that can develop from a mole; the most serious form of skin
cancer
c. another name for hives
d. skin lesion caused by a shallow scratch
e. another name for a skin boil
f. a rare skin cancer that usually develops in immune deficient individuals

Study Tips

continued from page 133

5. Take a photocopy of the illustrations of the membranes, the microscopic view of the skin, the hair, and the nails to your study group. Blacken out the labels and quiz each other on the location and function of various structures.

6. Make a chart of the different types of skin disorders. Your chart will be most helpful if you organize it according to *mechanisms*. Group the diseases by pathogenic organisms and by internal or external conditions.

7. Go over the questions at the end of the chapter and discuss possible test questions with your study group.

Case Studies

1. Dana is an intern who has just been assigned to the burn unit at St. John's Hospital. One patient in the unit has burns covering the lower half of each arm (front and back). How can Dana estimate the total percent of skin surface area affected by the burn? What should Dana's estimate be?

2. Uncle Ed, a light-skinned older gentleman, has just come from a visit to his physician and has news that the spot on his forehead is skin cancer. Of course, dark-skinned Aunt Gina is very upset. Before Uncle Ed gets around to explaining to the family what type of skin cancer he has, you examine the lesion and notice that it is a papule with an ulcer in the center. What type of skin cancer do you think Uncle Ed has? What do you know about this type of cancer that may help comfort Aunt Gina?

3. During your shift at the clinic, a young man arrives with a red, scaly rash formed into rings. What is this patient's diagnosis likely to be? What causes this condition? How can he avoid this type of rash in the future?

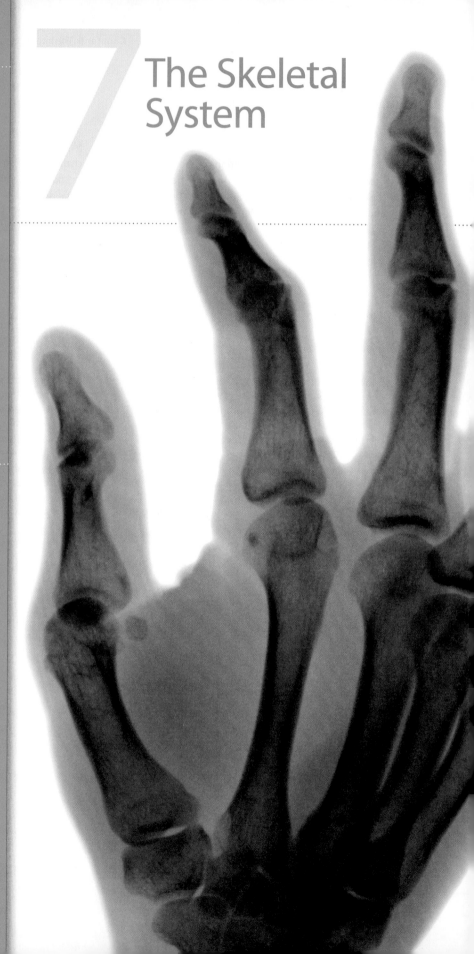

7 The Skeletal System

Objectives

After you have completed this chapter, you should be able to:

1. List and discuss the generalized functions of the skeletal system.

2. Identify the major anatomical structures found in a typical long bone.

3. Discuss the microscopic structure of bone and cartilage, including the identification of specific cell types and structural features.

4. Explain how bones are formed, how they grow, and how they are remodeled.

5. Identify the two major subdivisions of the skeleton and list the bones found in each area.

6. List and compare the major types of joints in the body and give an example of each.

7. Name and describe major disorders of bones and joints.

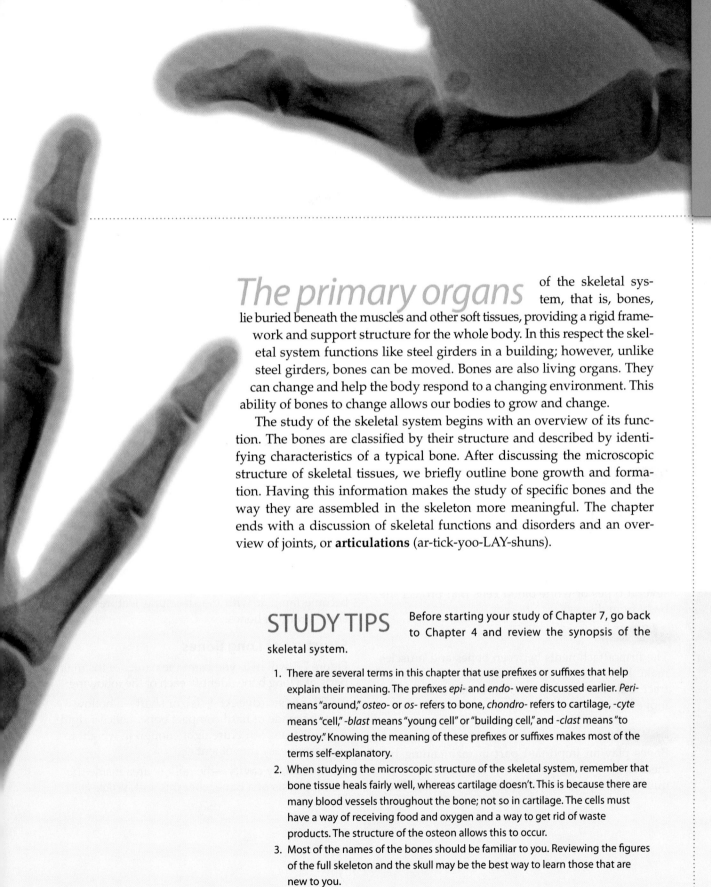

The primary organs of the skeletal system, that is, bones, lie buried beneath the muscles and other soft tissues, providing a rigid framework and support structure for the whole body. In this respect the skeletal system functions like steel girders in a building; however, unlike steel girders, bones can be moved. Bones are also living organs. They can change and help the body respond to a changing environment. This ability of bones to change allows our bodies to grow and change.

The study of the skeletal system begins with an overview of its function. The bones are classified by their structure and described by identifying characteristics of a typical bone. After discussing the microscopic structure of skeletal tissues, we briefly outline bone growth and formation. Having this information makes the study of specific bones and the way they are assembled in the skeleton more meaningful. The chapter ends with a discussion of skeletal functions and disorders and an overview of joints, or **articulations** (ar-tick-yoo-LAY-shuns).

STUDY TIPS

Before starting your study of Chapter 7, go back to Chapter 4 and review the synopsis of the skeletal system.

1. There are several terms in this chapter that use prefixes or suffixes that help explain their meaning. The prefixes *epi-* and *endo-* were discussed earlier. *Peri-* means "around," *osteo-* or *os-* refers to bone, *chondro-* refers to cartilage, *-cyte* means "cell," *-blast* means "young cell" or "building cell," and *-clast* means "to destroy." Knowing the meaning of these prefixes or suffixes makes most of the terms self-explanatory.

2. When studying the microscopic structure of the skeletal system, remember that bone tissue heals fairly well, whereas cartilage doesn't. This is because there are many blood vessels throughout the bone; not so in cartilage. The cells must have a way of receiving food and oxygen and a way to get rid of waste products. The structure of the osteon allows this to occur.

3. Most of the names of the bones should be familiar to you. Reviewing the figures of the full skeleton and the skull may be the best way to learn those that are new to you.

continued on page 205

An understanding of how bones articulate with one another in joints and how they relate to other body structures provides a basis for understanding the functions of many other organ systems. Coordinated movement, for example, is possible only because of the way bones are joined to one another and because of the way muscles are attached to those bones. In addition, knowing where specific bones are in the body will assist you in locating other body structures that are discussed later.

Functions of the Skeletal System

Support

The skeleton provides the internal framework of the body much like tent poles help maintain the structure of a tent. Skeletal muscles are attached to the bones and internal organs are found in the cavities surrounded by the bones and skeletal muscles. The skeletal system can provide this support only when the composition of the bone is strong enough to hold the weight and yet flexible enough to withstand twisting forces.

Protection

The skeletal system protects the soft tissues that are located inside of bony cavities. The skull protects the brain, and the ribs and breastbone protect vital organs in the chest (heart and lungs). Bone also contains a vital tissue (*red bone marrow*, the blood cell–forming tissue) that produces red blood cells and several types of white blood cells that protect the body from disease.

Movement

The firm attachments between bones and muscles make body movement possible. As muscles contract and shorten, they pull on bones and thereby move them.

Storage

Bones play an important part in maintaining homeostasis of blood calcium, a vital substance required for normal nerve and muscle function. They serve as a safety-deposit box for calcium. When the amount of calcium in blood increases above normal, calcium moves out of the blood and into the bones for storage. Conversely, when blood calcium decreases below normal, calcium moves in the opposite direction. It comes out of storage in bones and enters the blood.

Hematopoiesis

The term **hematopoiesis** (hee-mah-toh-poy-EE-sis) is used to describe the process of blood cell formation. It is a combination of two Greek words: *hemo* (HEE-moh) meaning "blood" and *poiesis* (poy-EE-sis) meaning "to make." Blood cell formation is a vital process carried on in red bone marrow. *Red bone marrow* is soft connective tissue found inside the hard walls of some bones that produces both red and white blood cells.

Types of Bones

There are four types of bones. Their names suggest their shapes: *long* (for example, humerus or upper arm bone), *short* (for example, carpals or wrist bones), *flat* (for example, frontal or skull bone), and *irregular* (for example, vertebrae or spinal bones). Some scientists recognize an additional category called *sesamoid* ("like a sesame seed"), or round, bones. An example of sesamoid bone is the kneecap (patella).

Many important bones in the skeleton are classified as long bones, and all have several common characteristics. By studying a typical long bone, you can become familiar with the structural features of the entire group of bones.

Structure of Long Bones

Figure 7-1 will help you learn the names of the main parts of a long bone. Identify each of the following:

1. **Diaphysis** (dye-AF-i-sis), or shaft—a hollow tube made of hard compact bone, hence a rigid and strong structure light enough in weight to permit easy movement

2. **Medullary cavity**—the hollow area inside the diaphysis of a bone; contains soft, *yellow bone*

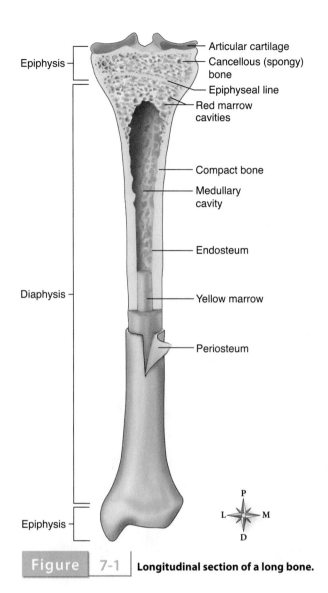

Figure 7-1 | **Longitudinal section of a long bone.**

5. **Periosteum**—a strong fibrous membrane covering a long bone everywhere except at joint surfaces, where it is covered by articular cartilage

6. **Endosteum**—a thin membrane that lines the medullary cavity

QUICK CHECK

1. Name some of the organs of the skeletal system.
2. What are the five major functions of the skeletal system?
3. What are the four categories of bones in the skeleton?
4. Describe the major features of a long bone.

Structure of Flat Bones (Figure 7-2)

1. **Compact** (dense) **bone** is a thin layer surrounding cancellous bone.

2. **Cancellous bone** (also known as *spongy bone* or *diploe* in flat bone) is on the inside of the thin layer of compact bone.

3. **Trabeculae** (trah-BEK-u-lee) are the bony portions of the spongy bone that surround the open spaces.

Microscopic Structure of Bone and Cartilage

The skeletal system contains two major types of connective tissue: **bone** and **cartilage.** Bone has different appearances and textures, depending on its

marrow, an inactive, fatty form of marrow found in the adult skeleton

3. **Epiphyses** (eh-PIF-i-sees), or the ends of the bone—red bone marrow fills in small spaces in the spongy bone composing the epiphyses

4. **Articular cartilage**—a thin layer of cartilage covering each epiphysis; functions like a small rubber cushion would if it were placed over the ends of bones where they form a joint

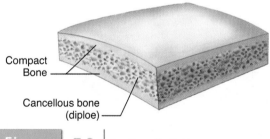

Figure 7-2 | **Section of a flat bone.**

The outer layers of compact bone surround cancellous bone called *diploe*.

location. In Figure 7-3, *A,* the outer layer of bone is hard and dense. Bone of this type is called **dense,** or **compact, bone.** The porous bone in the end of the long bone is cancellous bone—also called **spongy bone**. As the name implies, spongy bone contains many spaces that may be filled with marrow. Compact, or dense, bone appears solid to the naked eye. Figure 7-3, *B,* shows the microscopic appearance of both spongy and com-

pact bone. The needlelike threads of spongy bone that surround a network of spaces are called **trabeculae** (trah-BEK-yoo-lee).

As you can see in Figures 7-3, *B* and *C,* compact, or dense, bone does not contain a network of open spaces. Instead, the matrix (or intercellular substance) is organized into numerous structural units called **osteons** or **haversian systems**. Each circular and tubelike osteon is com-

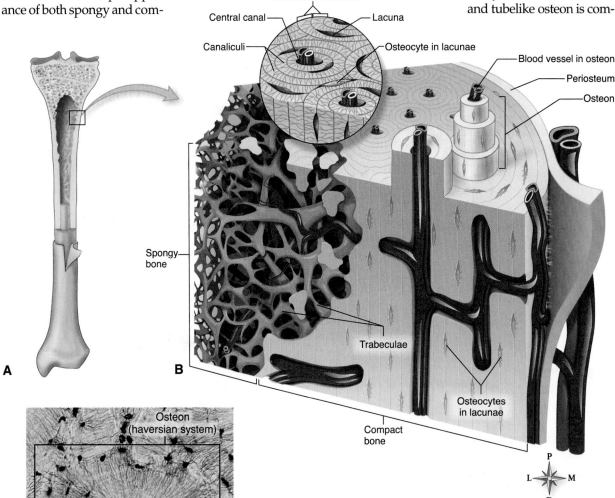

Figure 7-3   **Microscopic structure of bone.**

The longitudinal section of a long bone **(A)** shows the location of the microscopic section illustrated in **B.** Note that the compact bone forming the hard shell of the bone is constructed of cylindrical units called *osteons.* Spongy bone is constructed of bony projections called *trabeculae.* **C,** Photomicrograph shows osteon system of organization. The letter C shows the central canal and the arrow points to the lacunae or space that contains the mature osteocyte.

posed of calcified matrix arranged in multiple layers resembling the rings of an onion. Each ring is called a concentric **lamella** (lah-MEL-ah). The circular rings or lamellae surround the **central canal,** which contains blood vessels.

Within the hard bone matrix are mature bone cells called **osteocytes** (OS-tee-oh-sytes) that were formerly the active bone building cells called os-teoblasts (Figure 7-4, *B*). Osteocytes lie between the hard layers of the lamellae in little spaces called **lacunae** (lah-KOO-nee). Small passageways or canals called **canaliculi** (kan-ah-LIK-yoo-lye) contain cytoplasmic extentions of the osteocyte that connect the lacunae with one another and with the central (haversian) canal in each osteon (Figures 7-3, *B*, and 7-4). Nutrients pass from the blood vessel in the central canal through the canaliculi to the osteocytes. Numerous blood vessels from the outer **periosteum** (pair-ee-OS-tee-um) enter the bone and eventually pass through the central canals (Figure 7-3).

Cartilage both resembles and differs from bone. As with bone, it consists more of intercellular substance than of cells. Innumerable collagenous fibers reinforce the matrix of both tissues. However, in cartilage the fibers are embedded in a firm gel instead of in a calcified cement substance like they are in bone; hence cartilage has the flexibility of a firm plastic rather than the rigidity of bone. Cartilage cells, called **chondrocytes** (KON-droh-sytes), as with the osteocytes of bone, are located in lacunae (Figure 7-5). In cartilage, lacunae are suspended in the cartilage matrix much like air bubbles in a block of firm gelatin. Because there are no blood vessels in cartilage, nutrients must diffuse through the matrix to reach the cells. Because of this lack of blood vessels, cartilage rebuilds itself very slowly after an injury.

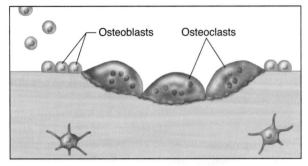

A

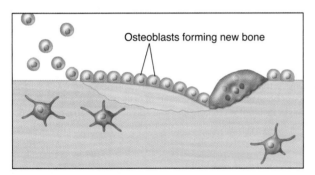

B

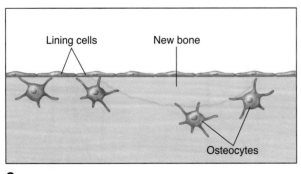

C

Figure 7-4 | **Bone cells.**

A, Osteoclasts are multinucleated cells that remove bone; **B,** osteoblasts are the bone-forming cells; and **C,** osteocytes are the mature bone cells that are located in the lacunae of compact bone.

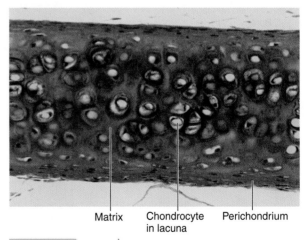

Matrix   Chondrocyte   Perichondrium
in lacuna

Figure 7-5 | **Cartilage tissue.**

Photomicrograph shows chondrocytes scattered around the tissue matrix in spaces called *lacunae.*

Bone Formation and Growth

When the skeleton begins to form in a baby before its birth, it consists not of bones but of cartilage and fibrous structures shaped like bones. Gradually these cartilage "models" are transformed into hardened bones as the cartilage is replaced with calcified bone matrix. This process of constantly "remodeling" a growing bone as it changes from a small cartilage model to the characteristic shape and proportion of the adult bone requires continuous activity by bone-forming cells called **osteoblasts** (OS-tee-oh-blasts) and bone-resorbing cells called **osteoclasts** (OS-tee-oh-clasts). Both the organic and inorganic bone matrix is deposited by osteoblasts. The osteoblasts surround themselves with new bone and become mature osteocytes located in lacunae.

The laying down of bone matrix is an ongoing process. Osteoblasts first lay down organic material followed by calcium salts. The organic material gives the bone the ability to withstand twisting and the calcification process makes bones as "hard as bone." The combined action of the osteoblasts and osteoclasts eventually results in bones transforming into their adult shapes (Figure 7-6). The process of remodeling by the bone-forming and bone-resorbing cells allows bones to respond to stress or injury by changing size, shape, and density. The stresses placed on certain bones during exercise increase the rate of bone deposition. When the body undergoes strain from the pull of a muscle, the osteoblasts lay down more bone to strengthen and resist the pull of muscles. For this reason, athletes or dancers may have denser, stronger bones than less active people. When bone is not under stress, as is the case when astronauts are in outer space, the osteoclasts begin breaking down bone.

Many bones of the body are formed from cartilage models as illustrated in Figures 7-6 and 7-7. This process is called **endochondral** (en-doh-KON-dral) **ossification** (os-i-fi-KAY-shun), meaning "formed in cartilage." Some bones are first formed as a membrane (such as flat bones of the

---

| **Figure** | **7-6** | **Endochondral ossification.** |

A, Bone formation begins with a cartilage model. **B** and **C,** Invasion of the diaphysis (shaft) by blood vessels and the combined action of osteoblast and osteoclast cells results in cavity formation, calcification, and the appearance of bone tissue. **D** and **E,** Centers of ossification also appear in the epiphyses (ends) of the bone. **F,** Note the epiphyseal plate, an indication that this bone is not yet mature and that additional growth is possible. **G,** In a mature bone, only a faint epiphyseal line marks where the cartilage has disappeared and the centers of ossification have fused together.

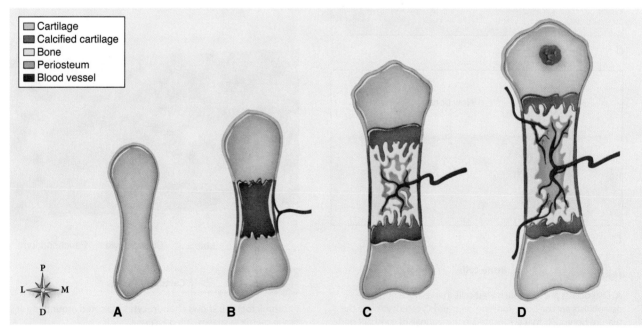

Cartilage
Calcified cartilage
Bone
Periosteum
Blood vessel

A   B   C   D

skull) that is eventually replaced by bone. The soft spot, or fontanel, on a newborn baby's skull is the remnant of such a membrane (Figure 7-7).

As you can see in Figure 7-6, a long bone grows and ultimately becomes "ossified" from small centers within a developing bone. Small centers of ossification are located in both ends *(epiphyses)* of the bone. A larger center of ossification is located in the shaft *(diaphysis)* of the bone. As long as a layer of cartilage, called an **epiphyseal plate,** remains between an epiphysis and the diaphysis, growth continues. Growth ceases when all epiphyseal cartilage is transformed into bone. All that remains then is an **epiphyseal line** that marks the location where the two centers of ossification have fused together. Physicians sometimes use this knowledge to determine whether a child is going to grow any more. If an x-ray study performed on the child's wrist shows a layer of epiphyseal cartilage, they know that additional growth will occur. However, if it shows no epiphyseal cartilage, they know that growth has stopped and that the individual has attained adult height.

 To learn more about bone formation and growth, go to **AnimationDirect** on your CD.

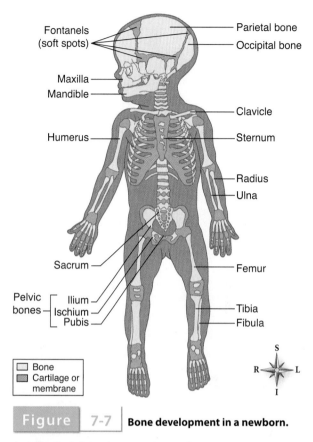

Figure 7-7 | **Bone development in a newborn.**

An infant's skeleton has many bones that are not yet completely ossified.

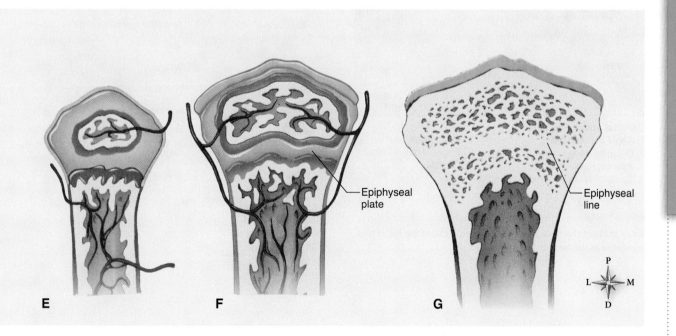

Epiphyseal plate

Epiphyseal line

E F G

1. What is the basic structural unit of compact bone tissue called?
2. What are osteocytes? Where would you find them in bone tissue?
3. How does cartilage differ from bone?
4. What is ossification? What is the role of the osteoblast?

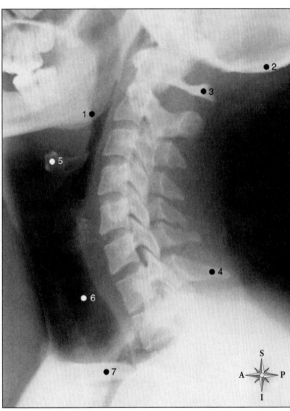

Cervical spine, lateral view
1. Angle of mandible
2. Occipital bone
3. Posterior arch of atlas
4. Spine of seventh cervical vertebra
5. Hyoid bone
6. Tracheal gas shadow
7. Clavicle

Figure   7-8   Hyoid bone.

X-ray study of the neck shows a small bone called the *hyoid* that is located at the base of the tongue.

Divisions of the Skeleton

The human skeleton has two divisions: the **axial skeleton** and the **appendicular skeleton.** Bones of the center or axis of the body make up the axial skeleton. The bones of the skull, spine, and chest and the hyoid bone in the neck are all in the axial skeleton (Figure 7-8). The bones of the upper and lower extremities or appendages make up the appendicular skeleton. The appendicular skeleton consists of the bones of the upper extremities (shoulder, pectoral girdles, arms, wrists, and hands) and the lower extremities (hip, pelvic girdles, legs, ankles, and feet) (Table 7-1). Locate the various parts of the axial skeleton and the appendicular skeleton in Figure 7-9.

Axial Skeleton

SKULL

The **skull** consists of 8 bones that form the **cranium,** 14 bones that form the **face,** and 6 tiny

Table 7-1	Main Parts of the Skeleton*	
AXIAL SKELETON†	**APPENDICULAR SKELETON‡**
Skull	Upper extremities
Ear bones	Shoulder (pectoral) girdle
Cranium	Arm
Face	Wrists
Spine	Hands
Vertebrae	Lower extremities
Thorax	Hip (pelvic) girdle
Ribs	Legs
Sternum	Ankles
Hyoid bone	Feet

*Total bones = 206.
†Total = 80 bones.
‡Total = 126 bones.

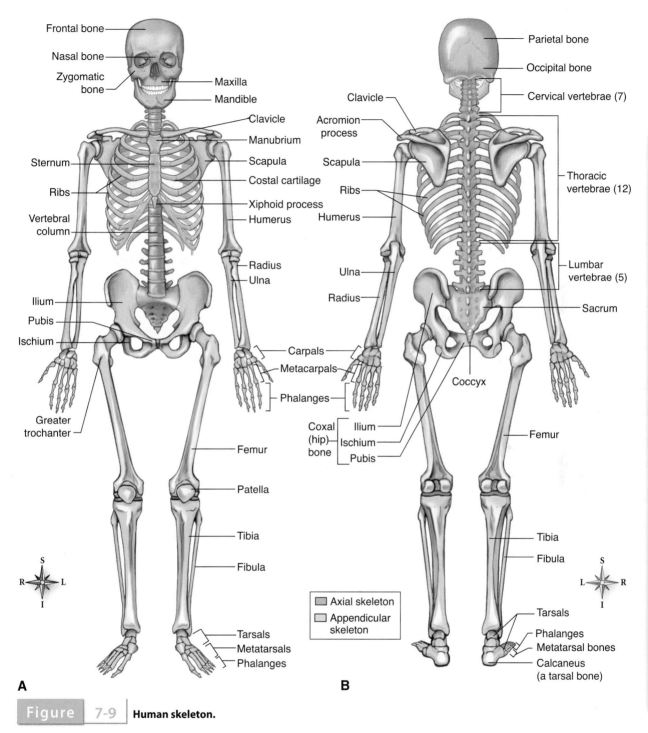

Frontal bone

Nasal bone

Zygomatic bone

Maxilla

Mandible

Clavicle

Manubrium

Sternum

Scapula

Ribs

Costal cartilage

Xiphoid process

Vertebral column

Humerus

Radius

Ulna

Ilium

Pubis

Ischium

Carpals

Metacarpals

Phalanges

Greater trochanter

Femur

Patella

Tibia

Fibula

Tarsals

Metatarsals

Phalanges

A

Parietal bone

Occipital bone

Clavicle

Cervical vertebrae (7)

Acromion process

Scapula

Ribs

Humerus

Thoracic vertebrae (12)

Ulna

Radius

Lumbar vertebrae (5)

Sacrum

Coccyx

Coxal (hip) bone

Ilium

Ischium

Pubis

Femur

Tibia

Fibula

Tarsals

Phalanges

Metatarsal bones

Calcaneus (a tarsal bone)

☐ Axial skeleton

☐ Appendicular skeleton

B

Figure 7-9 | **Human skeleton.**

The axial skeleton is distinguished by a blue tint. **A,** Anterior view. **B,** Posterior view.

bones in the **middle ear** (Table 7-2). It would be good for you to learn the names and locations of these bones to help in your study of these structures in relation to other body systems (Figure 7-10).

"My sinuses give me so much trouble." Have you ever heard this complaint or perhaps uttered it yourself? **Sinuses** are spaces or cavities inside some of the cranial bones. Four pairs of them (those in the frontal, maxillary, sphenoid,

Table 7-2 | Bones of the Skull

NAME	NUMBER	DESCRIPTION
CRANIAL BONES		
Frontal	1	Forehead bone; also forms front part of floor of cranium and most of upper part of eye sockets; cavity inside bone above upper margins of eye sockets (orbits) called *frontal sinus;* lined with mucous membrane
Parietal	2	Form bulging topsides of cranium
Temporal	2	Form lower sides of cranium; contain *middle and inner ear structures; mastoid sinuses* are mucosa-lined spaces in *mastoid process,* the protuberance behind ear; *external auditory canal* is tube leading into temporal bone; muscles attach to *styloid process*
Occipital	1	Forms back of skull; spinal cord enters cranium through large hole *(foramen magnum)* in occipital bone
Sphenoid	1	Forms central part of floor of cranium; pituitary gland located in small depression in sphenoid called *sella turcica (Turkish saddle);* muscles attach to *pterygoid process*
Ethmoid	1	Complicated bone that helps form floor of cranium, side walls and roof of nose and part of its middle partition (nasal septum—made up of the *vomer* and the *perpendicular plate*), and part of orbit; contains honeycomb-like spaces, the *ethmoid sinuses; superior* and *middle conchae* are projections of ethmoid bone; form "ledges" along side wall of each nasal cavity
FACE BONES		
Nasal	2	Small bones that form upper part of bridge of nose
Maxilla	2	Upper jawbones; also help form roof of mouth, floor, and side walls of nose and floor of orbit; large cavity in *maxillary* bone is *maxillary sinus*
Zygomatic	2	Cheek bones; also help form orbit
Mandible	1	Lower jawbone articulates with temporal bone at *condyloid process;* small anterior hole for passage of nerves and vessels is the *mental foramen*
Lacrimal	2	Small bones; help form medial wall of eye socket and side wall of nasal cavity
Palatine	2	Form back part of roof of mouth and floor and side walls of nose and part of floor of orbit
Inferior concha	2	Form curved "ledge" along inside of side wall of nose, below middle concha
Vomer	1	Forms lower back part of nasal septum
EAR BONES		
Malleus	2	Malleus, incus, and stapes are tiny bones in middle ear cavity in temporal bone; *malleus* means "hammer"—shape of bone
Incus	2	*Incus* means "anvil"—shape of bone
Stapes	2	Stapes means "stirrup"—shape of bone

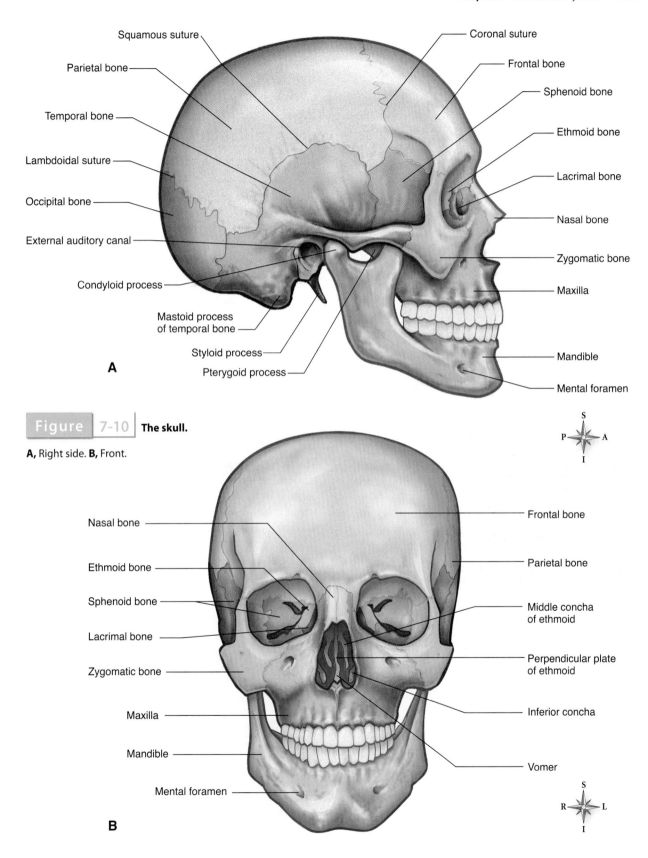

Squamous suture
Parietal bone
Temporal bone
Lambdoidal suture
Occipital bone
External auditory canal
Condyloid process
Mastoid process of temporal bone
Styloid process
Pterygoid process

Coronal suture
Frontal bone
Sphenoid bone
Ethmoid bone
Lacrimal bone
Nasal bone
Zygomatic bone
Maxilla
Mandible
Mental foramen

A

Figure 7-10 **The skull.**

A, Right side. **B,** Front.

Nasal bone
Ethmoid bone
Sphenoid bone
Lacrimal bone
Zygomatic bone
Maxilla
Mandible
Mental foramen

Frontal bone
Parietal bone
Middle concha of ethmoid
Perpendicular plate of ethmoid
Inferior concha
Vomer

B

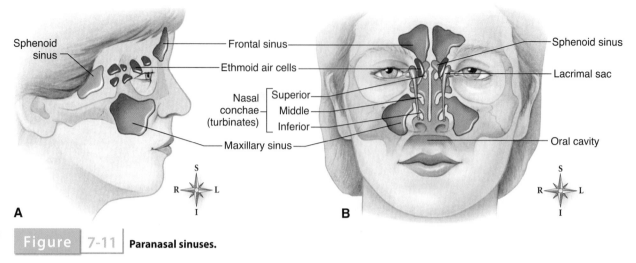

Figure 7-11 | **Paranasal sinuses.**

A, Lateral view of the face shows the position of the paranasal sinuses. **B,** Anterior view shows the relationship of the sinuses to each other and the nasal cavity.

and ethmoid bones) have openings into the nose and thus are referred to as **paranasal sinuses** (Figure 7-11)**.** Sinuses cause trouble when the mucous membrane that lines them becomes inflamed, swollen, and painful. For example, inflammation in the frontal sinus *(frontal sinusitis)* often begins as a result of a common cold. The word part *-itis* added to a word means "inflammation of."

Mastoiditis (mass-toyd-EYE-tis), inflammation of the air spaces within the mastoid portion of the temporal bone, can produce very serious medical problems if not treated promptly (Figure 7-12). Locate the mastoid process in Figure 7-10, *A*. Infectious material from middle ear infections sometimes finds its way into the mastoid air cells. These air cells do not drain into the nose like the paranasal sinuses do. Thus infectious material that accumulates may damage the thin, bony partition that separates the air cells from the brain. If this occurs, the infection may spread to the brain or the membranes covering the brain, a life-threatening situation. Chronic mastoiditis may be treated by surgically removing the affected tissue, including internal parts of the ear—rendering the individual deaf in the affected ear.

The two parietal bones, which give shape to the bulging topside of the skull, form immovable joints called **sutures** with several bones: the *lambdoidal suture* with the occipital bone, the *squamous suture* with the temporal bone and part of the sphenoid, and the *coronal suture* with the frontal bone (Figure 7-10).

You may be familiar with the "soft spots" on a baby's skull. These are six **fontanels,** or areas where ossi-

fication is incomplete at birth. You can see them depicted in Figure 7-7. Fontanels allow some compression of the skull during birth without much risk of breaking the skull bones. They also may be identified by a clinician as an important diagnostic indication of the position of the baby's head before delivery. The fontanels fuse to form sutures before a baby is 2 years old.

SPINE (VERTEBRAL COLUMN)

The term *vertebral column* may conjure up a mental picture of the **spine** as a single long bone shaped like a column in a building, but this is far from true. The vertebral column consists of a series of separate bones, or **vertebrae,** connected in such a way that they form a flexible curved rod (Figure 7-13). Different sections of the spine have different names: cervical region, thoracic

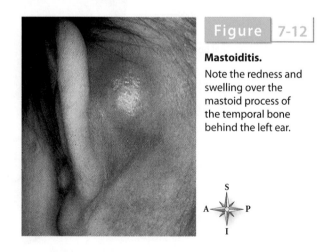

Figure 7-12

Mastoiditis.
Note the redness and swelling over the mastoid process of the temporal bone behind the left ear.

EPIPHYSEAL AND AVULSION FRACTURES

The point of articulation between the epiphysis and diaphysis of a growing long bone is susceptible to injury if overstressed, especially in the young child or preadolescent athlete. In these individuals the epiphyseal plate can be separated from the diaphysis or epiphysis, causing an epiphyseal fracture. This x-ray study shows such a fracture in a young boy. Without successful treatment, an **epiphyseal fracture** may inhibit normal growth. Stunted bone growth in turn may cause the affected limb to be shorter than the normal limb.

In addition to epiphyseal fractures, violent contraction or overstretching of a muscle in skeletally immature individuals also can cause a fragment of bone under the point of attachment to break away from the bone as a whole. The result is called an **avulsion** (ah-VUL-shen) **fracture** (see p. 197).

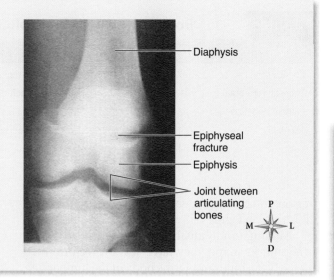

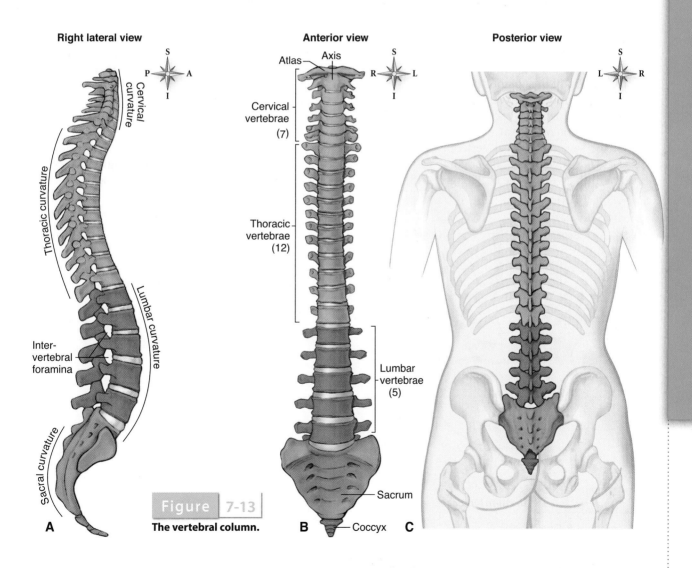

Right lateral view

Cervical curvature

Thoracic curvature

Lumbar curvature

Inter-vertebral foramina

Sacral curvature

A

Anterior view

Atlas — Axis

Cervical vertebrae (7)

Thoracic vertebrae (12)

Lumbar vertebrae (5)

Sacrum

B — Coccyx

Posterior view

C

Figure 7-13

The vertebral column.

Table 7-3		Bones of the Vertebral Column
NAME	**NUMBER**	**DESCRIPTION**
Cervical	7	Upper 7 vertebrae, in neck region; first cervical vertebra called *atlas;* second, *axis*
Thoracic vertebrae	12	Next 12 vertebrae; ribs attach to these
Lumbar vertebrae	5	Next 5 vertebrae; in small of back
Sacrum	1	In child, 5 separate vertebrae; in adult, fused into one
Coccyx	1	In child, 3 to 5 separate vertebrae; in adult, fused into one

region, lumbar region, sacrum, and coccyx. They are illustrated in Figure 7-13 and described in Table 7-3.

Although individual vertebrae are small bones, irregular in shape, they have several well-defined parts. Note, for example, the body of the lumbar vertebra shown in Figure 7-14, its spinous process (or spine), its two transverse processes, and the hole in its center, called the *vertebral foramen.* The superior and inferior articular processes permit limited and controlled movement between adjacent vertebrae. To feel the tip of the spinous process of one of your vertebrae, simply bend your head forward and run your fingers down the back of your neck until you feel a projection of bone at shoulder level. This is the tip of the seventh cervical vertebra's long spinous process. The seven cervical vertebrae form the supporting framework of the neck (Figure 7-8).

When viewed from the side, your neck and the small of your back curve slightly inward or forward, whereas the chest region of the spine and the lowermost portion curve in the opposite direction (Figure 7-13). The cervical and lumbar curves of the spine are called *concave curves,* and the thoracic and sacral curves are called *convex curves.* This configuration is not found in a newborn baby's spine. The newborn's spine forms a continuous convex curve from top to bottom (Figure 7-15). Gradually, as the baby learns to hold up his or her head, a reverse or concave curve develops in the neck (cervical region). Later, as the baby learns to stand, the lumbar region of the spine also becomes concave.

The normal curves of the spine have important functions. They give it enough strength to support the weight of the rest of the body. These curves also

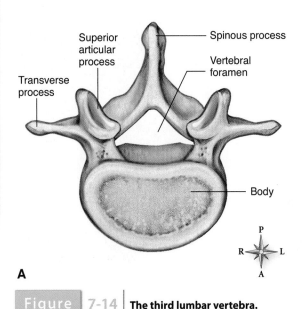

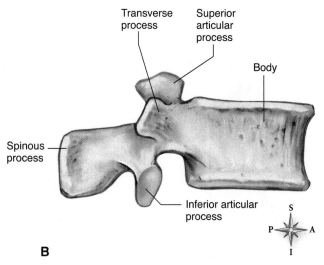

A, From above. **B,** From the side.

Figure 7-14 | **The third lumbar vertebra.**

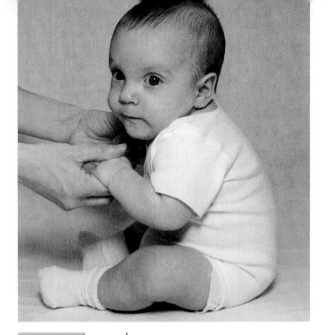

Figure | 7-15 | **Spinal curvature of an infant.**

The spine of the newborn baby forms a continuous convex curve.

provide the balance necessary for us to stand and walk on two feet instead of having to crawl on all fours. A curved structure has more strength than a straight one of the same size and materials. (The next time you pass a bridge, look to see whether or not its supports form a curve.) Clearly the spine needs to be a strong structure. It supports the head that is balanced on top of it, the ribs and internal organs

that are suspended from it in front, and the hips and legs that are attached to it below.

Poor posture or disease may cause the lumbar curve to become abnormally exaggerated, a condition known to some as *swayback* or **lordosis** (lor-DOH-sis). Abnormal thoracic curvature is **kyphosis** (ki-FOH-sis) or "hunchback." Abnormal side-to-side curvature is **scoliosis** (skoh-lee-OH-sis). Sometimes these abnormal curvatures (Figure 7-16) interfere with normal breathing and other vital functions. Scoliosis is a relatively common condition that appears before adolescence, usually of unknown cause. Treatments vary depending on the degree of lateral curvature and resulting deformity of individual vertebrae. Traditional treatments for scoliosis include long-term use of supportive braces, transcutaneous ("through-the-skin") muscle stimulation, and surgery. Electrical stimulation of muscles on one side of the spine over time helps pull the vertebrae into a more normal position. Surgical procedures to straighten the spine may involve bone grafts and the insertion of internal metal rods.

THORAX

Twelve pairs of ribs, the sternum (breastbone), and the thoracic vertebrae form the bony cage known as the **thorax** or **chest.** Each of the 12 pairs of ribs is attached posteriorly to a vertebra. Also, all the ribs except the lower two pairs are attached to the sternum and so have anterior and posterior anchors. Look

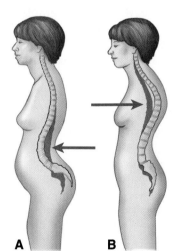
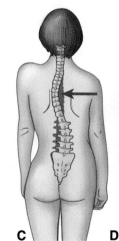
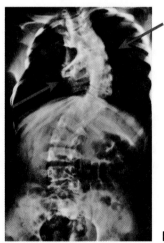
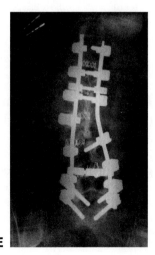

Figure | 7-16 | **Abnormal spinal curvatures.**

A, Lordosis. **B,** Kyphosis. **C,** Scoliosis. **D,** An x-ray showing pronounced scoliosis and **E,** an x-ray of an 11-year-old girl after corrective surgery for scoliosis.

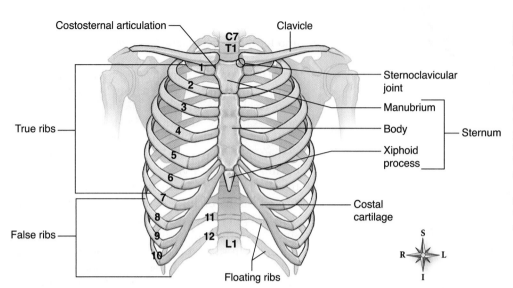

Costosternal articulation — Clavicle
C7
T1
True ribs
False ribs
Floating ribs
Sternoclavicular joint
Manubrium
Body
Xiphoid process
Sternum
Costal cartilage
S
R — L
I

Figure 7-17

Bones of the thorax.

Rib pairs 1 through 7, the *true ribs*, are attached by cartilage to the sternum. Rib pairs 8 through 10, the *false ribs*, are attached to the cartilage of the seventh pair. Rib pairs 11 and 12 are called *floating ribs* because they have no anterior cartilage attachments.

closely at Figure 7-17 and you can see that the first seven pairs of ribs (sometimes referred to as the *true ribs*) are attached to the sternum by costal cartilage. The eighth, ninth, and tenth pairs of ribs are attached to the cartilage of the seventh ribs and are sometimes called *false ribs.* The last two pairs of ribs, in contrast, are not attached to any costal cartilage but seem to float free in front, hence their descriptive name, *floating ribs* (Table 7-4).

QUICK CHECK

1. What is the difference between the axial skeleton and the appendicular skeleton?
2. What is a suture? A fontanel? A sinus?
3. What are the three major categories of vertebrae? How many bones in each?
4. How is a *false rib* different from a *true rib*?

Appendicular Skeleton

Of the 206 bones that form the skeleton as a whole, 126 are contained in the appendicular subdivision (Figure 7-9). Note that the bones in the shoulder, or **pectoral girdle,** connect the bones of the arm, forearm, wrist, and hands to the axial skeleton of the thorax, and the hip, or **pelvic girdle,** connects the bones of the thigh, leg, ankle, and foot to the axial skeleton of the pelvis.

UPPER EXTREMITY

The **scapula** (SKAP-yoo-lah), or shoulder blade, and the **clavicle** (KLAV-i-kul), or collar bone, compose the *shoulder,* or **pectoral girdle.** This connects the upper extremity to the axial skeleton. The only direct point

of attachment between bones occurs at the **sterno-clavicular** (ster-no-klah-VIK-yoo-lar) **joint** between the clavicle and the sternum or breastbone. As you can see in Figures 7-9 and 7-17, this joint is very small. Because the upper extremity is capable of a wide range of motion, great pressures can occur at or near the joint. As a result, fractures of the clavicle are very common.

The **humerus** (HYOO-mer-us) is the long bone of the arm and the second longest bone in the body. It is attached to the scapula at its proximal end and articulates with the two bones of the forearm at the elbow joint. The bones of the forearm are the **radius** and the **ulna.** The anatomy of the elbow is a good example of how structure determines function. Note in Figure 7-18 that the large bony process of the ulna, called the **olecranon** (oh-LEK-rah-non) **process,** fits nicely into a

Table	7-4	Bones of the Thorax
NAME	NUMBER	DESCRIPTION
True ribs	14	Upper seven pairs; attached to sternum by *costal cartilages*
False ribs	10	Lower five pairs; lowest two pairs do not attach to sternum; therefore, called *floating ribs;* next three pairs attached to sternum by costal cartilage of seventh ribs
Sternum	1	Breastbone; shaped like a dagger; piece of cartilage at lower end of bone called *xiphoid process;* superior portion called the *manubrium*

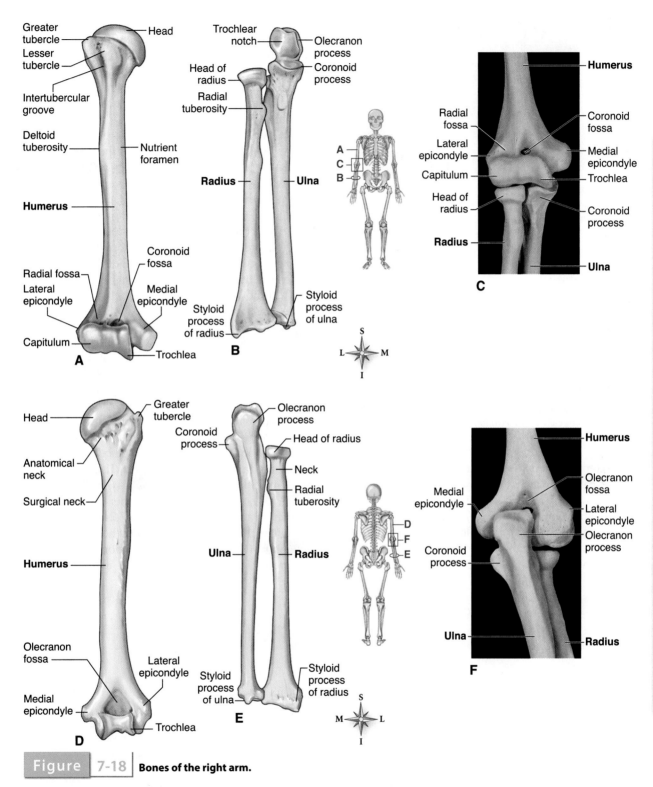

Figure 7-18 Bones of the right arm.

A, Humerus (upper part of the arm) anterior view. **B,** Radius and ulna (forearm) anterior view. **C,** Elbow joint (anterior view). **D,** Humerus (posterior view). **E,** Radius and ulna (posterior view). **F,** Elbow joint (posterior view). The insets show the relative position of the right arm bones within the entire skeleton.

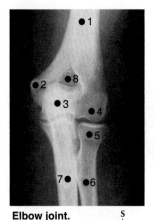
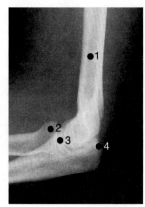

Elbow joint.

A, Anterior
1. Shaft of humerus
2. Medial epicondyle
3. Trochlea, overlain by upper end of ulna
4. Capitulum
5. Head of radius
6. Shaft of radius
7. Shaft of ulna
8. Coronoid fossa

B, Lateral
1. Shaft of humerus
2. Head of radius
3. Coronoid process of ulna
4. Olecranon process of ulna

Figure 7-19 | **X-ray of the elbow joint.**

Shows how the elbow acts as a hinge. When bent or flexed the coronoid process of the ulna fits in a depression in the humerus called the *coronoid fossa*. When the arm is straightened or extended, the olecranon process of the ulna fits into a depression on the humerus called the *olecranon fossa*.

large depression on the posterior surface of the humerus, called the **olecranon fossa.** The trochlea of the humerus fits into the trochlear notch of the ulna to make a hinge joint (Figure 7-19). The hinge joint of the trochlea allows the arm to be flexed or bent at the elbow while the olecranon process prevents the arm from being hyperextended.

The radius and the ulna of the forearm articulate with each other and with the distal end of the humerus at the elbow joint. In addition, they also touch each another distally where the ulna articulates with the bones of the wrist. In the anatomical position, with the arm at the side and the palm facing forward, the radius runs along the lateral side of the forearm, and the ulna is located along the medial border.

The wrist and the hand have more bones in them for their size than any other part of the body—8 **carpal** (KAR-pul), or wrist, bones; 5 **metacarpal** (met-ah-KAR-pul) bones that form the support structure for the palm of the hand; and 14 **phalanges** (fah-LAN-jeez), or finger bones—27 bones in all (Table 7-5). This composition is very important structurally. The presence of many small bones in the hand and wrist and the many movable joints between them makes the human hand highly maneuverable. Figure 7-20 shows the relationships between the bones of the wrist and hand.

LOWER EXTREMITY

The *hip,* or *pelvic girdle* connects the legs to the trunk. The hip girdle as a whole consists of two large **coxal,** or pelvic, **bones,** one located on each side of the pelvis. These two bones, with the sacrum and coccyx behind, provide a strong base of support for the torso and connect the lower extremities to the axial skeleton. In an infant's body each coxal bone consists of three separate bones—the **ilium** (ILL-ee-um), the **ischium** (IS-kee-um), and the **pubis** (PYOO-bis) (Figure 7-7). These bones grow together to become one bone in an adult (Figures 7-9 and 7-24).

Just as the humerus is the only bone in the arm, the **femur** (FEE-mur) is the only bone in the thigh (Figure 7-21). It is the longest bone in the body and

Table 7-5 | Bones of the Upper Extremities

NAME	NUMBER	DESCRIPTION
Clavicle	2	Collar bones; only joints between shoulder girdle and axial skeleton are those between each clavicle and sternum (*sternoclavicular joints*)
Scapula	2	Shoulder blades; scapula plus clavicle forms *shoulder girdle; acromion process*—tip of shoulder that forms joint with clavicle; *glenoid cavity*—arm socket
Humerus	2	Upper arm bone (muscles are attached to the *greater tubercle* and to the *medial* and *lateral epicondyles;* the trochlea articulates with the ulna; the *surgical neck* is a common fracture site)
Radius	2	Bone on thumb side of lower arm (muscles are attached to the *radial tuberosity* and to the *styloid process*)
Ulna	2	Bone on little finger side of lower arm; *olecranon process*—projection of ulna known as elbow or "funny bone" (muscles are attached to the *coronoid process* and to the *styloid process*)
Carpal bones	16	Irregular bones at upper end of hand; anatomical wrist
Metacarpals	10	Form framework of palm of hand
Phalanges	28	Finger bones; three in each finger, two in each thumb

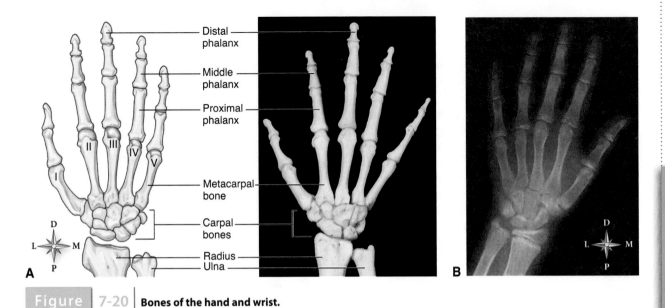

Figure 7-20 **Bones of the hand and wrist.**

A, Right hand. There are 14 phalanges in each hand. Each of these bones is called a *phalanx*. **B,** Left hand, x-ray.

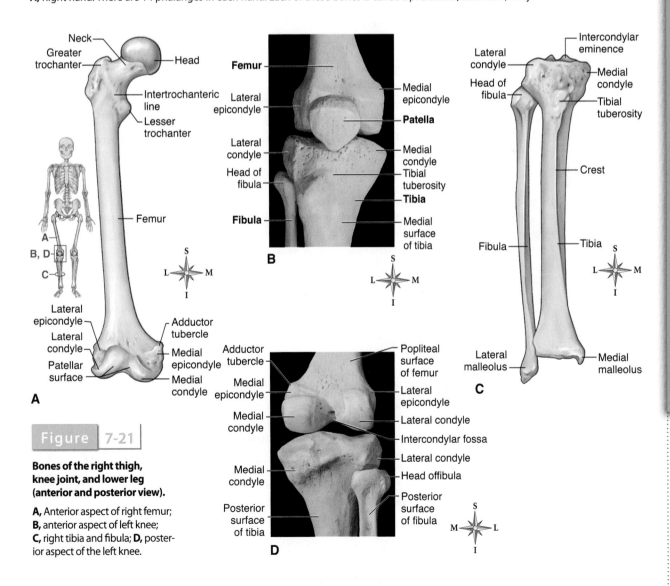

Figure 7-21

Bones of the right thigh, knee joint, and lower leg (anterior and posterior view).

A, Anterior aspect of right femur; **B,** anterior aspect of left knee; **C,** right tibia and fibula; **D,** posterior aspect of the left knee.

articulates proximally (toward the hip) with the coxal bone in a deep, cup-shaped socket called the **acetabulum** (ass-eh-TAB-yoo-lum). The articulation of the head of the femur in the acetabulum is more stable than the articulation of the head of the humerus with the scapula in the upper extremity. As a result, dislocation of the hip occurs less often than does disarticulation of the shoulder. Distally, the femur articulates with the kneecap, or **patella** (pah-TEL-ah) and the **tibia,** or "shinbone." The tibia forms a rather sharp edge or crest along the front of the lower leg. A slender, non–weight-bearing, and rather fragile bone named the **fibula** lies along the outer or lateral border of the lower leg.

Toe bones have the same name as finger bones—**phalanges.** There is the same number of toe bones as finger bones, a fact that might surprise you because toes are shorter than fingers. Foot bones comparable to the metacarpals and carpals of the hand have slightly different names. They are called **metatarsals** and **tarsals** in the foot (Figure 7-22). Just as each hand contains five metacarpal bones, each foot contains five metatarsal bones. However, the foot has only seven tarsal bones, in contrast to the hand's eight carpals. The largest tarsal bone is the **calcaneus,** or heel bone. The talus is the second

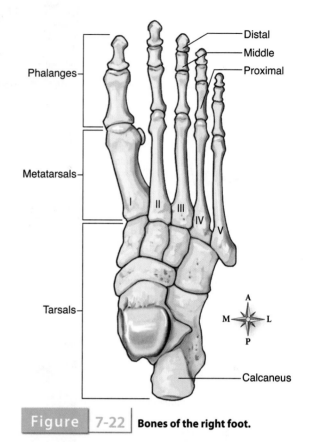

Figure 7-22 | **Bones of the right foot.**

Compare the names and numbers of foot bones (viewed here from above) with those of the hand bones shown in Figure 7-20.

| Table | 7-6 | Bones of the Lower Extremities |

NAME	NUMBER	DESCRIPTION
Coxal bone	2	Hipbones; *ilium*—upper flaring part of pelvic bone; *ischium*—lower back part; *pubic bone*—lower front part; *acetabulum*—hip socket; *symphysis pubis*—joint in midline between two pubic bones; *pelvic inlet*—opening into *true pelvis* or pelvic cavity; if pelvic inlet is misshapen or too small, infant skull cannot enter true pelvis for natural birth
Femur	2	Thigh or upper leg bones; *head of femur*—ball-shaped upper end of bone; fits into acetabulum (muscles are attached to the *greater* and *lesser trochanters* and to the *lateral* and *medial epicondyles;* the *lateral* and *medial condyles* form articulations at the knee)
Patella	2	Kneecap
Tibia	2	Shinbone; *medial malleolus*—rounded projection at lower end of tibia commonly called *inner anklebone;* muscles are attached to the *tibial tuberosity*
Fibula	2	Long slender bone of lateral side of lower leg; *lateral malleolus*—rounded projection at lower end of fibula commonly called *outer anklebone*
Tarsal bones	14	Form heel and back part of foot; anatomical ankle; largest is the *calcaneus*
Metatarsals	10	Form part of foot to which toes are attached; tarsal and metatarsal bones arranged so that they form three arches in foot; medial *(inner) longitudinal arch* and lateral *(outer) longitudinal arch,* which extend from front to back of foot, and transverse or *metatarsal arch,* which extends across foot
Phalanges	28	Toe bones; three in each toe, two in each great toe

CLINICAL APPLICATION

VERTEBROPLASTY

Vertebroplasty (ver-TEE-broh-plass-tee) is an orthopedic procedure that involves the injection of a "super glue" type of bone cement to repair fractured and compressed (collapsed) vertebrae (see illustration). In these patients the body of one or more vertebrae (generally lower thoracic and/or lumbar segments) have undergone a compression fracture due to trauma, tumors, or prolonged use of steroid drugs. In the procedure, bone cement is injected by needle into the area of compression, where it quickly hardens and thus stabilizes and seals the fracture. Vertebroplasty is cost effective, has a short recovery period, and in many cases may eliminate the need for difficult and expensive spinal surgery. The procedure is not intended for treatment of herniated disks and other types of vertebral pathology.

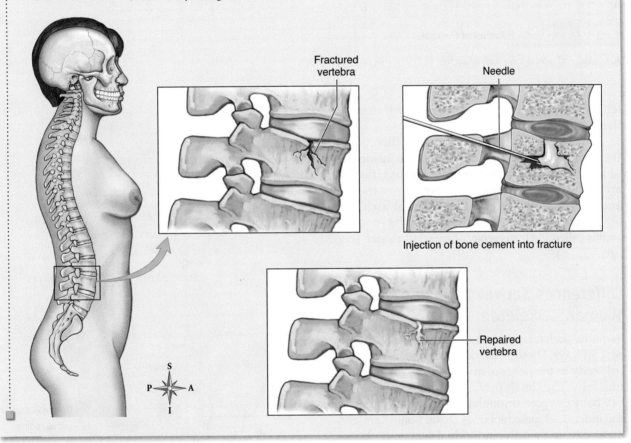

Fractured vertebra

Needle

Injection of bone cement into fracture

Repaired vertebra

largest tarsal bone and articulates with the tibia at the ankle joint. The bones of the lower extremities are summarized in Table 7-6.

You stand on your feet, so it's important that certain features of their structure make them able to support the body's weight. The great toe, for example, is considerably more solid and less mobile than the thumb. The foot bones are held together in such a way as to form springy lengthwise and crosswise arches. These provide great supporting strength and a highly stable base. Strong ligaments and leg muscle tendons normally hold the foot bones firmly in their arched positions. Frequently, however, the foot ligaments and tendons weaken. The arches then flat-

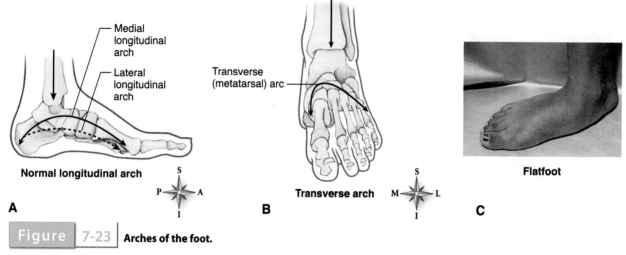

Figure 7-23 | **Arches of the foot.**

A, Medial and lateral longitudinal arches. **B,** Transverse arch. **C,** Flatfoot.

ten, a condition appropriately called *fallen arches,* or **flat feet** (Figure 7-23, *C*).

Two arches extend in a lengthwise direction in the foot (Figure 7-23, *A*). One lies on the inside part of the foot and is called the **medial longitudinal arch.** The other lies along the outer edge of the foot and is named the **lateral longitudinal arch.** Another arch extends across the ball of the foot; this arch is called the **transverse,** or **metatarsal, arch** (Figure 7-23, *B*).

Differences Between a Man's and a Woman's Skeleton

A man's skeleton and a woman's skeleton differ in several ways. These differences are the subject of careful study in the fields of anthropology and forensic medicine. The female pelvis is made so that the body of a baby can pass through it during birth. Although the individual male hipbones (coxal bones) are generally larger than the individual female hipbones, together the male hipbones form a narrower structure than do the female hipbones. A man's pelvis is shaped something like a funnel, but a woman's pelvis has a broader, shallower shape, more like a basin. (Incidentally, the word *pelvis* means "basin.") Another difference is that the pelvic inlet and pelvic outlet are both normally much wider in the female than in the male. Figure 7-24 shows this difference clearly. The pubic angle at the front of the female pelvis where the two pubic bones join is usually wider than it is in the male.

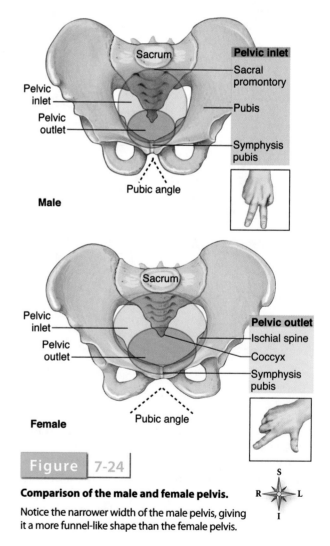

Figure 7-24

Comparison of the male and female pelvis.

Notice the narrower width of the male pelvis, giving it a more funnel-like shape than the female pelvis.

1. Name some of the bones of the upper extremity. And of the lower extremity.
2. What are the *phalanges?* Why are there two different sets of phalanges?
3. What are *metacarpal bones?* How do they differ from *metatarsal bones?*
4. How does the female pelvis differ from the male pelvis?

Joints (Articulations)

Every bone in the body, except one, connects to at least one other bone. In other words, every bone but one forms a joint with some other bone. (The exception is the hyoid bone in the neck, to which the tongue anchors.) Most of us probably never think much about our joints unless something goes wrong with them and they do not function properly. Then their tremendous importance becomes painfully clear. Joints hold our bones together securely and at the same time make it possible for movement to occur between the bones—between most of them, that is. Without joints we could not move our arms, legs, or any other of our body parts. Our bodies would, in short, be rigid, immobile hulks. Try, for example, to move your arm at your shoulder joint in as many directions as you can. Try to do the same thing at your elbow joint. Now examine the shape of the bones at each of these joints on a skeleton or in Figures 7-9 and 7-18. Do you see why you cannot move your arm at your elbow in nearly as many directions as you can at your shoulder?

Joint Types

One method classifies joints into three types according to the degree of movement they allow:

1. Synarthroses (no movement)
2. Amphiarthroses (slight movement)
3. Diarthroses (free movement)

Differences in joint structure account for differences in the degree of movement that is possible.

SYNARTHROSES

A **synarthrosis** (sin-ar-THROH-sis) is a joint in which fibrous connective tissue grows between the articulating (joining) bones holding them close together. Synarthroses do not allow any significant movement between the joined bones. The joints between cranial bones are synarthroses, commonly called *sutures* (Figure 7-25, *A*).

AMPHIARTHROSES

An **amphiarthrosis** (am-fee-ar-THROH-sis) is a joint in which cartilage connects the articulating bones. The symphysis pubis, the joint between the two pubic bones, is an amphiarthrosis (Figure 7-25, *B*).

Figure 7-25 | **Joints of the skeleton.**

A, Synarthrotic joint. **B,** Amphiarthrotic joint.

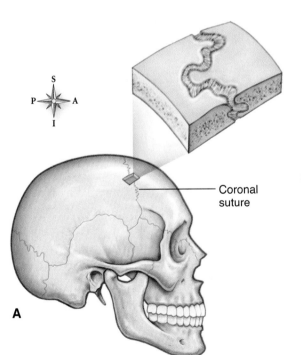

A — Coronal suture

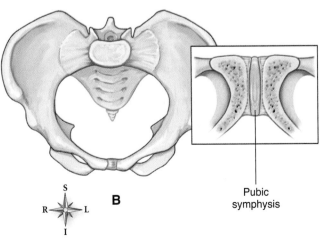

B — Pubic symphysis

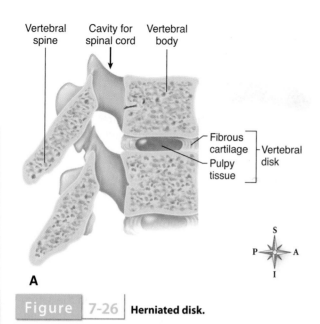

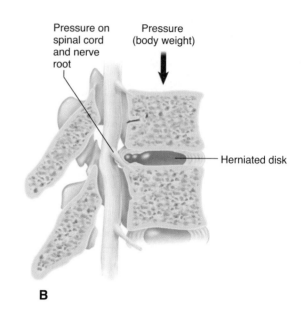

A

B

Figure 7-26 | **Herniated disk.**

Sagittal section of vertebrae showing **(A)** normal and **(B)** herniated disks.

Amphiarthroses allow slight movement between the joined bones.

Joints between the bodies of the vertebrae are also amphiarthroses. These joints make it possible to flex the trunk forward or sideways and even to circumduct and rotate it. Strong ligaments connect the bodies of the vertebrae, and fibrous disks lie between them. The central core of these intervertebral disks consists of a pulpy, elastic substance that loses some of its resiliency with age.

Damage to a disk caused by the pressure of sudden exertion or injury may push its wall into the spinal canal (Figure 7-26). Severe pain may result if the disk presses on the spinal cord. Popularly known as a *slipped disk,* this condition is known to health professionals as a **herniated disk**.

DIARTHROSES

The vast majority of our joints are diarthroses. Such joints allow considerable movement, sometimes in many directions and sometimes in only one or two directions.

Structure

Diarthroses (freely movable joints) are made alike in certain ways. All have a joint capsule, a joint cavity, and a layer of cartilage over the ends of two joining bones (Figure 7-27). The **joint cap-**

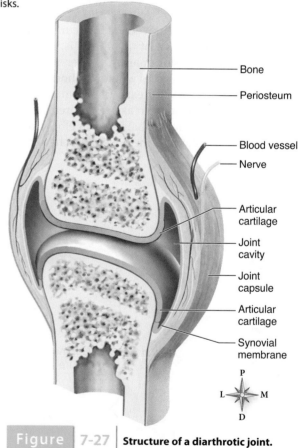

Figure 7-27 | **Structure of a diarthrotic joint.**

Each diarthrosis has a joint capsule, a joint cavity, and a layer of cartilage over the ends of the joined bones.

sule is made of the body's strongest and toughest material, fibrous connective tissue, and is lined with a smooth, slippery synovial membrane. The capsule fits over the ends of the two bones somewhat like a sleeve. Because it attaches firmly to the shaft of each bone to form its covering (called the *periosteum; peri* means "around," and *osteon* means "bone"), the joint capsule holds the bones securely together but at the same time permits movement at the joint. The structure of the joint capsule, in other words, helps make possible the joint's function.

Ligaments (cords or bands made of the same strong fibrous connective tissue as the joint capsule) also grow out of the periosteum and lash the two bones together even more firmly.

The layer of **articular cartilage** over the joint ends of bones acts like a rubber heel on a shoe—it absorbs jolts. The articular cartilage also provides a smooth surface that enables the bones of the joint to move with little friction. The **synovial membrane** secretes a lubricating fluid **(synovial fluid)** that allows easier movement with less friction.

There are several types of diarthroses, namely, ball-and-socket, hinge, pivot, saddle, gliding, and condyloid (Figure 7-28). Because they differ in structure, they differ also in their possible range of movement. In a ball-and-socket joint, a ball-shaped head of one bone fits into a concave socket of another bone. Shoulder and hip joints, for example, are ball-and-socket joints. Of all the joints in our bodies, these permit the widest range of movements. Think for a moment about how many ways you can move your upper arms. You can move them forward, backward, away from the sides of your body, and back down to your sides. You can also move them around so as to scribe a circle in the air with your hands.

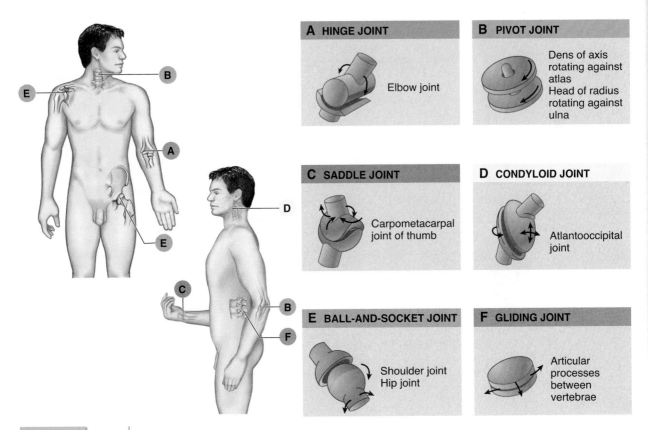

Figure 7-28 | **Types of diarthrotic joints.**

Notice that the structure of each type indicates its function (movement).

Hinge joints, like the hinges on a door, allow movements in only two directions, namely, flexion and extension. **Flexion** is bending a joint; **extension** is straightening it out (Table 7-7). Elbow and knee joints and the joints in the fingers are hinge joints.

Pivot joints are those in which a small projection of one bone pivots in an arch of another bone.

Table 7-7 | Types of Joint Movements

MOVEMENT	EXAMPLE	DESCRIPTION
Flexion (to flex a joint)	Flexion	Reduces the angle of the joint, as in bending the elbow
Extension (to extend a joint)	Extension	Increases the angle of a joint, as in straightening a bent elbow
Rotation (to rotate a joint)	Rotation	Spins one bone relative to another, as in rotating the head at the neck joint

MOVEMENT	EXAMPLE	DESCRIPTION
Circumduction (to circumduct a joint)	Circumduction	Moves the distal end of a bone in a circle, while circumducting a joint, keeping the proximal end relatively stable, as in moving the arm in a circle and thus circumducting the shoulder joint
Abduction (to abduct a joint)	Abduction	Increases the angle of a joint to move a part away from the midline, as in moving the arm to the side and away from the body
Adduction (to adduct a joint)	Adduction	Decreases the angle of a joint to move a part toward the midline, as in moving the arm in and down from the side

For example, a projection of the axis, the second vertebra in the neck, pivots (a motion referred to as **rotation**) in an arch of the atlas, the first vertebra in the neck. This *rotates* the head, which rests on the atlas.

Only one pair of saddle joints exists in the body—between the metacarpal bone of each thumb and a carpal bone of the wrist (the name of this carpal bone is the *trapezium*). Because the articulating surfaces of these bones are saddle-shaped, they make possible the human thumb's great mobility, a mobility no animal's thumb possesses. We can *flex, extend, abduct, adduct,* and *circumduct* our thumbs, and most important of all, we can move our thumbs to touch the tip of any one of our fingers. (This movement is called *opposing the thumb to the fingers.*) Without the saddle joints, we could not do simple acts such as picking up a pin or grasping a pencil between thumb and forefinger.

Gliding joints are the least movable diarthrotic joints. Their flat articulating surfaces allow limited gliding movements, such as that at the superior and inferior articulating processes between successive vertebrae.

Condyloid joints are those in which a condyle (an oval projection) fits into an elliptical socket. An example is the fit of the distal end of the radius into depressions in the carpal bones.

 To learn more about types of joint movement, go to **AnimationDirect** on your CD.

QUICK CHECK

1. What are the three major types of joints in the skeleton? Give an example of each.
2. What membrane in a diarthrotic joint provides lubrication for movement?
3. What is a ligament?
4. What is meant by "flexing" the elbow? Extending the elbow?

CLINICAL APPLICATION

PALPABLE BONY LANDMARKS

Health professionals often identify externally palpable bony landmarks when dealing with the sick and injured. **Palpable** bony landmarks are bones that can be touched and identified through the skin. They serve as reference points in identifying other body structures.

Try to identify as many of the externally palpable bones of the skeleton as possible on your own body. Using these as points of reference will make it easier for you to visualize the placement of other bones that cannot be touched or palpated through the skin.

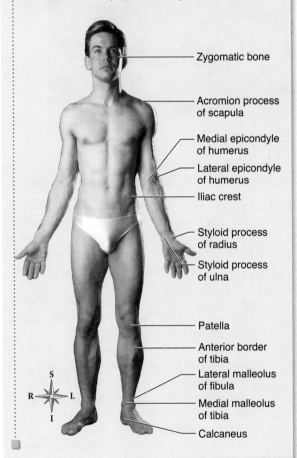

HEALTH & WELL-BEING

THE KNEE JOINT

The knee is the largest and most vulnerable joint. Because the knee is often subjected to sudden, strong forces during athletic activity, knee injuries are among the most common type of athletic injury. Sometimes, the articular cartilages on the tibia become torn when the knee twists while bearing weight. The ligaments holding the tibia and femur together also can be injured in this way. Knee injuries also may occur when a weight-bearing knee is hit by another person or a moving object such as a baseball bat.

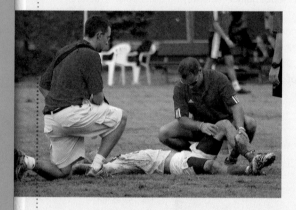

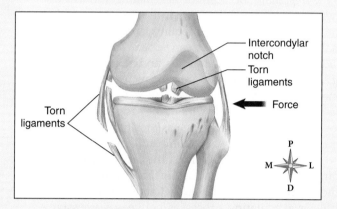

Women and Knee Injury

Women have a higher risk of knee injuries than men. There have been several proposed causes including the following:

1. The wider pelvis of a woman results in the femur angling toward the knee at a greater angle, called the Q angle (see figures at right). This results in the pull on the patella (kneecap) by the lateral quadriceps muscle, which pulls the patella out of alignment and may weaken the knee.
2. The female femoral intercondylar notch is narrow compared to the male femoral notch. This narrow notch may rub and weaken the ACL (anterior cruciate ligament) that stabilizes the knee.
3. An increase in the female hormone estrogen may cause the ligaments to be more flexible and more prone to overstretching and rupturing. This may cause an increased flexibility of ligaments when estrogen levels are higher, as occurs during ovulation or pregnancy.
4. Females tend to have stronger quadriceps (anterior thigh muscles) than hamstrings (posterior thigh muscles). The hamstring muscles keep the tibia in place when jumping or making sudden stops.

In order to avoid injury to the knee, it is recommended that (1) women wear shoes that prevent the pronation of the foot and knee, (2) exercise both the hamstrings and the quadriceps muscles, and (3) have a knowledgeable trainer teach them how to land after jumping and how to make quick turns without twisting the knee.

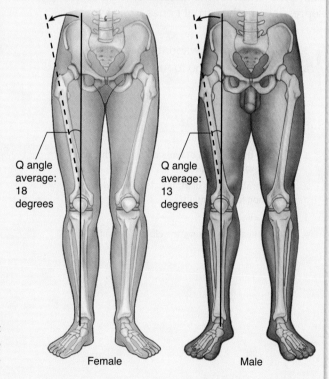

Female   Male

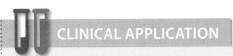

TOTAL HIP REPLACEMENT

Because total hip replacement (THR) is the most common orthopedic operation performed on older persons (more than 300,000 procedures per year in the United States), home health care professionals often are engaged to work with patients recovering from THR surgery.

The THR procedure involves replacement of the femoral head by a metal prosthesis and the acetabular socket by a polyethylene cup. The prostheses are usually coated with a porous material that allows natural growth of bone to mesh with the artificial material. Such meshing of tissue and prostheses ensures stability of the parts without the loosening that the use of glues in the past often allowed. First introduced in 1953, THR technique has advanced to the state that the procedure has a success rate of about 85% in older adults.

As patients recover at home after THR surgery, they can expect to progress through normal surgical healing and recovery, which includes stabilization of the prosthesis as new tissue grows into the porous coating that was applied to the prosthesis. Typically, THR patients can also expect to regain some previously lost function in the affected hip, including improved weight-bearing and walking movements.

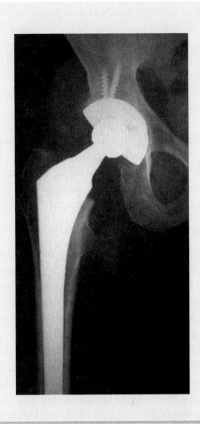

Skeletal Disorders

Skeletal disorders include pathologic conditions associated with bone, cartilage, ligaments, and joints.

Tumors of Bone and Cartilage

Two of the most serious skeletal disorders involve malignant tumors of bone tissue and cartilage. The most common and devastating malignant neoplasm of bone is called **osteosarcoma** (os-tee-oh-sar-KOH-mah). Twenty-five years ago nearly all patients diagnosed with this disease died within 3 years. Although still considered a very aggressive and destructive type of cancer, earlier diagnosis and newer treatment options are increasing survival rates and decreasing the need for immediate and complete amputation of affected limbs. Osteosarcomas occur most often in the distal femur (Figure 7-29, *A*) and proximal areas of the tibia and humerus. Nearly twice as many males are affected as females and most cases occur between 20 and 40 years

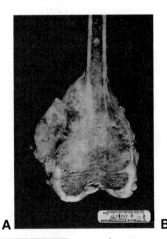
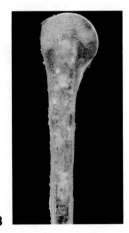

A   **B**

Figure 7-29 | **Tumors of bone and cartilage (surgical specimens sectioned longitudinally).**

A, Osteosarcoma of distal femur. The tumor has broken out of the medullary cavity and is growing on the surface of the bone. **B,** Chondrosarcoma of proximal humerus. Note the glistening appearance of the hyaline cartilage tumor in the medullary cavity.

of age. These tumors are characterized by severe, unrelenting pain. Treatment involves surgical removal of the tumor and both presurgical and postsurgical chemotherapy. **Chondrosarcoma** (KON-droh-sar-KOH-mah) is cancer of skeletal hyaline cartilage tissue and is the second most common type of cancer affecting bones. The most common tumor sites involve the medullary cavity of the humerus, femur, ribs and pelvic bones (Figure 7-29, *B*). Chondrosarcomas occur most often in adults between 40 and 70 years of age. Incidence is slightly higher in males. Pain is a common but not a universal symptom and when present is generally less severe than in osteosarcoma. Treatment is surgical removal of the lesion. Chemotherapy is not effective in treating chondrosarcoma.

Metabolic Bone Diseases

OSTEOPOROSIS

Osteoporosis (os-tee-oh-poh-ROH-sis) is the name of the disorder in which bones lose minerals and become less dense, as evidenced on scanning electron micrograph studies (Figure 7-30). It is one of the most common and serious bone diseases. Although the cause remains unknown, genetics play a part in the etiology, as do low estrogen levels and postmenopause status in women. Certain drugs, a diet low in calcium, lack of weight-bearing exercise, and smoking are also risk factors. Osteoporosis occurs most often in elderly white women. The disease is characterized by excessive loss of calcified bone matrix. A reduction in the number of needlelike trabeculae in spongy bone is particularly

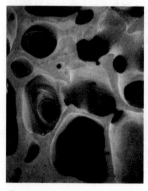 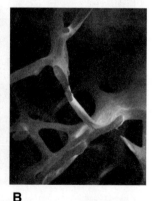

A   **B**

Figure 7-30 | **Comparison of normal and osteoporotic spongy bone.**

Scanning electron micrograph (SEM) of, **A,** normal bone and, **B,** bone with osteoporosis. Note the loss of trabeculae and appearance of enlarged pores in the osteoporotic bone.

noticeable. The name *osteoporosis* means "condition of bone pores" referring to the holes or pores formed as bone tissue is lost. Compare the appearance of normal and osteoporotic bone specimens in Figure 7-30.

A progressive increase in bone porosity causes the bones in people with osteoporosis to become brittle and easily broken. Fractures may be completely "spontaneous" or occur with even minor trauma or during routine activities. The most common fracture sites are the wrists, hips, and vertebrae. Compression fractures of the vertebrae result in a shortened stature and the classic kyphosis of the thoracic spine called **"dowager's hump"** in elderly women suffering from the disease. Treatment or preventive measures may include drug therapy, weight-bearing exercise, and dietary supplements of calcium and vitamin D to replace deficiencies or to offset intestinal malabsorption.

RICKETS AND OSTEOMALACIA

Rickets in young children and **osteomalacia** (os-tee-oh-mah-LAY-shah) in adults are metabolic skeletal diseases that affect significant numbers of individuals worldwide. Both diseases are characterized by demineralization, or loss of minerals, from bone related to vitamin D deficiency. Vitamin D helps the intestines absorb calcium from the diet. The loss of minerals is coupled to an increased production of unmineralized matrix. Rickets involves demineralization of developing bones in infants and young children before skeletal maturity. In osteomalacia, mineral content is lost from bones that have already matured. In rickets, the lack of rigidity caused by demineralization of developing bones results in gross skeletal changes including a classic "bowing of the legs" symptom (Figure 7-31). The demineralization of bones in osteomalacia does not generally affect overall skeletal contours but does result in increased susceptibility to fractures, especially in the vertebral bodies and femoral necks. Vitamin D is produced by the body when sunlight strikes the skin and is seldom produced during the winter months where people wear warmer clothing that covers more of their bodies. Vitamin D is added to some foods (milk and some juices) to help reduce this deficiency.

PAGET DISEASE

Paget (PAJ-et) **disease** of bone, also called *osteitis deformans*, was first described by British surgeon Sir James Paget in 1882. His remarkably detailed observations of a patient he treated repeatedly over a 20-year period for a deforming bone disease are consid-

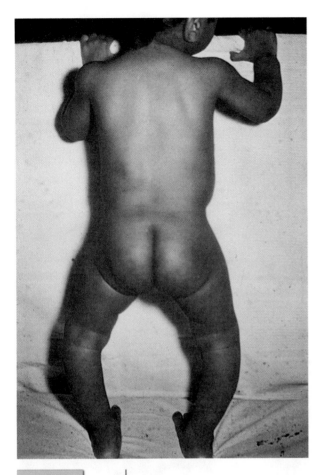

Figure 7-31 **Rickets.**

Bowing of legs in this toddler is due to poorly mineralized bones.

ered classic in the annals of surgery. The disease is characterized by localized, intermittent, and uncontrolled episodes of almost "frenzied" osteoclastic (bone resorbing) and osteoblastic (bone forming) activity. The faulty remodeling process results in bones that are deformed, unstable, and easily fractured. The disease is often asymptomatic early in its course but becomes painful as the weak but often thickened areas of defective bone cause deformity, arthritic symptoms, and fracture injuries. The disease may involve one or many bones. The spine, skull, pelvis, and long bones of the extremities are common sites. In addition to pain, the location of the lesion may produce additional unique symptoms. For example, deformity of skull bones may compress cranial nerves causing deafness, blindness, headaches, and facial paralysis. Unfortunately, areas of diseased bone develop into osteosarcomas in about

1% of affected individuals. Paget disease affects about 3% of people over 50 years of age. The disease has a genetic tendency and may be triggered by viral infections. Disease treatment includes mostly pain control and drugs that improve the strength of the bone (Figure 7-32).

Osteogenesis imperfecta (OS-tee-oh-jen-e-sis im-per-FEK-tah) is a genetic disease that can affect 1 in 30,000 births and is also called "brittle bone disease." The bones are brittle as the result of a lack of production of the organic matrix of bone. The organic material (mostly collagen) in bone gives it the ability to withstand twisting and compression forces without breaking. The same concept applies to the practice of placing metal rods inside of concrete in bridge or road construction. A bridge without metal rods would not be able to withstand the weight and vibration of traffic. Bones without organic material are thus very fragile and easily fractured. The diagnosis of this disease usually follows increased fracture rates and a blood test for the enzyme alkaline phosphatase. Treatment may include splinting of the bone to reduce fracture during growth and treat-

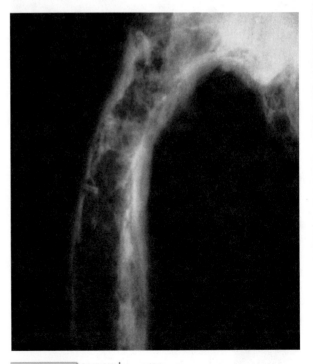

Figure 7-32 **Paget disease (osteitis deformans).**

Note the weakened and irregular cancellous bone overgrowth in the femur.

ment with drugs that decrease the activity of cells that break down bone (Figure 7-33).

Bone Infection

Osteomyelitis (os-tee-oh-my-el-EYE-tis) is the general name for bacterial infections of bone and marrow tissue. *Staphylococcus* bacteria are the most common pathogens found in this condition. They may reach bone via the bloodstream or from an adjacent soft tissue infection such as an abscess, or be introduced directly into the bone as a result of open fractures, penetrating wounds, or by flawed surgical aseptic techniques. On rare occasions, infections also may occur after insertion of infected donor tissues into bones or joints or by contaminated joint prostheses. Besides bacterial infections, bone tissue is also susceptible to damage by viruses, fungi, and other pathogens.

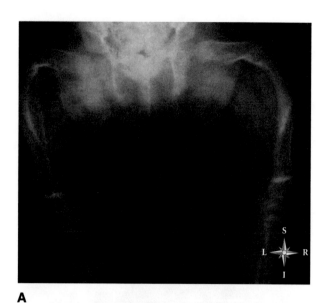

A

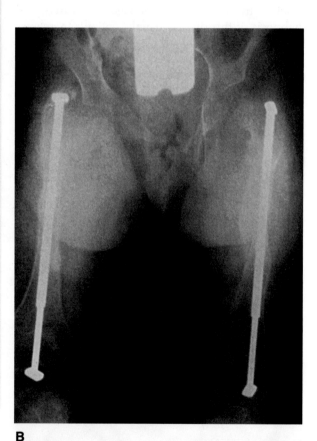

B

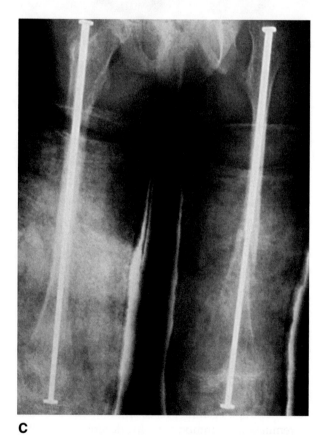

C

Figure 7-33 | **Osteogenesis imperfecta treatment of femurs.**

These x-ray films show the progression of treatment in the same individual with "brittle bone disease." A telescoping medullary rod is inserted and expanded while the individual grows. **A,** Shows original x-ray film; **B,** same individual with the rods in place; **C,** x-ray film of the same person 4 years later.

Any bone infection is difficult to treat because of the density of the bone and the slowness of the healing process compared with that of other tissues. Osteomyelitis produces persistent and severe pain, muscle spasm, swelling, and fever. Pus collecting in the confined space of the bone increases pressure, decreases blood flow, and in time will cause necrosis or death of bone tissue. Figure 7-34 shows a segment of infected bone in a severe case of chronic osteomyelitis. Even with intensive and repeated treatment using parenteral (IV) antibiotics, difficult cases of osteomyelitis may become chronic and reappear months or years after an assumed cure.

> **QUICK CHECK**
>
> 1. Name two types of malignant tumors that affect bones.
> 2. What metabolic bone disease is characterized by kyphosis of the thoracic spine called "dowager's hump"?
> 3. Identify the metabolic bone disease characterized by loss of bone minerals and vitamin D deficiency in children. What is the disease called in adults?
> 4. What is the general name for bacterial infections of bone and marrow tissue?

Bone Fractures

Excessive mechanical stress on bones can result in breaks or fractures (Figure 7-35). Sometimes bone

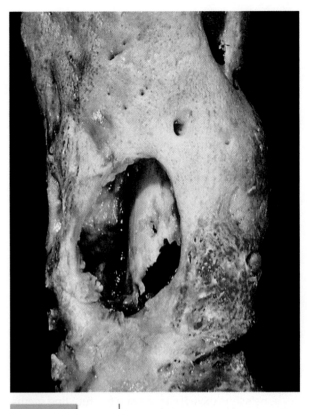

Figure 7-34 **Osteomyelitis.**

Segment of femur from a patient with chronic osteomyelitis.

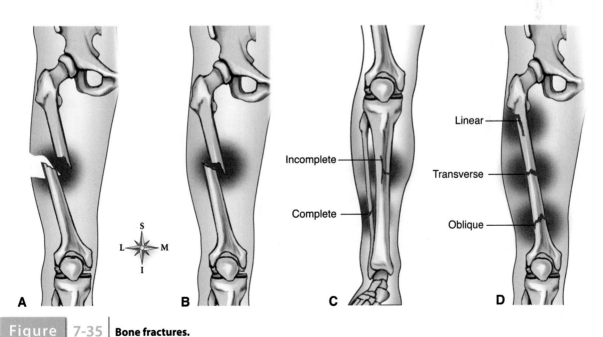

Figure 7-35 **Bone fractures.**

A, Open. **B,** Closed. **C,** Incomplete and complete. **D,** Linear, transverse, and oblique.

cancer or metabolic bone disorders weaken a bone to the point that it fractures with very little stress. **Open fractures,** or *compound fractures,* in which bone pierces the skin, invite the possibility of infection or osteomyelitis. **Closed fractures,** also known as *simple fractures,* do not pierce the skin and so do not pose an immediate danger of bone infection.

In **complete fractures** the bone fragments separate completely, whereas in **incomplete fractures** the bone fragments are still partially joined. Incomplete fractures in which a bone is bent but broken only on the outer curve of the bend are often called *greenstick fractures.* Greenstick fractures, common in children, usually heal rapidly. **Comminuted** (KOM-in-oot-ed) **fractures** are breaks that produce many fragments. **Impacted fractures** occur when bone fragments are driven into each other. Sometimes the angle of the fracture line or crack is used in labeling fracture types:

1. **Linear fracture**—fracture line is parallel to the bone's long axis.

2. **Transverse fracture**—fracture line is at a right angle to the bone's long axis.

3. **Oblique fracture**—fracture line is diagonal to the bone's long axis. If the oblique fracture line seems to spiral around a bone like the stripe on a candy cane, the fracture may be called a *spiral fracture.*

After a fracture occurs, a bone usually bleeds, becomes inflamed, and then forms a bony framework called a **callus** (KAL-us) around the injury (Figure 7-36). The callus tissue stabilizes the bone fragments and thus aids in the long healing and remodeling process.

 To learn more about bone fracture and repair, go to **AnimationDirect** on your CD.

Joint Disorders

Joint disorders can be classified as noninflammatory joint disease or inflammatory joint disease.

NONINFLAMMATORY JOINT DISEASE

Noninflammatory joint disease is distinguished from other joint conditions because it does not involve inflammation of the synovial membrane and does not produce systemic signs or symptoms.

Osteoarthritis (os-tee-oh-arth-RYE-tis), known also as *degenerative joint disease (DJD),* is the most common noninflammatory disorder of movable joints. Abnormal formation of new bone (*"bone spurs"*) at joint surfaces and degeneration of articular cartilage are characteristic features of osteoarthritis. Weight-bearing joints, such as the hips, lumbar spine, and

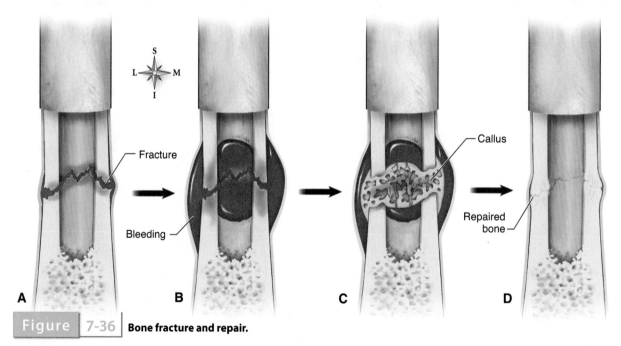

Figure 7-36 | Bone fracture and repair. After a fracture **(A),** there is bleeding and inflammation around the affected area **(B).** Special tissue forms a bony framework called a *callus* **(C)** that stabilizes the bone until the repair is complete.

knees are often involved. Localized tenderness over affected joints, morning stiffness, and pain on movement are frequent symptoms.

Figure 7-37, *A*, shows another common sign of osteoarthritis. The fingers of individuals with this form of DJD often show nodes at both the proximal interphalangeal joints (called **Bouchard nodes**) and the distal interphalangeal joints (called **Heberden nodes**). The etiology of most cases of DJD is unknown, but advanced age, joint damage caused by "wear and tear," and obesity are known risk factors. Advanced cases of osteoarthritis are the most common cause for partial or total hip and knee replacements.

Traumatic injury is often the cause of noninflammatory joint problems. **Dislocation,** or **subluxation** (sub-luks-AY-shun), occurs when the articular surfaces of bones forming the joint are no longer in proper contact with each other. A **sprain** is an acute injury to the ligaments around a joint. A common cause of sprains is a twisting or wrenching movement often associated with "whiplash"-type injuries.

The term **strain** is used to describe an injury involving the "*musculotendinous unit*" and may involve the muscle, the tendon, and the junction between the two, as well as their attachments to bone. Most strains occur in muscle tissue, often because of overstretching, or violent types of muscle contraction (see Chapter 8, p. 224). However, the portion of the unit injured depends on which component is weakest. In preadolescent athletes with incompletely ossified bones, the muscle component of the unit or the point of attachment of the muscle to the bone may be stronger than the developing bone itself or the union between its epiphysis and diaphysis. In these cases, violent muscle contractions can cause an **avulsion fracture** (often near a joint), in which a piece of bone is pulled free, or an **epiphyseal fracture** between the epiphysis and diaphysis of the involved bone (see box on p. 175).

INFLAMMATORY JOINT DISEASE (ARTHRITIS)

Arthritis (arth-RYE-tis) is a general name for many different inflammatory joint diseases. Arthritis can be caused by a variety of factors, including infection, injury, genetic factors, and autoimmunity. Here is a brief list of major types of arthritis:

1. **Rheumatoid** (ROO-mah-toyd) **arthritis—** believed to be a type of autoimmune disease, rheumatoid arthritis involves chronic inflammation of connective tissues. It begins in the

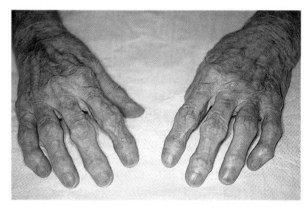

A

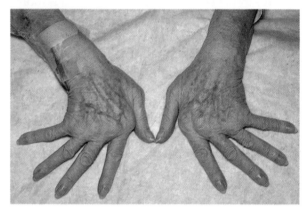

B

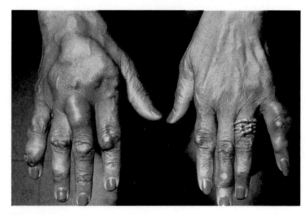

C

Figure 7-37 | **Types of arthritis.**

A, Osteoarthritis. Note the presence of nodes in the proximal interphalangeal joints (Bouchard nodes) and distal interphalangeal joints (Heberden nodes). **B,** Rheumatoid arthritis. Note the marked ulnar deviation of the wrists. **C,** Gouty arthritis. Note tophi filled with sodium urate crystals.

synovial membrane and spreads to cartilage and other tissues, often causing severe crippling. A characteristic deformity of the hands in rheumatoid arthritis is **ulnar deviation** of the fingers (Figure 7-37, *B*). The autoimmune nature of the disease may cause damage to many body organs, such as the blood vessels, eyes, lungs, and heart. Because it is a systemic disease, fever, anemia, weight loss, and profound fatigue are common. **Juvenile rheumatoid arthritis** is more severe than the adult form but involves similar deterioration and deformity of joints. The joint inflammatory process often destroys growth of cartilage, and growth of long bones is arrested. This form begins during childhood and is more common in girls.

2. **Gouty arthritis—Gout** is a metabolic condition in which uric acid, a nitrogenous waste, increases in the blood. Excess uric acid is deposited as sodium urate crystals in distal joints and other tissues (Figure 7-36, *C*). These crystals trigger the chronic inflammation and tissue damage characteristic of gouty arthritis.

3. **Infectious arthritis**—A variety of pathogens can infect synovial membrane and other joint tissues. One form of infectious arthritis, **Lyme arthritis,** or **Lyme disease,** has become a problem throughout most of the United States (U.S.) in only the last few decades. Lyme disease was identified in Old Lyme, Connecticut, in 1975 and is caused by a spirochete bacterium carried by deer ticks. This condition is characterized by inflammation in the knees or other joints accompanied by a variety of systemic signs and symptoms. Another group of bacteria called *Ehrlichia* is also carried by ticks and includes the agents that cause the various forms of **ehrlichiosis** (er-LICK-ee-oh-sis). This bacterial infection has some of the same symptoms as Lyme disease, but is more prevalent than Lyme arthritis in some parts of the U.S. One form of ehrlichiosis is more prevalent in the midwestern U. S. and another form is found mostly in the southern U. S. Both Lyme arthritis and ehrlichiosis are treated by the use of antibiotics (Figure 7-38).

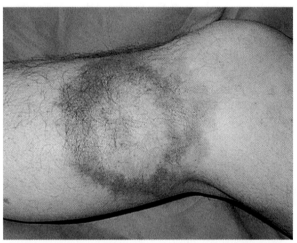

A

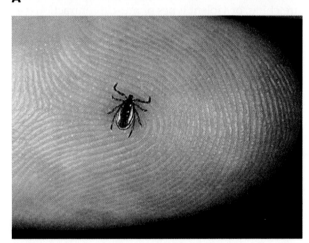

B

Figure 7-38 **Lyme disease.**

A, Circular, expanding rash caused by the spirochete bacteria *Borrelia burgdorferi*. **B,** Deer tick, vector for transmission of Lyme disease.

CLINICAL APPLICATION

ARTHROSCOPY

Arthroscopy is an imaging technique that allows a physician to examine the internal structure of a joint without the use of extensive surgery. As Figure **A** shows, a narrow tube with lenses and a fiberoptic light source is inserted into the joint space through a small puncture. Isotonic saline (salt) solution is injected through a needle to expand the volume of the synovial space. This spreads the joint structures and makes viewing easier **(B).**

Although arthroscopy is often used as a diagnostic procedure, it also can be used to perform joint surgery. While the surgeon views the internal structure of the joint through the arthroscope or on an attached video monitor, instruments can be inserted through puncture holes and used to repair or remove damaged tissue. Arthroscopic surgery is much less traumatic than previous methods in which the joint cavity was completely opened.

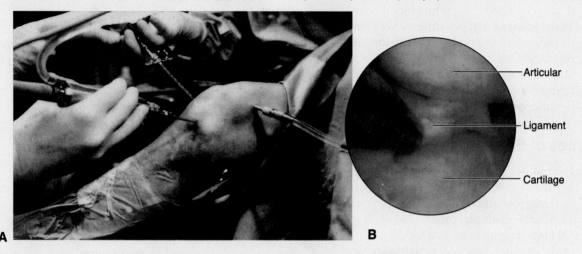

A

B

Articular

Ligament

Cartilage

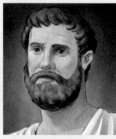

SCIENCE APPLICATIONS

BONES AND JOINTS

Ever since 400 BC, when Hippocrates (the Greek physician often regarded as a founder of the medical profession) first described treatments for human bone and joint disorders and injuries, many approaches to treating the human skeleton have been taken. For example, physical and occupational therapists help patients regain movement in joints through physical exercises, and orthopedic surgeons

Hippocrates (460-377 BC)

help their patients by means of surgical operations. Because the skeleton, with its many bones and joints, is the framework of the entire body, it is not surprising to learn that many different health professionals focus their attention on the skeleton. For example, podiatrists focus on solving problems associated with the bones and joints of the foot and ankle, sports trainers and physicians focus on maximizing and maintaining the health of many parts of the skeleton, and chiropractic physicians focus their treatments on alignment of the vertebral column. And, of course, radiographic technicians and radiologists are often called upon to make medical images of the bones and joints and then interpret the meaning of the images.

Outline Summary

 To download an MP3 version of the chapter summary for use with your iPod or portable media player, access the **Audio Chapter Summaries** on your CD.

Functions of the Skeletal System

A. Provides internal framework that supports the body
B. Protects internal organs and helps fight disease by producing white blood cells
C. Makes movement possible by working in concert with muscle contraction and relaxation
D. Stores calcium, a vital resource
E. Forms blood cells—the process called hematopoiesis

Types of Bones

A. **Four major t**ypes, according to overall shape of the bone
 1. Long—example: humerus (upper arm)
 2. Short—example: carpals (wrist)
 3. Flat—example: frontal (skull)
 4. Irregular—example: vertebrae (spinal bones)
 5. Some also recognize a sesamoid (round) bone category—example: patella (kneecap)
B. Structure of long bones (Figure 7-1)
 1. Diaphysis, or shaft—hollow tube of hard compact bone
 2. Medullary cavity—hollow space inside the diaphysis that contains yellow marrow
 3. Epiphyses, or ends, of the bone—made of spongy bone that contains red bone marrow
 4. Articular cartilage—thin layer that covers each epiphysis; provides as a cushion
 5. Periosteum—strong, fibrous membrane covering bone everywhere except at joint surfaces
 6. Endosteum—thin membrane that lines medullary cavity
C. Structure of flat bones (Figure 7-2)
 1. Thin layer of compact bone surrounding cancellous (spongy or diploe) bone
 2. Open spaces within spongy bone are surrounded by bony trabeculae

Microscopic Structure of Bone and Cartilage

A. Two major types of connective tissue: bone and cartilage (Figure 7-3)
B. Bone types
 1. Spongy
  a. Texture results from needlelike threads of bone called *trabeculae* surrounded by a network of open spaces
  b. Found in epiphyses of bones
  c. Spaces contain red bone marrow
 2. Compact (Figure 7-4)
  a. Structural unit is an osteon-calcified matrix arranged in multiple layers or rings called concentric lamella
  b. Bone cells, called *osteocytes*, are found inside spaces called *lacunae*, which are connected by tiny tubes called *canaliculi*
  c. Covered by periosteum
C. Cartilage (Figure 7-5)
 1. Cell type called chondrocytes located in lacunae
 2. Matrix is flexible gel-like substance and lacks blood vessels

Bone Formation and Growth (Figures 7-6 and 7-7)

A. Early bone development (before birth) consists of cartilage and fibrous structures.
B. Cartilage models gradually replaced by calcified bone matrix—process called endochondral ossification
C. Osteoblasts form new bone, and osteoclasts resorb bone

Divisions of the Skeleton (Figure 7-9 and Table 7-1)

A. Axial skeleton (80 bones)
 1. Skull (Figure 7-10 and Table 7-2)

2. Spine or vertebral column (Figures 7-13 and 7-14)
3. Thorax (Figure 7-17 and Table 7-4)
B. Appendicular skeleton (126 bones)
   1. Upper extremities, including shoulder (pectoral) girdle
   2. Lower extremities, including hip (pelvic) girdle

Differences Between a Man's and a Woman's Skeleton

A. Size—male skeleton generally larger (Figure 7-24)
B. Shape of pelvis—male pelvis deep and narrow, female pelvis broad and shallow
C. Size of pelvic inlet—female pelvic inlet generally wider, normally large enough for baby's head to pass through it
D. Pubic angle—angle between pubic bones of female generally wider

Joints (Articulations)

A. Every bone except the hyoid (which anchors the tongue) connects to at least one other bone.
B. Joint types (Figures 7-25 to 7-28)—classified by degree of movement
   1. Synarthroses (no movement)—fibrous connective tissue grows between articulating bones; for example, sutures of skull
   2. Amphiarthroses (slight movement)—cartilage connects articulating bones; for example, symphysis pubis
   3. Diarthroses (free movement)—most joints belong to this class
      a. Structures of freely movable joints—joint capsule and ligaments hold adjoining bones together but permit movement at joint
      b. Articular cartilage—covers joint ends of bones and absorbs jolts
      c. Synovial membrane—lines joint capsule and secretes lubricating fluid
      d. Joint cavity—space between joint ends of bones
C. Types of freely movable joints—ball-and-socket, hinge, pivot, saddle, gliding, and condyloid

Skeletal Disorders

A. Tumors of bone and cartilage
   1. Osteosarcoma (Figure 7-29, *A*)
      a. Most common and serious type of malignant bone neoplasm
      b. Frequent sites include distal femur and proximal tibia and humerus
   2. Chondrosarcoma (Figure 7-29, *B*)
      a. Cancer of skeletal hyaline cartilage
      b. Second most common cancer of skeletal tissues
      c. Frequent sites include medullary cavity of humerus, femur, ribs and pelvic bones
B. Metabolic bone diseases
   1. Osteoporosis (Figure 7-30)
      a. Characterized by loss of calcified bone matrix and reduction in number of trabeculae in spongy bone
      b. Bones fracture easily—especially in wrists, hips, and vertebrae
      c. Treatment includes drug therapy, exercise, and dietary supplements of calcium and vitamin D
   2. Rickets and osteomalacia—both diseases characterized by loss of bone minerals related to vitamin D deficiency
      a. Rickets (Figure 7-31)
         (1) Loss of bone minerals occurs in infants and young children before skeletal maturity
         (2) Lack of bone rigidity causes gross skeletal changes (bowing of legs)
         (3) Treated with vitamin D
      b. Osteomalacia
         (1) Mineral content is lost from bones that have already matured
         (2) Increases susceptibility to fractures
         (3) Treated with vitamin D
   3. Paget disease (osteitis deformans) (Figure 7-32)
         (1) Faulty remodeling results in deformed bones that fracture easily
         (2) Cause may be genetic or triggered by viral infections
   4. Osteogenesis imperfecta (also called *brittle bone disease*) (Figure 7-33)
         (1) Bones are brittle because of a lack of organic matrix

(2) Treatment may include splinting to reduce fracture and drugs that decrease cell activity

C. Bone infection
   1. Osteomyelitis (Figure 7-34)
      a. General term for bacterial (usually staphylococcal infection of bone)
      b. Treatment may involve surgery, drainage of pus, and IV antibiotic treatment—often over prolonged periods

D. Bone fractures (Figure 7-35)
   1. Open (compound) fractures pierce the skin and closed (simple) fractures do not
   2. Fracture types include complete and incomplete, linear, transverse, and oblique

E. Joint disorders
   1. Noninflammatory joint disorders—do not usually involve inflammation of the synovial membrane; symptoms tend to be local and not systemic
      a. Osteoarthritis, or *degenerative joint disease* (DJD) (Figure 7-37, *A*)
         (1) Most common noninflammatory disorder of movable joints—often called "wear and tear" arthritis
         (2) Symptoms include joint pain, morning stiffness, and appearance of Bouchard nodes (at proximal interphalangeal joints) and Heberden nodes (at distal interphalangeal joints) of the fingers
         (3) Most common cause for partial and total hip and knee replacements
      b. Traumatic injury

(1) Dislocation or subluxation—articular surfaces of bones in joint are no longer in proper contact
(2) Sprain—acute injury to *ligaments* around joints (example: whiplash-type injuries)
(3) Strain—acute injury to any part of the *"musculotendinous unit"* (muscle, tendon, junction between the two, and attachments to bone)

   2. Inflammatory joint disorders—the term *arthritis* is a general name for several types of inflammatory joint diseases that may be caused by infection, injury, genetic factors, and autoimmunity. Inflammation of the synovial membrane occurs, often with systemic signs and symptoms.
      a. Rheumatoid arthritis (Figure 7-37, *B*)—systemic autoimmune disease—chronic inflammation of synovial membrane with involvement of other tissues such as blood vessels, eyes, heart, and lungs
      b. Gouty arthritis (Figure 7-37, *C*)—synovial inflammation caused by gout, a condition in which sodium urate crystals form in joints and other tissues
      c. Infectious arthritis (Figure 7-38)—arthritis resulting from infection by a pathogen, as in Lyme arthritis and ehrlichiosis, caused by two different types of bacteria that are transmitted to humans by tick bites.

New Words

acetabulum	carpal	endochondral ossification	hematopoiesis
amphiarthrosis (*pl.,* amphiarthroses)	cartilage	endosteum	humerus
	central canal	epiphysis (*pl.,* epiphyses)	ilium
appendicular skeleton	chondrocyte	epiphyseal line	ischium
articular cartilage	clavicle	epiphyseal plate	joint capsule
articulation (joint)	compact (dense) bone	extension	lacuna (*pl.,* lacunae)
axial skeleton	coxal bone	femur	lamella (*pl.,* lamellae)
calcaneus	cranium	fibula	lateral longitudinal arch
canaliculi	diaphysis	flexion	ligament
cancellous (spongy) bone	diarthrosis (*pl.,* diarthroses)	fontanel	medial longitudinal arch

medullary cavity	sinus	avulsion fracture	Lyme arthritis
metacarpal	skull	Bouchard node	mastoiditis
metatarsal	spine	callus	oblique fracture
middle ear	sternoclavicular joint	chondrosarcoma	open fracture
olecranon fossa	suture	closed fracture	osteoarthritis
olecranon process	synarthrosis (*pl.*, synar-	comminuted fracture	osteogenesis imperfecta
osteoblast	throses)	complete fracture	osteomalacia
osteoclast	synovial fluid	dowager's hump	osteomyelitis
osteocyte	synovial membrane	ehrlichiosis	osteoporosis
osteon (haversian system)	tarsal	epiphyseal fracture	osteosarcoma
palpable	thorax (chest)	flatfeet	Paget disease
paranasal sinus	tibia	gout	rheumatoid arthritis
patella	trabeculae	Heberden node	rickets
pectoral girdle (shoulder)	transverse (metatarsal) arch	herniated disk	scoliosis
pelvic girdle (hip)	ulna	impacted fracture	sprain
periosteum	vertebra (*pl.*, vertebrae)	incomplete fracture	strain
phalanges (*sing.*, phalanx)		infectious arthritis	subluxation (dislocation)
pubis	**Diseases and Other**	juvenile rheumatoid arthritis	transverse fracture
radius	**Clinical Terms**	kyphosis	ulnar deviation
rotation	arthritis	linear fracture	
scapula		lordosis	

Review Questions

1. List and briefly describe the five functions of the skeletal system.
2. Describe the structure of the osteon.
3. Describe the structure of cartilage.
4. Explain briefly the process of endochondral ossification, including the function of the osteoblasts and osteoclasts.
5. Explain the importance of the epiphyseal plate.
6. In general, what bones are included in the axial skeleton? The appendicular skeleton?
7. The vertebral column is divided into five sections based on location. Name the sections and give the number of vertebrae in each section.
8. Distinguish between true, false, and floating ribs. How many of each are in the human body?
9. Describe and give an example of a synarthrotic joint.
10. Describe and give an example of an amphiarthrotic joint.
11. Describe and give two examples of a diarthrotic joint.
12. Briefly describe a joint capsule.
13. Describe open, closed, and comminuted fractures.
14. Describe the three types of arthritis.

Critical Thinking

15. When a patient receives a bone marrow transplant, what vital process is being restored?
16. Explain how the canaliculi allow bone to heal more efficiently than cartilage.
17. What effect does the task of childbearing have on the difference between the male and female skeleton?
18. Is it possible to tell whether a child is going to grow any taller? If so, how?
19. Compare and contrast the causes and changes associated with osteoporosis, osteomalacia, and Paget disease.
20. Why is mastoiditis potentially more dangerous than a paranasal sinus infection?

Chapter Test

1. The thin layer of cartilage on the ends of bones where they form joints is called the _____.

2. The hollow area in the shaft of a long bone where marrow is stored is called the _____.

3. The needlelike threads of spongy bone are called _____.

4. The structural units of compact bone are called either osteons or _____.

5. Osteocytes and chondrocytes live in small spaces in the matrix called _____.

6. Bone-resorbing cells are called _____.

7. Bone-forming cells are called _____.

8. The process of forming bone from cartilage is called _____.

9. If an _____ remains between the epiphysis and diaphysis, bone growth can continue.

10. The two major divisions of the human skeleton are the _____ skeleton and the _____ skeleton.

11. The three types of joints, named for the amount of movement they allow are _____, _____, and _____.

12. The _____ are cords or bands made of strong connective tissue that hold bones together.

13. Abnormal side-to-side curvature of the vertebral column is called _____.

14. The skeletal disorder characterized by excessive loss of calcified matrix and collagen fibers is called _____.

15. Microbial infection of the bone is called _____.

16. A _____ fracture invites the possibility of infection because the skin is pierced.

17. Degenerative joint disease, or _____, involves wearing away of articular cartilage.

18. Which of the following is not a function of the skeleton?
    a. Mineral storage
    b. Blood formation
    c. Heat production
    d. Protection

19. The strong fibrous membrane covering all of a long bone except the joint is called the
    a. endosteum
    b. periosteum
    c. ligament
    d. tendon

20. The fibrous lining of the hollow cavity in the long bone is called the
    a. endosteum
    b. periosteum
    c. medullary cavity
    d. ligament

21. The end of a long bone is called
    a. endosteum
    b. periosteum
    c. diaphysis
    d. epiphysis

22. The shaft of a long bone is called
    a. endosteum
    b. periosteum
    c. diaphysis
    d. epiphysis

23. Cancer of the cartilage is called
    a. osteosarcoma
    b. chondrosarcoma
    c. fibrosarcoma
    d. osteomalacia

24. The inflammatory joint disease that is caused by an increase of uric acid is
    a. osteoarthritis
    b. rheumatoid arthritis
    c. gouty arthritis
    d. infectious arthritis

Match the bones in Column A with their locations in Column B.

Column A
25. _____ ulna
26. _____ mandible
27. _____ humerus
28. _____ metatarsals
29. _____ tibia
30. _____ rib
31. _____ fibula
32. _____ sternum
33. _____ scapula
34. _____ femur
35. _____ metacarpals
36. _____ frontal bone
37. _____ patella
38. _____ zygomatic bone
39. _____ clavicle
40. _____ occipital bone
41. _____ carpals
42. _____ maxilla

Column B
 a. skull
 b. upper extremity (arm, forearm, wrist, and hand)
 c. trunk
 d. lower extremity (thigh, leg, ankle, and foot)

Study Tips

continued from page 163

4. The joints are named based on the amount of movement they allow (*arthro* means "joint"). The joint capsule is an example of a synovial membrane discussed in Chapter 5.
5. In your study group you can use flash cards to learn the terms in the bone structure and joints. Discuss the formation and structure of the osteon. A photocopy of the skeleton figures with the labels blackened out will help you learn the names and characteristics of the bones. There is no real shortcut to learning the names and locations of the bones, it's simply a memorization task, but quizzing each other will help you learn them faster.
6. Construct a table to help yourself learn the bone and joint disorders. Again, as in previous chapters, it would be helpful to organize them by mechanism or cause. The bone cancers should be easy to remember because they use the prefixes; *osteo-* for bone and *chondro-* for cartilage.

Case Studies

1. Andrew is a young boy who loves to climb trees. While attempting to climb his favorite oak tree, Andrew fell and fractured his humerus. The radiologist described Andrew's injury as a "greenstick fracture." What does this label tell you about the appearance of the fracture? If given proper medical care, is the injury likely to heal rapidly or slowly?
2. Christine is a young music student at the local college. One of her professors suggested that she analyze her conducting technique by videotaping herself as she conducts the choir. As she replays the tape, Christine notices that her hips and shoulders seem awkwardly bent—even when she is in a formal standing position. What condition might cause this abnormal curve of the trunk? What are some ways of treating this condition?
3. Agnes is an elderly woman with osteoporosis. She recently sustained a severe bone fracture for no apparent reason (she did not fall or otherwise injure herself). The fracture was not treated for some time, and as a result, Agnes developed osteomyelitis. Based on what you know of osteoporosis, how do you explain her mysterious fracture? How can a fracture progress to osteomyelitis?

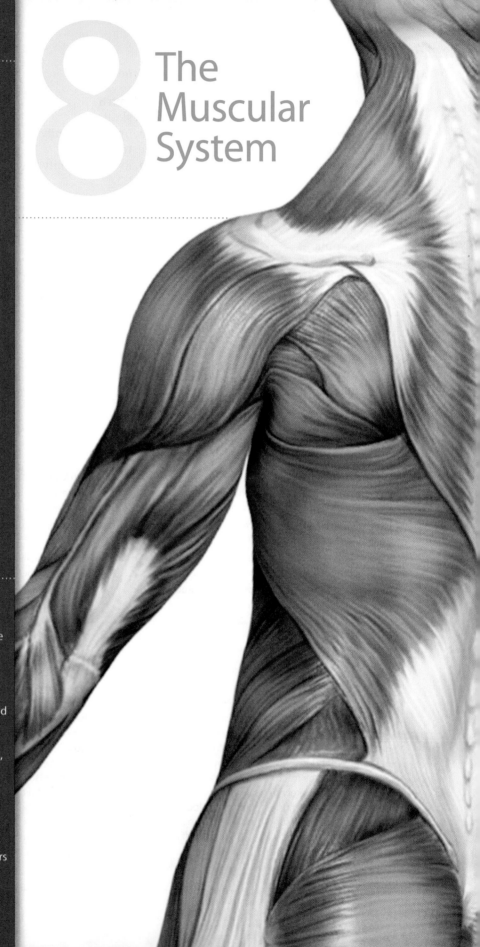

Outline

OBJECTIVES

**After you have completed this chapter,
you should be able to:**

1. List, locate in the body, and compare
   the structure and function of the three
   major types of muscle tissue.

2. Discuss the microscopic structure of a
   skeletal muscle sarcomere and motor
   unit.

3. Discuss how a muscle is stimulated and
   compare the major types of skeletal
   muscle contractions.

4. Name, identify on a model or diagram,
   and give the function of the major
   muscles of the body discussed in this
   chapter.

5. List and explain the most common
   types of movement produced by
   skeletal muscles.

6. Name and describe the major disorders
   of skeletal muscles.

8 The
Muscular
System

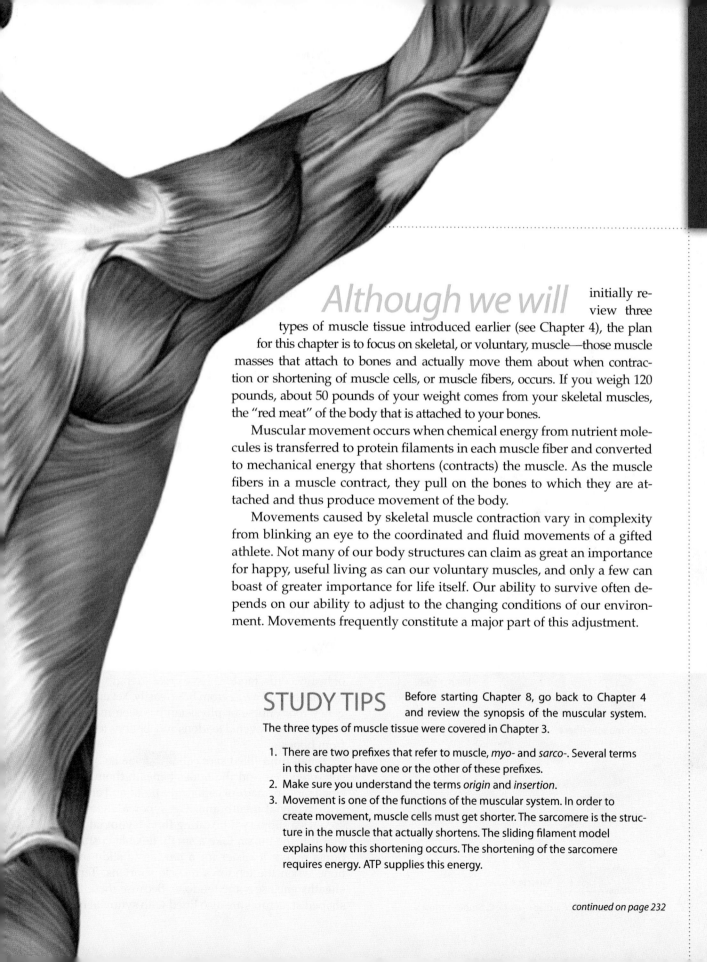

Although we will initially review three types of muscle tissue introduced earlier (see Chapter 4), the plan for this chapter is to focus on skeletal, or voluntary, muscle—those muscle masses that attach to bones and actually move them about when contraction or shortening of muscle cells, or muscle fibers, occurs. If you weigh 120 pounds, about 50 pounds of your weight comes from your skeletal muscles, the "red meat" of the body that is attached to your bones.

Muscular movement occurs when chemical energy from nutrient molecules is transferred to protein filaments in each muscle fiber and converted to mechanical energy that shortens (contracts) the muscle. As the muscle fibers in a muscle contract, they pull on the bones to which they are attached and thus produce movement of the body.

Movements caused by skeletal muscle contraction vary in complexity from blinking an eye to the coordinated and fluid movements of a gifted athlete. Not many of our body structures can claim as great an importance for happy, useful living as can our voluntary muscles, and only a few can boast of greater importance for life itself. Our ability to survive often depends on our ability to adjust to the changing conditions of our environment. Movements frequently constitute a major part of this adjustment.

STUDY TIPS

Before starting Chapter 8, go back to Chapter 4 and review the synopsis of the muscular system. The three types of muscle tissue were covered in Chapter 3.

1. There are two prefixes that refer to muscle, *myo-* and *sarco-*. Several terms in this chapter have one or the other of these prefixes.
2. Make sure you understand the terms *origin* and *insertion*.
3. Movement is one of the functions of the muscular system. In order to create movement, muscle cells must get shorter. The sarcomere is the structure in the muscle that actually shortens. The sliding filament model explains how this shortening occurs. The shortening of the sarcomere requires energy. ATP supplies this energy.

continued on page 232

Muscle Tissue

Under the microscope, threadlike and cylindrical **skeletal muscle** cells appear in bundles. They are characterized by many crosswise stripes and multiple nuclei (Figure 8-1, *A*). Each fine thread is a muscle cell—usually called a *muscle fiber.* This type of muscle tissue has three names: *skeletal muscle,* because it attaches to bone; *striated muscle,* because of its cross stripes or striations; and *voluntary muscle,* because its contractions can be controlled voluntarily.

In addition to skeletal muscle, the body also contains two other types of muscle tissue: cardiac muscle and smooth muscle. **Cardiac muscle** composes the bulk of the heart. Cells in this type of muscle tissue are also cylindrical, branch frequently (Figure 8-1, *B*), and then recombine into a continuous mass of interconnected tissue. As with skeletal muscle cells, they have cross striations. They also have unique dark bands called **intercalated disks** where the plasma membranes of adjacent cardiac fibers come in contact with each other. Cardiac muscle tissue demonstrates the principle that "form follows function." The interconnected nature of cardiac muscle fibers helps the tissue contract as a unit and increases the efficiency of the heart muscle in pumping blood.

Smooth muscle cells are tapered at each end and have a single nucleus (Figure 8-1, *C*). Because they lack cross stripes, or striations, they are sometimes called *nonstriated* muscle cells. They have a smooth, even appearance when viewed through a microscope. They are called *involuntary* because we normally do not have control over their contractions. Smooth, or involuntary, muscle forms an important part of blood vessel walls and of many hollow internal organs (viscera) such as the gut, urethra, and ureters. Because of its location in many visceral structures, it is sometimes also called *visceral muscle.* Although we cannot willfully control the action of smooth muscle, its contractions are highly regulated, which facilitates, for example, the passage of food through the digestive tract or urine through the ureters into the bladder.

All three muscle cell types—skeletal, cardiac, and smooth—specialize in contraction or shortening. Every movement we make is produced by contractions of skeletal muscle cells. Contractions of cardiac muscle cells pump blood through the heart, and smooth muscle contractions help pump liquids through our other hollow organs.

Structure of Skeletal Muscle

A skeletal muscle is an organ composed mainly of striated muscle cells and connective tissue. Most skeletal muscles attach to two bones that have a movable joint between them. In other words, most muscles extend from one bone across a joint to another bone. Also, one of the two bones is usually more stationary during a given movement than the other. The muscle's attachment to this more stationary bone is called its **origin.** Its attachment to the more movable bone is called the muscle's **insertion.** The rest of the muscle (all except its two ends) is called the *body* of the muscle (Figure 8-2).

Tendons anchor muscles firmly to bones. Being made of dense fibrous connective tissue in the shape of heavy cords, tendons have great strength. They do not tear or pull away from bone easily. Yet any emergency room nurse or physician has seen many tendon injuries—severed tendons and tendons torn loose from bones.

Small fluid-filled sacs called **bursae** lie between some tendons and the bones beneath them. These small sacs are made of connective tissue and are lined with **synovial membrane.** The synovial membrane secretes a slippery lubricating fluid **(synovial fluid)** that fills the bursa. Like a small, flexible cushion, a bursa makes it easier for a tendon to slide over a bone when the tendon's muscle shortens. **Tendon sheaths** enclose some tendons. Because these tube-shaped structures are also lined with synovial mem-

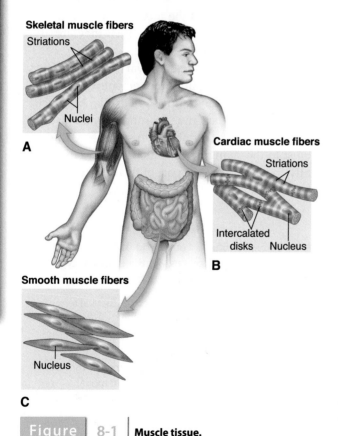

Skeletal muscle fibers
Striations
Nuclei
A

Cardiac muscle fibers
Striations
Intercalated disks
Nucleus
B

Smooth muscle fibers
Nucleus
C

| Figure | 8-1 | **Muscle tissue.** |

A, Skeletal muscle. **B,** Cardiac muscle. **C,** Smooth muscle.

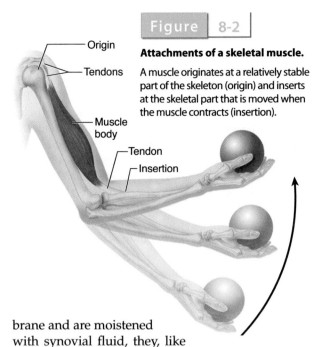

Figure 8-2

Attachments of a skeletal muscle.

A muscle originates at a relatively stable part of the skeleton (origin) and inserts at the skeletal part that is moved when the muscle contracts (insertion).

Origin
Tendons
Muscle body
Tendon
Insertion

brane and are moistened with synovial fluid, they, like the bursae, facilitate body movement.

Microscopic Structure and Function

Muscle tissue consists of elongated contractile cells, or **muscle fibers,** that are grouped together and arranged in a highly intricate way. Each skeletal muscle fiber is itself filled with two kinds of very fine and thread-like structures called **thick** and **thin myofilaments** (my-oh-FIL-ah-ments). The thick myofilaments are formed from a protein called **myosin,** and the thin myofilaments are composed mostly of the protein **actin.** Each shaftlike myosin molecule has a "head" that sticks out toward the actin molecules. At rest, the actin is blocked from connecting with the myosin heads. During contraction, however, actin is released and the myosin heads connect to form *cross bridges* between the thick and thin filaments.

Find the label **sarcomere** (SAR-koh-meer) in Figure 8-3. Think of the sarcomere as the basic functional, or *contractile,* unit of skeletal muscle. Recall that the osteon (haversian system) serves as the basic

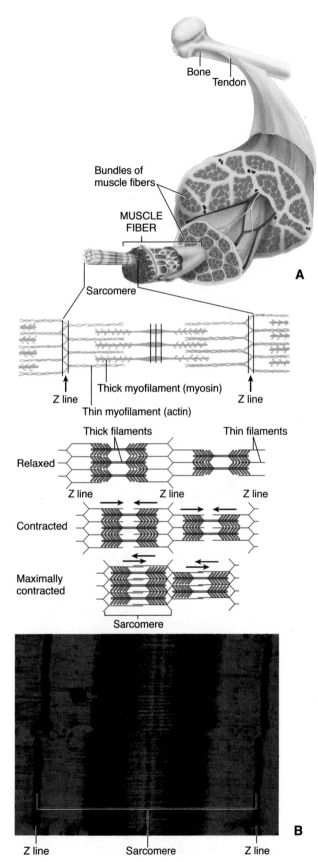

Bone
Tendon

Bundles of muscle fibers

MUSCLE FIBER

A

Sarcomere

Z line
Thick myofilament (myosin)
Z line
Thin myofilament (actin)

Thick filaments   Thin filaments
Relaxed
Z line   Z line   Z line

Contracted

Maximally contracted

Sarcomere

Z line   Sarcomere   Z line

B

Figure 8-3   **Structure of skeletal muscle.**

A, Each muscle organ has many muscle fibers, each containing many bundles of thick and thin myofilaments. The diagrams show the overlapping thick and thin filaments arranged to form adjacent segments called *sarcomeres*. During contraction, the thin filaments are pulled toward the center of each sarcomere, thereby shortening the whole muscle. **B,** This electron micrograph shows that the overlapping thick and thin filaments within each sarcomere create a pattern of dark striations in the muscle. The extreme magnification allowed by electron microscopy has revolutionized our concept of the structure and function of skeletal muscle and other tissues.

building block of compact bone; the sarcomere serves that function in skeletal muscle. The submicroscopic structure of a sarcomere consists of numerous actin and myosin myofilaments arranged so that when viewed under a microscope, dark and light stripes or cross striations are seen. The repeating units, or sarcomeres, are separated from each other by dark bands called Z *lines or Z disks.*

Although the sarcomeres in the upper portion (Figure 8-3, *A*) and in the electron photomicrograph (EM) of Figure 8-3, *B*, are in a relaxed state, the thick and thin myofilaments, which are lying parallel to each other, still overlap. Now look at the diagrams in the lower portion of Figure 8-3, *A*. Note that contraction of the muscle causes the two types of myofilaments to slide toward each other and shorten the sarcomere and thus the entire muscle. When the muscle relaxes, the sarcomeres can return to resting length, and the filaments resume their resting positions.

An explanation of how a skeletal muscle contracts is provided by the **sliding filament model.** According to this model, during contraction, the thick and thin myofilaments in a muscle fiber first attach to one another by forming cross bridges that then act as levers to ratchet or pull the myofilaments past each other.

The connecting bridges between the myofilaments form only if calcium is present. During the relaxed state, calcium ions (Ca^{++}) are stored within the endoplasmic reticulum (ER) in the muscle cell. When a nerve signal stimulates the muscle fiber, Ca^{++} are released from the ER into the cytoplasm. There, the Ca^{++} bind to the thin filaments and release actin to react with myosin. The myosin heads connect to actin, pull, release, then pull again. This ratcheting of myosin heads thus pulls the thin filaments toward the center of the sarcomere—producing the muscle contraction (Figure 8-4).

The contraction process of a muscle cell also requires energy. This energy is supplied by glucose and other nutrients.

The energy must be transferred to myosin heads by adenosine triphosphate (ATP) molecules, the energy-transfer molecules of the cell. Oxygen is required to transfer energy to ATP and make it available to the myosin heads, so it is not surprising that many muscles have high oxygen requirements. To supplement the oxygen carried to muscle fibers by the hemoglobin of blood, muscle fibers contain **myoglobin** (MY-oh-GLO-bin)—a red, oxygen-storing pigment similar to hemoglobin. We discuss the processes of transferring energy to ATP to cellular processes in Chapter 18.

 To learn more about the contraction and relaxation of sarcomeres, go to **AnimationDirect** on your CD.

QUICK CHECK

1. What are the three main types of muscle tissue? How do they differ?
2. What is a muscle's *origin*? Its *insertion*?
3. How do a muscle's myofilaments provide the mechanism for movement?

1 A nerve impulse travels to a muscle fiber through a motor neuron, triggering an electrical impulse that travels along the muscle fiber membrane.

2 The impulse triggers the release of calcium ions (Ca^{++}) from the endoplasmic reticulum and into the cytoplasm.

3 The Ca^{++} ions bind to thin filaments and release actin to react with myosin. Myosin heads form ratcheting cross-bridges with actin, which pull the thin filaments toward the middle of the sarcomere—thus producing a contraction.

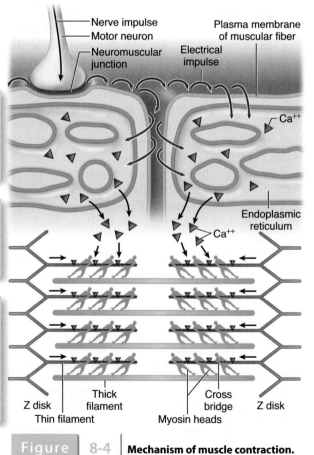

Figure 8-4 **Mechanism of muscle contraction.**

Functions of Skeletal Muscle

The three primary functions of the muscular system are as follows:

1. Movement
2. Posture or muscle tone
3. Heat production

Movement

Muscles move bones by pulling on them. Because the length of a skeletal muscle becomes shorter as its fibers contract, the bones to which the muscle attaches move closer together. As a rule, only the insertion bone moves. Look again at Figure 8-2. As the ball is lifted, the shortening of the muscle body pulls the insertion bone toward the origin bone. The origin bone stays put, holding firm, while the insertion bone moves toward it. One tremendously important function of skeletal muscle contractions therefore is to produce body movements. Remember this simple rule: a muscle's insertion bone moves toward its origin bone. It can help you understand muscle actions.

Voluntary muscular movement is normally smooth and free of jerks and tremors because skeletal muscles generally work in coordinated teams, not singly. Several muscles contract while others relax to produce almost any movement that you can imagine. Of all the muscles contracting simultaneously, the one that is mainly responsible for producing a particular movement is called the **prime mover** for that movement. The other muscles that help in producing the movement are called **synergists** (SIN-er-jists). As prime movers and synergist muscles at a joint contract, other muscles, called **antagonists** (an-TAG-eh-nists), relax. When antagonist muscles contract, they produce a movement opposite to that of the prime movers and their synergist muscles.

Locate the biceps brachii, brachialis, and triceps brachii muscles in Figure 8-7 on p. 216. All of these muscles are involved in bending and straightening the forearm at the elbow joint. The biceps brachii is the prime mover during bending, and the brachialis is its helper or synergist muscle. When the biceps brachii and brachialis muscles bend the forearm, the triceps brachii relaxes. Therefore while the forearm bends, the triceps brachii is the antagonistic muscle. While the forearm straightens, these three muscles continue to work as a team. However, during straightening, the triceps brachii becomes the prime mover and the biceps brachii and brachialis become the antagonistic muscles. This combined and coordinated activity is what makes our muscular movements smooth and graceful.

Posture

We are able to maintain our body position because of a specific type of skeletal muscle contraction called **tonic contraction.** Because relatively few of a muscle's fibers shorten at one time in a tonic contraction, the muscle as a whole does not shorten, and no movement occurs. Consequently, tonic contractions do not move any body parts. They do hold muscles in position, however. In other words, muscle tone maintains **posture.** Good posture is the definition of body positioning that favors best functioning of all body parts. Such positioning balances the distribution of weight and therefore puts the least strain on muscles, tendons, ligaments, and bones.

Skeletal muscle tone maintains posture by counteracting the pull of gravity. Gravity tends to pull the head and trunk down and forward, but the tone in certain back and neck muscles pulls just hard enough in the opposite direction to overcome the force of gravity and hold the head and trunk erect.

Heat Production

Healthy survival depends on our ability to maintain a constant body temperature. A fever, or elevation in body temperature, of only a degree or two above 37° C (98.6° F) is almost always a sign of illness. Just as serious is a fall in body temperature. Any decrease below normal, a condition called **hypothermia** (hye-poh-THER-mee-ah), drastically affects cellular activity and normal body function. The contraction of muscle fibers produces most of the heat required to maintain body temperature. Energy required to produce a muscle contraction is obtained from ATP. Some of the energy released during the breakdown of ATP during a muscular contraction is used to shorten the muscle fibers; however, much of the energy is lost as heat during the reaction. This heat helps us maintain our body temperature at a constant level.

Fatigue

If muscle cells are stimulated repeatedly without adequate periods of rest, the strength of the muscle contraction decreases, resulting in **fatigue.** If repeated stimulation occurs, the strength of the contraction continues to decrease, and eventually the muscle loses its ability to contract.

SCIENCE APPLICATIONS

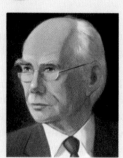

Andrew Huxley (b. 1917)

MUSCLE FUNCTION

The British physiologist Andrew F. Huxley (born 1917) is largely responsible for explaining how muscle fibers contract. After making pioneering discoveries in how nerves conduct impulses, a feat for which he shared the 1963 Nobel Prize in Medicine or Physiology, Huxley turned his attention to muscle fibers. It was he who in the 1950s proposed the sliding filament model, along with its mechanical explanation of muscle contraction.

Today, research physiologists continue to find out more about how muscle fibers work. These discoveries are being applied to many different professions. For example, nutritionists use this information in advising athletes and others what and when to eat to maximize muscular strength and endurance. Athletes themselves, along with their coaches and trainers, use current concepts of muscle science to help them improve their performance.

During exercise, the stored ATP required for muscle contraction becomes depleted. Formation of more ATP results in a rapid consumption of oxygen and nutrients, often outstripping the ability of the muscle's blood supply to replenish them. When oxygen supplies run low, the muscle cells switch to a type of energy conversion that does not require oxygen.

This process produces lactic acid that may result in a burning sensation in muscle during exercise. The term **oxygen debt** describes the continued increased metabolism that must occur in a cell to remove excess lactic acid that accumulates during prolonged exercise. Thus the depleted energy reserves are replaced. Labored breathing after the cessation of ex-

HEALTH & WELL-BEING

SLOW AND FAST MUSCLE FIBERS

Sports physiologists know there are three basic skeletal muscle fiber types in the body: slow, fast, and intermediate fibers. Each type is best suited to a particular style of muscular contraction—a fact that is useful when considering how different muscles are used in various athletic activities.

Slow fibers are also called "red fibers" because they have a high content of oxygen-storing myoglobin (a red pigment similar to hemoglobin). Slow fibers are best suited to endurance activities such as long-distance running (pictured) because they do not fatigue easily. Muscles that maintain body position—posture—have a high proportion of slow fibers.

Fast fibers are also called "white fibers" because they have a low red myoglobin content. Fast fibers are best suited for quick, powerful contractions because even though they fatigue quickly they can produce a great amount of ATP very quickly. Fast fibers are well suited to sprinting and weight-lifting events. Muscles that move the fingers have a high proportion of fast fibers—a big help when playing computer games or musical instruments.

Intermediate fibers have characteristics between the extremes of slow and fast fibers. This muscle type is found in muscles such as the calf muscle (gastrocnemius) that is used both for posture and occasional brief, powerful contractions such as jumping.

Each muscle of the body is a mixture of varying proportions of slow, fast, and intermediate fibers.

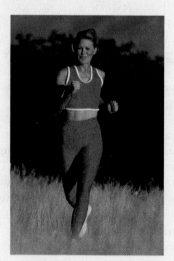

ercise is required to "pay the debt" of oxygen required for the metabolic effort. This mechanism is a good example of homeostasis at work. The body returns the cells' energy and oxygen reserves to normal resting levels.

Role of Other Body Systems in Movement

Remember that muscles do not function alone. Other structures such as bones and joints must function along with them. Most skeletal muscles cause movements by pulling on bones across movable joints. However, the respiratory, circulatory, nervous, muscular, and skeletal systems all play essential roles in producing normal movements. This fact has great practical importance.

For example, a person might have perfectly normal muscles and still not be able to move normally. He or she might have a nervous system disorder that shuts off impulses to certain skeletal muscles, which thereby results in **paralysis.** Multiple sclerosis creates paralysis in this way, but so do some other conditions such as a brain hemorrhage, a brain tumor, or a spinal cord injury. Skeletal system disorders, especially arthritis, have disabling effects on body movement. Muscle functioning, then, depends on the func-

tioning of many other parts of the body. This fact illustrates a principle that is repeated often in this book. It can be simply stated: Each part of the body is one of many components in a large, interactive system. The normal function of one part depends on the normal function of the other parts.

QUICK CHECK

1. What are the three primary functions of the muscular system?
2. When a *prime mover* muscle contracts, what does its *antagonist* do?
3. How would you define the term *posture*?
4. How does muscle function affect body temperature?
5. What is *oxygen debt*?

Motor Unit

Before a skeletal muscle can contract and pull on a bone to move it, the muscle must first be stimulated by nerve impulses. Muscle cells are stimulated by a nerve fiber called a **motor neuron** (Figures 8-4 and 8-5). The point of contact between the nerve ending and the muscle fiber is called a **neuromuscular junction.** Signal chemicals are released by the motor neuron in response to a nervous impulse. These chemicals then generate events within the muscle cell that result in contraction or shortening of the muscle cell. A single motor neuron, with the muscle cells it innervates, is called a **motor unit** (Figure 8-5).

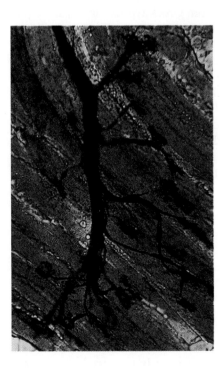

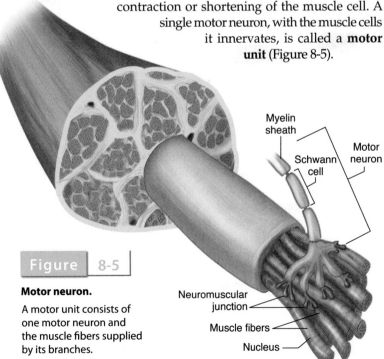

Myelin sheath

Schwann cell

Motor neuron

Neuromuscular junction

Muscle fibers

Nucleus

Figure 8-5

Motor neuron.

A motor unit consists of one motor neuron and the muscle fibers supplied by its branches.

Muscle Stimulus

In a laboratory setting, a single muscle fiber can be isolated and subjected to stimuli of varying intensities so that it can be studied. Such experiments show that a muscle fiber does not contract until an applied stimulus reaches a certain level of intensity. The minimal level of stimulation required to cause a fiber to contract is called the **threshold stimulus.**

When a muscle fiber is subjected to a threshold stimulus, it contracts completely. Because of this, muscle cells are said to respond **"all or none."** However, a muscle is composed of many muscle cells that are controlled by different motor units and that have different threshold-stimulus levels. Although each fiber in a muscle such as the biceps brachii responds in an *all or none* mode when subjected to a threshold stimulus, the muscle as a whole does not. This fact has tremendous importance in everyday life. It allows you to pick up a 2-liter bottle of soda or a 20-kg weight because different numbers of motor units can be activated for different loads. Once activated, however, each fiber always responds all or none.

Types of Skeletal Muscle Contraction

In addition to the tonic contraction of muscle that maintains muscle tone and posture, other types of contraction occur as well. These additional types of muscle contraction include the following:

1. Twitch contraction
2. Tetanic contraction
3. Isotonic contraction
4. Isometric contraction

Twitch and Tetanic Contractions

A **twitch** is a quick, jerky response to a stimulus. Twitch contractions can be seen in isolated muscles during research, but they play a minimal role in normal muscle activity. To accomplish the coordinated and fluid muscular movements needed for most daily tasks, muscles must contract not in a jerky fashion but in a smooth and sustained way.

A **tetanic contraction** is a more sustained and steady response than a twitch. It is produced by a series of stimuli bombarding the muscle in rapid succession. Contractions "melt" together to produce a sustained contraction or *tetanus*. About 30 stimuli per second, for example, evoke a tetanic contraction in certain types of skeletal muscle. Tetanic contraction is not necessarily a maximal contraction in which each muscle fiber responds at the same time. In most cases, only a few areas of the muscle fibers undergo contractions at any one time.

Isotonic Contraction

In most cases, **isotonic contraction** of muscle produces movement at a joint. With this type of contraction, the muscle changes length, and the insertion end moves relative to the point of origin (Figure 8-6, *A*). There are two types of isotonic contraction. One is *concentric contraction*, in which the muscle shortens. The other is *eccentric contraction*, in which the muscle lengthens but still provides work. For example lifting this book requires concentric contraction of the biceps muscle that flexes your elbow. Lowering the book slowly and safely requires eccentric contraction of the biceps muscle. Thus, what we call muscle "contraction" really means any pulling of the muscle whether it shortens or not.

Walking, running, breathing, lifting, twisting, and most body movements are examples of isotonic contraction.

Isometric Contraction

Contraction of a skeletal muscle does not always produce movement. Sometimes, it increases the tension within a muscle but does not change the length of the muscle. When the muscle contracts and no movement results, it is called an **isometric contraction**. The word *isometric* comes from Greek words that mean "equal measure." In other words, a muscle's length during an isometric contraction and during relaxation is about equal. Although muscles do not shorten (and thus produce no movement) during isometric contractions, tension within them increases (Figure 8-6, *B*). Because of this, repeated isometric contractions make muscles grow larger and stronger. Pushing against a wall or other immovable object is a good example of isometric exercise. Although no movement occurs and the muscle does not shorten, its internal tension increases dramatically.

 To learn more about types of skeletal muscle contractions, go to **AnimationDirect** on your CD.

Effects of Exercise on Skeletal Muscles

We know that exercise is good for us. Some of the benefits of regular, properly practiced exercise are

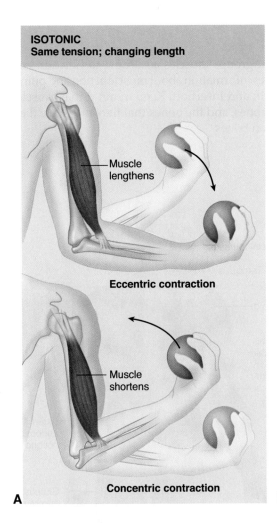

A

ISOTONIC
Same tension; changing length

- Muscle lengthens

Eccentric contraction

- Muscle shortens

Concentric contraction

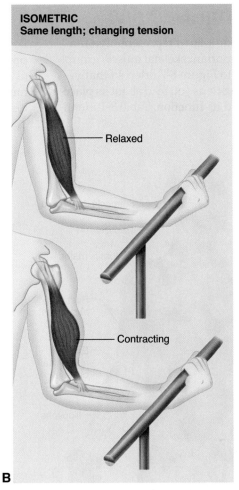

B

ISOMETRIC
Same length; changing tension

- Relaxed

- Contracting

Figure 8-6

Types of muscle contraction.

A, In isotonic contraction the muscle changes length, producing movement either by eccentric contraction (muscle lengthens) or concentric contraction (muscle shortens). **B,** In isometric contraction the muscle pulls forcefully against a load but does not shorten.

greatly improved muscle tone, better posture, more efficient heart and lung function, less fatigue, and looking and feeling better.

Skeletal muscles undergo changes that correspond to the amount of work that they normally do. During prolonged inactivity, muscles usually shrink in mass, a condition called **disuse atrophy.** Exercise, on the other hand, may cause an increase in muscle size called **hypertrophy.**

Muscle hypertrophy can be enhanced by **strength training,** which involves contracting muscles against heavy resistance. Isometric exercises and weight lifting are common strength-training activities. This type of training results in increased numbers of myofilaments in each muscle fiber. Although the number of muscle fibers stays the same, the increased number of myofilaments greatly increases the mass of the muscle.

Endurance training, often called **aerobic training,** does not usually result in muscle hypertrophy. Instead, this type of exercise program increases a muscle's ability to sustain moderate exercise over a long period. Aerobic activities such as running, bicycling, or other primarily isotonic movements increase the number of blood vessels in a muscle without significantly increasing its size. The increased blood flow allows a more efficient delivery of oxygen and glucose to muscle fibers during exercise. Aerobic training also causes an increase in the number of mitochondria in muscle fibers. This allows production of more ATP as a rapid energy source.

QUICK CHECK

1. What is a *motor unit?*
2. How does a muscle produce different levels of strength?
3. What is the difference between *isotonic* and *isometric* muscle contraction?
4. How does strength training affect a person's muscles?

Skeletal Muscle Groups

In the paragraphs that follow, representative muscles from the most important skeletal muscle groups are discussed. Refer to Figure 8-7 often so that you will be able to see a muscle as you read about its placement on the body and its function. Table 8-1 identifies and groups muscles according to function and provides information about muscle action and points of origin and insertion. Keep in mind that muscles move bones, and the bones that they move are their insertion bones.

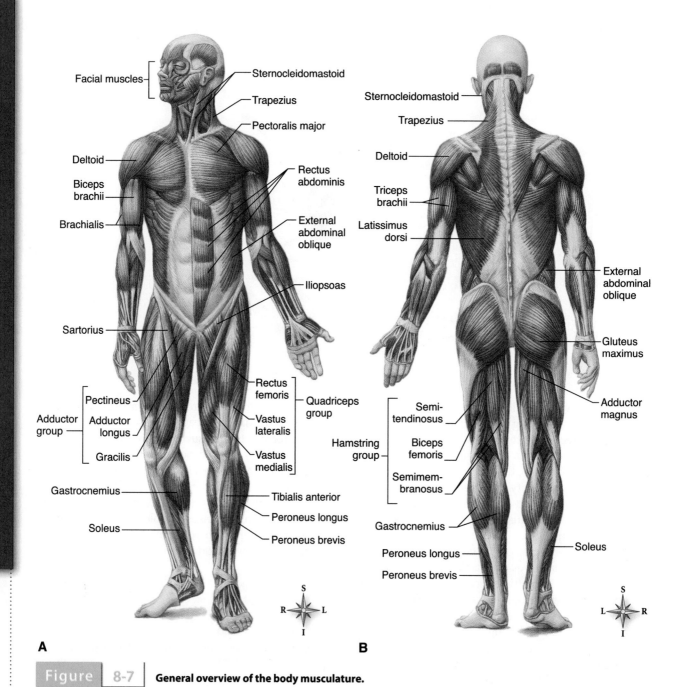

A, Anterior view. **B,** Posterior view.

Figure 8-7 **General overview of the body musculature.**

| Table | 8-1 | **Principal Muscles of the Body** |

MUSCLE	FUNCTION	INSERTION	ORIGIN
MUSCLES OF THE HEAD AND NECK			
Frontal	Raises eyebrow	Skin of eyebrow	Occipital bone
Orbicularis oculi	Closes eye	Maxilla and frontal bone	Maxilla and frontal bone (encircles eye)
Orbicularis oris	Draws lips together	Encircles lips	Encircles lips
Zygomaticus	Elevates corners of mouth and lips	Angle of mouth and upper lip	Zygomatic
Masseter	Closes jaws	Mandible	Zygomatic arch
Temporal	Closes jaw	Mandible	Temporal region of the skull
Sternocleidomastoid	Rotates and flexes head and neck	Mastoid process	Sternum and clavicle
Trapezius	Extends head and neck	Scapula	Skull and upper vertebrae
MUSCLES THAT MOVE THE UPPER EXTREMITIES			
Pectoralis major	Flexes and helps adduct upper arm	Humerus	Sternum, clavicle, and upper rib cartilages
Latissimus dorsi	Extends and helps adduct upper arm	Humerus	Vertebrae and ilium
Deltoid	Abducts upper arm	Humerus	Clavicle and scapula
Biceps brachii	Flexes elbow	Radius	Scapula
Triceps brachii	Extends elbow	Ulna	Scapula and humerus
MUSCLES OF THE TRUNK			
External oblique	Compresses abdomen	Midline of abdomen	Lower thoracic cage
Internal oblique	Compresses abdomen	Midline of abdomen	Pelvis
Transversus abdominis	Compresses abdomen	Midline of abdomen	Ribs, vertebrae, and pelvis
Rectus abdominis	Flexes trunk	Lower rib cage	Pubis
MUSCLES THAT MOVE THE LOWER EXTREMITIES			
Iliopsoas	Flexes thigh or trunk	Femur	Ilium and vertebrae
Sartorius	Flexes thigh and rotates lower leg	Tibia	Ilium
Gluteus maximus	Extends thigh	Femur	Ilium, sacrum, and coccyx
Adductor group			
Adductor longus	Adducts thigh	Femur	Pubis
Gracilis	Adducts thigh	Tibia	Pubis
Pectineus	Adducts thigh	Femur	Pubis
Hamstring group			
Semimembranosus	Flexes knee	Tibia	Ischium
Semitendinosus	Flexes knee	Tibia	Ischium
Biceps femoris	Flexes knee	Fibula	Ischium and femur
Quadriceps group			
Rectus femoris	Extends knee	Tibia	Ilium
Vastus lateralis, intermedius, and medialis	Extend knee	Tibia	Femur
Tibialis anterior	Dorsiflexes ankle	Metatarsals (foot)	Tibia
Gastrocnemius	Plantar flexes ankle	Calcaneus (heel)	Femur
Soleus	Plantar flexes ankle	Calcaneus (heel)	Tibia and fibula
Peroneus group			
Peroneus longus and brevis	Plantar flex ankle	Tarsal and metatarsals (ankle and foot)	Tibia and fibula

RESEARCH, ISSUES, AND TRENDS

ENHANCING MUSCLE STRENGTH

The most obvious and effective way of increasing skeletal muscle strength is by strength training, that is, regularly pulling against heavy resistance. The maximal amount of muscular strength one can achieve is determined mainly by genetics. However, there are a number of chemical enhancements athletes have tried over the centuries to improve strength. An early fad among athletes in the twentieth century was the overuse of vitamin supplements. Although moderate vitamin supplementation will ensure adequate intake of vitamins necessary for good muscle function, overuse may lead to *hypervitaminosis* and possibly serious consequences.

Another type of chemical often abused by athletes is *anabolic steroids*. Anabolic steroids are usually synthetic de-

rivatives of the male hormone *testosterone*. As with testosterone, they do in fact stimulate an increase in muscle size and strength, making them attractive to coaches and athletes wanting to win their events. However, inappropriate use of these hormones can cause serious, even life-threatening, hormonal imbalances. For this reason, anabolic steroids are banned from most organized sports.

Sports physiologists are now investigating a whole variety of chemicals that are reported to enhance strength or endurance. Always carefully review the latest research findings on such substances with the help of your reference librarian and discuss them with your physician before using them yourself, or you may suffer serious health consequences.

Muscles of the Head and Neck

The *muscles of facial expression* (Figure 8-8) allow us to communicate many different emotions nonverbally. Contraction of the **frontal muscle**, for example, allows you to raise your eyebrows in surprise and furrow the skin of your forehead into a frown. The **orbicularis** (or-bik-yoo-LAIR-iss) **oris** (OR-iss), called the *kissing muscle*, puckers the lips. The **zygomaticus** (zye-go-MAT-ik-us) elevates the corners of the mouth and lips and has been called the *smiling muscle*.

The muscles of **mastication** are responsible for closing the mouth and producing chewing movements. As a group, they are among the strongest muscles in the body. The two largest muscles of the group, identified in Figure 8-8, are the **masseter** (mas-SEE-ter), which elevates the mandible, and the **temporal** (TEM-pohral), which assists the masseter in closing the jaw.

The **sternocleidomastoid** (ster-no-klye-doh-MASStoyd) and **trapezius** (trah-PEE-zee-us) muscles are easily identified in Figures 8-7 and 8-8. The two sternocleidomastoid muscles are located on the anterior surface of the neck. They originate on the sternum and then pass up and cross the neck to insert on the mastoid process of the skull. Working together, they flex the head on the chest. If only one contracts, the head is both flexed and tilted to the opposite side. The triangular-shaped trapezius muscles form the line from each shoulder to the neck on its posterior surface. They have a wide line of origin extending from the base of the skull down the spinal column to the last thortacic vertebra. When contracted, the trapezius muscles help elevate the shoulders and extend the head backward.

Muscles That Move the Upper Extremities

The upper extremity is attached to the thorax by the fan-shaped **pectoralis** (pek-teh-RAH-lis) **major** muscle, which covers the upper chest, and by the **latissimus** (lah-TISS-i-mus) **dorsi** (dor-sye) muscle, which takes its origin from structures over the lower back (Figures 8-7 and 8-9). Both muscles insert on the hu-

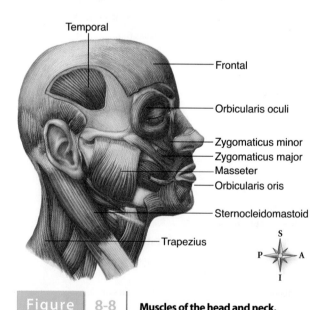

Figure 8-8 **Muscles of the head and neck.**

Muscles that produce most facial expressions surround the eyes, nose, and mouth. Large muscles of mastication stretch from the upper skull to the lower jaw. These powerful muscles produce chewing movements. The neck muscles connect the skull to the trunk of the body, rotating the head or bending the neck.

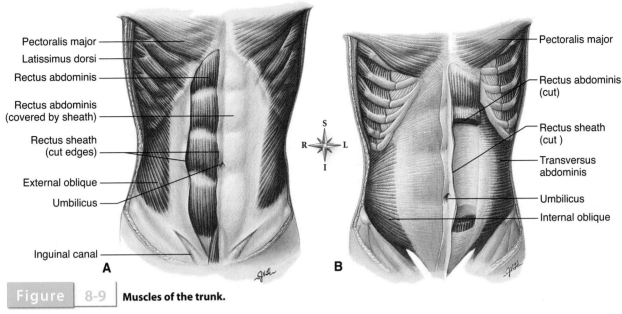

Pectoralis major
Latissimus dorsi
Rectus abdominis
Rectus abdominis (covered by sheath)
Rectus sheath (cut edges)
External oblique
Umbilicus
Inguinal canal

A

Pectoralis major
Rectus abdominis (cut)
Rectus sheath (cut)
Transversus abdominis
Umbilicus
Internal oblique

B

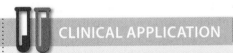

Figure 8-9 | **Muscles of the trunk.**

A, Anterior view showing superficial muscles. **B,** Anterior view showing deeper muscles.

CLINICAL APPLICATION

OCCUPATIONAL HEALTH PROBLEMS

Some epidemiologists specialize in the field of *occupational health,* the study of health matters related to work or the workplace. Many problems seen by occupational health experts are caused by repetitive motions of the wrists or other joints. Word processors (typists) and meat cutters, for example, are at risk of developing conditions caused by repetitive motion injuries.

One common problem often caused by such repetitive motion is **tenosynovitis** (ten-oh-sin-oh-VYE-tis)—inflammation of a tendon sheath. Tenosynovitis can be painful, and the swelling characteristic of this condition can limit movement in affected parts of the body. For example, swelling of the tendon sheath around tendons in an area of the wrist known as the *carpal tunnel* can limit movement of the wrist, hand, and fingers. The figure shows the relative positions of the tendon sheath and median nerve within the carpal tunnel. If this swelling, or any other lesion in the carpal tunnel, presses on the *median nerve,* a condition called **carpal tunnel syndrome** may result. Because the median nerve connects to the palm and radial side (thumb side) of the hand, carpal tunnel syndrome is characterized by weakness, pain, and tingling in that part of the hand. The pain and tingling also may radiate to the forearm and shoulder. Prolonged or severe cases of carpal tunnel syndrome may be relieved by injection of antiinflammatory agents. A permanent cure is sometimes accomplished by surgical cutting or removal of the swollen tissue pressing on the median nerve.

Repetitive motion and other types of trauma also may cause inflammation of a bursa, known as **bursitis** (ber-SYE-tis). For example, carpet layers, roofers, and others who work on their knees are prone to bursitis involving the knee joints. Bursitis is most often treated with antiinflammatory agents.

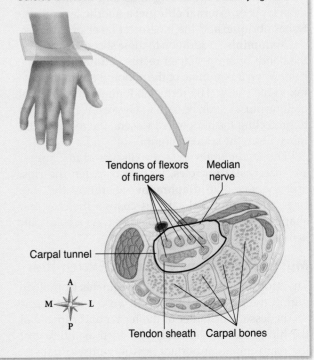

Tendons of flexors of fingers
Median nerve
Carpal tunnel
Tendon sheath
Carpal bones

merus. The pectoralis major is a flexor, and the latissimus dorsi is an extensor of the upper arm.

The **deltoid** muscle forms the thick, rounded prominence over the shoulder and upper arm (Figure 8-7). The muscle takes its origin from the scapula and clavicle and inserts on the humerus. It is a powerful abductor of the upper arm.

As the name implies, the **biceps** (bye-seps) **brachii** (BRAY-kee-eye) is a two-headed muscle that serves as a primary flexor of the forearm (Figure 8-7). It originates from the bones of the shoulder girdle and inserts on the radius in the forearm.

The **triceps brachii** is on the posterior or back surface of the upper arm. It has three heads of origin from the shoulder girdle and inserts into the olecranon process of the ulna. The triceps is an extensor of the elbow and thus performs a straightening function. Because this muscle is responsible for delivering blows during fights, it is often called the *boxer's muscle.*

Muscles of the Trunk

The muscles of the anterior, or front, side of the abdomen are arranged in three layers, with the fibers in each layer running in different directions much like the layers of wood in a sheet of plywood (Figure 8-9). The result is a very strong "girdle" of muscle that covers and supports the abdominal cavity and its internal organs.

The three layers of muscle in the anterolateral (side) abdominal walls are arranged as follows: the outermost layer or **external oblique;** a middle layer or **internal oblique;** and the innermost layer or **transversus abdominis.** In addition to these sheetlike muscles, the band- or strap-shaped **rectus abdominis** muscle runs down the midline of the abdomen from the thorax to the pubis. The rectus abdominis and external oblique muscles can be seen in Figure 8-9. In addition to protecting the abdominal viscera, the rectus abdominis flexes the spinal column.

The *respiratory muscles* are discussed in Chapter 14. **Intercostal muscles,** located between the ribs, and the sheetlike **diaphragm** separating the thoracic and abdominal cavities change the size and shape of the chest during breathing. As a result, air is moved into or out of the lungs.

Muscles That Move the Lower Extremities

The **iliopsoas** (ill-ee-oh-SO-us) originates from deep within the pelvis and the lower vertebrae to insert on the lesser trochanter of the femur and capsule of the hip joint. It is generally classified as a flexor of the thigh and an important postural muscle that sta-

bilizes and keeps the trunk from falling over backward when you stand. However, if the thigh is fixed so that it cannot move, the iliopsoas flexes the *trunk.* An example would be doing sit-ups.

The **gluteus** (GLOO-tee-us) **maximus** (MAX-i-mus) forms the outer contour and much of the substance of the buttock. It is an important extensor of the thigh (Figure 8-7) and supports the torso in the erect position.

The **adductor muscles** originate on the bony pelvis and insert on the femur. They are located on the inner or medial side of the thighs. These muscles adduct or press the thighs together.

The three **hamstring muscles** are called the *semimembranosus, semitendinosus,* and *biceps femoris.* Acting together, they serve as powerful flexors of the lower leg (Figure 8-7). They originate on the ischium and insert on the tibia or fibula.

The **quadriceps** (KWOD-reh-seps) **femoris** muscle group covers the upper thigh. The four thigh muscles—the *rectus femoris* and three *vastus* muscles—extend the lower leg (Figure 8-7 and Table 8-1). One component of the quadriceps group has its origin on the pelvis, and the remaining three originate on the femur; all four insert on the tibia. Only two of the vastus muscles are visible in Figure 8-7. The vastus intermedius is covered by the rectus femoris and is not visible. Functionally, the hamstrings (flexors) and quadriceps (extensors) act as powerful antagonists in movement of the lower leg.

The **tibialis** (tib-ee-AL-iss) **anterior** muscle (Figure 8-7) is located on the anterior, or front, surface of the leg. It dorsiflexes the foot. The **gastrocnemius** (gas-trok-NEE-mee-us) is the primary calf muscle. Note in Figure 8-7 that it has two fleshy components arising from both sides of the femur. It inserts through the Achilles tendon into the heel bone or calcaneus. The gastrocnemius is responsible for plantar flexion of the foot; because it is used to stand on tiptoe, it is sometimes called the *toe dancer's muscle.* A group of three muscles called the **peroneus** (pair-oh-NEE-us) **group** (Figure 8-7) is found along the sides of the lower leg. As a group, these muscles plantar flex the foot. A long tendon from one component of the group—the *peroneus longus* muscle tendon—forms a support arch for the foot (Figure 7-23).

QUICK CHECK

1. What function do the *muscles of mastication* make possible?
2. Why is the *triceps brachii* muscle sometimes called the "boxer's muscle"?
3. What action do the *hamstring muscles* perform?

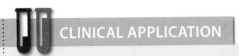

INTRAMUSCULAR INJECTIONS

Many drugs are administered by intramuscular injection. If the amount to be injected is 2 milliliters (ml) or less, the deltoid muscle is often selected as the site of injection. Note in Figure **A** that the needle is inserted into the muscle about two fingers' breadth below the acromion process of the scapula and lateral to the tip of the acromion. If the amount of medication to be injected is 2 to 3 ml, the gluteal area shown in Figure **B** is often used. Injections are made into the gluteus medius muscle near the center of the upper outer quadrant, as shown in the illustration. Another technique of locating the proper injection site is to draw an imaginary diagonal line from a point of reference on the back of the bony pelvis (posterior superior iliac spine) to the greater trochanter of the femur. The injection is given about three fingers' breadth above and one third of the way down the line. It is important that the sciatic nerve and the superior gluteal blood vessels be avoided during the injection. Proper technique requires knowledge of the underlying anatomy.

In addition to intramuscular injections, which are generally administered by a health care provider in an institutional setting, many individuals must self-administer injections of needed medications, such as insulin, on a regular basis in their homes. Educating these patients or their caregivers on how to correctly administer medication by injection is an important issue in the delivery of home health care services. Topics that must be covered include instruction on proper injection techniques, selection of needle length and gauge, identification of important anatomical landmarks when making injection site selections, and the preparation and rotation of selected injection sites.

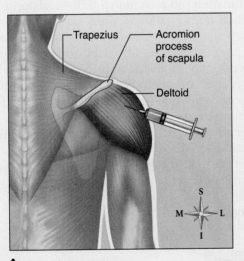

A

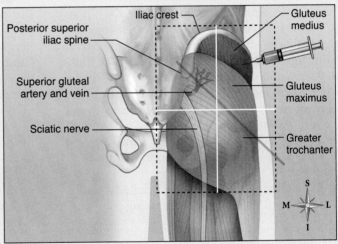

B

Movements Produced by Skeletal Muscle Contractions

The types of movement that may produce a muscle contraction at any joint depend largely on the shapes of the bones involved and the joint type (see Chapter 7). Muscles acting on some joints produce movement in several directions, whereas only limited movement is possible at other joints. The terms most often used to describe body movements are as follows:

1. Flexion
2. Extension
3. Abduction
4. Adduction
5. Rotation and circumduction
6. Supination and pronation
7. Dorsiflexion and plantar flexion

Flexion is a movement that makes the angle between two bones at their joint smaller than it was at

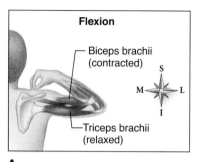

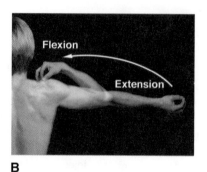

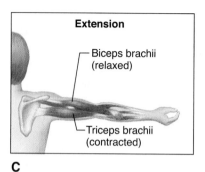

A   **B**   **C**

Figure 8-10   **Flexion and extension of the lower arm.**

A and **B,** When the lower arm is flexed at the elbow, the biceps brachii contracts while its antagonist, the triceps brachii, relaxes. **B** and **C,** When the lower arm is extended, the biceps brachii relaxes while the triceps brachii contracts.

the beginning of the movement. Most flexions are movements commonly described as bending. If you bend your elbow or your knee, you flex the lower arm or leg. **Extension** movements are the opposite of flexions. They make the angle between two bones at their joint larger than it was at the beginning of the movement. Therefore, extensions are straightening or stretching movements rather than bending movements. Figures 8-10 and 8-11 illustrate flexion and extension of the elbow and knee.

Abduction means moving a part away from the midline of the body, such as moving your arm out to the side. **Adduction** means moving a part toward the midline, such as bringing your arms down to your sides from an elevated position. Figure 8-12, *A*, shows abduction and adduction.

Rotation is movement around a longitudinal axis. You rotate your head and neck by moving your skull from side to side as in shaking your head "no" (Figure 8-12, *B*). **Circumduction** moves a part so that its distal end moves in a circle. When a pitcher winds up to throw a ball, she circumducts her arm.

Supination and **pronation** refer to hand positions that result from rotation of the forearm. (The term *prone* refers to the body as a whole lying face down. *Supine* means lying face up.) Supination results in a hand position with the palm turned to the anterior position (as in the anatomical position), and pronation occurs when you turn the palm of your hand so that it faces posteriorly (Figure 8-12, *C*).

Dorsiflexion and **plantar flexion** refer to ankle movements. In dorsiflexion the dorsum, or top, of the foot is elevated with the toes pointing upward. In plantar flexion the bottom of the foot is directed downward so that you are in effect standing on your toes (Figure 8-12, *D*).

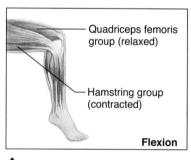

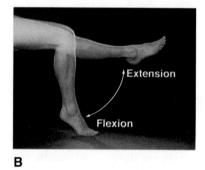

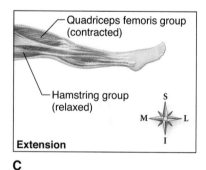

A   **B**   **C**

Figure 8-11   **Flexion and extension of the lower leg.**

A and **B,** When the lower leg flexes at the knee, muscles of the hamstring group contract while their antagonists in the quadriceps femoris group relax. **B** and **C,** When the lower leg extends, the hamstring muscles relax while the quadriceps femoris muscle contracts.

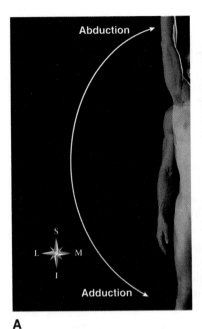

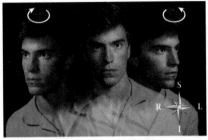

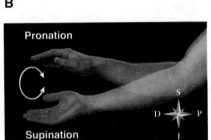

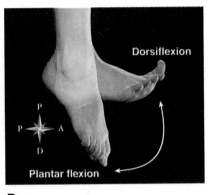

A

B

C

D

Figure 8-12

Examples of body movements.

A, Adduction and abduction. **B,** Rotation. **C,** Pronation and supination. **D,** Dorsiflexion and plantar flexion.

As you study the illustrations and learn to recognize the muscles discussed in this chapter, you should attempt to group them according to function, as in Table 8-2. You will note, for example, that flexors produce many of the movements used for walking, sitting, swimming, typing, and many other activities. Extensors also function in these activities but perhaps play their most important role in maintaining an upright posture.

 To learn more about movement produced by skeletal muscle contractions, go to **AnimationDirect** on your CD.

QUICK CHECK

1. When a person flexes the knee, what is the movement called?
2. What happens when a person abducts his or her arm?
3. How is *dorsiflexion* of the foot performed?

Major Muscular Disorders

As you might expect, muscle disorders, or **myopathies** (my-OP-ah-theez), generally disrupt the normal movement of the body. In mild cases, these disorders vary in degree of discomfort from merely inconvenient to slightly troublesome. Severe muscle disorders, however, can impair the muscles used in breathing—a life-threatening situation.

Table 8-2	Muscles Grouped According to Function			
PART MOVED	**FLEXORS**	**EXTENSORS**	**ABDUCTORS**	**ADDUCTORS**
Upper arm	Pectoralis major	Latissimus dorsi	Deltoid	Pectoralis major and latissimus dorsi contracting together
Lower arm	Biceps brachii	Triceps brachii	None	None
Thigh	Iliopsoas, sartorius, and rectus femoris	Gluteus maximus and hamstrings	Gluteus medius	Adductor group
Lower leg	Hamstrings	Quadriceps group	None	None
Foot	Tibialis anterior	Gastrocnemius and soleus	Peroneus longus	Tibialis anterior

Muscle Injury

Injuries to skeletal muscles resulting from overexertion or trauma usually result in a **muscle strain** (Figure 8-13). Muscle strains are characterized by muscle pain, or **myalgia** (my-AL-jee-ah), and involve overstretching or tearing of muscle fibers. If an injury occurs in the area of a joint and a ligament is damaged, the injury may be called a **sprain.** Any muscle inflammation, including that caused by a muscle strain, is termed **myositis** (my-oh-SYE-tis). If tendon inflammation occurs with myositis, as when one experiences a *charley horse,* the condition is termed **fibromyositis** (fye-broh-my-oh-SYE-tis). Although inflammation may subside in a few hours or days, it usually takes several weeks for damaged muscle fibers to re-

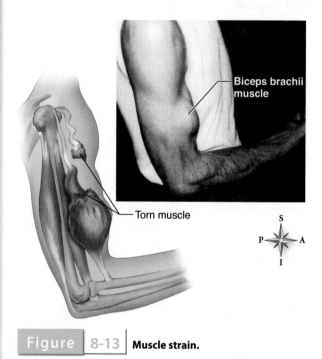

Figure 8-13 | **Muscle strain.**

Severe strain of the biceps brachii muscle. When a muscle is severely strained, it may break in two pieces, causing a visible gap in muscle tissue under the skin. Notice how the broken ends of the muscle reflexively contract (spasm) to form a knot of tissue.

pair themselves. Some damaged muscle cells may be replaced by fibrous tissue, forming scars. Occasionally, hard calcium is deposited in the scar tissue.

Cramps are painful muscle spasms (involuntary twitches). Cramps often result from mild myositis or fibromyositis, but can be a symptom of any irritation or of an ion and water imbalance.

Minor trauma to the body, especially a limb, may cause a muscle *bruise* or **contusion** (kon-TOO-zhun). Muscle contusions involve local internal bleeding and inflammation. Severe trauma to a skeletal muscle may cause a *crush injury.* Crush injuries not only greatly damage the affected muscle tissue but also cause the release of muscle fiber contents into the bloodstream, which can be life threatening. For example, the reddish muscle pigment *myoglobin* can accumulate in the blood and cause kidney failure.

Stress-induced muscle tension can result in myalgia and stiffness in the neck and back and is thought to be one cause of "stress headaches." Headache and back-pain clinics use a variety of strategies to treat stress-induced muscle tension. These treatments include massage, biofeedback, and relaxation training.

Muscle Infections

Several bacteria, viruses, and parasites are known to infect muscle tissue—often producing local or widespread myositis. For example, in trichinosis (see Appendix B on the CD that accompanies your book), widespread myositis is common. The muscle pain and stiffness that sometimes accompany influenza is another example.

Once a tragically common disease, **poliomyelitis** (poh-lee-oh-my-el-EYE-tis) is a viral infection of the nerves that control skeletal muscle movement. Although the disease can be asymptomatic, it often causes paralysis that may progress to death. Virtually eliminated in the United States as a result of a comprehensive vaccination program, it still affects millions in other parts of the world.

Muscular Dystrophy

Muscular dystrophy (DIS-troh-fee) is not a single disorder but a group of genetic diseases characterized by atrophy (wasting) of skeletal muscle tissues. Some, but not all, forms of muscular dystrophy can be fatal.

The most common form of muscular dystrophy is **Duchenne** (doo-SHEN) **muscular dystrophy (DMD).** This form of the disease is also called *pseudohypertrophy* (meaning "false muscle growth") because the atrophy of muscle is masked by excessive replacement of muscle by fat and fibrous tissue. DMD is characterized by mild leg muscle weakness that progresses rapidly to include the shoulder muscles. The first signs of DMD are apparent at about 3 years of age, and the stricken child is usually severely affected within 5 to 10 years. Death from respiratory or cardiac muscle weakness often occurs by the time the victim is 21 years old.

DMD is caused by a missing gene in the X chromosome. DMD occurs primarily in boys. Because girls have two X chromosomes and boys only one, genetic diseases involving X chromosome abnormalities are more likely to occur in boys than in girls. This is true because girls with one damaged X chromosome may not exhibit an "X-linked" disease if their other X chromosome is normal (see Chapter 24). The missing gene codes for a cell protein called *dystrophin*. In DMD, dystrophin is missing from muscle cells, which then become too weak to hold to-gether during muscle contraction. Immune system responses may add to the damage. Gene therapy (see Chapter 24) is now being tested for use in DMD patients, with the hope that the gene for dystrophin can be replaced by cells from a healthy donor.

Myasthenia Gravis

Myasthenia gravis (my-es-THEE-nee-ah GRAH-vis) is a chronic disease characterized by muscle weakness, especially in the face and throat. Most forms of this disease begin with mild weakness and chronic muscle fatigue in the face, then progress to wider muscle involvement. When severe muscle weakness causes immobility in all four limbs, a myasthenic crisis is said to have occurred. A person in *myasthenic crisis* is in danger of dying from respiratory failure because of weakness in the respiratory muscles.

Myasthenia gravis is an autoimmune disease in which the immune system attacks muscle cells at the neuromuscular junction (Figure 8-4). Nerve impulses from motor neurons are then unable to fully stimulate the affected muscle.

> **QUICK CHECK**
>
> 1. What does the term *myopathy* mean?
> 2. What is another term for muscle pain?
> 3. What is the cause of *Duchenne muscular dystrophy (DMD)*?
> 4. Describe the characteristics of *myasthenia gravis*.

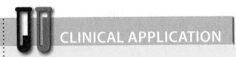

CLINICAL APPLICATION

RIGOR MORTIS

The term **rigor mortis** is a Latin phrase that means "stiffness of death." In a medical context, the term *rigor mortis* refers to the stiffness of skeletal muscles sometimes observed shortly after death. What causes rigor mortis? At the time of death, stimulation of muscle cells ceases. However, some muscle fibers may have been in mid-contraction at the time of death—when the myosin-actin cross bridges are still intact. ATP is required to release the cross bridges and "energize" them for their next attachment. Because the last of a cell's ATP supply is used up at the time it dies, many cross bridges may be left "stuck" in the contracted position. Thus muscles in a dead body may be stiff because individual muscle fibers ran out of the ATP required to "turn off" a muscle contraction.

Outline Summary

 To download an MP3 version of the chapter summary for use with your iPod or portable media player, access the **Audio Chapter Summaries** on your CD.

Introduction

A. Muscular tissue enables the body and its parts to move
   1. Movement caused by ability of muscle cells (called *fibers*) to shorten or contract
   2. Muscle cells shorten by converting chemical energy (obtained from food) into mechanical energy, which causes movement
   3. Three types of muscle tissue exist in the body (see Chapter 4)

Muscle Tissue

A. Skeletal muscle—also called *striated* or *voluntary* muscle (Figure 8-1, *A*)
   1. Is 40% to 50% of body weight ("red meat" attached to bones)
   2. Microscope reveals crosswise stripes, or striations
   3. Contractions can be voluntarily controlled
B. Cardiac muscle—composes bulk of heart (Figure 8-1, *B*)
   1. Cardiac muscle cells branch frequently
   2. Characterized by unique dark bands called *intercalated disks*
   3. Interconnected nature of cardiac muscle cells allows heart to contract efficiently as a unit
C. Smooth muscle—also called *nonstriated, involuntary,* or *visceral* muscle (Figure 8-1, *C*)
   1. Lacks cross stripes, or striations, when seen under a microscope; appears smooth
   2. Found in walls of hollow visceral structures such as digestive tract, blood vessels, and ureters
   3. Contractions not under voluntary control; movement caused by contraction is involuntary
D. Function—all muscle cells specialize in contraction (shortening)

Structure of Skeletal Muscle

A. Major structures
   1. Each skeletal muscle is an organ composed mainly of skeletal muscle cells and connective tissue
   2. Most skeletal muscles extend from one bone across a joint to another bone
   3. Parts of a skeletal muscle (Figure 8-2)
      a. Origin—attachment to the bone that remains relatively stationary or fixed when movement at the joint occurs
      b. Insertion—point of attachment to the bone that moves when a muscle contracts
      c. Body—main part of the muscle
   4. Muscles attach to bone by tendons—strong cords of fibrous connective tissue; some tendons are enclosed in synovial-lined tubes and are lubricated by synovial fluid; tubes are called *tendon sheaths*
   5. Bursae—small synovial-lined sacs containing a small amount of synovial fluid; located between some tendons and underlying bones
B. Microscopic structure and function (Figure 8-3)
   1. Contractile cells, or muscle fibers—grouped into bundles and intricately arranged
   2. Fibers contain thick myofilaments (containing the protein myosin) and thin myofilaments (composed of actin)
   3. Basic functional (contractile) unit called sarcomere
      a. Sarcomeres are separated from each other by dark bands called Z lines
      b. Sliding filament model explains mechanism of contraction

(1) Thick and thin myofilaments slide past each other as a muscle contracts

(2) Contraction requires calcium and energy-rich ATP molecules (Figure 8-4)

Functions of Skeletal Muscle

A. Movement
   1. Muscles produce movement by pulling on bones as a muscle contracts
      a. The insertion bone is pulled closer to the origin bone
      b. Movement occurs at the joint between the origin and the insertion
   2. Groups of muscles usually contract to produce a single movement
      a. Prime mover—muscle whose contraction is mainly responsible for producing a given movement
      b. Synergist—muscle whose contractions help the prime mover produce a given movement
      c. Antagonist—muscle whose actions oppose the action of a prime mover in any given movement
B. Posture
   1. A type of muscle contraction, called *tonic contraction*, enables us to maintain body position
      a. In tonic contraction, only a few of a muscle's fibers shorten at one time
      b. Tonic contractions produce no movement of body parts
      c. Tonic contractions maintain muscle tone called *posture*
   2. Good posture (optimum body positioning) favors best body functioning
   3. Skeletal muscle tone maintains posture by counteracting the pull of gravity
C. Heat production
   1. Survival depends on the body's ability to maintain a constant body temperature
      a. Fever—an elevated body temperature—often a sign of illness
      b. Hypothermia—body temperature below normal
   2. Contraction of muscle fibers produces most of the heat required to maintain normal body temperature
D. Fatigue
   1. Reduced strength of muscle contraction
   2. Caused by repeated muscle stimulation without adequate periods of rest
   3. Repeated muscular contraction depletes cellular ATP stores and outstrips the ability of the blood supply to replenish oxygen and nutrients
   4. Contraction in the absence of adequate oxygen produces lactic acid, which contributes to muscle burning
   5. *Oxygen debt*—term used to describe the metabolic effort required to burn excess lactic acid that may accumulate during prolonged periods of exercise
      a. Labored breathing after strenuous exercise is required to "pay the debt"
      b. This increased metabolism helps restore energy and oxygen reserves to pre-exercise levels

Role of Other Body Systems in Movement

A. Muscle functioning depends on the functioning of many other parts of the body
   1. Most muscles cause movements by pulling on bones across movable joints
   2. Respiratory, circulatory, nervous, muscular, and skeletal systems play essential roles in producing normal movements
B. Multiple sclerosis, brain hemorrhage, and spinal cord injury are examples of how pathological conditions in other body organ systems can dramatically affect movement

Motor Unit

A. Stimulation of a muscle by a nerve impulse is required before a muscle can shorten and produce movement
B. A motor neuron is the nerve cell that transmits an impulse to a muscle, causing contraction

C. A neuromuscular junction is the point of contact between a nerve ending and the muscle fiber it innervates

D. A motor unit is the combination of a motor neuron and the muscle cell or cells it innervates (Figure 8-5)

Muscle Stimulus

A. A muscle will contract only if an applied stimulus reaches a certain minimal level of intensity—called a threshold stimulus

B. Once stimulated by a threshold stimulus, a muscle fiber will contract completely, a response called *all or none*

C. Different muscle fibers in a muscle are controlled by different motor units having different threshold-stimulus levels

    1. Although individual muscle fibers always respond in an "all or none" mode to a threshold stimulus, the muscle as a whole does not

    2. Different motor units responding to different threshold stimuli permit a muscle as a whole to execute contractions of graded force

Types of Skeletal Muscle Contraction

A. Twitch and tetanic contractions

    1. Twitch contractions—quick, jerky responses to a stimulus—are laboratory phenomena and do not play a significant role in normal muscular activity

    2. Tetanic contractions are sustained and steady muscular contractions caused by a series of stimuli bombarding a muscle in rapid succession

B. Isotonic contractions (Figure 8-6)

    1. Contraction of a muscle that produces movement at a joint

    2. During isotonic contractions, the muscle changes length, causing the insertion end of the muscle to move relative to the point of origin

    3. Concentric contractions shorten muscles

    4. Eccentric contractions allow muscles to increase in length

    5. Most types of body movements such as walking and running are caused by isotonic contractions

C. Isometric contractions (Figure 8-6)

    1. Isometric contractions are muscle contractions that do not produce movement; the muscle as a whole does not shorten

    2. Although no movement occurs during isometric contractions, tension within the muscle increases

Effects of Exercise on Skeletal Muscles

A. Exercise, if regular and properly practiced, improves muscle tone and posture, results in more efficient heart and lung functioning, and reduces fatigue

B. Specific effects of exercise on skeletal muscles

    1. Muscles undergo changes related to the amount of work they normally do

        a. Prolonged inactivity causes disuse atrophy

        b. Regular exercise increases muscle size, called *hypertrophy*

    2. Strength training involves contraction of muscles against heavy resistance

        a. Strength training increases the numbers of myofilaments in each muscle fiber, and as a result, the total mass of the muscle increases

        b. Strength training does not increase the number of muscle fibers

    3. Endurance training increases a muscle's ability to sustain moderate exercise over a long period; it is sometimes called *aerobic training*

        a. Endurance training allows more efficient delivery of oxygen and nutrients to a muscle via increased blood flow

        b. Endurance training does not usually result in muscle hypertrophy

Skeletal Muscle Groups (Table 8-1)

A. Muscles of the head and neck (Figures 8-7 and 8-8)

    1. Facial muscles

        a. Orbicularis oculi

        b. Orbicularis oris

        c. Zygomaticus

    2. Muscles of mastication

        a. Masseter

        b. Temporal

    3. Sternocleidomastoid—flexes head

4. Trapezius—elevates shoulders and extends head
B. Muscles that move the upper extremities
 1. Pectoralis major—flexes upper arm
 2. Latissimus dorsi—extends upper arm
 3. Deltoid—abducts upper arm
 4. Biceps brachii—flexes forearm
 5. Triceps brachii—extends forearm
C. Muscles of the trunk (Figure 8-9)
 1. Abdominal muscles
  a. Rectus abdominis
  b. External oblique
  c. Internal oblique
  d. Transversus abdominis
 2. Respiratory muscles
  a. Intercostal muscles
  b. Diaphragm
D. Muscles that move the lower extremities
 1. Iliopsoas—flexes thigh
 2. Gluteus maximus—extends thigh
 3. Adductor muscles—adduct thighs
 4. Hamstring muscles—flex lower leg
  a. Semimembranosus
  b. Semitendinosus
  c. Biceps femoris
 5. Quadriceps femoris group—extend lower leg
  a. Rectus femoris
  b. Vastus muscles
 6. Tibialis anterior—dorsiflexes foot
 7. Gastrocnemius—plantar flexes foot
 8. Peroneus group—flexes foot
E. Movements produced by skeletal muscle contractions (Figures 8-10 through 8-12)
 1. Flexion—movement that decreases the angle between two bones at their joint: bending
 2. Extension—movement that increases the angle between two bones at their joint: straightening
 3. Abduction—movement of a part away from the midline of the body
 4. Adduction—movement of a part toward the midline of the body
 5. Rotation and circumduction—movement around a longitudinal axis
 6. Supination and pronation—hand positions that result from rotation of the forearm; supination results in a hand position with the palm turned to the anterior position;

pronation occurs when the palm faces posteriorly
 7. Dorsiflexion and plantar flexion—foot movements; dorsiflexion results in elevation of the dorsum or top of the foot; during plantar flexion, the bottom of the foot is directed downward

Major Muscular Disorders

A. Myopathies—muscle disorders; can range from mild to life threatening
B. Muscle injury
 1. Strain—injury from overexertion or trauma; involves stretching or tearing of muscle fibers
  a. Often accompanied by myalgia (muscle pain)
  b. May result in inflammation of muscle (myositis) or of muscle and tendon (fibromyositis)
  c. If injury is near a joint and involves ligament damage, it may be called a *sprain*
 2. Cramps are painful muscle spasms (involuntary twitches)
 3. Crush injuries result from severe muscle trauma and may release cell contents that ultimately cause kidney failure
 4. Stress-induced muscle tension can cause headaches and back pain
C. Muscle infections
 1. Several bacteria, viruses, and parasites can infect muscles
 2. Poliomyelitis is a viral infection of motor nerves that ranges from mild to life threatening
D. Muscular dystrophy
 1. A group of genetic disorders characterized by muscle atrophy
 2. Duchenne (pseudohypertrophic) muscular dystrophy is the most common type
  a. Characterized by rapid progression of weakness and atrophy
  b. X-linked inherited disease, affecting mostly boys
E. Myasthenia gravis—autoimmune muscle disease characterized by weakness and chronic fatigue

New Words

abduction	intercalated disk	prime mover	zygomaticus
actin	intercostal muscle	pronation	
adduction	internal oblique	quadriceps femoris	### Diseases and Other Clinical Terms
adductor muscle	isometric contraction	rectus abdominis	
aerobic training	isotonic contraction	rigor mortis	bursitis
all or none	latissimus dorsi	sarcomere	carpal tunnel syndrome
antagonist	masseter	sliding filament model	contusion
biceps brachii	mastication	sternocleidomastoid	cramps
bursa (*pl.,* bursae)	motor neuron	strength training	disuse atrophy
circumduction	motor unit	supination	Duchenne muscular
deltoid	muscle fiber	synergist	dystrophy (DMD)
dorsiflexion	myofilament	temporal	fibromyositis
endurance training	myoglobin	tendon	hypothermia
external oblique	myosin	tendon sheath	muscle strain
fatigue	neuromuscular junction	tetanic contraction	muscular dystrophy
frontal	orbicularis oris	threshold stimulus	myalgia
gastrocnemius	origin	tibialis anterior	myasthenia gravis
gluteus maximus	oxygen debt	tonic contraction	myopathy
hamstring muscle	pectoralis major	transverse abdominis	myositis
hypertrophy	peroneus group	trapezius	paralysis
iliopsoas	plantar flexion	triceps brachii	poliomyelitis
insertion	posture	twitch	tenosynovitis

Review Questions

1. Briefly describe the structure of cardiac muscle.
2. Briefly describe the structure of smooth muscle.
3. Give the function of tendons, bursae, and synovial membranes.
4. Explain how tonic contractions help maintain posture.
5. Give an example of how two body systems other than the muscular system contribute to the movement of the body.
6. Explain *twitch* and *tetanic* contractions.
7. Explain *isotonic* contractions.
8. Explain *isometric* contractions.
9. Name two muscles in the head or neck and give the origin, insertion, and function of each.
10. Name two muscles that move the upper extremity and give the origin, insertion, and function of each.
11. Name two muscles of the trunk and give the origin, insertion, and function of each.
12. Name three muscles of the lower extremity and give the origin, insertion, and function of each.
13. Describe the following movements: flexion, extension, abduction, adduction, and rotation.
14. What signs and symptoms are likely to accompany a moderate muscle strain?
15. What causes the signs and symptoms of myasthenia gravis?

Critical Thinking

16. Draw and label a relaxed sarcomere; explain the process that causes a sarcomere to contract.
17. Explain the interaction of the prime mover, the synergist, and the antagonist in efficient movement.
18. Describe the condition that causes a muscle to develop an "oxygen debt." How is this debt paid off?

19. Why can a spinal cord injury be followed by muscle paralysis?
20. Can a muscle contract very long if its blood supply is shut off? Give a reason for your answer.
21. Briefly explain changes that gradually take place in bones, joints, and muscles in a person who habitually gets too little exercise.
22. Briefly explain the progression of Duchenne muscular dystrophy.

Chapter Test

1. _____ is another name for muscle cell.
2. Cardiac muscle makes up the bulk of the tissue of the _____.
3. The muscle attachment to the more movable bone is called the _____.
4. The muscle attachment to the more stationary bone is called the _____.
5. _____ is the protein that makes up the thin myofilament.
6. _____ is the protein that makes up the thick myofilament.
7. The _____ is the basic functional unit of contraction in a skeletal muscle.
8. The three functions of the muscle system are _____, _____, and _____.
9. The molecule _____ supplies energy for muscle contraction.
10. _____ is the waste product produced when the muscle must switch to an energy-supplying process that does not require oxygen.
11. A single motor neuron with all the muscle cells it innervates is called a _____.
12. _____ is the minimal level of stimulation required to cause a muscle to contract.

13. _____ is a type of muscle contraction that produces movement in a joint and allows the muscle to shorten.
14. _____ is a type of muscle contraction that does not produce movement and does not allow the muscle to shorten but increases muscle tension.
15. _____ is a term that describes movement of a body part away from the midline of the body.
16. _____ is a term used to describe the movement that is opposite flexion.
17. _____ describes the hand position when the body is in anatomical position.
18. Excessive stretching or tearing of muscle fibers is called _____.
19. Inflammation of muscle and tendon is termed _____.
20. _____ is a viral infection of motor nerves that may progress to life-threatening paralysis of the respiratory muscles.
21. _____ is a group of muscle disorders characterized by muscle atrophy and that often progresses to death before age 21.
22. _____ is an autoimmune muscle disease characterized by weakness and chronic fatigue.

23. Skeletal muscles can also be called
   a. visceral muscle
   b. voluntary muscle
   c. cardiac muscle
   d. all of the above

24. Smooth muscle can also be called
   a. visceral muscle
   b. voluntary muscle
   c. cardiac muscle
   d. all of the above

Match each muscle in Column A with its corresponding location or function in Column B.

Column A
   25. _____ temporal muscle
   26. _____ biceps brachii
   27. _____ sartorius
   28. _____ masseter
   29. _____ gastrocnemius
   30. _____ pectoralis major
   31. _____ external oblique
   32. _____ gluteus maximus
   33. _____ sternocleidomastoid
   34. _____ rectus abdominis
   35. _____ rectus femoris
   36. _____ triceps brachii

Column B
   a. muscles of the head or neck
   b. muscles that move the upper extremity
   c. muscles of the trunk
   d. muscles that move the lower extremity

Study Tips

continued from page 207

4. ATP is most efficiently formed when oxygen is supplied to the muscle. When you can't supply the muscle with enough oxygen, your muscle uses a process that creates lactic acid and develops an oxygen debt.

5. The names of the muscles are probably less familiar to you than the names of the bones. But muscle names can give you information about the muscle. Muscles are named for their shape: *deltoid, trapezius.* They are named for the number of origins they have: *triceps* brachii, their points of attachment: *sternocleidomas-toid,* their size: gluteus *maximus,* and the direction of the muscle fibers: *rectus* abdominis (*rectus* means the muscle has fibers running parallel to the midline of the body). When you are learning the muscles, try to look for meaning in the muscle names.

6. Most of the terms for muscle movement are fairly straightforward. One way to remember the difference between *supination* and *pronation* is to picture your hand holding a bowl of soup—that's supination (silly, but an effective memory aid).

7. Draw a chart showing the mechanisms of muscular disorders by type: injury, infection, dystrophy, and myasthenia gravis.

8. Prepare flash cards to help you learn the terms in this chapter. Review them in your study group. Also discuss the process of contraction and fatigue, and be sure you understand the movement terms. If you are asked to learn the names and locations of the muscles, a photocopy of the muscle figures with the labels blackened out can be used to quiz each other. If you are asked to learn the function, origin, and insertion of the muscles, prepare and use flash cards along with the figures.

9. Go over the questions at the end of the chapter and discuss possible test questions in your study group.

Case Studies

1. Your nephew Tom has just been diagnosed with *pseudohypertrophic muscular dystrophy*. How did he get this disease? Is his twin sister, Geri, likely to develop the same condition? Are you likely to get this disease? (HINT: see Chapter 24) You know that muscular dystrophy typically causes atrophy or wasting of muscle tissue, yet Tom's leg muscles seem particularly well developed. Tom's physician said that the appearance of Tom's legs is typical for this form of muscular dystrophy. Can you explain this apparent contradiction?

2. Your friend Elena is suffering from a strain of her gastrocnemius muscle. What type of injury is this, and where in Elena's body is it located? What symptoms are likely to accompany Elena's injury? What movements should Elena avoid to prevent further injury to the gastrocnemius muscle?

3. Robert has decided to improve his appearance by exercising. He would like to build up his chest and shoulder muscles so that he looks better in the T-shirts he is so fond of wearing. He has decided to play racquetball every day as his primary training program because he knows that he uses his upper body muscles in this sport. After his first game of racquetball, you ask him how he likes his new sport and he can hardly answer you—he seems out of breath. Is Robert's plan likely to help him meet his goal? How do you explain his breathing difficulties?

Objectives

After you have completed this chapter, you should be able to:

1. List the organs and divisions of the nervous system and describe the generalized functions of the system as a whole.

2. Identify the major types of cells in the nervous system and discuss the function of each.

3. Identify the anatomical and functional components of a three-neuron reflex arc. Compare and contrast the propagation of a nerve impulse along a nerve fiber and across a synaptic cleft.

4. Identify the major anatomical components of the brain and spinal cord and briefly comment on the function of each.

5. Identify and discuss the coverings and fluid spaces of the brain and spinal cord.

6. Compare and contrast spinal and cranial nerves.

7. Discuss the structure and function of the two divisions of the autonomic nervous system.

8. Describe major nervous system disorders.

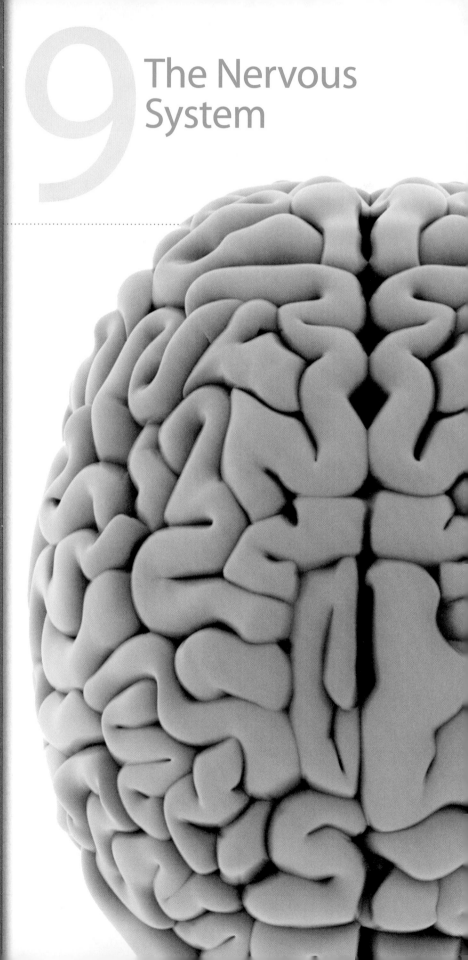

9 The Nervous System

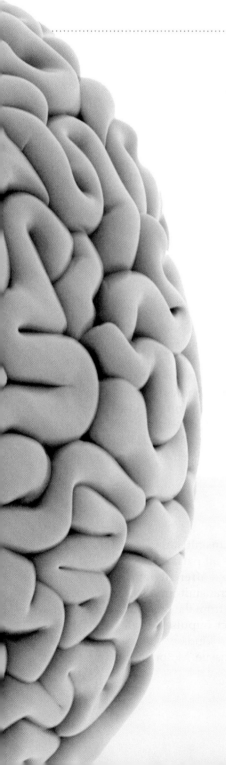

The normal body must accomplish a gigantic and enormously complex job—keeping itself alive and healthy. Each one of its billions of cells performs some activity that is a part of this function. Control of the body's billions of cells is accomplished mainly by two communication systems: the nervous system and the endocrine system. Both systems transmit information from one part of the body to another, but they do it in different ways. The nervous system transmits information very rapidly by nerve impulses conducted from one body area to another. The endocrine system transmits information more slowly by chemicals secreted by ductless glands into the bloodstream and then circulated from the glands to other parts of the body. Nerve impulses and hormones communicate information to body structures, increasing or decreasing their activities as needed for healthy survival. In other words, the communication systems of the body are also its control and integrating systems. They combine the body's hundreds of functions into its one overall function of keeping itself alive and healthy.

Recall that homeostasis is the balanced and controlled internal environment of the body that is basic to life itself. Homeostasis is possible only if our physiological control and integration systems function properly. Our plan for this chapter is to name the cells, organs, and divisions of

STUDY TIPS   Before beginning your study of Chapter 9, review the synopsis of the nervous system in Chapter 4. The amount of material presented in Chapter 9 may be overwhelming at first, but it can be somewhat easier to learn if you divide the chapter into three parts: the microscopic structure and function of the nervous system, the central nervous system, and the peripheral nervous system.

1. Keep in mind that the nervous system functions as one organized system. The function of the nervous system is accomplished by two processes: conduction of nerve impulses and passing of the nerve impulse across a synapse. Nerve impulses are an exchange of ions between the interior and exterior of the neuron.

continued on page 278

the nervous system; discuss the generation of nervous impulses; and then explain how these impulses move between one area of the body and another. We will not only study the major components of the nervous system, such as the brain, spinal cord, and nerves, but also learn how they function to maintain and regulate homeostasis or respond to disease. In Chapter 10, we will consider the senses.

Organs and Divisions of the Nervous System

The organs of the nervous system as a whole include the brain and spinal cord, the numerous nerves of the body, the special sense organs such as the eyes and ears, and the microscopic sense organs such as those found in the skin. The system as a whole consists of two principal divisions: the central nervous system and the peripheral nervous system (Figure 9-1). Because the brain and spinal cord occupy a midline or central location in the body, together they are called the **central nervous system,** or **CNS.** Similarly, the usual designation for the nerves of the body is the **peripheral nervous system,** or **PNS.** The term *peripheral* is appropriate because nerves extend to outlying or peripheral parts of the body. A subdivision of the peripheral nervous system, called the **autonomic nervous system,** or **ANS,** consists of structures that regulate the body's automatic or involuntary functions (for example, the heart rate, the contractions of the stomach and intestines, and the secretion of chemical compounds by glands).

 To learn more about the divisions of the nervous system, go to **AnimationDirect** on your CD.

Cells of the Nervous System

The two types of cells found in the nervous system are called **neurons** (NOO-rons), or nerve cells, and **glia** (GLEE-ah), which are support cells. Neurons conduct impulses, whereas glia support neurons.

Neurons

Each neuron consists of three parts: a main part called the neuron **cell body,** one or more branching projections called **dendrites** (DEN-drytes), and one elongated projection known as an **axon.** Identify each part on the neuron shown in Figure 9-2. Dendrites are the processes or projections that transmit impulses *to* the neuron cell bodies or axons, and axons are the processes that transmit impulses *away* from the neuron cell bodies or dendrites.

The three types of neurons are classified according to the direction in which they transmit impulses:

1. Sensory neurons
2. Motor neurons
3. Interneurons

Sensory neurons transmit impulses to the spinal cord and brain from all parts of the body. Sensory neurons are also called **afferent neurons**.

Motor neurons transmit impulses in the opposite direction—away from the brain and spinal cord. They do not conduct impulses to all parts of the body but only to two kinds of tissue—muscle and glandular epithelial tissue. Motor neurons are called **efferent neurons.**

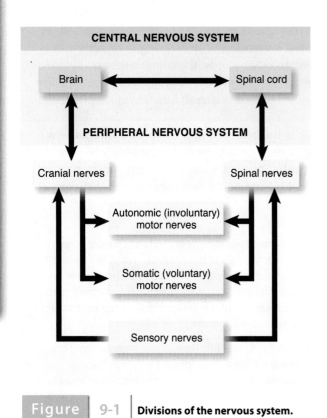

Figure 9-1 | **Divisions of the nervous system.**

Interneurons conduct impulses from sensory neurons to motor neurons. Interneurons are called *central* or *connecting* neurons.

The axon shown in Figure 9-2, *B,* is surrounded by a segmented wrapping of a material called **myelin** (MY-eh-lin). Myelin is a white, fatty substance formed by **Schwann cells** that wrap around some axons outside the central nervous system. Such fibers are called **myelinated fibers**. In Figure 9-2, *B,* one such axon has been enlarged to show additional detail. **Nodes of Ranvier** (rahn-vee-AY) are indentations between adjacent Schwann cells.

The outer cell membrane of a Schwann cell is called the **neurilemma** (noo-ri-LEM-mah). That axons in the brain and cord have no neurilemma is clinically significant because it plays an es-

sential part in the regeneration of cut and injured axons. Therefore the potential for regeneration in the brain and spinal cord is far less than it is in the peripheral nervous system.

Glia

Glia—or *neuroglia* (noo-ROG-lee-ah)—do not specialize in transmitting impulses. Instead, they are special types of supporting cells. Their name is appropriate because it is derived from the Greek word *glia* meaning "glue." One function of glia cells is to hold the functioning neurons together and protect them. An important reason for discussing glia is that one of the most common types of brain tumor—

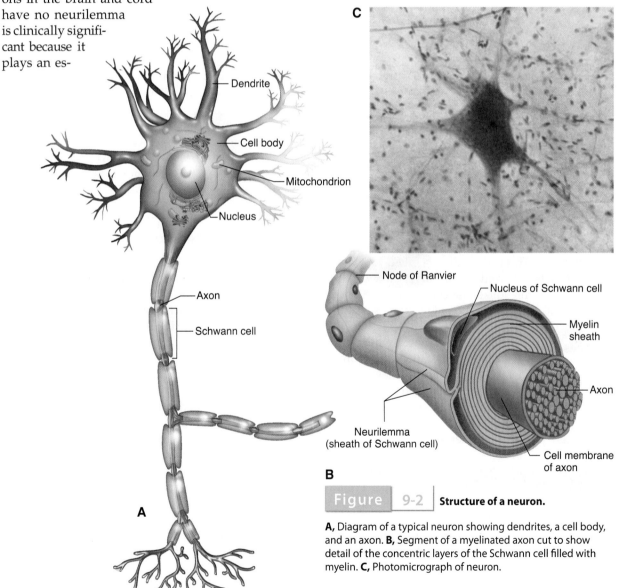

Figure 9-2 | **Structure of a neuron.**

A, Diagram of a typical neuron showing dendrites, a cell body, and an axon. **B,** Segment of a myelinated axon cut to show detail of the concentric layers of the Schwann cell filled with myelin. **C,** Photomicrograph of neuron.

CENTRAL NERVOUS SYSTEM NEUROGLIA

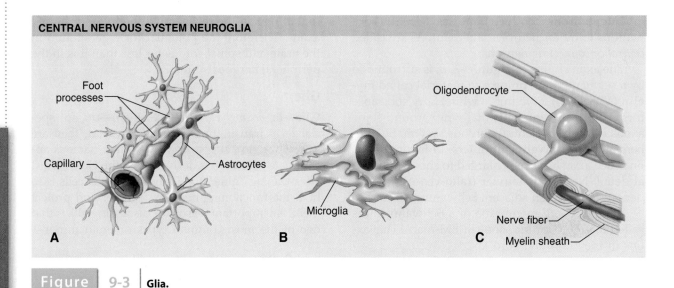

Foot processes

Capillary

Astrocytes

A

Microglia

B

Oligodendrocyte

Nerve fiber

Myelin sheath

C

Figure 9-3 | **Glia.**

A, Astrocytes have extensions attached to blood vessels in the brain. **B,** Microglia within the central nervous system can enlarge and consume microbes by phagocytosis. **C,** Oligodendrocytes have extensions that form myelin sheaths around axons in the central nervous system.

called **glioma** (glee-OH-mah)—develops from them. We now know that glia perform many different functions, including the regulation of neuron function. Therefore, they act not just as physical "glue" but also help bring the various functions of the nervous tissue together into a coordinated whole.

Glia vary in size and shape (Figure 9-3). Some are relatively large cells that look somewhat like stars because of the threadlike extensions that jut out from their surfaces. These glia cells are called **astrocytes** (ASS-troh-sytes), a word that means "star cells" (Figure 9-3). Their threadlike branches attach to neurons and to small blood vessels, holding these structures close to each other.

Microglia (my-KROG-lee-ah) are smaller than astrocytes. They usually remain stationary, but in inflamed or degenerating brain tissue, they enlarge, move about, and act as microbe-eating scavengers. They surround the microbes, draw them into their cytoplasm, and digest them. Recall from Chapter 3 that phagocytosis is the scientific name for this important cellular process.

The **oligodendrocytes** (ol-i-go-DEN-droh-sytes) help hold nerve fibers together and also serve another and probably more important function; they produce the fatty myelin sheath that envelops nerve fibers located in the brain and spinal cord. Recall that Schwann cells also form myelin sheaths but do so only in the peripheral nervous system.

QUICK CHECK

1. What is the difference between the central nervous system and the peripheral nervous system?
2. What are the major features of a neuron?
3. How are glia different from neurons?

Disorders of Nervous Tissue

MULTIPLE SCLEROSIS

A number of diseases are associated with disorders of the oligodendrocytes. Because these glial cells are involved in myelin formation, the diseases as a group are called *myelin disorders*. The most common primary disease of the CNS is a myelin disorder called **multiple sclerosis,** or **MS.** It is characterized by myelin loss and destruction accompanied by varying degrees of oligodendrocyte injury and death (Figure 9-4). The result is demyelination throughout the white matter of the CNS. Hard, plaquelike lesions replace the destroyed myelin, and affected areas are invaded by inflammatory cells. As the myelin around the axons is lost, nerve conduction is impaired, and weakness, incoordination, visual impairment, and speech disturbances occur. Although the disease occurs in both sexes and all age-groups, it is most common in women between the ages of 20 and 40 years.

The cause of multiple sclerosis is thought to be related to autoimmunity and to viral infections in

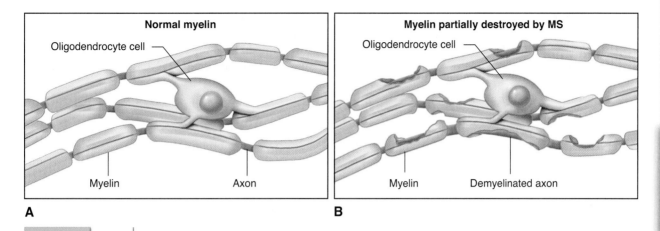

Normal myelin

Oligodendrocyte cell

Myelin   Axon

A

Myelin partially destroyed by MS

Oligodendrocyte cell

Myelin   Demyelinated axon

B

Figure 9-4 | **Effects of multiple sclerosis (MS).**

A, A normal myelin sheath allows rapid conduction. **B,** In those with MS, the myelin sheath is damaged, disrupting normal nerve conduction.

some individuals. MS is characteristically relapsing and chronic in nature, but some cases of acute and unremitting disease have been reported. In most instances the disease is prolonged, with remissions and relapses occurring over many years. Television personality and author Montel Williams reports that he lived with recurring episodes of MS for 20 years before he realized that he has the condition. Although there is not yet a cure for MS, early diagnosis and treatment can slow or stop its progression.

TUMORS

The general name for tumors arising in nervous system structures is **neuroma** (noo-ROH-mah). Tumors do not usually develop directly from neurons but instead from glia, membrane tissues, and blood vessels. As stated above, a common type of brain tumor—glioma—occurs in glia. Gliomas are usually benign but may still be life threatening. Patients usually show deficits reflecting damaged function of the area in which the tumor is located (Figure 9-13, *B*). Because these tumors often develop in deep areas of the brain, they are difficult to treat. Untreated gliomas may grow to a size that disrupts normal brain function, perhaps leading to death.

Multiple neurofibromatosis (noo-roh-fye-broh-mah-TOH-sis) is an inherited disease characterized by numerous fibrous neuromas throughout the body (Figure 9-5). The tumors are benign, appearing first as small nodules in the Schwann cells of cutaneous nerves. In some cases, involvement spreads as large, disfiguring fibrous tumors appear in many areas of the body, including muscles, bones, and internal organs.

Most malignant tumors of glia and other nervous tissues do not originate there but instead are secondary tumors resulting from metastasis of cancer cells from the breast, lung, or other organs.

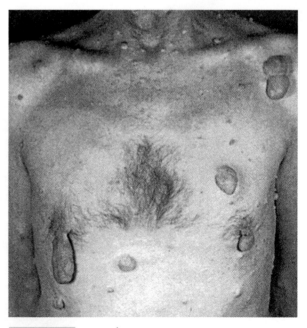

Figure 9-5 | **Multiple neurofibromatosis.**

This photo shows multiple tumors of Schwann cells in the nerves of the skin that are characteristic of this inherited condition.

QUICK CHECK

1. What is a *myelin disorder?* How does a myelin disorder disrupt nervous system function?

2. What is a *neuroma?*

Nerves

A **nerve** is a group of peripheral nerve fibers (axons) bundled together like the strands of a cable. Peripheral nerve fibers usually have a myelin sheath and because myelin is white, peripheral nerves often look white.

Bundles of axons in the CNS, called **tracts,** also may be myelinated and thus form the **white matter** of the brain and cord. Brain and cord tissue composed of cell bodies and unmyelinated axons and dendrites is called **gray matter** because of its characteristic gray appearance.

Figure 9-6 shows that each axon in a nerve is surrounded by a thin wrapping of fibrous connective tissue called the **endoneurium** (en-doh-NOO-ree-um).

Groups of these wrapped axons are called **fascicles.** Each fascicle is surrounded by a thin, fibrous **perineurium** (pair-i-NOO-ree-um). A tough, fibrous sheath called the **epineurium** (ep-i-NOO-ree-um) covers the whole nerve.

Reflex Arcs

During every moment of our lives, nerve impulses speed over neurons to and from our spinal cords and brains. If all impulse conduction ceases, life itself ceases. Only neurons can provide the rapid communication between cells that is necessary for maintaining life. Hormonal messages are the only other kind of communications the body can send, and they travel much more slowly than impulses. They can move from one part of the body to another only via circulating blood. Compared with impulse conduction, circulation is a very slow process.

Nerve impulses, sometimes called **action potentials,** can travel over trillions of routes—routes

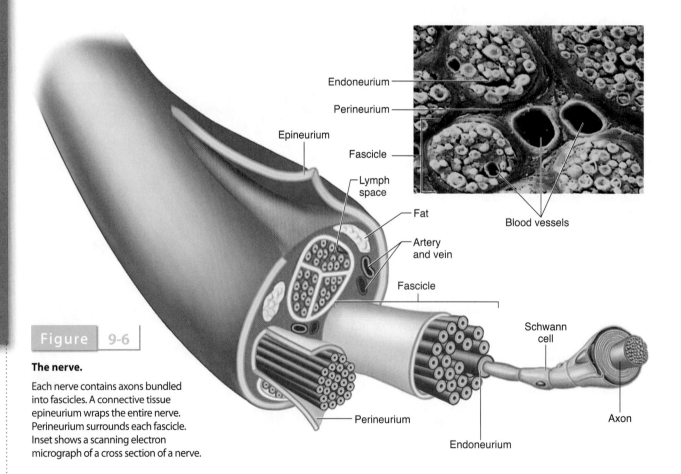

Figure 9-6

The nerve.

Each nerve contains axons bundled into fascicles. A connective tissue epineurium wraps the entire nerve. Perineurium surrounds each fascicle. Inset shows a scanning electron micrograph of a cross section of a nerve.

Endoneurium
Perineurium
Epineurium
Fascicle
Lymph space
Fat
Artery and vein
Fascicle
Blood vessels
Schwann cell
Axon
Perineurium
Endoneurium

made up of neurons because they are the cells that conduct impulses. Hence the routes traveled by nerve impulses are sometimes spoken of as *neuron pathways*. A basic type of neuron pathway, called a **reflex arc,** is important to nervous system functioning. The simplest kind of reflex arc is a two-neuron arc, so called because it consists of only two types of neurons: sensory neurons and motor neurons. Three-neuron arcs are the next simplest kind. They, of course, consist of all three kinds of neurons: sensory neurons, interneurons, and motor neurons. Reflex arcs are like one-way streets; they allow impulse conduction in only one direction. The next paragraph describes this direction in detail. Look frequently at Figure 9-7 as you read it.

Impulse conduction normally starts in receptors. **Receptors** are the beginnings of dendrites of sensory neurons. They are often located at some distance from the spinal cord (in tendons, skin, or mucous membranes, for example). In Figure 9-7 the sensory receptors are located in the quadriceps muscle group and in the patellar tendon. In the reflex that is illustrated there, stretch receptors are stimulated as a result of a tap on the patellar tendon from a rubber hammer used by a physician to elicit a reflex during a physical examination. The nerve impulse that is generated, its neurologic pathway, and its ultimate "knee-jerk" effect is an example of the simplest form of a two-neuron reflex arc.

In the knee-jerk reflex, only sensory and motor neurons are involved. The nerve impulse that is generated by stimulation of the stretch receptors travels along the length of the sensory neuron's dendrite to its cell body located in the *dorsal (posterior) root ganglion*. A **ganglion** (GANG-lee-on) is a group of nerve-cell bodies located in the PNS. This ganglion is located near the spinal cord. Each spinal ganglion contains not one sensory neuron cell body as shown in Figure 9-7, but hundreds of them. The axon of the sensory neuron travels from the cell body in the dorsal root ganglion and ends near the dendrites of another neuron located in the gray matter of the spinal cord. A microscopic space separates the axon ending of one neuron from the dendrites of another neuron. This space is called a **synapse.** The nerve impulse stops at the synapse, chemical signals are sent across the gap, and the impulse then continues along the dendrites, cell body, and axon of the motor neuron. The motor neuron axon forms a synapse with a structure called an *effector*, an organ that puts nerve signals "into effect."

Effectors are muscles or glands, and muscle contractions and gland secretion are the only kinds of reflexes operated by these effectors. The response to impulse conduction over a reflex arc is called a **reflex.**

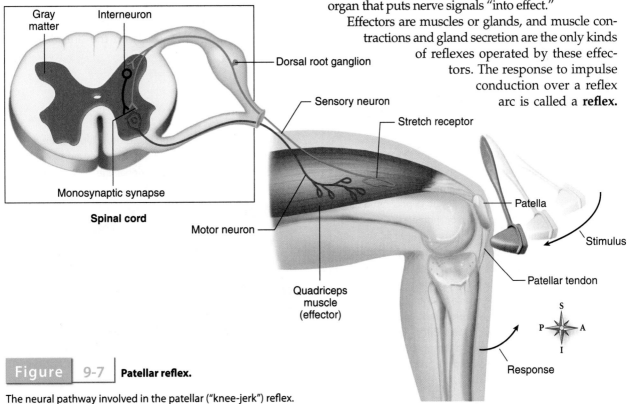

Figure 9-7 | **Patellar reflex.**

The neural pathway involved in the patellar ("knee-jerk") reflex.

In short, impulse conduction by a reflex arc causes a reflex to occur. In a patellar reflex, the nerve impulses that reach the quadriceps muscle (the effector) result in the "knee-jerk" response.

Now turn your attention to the *interneuron* shown in Figure 9-7. Some reflexes involve three rather than two neurons. In these more complex types of responses, an interneuron, in addition to the sensory and motor neurons, is involved. In three-neuron reflexes, the end of the sensory neuron's axon synapses first with an interneuron before chemical signals are sent across a second synapse, resulting in conduction through the motor neuron. For example, application of an irritating stimulus to the skin of the thigh initiates a three-neuron reflex response that causes contraction of muscles to pull the leg away from the irritant—a three-neuron arc reaction called the *withdrawal reflex*. All interneurons lie entirely within the gray matter of the brain or spinal cord. Gray matter forms the H-shaped inner core of the spinal cord. Because of the presence of an interneuron, three-neuron reflex arcs have two synapses. A two-neuron reflex arc, however, has only a sensory neuron and a motor neuron with one synapse between them.

Identify the motor neuron in Figure 9-7. Observe that its dendrites and cell body, like those of an interneuron, are located in the spinal cord's gray matter. The axon of this motor neuron, however, runs through the ventral (anterior) root of the spinal nerve and terminates in a muscle.

QUICK CHECK

1. How is *white matter* different from *gray matter*?
2. Can you explain the function of a *reflex arc*?
3. What is a *sensory receptor*? How does it relate to the reflex arc?
4. What is an *effector*? How does it relate to the reflex arc?

Nerve Impulses

What are nerve impulses? Here is one widely accepted definition: a nerve impulse is a self-propagating wave of electrical disturbance that travels along the surface of a neuron's plasma membrane. You might visualize this as a tiny spark sizzling its way along a fuse.

Nerve impulses do not continually race along every nerve cell's surface. First they have to be initiated by a stimulus, a change in the neuron's environment. Pressure, temperature, and chemical changes are the usual stimuli.

The membrane of each resting neuron has a slight positive charge on the outside and a negative charge on the inside, a state called *polarization*, as shown in Figure 9-8. This occurs because there is normally an excess of sodium ions (Na^+) on the outside of the

CLINICAL APPLICATION

ANTIDEPRESSANTS

Antidepressants are prescribed widely for outpatients suffering from depression associated with their ongoing illness. Depression also can be a distinct mental illness that can be caused by a variety of factors. Severe depression often occurs when a deficit of *serotonin* or another neurotransmitter exists at certain synapses in parts of the brain that affect one's mood. Some of the more commonly used antidepressants today are paroxetine (Paxil), fluoxetine (Prozac), and sertraline (Zoloft). These drugs produce their effects by blocking the uptake of serotonin back into presynaptic neurons. Drugs in this class of antidepressants are called *serotonin-specific reuptake inhibitors (SSRIs)*. Serotonin-uptake inhibition causes an increase in the amount of serotonin in the synapse, thereby reversing the serotonin deficit that contributes to feelings of depression. Other types of antidepressants increase serotonin levels in other ways or affect other neurotransmitters, such as dopamine or norepinephrine, also associated with depression.

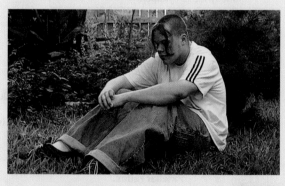

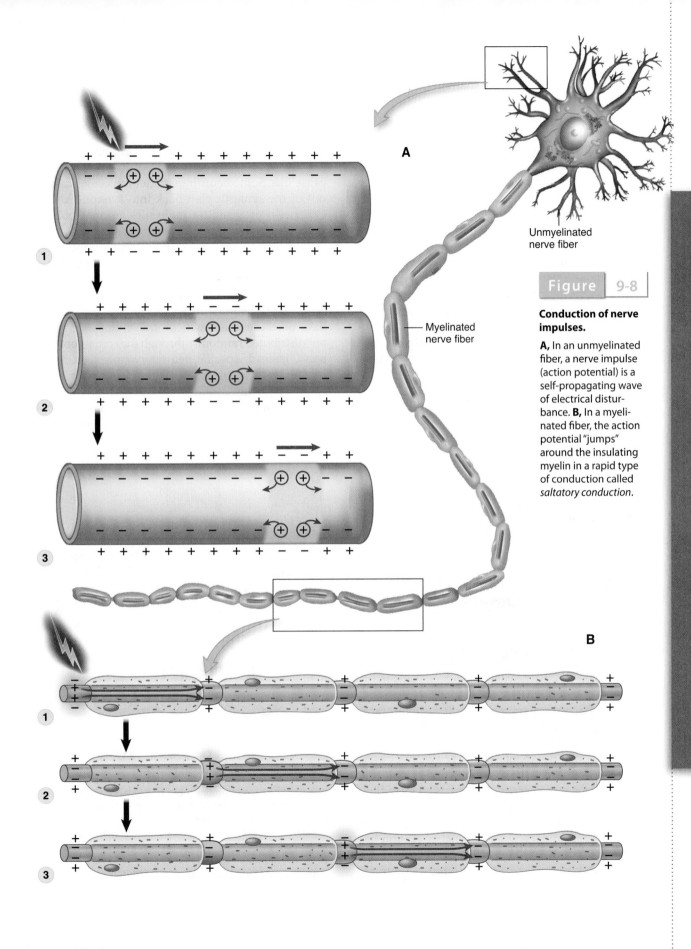

A

Unmyelinated
nerve fiber

Myelinated
nerve fiber

Figure 9-8

Conduction of nerve impulses.

A, In an unmyelinated fiber, a nerve impulse (action potential) is a self-propagating wave of electrical disturbance. **B,** In a myelinated fiber, the action potential "jumps" around the insulating myelin in a rapid type of conduction called *saltatory conduction.*

B

membrane. When a section of the membrane is stimulated, its Na⁺ channels suddenly open, and Na⁺ rushes inward. The inside of the membrane temporarily becomes positive, and the outside becomes negative—a process called *depolarization*. This section of the membrane then immediately recovers—a process called *repolarization*. However, the depolarization has already stimulated Na⁺ channels in the next section of the membrane to open. The impulse—or *action potential*—cannot go backward during the brief moment of repolarization and recovery of the previous section of membrane. Thus a self-propagating wave of electrical disturbance—a nerve impulse—travels in one direction across the neuron's surface (Figure 9-8, *A*).

If the traveling impulse encounters a section of membrane covered with insulating myelin, it simply "jumps" around the myelin. Called **saltatory conduction,** this type of impulse travel is much faster than is possible in nonmyelinated sections. Saltatory conduction is illustrated in Figure 9-8, *B*.

 To learn more about nerve impulses, go to **AnimationDirect** on your CD.

The Synapse

Transmission of signals from one neuron to the next—across the synapse—is an important part of the nerve conduction process. By definition, a synapse is the place where impulses are transmitted from one neuron, called the **presynaptic neuron,** to another neuron, called the **postsynaptic neuron.**

Three structures make up a synapse: a synaptic knob, a synaptic cleft, and the plasma membrane of a postsynaptic neuron. A **synaptic knob** is a tiny bulge at the end of a terminal branch of a presynaptic neuron's axon (Figure 9-9). Each synaptic knob contains many small sacs or vesicles. Each vesicle contains a very small quantity of a chemical compound called a **neurotransmitter.** When a nerve impulse arrives at the synaptic knob, neurotransmitter molecules are released from the vesicles into the **synaptic cleft.** The synaptic cleft is the space between a synaptic knob and the plasma membrane of a *postsynaptic neuron*. It is an incredibly narrow space—only about two millionths of a centimeter in width. Identify the synaptic cleft in Figure 9-9. The plasma membrane of a postsynaptic neuron has protein molecules embedded in it opposite each synaptic knob. These serve as receptors to which neurotrans-

mitter molecules bind. This binding can initiate an impulse in the postsynaptic neuron by opening ion channels in the postsynaptic membrane.

After impulse conduction by postsynaptic neurons is initiated, neurotransmitter activity is rapidly terminated. Either one or both of two mechanisms cause this. Some neurotransmitter molecules diffuse out of the synaptic cleft back into synaptic knobs. Other neurotransmitter molecules are metabolized into inactive compounds by specific enzymes.

Neurotransmitters are chemicals by which neurons communicate. As previously noted, at trillions of synapses in the CNS, presynaptic neurons release neurotransmitters that assist, stimulate, or inhibit postsynaptic neurons. At least 30 different compounds have been identified as neurotransmitters. They are not distributed randomly through the spinal cord and brain. Instead, specific neurotransmitters are localized in discrete groups of neurons and released in specific pathways.

For example, the substance named **acetylcholine** (ass-ee-til-KOH-leen) is released at some of the

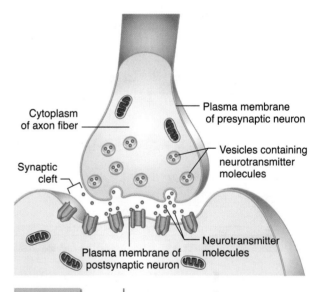

Cytoplasm of axon fiber

Synaptic cleft

Plasma membrane of presynaptic neuron

Vesicles containing neurotransmitter molecules

Plasma membrane of postsynaptic neuron

Neurotransmitter molecules

Figure 9-9 | **Components of a synapse.**

Diagram shows synaptic knob or axon terminal of presynaptic neuron, the plasma membrane of a postsynaptic neuron, and a synaptic cleft. On the arrival of an action potential at a synaptic knob, neurotransmitter molecules are released from vesicles in the knob into the synaptic cleft. The combining of neurotransmitter and receptor molecules in the plasma membrane of the postsynaptic neuron opens ion channels and thereby initiates impulse conduction in the postsynaptic neuron.

synapses in the spinal cord and at neuromuscular (nerve-muscle) junctions. Other well-known neurotransmitters include **norepinephrine** (nor-ep-i-NEF-rin), **dopamine** (DOH-pah-meen), and **serotonin** (sair-oh-TOH-nin). They belong to a group of compounds called **catecholamines** (kat-eh-KOL-ah-meens), which may play a role in sleep, motor function, mood, and pleasure recognition.

Two morphine-like neurotransmitters called **endorphins** (en-DOR-fins) and **enkephalins** (en-KEF-ah-lins) are released at various spinal cord and brain synapses in the pain conduction pathway. These neurotransmitters inhibit conduction of pain impulses. They are natural pain killers. Research shows that the release of endorphins increases during heavy exercise. Normally, pain is a warning signal that calls attention to injuries or dangerous circumstances. However, it is better to inhibit severe pain if it would stop us from continuing an activity that may be necessary for survival.

Very small molecules such as **nitric oxide (NO)** also have an important role as neurotransmitters. Unlike most other neurotransmitters, NO diffuses directly across the plasma membrane of neurons rather than being released from vesicles. NO is important during the male sexual response in regulating smooth muscles in the blood vessels of the penis to allow for penile erection. The drug sildenafil (Viagra) treats *male erectile dysfunction (MED)* by promoting the same response in the penis as NO.

Parkinson disease (PD) is a chronic nervous disorder resulting from a deficiency of the neurotransmitter *dopamine* in certain parts of the brain. The group of signs associated with this disorder, a syndrome called *parkinsonism,* includes rigidity and trembling of the head and extremities, a forward tilt of the trunk, and a shuffling manner of walking (Figure 9-10). You may have noticed these signs in former boxing champion Muhammad Ali, the actor Michael J. Fox, or in others you may know with PD. All of these characteristics result from lack of dopamine, leading to misinformation in the parts of the brain that normally prevents the skeletal muscles from being overstimulated. Dopamine injections and dopamine pills are not effective treatments because dopamine cannot cross the blood-brain barrier (see box on p. 246).

A breakthrough in the treatment of Parkinson disease came when the drug *levodopa* or L-dopa (Sinemet) was found to increase the dopamine levels in afflicted patients. Neurons use L-dopa, which can cross the blood-brain barrier, to make dopamine. For some reason, L-dopa does not always have the desired effects in individual patients or its effect may wear off over time, so a number of alternative treatments have been developed. For example, the drug apomorphine (Apokyn) has proved useful in treating individuals who no longer respond to L-dopa. One option that has shown some success is surgical grafting of normal dopamine-secreting neurons into the brains of individuals with PD. Another experimental option is an artificial implant that gives electrical stimulation to the brain, causing it to produce more dopamine.

 To learn more about Parkinson disease, go to **AnimationDirect** on your CD.

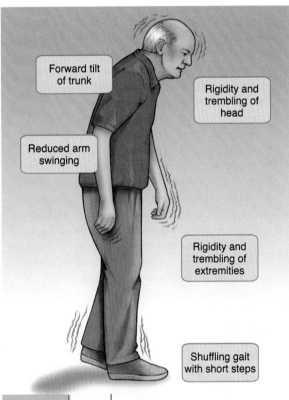

Figure 9-10 | **Parkinsonism.**

Parkinsonism is a syndrome typically found in individuals with Parkinson disease (PD). The signs include (but are not limited to) rigidity and trembling of the head and extremities, a forward tilt of the trunk, and a shuffling gait with short steps and reduced arm swinging.

1. How does *myelin* increase the speed of nerve impulse conduction?
2. What is a *synapse*?
3. How do *neurotransmitters* transmit signals across the synapse?
4. What are the characteristics of *parkinsonism*?

CLINICAL APPLICATION

THE BLOOD-BRAIN BARRIER

Astrocytes have an important function other than supporting neurons and blood vessels. Notice in the figure that the "feet" of the astrocytes form a wall around the outside of blood vessels in the nervous system. This astrocyte wall, along with the vessel wall, forms a structure known as the **blood-brain barrier (BBB).** The BBB allows water, oxygen, carbon dioxide, and a few other substances—such as alcohol—to move between the blood and the tissue of the brain. However, many toxins and pathogens that can enter other tissues through blood vessel walls cannot enter nervous tissue because of this barrier. This adaptation enhances survival because it protects vital brain and nerve tissues from damage. This protective function of the BBB has great clinical significance. Drugs used in other parts of the body to treat infections, cancer, and other disorders often cannot pass through the BBB. For example, penicillin and other antibiotics cannot enter the interstitial fluid of brain tissue from the blood. Obviously, this makes development of treatments for brain disorders sometimes very difficult. As discussed in the text (p. 245), parkinsonism resulting from a lack of dopamine in the brain cannot be treated with dopamine because it cannot cross the BBB. However, the dopamine precursor L-dopa *can* cross the BBB and be converted to dopamine in the brain in some patients.

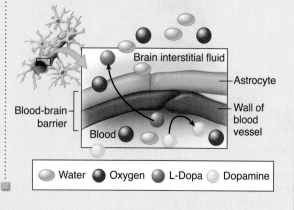

Central Nervous System

The CNS, as its name implies, is centrally located. Its two major structures, the brain and spinal cord, are found along the midsagittal plane of the body (Figure 9-11). The brain is protected in the cranial cavity of the skull, and the spinal cord is surrounded in the

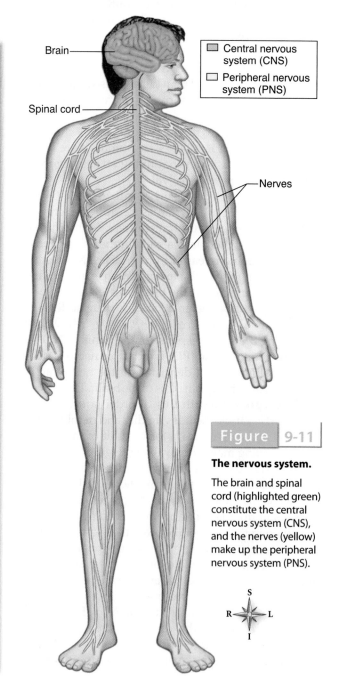

Brain

□ Central nervous system (CNS)
□ Peripheral nervous system (PNS)

Spinal cord

Nerves

Figure 9-11

The nervous system.

The brain and spinal cord (highlighted green) constitute the central nervous system (CNS), and the nerves (yellow) make up the peripheral nervous system (PNS).

spinal cavity by the vertebral column. In addition, the brain and spinal cord are covered by protective membranes called **meninges** (meh-NIN-jeez), which are discussed in a later section of the chapter.

Divisions of the Brain

The brain, one of our largest organs, consists of the following major divisions, named in ascending order beginning with the most inferior part:

I. Brainstem
   A. Medulla oblongata
   B. Pons
   C. Midbrain
II. Cerebellum
III. Diencephalon
   A. Hypothalamus
   B. Thalamus
IV. Cerebrum

Observe in Figure 9-12 the location and relative sizes of the medulla, pons, cerebellum, and cerebrum. Also identify the midbrain.

BRAINSTEM

The lowest part of the brainstem is the medulla oblongata. Immediately above the medulla lies the pons and above that the midbrain. Together these three structures are called the *brainstem* (Figure 9-12).

   The **medulla oblongata** (meh-DUL-ah ob-long-GAH-tah) is an enlarged, upward extension of the spinal cord. It lies just inside the cranial cavity above the large hole in the occipital bone called the *foramen magnum.* As with the spinal cord, the medulla consists of gray and white matter, but the arrangement differs in the two organs. In the medulla, bits of gray matter mix closely and intricately with white matter to form the *reticular formation* (*reticular* means "net-like"). In the spinal cord, gray and white matter do not intermingle; gray matter forms the interior core of the cord, and white matter surrounds it. The **pons** and **midbrain,** like the medulla, consist of white matter and scattered bits of gray matter.

   All three parts of the brainstem function as two-way conduction paths. Sensory fibers conduct impulses up from the cord to other parts of the brain, and motor fibers conduct impulses down from the brain to the cord. In addition, many important reflex centers lie in the brainstem. The cardiac, respiratory, and vasomotor centers (collectively called the *vital centers*), for example, are located in the me-

dulla. Impulses from these centers control heartbeat, respirations, and blood vessel diameter (which is important in regulating blood pressure).

CEREBELLUM

Structure

Look at Figure 9-12 to find the location, appearance, and size of the cerebellum. The cerebellum is the second largest part of the human brain. It lies under the occipital lobe of the cerebrum. In the cerebellum, gray matter composes the outer layer, and white matter composes the bulk of the interior.

Function

Most of our previous knowledge about cerebellar functions has come from observing patients who have some sort of disease of the cerebellum and from animals who have had the cerebellum removed. From such observations, we know that the cerebellum plays an essential part in the production of normal movements. Perhaps a few examples will make this clear. A patient who has a tumor of the cerebellum frequently loses his balance and topples over; he may reel like a drunken man when he walks. He cannot coordinate his muscles normally. He may complain, for instance, that he is clumsy in everything he does—that he cannot even drive a nail or draw a straight line. With the loss of normal cerebellar functioning, he has lost the ability to make precise movements. The most obvious functions of the cerebellum, then, are to produce smooth coordinated movements, maintain equilibrium, and sustain normal postures.

   Recent studies using new brain imaging methods show that the cerebellum may have far more functions than earlier observed. The cerebellum may assist the cerebrum and other parts of the brain, perhaps having an overall coordinating function for the whole brain.

DIENCEPHALON

The **diencephalon** (dye-en-SEF-ah-lon) is a small but important part of the brain located between the midbrain below and the cerebrum above. It consists of two major structures: the hypothalamus and the thalamus.

Hypothalamus

The **hypothalamus** (hye-poh-THAL-ah-muss), as its name suggests, is located below the thalamus. The posterior pituitary gland, the stalk that attaches it to the undersurface of the brain, and areas of gray matter located in the side walls of a fluid-filled space called the *third ventricle* are extensions of the hypothalamus.

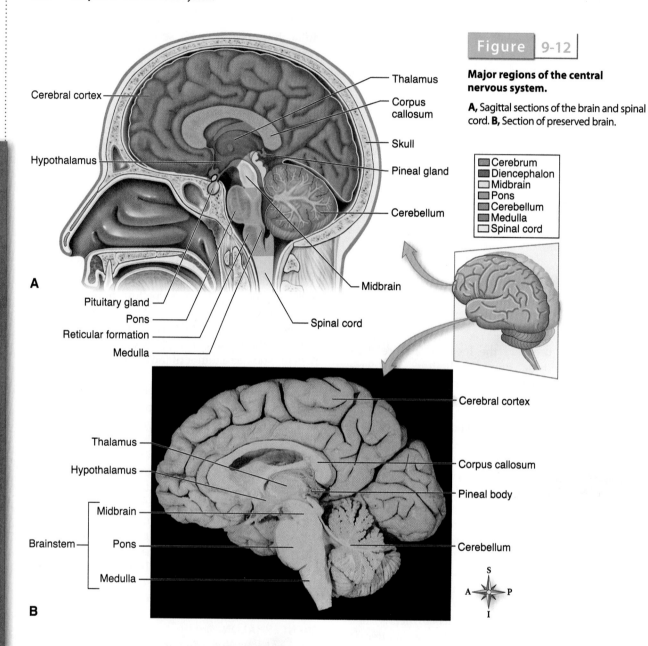

Figure   9-12

Major regions of the central nervous system.

A, Sagittal sections of the brain and spinal cord. **B,** Section of preserved brain.

- Cerebrum
- Diencephalon
- Midbrain
- Pons
- Cerebellum
- Medulla
- Spinal cord

A

B

Identify the pituitary gland and the hypothalamus in Figure 9-12.

The old adage, "Don't judge by appearances," applies well to appraising the importance of the hypothalamus. Measured by size, it is one of the least significant parts of the brain, but measured by its contribution to healthy survival, it is one of the most important brain structures. Impulses from neurons whose dendrites and cell bodies lie in the hypothalamus are conducted by their axons to neurons located in the spinal cord, and many of these impulses are then re-

layed to muscles and glands all over the body. Thus the hypothalamus exerts major control over virtually all internal organs. Among the vital functions that it helps control are the heartbeat, constriction and dilation of blood vessels, and contractions of the stomach and intestines.

Some neurons in the hypothalamus function in a surprising way; they make the hormones that the posterior pituitary gland secretes into the blood. Because one of these hormones (called *antidiuretic hormone,* or *ADH*) affects the volume of urine excreted, the hypothalamus plays an essential role in maintaining the body's water balance.

Some of the neurons in the hypothalamus function as endocrine (ductless) glands. Their axons secrete chemicals called *releasing hormones* into the blood, which then carries them to the anterior pituitary gland. Releasing hormones, as their name suggests, control the release of certain anterior pituitary hormones. These in turn influence the hormone secretion of other endocrine glands. Thus the hypothalamus indirectly helps control the functioning of every cell in the body.

The hypothalamus is a crucial part of the mechanism for maintaining body temperature. Therefore marked elevation in body temperature in the absence of disease often characterizes injuries or other abnormalities of the hypothalamus. In addition, this important center is involved in functions such as the regulation of water balance, sleep cycles, and the control of appetite and many emotions involved in pleasure, fear, anger, sexual arousal, and pain.

Thalamus

Just above the hypothalamus is a dumbbell-shaped section of gray matter called the **thalamus** (THAL-ah-muss). Each enlarged end of the dumbbell lies in a lateral wall of the third ventricle. The thin center section of the thalamus passes from left to right through the third ventricle. The thalamus is composed chiefly of dendrites and cell bodies of neurons that have axons extending up toward the sensory areas of the cerebrum. The thalamus performs the following functions:

1. It helps produce sensations. Its neurons relay impulses to the cerebral cortex from the sense organs of the body.

2. It associates sensations with emotions. Almost all sensations are accompanied by a feeling of some degree of pleasantness or unpleasantness. The way that these pleasant and unpleasant feelings are produced is unknown except that they seem to be associated with the arrival of sensory impulses in the thalamus.

3. It plays a part in the so-called *arousal*, or alerting mechanism.

CEREBRUM

The **cerebrum** (SAIR-eh-brum) is the largest and uppermost part of the brain. If you were to look at the outer surface of the cerebrum, the first features you would notice might be its many ridges and grooves. The ridges are called *convolutions*, or **gyri** (JYE-rye), and the grooves are called **sulci** (SUL-kye). The deepest sulci are called *fissures;* the longitudinal fissure divides the cerebrum into right and left halves or hemispheres. These halves are almost separate structures except for their lower midportions, which are connected by a structure called the **corpus callosum** (KOR-pus kah-LOH-sum) (see Figure 9-12). Two deep sulci subdivide each cerebral hemisphere into four major lobes and each lobe into numerous convolutions. The lobes are named for the bones that lie over them: the frontal lobe, the parietal lobe, the temporal lobe, and the occipital lobe. Identify these in Figure 9-13, *A.*

A thin layer of gray matter called the **cerebral cortex** is made up of neuron dendrites and cell bodies; this makes up the surface of the cerebrum. White matter, made up of bundles of nerve fibers (tracts), composes most of the interior of the cerebrum. Within this white matter, however, are a few islands of gray matter known as the **cerebral nuclei,** or **basal ganglia**, whose functioning is essential for producing automatic movements and postures. Parkinson disease (PD) is a disease of the cerebral nuclei. Because shaking or tremors are common symptoms of PD, it is also called "shaking palsy" (see discussion on p. 245).

What functions does the cerebrum perform? This is a hard question to answer briefly because the neurons of the cerebrum do not function alone. They function with many other neurons in many other parts of the brain and in the spinal cord. Neurons of these various structures continually bring impulses to cerebral neurons and also continually transmit impulses away from them. If all other neurons were functioning normally and only cerebral neurons were not functioning, here are some of the things that you could not do: You could not think or use your will. You could not remember anything that has ever happened to you. You could not decide to make the smallest movement, nor could you make it. You would not see or hear. You could not experience any of the sensations that make life so rich and varied. Nothing would anger or frighten you, and nothing would bring you joy or sorrow. You would, in short, be unconscious. These terms sum up cerebral functions: consciousness, thinking, memory, sensations, emotions, and willed movements. Figure 9-13, *B,* shows the areas of the cerebral cortex essential for willed movements, general sensations, vision, hearing, and normal speech.

It is important to understand that very specific areas of the cortex have very specific functions. For example, the temporal lobe's auditory areas interpret

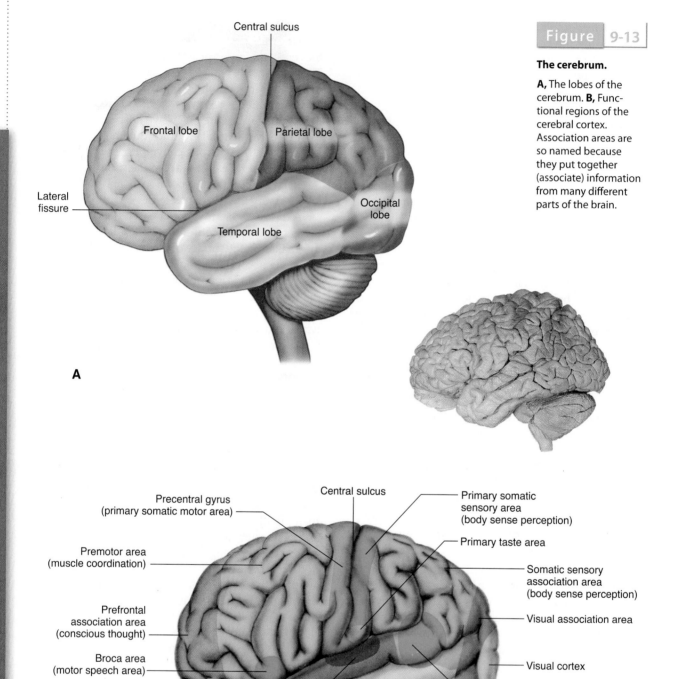

Central sulcus

Frontal lobe

Parietal lobe

Lateral fissure

Occipital lobe

Temporal lobe

A

Figure 9-13

The cerebrum.

A, The lobes of the cerebrum. **B,** Functional regions of the cerebral cortex. Association areas are so named because they put together (associate) information from many different parts of the brain.

Precentral gyrus
(primary somatic motor area)

Central sulcus

Primary somatic sensory area
(body sense perception)

Premotor area
(muscle coordination)

Primary taste area

Somatic sensory association area
(body sense perception)

Prefrontal association area
(conscious thought)

Visual association area

Broca area
(motor speech area)

Visual cortex

Auditory association area

Wernicke area
(sensory speech area)

Primary auditory area

B

S
A   P
I

Table 9-1	Functions of Major Divisions of the Brain		

BRAIN AREA	FUNCTION
Brainstem	
Medulla oblongata	Two-way conduction pathway between the spinal cord and higher brain centers; cardiac, respiratory, and vasomotor control center
Pons	Two-way conduction pathway between areas of the brain and other regions of the body; influences respiration
Midbrain	Two-way conduction pathway; relay for visual and auditory impulses
Cerebellum	Muscle coordination; maintenance of equilibrium and posture; assists cerebrum
Diencephalon	
Hypothalamus	Regulation of body temperature, water balance, sleep-cycle control, appetite, and sexual arousal
Thalamus	Sensory relay station from various body areas to cerebral cortex; emotions and alerting or arousal mechanisms
Cerebrum	Sensory perception, emotions, willed movements, consciousness, and memory

incoming nervous signals from the ear as very specific sounds. The visual area of the cortex in the occipital lobe helps you identify and understand specific images. Localized areas of the cortex are directly related to specific functions, as shown in Figure 9-13, *B*. This explains the very specific symptoms associated with an injury to localized areas of the cerebral cortex after a stroke or traumatic injury to the head. Table 9-1 summarizes the major components of the brain and their main functions.

 To learn more about areas of the brain that control body functions, go to **AnimationDirect** on your CD.

QUICK CHECK

1. What are the four main divisions of the brain?
2. What regions make up the *brainstem*?
3. Why is the *hypothalamus* said to be a link between the nervous system and the endocrine system?

Brain Disorders

DESTRUCTION OF BRAIN TISSUE

Injury or disease can destroy neurons. A common example is the destruction of neurons of the motor area of the cerebrum that results from a **cerebrovascular accident (CVA).** A CVA, or *stroke*, is a hemorrhage from or cessation of blood flow through cerebral blood vessels. When this happens, the oxygen supply to portions of the brain is disrupted, and neurons cease functioning. If the lack of oxygen is prolonged, the neurons die. If

the damage occurs in a motor control area of the brain (Figure 9-13, *B*), the victim can no longer voluntarily move the parts of the body controlled by the affected areas. Because the paths of motor neurons in the cerebrum cross over in the brainstem, paralysis appears on the side of the body opposite to the side of the brain on which the CVA occurred. The term **hemiplegia** (hem-ee-PLEE-jee-ah) refers to paralysis (loss of voluntary muscle control) of one whole side of the body.

One of the most common crippling diseases that can appear during childhood, **cerebral palsy (CP),** also results from damage to brain tissue. Cerebral palsy involves permanent, nonprogressive damage to motor control areas of the brain, which in turn causes abnormal muscle tension (spasticity) that hinders movement (Figure 9-14). Such damage is present at birth or occurs shortly after birth and remains throughout life.

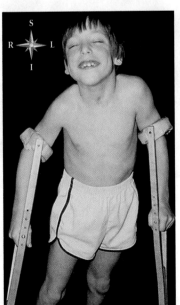

Figure 9-14

Cerebral palsy (CP).

This patient requires crutches to walk because abnormal tension (spasticity) in muscles prevents normal walking movements.

Possible causes of brain damage include prenatal infections or diseases of the mother; mechanical trauma to the head before, during, or after birth; nerve-damaging poisons; and reduced oxygen supply to the brain. The resulting impairment to voluntary muscle control can manifest itself in a variety of ways. Many people with cerebral palsy exhibit **spastic paralysis,** a type of paralysis characterized by involuntary contractions of affected muscles. In cerebral palsy, spastic paralysis may affect one entire side of the body **(hemiplegia),** both legs **(paraplegia),** both legs and one arm **(triplegia),** or all four extremities **(quadriplegia).**

A variety of degenerative diseases can result in destruction of neurons in the brain. This degeneration can progress to adversely affect memory, attention span, intellectual capacity, personality, and motor control. The general term for this syndrome is **dementia** (deh-MEN-shee-ah).

Dementia is characteristic of **Alzheimer** (ALZ-hye-mer) **disease (AD).** Its characteristic lesions develop in the cortex during the middle to late adult years (Figure 9-15). Exactly what makes dementia-causing lesions develop in the brains of individuals with Alzheimer disease is not known. There is some evidence that this disease has a genetic basis—at least in some families. Other evidence indicates that environmental factors may play a role. Because the exact cause of Alzheimer disease is still not known, development of an effective treatment has proved difficult. Currently, people diagnosed with AD are often treated with drugs such as donepezil (Aricept) for mild to moderate AD or with the drug memantine (Namenda) for moderate to advanced AD. In addition, treatment includes helping patients maintain their remaining mental abilities and looking after their hygiene, nutrition, and other aspects of personal health management.

Huntington disease (HD) is an inherited disease characterized by *chorea* (involuntary, purposeless movements) that progresses to severe dementia and death. The initial symptoms of this disease first appear between ages 30 and 40, with death occurring by age 55. Now that the gene responsible for Huntington disease has been located, researchers hope that an effective treatment will be found (see Chapter 24). The discovery of the HD gene poses an interesting question: if you could learn early in life that you will get HD, would you want to know?

The human immunodeficiency virus (HIV) that causes *acquired immunodeficiency syndrome (AIDS)* also can cause dementia. The immune deficiency char-

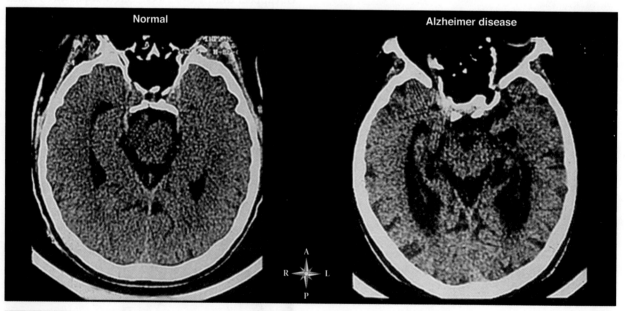

Figure 9-15 **Alzheimer disease (AD).**

The CT scan on the left shows a horizontal section of a normal brain. In the CT scan on the right, however, you can see the dark patches in the cerebral cortex that show damage to brain tissue typical of AD.

acteristic of AIDS results from HIV infection of white blood cells critical to the proper function of the immune system (see Chapter 15). However, HIV also infects neurons and can cause progressive degeneration of the brain, resulting in dementia.

SEIZURE DISORDERS

Some of the most common nervous system abnormalities belong to the group of conditions called *seizure disorders*. These disorders are characterized by **seizures**—sudden bursts of abnormal neuron activity that result in temporary changes in brain function. Seizures may be very mild, causing subtle changes in the level of consciousness, motor control, or sensory perception. On the other hand, seizures may be quite severe, resulting in jerky, involuntary muscle contractions called *convulsions* or even unconsciousness.

Recurring or chronic seizure episodes constitute a condition called **epilepsy.** Although some cases of epilepsy can be traced to specific causes such as tumors, trauma, or chemical imbalances, most epilepsy is idiopathic (of unknown cause). Those with epilepsy are often treated with well-known anticonvulsive drugs such as *phenobarbital, phenytoin (Dilantin),* or *valproic acid (Depakene)* that block neurotransmitters in affected areas of the brain. By thus blocking synaptic transmission, such drugs inhibit the explosive bursts of neuron activity associated with seizures. Continuing research has resulted in the release of several new epilepsy drugs that have provided improved treatment options for many patients. Newer drugs include gabapentin (Neurontin) and lamotrigine (Lamictal). With proper medication, many people with epilepsy lead normal lives without the fear of experiencing uncontrollable seizures.

Diagnosis and evaluation of epilepsy or any seizure disorder often rely on a graphic representation of brain activity called an **electroencephalogram** (eh-lek-troh-en-SEF-ah-loh-gram) **(EEG)** (Figure 9-16). In Figure 9-16, *B*, a normal EEG shows the chaotic rise and fall of the electrical activity in different parts of the brain as a series of wavy lines (the so-called *brain waves*). A seizure manifests itself as an explosive increase in the size and frequency of waves—as seen on the right side of Figure 9-16, *B*. Classifications of epilepsy are based on the locations in the brain and the duration of these changes in brain activity.

QUICK CHECK

1. What is a *CVA?* How does it affect the brain?
2. What disorders are characterized by *dementia?*
3. What is *epilepsy?*

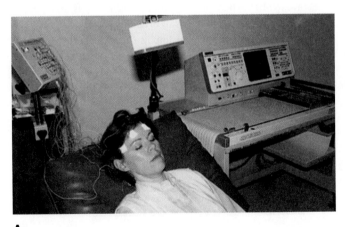

A

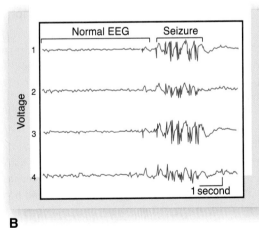

B

Figure 9-16 | **Electroencephalography.**

A, Photograph of a person with voltage-sensitive electrodes attached to her skull. Information from these electrodes is used to produce a graphic recording of brain activity—an electroencephalogram (EEG). **B,** An EEG tracing showing activity in four different places in the brain (obtained from four sets of electrodes). Compare the moderate chaotic activity identified as normal with the explosive activity that occurs during a seizure.

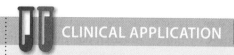

BRAIN STUDIES

Biotechnology has produced many methods for studying the brain without resorting to the trauma of exploratory surgery. Some of those methods are listed here.

X-Ray Photography

Traditional radiography (x-ray photography) of the head sometimes reveals tumors or injuries but does not show the detail of soft tissue necessary to diagnose many brain problems.

Computed Tomography (CT)

The CT imaging technique involves scanning the head with a revolving x-ray generator. X-rays that pass through tissue hit sensors, which send the information to a computer that constructs an image that appears as a "slice of brain" on a video screen (see Figure 5-12, *B*). Hemorrhages, tumors, and other lesions often can be detected with CT scanning.

Positron-Emission Tomography (PET)

PET scanning is a variation of CT scanning in which a radioactive substance is introduced into the blood supply of the brain. The radioactive material shows up as a bright spot on the image. Different substances are taken up by brain cells in different amounts, depending on the level of tissue activity, thereby enabling radiologists to determine the functional characteristics of specific parts of the brain (see figure).

Single-Photon Emission Computed Tomography (SPECT)

SPECT is similar to PET but uses more stable substances and different detectors. SPECT is used to visualize blood flow patterns in the brain, making it useful in diagnosing cerebrovascular accidents (CVAs) and brain tumors.

Ultrasonography

In ultrasonography, high-frequency sound (ultrasound) waves are reflected off anatomical structures to form images—similar to radar. Because it does not use harmful radiation, ultrasonography is often used in diagnosing hydrocephalus or brain tumors in infants.

Magnetic Resonance Imaging (MRI)

MRI, also called *nuclear magnetic resonance (NMR)* imaging, is a scanning method that also has the advantage of avoiding the use of harmful radiation. In MRI, a magnetic field surrounding the head induces brain tissues to emit radio waves that can be used by a computer to construct a sectional image. MRI has the added advantage of producing sharper images than CT scanning and ultrasound. This makes it very useful in detecting small brain lesions (see Figure 5–12, *C*).

Electroencephalography (EEG)

As discussed in this chapter, electroencephalography is the measurement of the electrical activity in the brain. Typically, changes in voltage are recorded as deflections of a continuous line drawn on graph paper (see Figure 9-16). EEGs are used to detect seizure disorders, sleeping disorders, and other brain abnormalities.

Evoked Potential (EP) Test

The EP test is similar to EEG, but the brain waves observed are caused (evoked) by specific stimuli, such as a flash of light or a sudden sound. This information is analyzed by a computer that generates a graphic image of the brain and displays it on a video screen—a *brain electric activity map (BEAM)*. Changes in color represent changes in brain activity evoked by each stimulus given. This technique is useful in diagnosing lesions of the visual or auditory systems because it reveals whether a sensory impulse is reaching the appropriate part of the brain.

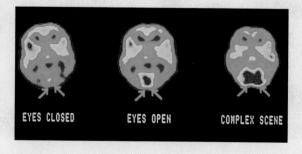

EYES CLOSED   EYES OPEN   COMPLEX SCENE

Spinal Cord

STRUCTURE

If you are of average height, your spinal cord is about 42 cm to 45 cm (17 or 18 inches) long (Figure 9-17). It lies inside the spinal column in the spinal cavity and extends from the occipital bone down to the bottom of the first lumbar vertebra. Place your hands on your hips, and they will line up with your fourth lumbar vertebra. Your spinal cord ends just above this level.

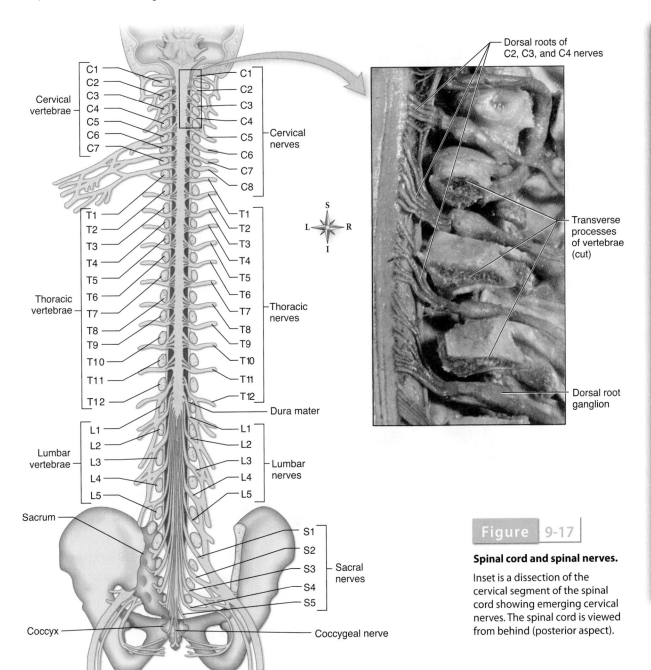

Figure 9-17

Spinal cord and spinal nerves.

Inset is a dissection of the cervical segment of the spinal cord showing emerging cervical nerves. The spinal cord is viewed from behind (posterior aspect).

Look now at Figure 9-18. Notice the H-shaped core of the spinal cord. It consists of gray matter and so is composed mainly of dendrites and cell bodies of neurons. Columns of white matter form the outer portion of the spinal cord, and bundles of myelinated nerve fibers—the **spinal tracts**—make up the white columns.

Spinal cord tracts provide two-way conduction paths to and from the brain. *Ascending tracts* conduct impulses up the cord to the brain. *Descending tracts* conduct impulses down the cord from the brain. Tracts are functional organizations in that all axons composing one tract serve one general function. For instance, fibers of the spinothalamic tracts serve a sensory function. They transmit impulses that produce sensations of crude touch, pain, and temperature. Other ascending tracts shown in Figure 9-18 include the gracilis and cuneatus tracts, which transmit sensations of touch and pressure up to the brain, and the anterior and posterior spino-cerebellar tracts, which transmit information about muscle length to the cerebellum. Descending tracts include the lateral and ventral corticospinal tracts, which transmit impulses controlling many voluntary movements.

FUNCTIONS

To try to understand spinal cord functions, think about a hotel telephone switching system. Suppose a guest in Room 108 calls the switching system and keys in the extension number for Room 520, and in a second or so, someone in that room answers. Very briefly, three events took place: a message traveled into the switching system, the system routed the message along the proper path, and the message traveled out from the switching system toward Room 520. The telephone switching system provided the network of connections that made possible the completion of the call. We might say that the switching system transferred the incoming call to an outgoing line. The spinal cord functions similarly. It contains the centers for thousands and thousands of reflex arcs. Look back at Figure 9-7. The interneuron shown there is an example of a spinal cord reflex center. It switches or transfers incoming sensory impulses to outgoing motor impulses, thereby making it possible for a reflex to occur. Reflexes that result from conduction over arcs whose centers lie in the spinal cord are called *spinal cord reflexes.*

Two common kinds of spinal cord reflexes are *withdrawal*

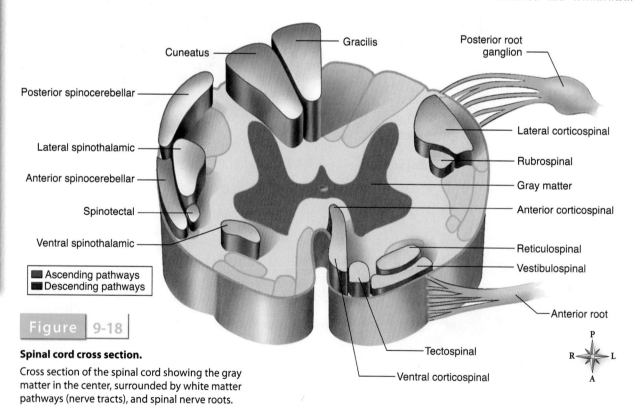

Cuneatus

Gracilis

Posterior root ganglion

Posterior spinocerebellar

Lateral spinothalamic

Anterior spinocerebellar

Spinotectal

Ventral spinothalamic

Lateral corticospinal

Rubrospinal

Gray matter

Anterior corticospinal

Reticulospinal

Vestibulospinal

Anterior root

Tectospinal

Ventral corticospinal

■ Ascending pathways
■ Descending pathways

Figure 9-18

Spinal cord cross section.

Cross section of the spinal cord showing the gray matter in the center, surrounded by white matter pathways (nerve tracts), and spinal nerve roots.

and *jerk reflexes*. An example of a withdrawal reflex is pulling one's hand away from a hot surface. The familiar knee jerk is an example of a jerk reflex.

In addition to functioning as the primary reflex center of the body, the spinal cord tracts, as previously noted, carry impulses to and from the brain. Sensory impulses travel up to the brain in ascending tracts, and motor impulses travel down from the brain in descending tracts. Therefore if an injury cuts the cord all the way across, impulses can no longer travel to the brain from any part of the body located below the injury, nor can they travel from the brain down to these parts. In short, this kind of spinal cord injury produces a loss of sensation, which is called **anesthesia** (an-es-THEE-zee-ah), and a loss of the ability to make voluntary movements, which is called **paralysis** (pah-RAL-i-sis).

Coverings and Fluid Spaces of the Brain and Spinal Cord

Nervous tissue is not a sturdy tissue. Even moderate pressure can kill nerve cells, so nature safeguards the chief organs made of this tissue—the spinal cord and the brain—by surrounding them with a tough, fluid-containing membrane called the **meninges** (meh-NIN-jeez). The meninges are then surrounded by bone. The spinal meninges form a tubelike covering around the spinal cord and line the bony vertebral foramen of the vertebrae that surround the cord. Look at Figure 9-19, and you can identify the three layers of the spinal meninges. They are the **dura mater** (DOO-rah MAH-ter), which is the tough outer layer that lines the vertebral canal, the **pia** (PEE-ah) **mater,** which is the innermost membrane covering the spinal cord itself, and the **arachnoid** (ah-RAK-noyd) **mater,** which is the membrane between the dura and the pia mater. The arachnoid mater resembles a cobweb with fluid in its spaces. The word *arachnoid* means "cobweb-like." It comes from *arachne,* the Greek word for spider.

The meninges that form the protective covering around the spinal cord also extend up and around the brain to enclose it completely (Figure 9-19).

Infection or inflammation of the meninges is termed **meningitis** (men-in-JYE-tis). This condition is most commonly caused by bacteria such as *Neisseria meningitidis* (meningococcus), *Strep-*

tococcus pneumoniae, or *Haemophilus influenzae* (see Appendix A on page A-1 of your book). However, viral infections, mycoses (fungal infections), and tumors also may cause inflammation of the meninges. Patients with meningitis usually complain of severe headaches and neck pain. Those experiencing symptoms should seek immediate attention to get the problem under control. Depending on the primary cause, meningitis may be mild and self-limiting or may progress to a severe, perhaps fatal, condition. If only the spinal meninges are involved, the condition is called *spinal meningitis.*

Fluid fills the subarachnoid spaces between the pia mater and arachnoid in the brain and spinal cord. This fluid is called **cerebrospinal fluid (CSF)** (sair-eh-broh-SPY-nal FLOO-id); it also fills spaces in the brain called cerebral **ventricles.** In Figure

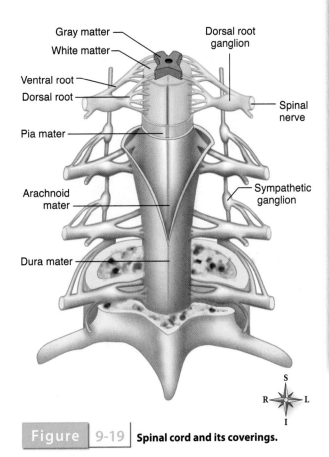

Gray matter
White matter
Ventral root
Dorsal root
Pia mater
Arachnoid mater
Dura mater

Dorsal root ganglion
Spinal nerve
Sympathetic ganglion

S
R — L
I

Figure 9-19 | **Spinal cord and its coverings.**

The meninges, spinal nerves, and sympathetic trunk are all depicted in this drawing.

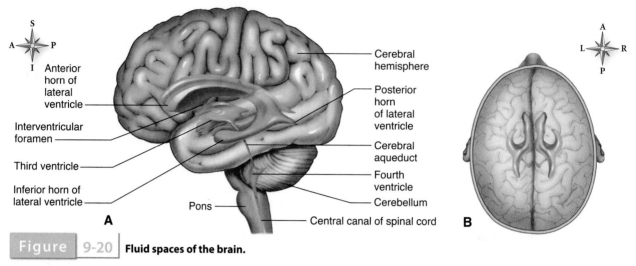

Anterior horn of lateral ventricle

Interventricular foramen

Third ventricle

Inferior horn of lateral ventricle

Pons

Cerebral hemisphere

Posterior horn of lateral ventricle

Cerebral aqueduct

Fourth ventricle

Cerebellum

Central canal of spinal cord

A

B

Figure 9-20 **Fluid spaces of the brain.**

A, The ventricles are highlighted within the brain in a left lateral view. **B,** The ventricles shown from above.

9-20, you can see the irregular shapes of the ventricles of the brain. These illustrations also can help you visualize the location of the ventricles if you remember that these large spaces lie deep inside the brain and that there are two lateral ventricles. One lies inside the right half of the cerebrum (the largest part of the human brain), and the other lies inside the left half.

CSF is one of the body's circulating fluids. It forms continually from fluid filtering out of the blood in a network of brain capillaries known as the **choroid plexus** (KOH-royd PLEK-sus) and into the ventricles.

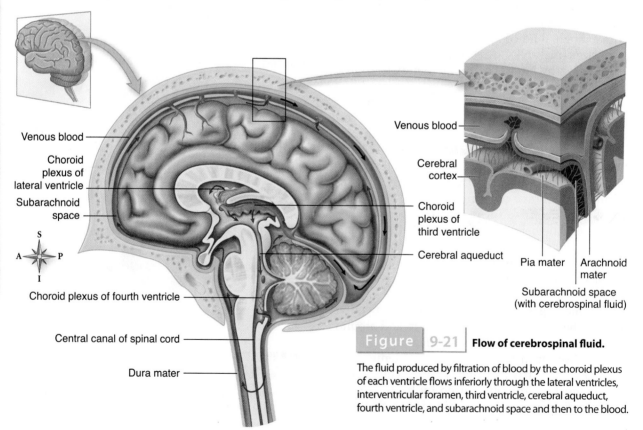

Venous blood

Choroid plexus of lateral ventricle

Subarachnoid space

Choroid plexus of fourth ventricle

Central canal of spinal cord

Dura mater

Venous blood

Cerebral cortex

Choroid plexus of third ventricle

Cerebral aqueduct

Pia mater | Arachnoid mater

Subarachnoid space (with cerebrospinal fluid)

Figure 9-21 **Flow of cerebrospinal fluid.**

The fluid produced by filtration of blood by the choroid plexus of each ventricle flows inferiorly through the lateral ventricles, interventricular foramen, third ventricle, cerebral aqueduct, fourth ventricle, and subarachnoid space and then to the blood.

CSF seeps from the lateral ventricles into the third ventricle and flows down through the cerebral aqueduct (find this in Figures 9-20 and 9-21) into the fourth ventricle. Most of the CSF moves through tiny openings from the fourth ventricle into the subarachnoid space near the cerebellum. Some of it moves into the small, tubelike central canal of the cord and then out into the subarachnoid spaces. Then it moves leisurely down and around the cord and up and around the brain (in the subarachnoid spaces of their meninges) and returns to the blood (in the veins of the brain).

Remembering that this fluid forms continually from blood, circulates, and is resorbed into blood can be useful. It can help you understand certain abnormalities. Suppose a person has a brain tumor that presses on the cerebral aqueduct. This blocks the way for the return of CSF to the blood. Because the fluid continues to form but cannot drain away, it accumulates in the ventricles or in the meninges. Other conditions can cause an accumulation of CSF in the ventricles. An example is **hydrocephalus** (hye-droh-SEF-ah-lus), or "water on the brain." One form of treatment involves surgical placement of a hollow tube or catheter through the blocked channel so that CSF can drain into another location in the body (Figure 9-22).

QUICK CHECK

1. What are the major functions of the spinal cord?
2. Name the three *meninges* that cover the brain and spinal cord.
3. What is *CSF?* What is its function?

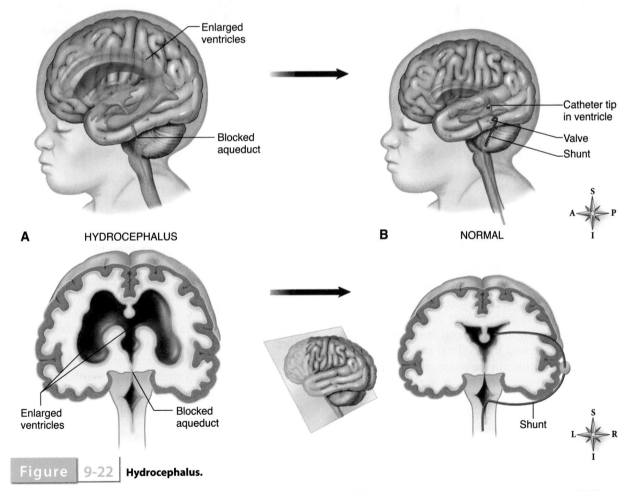

Figure 9-22 | **Hydrocephalus.**

A, Hydrocephalus is caused by narrowing or blockage of the pathways for CSF, causing the retention of CSF in the ventricles. **B,** This condition can be treated by surgical placement of a shunt or tube to drain the excess fluid. Notice in the cross sections of the brain how the ventricles and surrounding tissue return to their normal shapes and size after shunt placement.

LUMBAR PUNCTURE

The meninges, the fluid-containing membranes surrounding the brain and spinal cord, extend beyond the spinal cord, an anatomical fact that is most convenient in regard to being able to perform lumbar punctures without putting the spinal cord at risk of injury. A **lumbar puncture,** or "spinal tap," is the withdrawal of some cerebrospinal fluid (CSF) from the subarachnoid space in the lumbar region of the spinal cord. The physician inserts a needle just above or below the fourth lumbar vertebra, knowing that the spinal cord ends an inch or more above this level. The fourth lum-bar vertebra can be easily located because it lies on a line with the iliac crest. Placing an adult patient on his side and having him arch his back by drawing the knees and chest together separates the vertebrae sufficiently to introduce the needle. Lumbar punctures are often performed when CSF is needed for analysis or when it is necessary to reduce pressure caused by swelling of the brain or spinal cord after injury or disease. The normal sample of CSF from a lumbar puncture shown here is slightly yellowish and clear but the red color in the abnormal sample indicates bleeding (in this case, a hemorrhage in the subarachnoid space).

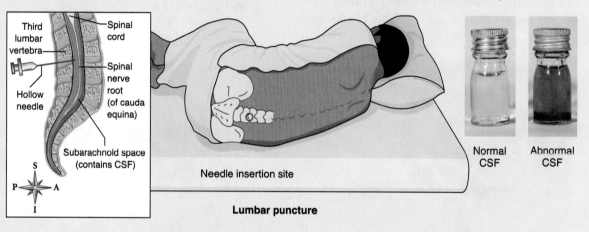

Normal CSF   Abnormal CSF

Needle insertion site

Lumbar puncture

Peripheral Nervous System

The nerves connecting the brain and spinal cord to other parts of the body constitute the peripheral nervous system (PNS). This system includes **cranial** and **spinal nerves** that connect the brain and spinal cord, respectively, to peripheral structures such as the skin surface and the skeletal muscles. In addition, other structures in the autonomic nervous system (ANS) are considered part of the PNS. These connect the brain and spinal cord to various glands in the body and to the cardiac and smooth muscle in the thorax and abdomen.

Cranial Nerves

Twelve pairs of cranial nerves are attached to the undersurface of the brain, extending mostly from the brainstem. Figure 9-23 shows the attachments of these nerves. Their fibers conduct impulses between the brain and structures in the head and neck and in the thoracic and abdominal cavities. For instance, the second cranial nerve (optic nerve) conducts impulses from the eye to the brain, where these impulses produce vision. The third cranial nerve (oculomotor nerve) conducts impulses from the brain to muscles in the eye, where they cause contractions that move the eye. The tenth cranial nerve (vagus nerve) conducts impulses between the medulla oblongata and structures in the neck and thoracic and abdominal cavities. The names of each cranial nerve and a brief description of their functions are listed in Table 9-2.

To learn more about cranial nerves, go to **AnimationDirect** on your CD.

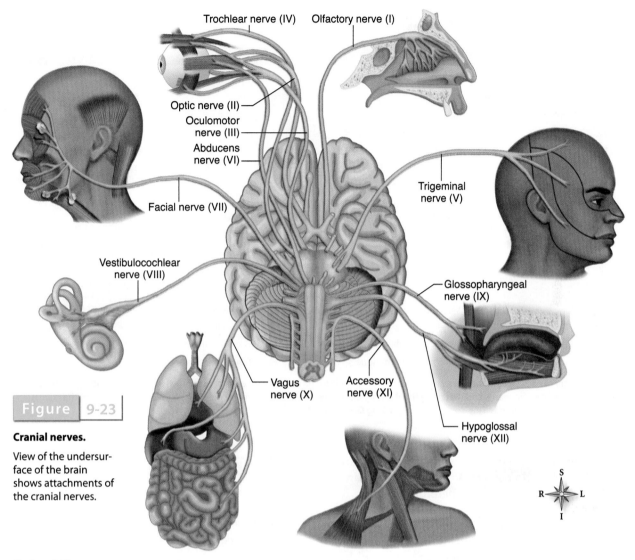

Trochlear nerve (IV)   Olfactory nerve (I)

Optic nerve (II)

Oculomotor
nerve (III)

Abducens
nerve (VI)

Facial nerve (VII)

Trigeminal
nerve (V)

Vestibulocochlear
nerve (VIII)

Glossopharyngeal
nerve (IX)

Vagus
nerve (X)

Accessory
nerve (XI)

Hypoglossal
nerve (XII)

Figure 9-23

Cranial nerves.

View of the undersur-
face of the brain
shows attachments of
the cranial nerves.

Spinal Nerves

STRUCTURE

Thirty-one pairs of nerves are attached to the spinal cord in the following
order: 8 pairs are attached to the cervical segments, 12
pairs are attached to the thoracic segments, 5 pairs are
attached to the lumbar segments, 5 pairs are attached
to the sacrospinal segments, and 1 pair is attached to
the coccygeal segment (Figure 9-17). Unlike cranial
nerves, spinal nerves have no special names; instead, a
letter and number identify each one. C1, for example,
indicates the pair of spinal nerves attached to the first
segment of the cervical part of the cord, and T8 indicates nerves attached to the eighth segment of the thoracic part of the spinal cord. In Figure 9-17 the cervical
area of the spine has
been dissected to show the
emerging spinal nerves in that area. Af-
ter spinal nerves exit from the spinal cord, they branch
to form the many peripheral nerves of the trunk and
limbs. Sometimes, nerve fibers from several spinal
nerves are reorganized to form a single peripheral
nerve. This reorganization can be seen as a network of
intersecting or "braided" branches called a **plexus.** Figure 9-17 shows several plexuses.

FUNCTIONS

Spinal nerves conduct impulses between the spinal cord and the parts of the body not supplied by

Table 9-2 | Cranial Nerves

NERVE*		IMPULSES	FUNCTIONS
I	Olfactory	From nose to brain	Sense of smell
II	Optic	From eye to brain	Vision
III	Oculomotor	From brain to eye muscles	Eye movements
IV	Trochlear	From brain to external eye muscles	Eye movements
VT	Trigeminal	From skin and mucous membrane of head and from teeth to brain; also from brain to chewing muscles	Sensations of face, scalp, and teeth; chewing movements
VI	Abducens	From brain to external eye muscles	Eye movements
VII	Facial	From taste buds of tongue to brain; from brain to face muscles	Sense of taste; contraction of muscles of facial expression
VIII	Vestibulocochlear	From ear to brain	Hearing; sense of balance
IX	Glossopharyngeal	From throat and taste buds of tongue to brain; also from brain to throat muscles and salivary glands	Sensations of throat, taste, swallowing movements, secretion of saliva
X	Vagus	From throat, larynx, and organs in thoracic and abdominal cavities to brain; also from brain to muscles of throat and to organs in thoracic and abdominal cavities	Sensations of throat and larynx and of thoracic and abdominal organs; swallowing, voice production, slowing of heartbeat, acceleration of peristalsis (gut movements)
XI	Accessory	From brain to certain shoulder and neck muscles	Shoulder movements; turning movements of head
XII	Hypoglossal	From brain to muscles of tongue	Tongue movements

* The first letter of each word in the following sentence corresponds to the first letter of each of the cranial nerves, in ascending order from I to XII. Many anatomy students find that using this memory aid, or one like it, helps in memorizing the names and numbers of the cranial nerves. It is "**O**n **O**ld **O**lympus' **T**iny **T**ops, **A** **F**riendly **V**iking **G**rew **V**ines **A**nd **H**ops."

cranial nerves. The spinal nerves shown in Figure 9-17 contain, as do all spinal nerves, sensory and motor fibers. Spinal nerves therefore function to make possible a range of sensations and movements. A disease or injury that prevents conduction by a spinal nerve thus results in a loss of feeling and a loss of movement in the part supplied by that nerve.

Detailed mapping of the skin's surface reveals a close relationship between the source on the spinal cord of each spinal nerve and the part of the body that it innervates (Figure 9-24). Knowledge of the segmental arrangement of spinal nerves is useful to physicians. For instance, a neurologist can identify the site of a spinal cord or nerve abnormality by determining which area of the body is insensitive to a pinprick. Skin surface areas that are supplied by a single spinal nerve are called **dermatomes** (DER-mah-tomes). A dermatome "map" of the body is shown in Figure 9-24.

QUICK CHECK

1. How many *cranial nerves* does a person have? How many *spinal nerves*?
2. What is a spinal nerve *plexus*?
3. What are *dermatomes*?

Peripheral Nerve Disorders

Many afflictions of peripheral nerves, or their branches, involve inflammation—or **neuritis** (noo-RYE-tis). You may know someone who suffers from a form of neuritis called **sciatica** (sye-AT-ik-ah). This is a painful inflammation of the spinal nerve branch in the thigh called the *sciatic nerve*—the largest nerve in the body. This condition is characterized by nerve pain, or **neuralgia** (noor-AL-jee-ah). In some cases, this condition may lead to atrophy of the leg muscles.

Compression or degeneration of the fifth cranial nerve, the trigeminal nerve, may result in a condition called **trigeminal neuralgia,** or *tic douloureux* (doo-

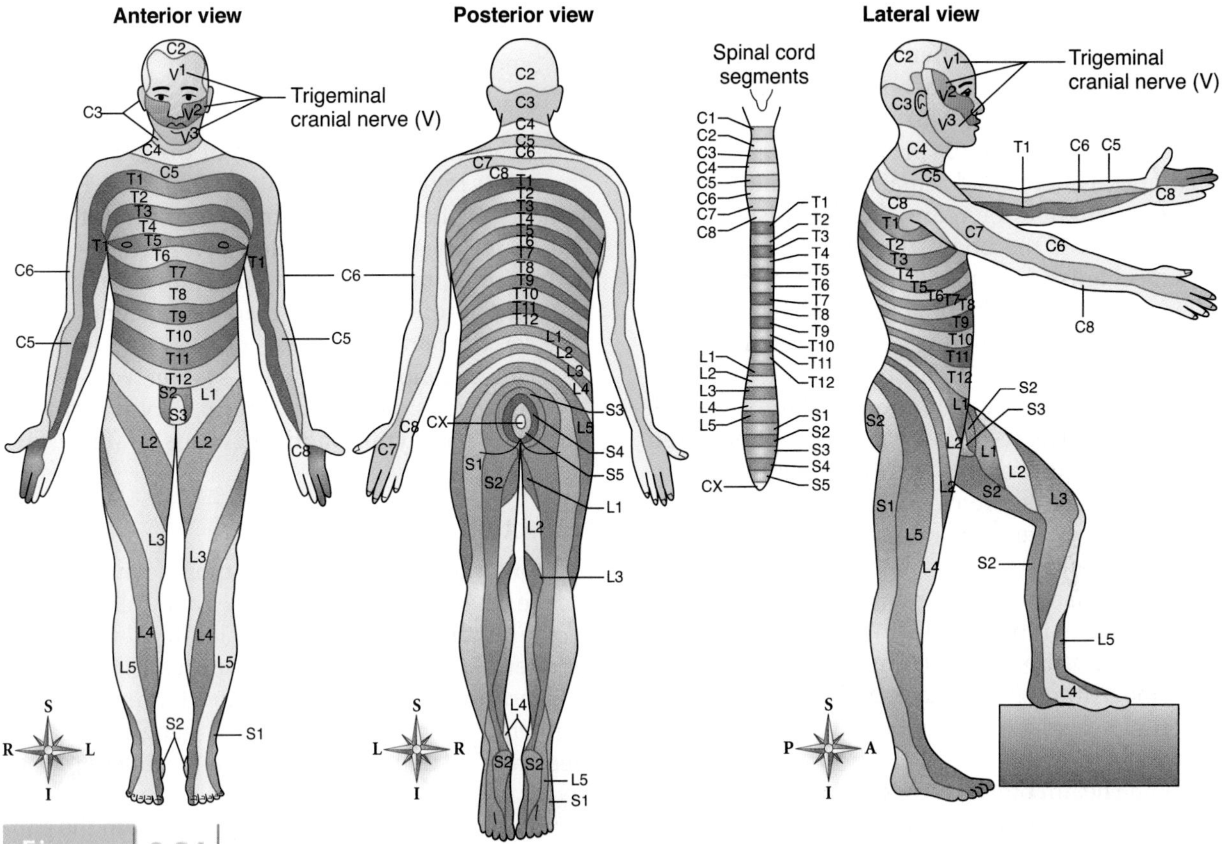
Anterior view
Posterior view
Lateral view
Trigeminal cranial nerve (V)
Spinal cord segments
Trigeminal cranial nerve (V)

Figure 9-24 **Dermatomes.**

Segmental dermatome distribution of spinal nerves to the front, back, and side of the body. *C*, Cervical segments; *T*, thoracic segments; *L*, lumbar segments; *S*, sacral segments; *CX*, coccygeal segment.

loo-ROO). This condition is characterized by recurring episodes of stabbing pain radiating from the angle of the jaw along a branch of the trigeminal nerve. Neuralgia of one branch occurs over the forehead and around the eyes. Pain along another branch is felt in the cheek, nose, and upper lip. Neuralgia of the third branch results in stabbing pains in the tongue and lower lip.

Compression, degeneration, or infection of the seventh cranial nerve, the facial nerve, may result in **Bell palsy.** Bell palsy is characterized by paralysis of some or all of the facial features innervated by the facial nerve, including the eyelids and mouth. This condition is often temporary but in some cases is irreversible. Plastic surgery is sometimes used to correct permanent disfigurement.

Herpes zoster, or **shingles**, is a unique viral infection that almost always affects the skin of a single dermatome (Figure 9-25). It is caused by a varicella

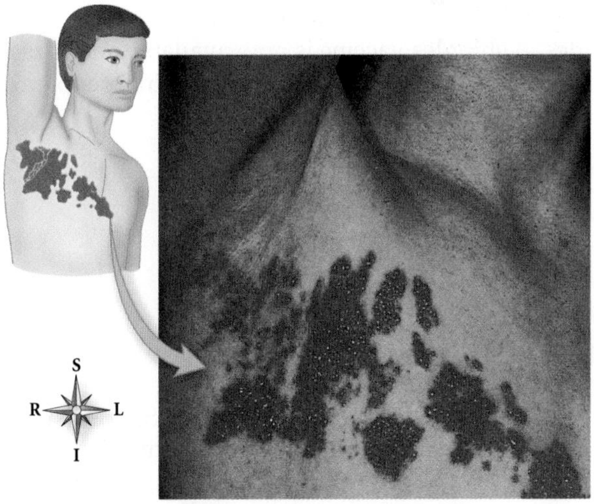

Figure 9-25 **Herpes zoster (shingles).**

Photograph of a 13-year-old boy with eruptions involving dermatome T4 (see Figure 9-24).

zoster virus (VZV) of chickenpox. Nearly 15% of the population will suffer from shingles at least once by the time they reach the age of 80. In most cases the disease results from reactivation of the varicella virus. The virus probably travels through a cutaneous nerve and remains dormant in a dorsal root ganglion for years after an episode of the chickenpox. If the body's immunological protective mechanism becomes diminished in the elderly after stress, or in individuals undergoing radiation therapy or taking immunosuppressive drugs, the virus may reactivate. If this occurs, the virus travels over the sensory nerve to the skin of a single dermatome. The result is a painful eruption of red, swollen plaques or vesicles that eventually rupture and crust before clearing in 2 to 3 weeks. In severe cases, extensive inflammation, hemorrhagic blisters, and secondary bacterial infection may lead to permanent scarring. In most cases, the eruption of vesicles is preceded by 4 to 5 days of preeruptive pain, burning, and itching in the affected dermatome. Although an attack of herpes zoster does not confer lasting immunity, only 5% of cases are recurrences.

Some health officials are concerned about a possible shingles epidemic among adults caused by widespread use of chickenpox vaccines in children. Apparently, adults who have not had occasional immune-boosting exposures to children with chickenpox have an increased risk of developing shingles. A shingles vaccine is now available and is recommended for adults at risk, including people 60 and older who have had chickenpox.

> **QUICK CHECK**
>
> 1. What is *neuralgia?*
> 2. What causes *shingles?*

Autonomic Nervous System

The autonomic nervous system (ANS) consists of certain motor neurons that conduct impulses from the spinal cord or brainstem to the following kinds of tissues:

1. Cardiac muscle tissue
2. Smooth muscle tissue
3. Glandular epithelial tissue

The ANS consists of the parts of the nervous system that regulate involuntary functions (for example, the heartbeat, contractions of the stomach and intestines, and secretions by glands). On the other hand, motor nerves that control the voluntary actions of skeletal muscles are sometimes called the *somatic nervous system.*

The autonomic nervous system consists of two divisions: the **sympathetic nervous system** and the **parasympathetic nervous system** (Figure 9-26).

Functional Anatomy

Autonomic neurons are the motor neurons that make up the ANS. The dendrites and cell bodies of some autonomic neurons are located in the gray matter of the spinal cord or brainstem. Their axons extend from these structures and terminate in peripheral "junction boxes" called **ganglia** (GANG-lee-ah). These autonomic neurons are called **preganglionic neurons** because they conduct impulses between the spinal cord and a ganglion. In the ganglia the axon endings of preganglionic neurons synapse with the dendrites or cell bodies of postganglionic neurons. **Postganglionic neurons**, as their name suggests, conduct impulses from a ganglion to cardiac muscle, smooth muscle, or glandular epithelial tissue.

Autonomic or **visceral effectors** are the tissues to which autonomic neurons conduct impulses. Specifically, visceral effectors are cardiac muscle that makes up the wall of the heart, smooth muscle that partially makes up the walls of blood vessels and other hollow internal organs, and glandular epithelial tissue that makes up the secreting part of glands.

Autonomic Conduction Paths

Conduction paths to visceral and somatic effectors from the CNS (spinal cord or brainstem) differ somewhat. Autonomic paths to visceral effectors,

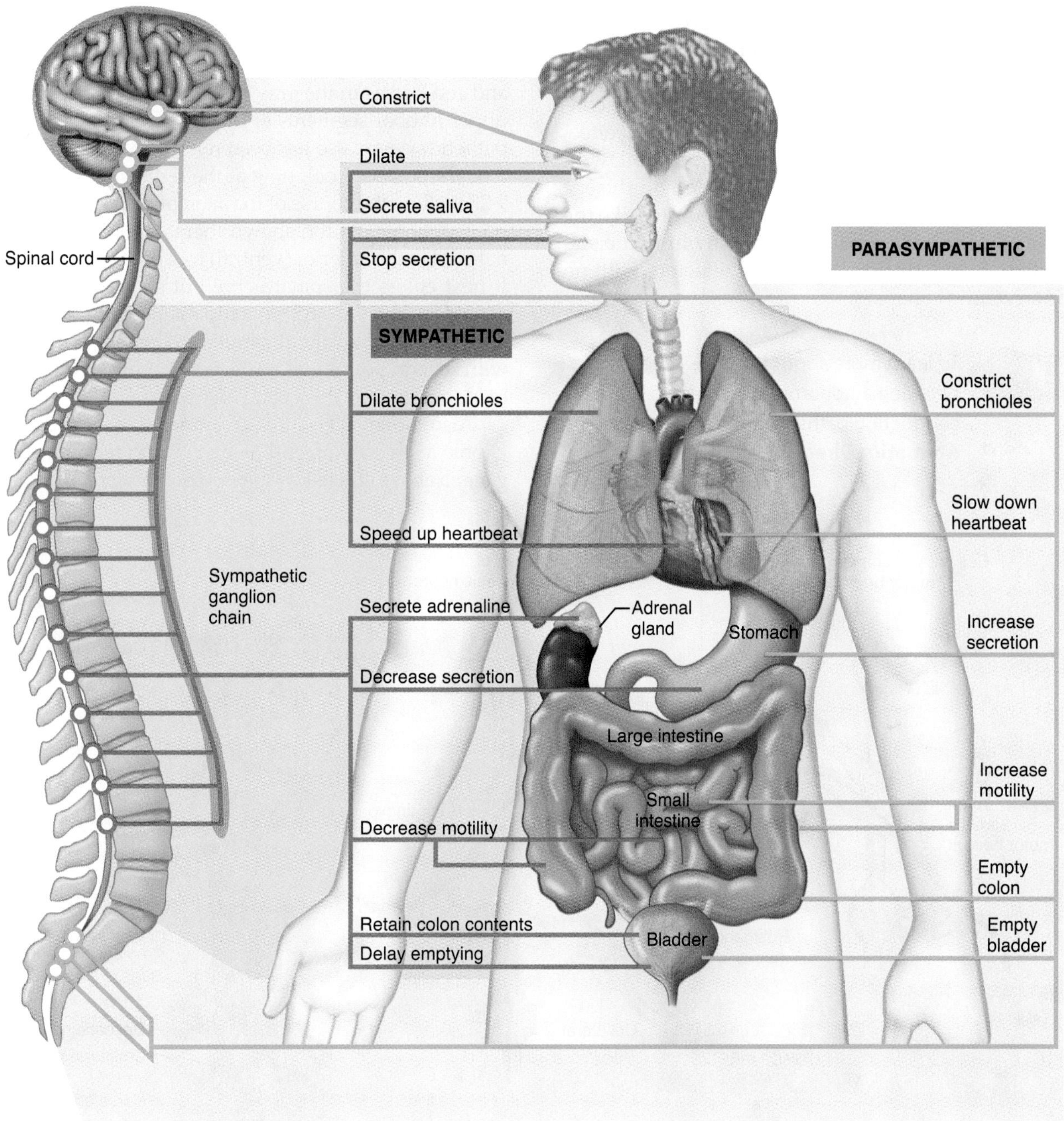

Constrict

Dilate

Secrete saliva

Stop secretion

Spinal cord

PARASYMPATHETIC

SYMPATHETIC

Dilate bronchioles

Constrict bronchioles

Speed up heartbeat

Slow down heartbeat

Sympathetic ganglion chain

Secrete adrenaline

Adrenal gland

Stomach

Increase secretion

Decrease secretion

Large intestine

Small intestine

Increase motility

Decrease motility

Empty colon

Retain colon contents

Bladder

Empty bladder

Delay emptying

Figure 9-26 **Innervation of the major target organs by the autonomic nervous system.**

The sympathetic pathways are highlighted with orange, and the parasympathetic pathways are highlighted with green.

as the right side of Figure 9-27 shows, consist of two-neuron relays. Impulses travel over preganglionic neurons from the spinal cord or brainstem to autonomic ganglia. There, they are relayed across synapses to postganglionic neurons, which then conduct the impulses from the ganglia to visceral effectors. Compare the autonomic conduction path with the somatic conduction path illustrated on the left side of Figure 9-27. Somatic motor neurons, like the ones shown here, conduct all the way from the spinal cord or brainstem to somatic effectors with no intervening synapses.

 To learn more about the difference between autonomic and somatic conduction paths, go to **AnimationDirect** on your CD.

Sympathetic Nervous System

STRUCTURE

Sympathetic preganglionic neurons have dendrites and cell bodies in the gray matter of the thoracic and upper lumbar segments of the spinal cord. The sympathetic system also has been referred to as the *thoracolumbar system*. Look now at the right side of Figure 9-27. Follow the course of the axon of the sympathetic preganglionic neuron shown there. It leaves the spinal cord in the anterior (ventral) root of a spinal nerve. It next enters the spinal nerve but soon leaves it to extend to and through a sympathetic ganglion and terminate in a collateral ganglion. There, it synapses with several postganglionic neurons whose axons extend to terminate in visceral effectors.

Also shown in Figure 9-27, branches of the preganglionic axon may ascend or descend to terminate in ganglia above and below their point of origin. All sym-

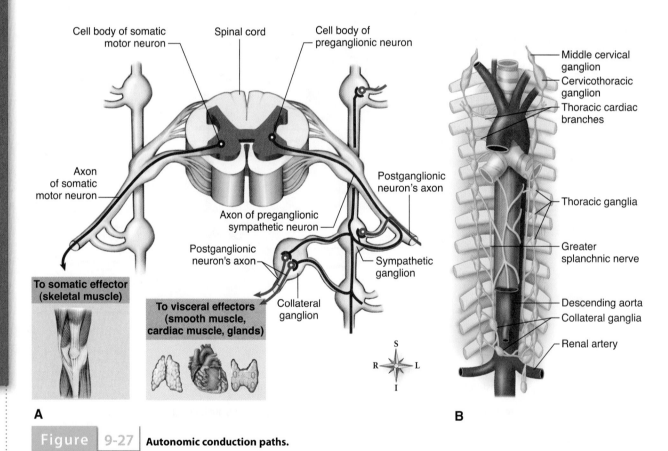

A, One somatic motor neuron conducts impulses all the way from the spinal cord to a somatic effector. Conduction from the spinal cord to any visceral effector, however, requires a relay of at least two autonomic motor neurons—a preganglionic and a postganglionic neuron. **B,** Location of the sympathetic chain ganglia.

Figure 9-27 | **Autonomic conduction paths.**

pathetic preganglionic axons therefore synapse with many postganglionic neurons, and these frequently terminate in widely separated organs. Hence sympathetic responses are usually widespread, involving many organs rather than just one.

Sympathetic postganglionic neurons have dendrites and cell bodies in sympathetic ganglia. Sympathetic ganglia are located in front of and at each side of the spinal column. Because short fibers extend between the sympathetic ganglia, they look a little like two chains of beads and are often referred to as the *sympathetic chain ganglia* (Figure 9-27, *B*). Axons of sympathetic postganglionic neurons travel in spinal nerves to blood vessels, sweat glands, and arrector hair muscles all over the body. Separate autonomic nerves distribute many sympathetic postganglionic axons to various internal organs.

FUNCTIONS OF THE SYMPATHETIC NERVOUS SYSTEM

The sympathetic nervous system functions as an emergency system. Impulses over sympathetic fibers take control of many internal organs when we exercise strenuously and when strong emotions—anger, fear, hate, anxiety—are elicited. In short, when we must cope with stress of any kind, sympathetic impulses increase to many visceral effectors and rapidly produce widespread changes within our bodies. The middle column of Table 9-3 lists many of the possible sympathetic responses. The heart beats faster. Most blood vessels constrict, causing blood pressure to increase. Blood vessels in skeletal muscles dilate, supplying the muscles with more blood. Sweat glands and adrenal glands secrete more abundantly. Salivary and other digestive glands secrete more sparingly. Digestive tract contractions (peristalsis) become sluggish, hampering digestion. Together, these sympathetic responses make us ready for strenuous muscular work, or they prepare us for *fight or flight.* The group of changes induced by sympathetic control is known as the **fight-or-flight response.**

Parasympathetic Nervous System

STRUCTURE

The dendrites and cell bodies of parasympathetic preganglionic neurons are located in the gray matter of the brainstem and the sacral segments of the spinal cord. The parasympathetic system also has been referred to as the *craniosacral system.* The preganglionic parasympathetic axons extend some distance

| Table | 9-3 | **Autonomic Functions** |

VISCERAL EFFECTORS	SYMPATHETIC CONTROL	PARASYMPATHETIC CONTROL
Heart muscle	Accelerates heartbeat	Slows heartbeat
Smooth muscle		
Of most blood vessels	Constricts blood vessels	None
Of blood vessels in skeletal muscles	Dilates blood vessels	None
Of the digestive tract	Decreases peristalsis; inhibits defecation	Increases peristalsis
Of the anal sphincter	Stimulates—closes sphincter	Inhibits—opens sphincter for defecation
Of the urinary bladder	Inhibits—relaxes bladder	Stimulates—contracts bladder
Of the urinary sphincters	Stimulates—closes sphincter	Inhibits—opens sphincter for urination
Of the eye		
Iris	Stimulates radial fibers—dilation of pupil	Stimulates circular fibers—constriction of pupil
Ciliary	Inhibits—accommodation for far vision (flattening of lens)	Stimulates—accommodation for near vision (bulging of lens)
Of hairs (pilomotor muscles)	Stimulates—"goose pimples"	No parasympathetic fibers
Glands		
Adrenal medulla	Increases epinephrine secretion	None
Sweat glands	Increases sweat secretion	None
Digestive glands	Decreases secretion of digestive juices	Increases secretion of digestive juices

before terminating in the parasympathetic ganglia located in the head and in the thoracic and abdominal cavities close to the visceral effectors that they control. The dendrites and cell bodies of parasympathetic postganglionic neurons lie in these outlying parasympathetic ganglia, and their short axons extend into the nearby structures. Therefore each parasympathetic preganglionic neuron synapses only with postganglionic neurons to a single effector. For this reason, parasympathetic stimulation frequently involves response by only one organ. This is not true of sympathetic responses; as noted, sympathetic stimulation usually results in responses by numerous organs.

FUNCTIONS OF THE PARASYMPATHETIC NERVOUS SYSTEM

The parasympathetic system dominates control of many visceral effectors under normal, everyday conditions. Impulses over parasympathetic fibers, for example, tend to slow heartbeat, increase peristalsis, and increase secretion of digestive juices and insulin (Table 9-3).

Autonomic Neurotransmitters

Turn your attention now to Figure 9-28. It illustrates information regarding autonomic neurotransmitters, the chemical compounds released from the axon terminals of autonomic neurons. Observe that three of the axons shown in Figure 9-28—the sympathetic preganglionic axon, the parasympathetic preganglionic axon, and the parasympathetic postganglionic axon—release acetylcholine. These axons are therefore classified as **cholinergic fibers.** Only one type of autonomic axon releases the neurotransmitter norepinephrine (noradrenaline). This is the axon of a sympathetic postganglionic neuron, and such neurons are classified as **adrenergic fibers.** That each division of the ANS signals its effectors with a different neurotransmitter explains how an organ can tell which division is stimulating it. The heart, for example, responds to acetylcholine from the parasympathetic division by slowing down. The presence of norepinephrine in the heart, on the other hand, is a signal from the sympathetic division, and the response is an increase in heart activity.

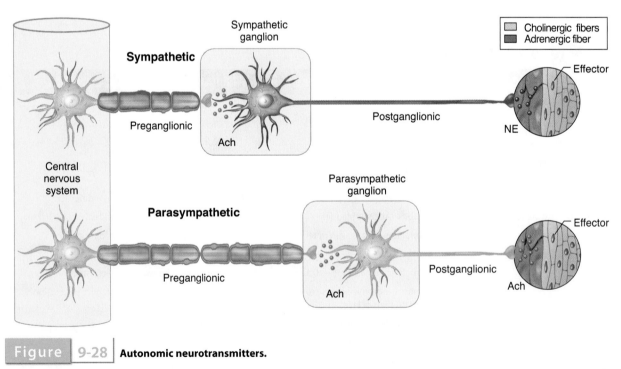

Figure 9-28 **Autonomic neurotransmitters.**

Three of the four fiber types are cholinergic, secreting the neurotransmitter acetylcholine (*Ach*) into a synapse. Only the sympathetic postganglionic fiber is adrenergic, secreting norepinephrine (*NE*) into a synapse.

Autonomic Nervous System as a Whole

The function of the autonomic nervous system is to regulate the body's automatic, involuntary functions in ways that maintain or quickly restore homeostasis. Many internal organs are doubly innervated by the ANS. In other words, they receive fibers from parasympathetic and sympathetic divisions. Parasympathetic and sympathetic impulses continually bombard them and, as Table 9-3 indicates, influence their function in opposite or antagonistic ways. For example, the heart continually receives sympathetic impulses that make it beat faster and parasympathetic impulses that slow it down. The ratio between these two antagonistic forces, determined by the ratio between the two different autonomic neurotransmitters, determines the actual heart rate.

The term *autonomic nervous system* is something of a misnomer. It seems to imply that this part of the nervous system is independent from other parts. But this is not true. Dendrites and cell bodies of preganglionic neurons are located, as observed in Figure 9-28, in the spinal cord and brainstem. They are continually influenced directly or indirectly by impulses from neurons located above them, notably by some in the hypothalamus and in the parts of the cerebral cortex called the **limbic system,** or *emotional brain.* Through conduction paths from these areas, emotions can produce widespread changes in the automatic functions of our bodies, in cardiac and smooth muscle contractions, and in secretion by glands. Anger and fear, for example, lead to increased sympathetic activity and the fight-or-flight response. According to some physiologists, the altered state of consciousness known as *meditation* leads to decreased sympathetic activity and a group of changes opposite those of the fight-or-flight response.

Disorders of the Autonomic Nervous System

STRESS-INDUCED DISEASE

Considering the variety and number of effectors innervated by the autonomic nervous system, it is no wonder that autonomic disorders have varied and far-reaching consequences. This is especially true of stress-induced diseases. Prolonged or excessive physiological response to stress, the fight-or-flight

response, can disrupt normal functioning throughout the body. Stress has been cited as an indirect cause or an important risk factor in a number of conditions. Only a few of those are listed here.

1. **Heart disease**—Although an extreme episode of stress can precipitate heart failure even in healthy people, chronic stress is known to increase the risk of certain heart disorders. One such condition is stress-induced high blood pressure, or *hypertension,* that can weaken the heart and blood vessels.

2. **Digestive problems**—Colitis (colon inflammation) and gastric ulcers, for example, may be precipitated by the changes in digestive secretion and movement, along with increased susceptibility to infection, that occur during prolonged or repeated stress responses.

3. **Reduced resistance to disease**—Hormones called *glucocorticoids* that are released by the adrenal glands during prolonged or repeated stress episodes depress the activity of the immune system. Depressed immune function leads to increased risk of infection and cancer.

Because both the nervous system and endocrine system are involved in stress disorders, they are usually thought of as *neuroendocrine* disorders.

NEUROBLASTOMA

Neuroblastoma (noo-roh-blast-OH-mah) is a malignant tumor of the sympathetic nervous system. It most often occurs in the developing nervous systems of young children and metastasizes rapidly to other parts of the body. Symptoms often include exaggerated or inappropriate sympathetic effects, including increased heart rate, sweating, and high blood pressure. As with some other forms of cancer, spontaneous remissions may occur.

QUICK CHECK

1. What are the two main divisions of the ANS?
2. Which division of the ANS produces the *fight-or-flight* response?
3. Which two neurotransmitters are used by the autonomic nerve pathways?
4. What problems in the body arise from ANS malfunctions?

SCIENCE APPLICATIONS

NEUROSCIENCE

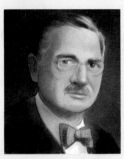

Otto Loewi (1873–1961)

The Austrian scientist Otto Loewi started his studies in the humanities, not science. Even after he did finally begin university studies in medicine, he often skipped his science classes to attend lectures in philosophy instead. But after Dr. Loewi turned his attention to human biology, his brilliance became evident. In 1921, while working to design an experiment that would unlock the mystery of how neurons communicate with other cells, he had a dream in which the answer was revealed to him. He rushed to his lab and performed a now famous experiment in which he discovered what we know as *acetylcholine*. For his work that showed that it is neurotransmitters that carry signals from neurons, Loewi shared a Nobel Prize in 1936. And, not surprisingly, Loewi later spent some of his time studying how dreams may help us understand subconscious thoughts.

Many professions depend on neuroscientists like Otto Loewi to provide information they need to help us improve our lives. For example, neurologists, psychiatrists, and other medical professionals use this information to treat disorders of the nervous system. Pharmacologists and pharmacy professionals use these ideas to develop drug treatments that affect the nervous system. Mental health professionals such as psychologists and counselors use concepts derived from neuroscience to better understand human emotions and behavior. Even people who specialize in business and marketing use some of the neuroscience discoveries—their focus is learning how to entice buyers to buy certain products or, perhaps, predict the behavior of crowds.

Outline Summary

To download an MP3 version of the chapter summary for use with your iPod or portable media player, access the **Audio Chapter Summaries** on your CD.

Organs and Divisions of the Nervous System (Figure 9-1)

A. Central nervous system (CNS)—brain and spinal cord
B. Peripheral nervous system (PNS)—all nerves
C. Autonomic nervous system (ANS)

Cells of the Nervous System

A. Neurons
  1. Consist of three parts
    a. Cell body of neuron—main part
    b. Dendrites—branching projections that conduct impulses to cell body of neuron
    c. Axon—elongated projection that conducts impulses *away from* cell body of neuron (Figure 9-2)

  2. Neurons classified according to function, or direction of impulse
    a. Sensory neurons: conduct impulses to the spinal cord and brain; also called *afferent neurons*
    b. Motor neurons: conduct impulses away from brain and spinal cord to muscles and glands; also called *efferent neurons*
    c. Interneurons: conduct impulses from sensory neurons to motor neurons; also called *central* or *connecting neurons*
B. Glia (neuroglia)
  1. Support cells, bringing the cells of nervous tissue together structurally and functionally
  2. Three main types of connective tissue cells of the CNS (Figure 9-3)

a. Astrocytes—star-shaped cells that anchor small blood vessels to neurons

b. Microglia—small cells that move in inflamed brain tissue carrying on phagocytosis

c. Oligodendrocytes—form myelin sheaths on axons in the CNS (Schwann cells form myelin sheaths in PNS only)

C. Disorders of nervous tissue

1. Multiple sclerosis—characterized by myelin loss in central nerve fibers and resulting conduction impairments (Figure 9-4)

2. Tumors

a. General name for nervous system tumors is *neuroma*

b. Most neuromas are gliomas, glial tumors

c. Multiple neurofibromatosis—characterized by numerous benign tumors (Figure 9-5)

Nerves

A. Nerve—bundle of peripheral axons (Figure 9-6)

1. Tract—bundle of central axons

2. White matter—brain or cord tissue composed primarily of myelinated axons (tracts)

3. Gray matter—brain or cord tissue composed primarily of cell bodies and unmyelinated fibers

B. Nerve coverings—fibrous connective tissue

1. Endoneurium—surrounds individual fibers within a nerve

2. Perineurium—surrounds a group (fascicle) of nerve fibers

3. Epineurium—surrounds the entire nerve

Reflex Arcs

A. Nerve impulses are conducted from receptors to effectors over neuron pathways or reflex arcs; conduction by a reflex arc results in a reflex (that is, contraction by a muscle or secretion by a gland)

B. The simplest reflex arcs are two-neuron arcs—consisting of sensory neurons synapsing in the spinal cord with motor neurons; three-neuron arcs consist of sensory neurons synapsing in the spinal cord with interneurons that synapse with motor neurons (Figure 9-7)

Nerve Impulses

A. Definition—self-propagating wave of electrical disturbance that travels along the surface of a neuron membrane (Figure 9-8); sometimes called *action potentials*

B. Mechanism

1. At rest, the neuron's membrane is slightly positive on the outside—polarized—from a slight excess of Na^+ on the outside

2. A stimulus triggers the opening of Na^+ channels in the plasma membrane of the neuron

3. Inward movement of Na^+ depolarizes the membrane by making the inside more positive than the outside at the stimulated point; this depolarization is a nerve impulse (action potential)

4. The stimulated section of membrane immediately repolarizes, but by that time the depolarization has already triggered the next section of membrane to depolarize, thus propagating a wave of electrical disturbances (depolarizations) all the way down the membrane

The Synapse

A. Definition—the place where impulses are transmitted from one neuron to another (the postsynaptic neuron) (Figure 9-9)

B. Synapse made of three structures—synaptic know, synaptic cleft, and plasma membrane

C. Neurotransmitters bind to specific receptor molecules in the membrane of a postsynaptic neuron, opening ion channels and thereby stimulating impulse conduction by the membrane

D. Names of neurotransmitters—acetylcholine, catecholamines (norepinephrine, dopamine, and serotonin), endorphins, enkephalins, nitric oxide (NO), and other compounds

E. Parkinson disease (PD)—characterized by abnormally low levels of dopamine in motor control areas of the brain; patients usually exhibit involuntary trembling and muscle rigidity (parkinsonism; Figure 9-10)

Central Nervous System (Figure 9-11)

A. Divisions of the brain (Figure 9-12 and Table 9-1)

1. Brainstem
   a. Consists of, named in ascending order, the medulla oblongata, pons, and midbrain
   b. Structure—white matter with bits of gray matter scattered through it
   c. Functions
      (1) All three parts of brainstem are two-way conduction paths
      (2) Sensory tracts in the brainstem conduct impulses to the higher parts of the brain
      (3) Motor tracts conduct from the higher parts of the brain to the spinal cord
      (4) Many important reflex centers lie in the brainstem
2. Cerebellum
   a. Second largest part of the human brain
   b. Helps control muscle contractions to produce coordinated movements so that we can maintain balance, move smoothly, and sustain normal postures
   c. Recent evidence shows the cerebellum also may have wider coordinating effects, assisting the cerebrum and other regions of the brain
3. Diencephalon
   a. Structure and function of the hypothalamus
      (1) Consists mainly of the posterior pituitary gland, pituitary stalk, and gray matter
      (2) Acts as the major center for controlling the ANS; therefore helps control the functioning of most internal organs
      (3) Controls hormone secretion by anterior and posterior pituitary glands; therefore it indirectly helps control hormone secretion by most other endocrine glands
      (4) Contains centers for controlling appetite, wakefulness, pleasure, etc.
   b. Structure and function of the thalamus

      (1) Dumbbell-shaped mass of gray matter extending into each cerebral hemisphere
      (2) Relays sensory impulses to cerebral cortex sensory areas
      (3) In some way produces the emotions of pleasantness or unpleasantness associated with sensations
4. Cerebrum
   a. Largest part of the human brain
   b. Outer layer of gray matter is the cerebral cortex; made up of lobes; composed mainly of dendrites and cell bodies of neurons
   c. Interior of the cerebrum composed mainly of white matter (that is nerve fibers arranged in bundles called *tracts*)
   d. Functions of the cerebrum—mental processes of all types, including sensations, consciousness, memory, and voluntary control of movements (Figure 9-13)

B. Brain disorders

1. Destruction of brain tissue
   a. Cerebrovascular accident (CVA)—hemorrhage from or cessation of blood flow through cerebral blood vessels; a "stroke"
   b. Cerebral palsy (CP)—condition in which damage to motor control areas of the brain before, during, or shortly after birth causes paralysis (usually spastic) of one or more limbs (Figure 9-14)
2. Dementia—syndrome that includes progressive loss of memory, shortened attention span, personality changes, reduced intellectual capacity, and motor control deficit
   a. Alzheimer disease (AD)—brain disorder of the middle and late adult years characterized by dementia (Figure 9-15)
   b. Huntington disease (HD)—inherited disorder characterized by chorea (purposeless movement) progressing to severe dementia
   c. HIV (also causes AIDS) can infect neurons and thus cause dementia
3. Seizure disorders

a. Seizure—sudden burst of abnormal neuron activity that results in temporary changes in brain function

b. Epilepsy—many forms, all characterized by recurring seizures

c. Electroencephalogram—graphic representation of voltage changes in the brain used to evaluate brain activity (Figure 9-16)

C. Spinal cord (Figure 9-17)

1. Columns of white matter, composed of bundles of myelinated nerve fibers, form the outer portion of the H-shaped core of the spinal cord; bundles of axons called *tracts*

2. Interior composed of gray matter made up mainly of neuron dendrites and cell bodies (Figure 9-18)

3. Spinal cord tracts provide two-way conduction paths—ascending and descending

4. Spinal cord functions as the primary center for all spinal cord reflexes; sensory tracts conduct impulses to the brain, and motor tracts conduct impulses from the brain

D. Coverings and fluid spaces of the brain and spinal cord

1. Coverings
   a. Cranial bones and vertebrae
   b. Cerebral and spinal meninges—the dura mater, arachnoid mater, and the pia mater (Figure 9-19)

2. Fluid spaces (Figures 9-20 to 9-22)
   a. Subarachnoid spaces of meninges
   b. Central canal inside cord
   c. Ventricles in brain

Peripheral Nervous System

A. Cranial nerves (Figure 9-23 and Table 9-2)

1. Twelve pairs—attached to undersurface of the brain

2. Connect brain with the neck and structures in the thorax and abdomen

B. Spinal nerves

1. Thirty-one pairs—contain dendrites of sensory neurons and axons of motor neurons

2. Conduct impulses necessary for sensations and voluntary movements (Figure 9-24)

3. Skin surface area supplied by a single nerve is called a *dermatome*

C. Peripheral nerve disorders

1. Neuritis—general term referring to nerve inflammation
   a. Sciatica is inflammation of the sciatic nerve that innervates the legs
   b. Neuralgia, or muscle pain, often accompanies neuritis

2. Trigeminal neuralgia—recurring episodes of stabbing pain along one or more branches of the trigeminal (fifth cranial) nerve in the head

3. Bell palsy—paralysis of facial features resulting from damage to the facial (seventh cranial) nerve

4. Herpes zoster, or shingles (Figure 9-25)
   a. Viral infection caused by chickenpox virus that has invaded the dorsal root ganglion and remained dormant until stress or reduced immunity precipitate an episode of shingles
   b. Usually affects a single dermatome, producing characteristic painful plaques or vesicles

Autonomic Nervous System

A. Functional anatomy

1. Autonomic nervous system—motor neurons that conduct impulses from the central nervous system to cardiac muscle, smooth muscle, and glandular epithelial tissue; regulates the body's automatic, or involuntary, functions (Figure 9-26)

2. Autonomic neurons—preganglionic autonomic neurons conduct from spinal cord or brainstem to an autonomic ganglion; postganglionic neurons conduct from autonomic ganglia to cardiac muscle, smooth muscle, and glandular epithelial tissue

3. Autonomic or visceral effectors—tissues to which autonomic neurons conduct impulses (that is, cardiac and smooth muscle and glandular epithelial tissue)

4. Composed of two divisions—the sympathetic system and the parasympathetic system

B. Autonomic conduction paths (Figure 9-27)
   1. Consist of two-neuron relays (that is, preganglionic neurons from the central nervous system to autonomic ganglia, synapses, postganglionic neurons from ganglia to visceral effectors)
   2. In contrast, somatic motor neurons conduct all the way from the CNS to somatic effectors with no intervening synapses

C. Sympathetic nervous systems
   1. Dendrites and cell bodies of sympathetic preganglionic neurons are located in the gray matter of the thoracic and upper lumbar segments of the spinal cord
   2. Axons leave the spinal cord in the anterior roots of spinal nerves, extend to sympathetic, or collateral, ganglia and synapse with several postganglionic neurons whose axons extend to spinal or autonomic nerves to terminate in visceral effectors
   3. A chain of sympathetic ganglia is in front of and at each side of the spinal column
   4. Functions of the sympathetic nervous system
      a. Serves as the emergency or stress system, controlling visceral effectors during strenuous exercise and when strong emotions (anger, fear, hate, or anxiety) are elicited
      b. Group of changes induced by sympathetic control is called the *fight-or-flight response*

D. Parasympathetic nervous system
   1. Structure
      a. Parasympathetic preganglionic neurons have dendrites and cell bodies in the gray matter of the brainstem and the sacral segments of the spinal cord
      b. Parasympathetic preganglionic neurons terminate in parasympathetic ganglia located in the head and the thoracic and abdominal cavities close to visceral effectors
      c. Each parasympathetic preganglionic neuron synapses with postganglionic neurons to only one effector
   2. Function—dominates control of many visceral effectors under normal, everyday conditions

E. Autonomic neurotransmitters (Figure 9-28)
   1. Cholinergic fibers—preganglionic axons of parasympathetic and sympathetic systems and parasympathetic postganglionic axons release acetylcholine
   2. Adrenergic fibers—axons of sympathetic postganglionic neurons release norepinephrine (noradrenaline)

F. Autonomic nervous system as a whole
   1. Regulates the body's automatic functions in ways that maintain or quickly restore homeostasis
   2. Many visceral effectors are doubly innervated (that is, they receive fibers from parasympathetic and sympathetic divisions and are influenced in opposite ways by the two divisions)

G. Disorders of the autonomic nervous system
   1. Stress-induced disease
      a. Prolonged or excessive response to stress can disrupt normal functioning throughout the body
      b. Examples of stress-induced conditions include heart disease, digestive problems, and reduced resistance to disease
   2. Neuroblastoma—highly malignant tumor of the sympathetic nervous system, primarily affecting young children

New Words

acetylcholine
action potential
adrenergic fiber
afferent
anesthesia
arachnoid mater
astrocyte
autonomic effect
autonomic nervous system (ANS)
autonomic neuron
blood-brain barrier (BBB)
catecholamines
central nervous system (CNS)
cerebral cortex
cerebral nuclei (basal ganglia)
cerebrospinal fluid
cerebrum
cholinergic fiber
choroid plexus
corpus callosum
cranial nerve
dermatome
diencephalon
dopamine
dura mater
efferent
endoneurium
endorphin
enkephalin

epineurium
fascicle
fight-or-flight response
ganglion (*pl.,* ganglia)
gray matter
gyri
hypothalamus
interneuron
limbic system
medulla oblongata
meninges
microglia
midbrain
motor neuron
myelin
myelinated fiber
nerve
neurilemma
neurotransmitter
nitric oxide (NO)
nodes of Ranvier
norepinephrine
oligodendrocyte
parasympathetic nervous system
perineurium
peripheral nervous system (PNS)
pia mater
plexus

pons
postganglionic neuron
postsynaptic neuron
preganglionic neuron
presynaptic neuron
receptor
reflex
reflex arc
saltatory conduction
Schwann cell
sensory neuron
serotonin
spinal nerve
spinal tract
sulci
sympathetic nervous system
synapse
synaptic cleft
synaptic knob
thalamus
tract
ventricles
visceral effector
white matter

Diseases and Other Clinical Terms

Alzheimer disease (AD)
anesthesia
Bell palsy

cerebral palsy (CP)
cerebrovascular accident (CVA)
dementia
electroencephalogram (EEG)
epilepsy
glioma
hemiplegia
herpes zoster (shingles)
Huntington disease (HD)
hydrocephalus
lumbar puncture
meningitis
multiple neurofibromatosis
multiple sclerosis (MS)
neuralgia
neuritis
neuroblastoma
neuroma
paraplegia
Parkinson disease (PD)
quadriplegia
sciatica
seizure
spastic paralysis
trigeminal neuralgia (tic douloureux)
triplegia

Review Questions

1. Draw and label the three parts of the neuron and explain the function of the dendrite and axon.
2. Name the three types of neurons classified according to the direction in which the impulse is being transmitted. Define or explain each of them.
3. Define or explain the following terms: *myelin, nodes of Ranvier,* and *neurolemma.*
4. Name and give the function of the three types of glia cells.
5. What occurs at the cellular level in multiple sclerosis? What effect does this have on the body?
6. From what type of cells or tissues do neuromas usually develop?
7. Define or explain the following terms: *epineurium, perineurium,* and *endoneurium.*
8. What causes gray matter to be gray and white matter to be white?
9. Explain how a reflex arc functions. What are the two types of reflex arc?
10. Explain what occurs during a nerve impulse. What is saltatory conduction?
11. Explain what occurs at a synapse. What are the two ways that neurotransmitter activity is terminated?
12. What is the cause of Parkinson disease? What are some treatment options?
13. Define dementia.
14. What is a seizure?
15. List two possible causes of Alzheimer disease.
16. List and describe the functions of the medulla oblongata.
17. List and describe the functions of the hypothalamus.
18. List and describe the functions of the thalamus.
19. List and describe the functions of the cerebellum.
20. Give the general function of the cerebrum. What are the specific functions of the occipital and temporal lobes?
21. List and describe the functions of the spinal cord.
22. Name and explain the three layers of the meninges.
23. What is the function of cerebrospinal fluid? Where and how is it produced?
24. How many nerve pairs are generated from the spinal cord? How many nerve pairs are generated from each section of the spinal cord? How are these nerves named? What is a plexus?
25. Define neuritis and neuralgia.
26. What is the cause of tic douloureux? What is the cause of Bell palsy?
27. Explain the structure and function of the sympathetic nervous system.
28. Explain the structure and function of the parasympathetic nervous system.

Critical Thinking

29. List the functional regions of the frontal, parietal, occipital, and temporal lobes.
30. Which of the cranial nerves deal primarily with motor function? Which deal primarily with sensory function?
31. There is a type of medication that inhibits the functioning of acetylcholinesterase (the enzyme that deactivates acetylcholine). Explain the effect this medication would have on the visceral effectors.

Chapter Test

1. _____ is the name of the nervous system division that includes the nerves that extend to the outlying parts of the body.
2. _____ is the name of the nervous system division that includes the brain and spinal cord.
3. A group of peripheral axons bundled together in an epineurium is called a _____.
4. The two types of cells found in the nervous system are _____ and _____.
5. The knee-jerk reflex is a type of neural pathway called a _____.

6. A _____ is a self-propagating wave of electrical disturbance that travels along the surface of a neuron's plasma membrane.

7. The exterior of the resting neuron has a slight _____ charge, whereas the interior has a slight _____ charge.

8. During a nerve impulse, _____ is the ion that rushes into the neuron.

9. The _____ is a place where impulses are passed from one neuron to another.

10. Acetylcholine and dopamine are examples of _____, which are chemicals used by neurons to communicate.

11. _____, _____, and _____ are the three membranes that make up the meninges.

12. There are _____ pairs of cranial nerves and _____ pairs of nerves that come from the spinal cord.

13. _____ are skin surface areas supplied by a single spinal nerve.

14. _____ is the part of the autonomic nervous system that regulates effectors during nonstress conditions.

15. _____ is the part of the autonomic nervous system that regulates effectors during the "fight-or-flight" response.

16. The preganglionic axons of the parasympathetic nervous system release the neurotransmitter _____. The postganglionic axons release _____.

17. The preganglionic axons of the sympathetic nervous system release the neurotransmitter _____. The postganglionic axons release _____.

18. The autonomic nervous system consists of neurons that conduct impulses from the brain or spinal cord to _____ tissue, _____ tissue, and _____ tissue.

Match each term in Column A with its corresponding function or description in Column B.

Column A
19. _____ dendrite
20. _____ axon
21. _____ myelin
22. _____ Schwann cells
23. _____ astrocyte
24. _____ microglia
25. _____ oligodendrocyte

Column B
a. cells that make myelin for axons outside the CNS
b. glia cells that help form the blood-brain barrier
c. a single projection that carries nerve impulses away from the cell body
d. cells that make myelin for axons inside the CNS
e. a white fatty substance that surrounds and insulates the axon
f. cells that act as microbe-eating scavengers in the CNS
g. a highly branched part of the neuron that carries impulses toward the cell body

Match each part of the central nervous system in Column A with its corresponding function in Column B.

Column A
26. _____ medulla oblongata
27. _____ pons
28. _____ midbrain
29. _____ hypothalamus
30. _____ thalamus
31. _____ cerebellum
32. _____ cerebrum
33. _____ spinal cord

Column B
a. part of the brainstem that is a conduction pathway between the brain and body; influences respiration
b. sensory relay station from various body areas to the cerebral cortex; also involved with emotion and alerting and arousal mechanisms
c. carries messages to and from the brain and the rest of the body; also mediates reflexes
d. part of the brainstem that contains cardiac, respiratory, and vasomotor centers
e. sensory perception, willed movements, consciousness, and memory are mediated here
f. regulates body temperature, water balance, sleep-wake cycle, and sexual arousal
g. regulates muscle coordination, maintenance of equilibrium and posture
h. part of the brainstem that contains relays for visual and auditory impulses

Match each disorder or disease in Column A with its description or cause in Column B.

Column A
34. _____ multiple sclerosis
35. _____ neuroma
36. _____ multiple neurofibromatosis
37. _____ Parkinson disease
37. _____ CVA
39. _____ dementia
40. _____ epilepsy
41. _____ meningitis
42. _____ tic douloureux
43. _____ Bell palsy
44. _____ neuroblastoma

Column B
a. inherited condition causing multiple benign tumors; the "elephant man" condition
b. cessation of blood flow to the brain; a stroke
c. syndrome that includes memory loss, short attention span, and reduced intellectual capacity
d. recurring or chronic seizure disorder
e. compression or degeneration of the seventh cranial nerve
f. disorder caused by the loss of myelin
g. a malignant tumor of the sympathetic nervous system
h. compression or degeneration of the fifth cranial nerve
i. infection or inflammation of the meninges
j. general term for a tumor in the nervous system
k. disease characterized by an abnormally low level of dopamine

Study Tips

continued from page 235

2. The synapse requires the production, release, and deactivation of neurotransmitters. Neurotransmitters function by stimulating receptors in the neuron on the other side of the synapse.

3. The material on the central nervous system can be learned best by using flash cards that match up the structure and function.

4. Make a chart showing the disorders of the nervous system. Organize them by type: myelin disorder, brain disorder, etc. Describe the damage done by the disorder and the effect it has on the body.

5. When studying the autonomic nervous system, remember the basic function of each part. The parasympathetic system tries to maintain a quiet homeostasis. The sympathetic system prepares the body for emergency situations—the "fight-or-flight" response.

6. In your study group, you should go over the terms presented in the first part of the chapter. Discuss the processes of nerve impulse transmission and what occurs at the synapse. Review the flash cards with the names and functions of the parts of the central nervous system. Remember that most of the structures in the central nervous system have more than one function. Go over the disorder chart. If you remember the general functions of the sympathetic and parasympathetic nervous systems, the specific effects will be easier to remember. Also review the questions at the end of the chapter and discuss possible test questions.

Case Studies

1. Tony's teachers describe him as a daydreamer. The teachers often find him staring off into space when they are trying to get his attention. When Tony's parents mentioned this to their family physician, the possibility of epilepsy was brought up by the physician. Could Tony's daydreaming be a sign of epilepsy? What test could help confirm such a diagnosis? What signs would one look for in such a test if epilepsy is present?

2. Over the last few years, your friend Angela has developed fibrous nodules in many areas of her skin. She recently confided that she has an inherited disorder of the nervous system that causes these bumps. What disease might Angela have? How can a nervous disorder cause skin lesions?

3. Baraka loves to dance. However, he and his friends notice that he misses easy steps more and more often. In fact, Baraka almost seems intoxicated his coordination is so badly affected. Baraka's physicians tell him that he has a myelin disorder. How would such a disorder cause Baraka's symptoms? Name a specific myelin disorder and explain how this disease causes similar problems.

Outline

Objectives

**After you have completed this chapter,
you should be able to:**

1. Classify sense organs as special
   or general and explain the basic
   differences between the two groups.

2. Discuss how a stimulus is converted
   into a sensation.

3. Discuss the general sense organs and
   their functions.

4. List the major senses.

5. Describe the structure of the eye and
   the functions of its components.

6. Name and describe the major visual
   disorders.

7. Discuss the anatomy of the ear and
   its sensory function in hearing and
   equilibrium.

8. Name and describe the major forms of
   hearing impairment.

9. Discuss the chemical receptors and
   their functions.

10 The Senses

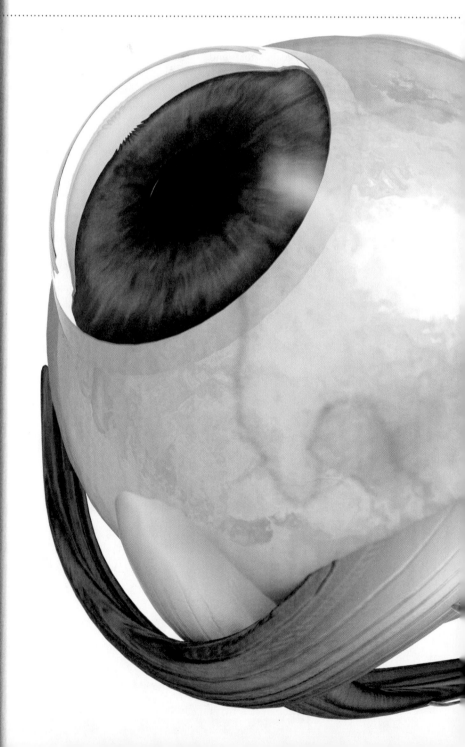

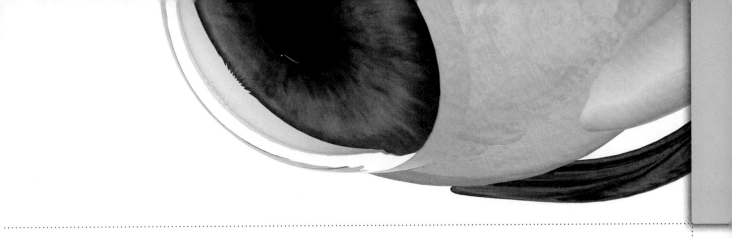

If you were asked to name the sense organs, what organs would you name? Can you think of any besides the eyes, ears, nose, and taste buds? Actually there are millions of other sense organs throughout the body in our skin, internal organs, and muscles. They constitute the many **sensory receptors** that allow us to respond to stimuli such as touch, pressure, temperature, and pain. These microscopic receptors are located at the tips of dendrites of sensory neurons.

Our ability to "sense" changes in our external and internal environments is a requirement for maintaining homeostasis and for survival itself. We can initiate protective reflexes important to homeostasis only if we can sense a change or danger. External dangers may be detected by sight or hearing. If the danger is internal, such as overstretching a muscle, detecting an increase in body temperature (fever), or sensing the pain caused by an ulcer, we have other receptors that make us aware of the problem, which makes it possible for us to then take appropriate action to maintain homeostasis.

STUDY TIPS

Each of the body's senses must go through the following processes to perform its function: (1) detect the physical stimulus to which it responds and (2) convert that stimulus into a nerve impulse. For example, the eye must let light in and focus it on a specific point; the receptors convert that stimulus into a nerve impulse and send it to the brain.

1. When you study structures and their specific function in a sensory system, focus on how they contribute to one of these two processes. Use flash cards to learn the specific structures and their functions in each sensory system. Link the disorders in the sensory system to their cause or mechanism. In the eye, these are refraction, retinal damage, or pathway damage. In the ear, conduction, infection, or nerve damage may cause disorders. A chart may be the best way to organize this information.

continued on page 307

Classification of Sense Organs

The sense organs are often classified as *special* sense organs and *general* sense organs. Special sense organs, such as the eye, are characterized by large and complex organs or by localized groupings of specialized receptors in areas such as the nasal mucosa or tongue. The general sense organs for detecting stimuli such as pain and touch are microscopic receptors widely distributed throughout the body.

Receptors are often classified according to the types of stimuli that activate them and whether they are *encapsulated* or *unencapsulated*, that is, whether they are covered by some sort of capsule or are "free" or "naked" of any such covering. Receptors in the retina of the eye are stimulated by light (*photoreceptors*), whereas taste and smell are activated by chemical stimuli (*chemoreceptors*). Still other receptors respond to physical damage or injury (*pain receptors*), changes in temperature (*thermoreceptors*), or mechanical stimuli that change their position or in some way deform the capsule that surrounds them (*mechanoreceptors*). Table 10-1 classifies the general sense organs, and Table 10-2 on p. 283 classifies the special sense organs.

Table 10-1	**General Sense Organs**		
TYPE		**MAIN LOCATIONS**	**GENERAL SENSES**
FREE NERVE ENDINGS			
(Naked nerve ending; several types exist)		Skin and mucosa (epithelial layers)	Pain, discriminative touch, tickle, and temperature
ENCAPSULATED NERVE ENDINGS			
Bulboid (Krause) corpuscle		Skin (dermal layer), subcutaneous tissue, mucosa of lips and eyelids, and external genitals	Touch and possibly cold
Lamellar (Pacini) corpuscle		Subcutaneous, submucous, and subserous tissues; around joints; in mammary glands and external genitals of both sexes	Pressure and high-frequency vibration
Tactile (Meissner) corpuscle		Skin (in papillae of dermis) and fingertips and lips (numerous)	Fine touch and low-frequency vibration
Bulbous (Ruffini) corpuscle		Skin (dermal layer) and subcutaneous tissue of fingers	Touch and pressure
Golgi tendon receptor		Near junction of tendons and muscles	Proprioception (sense of muscle tension)
Muscle spindle	Intrafusal fibers	Skeletal muscles	Proprioception (sense of muscle length)

Table 10-2 | Special Sense Organs

SENSE ORGAN	SPECIFIC RECEPTOR	TYPE OF RECEPTOR	SENSE
Eye	Rods and cones	Photoreceptor	Vision
Ear	Organ of Corti (spiral organ)	Mechanoreceptor	Hearing
	Cristae ampullares	Mechanoreceptor	Balance
Nose	Olfactory cells	Chemoreceptor	Smell
Taste buds	Gustatory cells	Chemoreceptor	Taste

Converting a Stimulus into a Sensation

All sense organs, regardless of size, type, or location, have in common some important functional characteristics. First, they must be able to sense or detect a stimulus in their environment. Of course, different sense organs detect different types of stimuli. Whether it is light, sound, temperature change, mechanical pressure, or the presence of chemicals ultimately identified as taste or smell, the stimulus must be changed into an electrical signal or nerve impulse. This signal is then transmitted over a nervous system "pathway" to the brain, where the sensation is actually perceived.

General Sense Organs

Groups of receptors within specific, complex sensory organs are typically associated with the special senses. In the general sense organs, however, receptors are found scattered within almost every part of the body. However, they are most concentrated in the skin (Figure 10-1). To demonstrate this fact, try touching your skin at any point over a fingertip with the tip of a toothpick. You can hardly miss stimulating at least one receptor and almost instantaneously experiencing a sensation of touch.

The ability to distinguish one touch stimulus from two is called "two-point discrimination." A neurological test that measures this function involves simultaneously touching two points on the skin over one area of the body to determine whether the ability to feel the two separate stimuli is present. The skin over different parts of the body will respond differently because of the differing numbers of touch receptors that are present. Touch receptors are distributed closely together over the fingertips (2-8 mm apart), relatively close together over the palms (8-12 mm), and quite far apart over the back of the torso (40-60 mm). Lesions to the parietal lobe of the brain will impair two-point discrimination.

Stimulation of some receptors leads to the sensation of vibration; stimulation of others gives the sensation of pressure, and stimulation of still others gives the sensation of pain or temperature. General sense receptors are listed in Table 10-1 and illustrated in Figure 10-1.

Some general sense receptors found near the point of junction between tendons and muscles and others found deep within skeletal muscle tissue are called **proprioceptors.** When stimulated, they provide us with information concerning the position or movement of the different parts of the body as well as the length and the extent of contraction of our muscles.

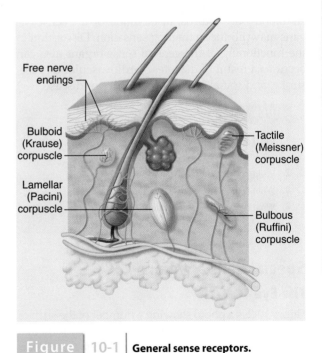

Free nerve endings

Bulboid (Krause) corpuscle

Lamellar (Pacini) corpuscle

Tactile (Meissner) corpuscle

Bulbous (Ruffini) corpuscle

Figure 10-1 | General sense receptors.

This section of skin shows the placement of a number of receptors described in Table 10-1.

The Golgi tendon receptors and muscle spindles identified in Table 10-1 are important proprioceptors.

Many general sense receptors are present deep in the body. For example, there are stretch receptors in your stomach that signal you when it is full. There are also stretch (pressure) receptors in most other hollow organs such as the stomach and intestines, arteries, vagina (birth canal), and urinary bladder that enable the normal functioning of those organs. There are also important chemical receptors in the aorta and other arteries that detect changes in pH and carbon dioxide levels in the blood—important information for regulating breathing and heart rate.

Disruption of general sense organs can occur by means of a variety of mechanisms. For example, third-degree burns can completely destroy general sense receptors throughout the affected area. Temporary impairment of general sense receptors occurs when the blood flow to them is slowed. This commonly occurs when you put your legs in a position (such as crossing them above the knee or folding a leg under yourself as you sit) that causes pressure to be applied to your legs in a way that reduces blood flow. When you try to stand up, you cannot feel your legs because the general sense organs are temporarily impaired. You may not even be able to walk at first because you cannot tell where your legs are without looking at them. As blood flow returns, reactivation of the sense organs may produce a tingling sensation. Disruption in the functioning of the general sense organs also can occur as a result of diabetes, cardiovascular disease, stroke, and spinal cord or brain injury or disease.

QUICK CHECK

1. What are different ways that sense organs can be classified into types?
2. Where is a sensation actually perceived?
3. What is the function of a *proprioceptor*?
4. What is *two-point discrimination*?

Special Sense Organs

The Eye

Figure 10-2 is a photo showing a number of the surface features of the eye. But when you actually look at a person's eye, as in this photo, you see only a small part of the whole eye. There is much more to this amazing and complex organ than can be seen from the outside.

Figure 10-3 shows that there are three layers of tissue forming the eyeball: the **sclera** (SKLEER-ah), the **choroid** (KOH-royd), and the **retina** (RET-i-nah).

The outer layer of sclera consists of tough fibrous tissue. The "white" of the eye is part of the front surface of the sclera (Figure 10-2). The other part of the front surface of the sclera is called the *cornea* and is sometimes spoken of as the "window" of the eye because of its transparency. The cornea is covered by a thin membrane that may be damaged by foreign objects, chemical irritants, or trauma. Wearing contact lenses that are dirty or left in longer than intended may increase the risk of developing *corneal ulcers* in otherwise healthy eyes. At a casual glance, the cornea does not look transparent but appears blue, brown, gray, or green because it lies over the **iris**, the circular colored part of the eye (Figures 10-2 and 10-3).

When the eyes are open, the *palpebral* (pal-PEH-brul) *fissure*—the opening outlined by the eyelash-lined upper and lower eyelids—is apparent. The upper eyelid partially overlaps the iris, whereas the lower lid touches the lower margin of the iris (Figure 10-2). Significant changes in the size of the palpebral fissure can be a sign of endocrine or nervous system disease.

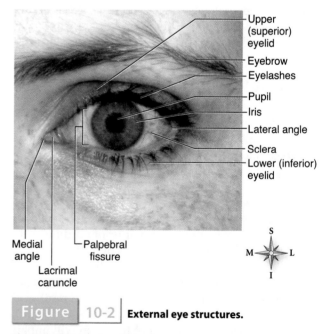

Medial angle · Lacrimal caruncle · Palpebral fissure · Upper (superior) eyelid · Eyebrow · Eyelashes · Pupil · Iris · Lateral angle · Sclera · Lower (inferior) eyelid

Figure 10-2 **External eye structures.**

Photo showing surface features.

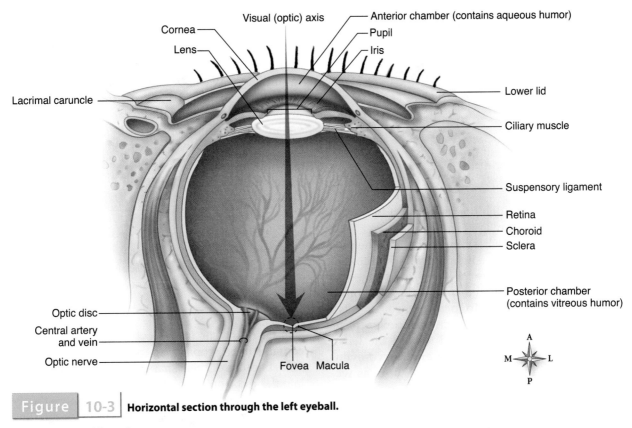

Visual (optic) axis

Cornea

Lens

Lacrimal caruncle

Anterior chamber (contains aqueous humor)

Pupil

Iris

Lower lid

Ciliary muscle

Suspensory ligament

Retina

Choroid

Sclera

Posterior chamber
(contains vitreous humor)

Optic disc

Central artery
and vein

Optic nerve

Fovea Macula

A

M — L

P

Figure 10-3 | **Horizontal section through the left eyeball.**

The eye as viewed from above.

Also visible in Figure 10-2 is the pink *lacrimal caruncle* (KAR-un-kul), a glandular structure located at the *medial angle*—the junction of the upper and lower lids near the nose. The lacrimal caruncle and the sebaceous secreting *tarsal*, or *meibomian* (mee-BOH-mee-an), *glands*, which line the inner surface of the eyelids, can sometimes become infected—frequently with staphylococcal organisms. One of the most common external eye infections involves the hair follicles of the eyelashes. The result is a painful swelling called a *sty* (Figure 10-4). A mucous membrane known as the **conjunctiva** (kon-JUNK-ty-vah) lines the underside of the eyelids and covers the sclera in front. The conjunctiva is kept moist by tears formed in the **lacrimal gland** located in the upper lateral portion of the orbit.

The middle layer of the eyeball, the *choroid*, contains a dark pigment that prevents the scattering of incoming light rays. Two involuntary muscles make up the front part of the choroid. One is the *iris*, the colored circular structure seen through the cornea, and the other is the *ciliary muscle* (Figure 10-3). The

black center of the iris is really a hole in this doughnut-shaped muscle; it is the **pupil** of the eye. Some of the fibers of the iris are arranged like spokes in a wheel. When they contract, the pupils dilate, letting in more light rays. Other fibers are circular. When they contract, the pupils constrict, letting in fewer

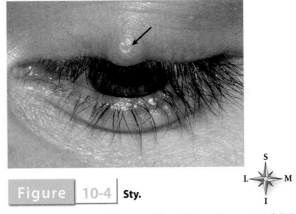

Figure 10-4 | **Sty.**

S

L — M

I

The arrow points to swelling caused by infection of an eyelash follicle.

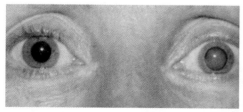

Figure 10-5 **Cataract.**

Notice the cloudiness of the left eye.

In most young people, the lens is both transparent and somewhat elastic, making it capable of easily changing shape. Unfortunately, in some individuals, longtime exposure to ultraviolet (UV) radiation in sunlight may cause the lens to become hard, lose its transparency, and become "milky" in appearance. This condition is called a **cataract** (Figure 10-5). Cataract formation may occur in one or both eyes, tends to be progressive, and may result in blindness. Cataracts can be removed surgically and the defective lens replaced with an artificial implant.

QUICK CHECK

1. What are the three layers of the eyeball?
2. What is the "hole" in the doughnut-shaped iris called?
3. What is an infection of a hair follicle in the eyelash called?
4. What eye structure is affected when a cataract forms?

---

light rays. Normally, the pupils constrict in bright light and dilate in dim light.

The **lens** of the eye lies directly behind the pupil. It is held in place by a ligament attached to the ciliary muscle. When we look at distant objects, the ciliary muscle is relaxed, and the lens has only a slightly curved shape. To focus on near objects, the ciliary muscle must contract. As it contracts, it pulls the choroid coat forward toward the lens, thus causing the lens to bulge and curve even more. Most of us become more farsighted as we grow older and lose the ability to focus on close objects because our lenses lose their elasticity and can no longer bulge enough to bring near objects into focus. **Presbyopia** or "old-sightedness" is the name for this condition.

The **retina,** or innermost layer, of the eyeball contains microscopic receptor cells, called *rods* and *cones* because of their shapes. Dim light can stimulate the rods, but fairly bright light is necessary to stimulate the cones. In other words, **rods** are the receptors for night vision and **cones** for daytime vision. There are three kinds of cones; each is sensitive to a different color: red, green, or blue. These three types of cones allow us to distinguish between different colors.

Rods and cones differ in number and distribution as well as function. Cones are less numerous than rods and are most

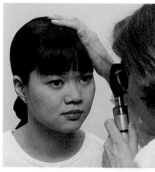

A

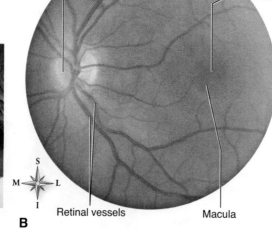

Optic disc

Fovea centralis

Retinal vessels

Macula

B

Figure 10-6

Using an ophthalmoscope to view the retina (fundus) of the left eye.

A, Ophthalmoscope examination.
B, Appearance of retinal structures.

densely concentrated in the **fovea,** a small depression in the center of a yellowish area called the **macula** found near the center of the retina (see Figure 10-3). This area of the retina serves as the site of acute image formation and color vision. Rods are absent entirely from the fovea and macula but are found in increasing numbers near the periphery of the retina.

The use of an **ophthalmoscope** (of-THAL-mahskop) makes it possible to examine the retinal surface, called the *fundus,* and internal eye structures (Figure 10-6). In addition to the macula and fovea, the ophthalmoscope allows the trained observer to see the creamy yellow optic disc and the retinal blood vessels. Nerve fibers exit the eye through the optic disc and then form the optic nerve (Figure 10-3). Rods or cones are not present in the optic disc area of the retina. The result is a *"blind spot"* in the visual field in both eyes (see box, Finding Your Blind Spot). Changes in the appearance of the fundus and retinal structures are signs used to diagnose such diverse conditions as increased intracranial pressure, diabetes, hypertension, and *shaken baby syndrome* (Figure 10-7).

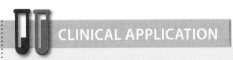

CLINICAL APPLICATION

FINDING YOUR BLIND SPOT

You can demonstrate the location of the blind spot in your visual field by covering your left eye and looking at the objects below. Begin by positioning your face about 35 cm (12 in) away from this page. Cover your left eye and stare continuously at the square with your right eye while slowly bringing your face closer and closer to the image. At one point, the circle will seem to disappear because its image has fallen on the blind spot.

Fluids fill the hollow inside of the eyeball. They maintain the normal shape of the eyeball and help refract light rays; that is, the fluids bend light rays in a way that focuses them on the retina. **Aqueous humor** is the name of the watery fluid found in front of the lens (in the anterior cavity of the eye), and **vitreous humor** is the name of the jelly-like fluid behind the lens (in the posterior cavity). Aqueous humor is constantly being formed, drained, and replaced in the anterior cavity. If drainage is blocked for any reason, the internal pressure within the eye will increase, and damage that could lead to blindness will occur. This condition is called **glaucoma** (glaw-KOH-mah).

VISUAL PATHWAY

Light is the stimulus that results in vision (that is, our ability to see objects as they exist in our environment). Light enters the eye through the pupil and is *refracted,* or bent, so that it is focused on the retina. Refraction occurs as light passes through the cornea, the aqueous humor, the lens, and the vitreous humor on its way to the retina.

The innermost layer of the retina contains the rods and cones, which are the **photoreceptor** cells

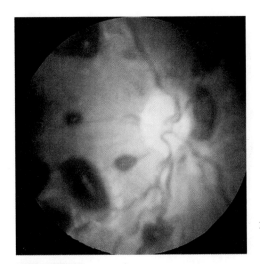

Figure 10-7 | **Shaken baby syndrome.**

Ophthalmoscope view shows multiple hemorrhages of the retina typical of this type of child abuse.

of the eye (Figure 10-8). They respond to a light stimulus by producing a nervous impulse. The rod and cone photoreceptor cells synapse with neurons in the bipolar and ganglionic layers of the retina. Nervous signals eventually leave the retina through the optic disc and form the optic nerve on the posterior surface of the eyeball (Figure 10-3).

After leaving the eye, the optic nerves enter the brain and travel to the visual cortex of the occipital lobe (Figure 10-9). In this area, *visual interpretation* of the nervous impulses generated by light stimuli in the rods and cones of the retina results in "seeing."

 To learn more about the process of seeing, go to **AnimationDirect** on your CD.

Visual Disorders

Healthy vision requires three basic processes: formation of an image on the

retina (refraction), stimulation of rods and cones, and conduction of nerve impulses to the brain. Malfunction of any of these processes can disrupt this chain of processes, producing a visual disorder.

REFRACTION DISORDERS

Focusing a clear image on the retina is essential for good vision. In the normal eye, light rays enter the eye and are focused into a clear, upside-down image on the retina (Figure 10-10, *A*). The brain can easily right the upside-down image in our conscious perception but cannot correct an image that is not sharply focused. If our eyeballs are elongated, the image focuses in front of the retina rather than on it. The retina receives only a fuzzy image. This condition, called **myopia** or *nearsightedness*, can be corrected by refractive eye surgery (see box on p. 293) or by using contact lenses or glasses (Figure 10-10, *B* and *C*). If our eyeballs are shorter (as measured from front to back) than normal, the image focuses behind the retina, also producing a fuzzy image. This

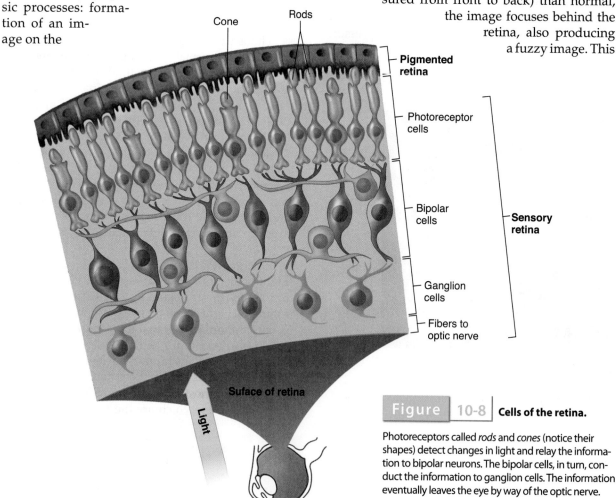

Figure 10-8 **Cells of the retina.**

Photoreceptors called *rods* and *cones* (notice their shapes) detect changes in light and relay the information to bipolar neurons. The bipolar cells, in turn, conduct the information to ganglion cells. The information eventually leaves the eye by way of the optic nerve.

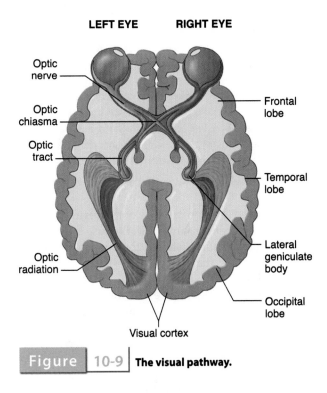

LEFT EYE   **RIGHT EYE**

Optic nerve

Optic chiasma

Optic tract

Optic radiation

Frontal lobe

Temporal lobe

Lateral geniculate body

Occipital lobe

Visual cortex

Figure 10-9 **The visual pathway.**

condition, called **hyperopia** or *farsightedness,* also can be corrected by eye surgery or lenses (Figure 10-10, *D* and *E*).

A variety of other conditions can prevent the formation of a clear image on the retina. For example, the inability to focus the lens properly as we age, referred to as *presbyopia,* has already been discussed. Older individuals can compensate for presbyopia by using "reading glasses" when near vision is needed. An irregularity (unequal curvature) in the cornea or lens, a condition called **astigmatism** (ah-STIG-mah-tiz-em) that distorts vision, also can be corrected with glasses or contact lenses. *Cataracts,* cloudy spots in the eye's lens that develop as we age, also may interfere with focusing (Figure 10-5). Cataracts are especially troublesome in dim light because weak beams of light cannot pass through the cloudy spots the way some brighter light can. This fact accounts for the trouble many older adults have with their "night vision." Although the tendency to develop cataracts is inherited, the disorder can be treated successfully with lens implant surgery.

Infections of the eye and its associated structures also have the potential to impair vision, sometimes permanently. Most eye infections start out in the con-

junctiva, producing an inflammation response known as "pink eye" or **conjunctivitis** (kon-junk-ti-VYE-tis). You may recall from Chapter 5 that a variety of different pathogens can cause conjunctivitis. For example, the bacterium *Chlamydia trachomatis* that commonly infects the reproductive tract can cause a chronic infection called *chlamydial conjunctivitis* or **trachoma.** Because chlamydia and other pathogens often inhabit the birth canal, antibiotics are routinely applied to the eyes of newborns to prevent conjunctivitis. Highly contagious *acute bacterial conjunctivitis,* characterized by drainage of a mucous pus

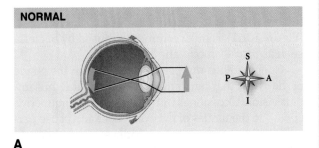

NORMAL

A

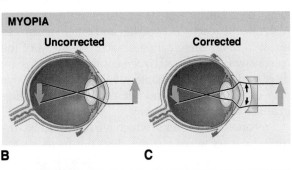

MYOPIA

Uncorrected   **Corrected**

B   **C**

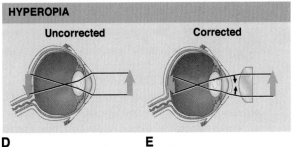

HYPEROPIA

Uncorrected   **Corrected**

D   **E**

Figure 10-10 **Refraction.**

A, Shows how light is refracted in the normal eye to form a well-focused image on the retina. **B** and **C,** The abnormal and corrected refraction observed in patients with myopia, or nearsightedness. **D** and **E,** Abnormal and corrected refraction in patients with hyperopia, or farsightedness.

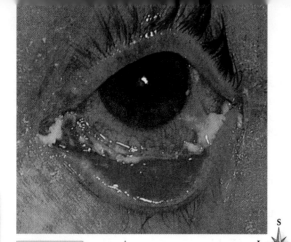

Figure 10-11 **Acute bacterial conjunctivitis.**

Notice the discharge of mucous pus characteristic of this highly contagious infection of the conjunctiva.

S
L — M
I

RESEARCH, ISSUES, AND TRENDS

CORNEAL RING IMPLANTS

One treatment of mild to moderate nearsightedness (myopia) involves implantation of tiny plastic rings around the edge of the cornea. These transparent rings, called *Intacs,* flatten the cornea without any actual cutting or shaving of the corneal surface or underlying tissue that occurs during incisional, radiofrequency energy, or laser-based refractive eye surgery techniques. If the result of Intac placement is not satisfactory, they can be removed and visual acuity will revert to preimplantation levels.

(Figure 10-11), is most commonly caused by bacteria such as *Staphylococcus* and *Haemophilus.*

Conjunctivitis may produce lesions on the inside of the eyelid that can damage the cornea and thus impair vision. Occasionally infections of the conjunctiva spread to the tissues of the eye proper and cause permanent injury—even total blindness. In addition to infection, conjunctivitis also may be caused by allergies. The red, itchy, watery eyes commonly associated with allergic reactions to pollen and other substances result from an allergic inflammation response of the conjunctiva. Allergy and hypersensitivity reactions are discussed further in Chapter 15. Trauma to the eye may cause bleeding below the conjunctiva resulting in a *subconjunctival hemorrhage.*

Yet another manner in which refraction can be disrupted occurs when one eye does not focus on the same object as the other eye. Normally, we use *binocu-* lar ("two-eyed") vision in which both eyes aim toward the same object at the same time. Because the eyes are separated by a short distance, the images formed in each eye do not match exactly—a fact that allows *depth perception.*

If the positioning of the eyes cannot be coordinated, a condition called **strabismus** (strah-BIS-mus) or "squint" results. In some cases, the eyes may diverge outward to the side, a condition called *divergent squint.* If one or both eyes converge toward the nose, the condition is called *convergent squint* or "cross-eye." The photo in Figure 10-12 shows a child with convergent left eye strabismus. Usually the brain compensates for missing or unusual elements in the visual field. However, in severe cases of strabismus, the eyes may be so far off in their center of focus that the brain cannot mesh the two resulting images into a single picture.

Strabismus is usually caused by paralysis, weakness, or another abnormality affecting the external muscles of the eye. Whatever the cause, strabismus often can be corrected by treatment in early childhood that forces the eyes to focus together, by means of cor-

---

RESEARCH, ISSUES, AND TRENDS

CORNEAL STEM CELL TRANSPLANTS

A new treatment for individuals who may be totally blind because of certain eye diseases or because of scarring caused by abrasion or chemical burns to their corneas may make it possible for them to see again. If, because of accident or disease, the clear membrane covering the cornea is permanently destroyed and cannot be regenerated, blindness results. In these cases, traditional corneal transplants are not possible because the clear membrane normally formed by the eye of the recipient, and necessary for survival of the transplanted tissue, has been damaged or destroyed. Research now indicates that **corneal stem cell transplants** can restore and maintain the clear covering membrane of the cornea that may have been destroyed by disease or injury.

In this procedure, adult stem cells that have the ability to develop into the clear covering membrane of the cornea are first harvested from the corneas of cadavers and then transplanted into and around the edges of the diseased or damaged corneas of the blind recipient. The new stem cells then produce the clear corneal surface membrane required for normal vision. This technique is still in the research stage and has limited applications so far. Problems associated with rejection of the foreign stem cells and suppression of the immune system of the recipient must still be resolved. However, when these hurdles have been surmounted, this exciting new development in clinical medicine will become an option for effectively treating blindness that was considered permanent in the past.

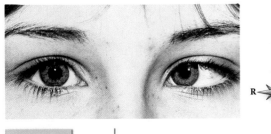

Figure 10-12 **Strabismus.**

This child exhibits convergent left eye strabismus.

rective lenses or by corrective surgery. If left untreated, by about 6 years of age the visual centers in the brain will learn to ignore information from one eye—causing a decrease in visual acuity and permanent blindness in the affected eye.

> **QUICK CHECK**
>
> 1. What are the humors of the eye?
> 2. How are rods and cones used in vision? How are they alike? How are they different?
> 3. How do myopia and hyperopia differ in terms of focusing an image on the retina?
> 4. What is trachoma?

DISORDERS OF THE RETINA

Damage to the retina impairs vision because even a well-focused image cannot be perceived if some or all of the light receptors do not function properly. For example, in a condition called *retinal detachment,* part of the retina falls away from the tissue supporting it. This condition often results from normal aging, eye tumors, or from sudden blows to the head—as in a sporting injury. Common warning signs include the sudden appearance of floating spots that may decrease over a period of weeks and odd "flashes of light" that appear when the eye moves. If left untreated, the retina may detach completely and cause total blindness in the affected eye. A number of treatments are available for correcting retinal detachment. A traditional approach is the use of laser therapy. Another approach involves placing a tight collar around the eyeball to increase pressure within the eye. The high pressure of the vitreous humor holds the retina in place against the rear of the eyeball.

Diabetes mellitus, a disorder involving the hormone insulin, may cause a condition known as **diabetic retinopathy** (ret-in-OP-ah-thee). In this disorder, diabetes causes small hemorrhages in retinal blood vessels that disrupt the oxygen supply to the photoreceptors. The eye responds by building new but abnormal vessels that block vision and may cause detachment of the retina. Diabetic retinopathy is considered one of the leading causes of blindness in the United States. Fortunately, treatments developed over the last two decades have improved the outlook in this regard. For example, a type of laser therapy in which laser beams are used to seal off hemorrhaging retinal vessels has been used successfully in many cases.

Another common condition that can damage the retina is **glaucoma**. Recall that glaucoma is excessive *intraocular* (in-trah-AHK-yoo-lar) *pressure* caused by abnormal accumulation of aqueous humor. As fluid pressure against the retina increases above normal, blood flow through the retina slows. Reduced blood flow causes degeneration of the retina and thus a loss of vision. Although acute forms of glaucoma can occur, most cases develop slowly over a period of years. This chronic form may not produce symptoms, especially in its early stages. For this reason, routine eye examinations typically include a screening test for glaucoma. As chronic glaucoma progresses, damage first appears at the edges of the retina, causing a gradual loss of peripheral vision resulting in a condition known commonly as "tunnel vision." Blurred vision and headaches also may occur. As the damage becomes more extensive, "halos" are seen around bright lights. If untreated, glaucoma eventually produces total, permanent blindness.

Degeneration of the retina can cause difficulty seeing at night or in dim light. This condition, called **nyctalopia** (nik-tah-LOH-pee-ah) or "night blindness," also can be caused by a deficiency of vitamin A. Vitamin A is needed to make *photopigment* in rod cells. Photopigment is a light-sensitive chemical that triggers stimulation of the visual nerve pathway. A lack of vitamin A may result in a lack of photopigment in rods, a condition that impairs dim-light vision.

The leading cause of permanent blindness in the elderly is progressive degeneration of the central part of the retina. Called *age-related* **macular degeneration**, this condition affects the part of the retina that is most essential to good vision—the central region called the *macula.* The exact cause of the degeneration is unknown, but the risk for developing this condition increases with age after reaching 50 (see box at bottom of p. 292). Other known risk factors include cigarette smoking and a family history of the disorder.

Retinal disorders are sometimes inherited. Most forms of **color blindness** are caused by genes on the X chromosome that produce abnormal photopigments in the cones. Each of three photopigments in cones is sensitive to one of the primary colors of light: green, blue, and red. In many color-blind individuals, the green-sensitive photopigment is missing or deficient; at other times, the red-sensitive photopigment is abnormal. (Deficiency of the blue-sensitive photopigment

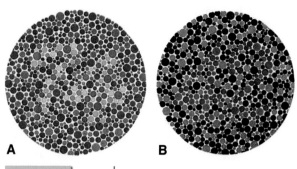

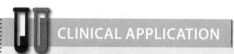

Figure 10-13 **Color vision screening figures.**

A, People with normal color vision can see *74* in this mosaic; people with red-green color blindness cannot. **B,** This mosaic is used to classify the type of red-green color blindness a patient has. If the patient sees only the *2,* the red-sensitive cones are abnormal. If only the *4* is seen, the green-sensitive cones are abnormal.

is very rare.) Color-blind individuals see colors, but they cannot distinguish between them normally. Because color blindness is an X-linked genetic trait, more men than women have this condition (see Chapter 24). Although color blindness is an abnormality, it is not usually considered a clinical disease.

Colored figures are often used to screen individuals for color blindness (Figure 10-13). A person with red-green color blindness cannot see the number 74 in

CLINICAL APPLICATION

VISUAL ACUITY

Visual acuity is the clearness or sharpness of visual perception. Acuity is affected by our focusing ability, the efficiency of the retina, and the proper function of the visual pathway and processing centers in the brain.

One common way to measure visual acuity is to use the familiar test chart on which letters or other objects of various sizes and shapes are printed. The subject is asked to identify the smallest object that he or she can see from a distance of 20 feet (6.1 m). The resulting determination of visual acuity is expressed as a double number such as "20-20." The first number represents the distance (in feet) between the subject and the test chart—the standard being 20. The second number represents the number of feet a person with normal acuity would have to stand away from the chart to see the same objects clearly. Thus a finding of 20-20 is normal because the subject can see at 20 feet what a person with normal acuity can see at 20 feet. A person with 20-100 vision can see objects at 20 feet that a person with normal vision can see at 100 feet away.

People whose acuity is worse than 20-200 after correction are considered to be *legally blind.* Legal blindness is the designation used to identify the severity of a wide variety of visual disorders so that laws that involve visual acuity can be enforced. For example, laws that govern the awarding of driving licenses require that drivers have a minimum level of visual acuity.

CLINICAL APPLICATION

MACULAR DEGENERATION

A serious and widespread visual problem affecting more than 1.5 million Americans over age 65 is called *age-related macular degeneration (AMD).* Nearly one third of people age 80 or older show some signs of the disease. AMD seldom (less than 3% of affected individuals) results in total blindness. Instead, as the disease progresses, the central visual field is lost and the ability to distinguish fine detail diminishes. Although varying amounts of peripheral vision remain, AMD patients are unable to read or drive and other daily activities are severely restricted because of the loss of clear "straight-ahead" sight.

The most common form of AMD is called *"dry"* AMD. This form of the disease causes gradual and progressive loss of central vision and no effective treatment is currently available. The less common (10% to 15% of cases) but more severe type of AMD is called *"wet"* AMD. In these patients, fragile and hemorrhage-prone blood vessels develop behind the macula (see Figure 10-3). Leaking blood vessels in pa-

tients with wet AMD damage the retina over the macula, and loss of central vision occurs.

In the past, treatment of wet AMD was limited to *photocoagulation therapy.* During this treatment, leaking blood vessels were sealed using a "hot" laser to coagulate the blood. Unfortunately, the treatment often damaged the sensitive retina and loss of vision occured. The subsequent development of *photodynamic therapy* resulted in the availability of a less damaging treatment option. In this procedure use of a "cool" laser beam activates a highly selective light-sensitive drug (verteporfin) that is injected intravenously. When the drug is activated it selectively destroys only the abnormal wet AMD blood vessels without damaging the overlying retina. Advances in wet AMD treatment now include the drug pegaptanib (Mucagen) and, more recently, introduction of ranibizumab (Lucentis) which is a monoclonal antibody produced pharmaceutical (see p. 431). The goal of current treatments is at least a reduction in continued vision loss if not actual improvement in straight-ahead vision that has already been damaged.

Figure 10-13, *A,* whereas a person with normal color vision can. To determine which photopigment is deficient, red or green, a color-blind person may be evaluated using a figure similar to Figure 10-13, *B.* Persons with a deficiency of red-sensitive photopigment can distinguish only the number *2;* those deficient in green-sensitive photopigment can see only the number *4.*

QUICK CHECK

1. How do the various types of refractory eye surgery improve eyesight? What is LASIK?
2. How does glaucoma harm the retina?
3. What is nyctalopia? What type of vitamin deficiency is associated with this condition?

CLINICAL APPLICATION

REFRACTIVE EYE SURGERY

A surgery technique used to treat myopia (nearsightedness) without the use of eyeglasses or contact lenses became available almost 25 years ago. The procedure, called **radial keratotomy (RK),** involves surgical placement of six or more radial slits (incisions) in a spokelike pattern around the cornea. As a result, the cornea flattens and the ability to focus improves. Other types of refractory eye surgery involving incisions include **astigmatic keratotomy (AK),** which involves treatment of astigmatism by placement of transverse cuts across the corneal surface, and **automated lamellar keratoplasty (ALK).** The ALK technique uses a special surgical device called a *microkeratome* to cut a thin cap off the corneal surface and then shave and reshape the underlying tissue. At the end of the procedure the corneal cap is put back in place and will heal without the need for sutures. ALK is used to treat both myopia and hyperopia (farsightedness).

More recent advances in refractory eye surgery involve the use of surgical lasers. **Excimer laser surgery,** also called **photorefractive keratectomy (PRK),** uses a "cool" excimer laser beam to vaporize corneal tissue. It is used to flatten the cornea to correct mild to moderate nearsightedness. An eye refractive surgery procedure often used to correct myopia is called **laser-assisted in situ keratomileusis (LASIK).** This procedure employs both PRK and ALK techniques. First, a microkeratome is used to create a hinged cap of tissue, which is lifted off the corneal surface **(A).** An excimer laser is then used to vaporize and reshape the underlying tissue **(B).** At the end of the procedure, the cap is replaced **(C).** Another laser surgery technique approved for treating hyperopia (farsightedness) is **laser thermal keratoplasty (LTK).** It employs ultra-short bursts of laser energy (about 3 seconds for each burst) to reshape the surface of the cornea, with no surgical cutting involved. Farsightedness is also treated by a technique called **conductive keratoplasty (CK);** it employs radiofrequency energy to heat hair-thin probes that are then used to change the shape of the cornea.

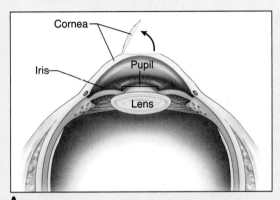

A

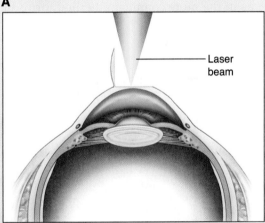

B

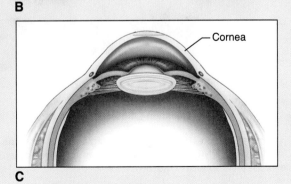

C

DISORDERS OF THE VISUAL PATHWAY

Damage or degeneration in the optic nerve, the brain, or any part of the visual pathway between them can impair vision (Figure 10-9). For example, the pressure associated with glaucoma also can damage the optic nerve. Diabetes, already cited as a cause of retina damage, also can cause degeneration of the optic nerve.

Damage to the visual pathway does not always result in total loss of sight. Depending on where the damage occurs, only a part of the visual field may be affected. For example, a certain form of neuritis often associated with multiple sclerosis can cause loss of only the center of the visual field—a condition called **scotoma** (skoh-TOH-mah).

A cerebrovascular accident (CVA), or stroke, can cause vision impairment when the resulting tissue damage occurs in one of the regions of the brain that process visual information (see Figure 9-13). For example, damage to an area that processes information about colors may result in a rare condition called *acquired cortical color blindness.* This condition is characterized by difficulty in distinguishing any color—not just one or two colors as in the more common inherited forms of color blindness.

The Ear

In addition to its role in hearing, the ear also functions as the sense organ of equilibrium and balance. As we shall later see, the stimulation, or "trigger," that activates receptors involved with hearing and equilibrium is mechanical, and the receptors themselves are called **mechanoreceptors** (mek-an-oh-ree-SEP-tors). Physical forces that involve sound vibrations and fluid movements are responsible for initiating nervous impulses that are eventually perceived as sound and balance.

The ear is more than an appendage on the side of the head. A large part of the ear and its most important part lies hidden from view deep inside the temporal bone. The ear is divided into the following anatomical areas (Figures 10-14 and 10-16):

1. External ear
2. Middle ear
3. Inner (internal) ear

EXTERNAL EAR

The external ear has two parts: the **auricle** (AW-ri-kul), or pinna, and the **external acoustic canal.** The auricle is the appendage on the side of the head surrounding the opening of the external acoustic

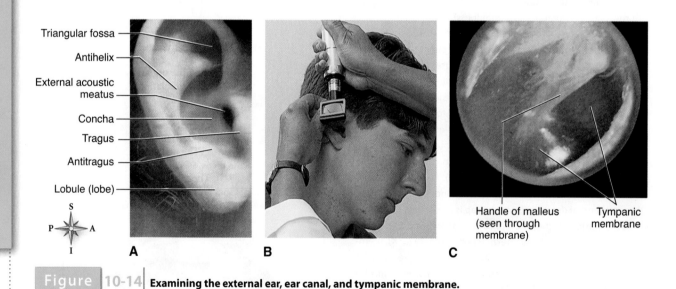

Triangular fossa
Antihelix
External acoustic meatus
Concha
Tragus
Antitragus
Lobule (lobe)

A **B** **C**

Handle of malleus (seen through membrane)   Tympanic membrane

Figure 10-14 **Examining the external ear, ear canal, and tympanic membrane.**

A, Anatomical structures of the auricle. **B,** Using a lighted otoscope to view the external ear canal and tympanic membrane. **C,** Note the translucent, pearly-gray appearance of a normal tympanic membrane. The "handle" of the malleus can be seen attaching near the center of the inner surface of the membrane.

canal. A number of the anatomical landmarks of the external ear are identified in Figure 10-14, *A*.

Because it lies exposed against the bony surface of the skull, the auricle is frequently injured by blunt trauma. Bruising may then cause an accumulation of blood and tissue fluid between the skin and underlying cartilage. If left untreated, the classic swelling of "cauliflower ear" may develop and become permanent. The skin in back of the ear is rich in sebaceous glands. And, if they become infected, painful cysts develop that must be drained. In people who suffer from gout, small nodules filled with uric acid called **tophi** (TOE-fi), often appear on the upper edge of the helix. Another type of nodule that may appear on the helix is called a *Darwin tubercle.* It is considered a variation of normal and requires no treatment. Although controversial, there is some evidence to suggest that the presence of oblique earlobe creases in individuals over the age of 50 may be related to coronary artery disease.

Note in Figure 10-14, *A*, that the *tragus* of the auricle lies just in front of the opening to the acoustic canal. The canal itself is a curving tube about 2.5 cm (1 inch) in length. It extends into the temporal bone and ends at the **tympanic** (tim-PAN-ik) **membrane,** or **eardrum,** which is a partition between the external and middle ear. The skin of the acoustic canal, especially in its outer one third, contains many short hairs and **ceruminous** (seh-ROO-mi-nus) **glands** that produce a waxy substance called **cerumen** that may collect in the canal and impair hearing by absorbing or blocking the passage of sound waves. Sound waves traveling through the external acoustic canal strike the tympanic membrane and cause it to vibrate.

Just as an ophthalmoscope is used to view the interior of the eyeball and examine the retina, a lighted instrument called an **otoscope** is used to examine the external ear canal and outer surface of the tympanic membrane (Figure 10-14, *B* and *C*). Changes in the appearance of the ear canal and tympanic membrane can provide a skilled observer with a great deal of information. For example, middle ear infections cause the eardrum to become red and inflamed and to bulge outward into the

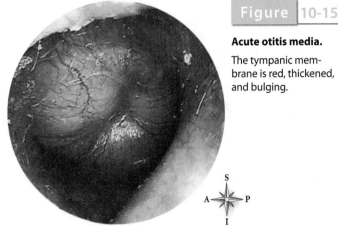

Figure 10-15

Acute otitis media.

The tympanic membrane is red, thickened, and bulging.

ear canal as pus and other fluids accumulate in the middle ear (Figure 10-15). Foreign objects or excess cerumen in the ear canal, inflammation of the lining of the canal caused by prolonged exposure to moisture or bacterial infection (swimmer's ear), and perforation of the eardrum itself are also easily observed using an otoscope.

HEALTH & WELL-BEING

SWIMMER'S EAR

External otitis, or *swimmer's ear,* is a common infection of the external ear in athletes. It can be bacterial or fungal in origin and is usually associated with prolonged exposure to water. The infection generally involves, at least to some extent, the acoustic canal and auricle. The ear as a whole is tender, red, and swollen. Treatment of swimmer's ear usually involves antibiotic therapy and prescription analgesics.

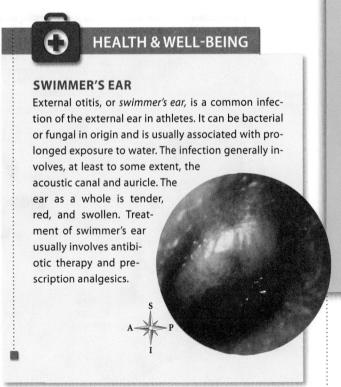

MIDDLE EAR

The middle ear is a tiny and very thin epithelium-lined cavity hollowed out of the temporal bone (Figure 10-16). It houses three very small bones. The names of these ear bones, called **ossicles** (OS-si-kuls), describe their shapes—**malleus** (hammer), **incus** (anvil), and **stapes** (stirrup). The "handle" of the malleus attaches to the inside of the tympanic membrane, and the "head" attaches to the incus (Figure 10-14, C). The incus attaches to the stapes, and the stapes presses against a membrane that covers a small opening, the *oval window.* The oval window separates the middle ear from the inner ear. When sound waves cause the eardrum to vibrate, that movement is transmitted and amplified by the ear ossicles as it passes through the middle ear. Movement of the stapes against the oval window causes movement of fluid in the inner ear.

A point worth mentioning, because it explains the frequent spread of infection from the throat to the ear, is that a tube—the **auditory,** or **eustachian** (yoo-STAY-shen), **tube**—connects the throat with the middle ear. The epithelial lining of the middle ears, auditory tubes, and throat are extensions of one continuous membrane. Consequently, infection causing a sore throat may spread to produce a middle ear infection called **otitis** (oh-TIE-tis) **media** (ME-dee-ah) (Figure 10-15).

The auditory tube serves a useful function: it makes possible equalization of pressure against inner and outer surfaces of the tympanic membrane and therefore prevents membrane rupture and the discomfort that marked pressure differences produce.

INNER EAR

The activation of mechanoreceptors in the inner ear generates nervous impulses that result in hearing and equilibrium. Anatomically, the inner ear consists of three spaces in the temporal bone, assembled in a complex maze called the **bony labyrinth** (LAB-i-rinth). This odd-shaped bony space is filled with a watery fluid called **perilymph** (PER-i-limf) and is divided into the following parts: **vestibule** (VES-ti-

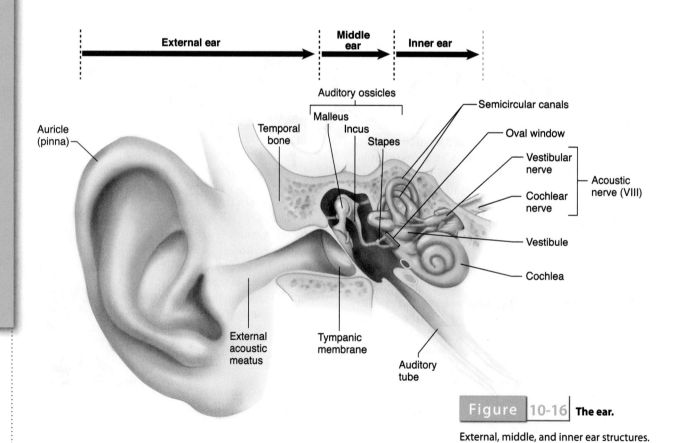

Figure 10-16 **The ear.**

External, middle, and inner ear structures.

byool), **semicircular canals,** and **cochlea** (KOHK-lee-ah) (Figure 10-16). The vestibule is adjacent to the oval window between the semicircular canals and the cochlea (Figure 10-17). Note in Figure 10-17 that a balloonlike membranous sac is suspended in the perilymph and follows the shape of the bony labyrinth much like a "tube within a tube." This is the **membranous labyrinth,** and it is filled with a thicker fluid called **endolymph** (EN-doh-limf).

The mechanoreceptors for balance and equilibrium are located in the three semicircular canals and the vestibule. The three half-circle semicircular canals are oriented at right angles to one another (Figure 10-17). Within each canal is a dilated area called the *ampulla* that contains a sensory structure called a **crista** (KRIS-tah) **ampullaris** (am-pyoo-LAIR-iss), which generates a nerve impulse when you move your head. The sensory cells in the cristae ampullaris have hairlike exten-

sions that are suspended in the endolymph. The sensory cells are stimulated when movement of the head causes the endolymph to move, thus causing the hairs to bend. Nerves from other receptors in the vestibule join those from the semicircular canals to form the **vestibular nerve,** which joins with the cochlear nerve to form the acoustic nerve, or cranial nerve VIII (Figure 10-17). Eventually, nervous impulses passing through this nerve reach the cerebellum and medulla. Other connections from these areas result in impulses reaching the cerebral cortex.

The organ of hearing, which lies in the snail-shaped cochlea, is the **organ of Corti** (KOR-tye). Also called the *spiral organ,* the organ of Corti is surrounded by endolymph, filling the membranous cochlea, or **cochlear duct,** which is the membranous tube within the bony cochlea. Sensory hair cells on the organ of Corti generate nerve

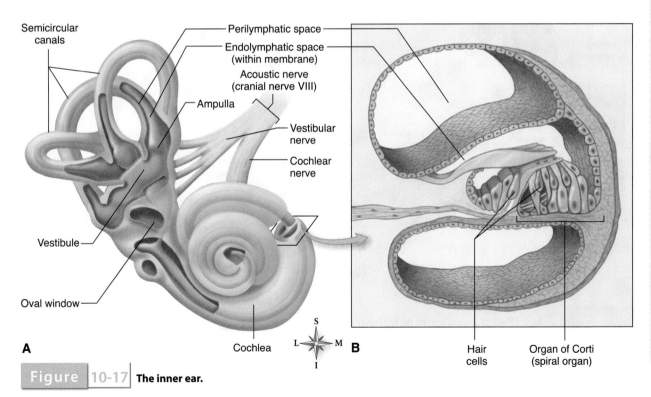

Semicircular canals

Perilymphatic space

Endolymphatic space (within membrane)

Acoustic nerve (cranial nerve VIII)

Ampulla

Vestibular nerve

Cochlear nerve

Vestibule

Oval window

Cochlea

Hair cells

Organ of Corti (spiral organ)

A   **B**

Figure 10-17 **The inner ear.**

A, The bony labyrinth (orange) is the hard outer wall of the entire inner ear and includes semicircular canals, vestibule, and cochlea. Within the bony labyrinth is the membranous labyrinth (purple), which is surrounded by perilymph and filled with endolymph. Each ampulla in the vestibule contains a crista ampullaris that detects changes in head position and sends sensory impulses through the vestibular nerve to the brain. The inset **(B)** shows a section of the membranous cochlea. Hair cells in the organ of Corti (spiral organ) detect sound and send the information through the cochlear nerve. The vestibular and cochlear nerves join to form cranial nerve VIII.

impulses when they are bent by the movement of endolymph set in motion by sound waves (Figures 10-17 and 10-18).

To learn more about the pathway of sound waves, go to **AnimationDirect** on your CD.

QUICK CHECK

1. What is another name for the eardrum?
2. Name the ear ossicles.
3. What fluid fills the membranous labyrinth? the organ of Corti?

Hearing Disorders

Hearing problems can be divided into two basic categories: *conduction impairment* and *nerve impairment*. Conduction impairment refers to the blocking of sound waves as they travel through the external and middle ear to the sensory receptors of the inner ear (the conduction pathway). Nerve impairment results in insensitivity to sound because of inherited or acquired nerve damage.

The most obvious cause of conduction impairment is blockage of the external auditory canal. Waxy buildup of cerumen commonly blocks conduction of sound toward the tympanic membrane. Foreign objects, tumors, and other matter can block conduction in the external or middle ear. An inherited bone

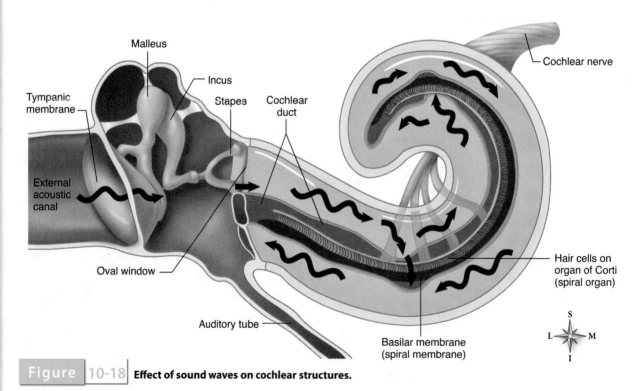

Malleus

Incus

Stapes

Cochlear duct

Tympanic membrane

External acoustic canal

Oval window

Auditory tube

Basilar membrane (spiral membrane)

Cochlear nerve

Hair cells on organ of Corti (spiral organ)

Figure 10-18 **Effect of sound waves on cochlear structures.**

Sound waves strike the tympanic membrane and cause it to vibrate. This vibration causes the membrane of the oval window to vibrate. Vibration of the oval window causes the perilymph in the bony labyrinth of the cochlea to move, which causes the endolymph in the membranous labyrinth of the cochlea or cochlear duct to move. This movement of endolymph stimulates hair cells on the organ of Corti (spiral organ) to generate a nerve impulse. The nerve impulse travels over the cochlear nerve, which becomes a part of cranial nerve VIII. Eventually, nerve impulses reach the auditory cortex and are interpreted as sound.

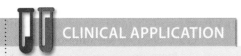

COCHLEAR IMPLANTS

Recent advances in electronic circuitry are now being used to correct some forms of nerve deafness. If the hairs on the organ of Corti are damaged, nerve deafness results—even if the vestibulocochlear nerve is healthy. A surgically implanted device can improve this form of hearing loss by eliminating the need for the sensory hairs. As you can see in the figure, a transmitter just outside the scalp sends external sound information to a receiver under the scalp (behind the auricle). The receiver translates the information into an electrical code that is relayed down an electrode to the cochlea. The electrode, wired to the organ of Corti, stimulates the vestibulocochlear nerve endings directly. Thus even though the cochlear hair cells are damaged, sound can still be perceived.

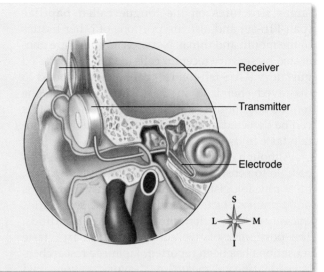

disorder called **otosclerosis** (oh-toh-skleh-ROH-sis) impairs conduction by causing structural irregularities in the stapes. Otosclerosis usually first appears during childhood or early adulthood as **tinnitus** (tin-EYE-tus), or "ringing in the ear."

Temporary conduction impairment often results from ear infection, or **otitis.** As stated earlier, the structure of the auditory tube makes the middle ear prone to bacterial or viral *otitis media.* Otitis media often produces swelling and pus formation that blocks the conduction of sound through the middle ear. Permanent damage to structures of the middle ear occasionally occurs in severe cases. Infectious organisms from a middle ear infection that invade the mastoid bone are often difficult to treat. They cause redness, inflammation, and swelling of the mastoid process that may push the auricle away from the skull. Hearing loss may be a complication in severe cases.

Hearing loss caused by nerve impairment is common in the elderly. Called **presbycusis** (pres-bi-KYOO-sis), this progressive hearing loss associated with aging results from degeneration of nerve tissue in the ear and the vestibulocochlear nerve. A similar type of hearing loss occurs after chronic exposure to loud noises that damages receptors in the organ of Corti. Because different sound *frequencies* (tones) stimulate different regions of the organ of Corti, hearing impairment is limited to only frequencies associated with the damaged portion of the organ of Corti. For example, the portion of the organ of Corti that degenerates first in presbycusis is normally stimulated by high-frequency sounds. Thus the inability to hear high-pitched sounds is common among the elderly.

Nerve damage also can occur in **Ménière** (men-YER) **disease,** a chronic inner ear disease of unknown cause. Ménière disease is characterized by tinnitus, progressive nerve deafness, and **vertigo** (sensation of spinning).

> **QUICK CHECK**
>
> 1. Name the two basic categories of hearing disorders.
> 2. Name the progressive hearing loss associated with aging.
> 3. Where are the receptor cells for hearing located?

The Taste Receptors

The chemical receptors, or **chemoreceptors**, that generate nervous impulses resulting in the sense of taste are called **taste buds.** About 10,000 of these microscopic receptors are found on the sides of much larger structures on the tongue called **papillae** (pah-PIL-ee) and also are portions of other tissues in the mouth and throat. Nervous impulses are generated by sensory receptor cells in taste buds, called **gustatory** (GUS-tah-toh-ree) **cells**. They respond to dissolved chemicals in the saliva that bathe the tongue and mouth tissues (Figure 10-19). All tastes can be detected in all areas of the tongue that contain taste buds.

Although current research suggests that we may be able to sense a large number of discrete tastes, most physiologists continue to list only four kinds of "primary" taste sensations—*sweet, sour, bitter, and salty*—that result from stimulation of taste buds. The possibility of two additional "primary" taste sensations has been reported. Japanese researchers have identified a "meaty" or "savory" flavor called **umami** (oh-MOM-me) that is triggered by the amino acid glutamate. Others have suggested that the metallic taste is also primary.

Most other flavors result from a combination of taste bud and olfactory receptor stimulation. In other words, the myriad tastes recognized are not tastes alone but tastes plus odors. For this reason, having a cold that interferes with the stimulation of the olfactory receptors by odors from foods in the mouth markedly dulls taste sensations. Nervous impulses that are generated by stimulation of taste buds travel primarily through two cranial nerves (VII and IX) to end in the taste area of the cerebral cortex.

The Smell Receptors

The chemoreceptors responsible for the sense of smell are located in a small area of epithelial tissue in the upper part of the nasal cavity (Figure 10-20). The location of the **olfactory receptors** is somewhat hidden, and we often have to forcefully sniff air to smell delicate odors. Each olfactory cell has a number of sensory cilia that sense different chemicals and cause the cell to respond by generating a nervous impulse. To be detected by olfactory receptors, chemicals must be dissolved in the watery mucus that lines the nasal cavity.

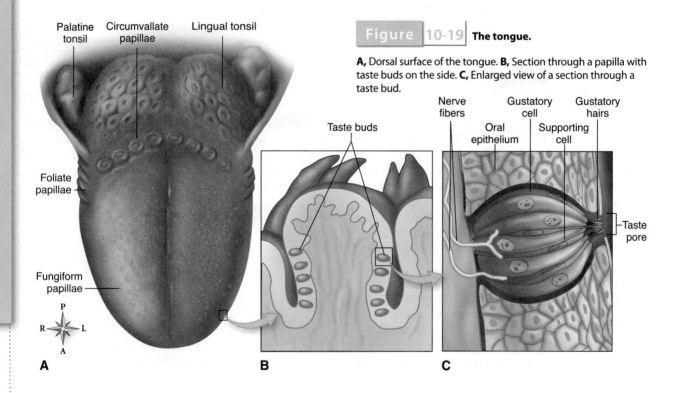

Figure **10-19**   **The tongue.**

A, Dorsal surface of the tongue. **B,** Section through a papilla with taste buds on the side. **C,** Enlarged view of a section through a taste bud.

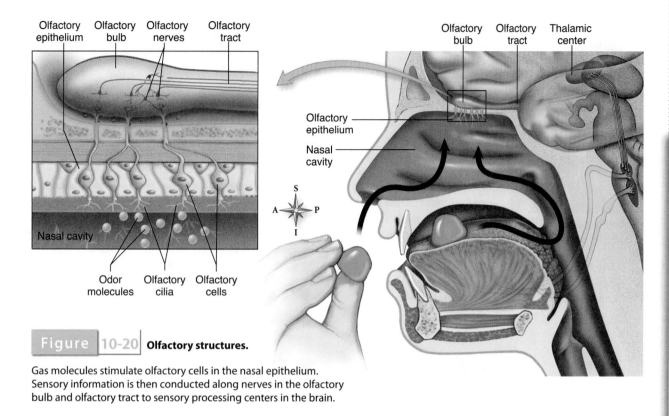

Olfactory epithelium Olfactory bulb Olfactory nerves Olfactory tract

Olfactory bulb Olfactory tract Thalamic center

Olfactory epithelium

Nasal cavity

S
A — P
I

Nasal cavity

Odor molecules Olfactory cilia Olfactory cells

Figure 10-20 **Olfactory structures.**

Gas molecules stimulate olfactory cells in the nasal epithelium. Sensory information is then conducted along nerves in the olfactory bulb and olfactory tract to sensory processing centers in the brain.

Although the olfactory receptors are extremely sensitive (that is, stimulated by even very slight odors), they are also easily fatigued—a fact that explains why odors that are at first very noticeable are not sensed at all after a short time. After the olfactory cells are stimulated by odor-causing chemicals, the resulting nerve impulse travels through the olfactory nerves in the olfactory bulb and tract and then enters the thalamic and olfactory centers of the brain, where the nervous impulses are interpreted as specific odors. The pathways taken by olfactory nerve impulses and the areas where these impulses are interpreted are closely associated with areas of the brain important in memory and emotion. For this reason, we may retain vivid and long-lasting memories of particular smells and odors.

Temporary reduction of sensitivity to smells often results from colds and other nasal infections. Progressive reduction of the sense of smell is often seen in smokers because of the damaging effects of the pollutants in tobacco smoke. In olfaction, as with all the special senses, advancing age often brings a structural degeneration that results in reduced function. It is no wonder that many older adults become isolated and depressed when their contact with the outside world, through the special senses, is gradually lost. Caring health professionals recognize these signs of aging and provide assistance needed by their aged patients to once again enjoy life.

To learn more about how the brain interprets odors, go to **AnimationDirect** on your CD.

QUICK CHECK

1. Where are taste receptors located?
2. Name the primary tastes that humans can perceive.
3. What is the job of olfactory receptors?

SCIENCE APPLICATIONS

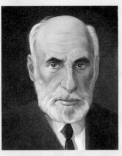

Santiago Ramón y Cajal
(1852–1934)

THE SENSES

Santiago Ramón y Cajal is considered by many to be the originator of the modern view of the nervous system's organization. He not only uncovered much information about sensory centers of the cortex and the structure of the retina but also made important discoveries about nearly every part of the nervous system. Most of this Spanish researcher's ideas about the nervous system are still intact today. Although Santiago wanted to be an artist, his father convinced him to follow in his footsteps and become an anatomist—a choice that led to a Nobel Prize in 1906.

Knowledge gained from the study of the sensory part of the nervous system and its relationship to the rest of the body is useful in many different fields. For example, the concepts and theories put into practice by optometrists and ophthalmologists, otologists and audiologists, and other professionals who assess and treat sensory disorders are based on neuroscience. People working in many other fields make indirect use of neuroscience as well. Artists use what we know of visual perception in creating their works, musicians and architects make use of our knowledge of sound perception when performing in or designing concert halls, and aerospace professionals use what we know of equilibrium and how it is perceived in the brain to understand what causes motion sickness.

Outline Summary

To download an MP3 version of the chapter summary for use with your iPod or portable media player, access the **Audio Chapter Summaries** on your CD.

Classification of Sense Organs

A. General sense organs (Table 10-1)
 1. Often exist as individual cells or receptor units
 2. Widely distributed throughout the body
 3. Different from *special* sense organs—groupings of receptors within highly complex organs
B. Classification by presence or absence of covering capsule
 1. Encapsulated
 2. Unencapsulated ("free" or "naked")
C. Classification by type of stimuli required to activate receptors
 1. Photoreceptors (light)
 2. Chemoreceptors (chemicals)
 3. Pain receptors (injury)
 4. Thermoreceptors (temperature change)
 5. Mechanoreceptors (movement or deforming of capsule)
 6. Proprioceptors (position of body parts or changes in muscle length or tension)

Converting a Stimulus into a Sensation

A. All sense organs have common functional characteristics
 1. All are able to detect a particular stimulus
 2. A stimulus is converted into a nerve impulse
 3. A nerve impulse is perceived as a sensation in the CNS

General Sense Organs

A. Distribution is widespread; single-cell receptors are common
B. Examples (Figure 10-1, Table 10-1)
 1. Skin receptors
  a. Free nerve endings (several types)—pain, discriminative touch, tickle, and temperature
  b. Tactile (Meissner) corpuscle—fine touch and vibration
  c. Bulbous (Ruffini) corpuscle—touch and pressure

       d. Lamellar (Pacini) corpuscle—pressure and vibration

       e. Bulboid (Krause) corpuscle—touch

  2. Muscle receptors

       a. Golgi tendon receptor—proprioception

       b. Muscle spindle—proprioception

  3. Deep receptors

       a. Stretch (pressure) receptors in hollow organs

       b. Chemical receptors—detect pH, carbon dioxide, other chemicals

Special Sense Organs

A. The eye (Figures 10-2 and 10-3)

  1. Layers of eyeball

       a. Sclera—tough outer coat; "white" of eye; cornea is transparent part of sclera over iris

       b. Choroid—pigmented vascular layer prevents scattering of light

          (1) Front part of this layer made of ciliary muscle and iris, the colored part of the eye

          (2) The pupil is the hole in the center of the iris

          (3) Contraction of iris muscle dilates or constricts pupil

       c. Retina (Figures 10-6 and 10-7)—innermost layer of the eye; contains rods (receptors for night vision) and cones (receptors for day vision and color vision)

  2. Conjunctiva—mucous membrane covering the front surface of the sclera and lining the eyelid

  3. Lens—transparent body behind the pupil; focuses light rays on the retina

  4. Eye fluids

       a. Aqueous humor—in the anterior cavity in front of the lens

       b. Vitreous humor—in the posterior cavity behind the lens

  5. Visual pathway

       a. Innermost layer of retina contains rods and cones

       b. Impulse travels from the rods and cones through the bipolar and ganglionic layers of retina (Figure 10-8)

       c. Nerve impulse leaves the eye through the optic nerve; the point of exit is free of receptors and is therefore called a *blind spot*

       d. Visual interpretation occurs in the visual cortex of the cerebrum (Figure 10-9)

B. Visual disorders

  1. Refraction disorders (Figure 10-10)

       a. Myopia (nearsightedness) is often caused by elongation of the eyeball

       b. Hyperopia (farsightedness) is often caused by a shortened eyeball

       c. Astigmatism is distortion caused by an irregularity of the cornea or lens

       d. Conjunctivitis (inflammation of the conjunctiva) can interfere with refraction

          (1) Trachoma—chronic chlamydial infection

          (2) Acute bacterial conjunctivitis—highly contagious infection that produces a discharge of mucous pus (Figure 10-11)

          (3) Conjunctivitis can be caused by allergies

       e. Strabismus—improper alignment of eyes (Figure 10-12)

          (1) Eyes can converge (cross) or diverge

          (2) If not corrected, can cause blindness

  2. Disorders of the retina

       a. Retinal detachment can be a complication of aging, eye tumors, or head trauma

       b. Diabetic retinopathy—damage to retina from hemorrhages and growth of abnormal vessels associated with diabetes mellitus

       c. Glaucoma—increased intraocular pressure decreases blood flow in retina and thus causes retinal degeneration

       d. Nyctalopia (night blindness) or the inability to see in dim light is caused by retinal degeneration or lack of vitamin A

       e. Macular degeneration—progressive degeneration of central part of retina; leading cause of permanent blindness in elderly

       f. Red-green color blindness is an X-linked genetic condition involving the inability to perceive certain colors; it is caused by an abnormality in the cones' photopigments

  3. Disorders of the visual pathway

       a. Degeneration of the optic nerve resulting from diabetes, glaucoma, and other causes can impair vision

       b. Scotoma is the loss of only the central visual field when only certain nerve pathways are damaged

       c. Cerebrovascular accidents (CVAs) can damage visual processing centers;

example is acquired cortical color blindness (Figure 10-13)

C. The ear

1. The ear functions as the sense organ of hearing and also of equilibrium and balance
2. Receptors for hearing and equilibrium are mechanoreceptors
3. Physical forces that create sound vibrations and fluid movement initiate nervous impulses in the ear
4. Divisions of the ear (Figure 10-16)
   a. External ear (Figure 10-14)
      (1) Auricle (pinna)—appendage on side of head
      (2) External acoustic canal
         (a) Curving tube 2.5 cm (1 inch) in length
         (b) Contains ceruminous glands
         (c) Ends at the tympanic membrane
   b. Middle ear
      (1) Epithelium-lined cavity that houses the ear ossicles—malleus, incus, and stapes
      (2) Ends in the oval window
      (3) The auditory (eustachian) tube connects the middle ear to the throat
      (4) Inflammation called *otitis media* (Figure 10-15)
   c. Inner ear (Figure 10-17)
      (1) Bony labyrinth filled with perilymph
      (2) Subdivided into the vestibule, semicircular canals, and cochlea
      (3) Membranous labyrinth filled with endolymph
      (4) The receptors for balance in the semicircular canals are called *cristae ampullaris*
      (5) Sensory hair cells on the organ of Corti (spiral organ) respond when bent by the movement of surrounding endolymph set in motion by sound waves (Figure 10-18)

D. Hearing disorders

1. Conduction impairment
   a. Can be caused by blockage of the external or middle ear (for example, by cerumen and tumors)
   b. Otosclerosis—inherited bone disorder involving irregularity of the stapes; it first appears as tinnitus (ringing), then progresses to hearing loss
   c. Otitis—ear inflammation caused by infection; can produce swelling and fluids that block sound conduction
2. Nerve impairment
   a. Presbycusis—progressive nerve deafness associated with aging
   b. Progressive nerve deafness also can result from chronic exposure to loud noise
   c. Ménière disease—chronic inner ear disorder characterized by tinnitus, nerve deafness, and vertigo

E. The taste receptors (Figure 10-19)

1. Receptors are chemoreceptors called *taste buds*
2. Cranial nerves VII and IX carry gustatory impulses
3. Most physiologists list only four kinds of primary taste sensations—sweet, sour, bitter, salty (umami and metallic tastes are sometimes included as primary taste sensations)
4. Gustatory and olfactory senses work together

F. The smell receptors (Figure 10-20)

1. Receptors for fibers of olfactory (cranial nerve I) lie in olfactory mucosa of nasal cavity
2. Olfactory receptors are extremely sensitive but easily fatigued
3. Odor-causing chemicals initiate a nervous signal that is interpreted as a specific odor by the brain

New Words

aqueous humor	bony labyrinth	choroid	conjunctiva
auditory (eustachian) tube	cerumen	cochlea	crista ampullaris
auricle	ceruminous gland	cochlear duct	endolymph
	chemoreceptor	cone	external acoustic canal

fovea	retina	automated lamellar	ophthalmoscope
gustatory cell	rod	keratoplasty (ALK)	otitis
incus	sclera	cataract	otitis media
iris	semicircular canal	color blindness	otosclerosis
lacrimal gland	sensory receptor	conductive keratoplasty (CK)	otoscope
lens	stapes	conjunctivitis	photorefractive
macula	taste buds	corneal stem cell transplant	keratectomy (PRK)
malleus	tympanic membrane	diabetic retinopathy	presbycusis
mechanoreceptor	(eardrum)	excimer laser surgery	presbyopia
membranous labyrinth	vestibular nerve	glaucoma	radial keratotomy (RK)
olfactory receptor	vestibule	hyperopia	scotoma
organ of Corti	vitreous humor	laser-assisted in situ	strabismus
ossicle		keratomileusis (LASIK)	tinnitus
papilla (*pl.,* papillae)	**Diseases and Other**	laser thermal keratoplasty	tophi
perilymph	**Clinical Terms**	macular degeneration	trachoma
photoreceptor		Ménière disease	umami
proprioceptor	astigmatic keratotomy (AK)	myopia	vertigo
pupil	astigmatism	nyctalopia	

Review Questions

1. Name the general senses found in the skin or subcutaneous tissue and list the type of stimuli to which each of them responds.
2. Name the two general senses of proprioception and give the location of each.
3. With what type of information do proprioceptors provide us?
4. Explain how the iris changes the size of the pupil.
5. Explain how the ciliary muscles allow the eye to focus on near and far objects.
6. What is *presbyopia* and what is its cause?
7. Name the two types of receptor cells in the retina. Explain the differences between the two receptors.
8. What is glaucoma and what is its cause?
9. What are cataracts, what causes them, and how can they be prevented?
10. What is meant by the *visual pathway*? Where is the *blind spot* and what causes it?
11. Explain how the disorder *strabismus* affects vision.
12. What causes diabetic retinopathy?
13. Briefly explain the structure of the external ear.
14. Explain how sound waves are transmitted through the middle ear.
15. Explain how sound waves are converted to an auditory impulse.
16. Explain how the structures in the inner ear help maintain balance or equilibrium.
17. What is Ménière disease?
18. Where are the gustatory cells located, and to what four "primary" tastes do they respond?
19. Explain how the sense of smell is stimulated.

Critical Thinking

20. Explain why food loses some of its taste when you have a bad cold or stuffy nose.
21. Explain why the longer you are in a newly painted room the less able you are to smell the paint.
22. Where in the eye is light sensed? Where is it perceived? (be specific)
23. Explain why the smell of a "doctor's office" or the smell of turkey cooking on Thanksgiving can easily generate an emotional response?
24. Why are there many more color-blind men than there are color-blind women?
25. Rock musicians sometimes lose their ability to hear high-frequency tones; explain how this can happen.

Chapter Test

1. The eye can be classified as a photoreceptor. Taste and smell can be classified as _____, and Golgi tendon receptors and muscle spindles can be classified as _____.

2. The specific mechanoreceptor for hearing is the _____.

3. The specific mechanoreceptor for balance is the _____.

4. The gustatory cells are involved with the sense of _____.

5. The four "primary" taste sensations that result from the stimulation of the taste buds are _____, _____, _____, and _____.

6. Taste buds can be found on much larger structures on the tongue called _____.

7. The chemoreceptors responsible for the sense of smell are the _____.

Match each structure of the eye in Column A with its corresponding function or description in Column B.

Column A
8. _____ sclera
9. _____ cornea
10. _____ iris
11. _____ pupil
12. _____ lacrimal
13. _____ lens
14. _____ rods
15. _____ cones
16. _____ choroid coat
17. _____ vitreous
18. _____ aqueous

Column B
a. gland in which tears are formed
b. hole in the eye that lets light in
c. receptors for night vision or dim light
d. thick jelly-like fluid or humor of the eye
e. tough, white outer layer of the eye
f. receptors for red, blue, and green color vision
g. structure on which ciliary muscles pull to help the eye focus
h. dark pigmented middle layer of the eye that prevents the scattering of incoming light
i. transparent part of the sclera, the window of the eye
j. colored part of the front of the eye
k. thin, watery humor of the eye

Match each structure of the ear in Column A with its corresponding function or description in Column B.

Column A
19. _____ tympanic membrane
20. _____ ossicles
21. _____ auditory tube
22. _____ perilymph
23. _____ endolymph
24. _____ cochlea
25. _____ organ of Corti

Column B
a. tube connecting the middle ear and the throat
b. watery fluid that fills the bony labyrinth
c. snail-shaped structure in the inner ear
d. organ of hearing
e. thick fluid in the membranous labyrinth
f. another term for eardrum
g. collective name for the incus, malleus, and stapes

Match each disorder in Column A with its description in Column B.

Column A

26. _____ myopia
27. _____ astigmatism
28. _____ conjunctivitis
29. _____ strabismus
30. _____ diabetic retinopathy
31. _____ glaucoma
32. _____ age-related macular degeneration
33. _____ color blindness
34. _____ otitis media
35. _____ Ménière disease

Column B

a. caused by increased fluid pressure in the eye
b. an inflammation of the conjunctiva, "pink eye"
c. progressive degeneration of the central part of the retina
d. nearsightedness caused by the elongation of the eyeball
e. an infection of the middle ear
f. an improper alignment of the eyes; can cause them to converge (cross)
g. chronic inner ear disorder of unknown cause; characterized by tinnitus, deafness, and vertigo
h. an X-linked genetic condition involving inability to perceive some colors
i. damage to the retina caused by hemorrhage and abnormal vessel growth
j. distortion of the image in the eye caused by irregularities of the cornea or lens

Study Tips

continued from page 281

2. In your study group, discuss how each of the sensory systems detect and respond to a stimulus. Photocopy the figures of the sense organs, blacken out the labels, and quiz each other on the name, location, and function of each structure.

3. Study your chart of the disorders of the sensory systems. Review the questions at the end of the chapter and discuss possible test questions in your study group.

Case Studies

1. Roger is legally blind. His vision impairment is a complication of diabetes mellitus. Can you describe what structural changes in Roger's eyes have caused his blindness? As you were helping him cross the street, a fellow pedestrian suddenly stumbled into your path. Without any signal from you, Roger jumped back to avoid hitting the other person. If Roger is blind, how could he have reacted this way?

2. As a child, Mrs. Stark was tested for color blindness and told that she had normal color vision. She never had any problems distinguishing colors until shortly after her retirement, when suddenly she lost her sense of color. She describes her perception of the world as being "like a black and white movie." She cannot distinguish yellows, oranges, blues, greens, reds, or any other colors. What might have caused Mrs. Stark's problems?

3. You have just been diagnosed with otitis media. Describe what has happened to your body to produce this condition. If left untreated, what are the possible outcomes of this condition?

Outline

Objectives

After you have completed this chapter, you should be able to:

1. Distinguish between endocrine and exocrine glands and define the terms *hormone* and *prostaglandin*.

2. Identify and locate the primary endocrine glands and list the major hormones produced by each gland.

3. Describe the mechanisms of steroid and nonsteroid hormone action.

4. Explain how negative and positive feedback mechanisms regulate the secretion of endocrine hormones.

5. Explain the primary mechanisms of endocrine disorders.

6. Identify the principal functions of each major endocrine hormone and describe the conditions that may result from hyposecretion or hypersecretion.

7. Define diabetes insipidus, diabetes mellitus, gigantism, goiter, cretinism, and glycosuria.

11 The Endocrine System

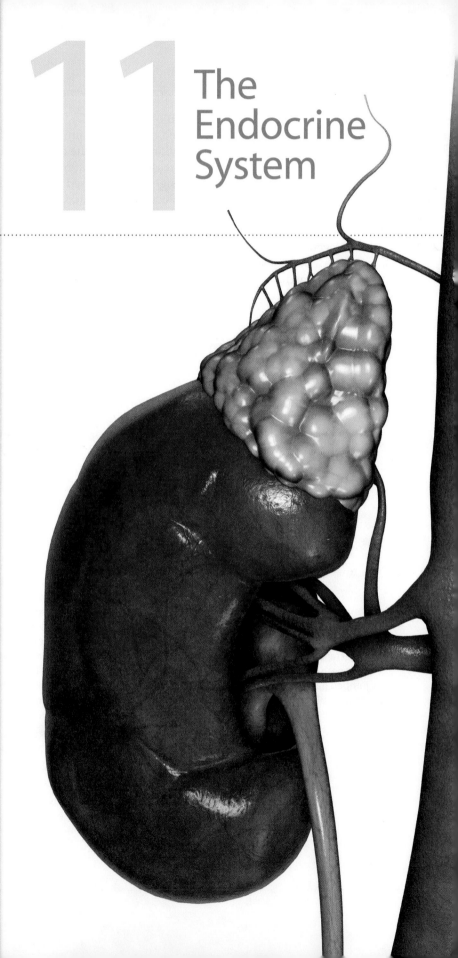

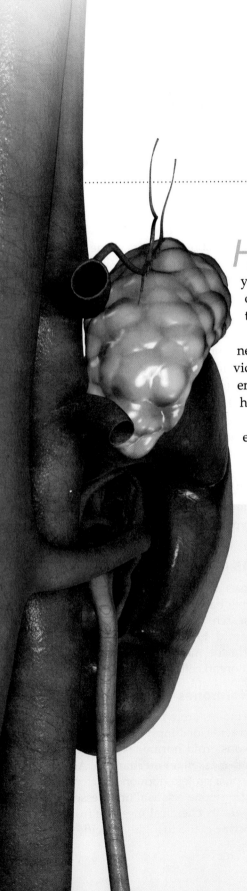

Have you ever known anyone with thyroid problems or diabetes? Surely you've seen the dramatic changes that happen to a person's body as he or she goes through puberty. These are all proof of the importance of the endocrine system for normal development and health.

The **endocrine system** performs the same general functions as the nervous system: communication and control. The nervous system provides rapid, brief control by way of fast-traveling nerve impulses. The endocrine system provides slower but longer-lasting control by way of hormones (chemicals) secreted into and circulated by the blood.

The organs of the endocrine system are located in widely separated parts of the body—in the neck; in the cranial, thoracic, abdominal,

STUDY TIPS

Before studying Chapter 11, review the synopsis of the endocrine system in Chapter 4. The function of the endocrine system is the same as that of the nervous system. The differences are in the methods used and the extent of their effects. The endocrine system uses chemicals in the blood (hormones) rather than nerve impulses. Hormones can have a direct effect on almost every cell in the body, an impossible task for the nervous system. Steroid hormones can act directly because they can enter the cell; protein hormones can't, so they need a second-messenger system.

1. Reviewing material from earlier chapters such as receptor proteins in the cell membrane, ATP, homeostasis, and negative feedback loops will help you understand the material in this chapter.
2. Use flash cards to learn the names of the hormones, what they do, and the names and locations of the glands that produce them.
3. Remember that hormones released by the posterior pituitary gland are made in the hypothalamus.
4. When studying the disorders of the endocrine system, make a chart that identifies the disorders as a hyposecretion or hypersecretion of a specific gland. This may be more difficult than you think because many of the disorders are named after people, so the names themselves are not helpful

continued on page 339

and pelvic cavities; and also outside of the body cavities. Note the names and locations of the endocrine glands shown in Figure 11-1.

All organs of the endocrine system are glands, but not all glands are organs of the endocrine system. Of the two types of glands in the body—**exocrine glands** and **endocrine glands**—only endocrine glands belong to this system. Exocrine glands secrete their products into ducts that empty onto a surface or into a cavity. For example, sweat glands produce a watery secretion that empties onto the surface of the skin. Salivary glands are also exocrine glands; they secrete saliva that flows into the mouth. Endocrine glands are ductless glands. They secrete chemicals known as **hormones** into intercellular spaces. From there, the hormones diffuse directly into the blood and are carried throughout the body. Each hormone molecule may then bind to a cell that has specific receptors for that hormone, triggering a reaction in the cell. Such a cell is called a **target organ cell.** The list of endocrine glands and their target organs continues to grow thanks to ongoing research. The names, locations, and functions of the well-known endocrine glands are shown in Figure 11-1 and Table 11-1.

In this chapter you will read about the functions of the main endocrine glands and discover why their importance is almost impossible to exaggerate. Hormones are the main regulators of metabolism, growth and development, reproduction, and many other body activities. They play important roles in maintaining homeostasis—fluid and electrolyte, acid-base, and energy balances, for example. Hormones make the difference between normalcy and many kinds of abnormalities such as dwarfism, gigantism, and sterility. They are important not only for the healthy survival of each one of us but also for the survival of the human species.

Diseases of the endocrine glands are numerous, varied, and sometimes spectacular. Tumors or other abnormalities often cause a gland to secrete too much or too little hormone. Production of too much hormone by a diseased gland is called **hypersecretion.** If too little hormone is produced, the condition is called **hyposecretion.**

Mechanisms of Hormone Action

A hormone causes its target cells to respond in particular ways; this has been the subject of intense interest and research. The two major classes of hormones—**nonsteroid hormones** and **steroid hormones**—differ in the mechanisms by which they influence target organ cells.

Nonsteroid Hormones

Nonsteroid hormones are whole proteins, shorter chains of amino acids, or simply versions of single amino acids. Nonsteroid hormones work according to the **second-messenger mechanism.** According to this concept, a protein hormone, such as thyroid-stimulating hormone, acts as a "first messenger" (that is, it delivers its chemical message from the cells of an endocrine gland to highly specific mem-

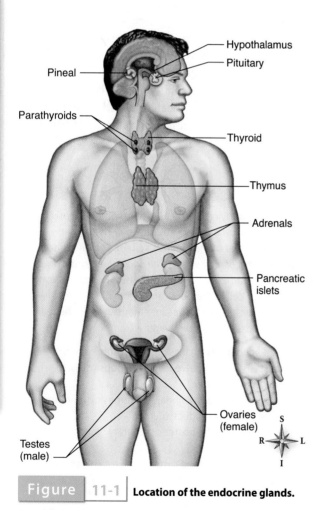

Hypothalamus
Pituitary
Pineal
Parathyroids
Thyroid
Thymus
Adrenals
Pancreatic islets
Ovaries (female)
Testes (male)

S
R — L
I

Figure 11-1 **Location of the endocrine glands.**

Thymus gland is shown at maximum size at puberty.

brane receptor sites on the cells of a target organ). This interaction between a hormone and its specific receptor site on the cell membrane of a target organ cell is often compared to the fitting of a unique key into a lock. (This idea is the *lock-and-key model* of chemical activity.) After the hormone is attached to its specific receptor site, a number of chemical reactions occur. These reactions activate molecules within the cell called *second messengers.* One example of this mechanism occurs when the hormone-receptor interaction changes energy-rich ATP molecules inside the cell into **cyclic AMP** (adenosine monophosphate). Cyclic AMP serves as the second messenger, delivering information inside the cell that regulates the cell's activity. For example, cyclic AMP causes thyroid cells to respond to thyroid-stimulating hormone by secreting a thyroid hormone such as *thyroxine.* Cyclic AMP is only one of several second messengers that have been discovered.

In summary, nonsteroid hormones serve as first messengers, providing communication between endocrine glands and target organs. Another molecule, such as cyclic AMP, then acts as the second messenger, providing communication within a hormone's target cells. Figure 11-2 summarizes the mechanism of nonsteroid hormone action.

Steroid Hormones

The primary actions of small, lipid-soluble steroid hormones such as estrogen do not occur by the second-

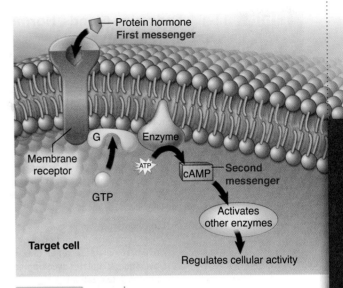

Figure 11-2 | **Mechanism of protein hormone action.**

The hormone acts as "first messenger," delivering its message via the bloodstream to a membrane receptor in the target organ cell much like a key fits into a lock. The "second messenger" causes the cell to respond and perform its specialized *function.*

messenger mechanism. Because they are lipid soluble, steroid hormones can pass intact directly through the cell membrane of the target organ cell. Once inside the cell, steroid hormones pass through the cytoplasm and enter the nucleus, where they bind with a receptor (according to the lock-and-

---

RESEARCH, ISSUES, AND TRENDS

SECOND-MESSENGER SYSTEMS

Rapid and revolutionary discoveries about how nonsteroid hormones act on their target cells began with the pioneering work of Earl Sutherland, who received the 1971 Nobel Prize for formulating the second-messenger hypothesis, and new discoveries continue to be made even today. Later, the important role of the so-called *G protein* in getting the signal from the receptor to the enzyme that forms cyclic AMP (cAMP) was discovered. Look for the G protein in Figure 11-2. More recently, the role of nitric oxide (NO) in second-messenger systems has been worked out. All of these discoveries resulted in Nobel Prizes, which shows the importance the scientific community has placed on them. Why? By working out

the details of how hormones work, we can more clearly understand how and why things can go wrong that affect endocrine disorders. Perhaps we may even gain new knowledge about disorders that we previously did not even know involved hormone mechanisms. Once the processes of disease mechanisms are figured out, we hope scientists will be able to design tests that can screen for such problems. Or perhaps they can develop drugs that will "fix" the broken mechanisms and cure the disease. Although this complex subject may seem like too much for you to comprehend now, you will discover that understanding how hormones act on target cells **(signal transduction)** will prepare you for the revolution in medicine that is now upon us.

Table 11-1	**Endocrine Glands, Hormones, and Their Functions**	
GLAND/HORMONE	**FUNCTION**	**DYSFUNCTION***
ANTERIOR PITUITARY		
Thyroid-stimulating hormone (TSH)	Tropic hormone Stimulates secretion of thyroid hormones	*Hypersecretion:* overstimulation of thyroid *Hyposecretion:* understimulation of thyroid
Adrenocorticotropic hormone (ACTH)	Tropic hormone Stimulates secretion of adrenal cortex	*Hypersecretion:* overstimulation of adrenal cortex hormones
Follicle-stimulating hormone (FSH)	Tropic hormone *Female:* stimulates development of ovarian follicles and secretion of estrogens *Male:* stimulates seminiferous tubules of testes to grow and produce sperm	*Hyposecretion:* understimulation of adrenal cortex hormones *Hyposecretion:* lack of sexual development and sterility
Luteinizing hormone (LH)	Tropic hormone *Female:* stimulates maturation of ovarian follicle and ovum; stimulates secretion of estrogen; triggers ovulation; stimulates development of corpus luteum (luteinization) *Male:* stimulates interstitial cells of the testes to secrete testosterone	*Hyposecretion:* lack of sexual development and sterility
Growth hormone (GH)	Stimulates growth in all organs; mobilizes food molecules, causing an increase in blood glucose concentration	*Hypersecretion:* gigantism (pre-adult); acromegaly (mature adult) *Hyposecretion:* dwarfism (pre-adult)
Prolactin (lactogenic hormone)	Stimulates breast development during pregnancy and milk secretion (milk letdown) after pregnancy	*Hypersecretion:* inappropriate lactation in men or nonnursing women *Hyposecretion:* insufficient lactation in nursing women
POSTERIOR PITUITARY†		
Antidiuretic hormone (ADH)	Stimulates retention of water by the kidneys	*Hypersecretion:* abnormal water retention *Hyposecretion:* diabetes insipidus
Oxytocin (OT)	Stimulates uterine contractions at the end of pregnancy; stimulates the release of milk into the breast ducts	*Hypersecretion:* inappropriate ejection of milk in lactating women *Hyposecretion:* prolonged or difficult labor and delivery (uncertain)
HYPOTHALAMUS		
Releasing hormones (RHs) (several)	Stimulate the anterior pituitary to release hormones	*Hypersecretion:* hypersecretion by anterior pituitary *Hyposecretion:* hyposecretion by anterior pituitary
Inhibiting hormones (IHs) (several)	Inhibit the anterior pituitary's secretion of hormones	*Hypersecretion:* hypersecretion by anterior pituitary *Hyposecretion:* hyposecretion by anterior pituitary
THYROID		
Thyroxine (T_4) and triiodothyronine (T_3)	Stimulate the energy metabolism of all cells	*Hypersecretion:* hyperthyroidism, Graves disease *Hyposecretion:* hypothyroidism, cretinism (pre-adult); myxedema (adult); goiter
Calcitonin (CT)	Inhibits the breakdown of bone; causes a decrease in blood calcium concentration	*Hypersecretion:* possible hypocalcemia *Hyposecretion:* possible hypercalcemia
PARATHYROID		
Parathyroid hormone (PTH)	Stimulates the breakdown of bone; causes an increase in blood calcium concentration	*Hypersecretion:* possible hypercalcemia *Hyposecretion:* possible hypocalcemia

ADRENAL CORTEX

Mineralocorticoids: aldosterone	Regulate electrolyte and fluid homeostasis	*Hypersecretion:* increased water retention *Hyposecretion:* abnormal water loss (dehydration)
Glucocorticoids: cortisol (hydrocortisone)	Stimulate gluconeogenesis, causing an increase in blood glucose concentration; also have antiinflammatory, antiimmunity, and antiallergy effects	*Hypersecretion:* Cushing syndrome *Hyposecretion:* Addison disease
Sex hormones	Stimulate sexual drive in the female but have negligible effects in the male	*Hypersecretion:* premature sexual (androgens) development; masculinization of female *Hyposecretion:* no significant effect

ADRENAL/MEDULLA

Epinephrine (Epi) and norepinephrine (NR)	Prolong and intensify the sympathetic nervous response during stress	*Hypersecretion:* stress effects (adrenaline) *Hyposecretion:* no significant effect

PANCREATIC ISLETS

Glucagon	Stimulates glycogenolysis in liver, causing an increase in blood glucose concentration	(Uncertain)
Insulin	Promotes glucose entry into all cells, causing a decrease in blood glucose concentration	*Hypersecretion:* severe hypoglycemia (insulin shock) *Hyposecretion:* diabetes mellitus

OVARY

Estrogens	Promote development and maintenance of female sexual characteristics (see Chapter 22)	*Hypersecretion:* premature sexual development (female) and infertility *Hyposecretion:* lack of sexual development (female), infertility, and osteoporosis
Progesterone	Promotes conditions required for pregnancy (see Chapter 22)	*Hyposecretion:* sterility

TESTIS

Testosterone	Promotes development and maintenance of male sexual characteristics	*Hypersecretion:* premature sexual development (male); muscle hypertrophy *Hyposecretion:* lack of sexual development (male)

THYMUS

Thymosin	Promotes development of immune-system cells	*Hyposecretion:* depression of immune system functions

PLACENTA

Chorionic gonadotropin, estrogens, progesterone	Promote conditions required during early pregnancy	*Hyposecretion:* spontaneous abortion (miscarriage)

PINEAL

Melatonin	Inhibits tropic hormones that affect the ovaries; may be involved in the body's internal clock and sleep cycle	*Hypersecretion:* winter depression, sleep disorders, and other possible effects

HEART (ATRIA)

Atrial natriuretic hormone (ANH)	Regulates fluid and electrolyte homeostasis	(Uncertain)

GASTROINTESTINAL (GI) TRACT

Ghrelin	Affects energy balance (metabolism)	Possible obesity; increase in hunger and suppression of fat utilization

FAT-STORING CELLS

Leptin	Controls how hungry or full we feel	Possible obesity, other metabolic disorders

*In some cases, signs of hyposecretion result from target cell abnormality rather than from actual hyposecretion of a hormone.
†Posterior pituitary hormones are synthesized in the hypothalamus but released from axon terminals in the posterior pituitary.

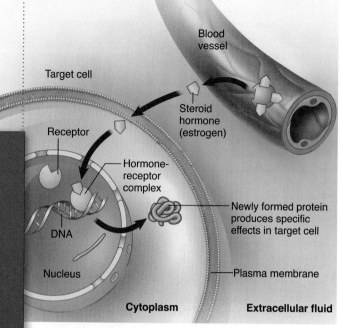

Blood vessel

Target cell

Steroid hormone (estrogen)

Receptor

Hormone-receptor complex

Newly formed protein produces specific effects in target cell

DNA

Nucleus

Plasma membrane

Cytoplasm **Extracellular fluid**

Figure 11-3 Mechanism of steroid hormone action.

Steroid hormones pass through the plasma membrane and enter the nucleus to form a hormone receptor complex that acts on DNA. As a result, a new protein is formed in the cytoplasm that produces specific effects in the target cell.

key model) to form a hormone-receptor complex. This complex acts on DNA, which ultimately causes the formation of a new protein in the cytoplasm that then produces specific effects in the target cell. In the case of estrogen, for example, that effect might be breast development in the female adolescent.

Figure 11-3 summarizes this mechanism of steroid hormone action. Because it takes some time to accomplish all of the steps illustrated in the diagram, steroid hormone responses typically are slow compared to responses triggered by nonsteroid hormones.

Besides the primary effects of steroids produced by the DNA-triggering mechanism just described, steroid hormones may also trigger membrane receptors to produce a variety of secondary effects. These secondary effects usually appear much more rapidly than do the primary steroid effects.

 To learn more about reasons cells may fail to respond to hormones, go to **AnimationDirect** on your CD.

QUICK CHECK

1. What is the chemical messenger used by the endocrine system?
2. How do *nonsteroid* hormones and *steroid* hormones differ? How are they alike?
3. What is a *second-messenger* system?

Regulation of Hormone Secretion

Regulation of hormone levels in the blood depends on a homeostatic mechanism called *negative feedback*—a concept first introduced in Chapter 1. The principle of **negative feedback** in the endocrine system can be illustrated by using the hormone insulin as an example. When released from endocrine cells in the pancreas, insulin lowers blood sugar levels. Normally,

HEALTH & WELL-BEING

STEROID ABUSE

Some steroid hormones are called **anabolic steroids** because they stimulate the building of large molecules (anabolism). Specifically, they stimulate the building of proteins in muscle and bone. Steroids such as testosterone and its synthetic derivatives are often abused by athletes and others who want to increase their athletic performance. The anabolic effects of the hormones increase the mass and strength of skeletal muscles.

Unfortunately, steroid abuse has other consequences that are not desirable. It disrupts the normal negative feedback control of hormones throughout the body and may result in tissue damage, sterility, mental imbalance, and many life-threatening metabolic problems. Abuse of steroids, other performance-enhancing drugs, or blood products in athletics is called *doping*. Such practices are outlawed in sports worldwide (see also the boxed essay on p. 350).

elevated blood sugar levels occur after a meal, after the absorption of sugars from the digestive tract takes place. The elevated blood sugar stimulates the release of insulin from the pancreas. Insulin then assists in the transfer of sugar from the blood into cells, causing blood sugar levels to drop. Low blood sugar levels then cause endocrine cells in the pancreas to cease the production and release of insulin. These responses are *negative*. Therefore the homeostatic mechanism is called a *negative feedback control mechanism* because it reverses the change in blood sugar level (Figure 11-4).

Positive feedback mechanisms, which are uncommon, amplify changes rather than reverse them. Usually, such amplification threatens homeostasis, but in some situations it can help the body maintain its stability. For example, during labor, the muscle contractions that push the baby through the birth canal become stronger and stronger by means of a positive feedback mechanism that regulates secretion of the hormone oxytocin (OT).

Mechanisms of Endocrine Disease

Diseases of the endocrine system are numerous, varied, and sometimes catastrophic. Tumors or other abnormalities frequently cause the glands to secrete too much or too little of their hormones. Production of too much hormone by a diseased gland is called **hypersecretion.** If too little hormone is produced, the condition is called **hyposecretion.**

A variety of endocrine disorders that appear to result from hyposecretion are actually caused by a problem in the target cells. If the usual target cells of a particular hormone have damaged receptors, too

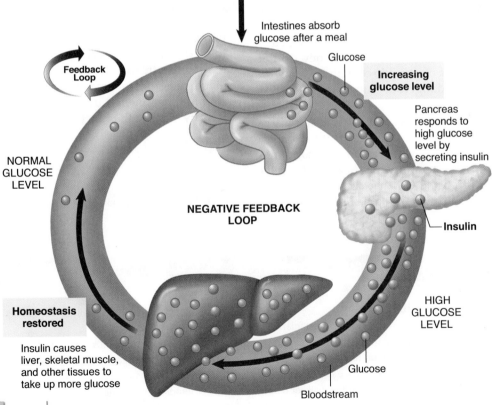

Intestines absorb
glucose after a meal

Glucose

**Feedback
Loop**

**Increasing
glucose level**

Pancreas
responds to
high glucose
level by
secreting insulin

NORMAL
GLUCOSE
LEVEL

**NEGATIVE FEEDBACK
LOOP**

Insulin

HIGH
GLUCOSE
LEVEL

**Homeostasis
restored**

Insulin causes
liver, skeletal muscle,
and other tissues to
take up more glucose

Glucose

Bloodstream

Figure 11-4 | **Negative feedback.**

The secretion of most hormones is regulated by negative feedback mechanisms that tend to reverse any deviations from normal. In this example, an increase in blood glucose triggers secretion of insulin. Because insulin promotes glucose uptake by cells, the blood glucose level is restored to its lower, normal level.

few receptors, or some other abnormality, they will not respond to that hormone properly. In other words, lack of target cell response could be a sign of hyposecretion or a sign of target cell insensitivity. *Diabetes mellitus,* for example, can result from insulin hyposecretion or from the target cells' insensitivity to insulin.

Disorders that result from the hypersecretion or hyposecretion of several hormones are often called **polyendocrine disorders**. Imbalances of one type of hormone often affect other hormones as well.

Endocrinologists, scientists who specialize in endocrine function, or **endocrinology** (en-doh-krin-AHL-ah-jee), have developed a variety of strategies for treating endocrine disorders. Surgical or chemical treatment of tumors or damaged tissue is useful in some cases. Another common strategy is the use of pharmacological preparations of hormones. For example, insulin injections are used in treating some forms of diabetes mellitus. The availability of synthetic hormones produced with genetic engineering technology has revolutionized the treatment of many endocrine disorders. Synthetic hormones are cheaper and more widely available than natural human hormones, and they do not carry the same risk of possible contamination with viruses or other dangerous substances (see box on p. 330).

Table 11-1 summarizes some of the major disorders of the endocrine system. Refer to this table often as you study the individual glands and hormones of the endocrine system. You may also want to refer to Appendix B on the CD that accompanies your book, which also contains a table listing major endocrine disorders.

Prostaglandins

Prostaglandins (PGs), or tissue hormones, are important and extremely powerful substances found in a wide variety of tissues. They play an important role in communication and in the control of many body functions but do not meet the definition of a typical hormone. The term *tissue hormone* is appropriate because in many instances a prostaglandin is produced in a tissue and then diffuses only a short distance to act on cells within that tissue. Typical hormones influence and control activities of widely separated organs; typical prostaglandins influence activities of neighboring cells.

The prostaglandins in the body can be divided into several groups. Three classes of prostaglandins—prostaglandin A (PGA), prostaglandin E (PGE), and prostaglandin F (PGF)—are among the best known. PGs have profound effects on many body functions. They influence respiration, blood pressure, gastrointestinal secretions, inflammation, and the reproductive system. Researchers believe that most PGs regulate cells by influencing the production of cyclic AMP. Although much research is yet to be done, PGs are already playing an important role in the treatment of conditions such as high blood pressure, asthma, and ulcers. In fact, many common treatments such as aspirin create their effects by altering the functions of PGs in the body.

> **QUICK CHECK**
>
> 1. How does negative feedback affect hormone levels in the blood?
> 2. Why are prostaglandins called *tissue hormones*?

RESEARCH, ISSUES, AND TRENDS

PROSTAGLANDIN THERAPY

Although much research is yet to be done, prostaglandins are already playing an important role in the treatment of diverse conditions such as high blood pressure, asthma, and ulcers. Because some prostaglandins have local muscle-relaxing effects, they can relax muscles in the walls of blood vessels to reduce blood pressure. In asthma, prostaglandins administered in a nebulizer (mist applicator) relax the muscles that constrict airflow during an asthma attack. Some gastric ulcers can be treated with prostaglandins that decrease stomach acid secretion.

Pharmacologists, scientists who study drug actions, or **pharmacology** (farm-ah-KAHL-ah-jee), have discovered that prostaglandins may also be involved in some traditional therapies. For example, evidence indicates that aspirin and its derivatives *(salicylates)* produce some of their effects by blocking prostaglandins involved in the inflammation response.

Pituitary Gland

The **pituitary** (pi-TOO-i-tair-ee) **gland** is a small but mighty structure. Although no larger than a pea, it is really two endocrine glands. One is called the anterior pituitary gland or **adenohypophysis** (ad-eh-no-hye-POF-i-sis), and the other is called the posterior pituitary gland or **neurohypophysis** (noo-roh-hye-POF-i-sis). Differences between the two glands are indicated by their names—*adeno* means "gland," and *neuro* means "nervous." The adenohypophysis has the structure of an endocrine gland, whereas the neurohypophysis has the structure of nervous tissue. Hormones secreted by the adenohypophysis serve very different functions from those released from the neurohypophysis.

The protected location of this dual gland suggests its importance. The pituitary gland lies buried deep in the cranial cavity, in the small depression of the sphenoid bone that is shaped like a saddle and called the **sella turcica** (Turkish saddle). A stemlike structure, the pituitary stalk, attaches the gland to the undersurface of the brain. More specifically, the stalk attaches the pituitary body to the hypothalamus.

Anterior Pituitary Gland Hormones

The anterior pituitary gland secretes several major hormones. Each of the four hormones listed as a **tropic** (TRO-pik) **hormone** in Table 11-1 stimulates another endocrine gland to grow and secrete its hormones. Because the anterior pituitary gland exerts this control over the structure and function of the thyroid gland, the adrenal cortex, the ovarian follicles, and the corpus luteum, in the past it was sometimes called the *master gland*. However, because its secretions are in turn controlled by the hypothalamus and other mechanisms, the anterior pituitary is hardly the master of body function it was once thought to be.

Thyroid-stimulating hormone (TSH) acts on the thyroid gland. As its name suggests, it stimulates the thyroid gland to increase secretion of thyroid hormone.

The **adrenocorticotropic** (ad-re-no-kor-ti-koh-TROH-pik) **hormone (ACTH)** acts on the adrenal cortex. It stimulates the adrenal cortex to increase in size and to secrete larger amounts of its hormones, especially larger amounts of cortisol (hydrocortisone).

Follicle-stimulating hormone (FSH) stimulates the primary ovarian follicles in an ovary to start growing and to continue developing to maturity (that is, to the point of ovulation). FSH also stimulates follicle cells to secrete estrogens. In the male, FSH stimulates the seminiferous tubules to grow and form sperm.

Luteinizing (LOO-teh-nye-zing) **hormone (LH)** acts with FSH to perform several functions. It stimulates a follicle and ovum to complete their growth to maturity, it stimulates follicle cells to secrete estrogens, and it causes ovulation (rupturing of the mature follicle with expulsion of its ripe ovum). Because of this function, LH is sometimes called the *ovulating hormone*. Finally, LH stimulates the formation of a golden body, the corpus luteum, in the ruptured follicle; the process is called **luteinization**. This function, of course, is the one that earned LH its title of *luteinizing hormone*. As it promotes luteinization, LH stimulates the corpus luteum to produce the hormone progesterone. The male pituitary gland also secretes LH. In males LH stimulates interstitial cells in the testes to develop and secrete testosterone, the male sex hormone.

Another important hormone secreted by the anterior pituitary gland is *growth hormone*. **Growth hormone (GH)** speeds up the movement of digested proteins (amino acids) out of the blood and into the cells, and this accelerates the cells' anabolism (buildup) of amino acids to form tissue proteins; hence this action promotes normal growth. Growth hormone also affects fat and carbohydrate metabolism; it accelerates fat catabolism (breakdown) but slows glucose catabolism. This means that less glucose leaves the blood to enter cells, and therefore the amount of glucose in the blood increases. Thus growth hormone and insulin have opposite effects on blood glucose. Insulin decreases blood glucose, and growth hormone increases it. Too much insulin in the blood produces **hypoglycemia** (hye-poh-glye-SEE-mee-ah) (lower than normal blood glucose concentration). Too much growth hormone produces **hyperglycemia** (higher than normal blood glucose concentration).

Hypersecretion of growth hormone during the early years of life produces a condition called **gigantism** (jye-GAN-tiz-em). The name suggests the obvious characteristics of this condition. The child grows to a giant size. If the anterior pituitary gland secretes too much growth hormone after the normal growth years, the disease called **acromegaly** (ak-roh-MEG-ah-lee) develops. Characteristics of this disease are enlargement of the bones of the hands, feet, jaws, and cheeks. The facial appearance that is typical of acromegaly results from the combination of bone and soft tissue overgrowth. A prominent forehead and large nose are characteristic. In addition, patients with acromegaly may have enlarged skin pores and an overgrown mandible. Figure 11-5 illustrates the major characteristics of gigantism and acromegaly.

Hyposecretion of growth hormone during the growth years often produces pituitary **dwarfism.** Pituitary dwarfs usually have a body frame of normal proportions but are much smaller in overall size. Dwarfism caused by other conditions may produce an oddly proportioned body frame. Figure 11-5, *A*, illustrates both gigantism and pituitary dwarfism.

The anterior pituitary gland also secretes **prolactin** (pro-LAK-tin), or lactogenic hormone. During pregnancy, prolactin stimulates the breast de-velopment necessary for eventual lactation (milk secretion). Also, soon after delivery of a baby, prolactin stimulates the breasts to start secreting milk, a function suggested by prolactin's other name, *lactogenic hormone.*

For a brief summary of anterior pituitary hormone target organs and functions, see Figure 11-6.

Posterior Pituitary Gland Hormones

The posterior pituitary gland releases two hormones— **antidiuretic** (an-tye-dye-yoo-RET-ik) **hormone (ADH)** and **oxytocin** (ok-see-TOH-sin), or **OT.** ADH accelerates the reabsorption of water from urine in kidney tubules back into the blood. With more water moving out of the tubules into the blood, less water remains in the tubules, and therefore less urine leaves the body. The name *antidiuretic hormone* is appropriate because *anti-* means "against" and **diuretic** means "increasing the volume of urine excreted." Therefore antidiuretic means "acting against an increase in urine volume"; in other words, ADH acts to decrease urine volume.

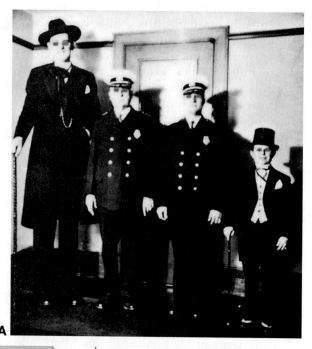

A

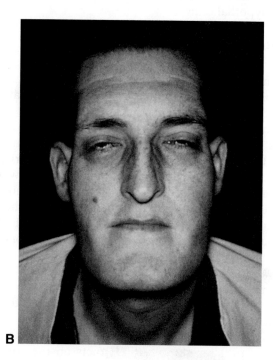

B

Figure **11-5** **Growth hormone abnormalities.**

A, Generations of students have viewed this photo of growth hormone abnormalities. The man to the far left exhibits gigantism caused by hypersecretion of growth hormone. The man on the far right exhibits pituitary dwarfism caused by hyposecretion of growth hormone. **B,** Acromegaly. Notice the large head, exaggerated projection of the lower jaw, and protrusion of the frontal bone.

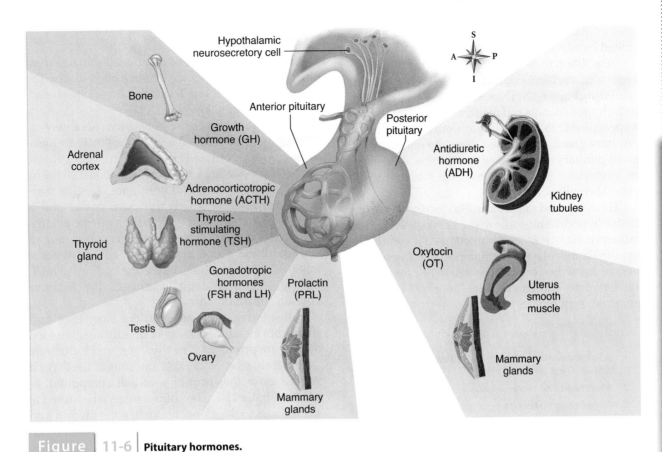

Hypothalamic
neurosecretory cell

Bone

Anterior pituitary

Posterior
pituitary

Growth
hormone (GH)

Adrenal
cortex

Antidiuretic
hormone
(ADH)

Adrenocorticotropic
hormone (ACTH)

Kidney
tubules

Thyroid-
stimulating
hormone (TSH)

Thyroid
gland

Oxytocin
(OT)

Gonadotropic
hormones
(FSH and LH)

Prolactin
(PRL)

Uterus
smooth
muscle

Testis

Ovary

Mammary
glands

Mammary
glands

Figure | 11-6 | **Pituitary hormones.**

Principal anterior and posterior pituitary hormones and their target organs.

The posterior pituitary hormone oxytocin is secreted by a woman's body before and after she has a baby. Oxytocin stimulates contraction of the smooth muscle of the pregnant uterus and is believed to initiate and maintain labor. This is why physicians sometimes prescribe oxytocin injections to induce or increase labor. Oxytocin also performs a function important to a newborn baby. It causes the glandular cells of the breast to release milk into ducts from which a baby can obtain it by sucking. In short, oxytocin stimulates "milk letdown." Oxytocin is also thought to enhance social bonding—a function helpful in supporting the mother-infant bond. The right side of Figure 11-6 summarizes posterior pituitary functions.

Diabetes insipidus (dye-ah-BEE-teez in-SIP-i-dus) is the name of the disease caused by hyposecretion of antidiuretic hormone. This condition is marked by the elimination of extremely large volumes of urine each day. In untreated cases, patients may excrete as much as 25 to 30 L of urine in a 24-hour period. In addition to voiding an abnormally large quantity of urine, these individuals suffer from great thirst, dehydration, and serious electrolyte imbalances. Treatment of diabetes insipidus requires the administration of replacement quantities of antidiuretic hormone orally, by injection, or by absorption of the hormone through the mucosa of the nose when given as a nasal spray.

Disorders of the anterior and posterior pituitary are summarized in Table 11-1.

Hypothalamus

In discussing ADH and oxytocin, we noted that these hormones were *released* from the posterior lobe of the pituitary. Actual production of these two hormones occurs in the hypothalamus. Two groups of specialized neurons in the hypothalamus synthesize the posterior pituitary hormones, which then pass down along axons into the pituitary gland. Release of ADH and oxytocin into the blood is controlled by nervous stimulation.

In addition to oxytocin and ADH, the hypothalamus also produces substances called **releasing** and **inhibiting hormones.** These substances are produced in the hypothalamus and then travel directly through a specialized blood capillary system to the anterior pituitary gland, where they cause the release of anterior pituitary hormones or, in a number of instances, inhibit their production and their release into the general circulation.

The combined nervous and endocrine functions of the hypothalamus allow the nervous system to influence many endocrine functions. Therefore, the hypothalamus plays a dominant role in the regulation of many body functions related to homeostasis. Examples include the regulation of body temperature, appetite, and thirst.

QUICK CHECK

1. How are the anterior pituitary and posterior pituitary different? How are they alike?
2. What makes a hormone a *tropic* hormone?
3. Can you name the hormones produced by the pituitary gland?
4. How does the hypothalamus control the pituitary gland?

Thyroid Gland

Earlier in this chapter, we mentioned that some endocrine glands are not located in a body cavity. The thyroid is one of these. It lies in the neck just below the larynx (Figure 11-7).

The thyroid gland secretes two thyroid hormones, **thyroxine** (thye-ROK-sin), or T_4, and **triiodothyronine** (try-eye-oh-doh-THY-roh-neen), or T_3. It also secretes the hormone **calcitonin** (kal-si-TOH-nin), or **CT**. Of the two thyroid hormones, T_4 is the more abundant; however, T_3 is the more potent and is considered by physiologists to be the principal thyroid hormone. One molecule of T_4 contains four atoms of iodine, and one molecule of T_3, as its name suggests, contains three iodine atoms. For T_4 and T_3 to be produced in adequate amounts, the diet must contain sufficient iodine.

Most endocrine glands do not store their hormones but instead secrete them directly into the blood as they are produced. The thyroid gland is different in that it stores considerable amounts of the thyroid hormones in the form of a colloid compound, as seen in Figure 11-8. The colloid material is stored in the follicles of the gland, and when the thyroid hormones are needed, they are released from the colloid and secreted into the blood.

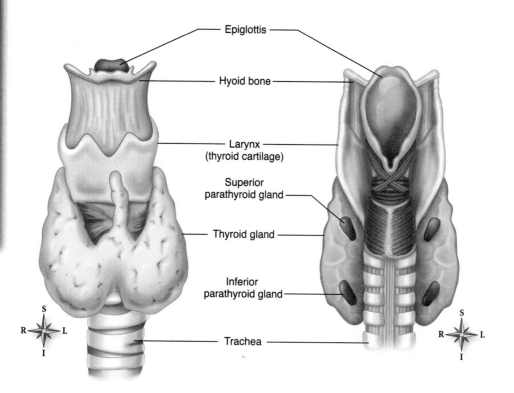

Epiglottis

Hyoid bone

Larynx (thyroid cartilage)

Superior parathyroid gland

Thyroid gland

Inferior parathyroid gland

Trachea

Figure 11-7

Thyroid and parathyroid glands.

Note their relationship to each other and to the larynx (voice box) and trachea.

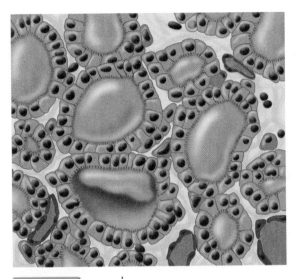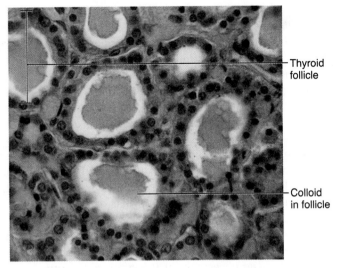

Thyroid
follicle

Colloid
in follicle

Figure 11-8 **Thyroid gland tissue.**

Note that each of the follicles is filled with colloid. The colloid serves as a storage medium for the thyroid hormones.

T_4 and T_3 influence every one of the trillions of cells in our bodies. They make them speed up their release of energy from foods. In other words, these thyroid hormones stimulate cellular metabolism. This has far-reaching effects. Because all body functions depend on a normal supply of energy, they all depend on normal thyroid secretion. Even normal mental and physical growth and development depend on normal thyroid functioning.

Calcitonin decreases the concentration of calcium in the blood by first acting on bone to inhibit its breakdown. With less bone being resorbed, less calcium moves out of bone into blood, and, as a result, the concentration of calcium in blood decreases. An increase in calcitonin secretion quickly follows any increase in blood calcium concentration, even if it is a slight one. This causes blood calcium concentration to decrease to its normal level. Calcitonin thus helps maintain homeostasis of blood calcium. It prevents a harmful excess of calcium in the blood, a condition called **hypercalcemia** (hye-per-kal-SEE-mee-ah), from developing.

Hyperthyroidism (hye-per-THYE-royd-iz-em), or oversecretion of the thyroid hormones, dramatically increases the metabolic rate. Food material is burned by the cells at an excessive rate, and individuals who suffer from this condition lose weight, have an increased appetite, and show signs of nervous irritability. They appear restless, jumpy, and excessively active. Many patients with hyperthyroidism also have very prominent, almost protruding eyes—a condition called **exophthalmos** (Figure 11-9).

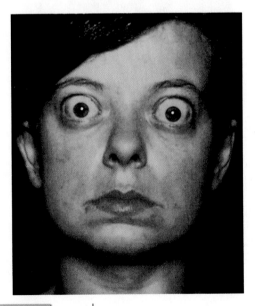

Figure 11-9 **Hyperthyroidism.**

Note the prominent, protruding eyes (exophthalmos) of this woman with Graves disease.

Hyperthyroidism with exophthalmos is characteristic of **Graves disease,** an inherited condition that occurs five times more frequently in women than in men.

Hypothyroidism (hye-poh-THYE-royd-iz-em) or undersecretion of thyroid hormones can be caused by and result in a number of different conditions. Low dietary intake of iodine causes a painless enlargement of the thyroid gland called **goiter** (GOY-ter), shown in Figure 11-10. This condition was once common in areas of the United States where the iodine content of the soil and water was inadequate. The use of iodized salt has dramatically reduced the incidence of goiters caused by low iodine intake. To produce a goiter, the gland enlarges in an attempt to compensate for the lack of iodine in the diet necessary for the synthesis of thyroid hormones.

Hyposecretion of thyroid hormones during the formative years leads to a condition called **cretinism** (KREE-tin-iz-em). It is characterized by a low metabolic rate, retarded growth and sexual development, and often, mental retardation. Fortunately, health screening for low thyroid function can lead to treatment before cretinism develops. Later in life, deficient thyroid hormone secretion produces the disease called **myxedema** (mik-seh-DEE-mah). The low metabolic rate that characterizes myxedema leads to lessened mental and physical vigor, weight gain, loss of hair, and an accumulation of mucous fluid in the subcutaneous tissue that is often most noticeable around the eyes (Figure 11-11).

Disorders of thyroid secretion are summarized in Table 11-1.

 To learn more about thyroid secretion, go to **AnimationDirect** on your CD.

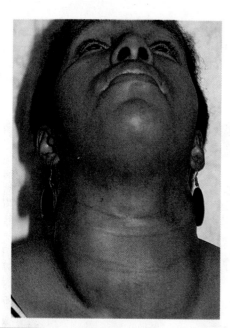

The enlarged thyroid gland appears as a swelling of the neck. This condition results from a low dietary intake of iodine.

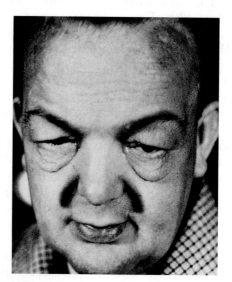

This condition results from hyposecretion of the thyroid gland during the adult years. Note the edema around the eyes and the facial puffiness.

To learn more about the pathophysiology of hypothyroidism, go to **AnimationDirect** on your CD.

Parathyroid Glands

The **parathyroid glands** are small glands. There are usually four of them, and they are found on the back of the thyroid gland (see Figure 11-7). The parathyroid glands secrete **parathyroid hormone (PTH).**

PTH increases the concentration of calcium in the blood—the opposite effect of the thyroid gland's calcitonin. Whereas calcitonin acts to decrease the amount of calcium being resorbed from bone, PTH acts to increase it. PTH stimulates bone-resorbing cells or osteoclasts to increase their breakdown of bone's hard matrix, a process that frees the calcium stored in the matrix. The released calcium then moves out of bone into blood, and this in turn increases the blood's calcium concentration. For a summary of the antagonistic effects of calcitonin and parathyroid hormone, see Figure 11-12. This is a matter of life-and-death importance because our cells are extremely sensitive to changing amounts of blood calcium. They cannot function normally with either too much or too little calcium. For example, with too much blood calcium, brain cells and heart cells soon do not function normally; a person becomes mentally disturbed, and the heart may stop altogether. However, with too little blood calcium, nerve cells become overactive, sometimes to such a degree that they bombard muscles with so many impulses that the muscles go into spasms.

Disorders of parathyroid secretion are summarized in Table 11-1.

> ### QUICK CHECK
>
> 1. Where are the thyroid and parathyroid glands located?
> 2. What gland is the only one that stores its hormones for later use?
> 3. Calcitonin and parathyroid hormone both regulate the blood concentration of what important ion?
> 4. Explain how a goiter develops.

Adrenal Glands

As you can see in Figures 11-1 and 11-13, an adrenal gland curves over the top of each kidney. From the surface an adrenal gland appears to be only one organ, but it is actually two separate endocrine glands: the **adrenal cortex** and the **adrenal**

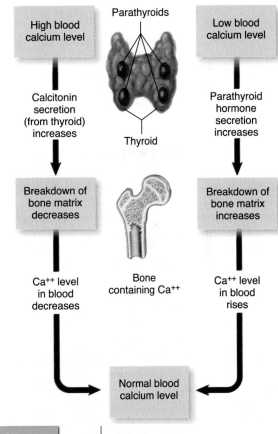

Figure 11-12 **Regulation of blood calcium levels.**

Calcitonin and parathyroid hormones have antagonistic (opposite) effects on calcium concentration in the blood. Both are negative feedback effects because they reverse a trend away from normal blood calcium levels.

medulla. Does this two-glands-in-one structure remind you of another endocrine organ? (See pp. 317-319.) The adrenal cortex is the outer part of an adrenal gland, and the medulla is its inner part. Adrenal cortex hormones have different names and quite different actions from adrenal medulla hormones.

Adrenal Cortex

Three different zones or layers of cells make up the **adrenal cortex** as you can see in Figure 11-13. Follow this diagram carefully as you read the following paragraph, and you will easily see the special function of each layer of the adrenal cortex.

Hormones secreted by the three cell layers or zones of the adrenal cortex are called **corticoids** (KOR-ti-koyds). The outer zone of adrenal cortex cells secretes hormones called **mineralocorticoids** (min-er-al-o-KOR-ti-koyds), or **MCs** for short. The main mineralocorticoid is the hormone **aldosterone** (al-DOS-ste-rone). The middle zone secretes **glucocorticoids** (gloo-ko-KOR-ti-koyds), or **GCs. Cortisol**, or **hydrocortisone,** the name given when cortisol is used as a pharmaceutical, is the chief glucocorticoid. The innermost or deepest zone of the cortex secretes small amounts of **sex hormones.** Sex hormones secreted by the adrenal cortex resemble testosterone. We shall now discuss briefly the functions of these three kinds of adrenal cortical hormones.

As their name suggests, **mineralocorticoids** help control the amount of certain mineral salts (mainly sodium chloride) in the blood. Aldosterone is the chief mineralocorticoid. Remember its main functions—to increase the amount of sodium and decrease the amount of potassium in the blood—because these changes lead to other profound changes. Aldosterone increases blood sodium and decreases blood potassium by influencing the kidney tubules. It causes them to speed up their reabsorption of sodium back into the blood so that less of it will be lost in the urine. At the same time, aldosterone causes the tubules to increase their secretion of potassium so that more of this mineral will be lost in the urine. The effects of aldosterone speed up kidney reabsorption of water.

One of the important functions of glucocorticoids is to help maintain normal blood glucose concentration. Glucocorticoids increase **gluconeogenesis** (gloo-koh-nee-oh-JEN-eh-sis), a process that converts amino acids or fatty acids to glucose and that is performed mainly by liver cells. Glucocorticoids act in several ways to increase gluconeogenesis. They promote the breakdown of tissue proteins to amino acids, especially in muscle cells. Amino acids thus formed move out of the tissue cells into blood and circulate to

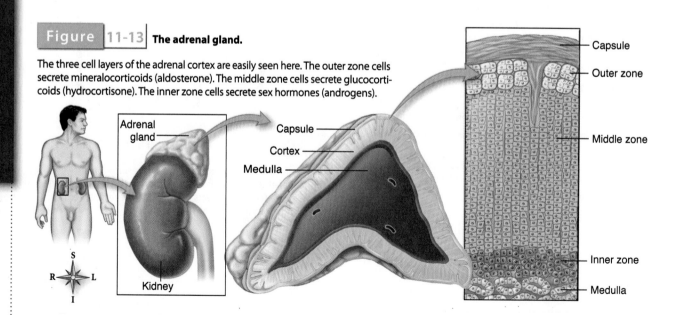

Figure 11-13 **The adrenal gland.**

The three cell layers of the adrenal cortex are easily seen here. The outer zone cells secrete mineralocorticoids (aldosterone). The middle zone cells secrete glucocorticoids (hydrocortisone). The inner zone cells secrete sex hormones (androgens).

Adrenal gland

Kidney

Capsule
Cortex
Medulla

Capsule
Outer zone
Middle zone
Inner zone
Medulla

the liver. Liver cells then change them to glucose by the process of gluconeogenesis. The newly formed glucose leaves the liver cells and enters the blood. This action increases blood glucose concentration.

In addition to performing functions that are necessary for maintaining normal blood glucose concentration, glucocorticoids also play an essential part in maintaining normal blood pressure. They act in a complicated way to make it possible for two other hormones secreted by the adrenal medulla to partially constrict blood vessels, a condition necessary for maintaining normal blood pressure. Also, glucocorticoids act with these hormones from the adrenal medulla to produce an antiinflammatory effect. They bring about a normal recovery from inflammations produced by many kinds of agents. The use of hydrocortisone to relieve skin rashes, for example, is based on the antiinflammatory effect of glucocorticoids.

Another effect produced by glucocorticoids is called their *antiimmunity, antiallergy effect.* Glucocorticoids bring about a decrease in the number of certain cells that produce antibodies, substances that make us immune to some factors and allergic to others.

When extreme stimuli act on the body, they produce an internal state or condition known as **stress.** Surgery, hemorrhage, infections, severe burns, and intense emotions are examples of extreme stimuli that bring on stress. The normal adrenal cortex responds to the condition of stress by quickly increasing its secretion of glucocorticoids. This fact is well established. What is still not known, however, is whether the increased amount of glucocorticoids helps the body cope successfully with stress. Increased glucocorticoid secretion is only one of many ways in which the body responds to stress, but it is one of the first stress responses, and it brings about many of the other stress responses. Examine Figure 11-14 to discover what stress responses are produced by a high concentration of glucocorticoids in the blood.

The sex hormones that are secreted by the inner zone are male hormones (androgens) similar to testosterone. These hormones are secreted in small amounts in both males and females. In females, these androgens stimulate the female sexual drive. In males, so much testosterone is secreted by the testes that adrenal androgens are usually not very important.

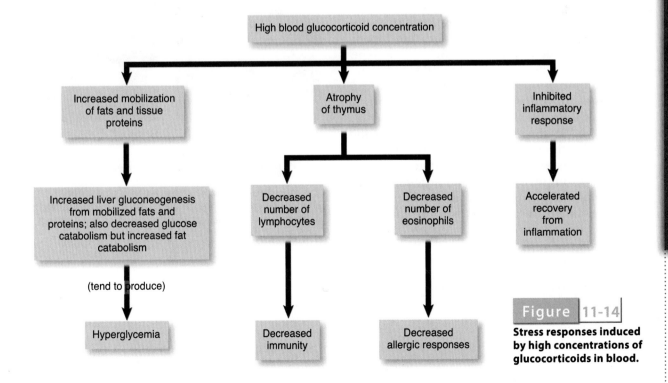

Figure 11-14

Stress responses induced by high concentrations of glucocorticoids in blood.

Adrenal Medulla

The **adrenal medulla,** or inner portion of the adrenal gland shown in Figure 11-13, secretes the hormones **epinephrine** (ep-i-NEF-rin) **(Epi)** and **norepinephrine** (nor-ep-i-NEF-rin) **(NR).**

Our bodies have many ways to defend themselves against enemies that threaten their well-being. A physiologist might say that the body resists stress by making many stress responses. We have just discussed increased glucocorticoid secretion. An even faster-acting stress response is increased secretion by the adrenal medulla. This occurs very rapidly because nerve impulses conducted by sympathetic nerve fibers stimulate the adrenal medulla. When stimulated, it literally squirts epinephrine and norepinephrine into the blood. As with glucocorticoids, these hormones may help the body resist or avoid stress. In other words, these hormones produce the body's "fight-or-flight" response to danger (stress). However, epinephrine and norepinephrine are not essential for maintaining life.

Suppose you suddenly faced some threatening situation. Imagine that a gunman threatened to kill you or that your doctor told you that you had to have a dangerous operation. Almost instantaneously, the medullas of your two adrenal glands would be galvanized into feverish activity. They would quickly secrete large amounts of epinephrine (adrenaline) into your blood. Many of your body functions would seem to be supercharged. Your heart would beat faster; your blood pressure would rise; more blood would be pumped to your skeletal muscles; your blood would contain more glucose for more energy, and so on. In short, you would be geared for strenuous activity, for "fight or flight." Epinephrine prolongs and intensifies changes in body function brought about by the stimulation of the sympathetic subdivision of the autonomic nervous system. Recall from Chapter 9 that sympathetic, or adrenergic, fibers release epinephrine and norepinephrine as neurotransmitter substances.

The close functional relationship between the nervous and the endocrine systems is perhaps most noticeable in the body's response to stress. In stress conditions, the hypothalamus acts on the anterior pituitary gland to cause the release of ACTH, which stimulates the adrenal cortex to secrete glucocorticoids. In addition, the sympathetic subdivision of the autonomic nervous system is stimulated with the adrenal medulla, so the release of epinephrine and norepinephrine occurs to assist the body in responding to the stressful stimulus. Unfortunately, during periods of prolonged stress, glucocorticoids may have harmful side effects because they are antiinflammatory and cause blood vessels to constrict. For example, decreased immune activity in the body may promote the spread of infections and cancer, and prolonged blood vessel constriction may lead to increased blood pressure.

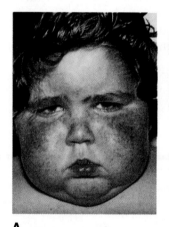 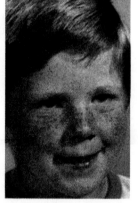

A   **B**

Figure **11-15** **Cushing syndrome.**

This condition results from hypersecretion of glucocorticoid hormone by a tumor of the middle zone of the adrenal cortex. **A,** Photo taken when patient was first diagnosed with Cushing syndrome. **B,** Taken 4 months after treatment.

To learn more about adrenal function, go to **AnimationDirect** on your CD.

Adrenal Abnormalities

Injury, disease states, or malfunction of the adrenal glands can result in hypersecretion or hyposecretion of several different hormones.

Tumors of the adrenal cortex located in the middle zone often result in the production of abnormally large amounts of glucocorticoids. The medical name for the collection of symptoms that characterize hypersecretion of glucocorticoids is **Cushing syndrome.** For some reason more women than men develop Cushing syndrome. Its most noticeable features are the so-called *moon face* (Figure 11-15) and the *buffalo hump* on the upper back that develop because of the redistribution of body fat. Individuals with Cushing syndrome also have elevated blood sugar levels and suffer frequent infections. Surgical removal of a glucocorticoid-producing tumor may result in dramatic improvement of the moon-face symptom within only 4 months.

Tumors that affect the inner zone of the adrenal cortex often produce testosterone-like sex hormones called *androgens.* As a result, the symptoms of hypersecretion often resemble the male secondary sexual characteristics such as beard growth, development of body hair, and increased muscle mass. If these masculinizing symptoms appear in a woman (Figure 11-16), the cause is frequently a **virilizing** (VEER-il-eye-zing) **tumor** of the adrenal cortex. The term *virile* is from the Latin word *virilis* meaning "male" or "masculine."

Deficiency or hyposecretion of adrenal cortex hormones results in a condition called **Addison disease.** President John F. Kennedy suffered from Addison disease, which causes reduced cortical hormone levels that result in muscle weakness, reduced blood sugar, nausea, loss of appetite, and weight loss.

Disorders of adrenal secretion are summarized in Table 11-1.

QUICK CHECK

1. Why is the adrenal gland often thought of as two separate glands?
2. Name the hormones produced by the adrenal gland.
3. How does the pituitary gland influence adrenal function?
4. Addison disease is caused by hyposecretion of which hormone?

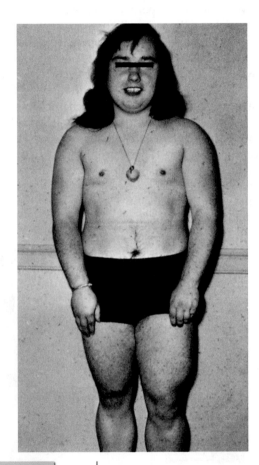

Figure 11-16 **Results of a virilizing tumor.**
This young girl has a virilizing tumor of the inner zone of the adrenal cortex. The tumor secretes androgens, thereby producing masculinizing effects that resemble the secondary sex characteristics of men.

Pancreatic Islets

All the endocrine glands discussed so far are big enough to be seen without a magnifying glass. The **pancreatic islets,** or **islets of Langerhans,** in contrast, are too tiny to be seen without a microscope. These glands are merely little clumps of cells scattered like islands in a sea among the pancreatic cells that secrete the pancreatic digestive juice (Figure 11-17).

Two of the most important kinds of cells in the pancreatic islets are the *alpha cells* (or *A cells*) and *beta cells* (or *B cells*). Alpha cells secrete a hormone called **glucagon,** whereas beta cells secrete one of the most well known of all hormones, **insulin.** Glucagon accelerates a process called **glycogenolysis** (glye-ko-jen-OL-i-sis) in the liver. Glycogenolysis is a chemical process by which the glucose stored in the liver cells in the form of glycogen is converted to glucose. This glucose then leaves the liver cells and enters the blood. Glucagon therefore increases blood glucose concentration.

Insulin and glucagon are antagonists. In other words, insulin decreases blood glucose concentration; glucagon increases it. Insulin is the only hormone that can decrease blood glucose concentration. Other hormones, however, increase its concentration, including glucocorticoids, growth hormone, and glucagon. Insulin decreases blood glucose by accelerating its movement out of the blood, through cell membranes, and into cells. As glucose enters the cells at a faster rate, the cells increase their metabolism of glucose. Briefly then, insulin decreases blood glucose and increases glucose metabolism.

If the pancreatic islets secrete a normal amount of insulin, a normal amount of glucose enters the cells, and a normal amount of glucose stays behind in the blood. ("Normal" blood glucose is about 80 to 110 mg of glucose in every 100 ml of blood during fasting.) If the pancreatic islets secrete too much insulin, as they sometimes do when a person has a tumor of the pancreas, more glucose than usual leaves the blood to enter the cells, and blood glucose decreases. If the pancreatic islets secrete too little insulin, as they do in **type 1 diabetes** (dye-ah-BEE-tes) **mellitus** (mell-EYE-tus), less glucose leaves the blood to enter the cells,

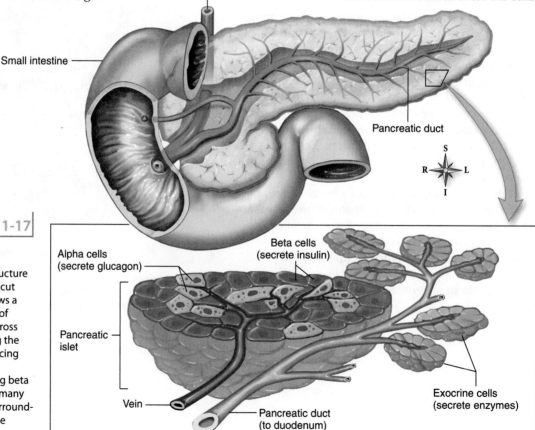

Figure 11-17

Pancreas.

Location and structure of the pancreas (cut open). Inset shows a pancreatic islet (of Langerhans) in cross section, showing the glucagon-producing alpha cells and insulin-producing beta cells. Notice the many exocrine cells surrounding the endocrine pancreatic islet.

Common bile duct

Small intestine

Pancreatic duct

S
R — L
I

Alpha cells (secrete glucagon)

Beta cells (secrete insulin)

Pancreatic islet

Vein

Pancreatic duct (to duodenum)

Exocrine cells (secrete enzymes)

so the blood glucose increases, sometimes to even three or more times the normal amount. Most cases of **type 2 diabetes mellitus** result from an abnormality of the insulin receptors, preventing the normal effects of insulin on its target cells and thus also raising blood glucose levels.

Screening tests for all types of diabetes mellitus are based on the fact that the blood glucose level is elevated in this condition. Today, most screening is done with a simple test that requires only a drop of blood. Subjects with a high blood glucose level are suspected

of having diabetes mellitus. Testing for sugar in the urine is another common screening procedure. In diabetes mellitus, excess glucose is filtered out of the blood by the kidneys and lost in the urine, producing the condition **glycosuria** (glye-koh-SOO-ree-ah). Figure 11-18 summarizes some of the many problems that can be caused by diabetes mellitus. A quick look at these problems underscores the importance of insulin and insulin receptors in healthy bodies.

Disorders of pancreatic islet secretion are summarized in Table 11-1.

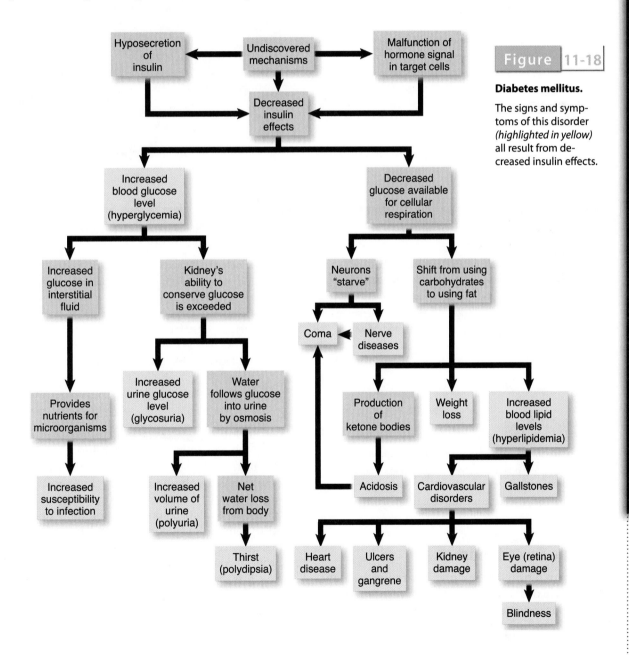

Figure 11-18

Diabetes mellitus.

The signs and symptoms of this disorder *(highlighted in yellow)* all result from decreased insulin effects.

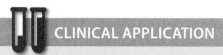

CLINICAL APPLICATION

SYNTHETIC HUMAN INSULIN

Advances in biotechnology and genetic engineering have made several types of synthetic human insulin available for treatment of diabetes. Genetically engineered human insulin was one of the first "artificial hormones" developed for use in clinical medicine. Prior to its release, pork and beef pancreases were harvested from animals to produce the only form of insulin available for human use. This form of insulin is still widely used. However, in some individuals, small but important differences in the chemical makeup of animal and human insulin (one to three amino acids) results in immune system or allergic reactions. For these individuals, development of synthetic human insulin was a major medical breakthrough.

Today, synthetic insulin is administered in different ways, depending on individual circumstances. For example, it can be injected with small needles in various forms, such as in a small syringe "pen." Or it can be injected through a timed, implantable insulin pump. Other methods of insulin delivery are also available or being investigated. For example, powdered or liquid insulin can be inhaled using an inhaler, then absorbed through respiratory mucous membranes. Patches containing insulin may be used to absorb insulin through the skin. Researchers have also developed insulin pills that could dramatically improve diabetes care for millions if in the long run they prove to be safe and effective.

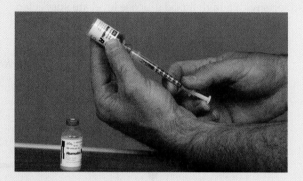

HEALTH & WELL-BEING

EXERCISE AND DIABETES MELLITUS

Type 1 diabetes mellitus is characterized by high blood glucose concentration because the lack of sufficient insulin prevents glucose from entering cells. However, exercise physiologists have found that aerobic training increases the number of insulin receptors in target cells and the insulin affinity (attraction) of the receptors. This condition allows a small amount of insulin to have a greater effect than it would have otherwise had. Thus exercise reduces the severity of the diabetic condition.

All forms of diabetes benefit from properly planned exercise therapy. Not only is this form of treatment natural and cost-effective, but it also helps reduce or prevent other problems such as obesity and heart disease.

QUICK CHECK

1. Name the two primary hormones of the pancreatic islets.
2. What effect does insulin have on the blood's glucose concentration?
3. How does diabetes produce glucose in the urine?

Female Sex Glands

A woman's primary sex glands are her two ovaries. Each ovary contains two different kinds of glandular structures: the ovarian follicles and the corpus luteum. **Ovarian follicles** are little pockets in which egg cells, or **ova,** develop. Ovarian follicles also secrete estrogen, the "feminizing hormone." Estrogen is involved in the development and maturation of the breasts and external genitals. This hormone is also responsible for development of adult female body contours and initiation of the menstrual cycle. The **corpus luteum** chiefly secretes progesterone but also some estrogen. We shall save our discussion of the structure of these endocrine glands and the functions of their hormones for Chapter 22.

Male Sex Glands

Some of the cells of the testes produce the male sex cells called **sperm.** Other cells in the testes, male reproductive ducts, and glands produce the liquid portion of the male reproductive fluid called *semen.* The interstitial cells in the testes secrete the male sex hormone called **testosterone** directly into the blood. These cells of the testes are therefore the male endocrine glands. Testosterone is the "masculinizing hormone." It is responsible for the maturation of the external genitals, beard growth, changes in voice at puberty, and for the muscular development and body contours typical of the male. Chapter 22 contains more information about the structure of the testes and the functions of testosterone.

Thymus

The thymus is located in the mediastinum (see Figure 11-1), and in infants it may extend up into the neck as far as the lower edge of the thyroid gland. Like the adrenal gland, the thymus has a cortex and medulla. Both portions are composed largely of lymphocytes (white blood cells). As part of the body's immune system, the endocrine function of the thymus is not only important but also essential. This small structure (it weighs a little more than an ounce) plays a critical part in the body's defenses against infections—its vital immunity mechanism.

The hormone **thymosin** (THY-moh-sin) is actually a group of several hormones that together play an important role in the development and function of the body's immune system.

Placenta

The placenta functions as a temporary endocrine gland. During pregnancy, it produces **chorionic** (koh-ree-ON-ik) **gonadotropins** (go-nah-doh-TROH-pins), so called because they are tropic hormones secreted by cells of the **chorion** (KOH-ree-on), the outermost membrane that surrounds the baby during development in the uterus. In addition to chorionic gonadotropins, the placenta also produces estrogen and progesterone. During the earliest weeks of pregnancy, the kidneys excrete large amounts of chorionic gonadotropins in the urine. This fact, discovered more than a half century ago, led to the development of early pregnancy tests.

Pineal Gland

The pineal gland is a small gland near the roof of the third ventricle of the brain (see Figure 9-12). It is named "pineal" because it resembles the pine nut (which looks like a small kernel of corn). The pineal gland is easily located in a child but becomes fibrous and encrusted with calcium deposits as a person ages. The pineal gland produces a number of hormones in very small quantities, with **melatonin** being the most significant. Melatonin inhibits the tropic hormones that affect the ovaries, and it is thought to be involved in regulating the onset of puberty and the menstrual cycle in women. Because the pineal gland receives and responds to sensory information from the optic nerves, it is sometimes called the *third eye.* The pineal gland uses information regarding changing light levels to adjust its output of melatonin; melatonin levels increase during the night and decrease during the day. This cyclic variation is thought to be an important timekeeping mechanism for the body's internal clock and sleep cycle. Melatonin supplements are now widely used as an aid to induce sleep or to "reprogram" the sleep cycle as a treatment for jet lag.

Abnormal secretion of or sensitivity to melatonin is implicated in a number of disorders. One dramatic example is *seasonal affective disorder (SAD).* Patients with this condition exhibit signs of clinical depression only during the winter months, when nights are long. Apparently, unusually high melatonin levels associated with long winter nights cause psychological effects in these patients. A treatment that has been successful in some cases involves the use of bright lights in the person's indoor environment for a few hours each day after sundown. The pineal gland seems to be tricked into responding as if the patient were experiencing a long summer day, thus secreting less melatonin (see Table 11-1).

Other Endocrine Structures

Continuing research into the endocrine system has shown that nearly every organ and system has an endocrine function. Tissues in the kidneys, stomach, intestines, and other organs secrete hormones that regulate a variety of essential human functions. For example, **ghrelin** (GRAY-lin) is secreted by epithelial cells lining the stomach and boosts appetite, slows metabolism, and reduces fat burning. Ghrelin may, therefore, be involved in the development of obesity. Another example is **atrial natriuretic hormone (ANH),** which is secreted by cells in the wall of the heart's atria (upper chambers). ANH is an important regulator of fluid and electrolyte homeostasis. ANH is an antagonist to aldosterone. Aldosterone stimulates the kidney to retain sodium ions and water, whereas ANH stimulates loss of sodium ions and water.

A more recently discovered hormone is **leptin,** which is secreted by fat-storing cells throughout the body. Leptin seems to regulate how hungry or full we feel and how fat is metabolized by the body. Researchers are now looking at how leptin works with other hormones, such as ghrelin, in the hopes of finding ways to treat patients with obesity, diabetes mellitus, and other disorders involving fat storage.

QUICK CHECK

1. Which hormones are produced by the male and female sex glands?
2. Why is the placenta considered to be a gland?
3. Why is the pineal gland sometimes called a timekeeper of the body?

SCIENCE APPLICATIONS

ENDOCRINOLOGY

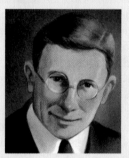

Banting (1891–1941)

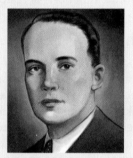

Best (1899–1978)

The undisputed heroes of endocrinology are Canadian surgeon Frederick Banting and his assistant Charles Best. Until the early twentieth century, children with type 1 diabetes mellitus died a slow, horrible death as a result of their cells literally starving to death from lack of glucose. Acting on Banting's idea for removing insulin from the pancreatic islets of dogs, the two were the first to successfully isolate this important hormone. Chemist James Collip was able to purify the insulin sufficiently so that in 1921 their colleague, Scots physiologist John Macleod, could administer the insulin to a 14-year-old boy with diabetes. It worked! The treatment not only relieved the boy's suffering, but it also gave him a healthy, long life. This breakthrough, for which Banting and Macleod received the 1923 Nobel Prize, was the start of a century of rapid progress in understanding and treating endocrine disorders.

Because hormones affect so many different body functions, nearly every kind of health professional, from medical doctors to nurses to dietitians, needs to be aware of their functions. Of course, hormones and chemicals that influence hormone actions are often used in treatments, so pharmacologists and pharmacists also must have an excellent knowledge of endocrinology. Some scientists have applied principles of endocrinology in a variety of unexpected ways, including the development of early pregnancy test kits and ovulation test kits, to the use of synthetic hormones in healthy people to help them control their fertility.

Outline Summary

To download an MP3 version of the chapter summary for use with your iPod or portable media player, access the **Audio Chapter Summaries** on your CD.

Mechanisms of Hormone Action

A. Endocrine glands secrete chemicals (hormones) into the blood (Figure 11-1)

B. Hormones perform general functions of communication and control but a slower, longer-lasting type of control than that provided by nerve impulses

C. Cells acted on by hormones are called *target organ cells*

D. Nonsteroid hormones (first messengers) bind to receptors on the target cell membrane, triggering second messengers to affect the cell's activities (Figure 11-2)

E. Steroid hormones
1. Primary effects produced by binding to receptors within the target cell nucleus and influence cell activity by acting on DNA—a slower process than nonsteroid action (Figure 11-3)
2. Secondary effects may occur when steroid hormones bind to membrane receptors to rapidly trigger functional changes in the target cell

Regulation of Hormone Secretion

A. Hormone secretion is controlled by homeostatic feedback
B. Negative feedback—mechanisms that reverse the direction of a change in a physiological system (Figure 11-4)
C. Positive feedback—(uncommon) mechanisms that amplify physiological changes

Mechanisms of Endocrine Disease (Table 11-1)

A. Hypersecretion—secretion of an excess of hormone
B. Hyposecretion—insufficient hormone secretion
C. Polyendocrine disorders—hyper- or hyposecretion of more than one hormone
D. Target cell insensitivity produces results similar to hyposecretion
E. Endocrinologists have developed many different strategies for treatment (for example, surgery and hormone therapy)

Prostaglandins

A. Prostaglandins (PGs) are powerful substances found in a wide variety of body tissues
B. PGs are often produced in a tissue and diffuse only a short distance to act on cells in that tissue
C. Several classes of PGs include prostaglandin A (PGA), prostaglandin E (PGE), and prostaglandin F (PGF)
D. PGs influence many body functions, including respiration, blood pressure, gastrointestinal secretions, and reproduction

Pituitary Gland (Figure 11-6)

A. Anterior pituitary gland (adenohypophysis)
1. Names of major hormones
   a. Thyroid-stimulating hormone (TSH)
   b. Adrenocorticotropic hormone (ACTH)
   c. Follicle-stimulating hormone (FSH)
   d. Luteinizing hormone (LH)
   e. Growth hormone (GH)
   f. Prolactin (lactogenic hormone)
2. Functions of major hormones
   a. TSH—stimulates growth of the thyroid gland; also stimulates it to secrete thyroid hormone
   b. ACTH—stimulates growth of the adrenal cortex and stimulates it to secrete glucocorticoids (mainly cortisol)
   c. FSH—initiates growth of ovarian follicles each month in the ovary and stimulates one or more follicles to develop to the stage of maturity and ovulation; FSH also stimulates estrogen secretion by developing follicles; stimulates sperm production in the male
   d. LH—acts with FSH to stimulate estrogen secretion and follicle growth to maturity; causes ovulation; causes luteinization of the ruptured follicle and stimulates progesterone secretion by corpus luteum; causes interstitial cells in the testes to secrete testosterone in the male
   e. GH—stimulates growth by accelerating protein anabolism; also accelerates fat catabolism and slows glucose catabolism; by slowing glucose catabolism, tends to increase blood glucose to higher than normal level (hyperglycemia)
      (1) Hypersecretion during childhood results in gigantism and during adulthood results in acromegaly
      (2) Hyposecretion during childhood results in pituitary dwarfism
   f. Prolactin or lactogenic hormone—stimulates breast development during pregnancy and secretion of milk after the delivery of the baby
B. Posterior pituitary gland (neurohypophysis)
1. Names of hormones
   a. Antidiuretic hormone (ADH)

(1) Hyposecretion causes diabetes insipidus, characterized by excessive volume of urine
  b. Oxytocin (OT)
 2. Functions of hormones
  a. ADH—accelerates water reabsorption from urine in the kidney tubules into the blood, thereby decreasing urine secretion
  b. Oxytocin—stimulates the pregnant uterus to contract; may initiate labor; causes glandular cells of the breast to release milk into ducts

Hypothalamus

A. Actual production of ADH and oxytocin occurs in the hypothalamus
B. After production in the hypothalamus, hormones pass along axons into the pituitary gland
C. The secretion and release of posterior pituitary hormones are controlled by nervous stimulation
D. The hypothalamus controls many body functions related to homeostasis (temperature, appetite, and thirst)

Thyroid Gland (Figure 11-7)

A. Names of hormones
 1. Thyroid hormone—thyroxine (T_4) and triiodothyronine (T_3)
 2. Calcitonin (CT)
B. Functions of hormones
 1. Thyroid hormones—accelerate catabolism (increase the body's metabolic rate)
 2. Calcitonin—decreases the blood calcium concentration by inhibiting breakdown of bone, which would release calcium into the blood
C. Hyperthyroidism (hypersecretion of thyroid hormones) increases metabolic rate
 1. Characterized by restlessness and exophthalmos (protruding eyes)
 2. Graves disease is an inherited form of hyperthyroidism
D. Hypothyroidism (hyposecretion of thyroid hormones)
 1. May result from different conditions
 2. Goiter—painless enlargement of thyroid caused by dietary deficiency of iodine
 3. Hyposecretion during early development may result in cretinism (retardation) and

during adulthood in myxedema (characterized by edema and sluggishness)

Parathyroid Glands (Figure 11-7)

A. Name of hormone—parathyroid hormone (PTH)
 1. Function of hormone—increases blood calcium concentration by increasing the breakdown of bone with the release of calcium into the blood

Adrenal Glands (Figure 11-13)

A. Adrenal cortex
 1. Names of hormones (corticoids)
  a. Glucocorticoids (GCs)—chiefly cortisol (hydrocortisone)
  b. Mineralocorticoids (MCs)—chiefly aldosterone
  c. Sex hormones—small amounts of male hormones (androgens) secreted by adrenal cortex of both sexes
 2. Three cell layers (zones)
  a. Outer layer—secretes mineralocorticoids
  b. Middle layer—secretes glucocorticoids
  c. Inner layer—secretes sex hormones
 3. Mineralocorticoids—increase blood sodium and decrease body potassium concentrations by accelerating kidney tubule reabsorption of sodium and excretion of potassium
 4. Functions of glucocorticoids
  a. Help maintain normal blood glucose concentration by increasing gluconeogenesis—the formation of "new" glucose from amino acids produced by the breakdown of proteins, mainly those in muscle tissue cells; also the conversion to glucose of fatty acids produced by the breakdown of fats stored in adipose tissue cells
  b. Play an essential part in maintaining normal blood pressure—make it possible for epinephrine and norepinephrine to maintain a normal degree of vasoconstriction, a condition necessary for maintaining normal blood pressure
  c. Act with epinephrine and norepinephrine to produce an antiinflammatory effect, to bring about normal recovery from inflammations of various kinds

  d. Produce antiimmunity, antiallergy effect; bring about a decrease in the number of lymphocytes and plasma cells and therefore a decrease in the amount of antibodies formed
  e. Secretion of glucocorticoid quickly increases when the body is thrown into a condition of stress; high blood concentration of glucocorticoids, in turn, brings about many other stress responses (Figure 11-14)

B. Adrenal medulla
  1. Names of hormones—epinephrine (Epi), or adrenaline, and norepinephrine (NR)
  2. Functions of hormones—help the body resist stress by intensifying and prolonging the effects of sympathetic stimulation; increased epinephrine secretion is the first endocrine response to stress

C. Adrenal abnormalities
  1. Hypersecretion of glucocorticoids causes Cushing syndrome: moon face, hump on back, elevated blood sugar levels, frequent infections
  2. Hypersecretion of adrenal androgens may result from a virilizing tumor and cause masculinization of affected women
  3. Hyposecretion of cortical hormones may result in Addison disease: muscle weakness, reduced blood sugar, nausea, loss of appetite, and weight loss

Pancreatic Islets (Figure 11-17)

A. Names of hormones
  1. Glucagon—secreted by alpha cells
  2. Insulin—secreted by beta cells

B. Functions of hormones
  1. Glucagon increases the blood glucose level by accelerating glycogenolysis in liver (conversion of glycogen to glucose)
  2. Insulin decreases the blood glucose by accelerating the movement of glucose out of the blood into cells, which increases glucose metabolism by cells

C. Diabetes mellitus (Figure 11-18)
  1. Type 1 results from hyposecretion of insulin
  2. Type 2 results from target cell insensitivity to insulin

  3. Glucose cannot enter cells and thus blood glucose levels rise, producing glycosuria (glucose in the urine)

Female Sex Glands

A. The ovaries contain two structures that secrete hormones—the ovarian follicles and the corpus luteum; see Chapter 22
  1. Effects of estrogen (feminizing hormone)
    a. Development and maturation of breasts and external genitals
    b. Development of adult female body contours
    c. Initiation of menstrual cycle

Male Sex Glands

A. The interstitial cells of testes secrete the male hormone testosterone; see Chapter 22
  1. Effects of testosterone (masculinizing hormone)
    a. Maturation of external genitals
    b. Beard growth
    c. Voice changes at puberty
    d. Development of musculature and body contours typical of the male

Thymus

A. Name of hormone—thymosin
B. Function of hormone—plays an important role in the development and function of the body's immune system

Placenta

A. Name of hormones—chorionic gonadotropins, estrogens, and progesterone
B. Functions of hormones—maintain the corpus luteum during pregnancy

Pineal Gland

A. A small gland near the roof of the third ventricle of the brain
  1. Glandular tissue predominates in children and young adults
  2. Becomes fibrous and calcified with age

B. Called third eye because its influence on secretory activity is related to the amount of light entering the eyes
C. Secretes melatonin, which
   1. Inhibits ovarian activity
   2. Regulates the body's internal clock
D. Abnormal secretion of (or sensitivity to) melatonin may produce seasonal affective disorder (SAD) or winter depression, a form of depression that occurs when exposure to sunlight is low and melatonin levels are high

Other Endocrine Structures

A. Many organs (for example, the stomach, intestines, and kidneys) produce endocrine hormones
   1. Stomach lining produces ghrelin, which affects appetite and metabolism
B. The atrial wall of the heart secretes atrial natriuretic hormone (ANH), which stimulates sodium loss from the kidneys
C. Fat-storing cells secrete leptin, which controls how full or hungry we feel

New Words

adenohypophysis	ghrelin	positive feedback	cretinism
adrenal cortex	glucagon	prolactin	Cushing syndrome
adrenal medulla	glucocorticoid (GC)	prostaglandin (PG)	diabetes insipidus
adrenocorticotropic hormone (ACTH)	gluconeogenesis	releasing hormone (RH)	dwarfism
aldosterone	glycogenolysis	second-messenger mechanism	exophthalmos
antidiuretic hormone (ADH)	growth hormone (GH)	sella turcica	gigantism
atrial natriuretic hormone (ANH)	hormone	sex hormone	glycosuria
calcitonin (CT)	inhibiting hormone (IH)	signal transduction	goiter
chorion	insulin	steroid hormone	Graves disease
chorionic gonadotropin	leptin	stress	hypercalcemia
corticoid	luteinization	target organ cell	hyperglycemia
cortisol (hydrocortisone)	luteinizing hormone (LH)	thymosin	hypersecretion
cyclic AMP	melatonin	thyroid-stimulating hormone (TSH)	hyperthyroidism
diuretic	mineralocorticoid (MD)	thyroxine (T_4)	hypoglycemia
endocrine gland	negative feedback	triiodothyronine (T_3)	hyposecretion
endocrine system	neurohypophysis	tropic hormone	hypothyroidism
endocrinology	nonsteroid hormone		myxedema
epinephrine (Epi)	norepinephrine (NR)	**Diseases and Other Clinical Terms**	pharmacology
exocrine gland	oxytocin (OT)		polyendocrine disorder
follicle-stimulating hormone (FSH)	pancreatic islet (islet of Langerhans)	acromegaly	type 1 diabetes mellitus
	parathyroid gland	Addison disease	type 2 diabetes mellitus
	parathyroid hormone (PTH)		virilizing tumor
	pituitary gland		

Review Questions

1. Differentiate between endocrine and exocrine glands.
2. Define or explain the following terms: *hormone, target organ, hypersecretion,* and *hyposecretion.*
3. Explain the mechanism of action of nonsteroid hormones.
4. Explain the mechanism of action of steroid hormones.

5. Explain and give an example of a negative feedback loop for the regulation of hormone secretion.
6. Explain and give an example of a positive feedback loop for the regulation of hormone secretion.
7. Explain the difference between prostaglandins and hormones. List some of the body functions that can be influenced by prostaglandins.
8. Describe the structure of the pituitary gland and where it is located.
9. Name the four tropic hormones released by the anterior pituitary gland and briefly explain their functions.
10. Explain the function of growth hormone.
11. Gigantism and acromegaly have the same cause; what is the cause and what causes the difference in effect between the two conditions?
12. Explain the function of ADH.
13. What is the cause of diabetes insipidus? What are the signs and symptoms of the condition?
14. Explain the function of prolactin and oxytocin.
15. Explain the function of the hypothalamus in the endocrine system.
16. Explain the difference between T_3 and T_4. What is unique about the thyroid gland?
17. Distinguish between *cretinism* and *myxedema*.

18. Name the hormones produced by the zones or areas of the adrenal cortex.
19. What are the signs and symptoms of Cushing syndrome? Of Addison disease?
20. Explain the function of aldosterone.
21. Explain the function of glucocorticoids.

Critical Thinking

22. Explain why a secondary messenger system is needed for nonsteroid hormones but not for steroid hormones.
23. Pick a body function (regulation of glucose or calcium levels in the blood) and explain how the interaction of hormones is used to help maintain homeostasis.
24. Why is a goiter usually more of a dietary problem rather than an endocrine problem?
25. A doctor discovered a patient had very low levels of thyroxine by noting high levels of TSH. Is the patient's problem in the thyroid gland or the pituitary gland? Explain your answer.
26. If a person diagnosed with diabetes mellitus were found to be producing a normal amount of insulin, what other cause could explain the diabetes?

Chapter Test

1. _____ glands secrete their products into ducts that empty onto a surface or into a cavity.
2. _____ glands are ductless and secrete their products, called _____, into intercellular space, where they diffuse into the blood.
3. The two major classes of hormones are _____ and _____.
4. A cell or body organ that has receptors for a hormone that triggers a reaction is called a _____.
5. One example of a second-messenger system involves the conversion of ATP into _____.
6. The hormone receptors for a nonsteroid hormone are located in the _____, whereas the receptors for a steroid hormone are located in the _____.

7. "Tissue hormones" is another name for _____.
8. What part of the pituitary gland is made of nervous tissue? _____
9. What part of the pituitary gland is made of glandular tissue? _____
10. The hormone oxytocin is released by the _____ but is made in the _____.
11. A tropic hormone secreted by the anterior pituitary gland is:
    a. thyroid-stimulating hormone
    b. adrenocorticotropic hormone
    c. luteinizing hormone
    d. all of the above
12. Antidiuretic hormone (ADH)
    a. is made in the posterior pituitary gland
    b. accelerates water reabsorption in the kidney
    c. in high concentration causes diabetes insipidus

d. all of the above

13. Which of the following hormones is released by the anterior pituitary gland and stimulates breast development during pregnancy necessary for eventual milk production?
    a. Estrogen
    b. Oxytocin
    c. Prolactin
    d. Progesterone

14. Which hormone released by the posterior pituitary gland stimulates the contraction of the pregnant uterus?
    a. Estrogen
    b. Oxytocin

c. Prolactin
d. Progesterone

15. Thyroxine:
    a. is symbolized by T_3
    b. is made in the thyroid gland
    c. contains less iodine than triiodothyronine
    d. all of the above

16. Calcitonin:
    a. decreases the level of calcium in the blood
    b. increases the level of calcium in the blood
    c. stimulates the release of calcium from bone tissue
    d. both b and c

Match each hormone in Column A with its function or source in Column B.

Column A
17. _____ parathyroid hormone
18. _____ mineralocorticoids
19. _____ glucocorticoids
20. _____ epinephrine
21. _____ glucagons
22. _____ insulin
23. _____ chorionic gonadotropins
24. _____ melatonin
25. _____ atrial natriuretic hormone

Column B
a. released by the adrenal medulla; prolongs the effect of the sympathetic nervous system
b. made in the heart; helps regulate blood sodium
c. made in the pancreatic islets; decreases blood glucose levels
d. has the opposite effect of calcitonin
e. made by the alpha cells in the pancreatic islets
f. made in the outermost layer of the adrenal cortex
g. the most significant hormone released by the pineal gland
h. the hormone made in the placenta and detected by home pregnancy tests
i. made by the middle layer of the adrenal cortex

Match each description or signs and symptoms in Column B with its corresponding endocrine disorder in Column A.

Column A
26. _____ giantism
27. _____ acromegaly
28. _____ diabetes insipidus
29. _____ Graves disease
30. _____ myxedema
31. _____ goiter
32. _____ cretinism
33. _____ Cushing syndrome
34. _____ diabetes mellitus
35. _____ seasonal affective disorder

Column B
a. an inherited hyperthyroidism with exophthalmos
b. hyposecretion of thyroid hormone in later life leading to lessened physical and mental vigor
c. hyposecretion of insulin causing an increased blood glucose level
d. hypersecretion of growth hormone after the normal growth years
e. an enlarged thyroid gland as a result of dietary deficiency of iodine
f. a condition caused by a hypersecretion of glucocorticoids
g. hypersecretion of growth hormone in the early years of life
h. hyposecretion of thyroid hormone in the formative years resulting in physical, mental, and sexual retardation
i. a condition caused by high secretions of melatonin, causing depression in winter
j. hyposecretion of ADH, causing the production of a large volume of urine

Study Tips

continued from page 309

in explaining the disorders. Usually, if you know the normal function of the hormone, you should be able to figure out what effect on the body hyposecretion or hypersecretion would have.

5. In your study group, discuss the hormone mechanisms and negative feedback loops involved in hormone regulation. Review the hormone flash cards. A photocopy of Table 11-1 would be a good way to organize almost all the information in the chapter. Go over the chart of endocrine disorders and the questions at the end of the chapter, and discuss possible test questions.

Case Studies

1. George, the chief executive officer of a major institution, was jogging around his summer home when he became distressed at what seemed to be an irregularity of his heart rhythm. His assistants immediately rushed George to a hospital, where he was diagnosed as having atrial fibrillation (uncoordinated contractions of the upper heart chambers). George was even more distressed to hear that he had a specific heart condition, fearing it might disrupt his very active lifestyle. His physicians informed him that the overactivity of his heart—and perhaps other organs—was caused by hyperthyroidism. Explain how hyperthyroidism could cause George's problems. What strategies might his physicians have available for treating him?

2. In George's case (see case study #1), the attending physicians chose to surgically remove part of the thyroid in an attempt to control George's hyperthyroidism. What precautions ought George's surgeons take in removing this tissue? (HINT: What anatomical structures in the thyroid area should they avoid cutting or removing?)

3. Your friend Lynn has type 1 diabetes mellitus. What therapy is likely to help her regain control of her metabolism and thus avoid possible tissue or organ damage? Lynn has told you that her condition, if untreated, results in "starvation" of cells in her body. This condition is characterized by hyperglycemia (elevated blood glucose), so you might wonder how the cells could starve if they have an excess of nutrients available. What is the explanation for this seemingly contradictory fact?

Outline

Objectives

After you have completed this chapter, you should be able to:

1. Describe the primary functions of blood.
2. Describe the characteristics of blood plasma.
3. List the formed elements of blood and identify the most important function of each.
4. Discuss anemia in terms of red blood cell numbers and hemoglobin content.
5. Explain the steps involved in blood clotting.
6. Describe ABO and Rh blood typing.
7. Define the following medical terms associated with blood: *hematocrit, leukocytosis, leukopenia, polycythemia, sickle cell, phagocytosis, acidosis, thrombosis, erythroblastosis fetalis, serum, fibrinogen, Rh factor, anemia, hemophilia, thrombocytopenia.*
8. Name two common disorders associated with each type of blood cell.

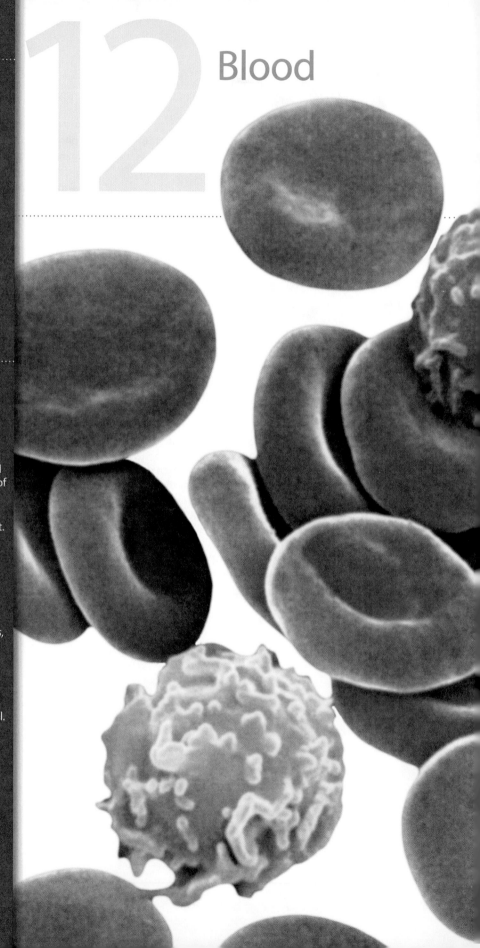

12 Blood

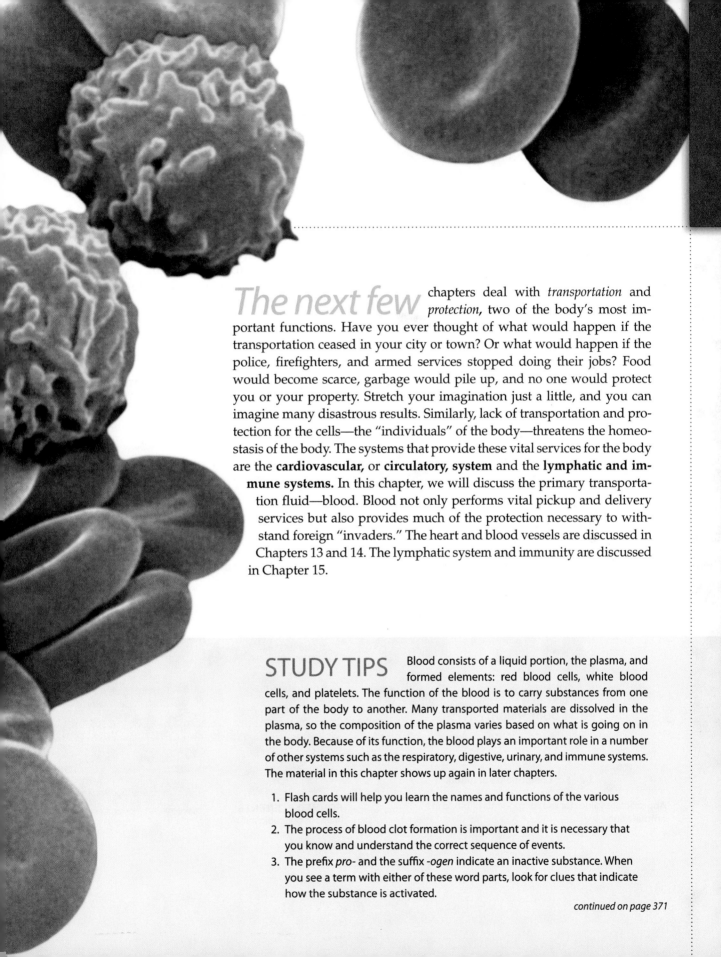

The next few chapters deal with *transportation* and *protection*, two of the body's most important functions. Have you ever thought of what would happen if the transportation ceased in your city or town? Or what would happen if the police, firefighters, and armed services stopped doing their jobs? Food would become scarce, garbage would pile up, and no one would protect you or your property. Stretch your imagination just a little, and you can imagine many disastrous results. Similarly, lack of transportation and protection for the cells—the "individuals" of the body—threatens the homeostasis of the body. The systems that provide these vital services for the body are the **cardiovascular,** or **circulatory, system** and the **lymphatic and immune systems.** In this chapter, we will discuss the primary transportation fluid—blood. Blood not only performs vital pickup and delivery services but also provides much of the protection necessary to withstand foreign "invaders." The heart and blood vessels are discussed in Chapters 13 and 14. The lymphatic system and immunity are discussed in Chapter 15.

STUDY TIPS

Blood consists of a liquid portion, the plasma, and formed elements: red blood cells, white blood cells, and platelets. The function of the blood is to carry substances from one part of the body to another. Many transported materials are dissolved in the plasma, so the composition of the plasma varies based on what is going on in the body. Because of its function, the blood plays an important role in a number of other systems such as the respiratory, digestive, urinary, and immune systems. The material in this chapter shows up again in later chapters.

1. Flash cards will help you learn the names and functions of the various blood cells.
2. The process of blood clot formation is important and it is necessary that you know and understand the correct sequence of events.
3. The prefix *pro-* and the suffix *-ogen* indicate an inactive substance. When you see a term with either of these word parts, look for clues that indicate how the substance is activated.

continued on page 371

Blood Composition and Volume

Blood is a fluid tissue that has many kinds of chemicals dissolved in it and millions upon millions of cells floating in it (Figure 12-1). The liquid (extracellular) part is called **plasma.** Suspended in the plasma are many different types of cells and cell fragments that make up the **formed elements** of blood.

Many people are curious about just how much blood they have. The amount depends on how big they are and whether they are male or female. A big person has more blood than a small person, and a man has more blood than a woman. But as a general rule, most adults probably have between 4 and 6 L of blood. It normally accounts for about 7% to 9% of the total body weight.

The volume of the plasma part of blood is usually a little more than half the entire volume of whole blood. An example of normal blood volumes for a person follows:

	Plasma	2.6 L
+	Formed elements	2.4 L
	Whole blood	5.0 L

Blood is alkaline, with a pH between 7.35 and 7.45—always staying just above the neutral point of 7.00 (see Chapter 2). If the alkalinity of your blood decreases toward neutral, you are a very sick person; in fact, you have **acidosis.** But even in this condition, blood almost never becomes the least bit acid; it just becomes less alkaline than normal.

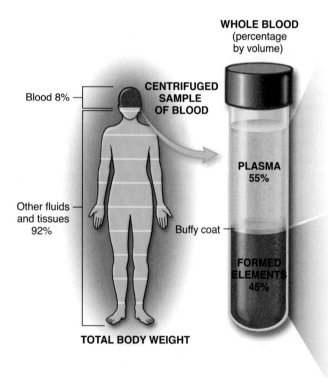

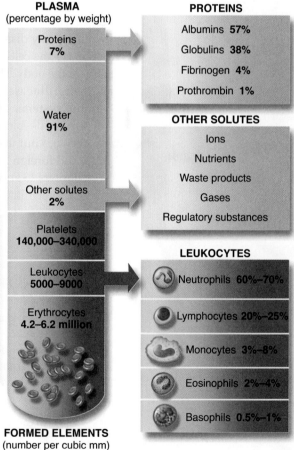

Figure 12-1 | Components of blood.

Approximate values for the components of blood in a normal adult.

Whole blood is a precious commodity in regard to human life, in the case of major injury, often a lifesaving commodity. Until such time as a safe and effective blood substitute (see box below) is developed, being able to treat major blood loss will depend on the availability of donated blood. To fill that need, each year more than 14 million units of whole blood are donated to blood banks in the United States. Unfortunately, blood can be stored for only 6 weeks, and the donated blood must be "cross-matched" and "typed" before it can be infused into a needy recipient. Because severe blood loss often occurs as a result of accidental trauma, the time required to type and cross-match donor and recipient blood to ensure compatibility often delays blood transfusion beyond the time when such treatment has its greatest value. In cases of severe blood loss, the first hour—the "golden hour"—is critical, and the availability of blood truly can be lifesaving. So-called *plasma volume expanders*, such as albumin solutions, may help maintain blood volume in the body for short periods after acute losses, but unlike whole blood, these solutions do not contain the needed components found in the formed elements and plasma that are required to maintain homeostasis over time. Safety concerns related to viral contamination of blood, the time delays required to first cross-match donor and recipient blood, especially detrimental in crisis situations, and the possibility of errors being made in the process are powerful incentives that are propelling research in the direction of developing an "artificial blood."

QUICK CHECK

1. Name the liquid (extracellular) fraction of whole blood.
2. Blood accounts for what percent (%) of total body weight?
3. How do *plasma volume expanders* differ from whole blood?

Blood Types

Blood is identified as a specific "type" by using the **ABO** and **Rh systems** of classification.

RESEARCH, ISSUES, AND TRENDS

ARTIFICIAL BLOOD

One of the primary benefits of blood transfusion is an increase in oxygen-carrying capacity caused by increases in hemoglobin levels. However, blood is a complex liquid tissue, and transfusion always carries with it certain risks. For years medical researchers have worked to develop "artificial blood" or a "blood substitute" that could duplicate one or more blood functions without subjecting a recipient to transfusion reactions, infections, or other health dangers.

At the present time several blood substitutes are in various stages of development. As a group they are sometimes called *oxygen therapeutics*. Ultimately, to be successful and approved for use, these experimental products must be proven in clinical trials to be safe and effective in transporting oxygen in individuals who are seriously sick or injured. Availability of an oxygen therapeutic in circumstances where blood is not available could well be lifesaving. Ideally, the drug manufacturing process should result in an oxygen-carrying blood substitute that can be transfused into any blood-type recipient without typing and that is free of blood-borne viruses such as HIV and hepatitis C. Another "second-generation" artificial blood product is also under development. If efforts are successful, it will be produced using recombinant hemoglobin technology. By using genetic engineering techniques, production of this type of product would not require the use of existing human blood or blood products.

Artifical blood products would likely be easier to store and transport than natural blood, and thus more readily available in emergencies or remote locations. They may also prove to be safer—at least in terms of blood-borne infections and transfusion reactions. When available, artificial blood substitutes will be viewed as exciting and welcome developments in transfusion medicine.

Blood types are identified by certain antigens in red blood cells (RBCs) (Figure 12-2). An **antigen** (AN-ti-jen) is a substance that can stimulate the body to make antibodies. Almost all substances that act as antigens are foreign proteins. That is, they are not the body's own natural proteins but instead are proteins that have entered the body from the outside by means of infection, transfusion, or some other method.

The word *antibody* can be defined in terms of what causes its formation or in terms of how it functions. Defined the first way, an **antibody** (AN-ti-bod-ee) is a substance made by the body in response to stimulation by an antigen. Defined according to its functions, an antibody is a substance that reacts with the antigen that stimulated its formation. Many antibodies react with their antigens to cause clumping; that is, they **agglutinate** (ah-GLOO-tin-ayt) the antigens. In other words, the antibodies cause their targeted antigens to stick together in little clusters.

ABO SYSTEM

Every person's blood is one of the following blood types in the ABO system of typing:

1. Type A
2. Type B
3. Type AB
4. Type O

Suppose that you have type A blood (as do about 41% of Americans). The letter *A* stands for a certain type of antigen (a protein) in the plasma membrane of your RBCs that has been present since birth. Because you were born with type A antigen, your body does not form antibodies to react with it. In other words, your blood plasma contains no anti-A antibodies. It does, however, contain anti-B antibodies. For some unknown reason, these antibodies are present naturally in type A blood plasma. The body

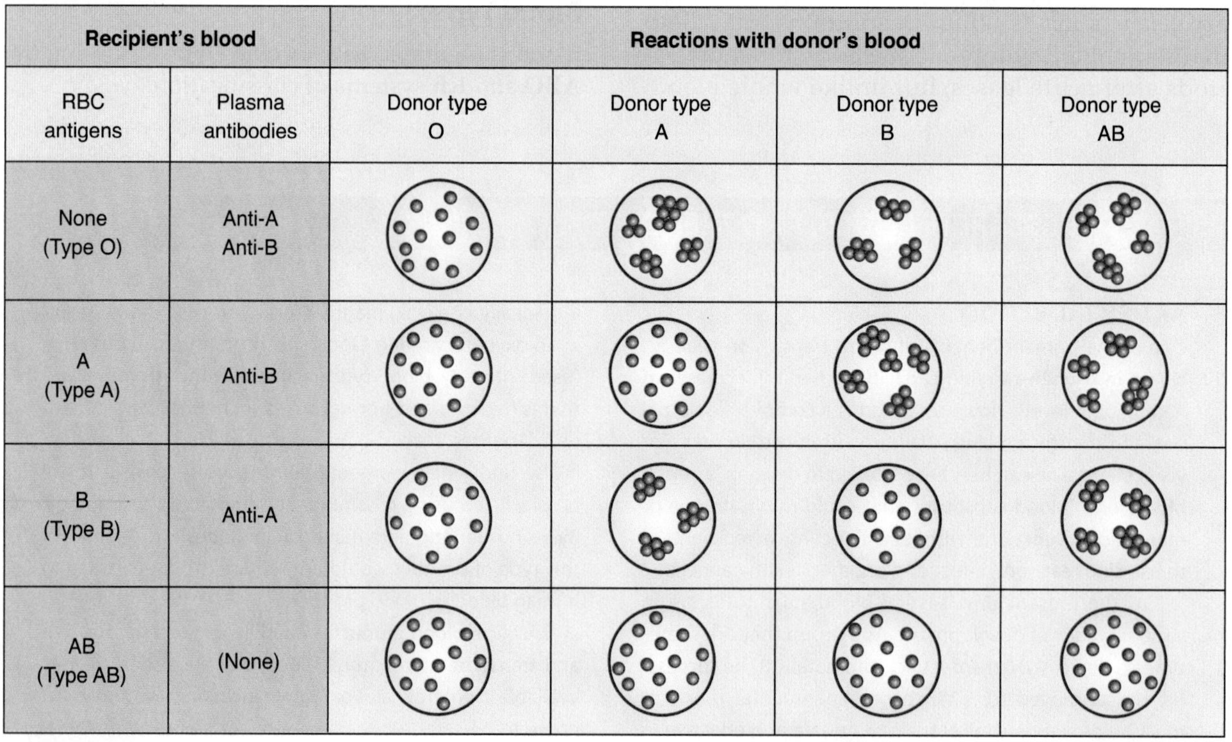

Recipient's blood		Reactions with donor's blood			
RBC antigens	Plasma antibodies	Donor type O	Donor type A	Donor type B	Donor type AB
None (Type O)	Anti-A Anti-B				
A (Type A)	Anti-B				
B (Type B)	Anti-A				
AB (Type AB)	(None)				

Figure 12-2

Results of different combinations of donor and recipient blood.
The left columns show the recipient's blood characteristics and the top row shows the donor's blood type. *Inset,* photo showing samples of agglutinated and nonagglutinated blood.

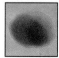

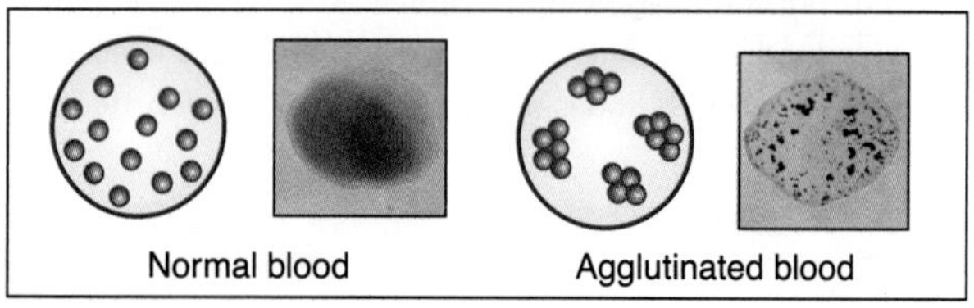

Normal blood   Agglutinated blood

did not form them in response to the presence of the B antigen; they are simply part of the body's genetic makeup. In summary, in type A blood the RBCs contain type A antigen and the plasma contains anti-B antibodies.

Similarly, in type B blood, the RBCs contain type B antigen, and the plasma contains anti-A antibodies. In type AB blood, as its name indicates, the RBCs contain both type A and type B antigens, and the plasma contains neither anti-A nor anti-B antibodies. The opposite is true of type O blood; its RBCs contain neither type A nor type B antigens, and its plasma contains both anti-A and anti-B antibodies.

Harmful effects or even death can result from a blood transfusion if the donor's RBCs become agglutinated by antibodies in the recipient's plasma. If a donor's RBCs do not contain any A or B antigen, they of course cannot be clumped by anti-A or anti-B antibodies. For this reason the type of blood that contains neither A nor B antigens—namely, type O blood—can be used in an emergency as donor blood with only minimal danger of anti-A or anti-B antibodies clumping its RBCs. Type O blood has therefore been called **universal donor blood** and is always in short supply. Similarly, blood type AB has been called **universal recipient blood** because it contains neither anti-A nor anti-B antibodies in its plasma. Therefore it does not clump any donor's RBCs containing A or B antigens. In a normal clinical setting, however, all blood intended for transfusion is matched carefully to the blood of the recipient for a variety of factors.

Figure 12-2 shows the results of different combinations of donor and recipient blood.

 To learn more about blood grouping, go to AnimationDirect on your CD.

RH SYSTEM

You may be familiar with the term **Rh-positive** blood. It means that the RBCs of this blood type contain an antigen called the *Rh factor*. If, for example, a person has type AB, Rh-positive blood, his red blood cells contain type A antigen, type B antigen, and the Rh factor antigen. The term *Rh* is used because this important blood cell antigen was first discovered in the blood of Rhesus monkeys.

In **Rh-negative** blood the RBCs do not have the Rh antigens on their surfaces. Plasma never naturally contains anti-Rh antibodies. But if Rh-positive blood cells are introduced into an Rh-negative person's body, anti-Rh antibodies soon appear in the recipient's (in this case, the mother's) blood plasma. In this fact lies the danger for a baby born to an Rh-negative mother and an Rh-positive father. If the baby inherits the Rh-positive trait from his father, the Rh factor on his RBCs may stimulate the mother's body to form anti-Rh antibodies. Then, if she later carries another Rh-positive fetus, he may develop a type of hemolytic anemia called **erythroblastosis** (e-rith-roh-blas-TOH-sis) **fetalis** (feh-TAL-iss), caused by the mother's Rh antibodies reacting with the baby's Rh-positive cells (see pp. 354-355 and Figure 12-8).

All Rh-negative mothers who carry an Rh-positive baby should be treated with a protein marketed as **RhoGAM**. RhoGAM stops the mother's body from forming anti-Rh antibodies and thus prevents the possibility of harm to the next Rh-positive baby.

Likewise, a person with Rh-negative blood who receives a transfusion of Rh-positive blood will also develop anti-Rh antibodies and be at risk of an immune reaction if exposed to Rh-positive blood again later.

 To learn more about hemolytic disease of the newborn, go to **AnimationDirect** on your CD.

QUICK CHECK

1. Name the blood types identified in the ABO system of typing.
2. What blood type is called universal donor blood? Universal recipient blood?
3. What is meant when a person's blood is described as "Rh-negative"?

Blood Plasma

Blood plasma is the liquid part of the blood, or blood minus its formed elements. It consists of water with many substances dissolved in it. All of the chemicals needed by cells to stay alive—food, oxygen, and salts, for example—have to be brought to them by the blood. Food and salts are dissolved in plasma; so, too, is about 3% of the total amount of oxygen (O_2) transported in the blood. Wastes that cells must get rid of are dissolved in plasma and transported to the excretory organs. Approximately

5% of the total amount of the waste product carbon dioxide (CO_2) that is carried in the blood is dissolved in the plasma. In addition to the relatively small amounts of O_2 and CO_2 dissolved in plasma, other mechanisms are involved in the transportation of these important gases in the blood and are described below. The hormones and other regulatory chemicals that help control cells' activities are also dissolved in plasma.

As Figure 12-1 shows, the most abundant type of solute in the plasma is a group of **plasma proteins.** These proteins include **albumins**, which help retain water in the blood; **globulins,** which include the antibodies that help protect us from infections; and *fibrinogen* and *prothrombin,* which are necessary for blood clotting.

Intravenous administration of albumin is sometimes used as a plasma volume expander in people with abnormally low blood volume. The injected albumin will draw about three to four times its volume of fluid into the blood through the process of osmosis. The result is an expansion of blood volume that can be lifesaving in cases of hemorrhage, severe burns, or kidney disease.

Blood **serum** is plasma minus its clotting factors, such as fibrinogen and prothrombin. Serum is obtained from whole blood by allowing the blood

to first clot in the bottom of a tube; then the liquid serum that remains at the top is poured off. Serum still contains antibodies, so it can be used to treat patients who have a need for specific antibodies.

Formed Elements

There are three main types and several subtypes of formed elements:

1. Red blood cells (RBCs), or erythrocytes (eh-RITH-roh-sytes)
2. White blood cells (WBCs), or leukocytes (LOO-koh-sytes)
   a. Granular leukocytes (have granules in their cytoplasm)
      (1) Neutrophils
      (2) Eosinophils
      (3) Basophils
   b. Nongranular leukocytes (do not have granules in their cytoplasm)
      (1) Lymphocytes
      (2) Monocytes
3. Platelets, or thrombocytes (THROM-boh-sytes)

Figure 12-1 shows the breakdown of numbers and percentages of the formed elements. Table 12-1 lists the functions of these different kinds of blood cells and shows what each looks like under the microscope.

CLINICAL APPLICATION

CARDIAC BLOOD TESTS

Sometimes blood plasma contains excesses of normal substances or low amounts of abnormal substances that may indicate disease. For example, when the heart muscle is damaged, enzymes contained within the muscle cells are released into the bloodstream, causing increased plasma levels of these enzymes. Blood tests for a number of cardiac enzymes, including creatine kinase (CK), lactic dehydrogenase (LD), and serum glutamic-oxaloacetic transaminase (SGOT), are useful in confirming a *myocardial infarction (MI),* or "heart attack."

The *troponins test* is another very valuable diagnostic aid. Rather than making an enzymatic determination, it identifies a specific biochemical marker present in cardiac disease. The presence of cardiac troponins is particularly useful in differentiating cardiac from noncardiac chest pain and in evaluating angina and suspected coronary ischemic syndrome.

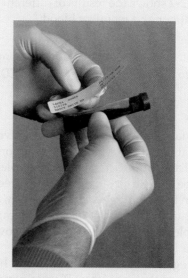

Table 12-1	Classes of Blood Cells
BODY CELL	**FUNCTION**
Erythrocyte	Oxygen and carbon dioxide transport
Neutrophil	Immune defense (phagocytosis)
Eosinophil	Defense against parasites
Basophil	Inflammatory response and heparin secretion
B lymphocyte	Antibody production (precursor of plasma cells)
T lymphocyte	Cellular immune response
Monocyte	Immune defenses (phagocytosis)
Thrombocyte	Blood clotting

It is difficult to believe just how many blood cells and cell fragments are in the human body. For instance, 5,000,000 RBCs, 7500 WBCs, and 300,000 platelets in 1 cubic millimeter (mm^3) of blood (approximately one drop) would be considered normal RBC, WBC, and platelet counts. Because RBCs, WBCs, and platelets are continually being destroyed, the body also must continually make new ones to take their place at a really staggering rate; a few million RBCs are manufactured *each second!*

Two kinds of connective tissue—**myeloid tissue** and **lymphatic tissue**—make blood cells for the body. Recall that formation of new blood cells is called *hematopoiesis.* Myeloid tissue is better known as *red bone marrow.* In the adult, it is found chiefly in the sternum, ribs, and hip bones. A few other bones such as the vertebrae, clavicles, and cranial bones also contain small amounts of this valuable substance. Red bone marrow forms all types of blood cells except some lymphocytes and monocytes. Most of these others are formed by lymphatic tissue, which is located chiefly in the lymph nodes, thymus, and spleen.

As blood cells mature, they move into the circulatory vessels. Erythrocytes circulate up to 4 months before they break apart and their components are removed from the bloodstream by the spleen and liver. Granular leukocytes often have a life span of only a few days, but nongranular leukocytes may live more than 6 months.

QUICK CHECK

1. What is the most abundant type of solute in plasma? Give examples.
2. List the formed elements of blood.

Mechanisms of Blood Disease

Most blood diseases are disorders of the formed elements. Thus it is not surprising that the basic mechanism of many blood diseases is the failure of the blood-producing myeloid and lymphatic tissues to form blood cells properly. In many cases, this failure is the result of damage by toxic chemicals or radiation. In other cases, it results from an inherited defect, viral infection, or even cancer.

If bone marrow failure is the suspected cause of a particular blood disorder, a sample of myeloid tissue may be drawn into a syringe from inside the pelvic bone (iliac crest) or the sternum. This procedure, called *aspiration biopsy cytology (ABC),* allows examination of the tissue that may help confirm or reject a tentative diagnosis. If the bone marrow is severely damaged, the choice of a **bone marrow transplant** may be offered to the patient. In this procedure, myeloid tissue from a compatible donor is introduced into the recipient intravenously. Transplantation also may involve infusion of blood-forming, or *hematopoietic, stem cells,* harvested from the individual being treated, from a compatible donor, or from umbilical cord blood (see box p. 469). If the recipient's immune system does not reject the new tissue or stem cells, always a danger in transplant procedures, a new colony of healthy tissue may become established in the bone marrow. As a result, myeloid tissue destroyed by disease, high-dose irradiation, or chemotherapy will be replaced and begin again to produce normal, functioning blood cells.

Red Blood Cells (Erythrocytes)

The red blood cell, or erythrocyte, is an elegant example of how structural adaptation can impact biological function. Note in Figure 12-3 that the RBC, which is surrounded by a tough and flexible plasma membrane, is "caved in" on both sides so that each one has a thin center and thicker edges. Mature RBCs have no nucleus or cytoplasmic organelles. Because of this they are unable to reproduce themselves or replace lost or damaged cellular components. The result is a relatively short life span of about 80 to 120 days. However, the addi-

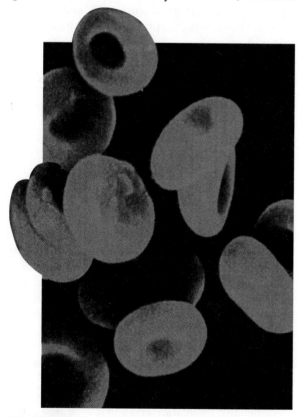

Figure 12-3 | **RBCs.**

Color-enhanced scanning electron micrograph shows the detailed structure of normal RBCs.

tional intracellular space that becomes available in each cell when the nucleus and cytoplasmic organelles are lost is filled to capacity with an important red pigment called **hemoglobin (Hb)** (HEE-moh-gloh-bin).

The unique chemical properties of hemoglobin permit the RBC to perform several critically important functions required for maintenance of homeostasis. The exchange of oxygen and carbon dioxide between the blood and the body's cells and its role in maintenance of acid-base balance are among the most vital. Iron (Fe) is an essential nutrient needed to give hemoglobin its oxygen-carrying ability. Vitamin B_{12} and folate (also a B vitamin) are also among the critical nutrients needed by the red bone marrow to manufacture enough hemoglobin to maintain survival.

In peripheral blood smears, an RBC of normal size is about 7 to 9 µm in diameter and is called a *normocytic RBC* (*normo-* normal, *-cyte* cell). A normocytic RBC is approximately the same size as the nucleus of a small lymphocyte (Figure 12-4). Abnormally small RBCs are called *microcytes* (*micro-* small, *-cyte* cell) and larger RBCs are called *macrocytes* (*macro-* large, *-cyte* cell).

Figure 12-4 also compares the appearance of RBCs with normal amounts of the red pigment hemoglobin, called *normochromic RBCs* (*normo-* normal + *chromic* color) with those that are deficient in hemoglobin, called *hypochromic RBCs* (*hypo-* low + *chromic* color), and those that have an excess of hemoglobin, called *hyperchromic RBCs* (*hyper-* high + *chromic* color). Production of *macrocytic hyperchromic RBCs* during periods of chronic blood loss is a good example of a "compensatory response" intended to maintain homeostasis. Because the body is unable to produce adequate numbers of RBCs with normal levels of hemoglobin in each cell to replace those lost by hemorrhage, the body increases the size and amount of hemoglobin in those cells it can produce to help maintain the oxygen-carrying capacity of the blood.

During a short life span, each RBC travels around the entire circulatory system more than 100,000 times! It is the flexible plasma membrane that permits each cell to "deform" and undergo drastic changes in shape as it repeatedly passes through capillaries whose lumen is smaller than the RBC cells' diameter. Because of the large numbers of RBCs and their unique shape, the total surface

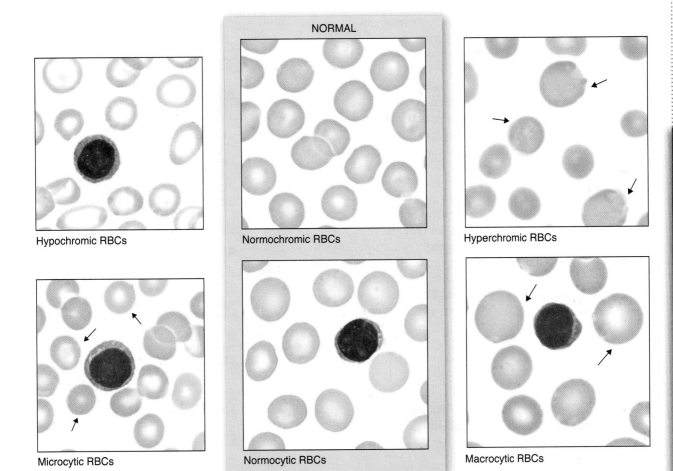

	NORMAL	
Hypochromic RBCs	Normochromic RBCs	Hyperchromic RBCs
Microcytic RBCs	Normocytic RBCs	Macrocytic RBCs

Figure 12-4 | **RBC abnormalities.**

Micrographs showing normal red blood cells (RBCs) in a smear compared to abnormal RBCs. The cells with a large, dark nucleus shown in some of the images are lymphocytes—a type of white blood cell similar in size to an RBC.

area available for them to perform their biological functions is enormous. Oxygen unites with hemoglobin to form an oxygen-hemoglobin complex called **oxyhemoglobin** (OK-see-HEE-moh-gloh-bin). Oxyhemoglobin makes possible the efficient transport of nearly 97% of all of the oxygen required for the body cells (3% is dissolved in plasma). Hemoglobin also combines with carbon dioxide to form **carbaminohemoglobin** (karb-am-ee-no-HEE-moh-GLOH-bin). It functions to transport about 20% of the carbon dioxide produced as a waste product of cellular metabolism to the lungs for disposal into the external environment. Recall that about 5% of CO_2 is transported in the blood dissolved in plasma. The majority of CO_2 (75%) carried in the blood

is converted in RBCs to bicarbonate for its journey to the lungs for excretion (see Chapter 16).

The **CBC,** or **complete blood cell count,** is a battery of tests used to measure the amounts or levels of many blood constituents and is often ordered as a routine part of the physical examination (see box on p. 350). Measuring the actual *numbers* of circulating RBCs per unit of blood volume is a valuable part of the CBC. Values listed in CBC results as "normal" will vary slightly between different laboratories and reference texts. For RBCs, a range of 4.2 to 6.2 million per cubic millimeter of blood (mm^3), with males generally having a higher number than females, is common. Normal deviations from average ranges often occur with age differences, level of hydration, altitude of residence, and other variables. Originally RBC counts were done with a *hemocytometer*, a microscope slide with a counting grid etched on it. The current practice is to use a faster, more accurate automated blood cell counter.

The **hematocrit** (hee-MAT-oh-crit) component of the CBC provides information about the *volume* of RBCs in a blood sample. If whole blood is placed in a special centrifuge tube and then "spun down," the heavier formed elements will quickly settle to the bottom of the tube. During the procedure, RBCs are forced to the bottom of the tube first. The WBCs and platelets then settle out in a layer called the **buffy coat.** In Figure 12-5 the buffy coat can be seen between the packed RBCs on the bottom of the hematocrit tube and the liquid layer of plasma above. Thus the hematocrit test—also called packed-cell volume (PCV) test—gives an estimate of the proportion of RBCs to plasma. Such information could help screen for dehydration, hemorrhaging, or other

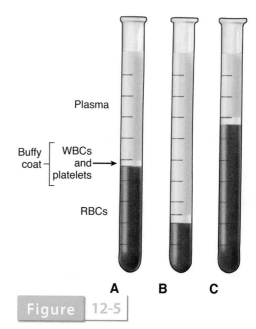

Figure 12-5

A depiction of hematocrit tubes showing the proportions of blood components in normal blood, anemia, and polycythemia.

Note the buffy coat located between the packed RBCs and the plasma. **A,** Normal blood with the typical percent of RBCs. **B,** Anemia (a low percent of RBCs). **C,** Polycythemia (a high percent of RBCs).

circumstances that affect the RBC ratio. Normally about 45% of the blood volume consists of RBCs (Figure 12-1).

 To learn more about red blood cells, go to **AnimationDirect** on your CD.

HEALTH & WELL-BEING

BLOOD DOPING

A number of athletes have reportedly improved their performance by a practice called *blood boosting* or **blood doping.** A few weeks before an important event, an athlete has some blood drawn. The RBCs in this sample are separated and frozen. Just before competition, the RBCs are thawed and injected back into the athlete. The increased hematocrit that results slightly improves the oxygen-carrying capacity of the blood, which theoretically improves performance. However, in practice the effects are slight. This method is judged to be an unfair and unwise practice in athletics.

In addition to blood transfusions, injection of substances such as hormones that increase RBC levels in an attempt to improve athletic performance has also been condemned by leading authorities in the area of sports medicine and by athletic organizations around the world. "Doping" with either the naturally occurring hormone erythropoietin (EPO) or with synthetic drugs that have similar biological effects—such as Epogen and Procrit—can result in devastating medical outcomes.

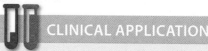

CLINICAL APPLICATION

COMPLETE BLOOD CELL COUNT

One of the most useful and frequently performed clinical blood tests is called the *complete blood cell count,* or simply the CBC. The CBC is a collection of tests whose results, when interpreted as a whole, can yield an enormous amount of information regarding a person's health. Standard RBC, WBC, and thrombocyte counts, the differential WBC count, hematocrit, hemoglobin content, and other characteristics of the formed elements are usually included in this battery of tests. Normal ranges for blood values included in most CBC tests are found in Appendix C on the CD that accompanies your book.

Red Blood Cell Disorders

Red blood cell disorders are most often related to either overproduction of RBCs—a condition called **polycythemia** (pol-ee-sye-THEE-mee-ah)—or to a group of disorders that result in low oxygen-carrying capacity of the blood called **anemia** (ah-NEE-me-ah).

QUICK CHECK

1. List the terms used to describe RBCs of different sizes and hemoglobin content.
2. What is the CBC, or complete blood cell count?

Polycythemia

Polycythemia is a serious blood disorder characterized by dramatic increases in RBC numbers. The cause is generally a cancerous transformation of elements in the red bone marrow. Whole blood RBC counts may reach or exceed levels of 10 million/mm^3. The disease increases blood viscosity or thickness. Thicker than normal blood resists flow—just as thicker than normal ketchup resists flow out of the bottle. This increased flow resistance often causes hypertension (high blood pressure), coagulation problems, excessive distention of blood vessels, and hemorrhaging.

In polycythemia, the hematocrit (RBC %) may reach 60%—way above the normal 45% average (Figure 12-5, *C*). Treatment involves blood removal (bleeding), irradiation of bone marrow, and chemotherapy treatment to suppress RBC production.

Anemia

Anemia can result from inadequate numbers of RBCs (Figure 12-5, *B*), a deficiency in the production of normal hemoglobin, or production of hemoglobin that is in some way defective. Thus anemia can occur if the hemoglobin in RBCs is inadequate or defective, even if adequate numbers of RBCs are present. Many of the clinical signs and symptoms of anemia, regardless of type or cause, are related to low tissue oxygen levels. Anemic individuals often feel fatigued or "tired all the time," and suffer from weakness, skin pallor, headache, and faintness. Some symptoms are caused by the body's attempts to increase or "compensate" for low tissue oxygen levels by speeding up the heart and respiratory rates. These compensatory mechanisms are examples of homeostasis at work—the body attempting to return tissue oxygen levels to normal despite the low oxygen-carrying capacity of the blood in anemia. A number of the more common types of anemia are described below and in Table 12-2.

Table 12-2 | Laboratory Results for Types of Anemia

ANEMIA	FOLATE CONTENT	HEMOGLOBIN	HEMATOCRIT CONTENT	IRON CONTENT	RBC SIZE (VOLUME)	VITAMIN B$_{12}$ CONTENT
Aplastic anemia	Normal	Low to normal	Low to normal	High	Normal to slightly high	Normal
Pernicious anemia	Normal	Low	Low	High	High	Low
Hemorrhagic anemia						
Acute blood-loss anemia	Normal	Low to normal	Low to normal	Normal	Slightly low	Normal
Chronic blood-loss anemia	Normal	Low	Low	Low	Low to normal	Normal
Iron deficiency anemia	Normal	Low	Low	Low	Low	Normal
Hemolytic anemia (sickle cell anemia and thalassemia)	Normal	Low	Low	Normal to high	Normal to high	Normal

RESEARCH, ISSUES, AND TRENDS

CHELATION THERAPY

The term *chelation therapy* is used to describe a procedure once used almost exclusively to treat lead poisoning. Although still used in cases of lead poisoning, the process is now widely employed as an "alternative" medical treatment for atherosclerosis and other types of cardiovascular disease. Chelation therapy involves intravenous injection of chemicals (generally EDTA, or ethylenediaminetetraacetic acid), which then bind with heavy metal ions. The resulting chemical complex is rapidly excreted in the urine. Chelation therapists claim that by binding with and removing calcium ions from the blood, repeated treatments (often 50 separate injections) will help reverse the buildup of calcium-dense atherosclerotic plaques from diseased artery walls. The process is highly controversial and rejected by most mainstream cardiologists as being ineffective and potentially dangerous.

To learn more about the clinical manifestations of anemias, go to **AnimationDirect** on your CD.

HEMORRHAGIC ANEMIA

Hemorrhagic anemia is caused by an actual decrease in the number of circulating RBCs lost because of hemorrhage or bleeding. It is referred to as either *acute blood-loss anemia* resulting, for example, from extensive surgery or sudden trauma, or *chronic blood-loss anemia* caused by slow but continuous loss of blood over time from diseases such as cancer or ulcers. As noted above, although fewer RBCs are present in circulating blood because of the hemorrhage, those RBCs that are produced during this time are both macrocytic and hyperchromic—an attempt to restore homeostasis by compensating for the low oxygen-carrying capacity caused by the hemorrhagic anemia. Once the actual bleeding is stopped, transfusion of whole blood or red cells and successful treatment of the underlying reason for chronic blood loss are curative.

APLASTIC ANEMIA

Aplastic (ay-PLAS-tik) **anemia** is characterized by abnormally low RBC counts and destruction of bone marrow. The cause is often related to high-dose exposure to certain toxic chemicals such as benzene or mercury, irradiation, and in susceptible individuals, certain drugs including chloramphenicol. Acute cases of the disease are very serious, with death rates reaching 70% at 3 or 4 months after diagnosis. Bone marrow or stem cell transplants provide the most effective treatment.

DEFICIENCY ANEMIAS

Deficiency anemias are caused by an inadequate supply of some substance, such as vitamin B_{12} or iron, required for red blood cell or hemoglobin production. In addition to adequate numbers of normally functioning RBCs, the amount and quality of hemoglobin are critical factors in maintaining the oxygen-carrying capacity of the blood. Normal hemoglobin ranges from 12 to 14 grams per 100 milliliters (g/100 ml) of whole blood for adult females and from 14 to 17 g/100 ml for adult males. A hemoglobin value less than 9 g/100 ml indicates anemia. Figure 12-6 shows the relationship of the four iron-containing groups and four protein subunits or chains in the hemoglobin molecule. Chemical changes in the hemoglobin molecule can result in development of defective hemoglobin and red cells and thus impair the ability of the blood to deliver adequate oxygen to the body tissues.

Pernicious (per-NISH-us) **anemia** results from a dietary deficiency of vitamin B_{12} or from the failure of the stomach lining to produce "intrinsic factor"—the substance that allows vitamin B_{12} to be absorbed. Genetics plays a role in development of pernicious anemia, and research evidence suggests that it is an autoimmune disease. Vitamin B_{12} deficiency impairs the bone marrow and results in decreased RBC production as well as a reduction in WBC and platelet numbers. The reduced number of red cells that do enter the circulation are macrocytes and are much larger than normal RBCs.

In addition to the classic symptoms of anemia caused by low oxygen delivery to tissues, patients with pernicious anemia develop numerous nervous system problems such as numbness, tingling, and burning in the feet and hands. Mental impairment, delusions, irritability, and depression are also common. Pernicious anemia is successfully treated by repeated injections of vitamin B$_{12}$.

Folate deficiency anemia is similar to pernicious anemia because it also causes a decrease in the RBC count resulting from a vitamin deficiency. In this condition, it is *folic acid* (vitamin B$_9$) that is deficient. Folic acid deficiencies are common among individuals with alcoholism and other malnourished individuals. Treatment for acute folate deficiency anemia involves taking vitamin supplements until a balanced diet can be restored.

Iron deficiency anemia, as the name suggests, is caused by a deficiency of iron, which is required for hemoglobin synthesis. Although the body carefully protects its iron reserves, they may be depleted through hemorrhage, increased requirements such as wound healing or pregnancy, or by low intake. Unfortunately, iron deficiency is the most common nutritional deficiency in the world. The tragic result is that an estimated 10% of the population in some developed countries and up to 50% in developing countries suffer from iron deficiency anemia. In most cases the RBC numbers are only slightly below normal. However, the cells are small (microcytic) and appear pale due to the reduction in hemoglobin content. A low hematocrit value is common in iron deficiency anemia. Can you explain how this can be if the RBC numbers are near normal? The reason is that the *size* of the RBCs is small (microcytic) so the red cell *volume* and therefore the hematocrit value are both decreased. Oral administration of iron-containing compounds, such as ferrous sulfate or ferrous gluconate, is very effective in treating the basic iron deficiency seen in the disease. The probability of a complete cure is excellent if, in addition to administration of iron, any underlying causes such as chronic bleeding or iron malabsorption problems are corrected.

HEMOLYTIC ANEMIAS

Hemolytic anemias as a group are all associated with a decreased RBC life span caused by an in-creased rate of destruction. Frequently, an abnormal hemoglobin will cause red blood cells to become distorted and easily broken. The hemolytic anemias have some distinguishing symptoms in addition to those expected because of low oxygen delivery to tissues. Many are related to the fact that the body retains many of the breakdown products of the excess numbers of RBCs that are destroyed, including iron and pigments. The result may be *jaundice,* a yellow skin appearance caused by the conversion of the heme pigment of hemoglobin in the liver. Swelling of the spleen, problems associated with excess iron storage, and gallstone formation are also common. Some symptoms are unique to a particular type of hemolytic anemia, as discussed below.

Sickle cell anemia is a genetic disease that results in the formation of limited amounts of an abnormal type of hemoglobin called *sickle hemoglobin,* or hemoglobin S (HbS). The genetic defect produces a change in one of the protein chains (see Figure 12-6), causing the resulting HbS to be less stable and less soluble than normal hemoglobin. The defective hemoglobin forms crystals and causes the red cell to become fragile and as-

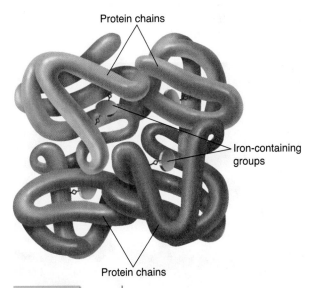

Protein chains

Iron-containing groups

Protein chains

Figure 12-6 | **The hemoglobin molecule.**

This large molecule is composed of four protein subunits or chains that each hold an iron-containing chemical group at its core. The iron gives hemoglobin its oxygen-carrying capacity.

sume a sickled shape when the blood oxygen level is low (Figure 12-7).

A person who inherits only one defective gene develops only a small amount of HbS and has a form of the disease called *sickle cell trait*. Those with sickle cell trait often have no symptoms at all. However, in some stressful or high-exertion situations, a person with sickle cell trait could become ill.

If two defective genes are inherited (one from each parent), then more HbS is produced and a much more severe condition called *sickle cell disease* develops. In addition to RBC sickling and rupture, high levels of HbS may cause reduction in blood flow, blood clotting, and in episodes of "crisis," severe pooling of red cells, particularly in the spleen, causing sudden death. Treatment is primarily supportive because no effective anti-sickling drugs are currently available. However, patient education, early diagnosis, preventive measures to reduce dehydration and infection, and limited use of blood transfusions to treat episodes of crisis are improving survival rates. This type of anemia is found almost entirely in those of black African descent, and in the United States nearly 1 in every 600 African-American newborns are affected with sickle cell trait or disease.

Thalassemia (thal-ah-SEE-mee-ah) refers to a group of inherited hemolytic anemias. The most common type, which occurs most often in individuals of Mediterranean descent, is characterized by production of abnormal hemoglobin and inadequate numbers of small (microcytic) and often oddly shaped RBCs that are short lived.

Thalassemia, like sickle cell anemia, occurs in two forms, mild and severe. In both forms, flawed protein syntheses in the RBCs results in defective hemoglobin production and early hemolysis, or death, of defective red cells. *Thalassemia minor,* or *thalassemia trait,* occurs when only one defective gene is inherited and is characterized by mild anemia, minimal RBC changes, and few symptoms.

Thalassemia major, which occurs when two defective genes are inherited, is a very serious and life-threatening hemolytic anemia. Red cells are quickly destroyed, hemoglobin levels often fall below 7 g/100 ml of blood, low blood and tissue oxygen levels cause multiple problems, bone marrow mass expands causing crippling and skeletal deformities, and swelling of the spleen and liver occurs. If adequate and ongoing treatment is not initiated, iron released as a result of RBC hemolysis accumulates in pathological tissue deposits throughout the body. Bone marrow and stem cell transplantation and experimental gene manipulation initiatives hold the most promise for long-term treatment success. Because thalassemia is a genetically transmitted disease, genetic counseling is appropriate.

Hemolytic disease of the newborn begins during pregnancy if fetal RBCs of a different ABO type (see p. 345) than the mother cross the placenta and enter the mother's circulation. This can happen during delivery as blood cells leak from placenta as it pulls away from the lining of the uterus (womb). If this should occur, antibodies against them will be formed because antigens on the fetal RBCs are "foreign" to the mother. The process is called *fetal-maternal ABO incompatibility.* (Antigen-antibody reactions will be discussed in more depth in Chapter 15.) Problems for the unborn baby begin if the maternal antibodies against the "foreign" fetal RBCs cross the placental barrier and enter the fetal circulation. If this occurs, the maternal antibodies will attack and destroy the unborn baby's red cells, causing a hemolytic anemia to develop.

Rh factor incompatibility between an Rh-positive unborn baby and its Rh-negative mother (Figure 12-8) results in hemolytic anemia called **erythroblastosis** (e-rith-roh-blas-TOH-sis) **fetalis** (feh-TAL-iss). Rh factor incompatibility is clinically more important than ABO incompatibility because the hemolytic response, although it occurs less frequently, is

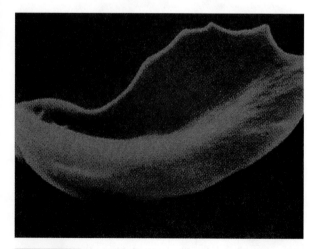

Figure 12-7 | **Sickle cell.**

A sickle-shaped red blood cell typical of sickle cell anemia.

generally more severe. Fortunately, infant mortality caused by Rh incompatibility has been drastically reduced following introduction and widespread use of a product called RhoGAM in Rh-negative mothers (see p. 345).

Hemolytic disease in the newborn caused by either ABO or Rh incompatibility may occur early in pregnancy or become apparent only at birth. Red cell numbers and hemoglobin levels decline. Jaundice, intravascular coagulation, heart and lung damage, and swelling of the liver and spleen are common. If problems are detected by laboratory tests of amniotic fluid or from fetal or maternal blood sampling prior to birth, in utero exchange transfusions and early delivery may be needed to save the life of the infant.

White Blood Cells (Leukocytes)

Recall from the listing of formed elements found in the blood (see p. 346) that the *white blood cells* (WBCs), or **leukocytes,** are categorized by the presence of granules *(granulocytes)* or absence of granules *(agranulocytes)* in their cytoplasm. The granulocytic WBCs include

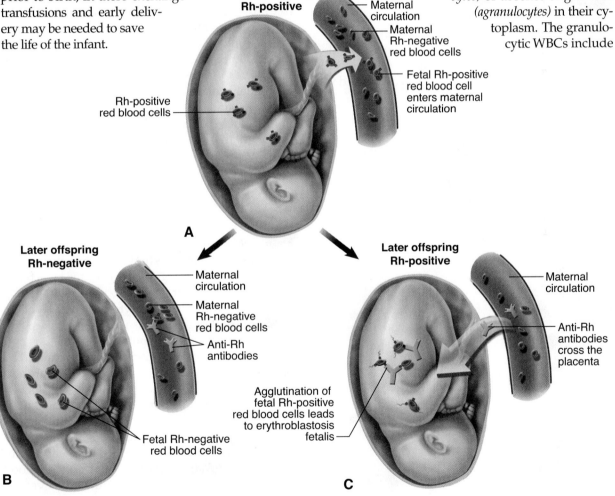

Earlier offspring Rh-positive

Maternal circulation

Maternal Rh-negative red blood cells

Fetal Rh-positive red blood cell enters maternal circulation

Rh-positive red blood cells

A

Later offspring Rh-negative

Maternal circulation

Maternal Rh-negative red blood cells

Anti-Rh antibodies

Fetal Rh-negative red blood cells

B

Later offspring Rh-positive

Maternal circulation

Anti-Rh antibodies cross the placenta

Agglutination of fetal Rh-positive red blood cells leads to erythroblastosis fetalis

C

Figure 12-8 **Erythroblastosis fetalis.**

A, Rh-positive blood cells enter the mother's bloodstream during delivery of an Rh-positive baby. If not treated, the mother's body will produce anti-Rh antibodies. **B,** A later pregnancy involving an Rh-negative baby is normal because there are no Rh antigens in the baby's blood. **C,** A later pregnancy involving an Rh-positive baby may result in erythroblastosis fetalis. Anti-Rh antibodies enter the baby's blood supply and cause agglutination of RBCs that have the Rh antigen.

the **neutrophils** (NOO-troh-fils), **eosinophils** (ee-oh-SIN-oh-fils), and **basophils** (BAY-so-fils) (Figure 12-9 *A, B,* and *C*). The **lymphocytes** (LIM-foh-sytes) and **monocytes** (MON-oh-sytes) (Figure 12-9, *D* and *E*) are agranulocytes.

 To learn more about white blood cells, go to **AnimationDirect** on your CD.

WBC Count

Normally, the total number of WBCs per cubic millimeter of whole blood (mm³) ranges between 5000 and 10,000. The term **leukopenia** (loo-koh-PEE-nee-ah) is used to describe an abnormally *low* WBC count (less than 5000 WBCs/mm³ of blood). Leukopenia does not occur often. However, malfunction of blood-forming tissues and cells and some diseases affecting the immune system, such as AIDS (discussed in Chapter 15), may lower WBC numbers.

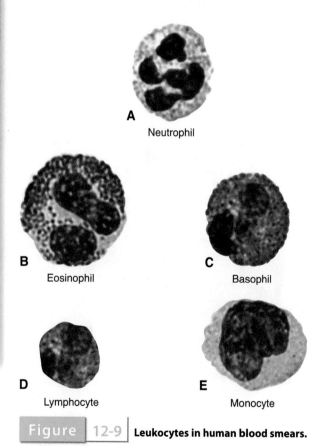

A
Neutrophil

B
Eosinophil

C
Basophil

D
Lymphocyte

E
Monocyte

Figure 12-9 | **Leukocytes in human blood smears.**

Each light micrograph shows a different type of stained WBC surrounded by several smaller RBCs.

Leukocytosis (loo-koh-sye-TOH-sis) refers to an abnormally *high* WBC count (that is, more than 10,000 WBCs/mm³ of blood). It is a much more common problem than leukopenia and almost always accompanies bacterial infections. In addition, leukocytosis is also seen in many forms of blood cancer (described below), which are often diagnosed when tremendous increases in WBC numbers are detected in blood tests.

A special type of white blood cell count called a **differential WBC count** reveals more information than simply counting the total number of all of the different types of WBCs in a blood sample. In a differential WBC count, a component test in the CBC (see box, p. 350), the *proportions* of each type of white blood cell are reported as percentages of the total WBC count. Normal percentages are shown in Figure 12-1. Because all disorders do not affect each WBC type the same way, the differential WBC count is a valuable diagnostic tool. For example, although some parasite infestations do not cause an increase in the total WBC count, they often do cause an increase in the proportion of eosinophils that are present. The reason? This type of WBC specializes in defending against parasites (Table 12-1).

Leukocyte Types and Functions

GRANULOCYTES

Neutrophils are the most numerous of the active WBCs, called **phagocytes** (FAG-oh-sytes), that protect the body from invading microorganisms by actually taking them into their own cell bodies and digesting them in the process of phagocytosis (Figure 12-10).

Eosinophils also serve as weak phagocytes. Perhaps one of their most important functions, as noted, involves protection against infections caused by certain parasites and parasitic worms. They are also involved in allergic reactions.

Basophils, in peripheral blood, and related **mast cells** found in the tissues, both secrete the chemical **histamine,** which is released during inflammatory reactions. Basophils also produce a potent anticoagulant called **heparin,** which helps prevent blood from clotting as it flows through the blood vessels of the body.

AGRANULOCYTES

Monocytes are the largest leukocytes. Like neutrophils, they are aggressive phagocytes. Because of their size, they are capable of engulfing larger bac-

Foreign particle
about to be consumed

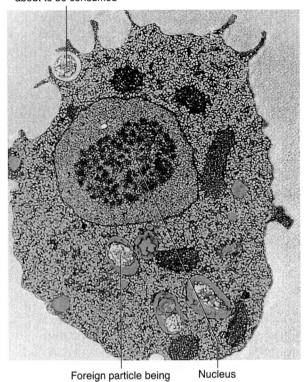

Foreign particle being
digested by the cell

Nucleus

Figure 12-10 **Phagocytosis.**

This transmission electron micrograph shows a phagocytic cell
consuming a foreign particle in a manner similar to that used
by human WBCs. Extensions of the plasma membrane literally
reach out and grab a particle and then digest the particle
within an intracellular vesicle (also see Figure 15-12).

terial organisms and cancerous cells. **Macrophages**
(meaning "large eater") are monocytes that have
grown to several times their original size after mi-
grating out of the bloodstream. They are discussed
further in Chapter 15 (see Figure 15-12).

Lymphocytes help protect us against infections,
but they do it by a process different from phagocytosis. Lymphocytes function in the immune mechanism, the complex process that makes us immune
to infectious diseases. Lymphocytes called *B lym-*
phocytes secrete chemical compounds, called *anti-*
bodies, that specifically act to destroy particular
bacteria, viruses, chemical toxins, or other foreign
substances. Mature B lymphocytes, called **plasma**
cells, are formed in large numbers in a type of bone
marrow cancer called *multiple myeloma,* which is
described below. Other lymphocytes, called *T lym-*

phocytes, do not secrete antibodies but instead protect us by directly attacking bacteria or cancerous
cells. Details of the immune system are discussed in
Chapter 15.

White Blood Cell Disorders

Two major groups of disease conditions constitute a
majority of WBC and blood-related cancers, or neoplasms. **Lymphoid neoplasms** arise from lymphoid
precursor cells that normally produce B lymphocytes,
T lymphocytes, or their descendent cell types. **My-**
eloid neoplasms appear as a result of malignant transformation of myeloid stem or precursor cells that
normally produce granulocytic WBCs, monocytes,
RBCs, and platelets (Table 12-1).

Multiple Myeloma

Multiple myeloma (my-el-OH-mah) is cancer of mature, antibody-secreting B lymphocytes called *plasma*
cells (Figure 12-11). It is the most common and one of
the most deadly forms of blood-related cancers in
people older than 65 years of age. The
cancerous transformation of plasma cells results in impairment of
bone marrow function, production of defective antibodies,

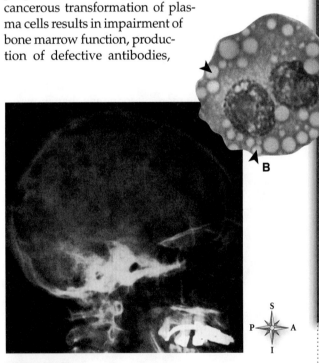

B

Figure 12-11 **Multiple myeloma.**

A, X-ray film of skull showing "honeycomb" or "punched-out" bone
defects caused by diseased antibody from plasma cells. **B,** Malignant
plasma cell. Vacuoles *(arrowheads)* contain defective antibodies.

recurrent infections, anemia, and the painful destruction and fracture of bones in the skull, vertebrae, and throughout the skeletal system. The x-ray photo in Figure 12-11 shows typical "honeycomb"- or "punched-out"–appearing defects in skull bones caused by the defective myeloma antibody. Treatment may lengthen life and help relieve symptoms but does not cure the disease. Chemotherapy, marrow and stem cell transplantation, and certain drug and antibody treatments are being used with varying degrees of success.

Leukemia

Leukemia (loo-KEE-mee-ah) is the term used to describe a number of blood cancers affecting the WBCs. In almost every form of leukemia, marked leukocytosis, or elevated WBC levels, occur. Leukocyte counts in excess of 100,000/mm³ in circulating blood are common. The different types of leukemia are identified as either *acute* or *chronic*, based on how quickly symptoms appear after the disease begins, and as *lymphocytic* or *myeloid* depending on the cell type involved. Four of the most common leukemias are briefly described below.

CHRONIC LYMPHOCYTIC LEUKEMIA

Chronic lymphocytic leukemia (CLL) most often affects older adults and is rare in individuals younger than 30 years of age. Average age of onset is about 65 years, appearing more often in men than in women. In those with CLL, malignant precursor B lymphocytes are produced in great numbers (Figure 12-12).

They are long lived but do not produce normal antibodies and, as a result, some increase in infections may occur. However, early in the disease few symptoms are apparent, and many patients are diagnosed inadvertently as part of routine physical examinations when results of blood tests become available. When symptoms do appear, they are often quite mild. Anemia, fatigue, and development of enlarged but generally painless lymph nodes is common. Many patients with CLL live many years after diagnosis with little or no treatment. More severe cases often benefit from chemotherapy and irradiation.

ACUTE LYMPHOCYTIC LEUKEMIA

Acute lymphocytic leukemia (ALL) is primarily a disease of children and constitutes the most common form of "blood cancer" in children between 3 and 7 years of age (Figure 12-13). Fully 80% of children who develop leukemia have this form of the disease. Although always a serious condition, it is highly curable in children but less so when it occurs in adults. Onset of the disease is sudden and often marked by fever, bone pain, and increased rates of infection. Cancerous cells crowd out other bone marrow cells and decrease the production of RBCs, platelets, and other nonmalignant lymphocyte precursor cells, thereby producing anemia. As cancerous transformation of B lymphocytes continues, their numbers increase in circulating blood and swelling often occurs in lymph nodes, spleen, and liver. Treatment may involve chemotherapy, irradiation, and bone marrow or stem cell transplants.

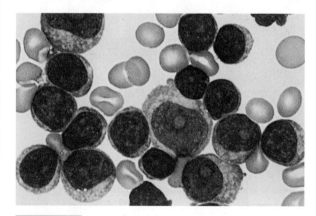

Figure 12-12 **Chronic lymphocytic leukemia (CLL).**
Peripheral blood smear showing large numbers of diseased B lymphocytes.

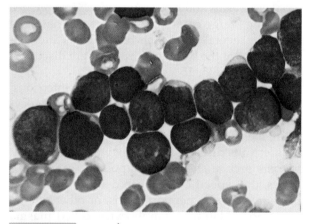

Figure 12-13 **Acute lymphocytic leukemia (ALL).**
Appearance of B lymphocytes in acute lymphocytic leukemia.

CHRONIC MYELOID LEUKEMIA

Chronic myeloid leukemia (CML) accounts for about 20% of all cases of leukemia and occurs most often in adults between 25 and 60 years of age. CML results from cancerous transformation of granulocytic (neutrophil, eosinophil, and basophil) precursor cells in the bone marrow. Onset is slow and early symptoms, such as fatigue, weakness, and weight loss, tend to be nonspecific. Once established, the disease progresses slowly. Diagnosis is often made by discovery of marked elevations of granulocytic WBCs in peripheral blood (Figure 12-14) and by extreme spleen enlargement. Bone marrow transplants are curative in up to 70% of cases. The recent introduction of a new "rational" or "designer" drug called *Gleevec* constitutes a major advance in treatment of CML. It specifically seeks out and blocks the flawed signals in CML cancer cells that cause runaway proliferation.

ACUTE MYELOID LEUKEMIA

The pathological transformation of myeloid stem cells resulting in **acute myeloid leukemia (AML)** accounts for 80% of all cases of acute leukemia in adults and 20% of acute leukemia in children. As the name suggests, onset is sudden, and once symptoms appear, the disease progresses rapidly. Patients most often seek help because of fatigue, bone and joint pain, spongy bleeding gums, symptoms of anemia, and recurrent infections. The prognosis in AML is poor, with only about 50% of children and 30% of adults achieving long-term survival. Advances in bone marrow and stem cell transplantation have increased cure rates in selected patients.

Infectious Mononucleosis

Infectious mononucleosis (MON-oh-NEW-clee-oh-sis) is a common noncancerous WBC disorder appearing most often in adolescents and young adults between 15 and 25 years of age. The disease is usually caused by the *Epstein-Barr virus (EBV)*, found in the saliva of infected individuals. "Mono," as it is often called, can be spread by kissing or any other direct contact with an infected person's saliva, such as sharing a straw, toothbrush, or eating utensil. Leukocytosis is common early in the disease, with total WBC counts averaging between 12,000 to 18,000/mm[3]. More than 60% of the leukocytes can be identified in a differential WBC count as large, *atypical* (abnormal) *lymphocytes,* which have abundant cytoplasm and a large nucleus (Figure 12-15).

Symptoms of "mono" vary greatly but, in addition to the leukocytosis and atypical lymphocytes seen in peripheral blood, fever, sore throat, rash, severe fatigue, and enlargement of lymph nodes and the spleen are common findings. Infectious mononucleosis is generally self-limited and resolves without complications in about 4 to 6 weeks, although fatigue may last for longer periods. Occasionally, severe complications affecting almost any body organ system may occur in individuals with weakened immune systems.

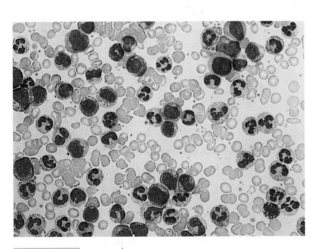

Figure 12-14 **Chronic myeloid leukemia (CML).**

Severe granulocytic leukocytosis typical of CML.

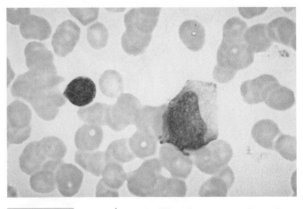

Figure 12-15 **Atypical lymphocyte seen in patient with infectious mononucleosis.**

The cell on the left is a typical small lymphocyte with its nucleus almost filling the cell. The larger atypical lymphocyte on the right has much more cytoplasm and a larger nucleus.

Platelets and Blood Clotting

Platelets, the third main type of formed element, play an essential part in blood clotting. Your life might someday be saved just because your blood can clot. A clot plugs up torn or cut vessels and stops bleeding that otherwise might prove fatal.

The story of how blood clots is the story of a chain of rapid-fire reactions. The first step in the chain is some kind of an injury to a blood vessel that makes a rough spot in its lining. (Normally the lining of blood vessels is extremely smooth.) Almost immediately, damaged tissue cells release particular clotting factors into the plasma. These factors rapidly react with other factors already present in the plasma to form **prothrombin activator** (proh-THROM-bin AK-ti-vay-ter). At the same time this is happening, platelets become "sticky" at the point of injury and soon accumulate near the opening in the broken blood vessel, forming a soft, temporary *platelet plug*. As the platelets accumulate, they release additional clotting factors, forming even more prothrombin activator. If the normal amount of blood calcium is present, prothrombin activator triggers the next step of clotting by converting **prothrombin** (a protein in normal blood) to **thrombin** (THROM-bin). In the last step, thrombin reacts with **fibrinogen** (fi-BRIN-oh-jen) (a normal plasma protein) to change it to a fibrous gel called **fibrin.** Under the microscope, fibrin looks like a tangle of fine threads with RBCs caught in the tangle. Figure 12-16 illustrates the steps in the blood-clotting mechanism.

The clotting mechanism contains clues for ways to stop bleeding by speeding up blood clotting. For example, you might simply apply gauze to a bleed-

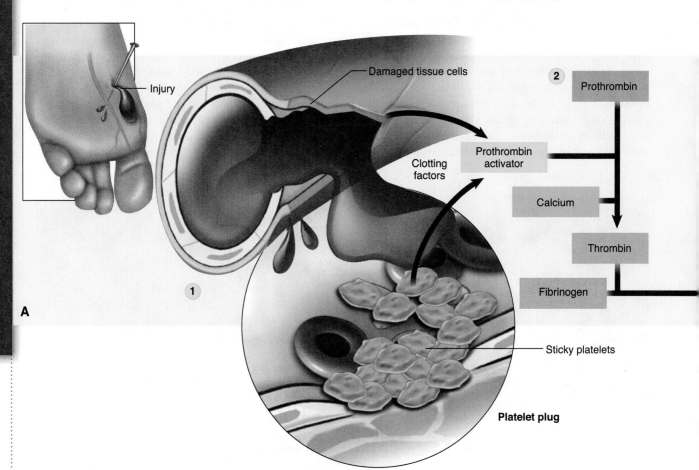

A

ing surface. Its slight roughness would cause more platelets to stick together and release more clotting factors. These additional factors would then make the blood clot more quickly.

Physicians sometimes prescribe vitamin K before surgery to make sure that the patient's blood will clot fast enough to prevent hemorrhage. Vitamin K stimulates liver cells to increase the synthesis of prothrombin. More prothrombin in blood allows faster production of thrombin during clotting and thus faster clot formation. The anticoagulant warfarin sodium (Coumadin) acts by inhibiting the synthesis of prothrombin and other vitamin K–dependent clotting factors. By doing so, warfarin decreases the ability of blood to clot and is effective in preventing repeat

thromboses following a heart attack or the formation of clots after surgical replacement of heart valves. Heparin also can be used to prevent excessive blood clotting. Heparin inhibits the conversion of prothrombin to thrombin, thus preventing formation of a thrombus. A clot-dissolving substance called *tissue plasminogen activator (TPA or t-PA)* is often used to dissolve clots that block the arteries that supply the heart muscle.

A laboratory test called the *prothrombin time* is used to regulate dosage of anticoagulant drugs. In this test thromboplastin and calcium are added simultaneously to a tube of the patient's plasma and a tube containing a normal control solution, and the time required for clot formation in both tubes is determined. A patient's prothrombin time in excess

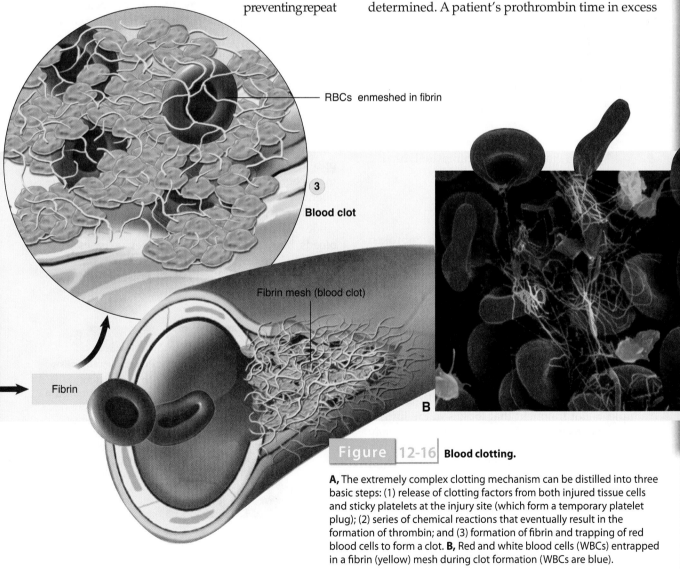

RBCs enmeshed in fibrin

3

Blood clot

Fibrin mesh (blood clot)

Fibrin

B

Figure 12-16 **Blood clotting.**

A, The extremely complex clotting mechanism can be distilled into three basic steps: (1) release of clotting factors from both injured tissue cells and sticky platelets at the injury site (which form a temporary platelet plug); (2) series of chemical reactions that eventually result in the formation of thrombin; and (3) formation of fibrin and trapping of red blood cells to form a clot. **B,** Red and white blood cells (WBCs) entrapped in a fibrin (yellow) mesh during clot formation (WBCs are blue).

of the standard control value (7 to 10 seconds) indicates the level of anticoagulant effect caused by the administered drug. This information allows the physician to adjust the dose required to maintain an appropriate level of anticoagulant effect.

Unfortunately, prothrombin time test results may vary among different clinical laboratories. Variability is often caused by differing techniques or differences in the sensitivity of reagents used. In order to minimize the effects of these and other variables and standardize the results of anticoagulation testing, a system called the **INR** (abbreviation for **I**nternational **N**ormalized **R**atio) has been developed. Prothrombin time is reported in seconds. The INR is a mathematical calculation and is reported as a number. An INR of 0.8 to 1.2 is considered normal. In regulating anticoagulant therapy, keeping the INR between 2 and 3 will help ensure the prevention of unwanted blood coagulation in conditions such as atrial fibrillation (see p. 387) or will prevent further clotting in coronary blood vessels after a heart attack.

 To learn more about platelets and blood clotting, go to AnimationDirect on your CD.

Clotting Disorders

Unfortunately, clots sometimes form in unbroken blood vessels of the heart, brain, lungs, or some other organ—a dreaded thing because clots may produce sudden death by shutting off the blood supply to a vital organ. When a clot stays in the place where it formed, it is called a **thrombus** (THROM-bus) and the condition is spoken of as **thrombosis** (throm-BO-sus). If part of the clot dislodges and circulates through the bloodstream, the dislodged part is then called an **embolus** (EM-bo-lus), and the condition is called an **embolism** (EM-bo-liz-em). For example, a clot fragment that lodges in the lung is called a *pulmonary embolism*—a situation that may prove fatal (Figure 12-17).

Suppose that your doctor told you that you had a clot in one of your coronary arteries. Which diagnosis would he make—coronary thrombosis or coronary embolism—if he thought that the clot had formed originally in the coronary artery as a result of the accumulation of fatty material in the vessel wall?

HEMOPHILIA

Hemophilia (hee-moh-FIL-ee-ah) is an X-linked (see Chapter 24, pp. 670-671) inherited disorder that affects more than 300,000 people around the world. Typically, it is transmitted from a symptom-free "carrier mother" to an affected son. Hemophilia is a "bleeding disorder" that results from a failure to produce one or more plasma proteins responsible for blood clotting—a process illustrated in Figure 12-16.

The most common form of the disease, called *hemophilia A*, is caused by absence of **factor VIII**. This serious coagulation disorder has plagued the royal families of Europe for hundreds of years and, as a result, its signs and symptoms and the genetics of its transmission are well known. Simply stated, people with hemophilia are relatively unable to form blood clots.

Because minor blood vessel injuries are common in ordinary life, hemophilia can be a life-threatening condition. Mild forms may not be apparent until the individual is subjected to surgery or trauma, whereas more severe cases may result in frequent and even spontaneous episodes of extensive bleeding. The most common signs of the disease include easy bruising, deep muscle hemorrhage, nosebleeds, blood in the urine, and in severe cases, even bleeding into the brain. Perhaps the most characteristic sign is repeated episodes of bleeding into the

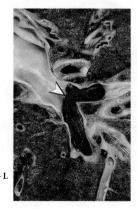

Figure 12-17

Pulmonary embolism. An embolus (clot fragment) that formed in the leg but broke away and lodged in a branch of the pulmonary artery within the lung. Arrowhead shows the embolus blocking the artery, thus drastically reducing gas exchange in the affected lung.

joints—especially the elbows, knees, and ankles. The result is chronic pain and progressive joint deformity.

Treatment of hemophilia involves initiation of lifestyle changes that help prevent injury, prompt response to bleeding episodes, avoiding drugs such as aspirin that alter the clotting mechanism, and administration of factor VIII.

Historically, only small amounts of factor VIII could be obtained by fractionation of large quantities of plasma obtained from many donors. Given the shortage of donated blood, this method could not meet demand as physicians prescribed more factor VIII to prevent as well as treat bleeding episodes. Further, even with new and more effective blood banking safety precautions, purification methods and diagnostic tests, pooling and fractionating donated blood and plasma still involve some risk of disease transmission—especially the viruses associated with AIDS and hepatitis. Currently, recombinant methods eliminate these risks and are used to produce enough recombinant antihemophilic factor VIII (rAHF) to meet the needs of the world's hemophiliac population.

THROMBOCYTOPENIA

A more common type of clotting disorder results from a decrease in the platelet count—a condition called **thrombocytopenia** (throm-boh-sye-toh-PEE-nee-ah). This condition is characterized by bleeding from many small blood vessels throughout the body, most visibly in the skin and mucous membranes. If the number of thrombocytes falls to 20,000/mm^3 or less (normal range is 150,000 to 400,000/mm^3), catastrophic bleeding may occur. A number of different mechanisms can result in thrombocytopenia. For example, platelet numbers below 50,000/mm^3 may result from mechanical destruction as blood passes over artificial heart valves. The usual cause, however, is bone marrow destruction by drugs, chemicals, radiation, or cancer. Reduced platelet counts are also common in immune system diseases such as lupus and HIV/AIDS, in which a reduction in platelets occurs early in the course of infection. Some drugs, such as aspirin, may cause thrombocytopenia as a side effect. In such cases, stopping the use of the drug usually solves the problem. Active treatment options include administration of corticosteroid-type drugs, which increase platelet production, transfusion of platelets, and in severe cases, removal of the spleen, which is a major site of platelet destruction.

> **QUICK CHECK**
>
> 1. What is the difference between a thrombus and an embolus?
> 2. What is the role of *prothrombin, thrombin, fibrinogen,* and *fibrin* in the blood clotting mechanism?
> 3. Identify two types of clotting disorders.

SCIENCE APPLICATIONS

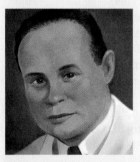

Charles Richard Drew (1904–1950)

HEMATOLOGY

American physician Charles Richard Drew was a pioneer in hematology, the study of blood. During World War II, he developed the idea of blood banks and researched the best way to store blood to be used for transfusions in wounded soldiers. In New York, he set up the first ever blood bank in 1941—one that served as the model for a network of blood banks later opened by the American Red Cross.

Many hematologists continue in Drew's footsteps, refining and perfecting the practice of blood science. Many professions benefit from this research. Phlebotomists collect blood for testing or storage, clinical laboratory technicians analyze blood samples, and many different health professionals use blood analysis and blood transfusions to help their patients.

Outline Summary

To download an MP3 version of the chapter summary for use with your iPod or portable media player, access the **Audio Chapter Summaries** on your CD.

Blood Composition and Volume

A. Blood components
  1. Liquid fraction of whole blood (extracellular part) called *plasma* (Figure 12-1)
  2. Cellular components suspended in the plasma make up formed the elements
B. Normal volumes of blood
  1. Plasma—2.6 L
  2. Formed elements—2.4 L
  3. Whole blood—4 to 6 L average or 7% to 9% of total body weight
C. Blood pH
  1. Blood is alkaline—pH 7.35 to pH 7.45
  2. Blood pH decreased toward neutral creates a condition called *acidosis*
D. Blood donations
  1. Approximately 14 million units donated annually
  2. Plasma volume expanders (such as albumin) can maintain blood volume after hemorrhage for only short periods
  3. Storage of donated blood limited to 6 weeks
E. Blood types
  1. ABO system (Figure 12-2)
    a. Type A blood—type A antigens in RBCs; anti-B type antibodies in plasma
    b. Type B blood—type B antigens in RBCs; anti-A type antibodies in plasma
    c. Type AB blood—type A and type B antigens in RBCs; no anti-A or anti-B antibodies in plasma; called *universal recipient blood*
    d. Type O blood—no type A or type B antigens in RBCs; both anti-A and anti-B antibodies in plasma; called *universal donor blood*
  2. Rh system
    a. Rh-positive blood—Rh factor antigen present in RBCs
    b. Rh-negative blood—no Rh factor present in RBCs; no anti-Rh antibodies present naturally in plasma; anti-Rh antibodies, however, appear in the plasma of Rh-negative persons if Rh-positive RBCs have been introduced into their bodies
    c. Erythroblastosis fetalis—may occur when Rh-negative mother carries a second Rh-positive fetus; caused by mother's Rh antibodies reacting with baby's Rh-positive cells (Figure 12-8)
F. Blood plasma
  1. Liquid fraction of whole blood minus formed elements (Figure 12-1)
  2. Composition—water containing many dissolved substances including:
    a. Foods, salts
    b. About 3% of total O_2 transported in blood
    c. About 5% of total CO_2
    d. Most abundant solutes dissolved in plasma are plasma proteins
      (1) Albumins
      (2) Globulins
      (3) Fibrinogen
      (4) Prothrombin
  3. Plasma minus clotting factors is called *serum*
    a. Serum is liquid remaining after whole blood clots
    b. Serum contains antibodies
G. Formed elements
  1. Types (Figure 12-1)
    a. RBCs (erythrocytes)
    b. WBCs (leukocytes)
      (1) Granular leukocytes—neutrophils, eosinophils, and basophils
      (2) Nongranular leukocytes—lymphocytes and monocytes
    c. Platelets, or thrombocytes
  2. Number
    a. RBCs—4.2 to 6.2 million/mm^3 of blood
    b. WBCs—5000 to 10,000/mm^3 of blood
    c. Platelets—150,000 to 400,000/mm^3 of blood
  3. Formation
    a. Red bone marrow (myeloid tissue) forms all blood cells except some lymphocytes and monocytes.

    b. Most other cells are formed by lymphatic (lymphoid) tissue in the lymph nodes, thymus, and spleen

Mechanisms of Blood Disease

A. Most blood diseases result from failure of myeloid and lymphatic tissues
B. Causes include toxic chemicals, radiation, inherited defects, nutritional deficiencies and cancers, including leukemia
C. Aspiration biopsy cytology (ABC) permits examination of blood-forming tissues to assist in diagnosis of blood diseases
D. Bone marrow, cord blood, and hematopoietic stem cell transplants may be used to replace diseased or destroyed blood-forming tissues

Red Blood Cells (Erythrocytes)

A. Excellent example of how structural adaptation affects biological function
    1. Tough and flexible plasma membrane deforms easily allowing RBCs to pass through small-diameter capillaries
    2. Biconcave disk shape (thin center and thicker edges) results in large cellular surface area (Figure 12-3)
    3. Absence of nucleus and cytoplasmic organelles limits life span to about 120 days but provides more cellular space for red pigment called *hemoglobin (Hb)* (Figure 12-6)
    4. Iron (Fe), folate (a B vitamin), and vitamin B_{12} are among the critical nutrients needed to manufacture red blood cells in the red bone marrow
    5. Named according to size: normocytes (normal size about 7-9 μm in diameter); microcytic (small size); macrocytic (large size) (Figure 12-4)
    6. Named according to hemoglobin content of cell: normochromic (normal Hb content); hypochromic (low Hb content); hyperchromic (high Hb content) (Figure 12-4)
B. General functions
    1. Transport of respiratory gases (O_2 and CO_2)
        a. Combined with hemoglobin
            (1) Oxyhemoglobin ($Hb + O_2$)
            (2) Carbaminohemoglobin ($Hb + CO_2$)
        b. CO_2 inside the RBC as bicarbonate

    2. Important role in homeostasis of acid-base balance
    3. Complete blood cell count (CBC)—battery of laboratory tests used to measure the amounts or levels of many blood constituents
    4. Hematocrit (packed cell volume or PCV) is the percentage of whole blood that is RBCs (Figure 12-5)

Red Blood Cell Disorders

A. Most often related to either overproduction of RBCs—called *polycythemia*; or to low oxygen-carrying capacity of blood—called *anemia*
B. Polycythemia
    1. Cause is generally cancerous transformation of red bone marrow
    2. Dramatic increase in RBC numbers—often in excess of 10 million/mm^3 of blood; hematocrit may reach 60%
    3. Signs and symptoms include:
        a. Increased blood viscosity or thickness
        b. Slow blood flow and coagulation problems
        c. Frequent hemorrhages
        d. Distention of blood vessels and hypertension
    4. Treatment may include:
        a. Blood removal
        b. Irradiation and chemotherapy to suppress RBC production
C. Anemia
    1. Caused by low numbers or abnormal RBCs or by low levels or defective types of hemoglobin
        a. Normal Hb levels 12 to 14 g/100 ml of blood
        b. Low Hb level (below 9 g/100 ml of blood) classified as anemia
    2. Majority of clinical signs of anemia related to low tissue oxygen levels
        a. Fatigue; skin pallor
        b. Weakness; faintness; headache
        c. Compensation results in increased heart and respiratory rates
    3. Hemorrhagic anemia
        a. Acute—blood loss is immediate (for example, surgery or trauma)
        b. Chronic—blood loss occurs over time (for example, ulcers or cancer)

4. Aplastic anemia
   a. Characterized by low RBC numbers and destruction of bone marrow
   b. Often caused by toxic chemicals, irradiation, or certain drugs
5. Deficiency anemias—caused by inadequate supply of some substance needed for RBC or hemoglobin production
   a. Pernicious anemia
      (1) Caused by vitamin B_{12} deficiency
      (2) Genetic-related autoimmune disease
      (3) Decreased RBC, WBC, and platelet numbers
      (4) RBCs are macrocytic
      (5) Classic symptoms of anemia coupled with CNS impairment
      (6) Treatment is repeated vitamin B_{12} injections
   b. Folate deficiency anemia
      (1) Caused by folate (vitamin B_9) deficiency
      (2) Decreased RBC count
      (3) Common in alcoholism and malnutrition
   c. Iron deficiency anemia
      (1) Caused by deficiency or inability to absorb iron needed for Hb synthesis (dietary iron deficiency is common worldwide)
      (2) RBCs are microcytic and hypochromic
      (3) Hematocrit is decreased
      (4) Treatment is oral administration of iron compounds
6. Hemolytic anemias
   a. Caused by decreased RBC life span or increased RBC rate of destruction
   b. Symptoms—such as jaundice, swelling of spleen, gallstone formation and tissue iron deposits—are related to retention of RBC breakdown products
   c. Sickle cell anemia (Figure 12-7)
      (1) Genetic disease resulting in formation of abnormal hemoglobin (HbS); primarily found in black people
      (2) RBCs become fragile and assume sickled shape when blood oxygen levels decrease
      (3) Mild sickle cell trait—result of one defective gene
      (4) More severe sickle cell disease—result of two defective genes; causes

blood stasis, clotting, and "crises" that may be fatal
      (5) Affects 1 in every 600 African American newborns
   d. Thalassemia
      (1) Group of inherited hemolytic anemias occurring primarily in people of Mediterranean descent
      (2) RBCs microcytic and short lived
      (3) Present as mild thalassemia trait and severe thalassemia major
      (4) Hb levels often fall below 7 g/100 ml of blood in thalassemia major
      (5) Classic symptoms of anemia coupled with skeletal deformities and swelling of spleen and liver
   e. Hemolytic disease of newborn and erythroblastosis fetalis (Figure 12-8)
      (1) Caused by blood ABO or Rh factor incompatibility during pregnancy between developing baby and mother
      (2) Maternal antibodies against "foreign" fetal RBCs or Rh factor can cross placenta, enter the fetal circulation, and destroy the unborn baby's red cells
      (3) Symptoms in developing fetus related to decline in RBC numbers and Hb levels; jaundice, intravascular coagulation, and heart and lung damage are common
      (4) Treatment may include in utero blood transfusions and premature delivery of the baby
      (5) Prevention of Rh factor incompatibility now possible by administration of RhoGAM to Rh negative mothers

White Blood Cells (Leukocytes)

A. Categorized by presence of granules (granulocytes) or absence of granules (agranulocytes)
B. WBC count—normal range is 5000 to 10,000/mm^3 of blood
   1. Leukopenia—abnormally low WBC count (below 5000/mm^3 of blood)
      a. Occurs infrequently
      b. May occur with malfunction of blood-forming tissues or diseases affecting immune system, such as AIDS

2. Leukocytosis—abnormally high WBC count (over 10,000/mm^3 of blood)
  a. Frequent finding in bacterial infections
  b. Classic sign in blood cancers (leukemia)
3. Differential WBC count—component test in CBC; measures proportions of each type of WBC in blood sample (Figures 12-1 and 12-9)

C. Leukocyte types and functions
  1. Granulocytes—neutrophils; eosinophils; basophils
    a. Neutrophils
      (1) Most numerous type of phagocyte
      (2) Numbers increase in bacterial infections
    b. Eosinophils
      (1) Weak phagocyte
      (2) Active against parasites and parasitic worms
      (3) Involved in allergic reactions
    c. Basophils
      (1) Related to mast cells in tissue spaces
      (2) Both mast cells and basophils secrete histamine (related to inflammation)
      (3) Basophils also secrete heparin (an anticoagulant)
  2. Agranulocytes—monocytes in peripheral blood (macrophages in tissues); lymphocytes—B lymphocytes (plasma cells) and T lymphocytes
    a. Monocytes
      (1) Largest leukocyte
      (2) Aggressive phagocyte—capable of engulfing larger bacteria and cancer cells
      (3) Develop into much larger cells called *macrophages* after leaving blood to enter tissue spaces
    b. Lymphocytes
      (1) B lymphocytes involved in immunity against disease by secretion of antibodies
      (2) Mature B lymphocytes called *plasma cells*
      (3) T lymphocytes involved in direct attack on bacteria or cancer cells (not antibody production)

White Blood Cell Disorders

A. Two major types of WBC cancers or neoplasms
  1. Lymphoid neoplasms—result from B and T lymphocyte precursor cells or their descendent cell types

  2. Myeloid neoplasms—result from malignant transformation of precursor cells of granulocytic WBCs, monocytes, RBCs, and platelets
B. Multiple myeloma (Figure 12-11)
  1. Cancer of B lymphocytes called *plasma cells*
  2. Most deadly blood cancer in people older than age 65
  3. Causes bone marrow dysfunction and production of defective antibodies
  4. Characterized by:
    a. Recurrent infections and anemia
    b. Destruction and fracture of bones
  5. Treatment includes chemotherapy, drug, antibody therapy, and marrow and stem cell transplantation
C. Leukemias—WBC-related blood cancers
  1. Characterized by marked leukocytosis
  2. Identified as:
    a. Acute—rapid development of symptoms
    b. Chronic—slow development of symptoms
    c. Lymphoid
    d. Myeloid
  3. Chronic lymphocytic leukemia (CLL) (Figure 12-12)
    a. Average age at onset is 65; rare before age 30
    b. More common in men than in women
    c. Often diagnosed unexpectedly in routine physical exams with discovery of marked B lymphocytic leukocytosis
    d. Generally mild symptoms include anemia, fatigue, and enlarged—often painless—lymph nodes
    e. Most patients live many years following diagnosis
    f. Treatment of severe cases involves chemotherapy and irradiation
  4. Acute lymphocytic leukemia (ALL) (Figure 12-13)
    a. Primarily a disease of children between 3 and 7 years of age; 80% of children who develop leukemia have this form of the disease
    b. Highly curable in children but less so in adults
    c. Onset is sudden—marked by fever, leukocytosis, bone pain, and increases in infections
    d. Lymph node, spleen, and liver enlargement is common

e. Treatment includes chemotherapy, irradiation, and bone marrow or stem cell transplantation

5. Chronic myeloid leukemia (CML) (Figure 12-14)

a. Accounts for about 20% of all cases of leukemia

b. Occurs most often in adults between 25 and 60 years of age

c. Caused by cancerous transformation of granulocytic precursor cells in the bone marrow

d. Onset and progression of disease is slow with symptoms of fatigue, weight loss, and weakness

e. Diagnosis often made by discovery of marked granulocytic leukocytosis and extreme spleen enlargement

f. Treatment by new "designer drug" Gleevec or bone marrow transplantation is curative in more than 70% of cases

6. Acute myeloid leukemia (AML)

a. Accounts for 80% of all cases of acute leukemia in adults and 20% of acute leukemia in children

b. Characterized by sudden onset and rapid progression

c. Symptoms include leukocytosis, fatigue, bone and joint pain, spongy bleeding gums, anemia, and recurrent infections

d. Prognosis is poor with only about 50% of children and 30% of adults achieving long-term survival

e. Bone marrow and stem cell transplantation has increased cure rates in selected patients

D. Infectious mononucleosis (Figure 12-15)

1. Noncancerous WBC disorder

2. Highest incidence between 15 and 25 years of age

3. Caused by virus present in saliva of infected individuals

4. Leukocytosis of atypical lymphocytes with abundant cytoplasm and large nuclei

5. Symptoms include fever, severe fatigue, sore throat, rash, and enlargement of lymph nodes and spleen

6. Generally self-limited and resolves without complications in about 4 to 6 weeks.

Platelets and Blood Clotting

A. Platelets

1. Play essential role in blood clotting

a. Blood vessel damage causes platelets to become sticky and form a "platelet plug"

b. Accumulated platelets release additional clotting factors that enter into the clotting mechanism

c. Platelets ultimately become a part of the clot itself

B. Clotting mechanism (Figure 12-16)

1. Damaged tissue cells release clotting factors leading to formation of prothrombin activator, which combines with platelet-produced prothrombin activator

2. Prothrombin activator and calcium convert prothrombin to thrombin

3. Thrombin reacts with fibrinogen to form fibrin

4. Fibrin threads form a tangle to trap RBCs (and other formed elements) to produce a blood clot

C. Altering the blood clotting mechanism

1. Application of gauze (rough surface) to wound causes platelet aggregation and release of clotting factors

2. Administration of vitamin K will increase synthesis of prothrombin

3. Drug warfarin sodium will delay clotting by inhibiting prothrombin synthesis

4. Heparin delays clotting by inhibiting conversion of prothrombin to thrombin

5. Laboratory tests used to monitor effectiveness of anticoagulant therapy include:

a. Prothrombin time—reported in seconds (7 to 10 seconds is normal)

b. INR (International Normalized Ratio)—a calculated value reported as a number (0.8 to 1.2 is normal)

D. Clotting disorders

1. Thrombus—stationary blood clot

2. Embolus—circulating blood clot (drug called *tissue plasminogen activator [TPA]* used to dissolve clots that have already formed) (Figure 12-17)

3. Hemophilia—X-linked inherited disorder that results from inability to produce factor VIII (a plasma protein) responsible for blood clotting

a. Most serious "bleeding disease" worldwide; hemophilia A most common form

b. Characterized by easy bruising, deep muscle hemorrhage, blood in urine, and repeated episodes of bleeding into joints causing pain and deformity

c. Treatment includes administration of factor VIII, injury prevention, and avoiding drugs such as aspirin that alter the clotting mechanism

4. Thrombocytopenia—caused by reduced platelet counts

a. Characterized by bleeding from small blood vessels, most visibly in the skin and mucous membranes

b. Platelet count below 20,000/mm^3 may cause catastrophic bleeding (normal platelet count 150,000 to 400,000/mm^3)

c. Most common cause is bone marrow destruction by drugs, chemicals, radiation, and diseases such as cancer, lupus, and HIV/AIDS

d. Treatment may involve transfusion of platelets, corticosteroid-type drugs, or removal of the spleen

New Words

ABO system	monocyte	anemia	INR (International
agglutinate	myeloid tissue	aplastic anemia	Normalized Ratio)
albumin	neutrophil	blood doping	iron deficiency anemia
antibody	oxyhemoglobin	bone marrow transplant	leukemia
antigen	phagocyte	chronic lymphocytic	leukocytosis
basophil	plasma	leukemia (CLL)	leukopenia
buffy coat	plasma cell	chronic myeloid leukemia	lymphoid neoplasm
carbaminohemoglobin	plasma protein	(CML)	multiple myeloma
eosinophil	prothrombin	complete blood cell count	myeloid neoplasm
erythrocyte (red blood cell)	prothrombin activator	(CBC)	pernicious anemia
fibrin	Rh system	differential WBC count	polycythemia
fibrinogen	serum	embolism	Rh-negative
formed element	thrombin	embolus	RhoGAM
globulin	thrombocyte	erythroblastosis fetalis	Rh-positive
hemoglobin (Hb)		factor VIII	sickle cell anemia
heparin	**Diseases and Other**	folate deficiency anemia	thalassemia
histamine	**Clinical Terms**	hematocrit	thrombocytopenia
leukocyte	acidosis	hemolytic anemia	thrombosis
lymphatic tissue	acute lymphocytic	hemophilia	thrombus
lymphocyte	leukemia (ALL)	hemorrhagic anemia	universal donor blood
macrophage	acute myeloid leukemia	infectious	universal recipient blood
mast cell	(AML)	mononucleosis	

Review Questions

1. Name several substances found in blood plasma.
2. Explain the function of albumins, globulins, and fibrinogen.
3. What is the difference between serum and plasma?
4. What two types of connective tissue form blood cells? Where are they found and what do each of them form?
5. Describe the structure of a red blood cell. What advantage does this unique shape give the red blood cell that helps it perform its function?

6. Both aplastic anemia and pernicious anemia are characterized by low red blood cell count; explain the difference in their causes.
7. What is the buffy coat?
8. Explain the function of neutrophils and monocytes.
9. Explain the function of lymphocytes.
10. Explain the function of eosinophils and basophils.
11. Distinguish between leukopenia and leukocytosis.
12. How is hemophilia transmitted? What blood clotting factors can be affected?
13. Explain the process of blood clot formation.
14. Differentiate between a thrombus and an embolus.

15. Explain how type A blood differs from type B blood.
16. Explain the cause of erythroblastosis fetalis.

Critical Thinking

17. Explain how heparin inhibits blood clot formation.
18. Differentiate between the process of blood clot formation and the process of blood agglutination.
19. Why is the first Rh-positive baby born to an Rh-negative mother usually unaffected?

Chapter Test

1. The liquid part of the blood is called _____.
2. Three important plasma proteins are _____, _____, and _____.
3. Blood plasma without the clotting factors is called _____.
4. The three formed elements of the blood are _____, _____, and _____.
5. The two types of connective tissue that make blood cells are _____ and _____.
6. The red pigment in red blood cells that carries oxygen is called _____.
7. The term _____ is used to describe a number of disease conditions caused by the inability of red blood cells to carry a sufficient amount of oxygen.
8. If the body produces an excess of red blood cells, the condition is called _____.
9. Which white blood cells are the most numerous of the phagocytes? _____.
10. Which white blood cells produce antibodies to fight microbes? _____.
11. Prothrombin activator and the mineral _____ in the blood convert prothrombin into thrombin in the formation of a blood clot.

12. Thrombin converts the inactive plasma protein _____ into a fibrous gel called _____.
13. Vitamin _____ stimulates the liver to increase synthesis of prothrombin.
14. A _____ is a pathological rather than curative blood clot that stays in the place where it was formed.
15. If a part of a blood clot is dislodged and circulates through the bloodstream, it is called _____.
16. _____ is a foreign substance that can cause the body to produce an antibody.
17. A person with type AB blood has _____ antigens on the blood cell and _____ antibodies in the plasma.
18. A person with type B blood has _____ antigens on the blood cell and _____ antibodies in the plasma.
19. Type _____ blood is considered the universal donor.
20. Type _____ blood is considered the universal recipient.
21. A condition called _____ can develop if an Rh-negative mother produces antibodies against the blood of an Rh-positive fetus.

Match each blood disorder in Column A with its corresponding description or cause in Column B.

Column A
22. _____ pernicious anemia
23. _____ sickle cell anemia
24. _____ thalassemia
25. _____ hemophilia
26. _____ thrombocytopenia
27. _____ leukocytosis
28. _____ leukopenia
29. _____ aplastic anemia

Column B
a. a type of inherited anemia that produces abnormal hemoglobin and red blood cell deformities
b. an abnormally low white blood cell count
c. an inherited disorder in which a small amount of hemoglobin is produced; can be major or minor
d. an inherited inability to form some blood clotting factors
e. an abnormally low number of platelets
f. a low number of red blood cells because of a lack of vitamin B_{12}
g. a low number of red blood cells related to destruction of bone marrow
h. an abnormally high white blood cell count

Study Tips

continued from page 341

4. When studying the blood disorders, make a chart that identifies the type of disorder: red blood cell, white blood cell, or clotting disorder. List the name and the specific cause of each disorder.

5. As you study the ABO blood typing system, be sure you give extra attention to learning what antigens are on the red blood cells and what antibodies are in the plasma. The antigens give a blood type its name, that is, type A blood has A antigens. Antibodies are the opposite of the blood type. Type A blood has anti-B antibodies. Type O has no antigens and both antibodies; type AB has both antigens and no antibodies.

6. In your study group, review the flash cards you made for studying the function of the blood cells. Discuss the process of blood clot formation. Go over the blood disorder chart. Review the antigens and antibodies of the various blood types. Go over the questions at the end of the chapter and discuss possible test questions.

Case Studies

1. Angela's physician suspects that Angela has just suffered a *myocardial infarction,* or heart attack. She tells Angela that she is going to take a blood sample so that the hospital lab can perform a test to confirm her diagnosis. What information can Angela's blood yield to help the physician?

2. Yvonne has just been told that she has a condition called *pernicious anemia.* She looked up the definition of this disease in a dictionary and learned that it is caused by a decreased availability of vitamin B_{12} needed for manufacturing RBCs. Yvonne promptly went to the local pharmacy to buy some vitamin B_{12} tablets to help her overcome this condition. Is this a wise course of action?

3. Your brother has just been diagnosed as having anemia, but your mother cannot seem to remember the specific type. She shows you a copy of your young brother's CBC results, but no diagnosis is stated. Based on the results given below, what would you guess is your brother's condition? (HINT: see Table 12-2.) Are you likely to develop this condition?

Folate content: normal
Hematocrit: low
Hemoglobin content: low
Iron content: slightly high
RBC size (mean corpuscular volume): high
Vitamin B_{12} content: normal

Outline

Objectives

After you have completed this chapter, you should be able to:

1. Discuss the location, size, and position of the heart in the thoracic cavity and identify the heart chambers, sounds, and valves.

2. Describe the major types of cardiac valve disorders.

3. Trace blood through the heart and compare the functions of the heart chambers on the right and left sides.

4. Explain how a myocardial infarction might occur.

5. List the anatomical components of the heart conduction system and discuss the features of the normal electrocardiogram.

6. Describe the major types of cardiac dysrhythmia.

7. List and describe the possible causes of heart failure.

13 The Heart and Heart Disease

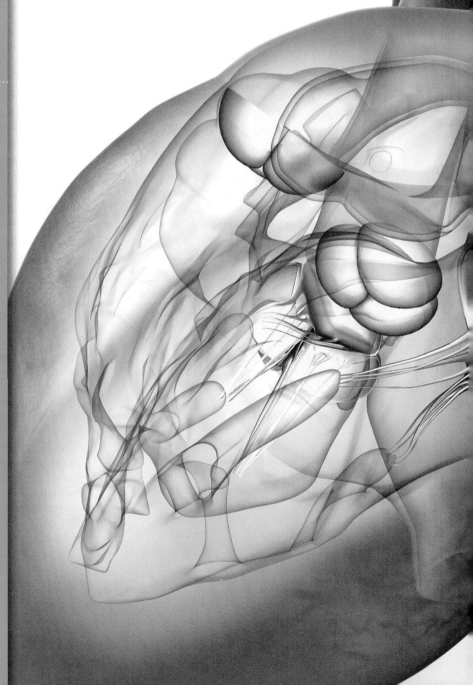

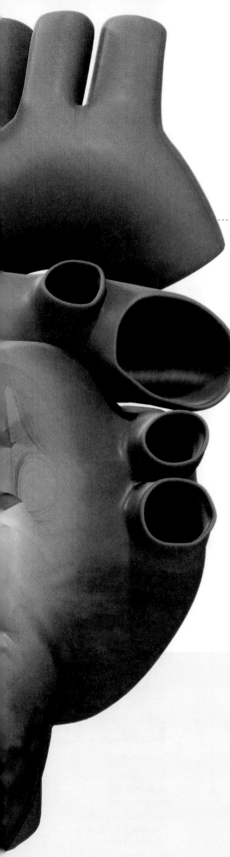

Differing amounts of nutrients and waste products enter and leave the fluid surrounding each body cell continually. In addition, requirements for hormones, body salts, water, and other critical substances constantly change. However, homeostasis or constancy of the body fluid contents surrounding the billions of cells that make up our bodies is required for survival. The system that supplies our cells' transportation needs is the **cardiovascular system.** The levels of dozens of substances in the blood can remain constant even though the absolute amounts that are needed or produced may change because we have this extremely effective system that transports these substances to or from each cell as circumstances change.

In this chapter, we discuss the heart—the pump that keeps blood moving around a closed circuit of blood vessels. As appropriate, we include discussions of **heart disease,** a group of disorders that together constitute the leading cause of death for both men and women in the United States. Chapter 14 continues the study of the cardiovascular system by discussing the blood vessels in health and disease.

STUDY TIPS

Before studying Chapter 13, review the synopsis of the cardiovascular system in Chapter 4. Chapter 13 deals with the heart, the pump that moves the blood through the blood vessels.

1. Make flash cards to help you learn the structures of the heart.
2. The location of the semilunar valves should be easy to remember because their names tell you where they are. It is harder to remember where the tricuspid and mitral valves are because their names don't give any clues to their locations. An easier way to remember them is to use their other names, the right and left atrioventricular valves. These names tell you exactly where they are, between the atria and ventricles on the right or left side.
3. Blood moves through the heart in one direction: from the right heart, to the lungs, to the left heart, and out the aorta. Heart conduction may make more sense if you remember that atria contract from the top down

continued on page 393

Location, Size, and Position of the Heart

No one needs to be told where the heart is or what it does. Everyone knows that the heart is in the chest, that it beats night and day to keep the blood flowing, and that if it stops, life stops.

Most of us probably think of the heart as being located on the left side of the body. As you can see in Figure 13-1, the heart is located between the lungs in the lower portion of the mediastinum. Draw an imaginary line through the middle of the trachea in Fig-

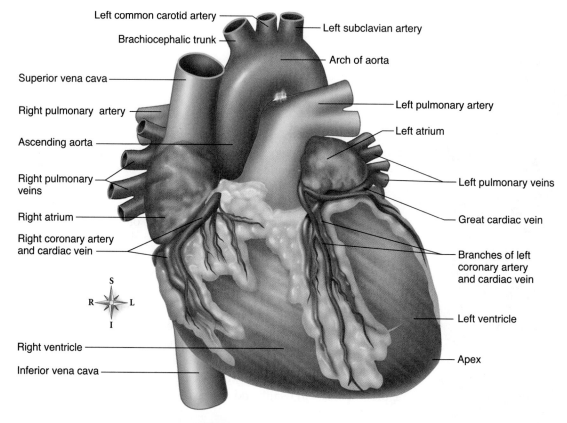

Left common carotid artery — Left subclavian artery
Brachiocephalic trunk —
— Arch of aorta
Superior vena cava —
Right pulmonary artery — — Left pulmonary artery
Ascending aorta — — Left atrium
Right pulmonary veins — — Left pulmonary veins
Right atrium — — Great cardiac vein
Right coronary artery and cardiac vein — — Branches of left coronary artery and cardiac vein
— Left ventricle
Right ventricle — — Apex
Inferior vena cava —

S
R — L
I

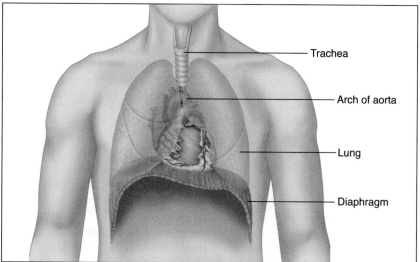

Trachea

Arch of aorta

Lung

Diaphragm

Figure 13-1

The heart.

The heart and major blood vessels viewed from the front (anterior). Inset shows the relationship of the heart to other structures in the thoracic cavity.

ure 13-1 and continue the line down through the thoracic cavity to divide it into right and left halves. Note that about two thirds of the mass of the heart is to the left of this line and one third is to the right.

The heart is often described as a triangular organ, shaped and sized roughly like a closed fist. In Figure 13-1 you can see that the apex, or blunt point, of the lower edge of the heart lies on the diaphragm, pointing toward the left. Physicians and nurses often listen to the heart sounds by placing a stethoscope on the chest wall directly over the apex of the heart. Sounds of the so-called *apical beat* are easily heard in this area (that is, in the space between the fifth and sixth ribs on a line even with the midpoint of the left clavicle).

The heart is positioned in the thoracic cavity between the sternum in front and the bodies of the thoracic vertebrae behind. Because of this placement, it can be compressed or squeezed by application of pressure to the lower portion of the body of the sternum using the heel of the hand. Rhythmic compression of the heart in this way can maintain blood flow in cases of cardiac arrest and, if combined with effective artificial respiration, the resulting procedure, called **cardiopulmonary resuscitation (CPR),** can be lifesaving. The exact procedures for CPR change frequently as new research data become available, so it is important for individuals certified in CPR to re-certify on a regular basis.

 To learn more about the location of the heart, go to **AnimationDirect** on your CD.

Anatomy of the Heart

Heart Chambers

If you cut open a heart, you can see many of its main structural features (Figure 13-2). This organ is hol-

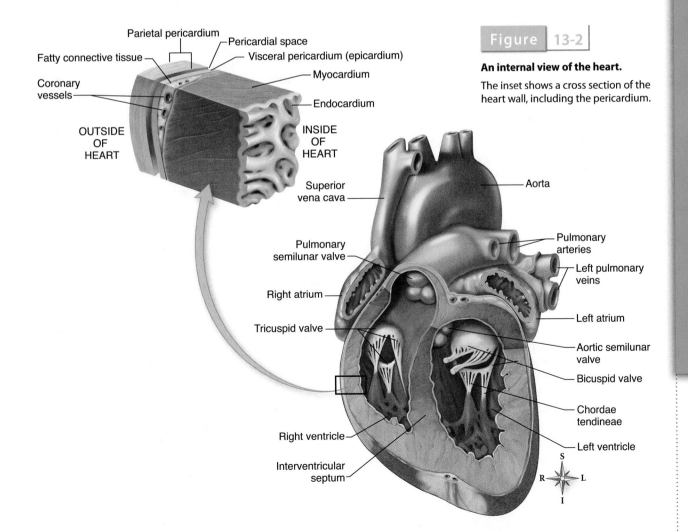

Figure 13-2

An internal view of the heart.

The inset shows a cross section of the heart wall, including the pericardium.

Parietal pericardium
Pericardial space
Fatty connective tissue
Visceral pericardium (epicardium)
Coronary vessels
Myocardium
Endocardium

OUTSIDE OF HEART
INSIDE OF HEART

Superior vena cava
Aorta
Pulmonary semilunar valve
Pulmonary arteries
Left pulmonary veins
Right atrium
Left atrium
Tricuspid valve
Aortic semilunar valve
Bicuspid valve
Chordae tendineae
Right ventricle
Left ventricle
Interventricular septum

S
R — L
I

low, not solid. A partition divides it into right and left sides. The heart contains four cavities, or hollow chambers. The two upper chambers are called **atria** (AY-tree-ah) (*singular,* **atrium**), and the two lower chambers are called **ventricles** (VEN-tri-kuls).

The atria are smaller than the ventricles, and their walls are thinner and less muscular. Atria are often called *receiving chambers* because blood enters the heart through veins that open into these upper cavities. Eventually, blood is pumped from the heart into arteries that exit from the ventricles; therefore the ventricles are sometimes referred to as the *discharging chambers* of the heart.

Each heart chamber is named according to its location. Thus there are right and left atrial chambers above and right and left ventricular chambers below.

The wall of each heart chamber is composed of cardiac muscle tissue usually referred to as the **myocardium** (my-oh-KAR-dee-um). The septum between the atrial chambers is called the *interatrial septum;* the *interventricular septum* separates the ventricles.

Each chamber of the heart is lined by a thin layer of very smooth tissue called the **endocardium** (en-doh-KAR-dee-um) (Figure 13-2). Inflammation of this lining is referred to as **endocarditis** (en-doh-kar-DYE-tis). If inflamed, the endocardial lining can become rough and abrasive to RBCs passing over its surface. Blood flowing over a rough surface is subject to clotting, and a **thrombus** (THROM-bus), or clot, may form (see Chapter 12). Unfortunately, rough spots caused by endocarditis or injuries to blood vessel walls often cause the release of platelet factors. The result is often the formation of a fatal blood clot.

 To learn more about the chambers of the heart, go to **AnimationDirect** on your CD.

The Pericardium and Pericarditis

The heart has a covering and a lining. Its covering, called the **pericardium** (pair-i-KAR-dee-um), consists of two layers of fibrous tissue with a small space in between them. The inner layer of the pericardium is called the **visceral pericardium,** or **epicardium** (ep-i-KAR-dee-um). It covers the heart the way an apple skin covers an apple. The outer layer of pericardium is called the **parietal pericardium.** It

fits around the heart like a loose-fitting sack, allowing enough room for the heart to beat.

It is easy to remember the difference between the *endocardium,* which lines the heart chambers, and the *epicardium,* which covers the surface of the heart (Figure 13-2), if you understand the meaning of the prefixes *endo-* and *epi-*. *Endo-* comes from the Greek word meaning "inside" or "within," and *epi-* comes from the Greek word meaning "upon" or "on."

The two pericardial layers slide against each other without friction when the heart beats because these are serous membranes with moist, not dry, surfaces. A thin film of pericardial fluid furnishes the lubricating moistness between the heart and its enveloping pericardial sac.

If the pericardium becomes inflamed, a condition called **pericarditis** (pair-i-kar-DYE-tis) results. Pericarditis may be caused by a variety of factors: trauma, viral or bacterial infection, tumors, and other factors. The pericardial edema that characterizes this condition often causes the visceral and parietal pericardia to rub together—causing severe chest pain. Pericardial fluid, pus, or blood (in the case of an injury) may accumulate in the space between the two pericardial layers and impair the pumping action of the heart. This is termed *pericardial effusion* and may develop into a serious compression of the heart called **cardiac tamponade** (tam-poh-NAHD).

QUICK CHECK

1. What are the functions of the atria and ventricles of the heart?
2. What coverings does the heart have? What is the heart's lining called?
3. What is *pericarditis?*

Heart Action

The heart serves as a muscular pumping device for distributing blood to all parts of the body. Contraction of the heart is called **systole** (SISS-toh-lee), and relaxation is called **diastole** (dye-ASS-toh-lee). When the heart beats (that is, when it contracts), the atria contract first (atrial systole), forcing blood into the ventricles. Once filled, the two ventricles contract (ventricular systole) and force blood out of the heart (Figure 13-3). For the heart to be efficient in its pumping action, more than just the rhythmic contraction of its muscular fibers is required. The direction of blood flow must be directed and controlled. This is accom-

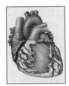

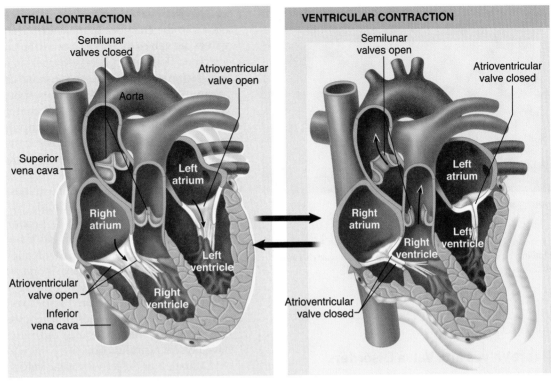

ATRIAL CONTRACTION

Semilunar valves closed

Atrioventricular valve open

Aorta

Superior vena cava

Left atrium

Right atrium

Atrioventricular valve open

Left ventricle

Inferior vena cava

Right ventricle

VENTRICULAR CONTRACTION

Semilunar valves open

Atrioventricular valve closed

Left atrium

Right atrium

Right ventricle

Left ventricle

Atrioventricular valve closed

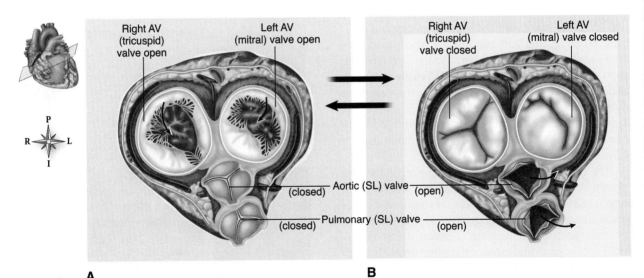

Right AV (tricuspid) valve open

Left AV (mitral) valve open

Right AV (tricuspid) valve closed

Left AV (mitral) valve closed

(closed) Aortic (SL) valve (open)

(closed) Pulmonary (SL) valve (open)

A

B

Figure 13-3 | **Heart action.**

A, During atrial systole (contraction), cardiac muscle in the atrial wall contracts, forcing blood through the atrioventricular (AV) valves and into the ventricles. Bottom illustration shows superior view of all four valves, with semilunar (SL) valves closed and AV valves open. **B,** During ventricular systole that follows, the AV valves close, and blood is forced out of the ventricles through the semilunar valves and into the arteries. Bottom illustration shows superior view of SL valves open and AV valves closed.

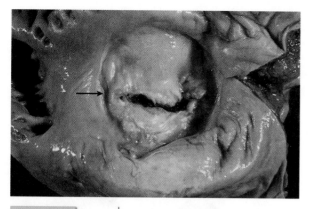

Figure | 13-4 | **Mitral valve stenosis.**

Stenosed valves are valves that are narrower than normal, slowing blood flow from a heart chamber. Compare this valve with the normal valve shown in Figure 13-3, *A*.

plished by four sets of valves located at the entrance and near the exit of the ventricles.

Heart Valves and Valve Disorders

The two valves that separate the atrial chambers above from the ventricles below are called **AV,** or **atrioventricular** (ay-tree-oh-ven-TRIK-yoo-lar), **valves.** The two AV valves are called the **bicuspid,** or **mitral** (MY-tral), **valve,** located between the left atrium and ventricle, and the **tricuspid valve,** located between the right atrium and ventricle. The AV valves prevent backflow of blood into the atria when the ventricles contract. Locate the AV valves in Figures 13-2 and 13-3. Note that a number of stringlike structures called **chordae tendineae** (KOR-dee ten-DIN-ee) attach the AV valves to the wall of the heart.

The **SL,** or **semilunar** (sem-i-LOO-nar), **valves** are located between the two ventricular chambers and the large arteries that carry blood away from the heart when contraction occurs (Figure 13-3). The ventricles, like the atria, contract together. Therefore the two semilunar valves open and close at the same time. The **pulmonary semilunar valve** is located at the beginning of the pulmonary artery and allows blood going to the lungs to flow out of the right ventricle but prevents it from flowing back into the ventricle. The **aortic semilunar valve** is located at the beginning of the aorta and allows blood to flow out of the left ventricle up into the aorta but prevents backflow into this ventricle.

Disorders of the cardiac valves can have several effects. For example, a congenital defect in valve structure can result in mild to severe pumping inefficiency.

Incompetent valves leak, allowing some blood to flow back into the chamber from which it came. **Stenosed valves** are valves that are narrower than normal, slowing blood flow from a heart chamber (Figure 13-4).

Rheumatic heart disease is cardiac damage resulting from a delayed inflammatory response to streptococcal infection that occurs most often in children. A few weeks after an untreated or improperly treated streptococcal infection, the cardiac valves and other tissues in the body may become inflamed—a condition called *rheumatic fever.* If severe, the inflammation can result in stenosis or other deformities of the valves, chordae tendineae, or myocardium.

Mitral valve prolapse (MVP), a condition affecting the bicuspid, or mitral, valve, has a genetic basis in some cases but can result from rheumatic fever or other factors. A prolapsed mitral valve is one whose flaps extend back into the left atrium, causing incompetence (leaking) of the valve (Figure 13-5). This condition was once thought to be common, but recent studies show that many patients previously diagnosed with MVP have normal heart function.

Damaged or defective cardiac valves often can be replaced surgically. Animal valves and artificial valves made from synthetic materials are commonly used in valve replacement procedures.

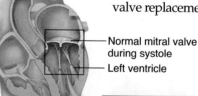

Normal mitral valve during systole
Left ventricle

Left atrium

Prolapsed mitral valve

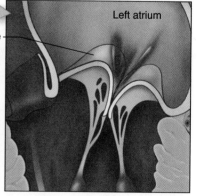

Figure | 13-5 | **Mitral valve prolapse.**

The normal mitral valve *(upper left)* prevents backflow of blood from the left ventricle into the left atrium during ventricular systole (contraction). The prolapsed mitral valve *(right)* permits leakage because the valve flaps billow backward, parting slightly. The photo inset shows the ballooning *(arrow)* of the mitral valve into the atrium.

To learn more about heart valve disorders, go to **AnimationDirect** on your CD.

Heart Sounds

If a stethoscope is placed on the anterior chest wall, two distinct sounds can be heard. They are rhythmical and repetitive sounds that are often described as *lub dup*. Disorders of the cardiac valves are often diagnosed by detecting changes in these normal valve sounds of the heart.

The first, or *lub*, sound is caused by the vibration and abrupt closure of the AV valves as the ventricles contract. Closure of the AV valves prevents blood from rushing back up into the atria during contraction of the ventricles. This first sound is of longer duration and lower pitch than the second. The pause between this first sound and the *dup*, or second sound, is shorter than that after the second sound and the *lub dup* of the next systole. The second

heart sound is caused by the closing of both the semilunar valves when the ventricles undergo diastole (relax) (Figure 13-3).

Abnormal heart sounds called **heart murmurs** are often caused by disorders of the valves. For example, incompetent valves may cause a swishing sound as a "lub" or "dup" ends. Stenosed valves, on the other hand, often cause swishing sounds just before a "lub" or "dup."

Blood Flow Through the Heart

The heart acts as two separate pumps. The right atrium and the right ventricle perform a task quite different from the left atrium and the left ventricle. When the heart "beats," first the atria contract simultaneously. This is atrial systole. Then the ventricles fill with blood, and they, too, contract together during ventricular systole. Although the atria contract as a unit followed by the ventricles below, the right and left sides of the heart act as separate pumps. As we study the blood flow through the heart, the separate functions of the two pumps will become clearer.

Note in Figure 13-6 that blood enters the right atrium through

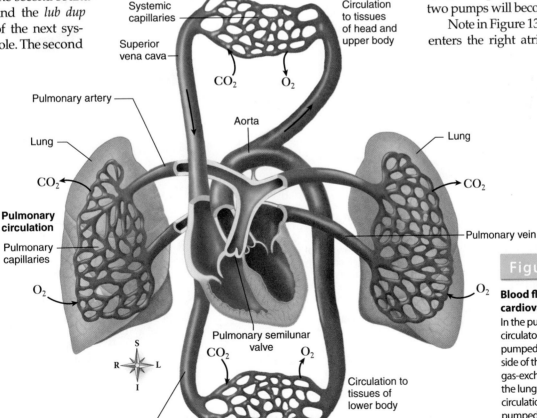

Figure 13-6

Blood flow through the cardiovascular system. In the pulmonary circulatory route, blood is pumped from the right side of the heart to the gas-exchange tissues of the lungs. In the systemic circulation, blood is pumped from the left side of the heart to all other tissues of the body.

two large veins called the **superior vena** (VEE-nah) **cava** (KAY-vah) and **inferior vena cava.** The right heart pump receives oxygen-poor blood from the veins. After entering the right atrium, it is pumped through the right AV, or tricuspid, valve and enters the right ventricle. When the ventricles contract, blood in the right ventricle is pumped through the pulmonary semilunar valve into the **pulmonary artery** and eventually to the lungs, where oxygen is added and carbon dioxide is lost.

As you can see in Figure 13-6, blood rich in oxygen returns to the left atrium of the heart through four **pulmonary veins.** It then passes through the left AV, or bicuspid, valve into the left ventricle. When the left ventricle contracts, blood is forced through the aortic semilunar valve into the **aorta** (ay-OR-tah) and is distributed to the body as a whole.

As you can tell from Figure 13-6, the two sides of the heart actually pump blood through two separate "circulations" and function as two separate pumps. The **pulmonary circulation** involves movement of blood from the right ventricle to the lungs, and the **systemic circulation** involves movement of blood from the left ventricle throughout the body

as a whole. The pulmonary and systemic circulations are discussed in Chapter 14.

Coronary Circulation and Coronary Heart Disease

To sustain life, the heart must pump blood throughout the body on a regular and ongoing basis. As a result, the heart muscle or myocardium requires a constant supply of blood containing nutrients and oxygen to function effectively. The delivery of oxygen and nutrient-rich arterial blood to cardiac muscle tissue and the return of oxygen-poor blood from this active tissue to the venous system is called the **coronary circulation** (Figure 13-7).

Blood flows into the heart muscle by way of two small vessels—the **right** and **left coronary arteries.** The coronary arteries are the aorta's first branches, as you can see in Figure 13-7, *A*. The openings into these small vessels lie behind the flaps of the aortic semilunar valves. During ventricular diastole, blood in the aorta that backs up behind the closed aortic SL valve can flow into the coronary arteries.

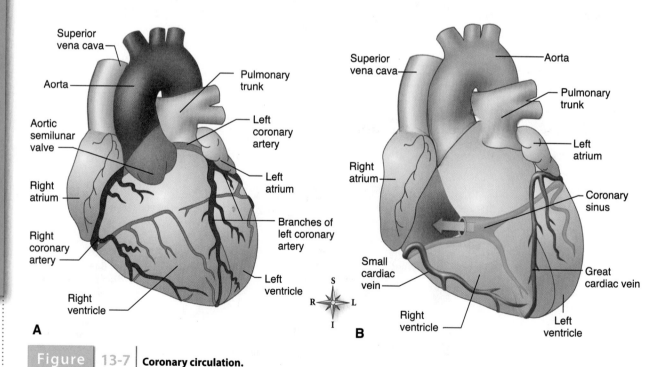

Figure 13-7 | **Coronary circulation.**

A, Arteries. **B,** Veins. Both are anterior views of the heart. Vessels near the anterior surface are more darkly colored than vessels of the posterior surface seen through the heart.

In both coronary thrombosis and coronary **embolism** (EM-boh-liz-em), a blood clot occludes or plugs up some part of a coronary artery. Blood cannot pass through the occluded vessel and so cannot reach the heart muscle cells it normally supplies. Deprived of oxygen, these cells soon become damaged. In medical terms, **myocardial** (my-oh-KAR-dee-all) **infarction** (in-FARK-shun) **(MI)**, or tissue death, occurs.

Myocardial infarction, also referred to as a "heart attack," is a common cause of death during middle and late adulthood. Recovery from a myocardial infarction is possible if the amount of heart tissue damaged was small enough so that the remaining undamaged heart muscle can still pump blood effectively enough to supply the needs of the rest of the heart and the body.

Coronary arteries also may become blocked as a result of **atherosclerosis,** a type of "hardening of the arteries" in which lipids and other substances build up on the inside wall of blood vessels. Mechanisms of atherosclerosis are discussed further in Chapter 14. Coronary atherosclerosis has increased dramatically over the last few decades to become the leading cause of death in western countries. Many pathophysiologists believe this increase results from a change in lifestyle. They cite several important risk factors associated with coronary atherosclerosis: physical inactivity, cigarette smoking, high-fat and high-cholesterol diets, obesity, hypertension (high blood pressure), and diabetes.

The term **angina** (an-JYE-nah) **pectoris** (PEK-tor-iss) is used to describe the severe chest pain that occurs when the myocardium is deprived of adequate oxygen. It is often a warning that the coronary arteries are no longer able to supply enough blood and oxygen to the heart muscle.

Coronary bypass surgery is a common treatment for those who suffer from severely restricted coronary artery blood flow. In this procedure, veins are "harvested" or removed from other areas of the body and used to bypass partial blockages in coronary arteries (Figure 13-8). A therapy called *coronary angioplasty* also may be used to treat blockages to coronary blood flow. Angioplasty is described in greater detail in Chapter 14, p. 401.

After blood has passed through the capillary beds in the myocardium, it flows into cardiac veins, which empty into the **coronary sinus** and finally into the right atrium.

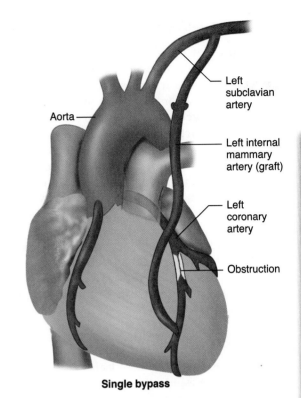

Single bypass

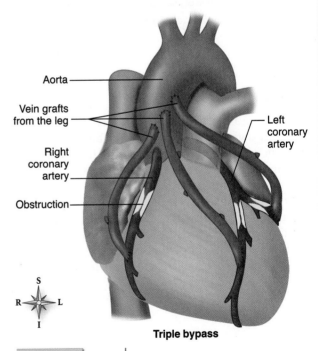

Triple bypass

Figure 13-8 **Coronary bypass.**

In coronary bypass surgery, blood vessels are "harvested" from other parts of the body and used to construct detours around blocked coronary arteries. Artificial vessels also can be used.

Cardiac Cycle

The beating of the heart is a regular and rhythmic process. Each complete heartbeat is called a **cardiac cycle** and includes the contraction (systole) and relaxation (diastole) of atria and ventricles. Each cycle takes about 0.8 second to complete if the heart is beating at an average rate of about 72 beats per minute. The term **stroke volume** refers to the volume of blood ejected from the ventricles during each beat. **Cardiac output,** or the volume of blood pumped by one ventricle per minute, averages about 5 L in a normal, resting adult.

Valve disorders, coronary artery blockage, or myocardial infarction can all decrease stroke volume and thus may decrease cardiac output. Decreased cardiac output can result in fatigue or even death.

> **QUICK CHECK**
>
> 1. What are systole and diastole of the heart?
> 2. What are the two major "circulations" of the body?
> 3. What causes each of the two major *heart sounds?*
> 4. What is the medical term for *heart attack?* What is the mechanism?

Conduction System of the Heart

Cardiac muscle fibers can contract rhythmically on their own. However, they must be coordinated by electrical signals (impulses) if the heart is to pump effectively. Although the rate of the cardiac muscle's rhythm is controlled by autonomic nerve signals, the heart has its own built-in conduction system for coordinating contractions during the cardiac cycle (Figure 13-9). The most important thing to realize about this conduction system is that all of the cardiac muscle fibers in each region of the heart are electrically linked together. The *intercalated disks* that were first introduced in Chapter 3 (see Figure 3-24, p. 68) are actually electrical connectors that join muscle fibers into a single unit that can conduct an impulse through the entire wall of a heart chamber without stopping. Thus both atrial walls will contract at about the same time because all their fibers are electrically linked. Likewise, both ventricular walls will contract at about the same time.

Four structures embedded in the wall of the heart specialize in generating strong impulses and conducting them rapidly to certain regions of the heart wall. Thus they make sure that the atria contract and then the ventricles contract in an efficient manner. The structures that make up this conduction system of the heart are as follows:

1. **Sinoatrial** (sye-no-AY-tree-al) **node,** which is sometimes called the SA node or the **pacemaker**
2. **Atrioventricular** (ay-tree-oh-ven-TRIK-yoo-lar) **node,** or **AV node**
3. **AV bundle,** or **bundle of His**
4. **Purkinje** (pur-KIN-jee) **fibers**

Impulse conduction normally starts in the heart's pacemaker, namely, the SA node. From there, it spreads, as you can see in Figure 13-9, in all directions through the atria. This causes the atrial fibers to contract. When impulses reach the AV node, it relays them by way of the bundle of His and Purkinje fibers to the ventricles, causing them to contract. Normally, therefore, a ventricular beat follows each atrial beat.

 To learn more about the conduction of heart impulses, go to **AnimationDirect** on your CD.

Electrocardiography

The specialized structures of the heart's conduction system generate tiny electrical currents that spread through surrounding tissues to the surface of the body. This fact is of great clinical significance because these electrical signals can be picked up from the body surface and transformed into visible tracings by an instrument called an **electrocardiograph** (ee-lek-troh-KAR-dee-oh-graf).

The **electrocardiogram** (ee-lek-troh-KAR-dee-oh-gram), or **ECG,** is the graphic record of the heart's electrical activity. Skilled interpretation of these ECG records may sometimes make the difference be-

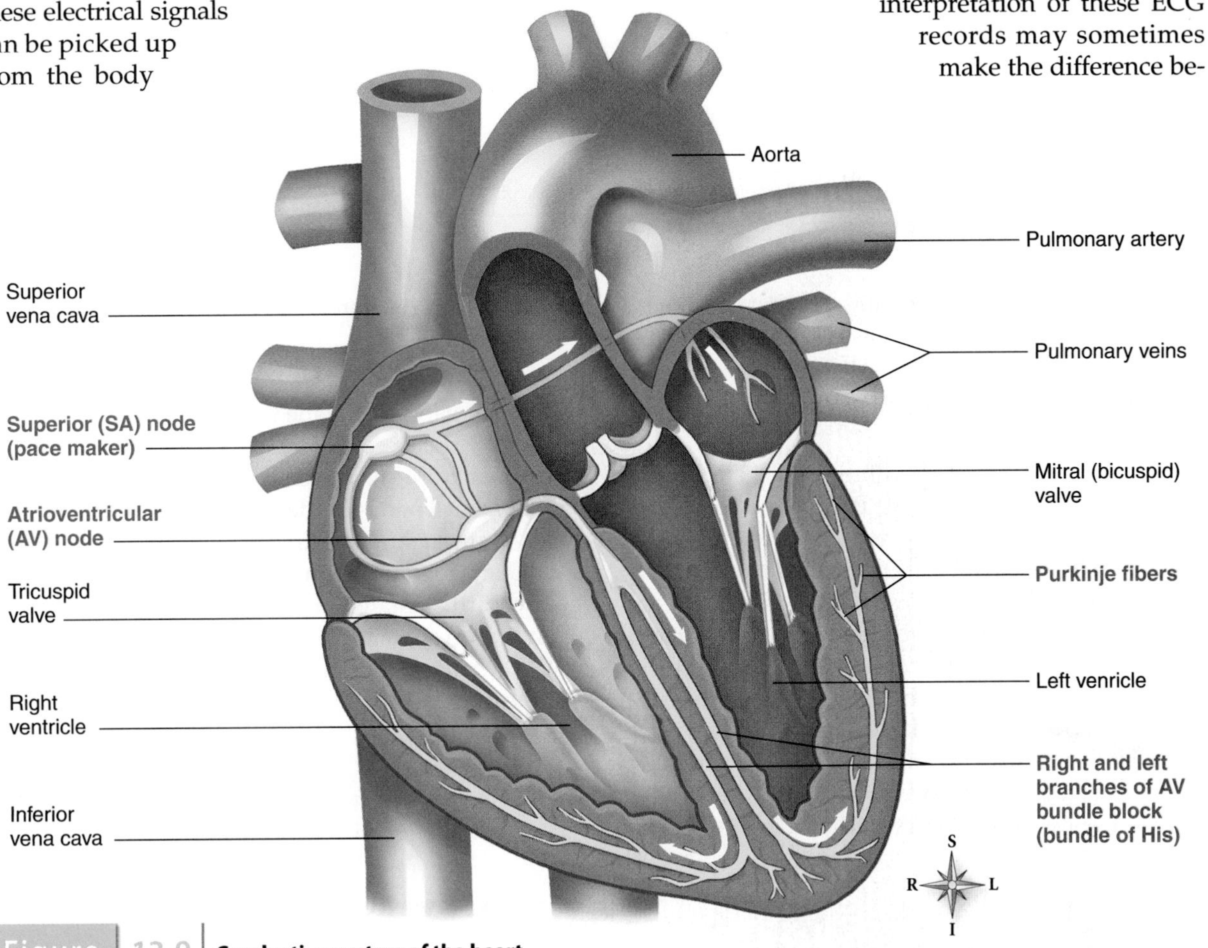

Label (left)	Label (right)
Superior vena cava	Aorta
Superior (SA) node (pace maker)	Pulmonary artery
Atrioventricular (AV) node	Pulmonary veins
Tricuspid valve	Mitral (bicuspid) valve
Right ventricle	Purkinje fibers
Inferior vena cava	Left venricle
	Right and left branches of AV bundle block (bundle of His)

Figure 13-9 | **Conduction system of the heart.**

Specialized cardiac muscle cells (yellow) in the wall of the heart rapidly conduct an electrical impulse throughout the myocardium. The signal is initiated by the sinoatrial (SA) node (pacemaker) and spreads to the rest of the atrial myocardium and to the atrioventricular (AV) node. The AV node then initiates a signal that is conducted through the ventricular myocardium by way of the AV bundle (of His) and Purkinje fibers. Labels for parts of the heart's conduction system are highlighted in red.

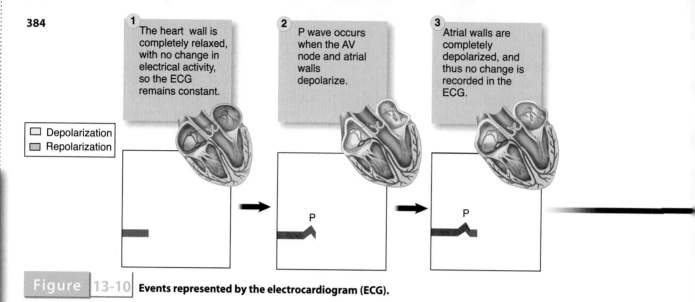

1 The heart wall is completely relaxed, with no change in electrical activity, so the ECG remains constant.

2 P wave occurs when the AV node and atrial walls depolarize.

3 Atrial walls are completely depolarized, and thus no change is recorded in the ECG.

□ Depolarization
▨ Repolarization

Figure 13-10 **Events represented by the electrocardiogram (ECG).**

It is nearly impossible to illustrate the invisible, dynamic events of heart conduction in a few cartoon panels or "snapshots," but the sketches here give you an idea of what is happening in the heart as an ECG is recorded.

tween life and death. A normal ECG tracing is shown in Figure 13-10.

A normal ECG tracing has three very characteristic deflections, or waves, called the **P wave,** the **QRS complex,** and the **T wave.** These deflections represent the electrical activity that regulates the contraction or relaxation of the atria or ventricles. The term *depolarization* describes the electrical activity that triggers contraction of the heart muscle. *Repolarization* begins just before the relaxation phase of cardiac muscle activity. In the normal ECG shown in Figure 13-10, the small P wave occurs with depolarization of the atria. The QRS complex occurs as a result of depolarization of the ventricles, and the T wave results from electrical activity generat-

ed by repolarization of the ventricles. You may wonder why no visible record of atrial repolarization is noted in a normal ECG. The reason is simply that the deflection is very small and is hidden by the large QRS complex that occurs at the same time.

Damage to cardiac muscle tissue that is caused by a myocardial infarction or disease affecting the heart's conduction system results in distinctive changes in the ECG. Therefore ECG tracings are extremely valuable in the diagnosis and treatment of heart disease.

QUICK CHECK

1. What structure is called the natural "pacemaker" of the heart?
2. What information is in an electrocardiogram?

Cardiac Dysrhythmia

Various conditions such as endocarditis or myocardial infarction can damage the heart's conduction system and thereby disturb the rhythmic beating of the heart. The term **dysrhythmia** (dis-RITH-mee-ah) refers to an abnormality of heart rhythm. The term *arrhythmia* (ay-RITH-mee-ah) is still sometimes used to refer to rhythm abnormalities.

One kind of dysrhythmia is called a **heart block.** In *AV node block,* impulses are blocked from getting through to the ventricular myocardium, resulting in the ventricles contracting at a much slower rate than normal. On an ECG, there may be a large distance between the P wave and the R peak of the QRS complex. *Complete heart block* occurs when the P waves do not match up with the QRS complexes at all—as in an ECG that shows two or more P waves for every QRS complex (Figure 13-11, *A*). A

CLINICAL APPLICATION

ECHOCARDIOGRAPHY

Although the stethoscope is still the basic tool of the **cardiologist,** or heart specialist, more sophisticated methods for detecting abnormalities in heart valve function are available. One widely used technique is **echocardiography** (ek-oh-kar-dee-OG-rah-fee). Ultrasound (extremely high-pitched sound) directed toward the heart is reflected back (echoed) by the tissues. Like an airport's radar, a detector picks up the echoed ultrasound and produces an image showing different regions of blood and heart tissues. As the valves and other structures move during a series of heartbeats, the image changes. A cardiologist can examine a continuous recording called an *echocardiogram* and determine the nature of a valve problem or other heart disorder.

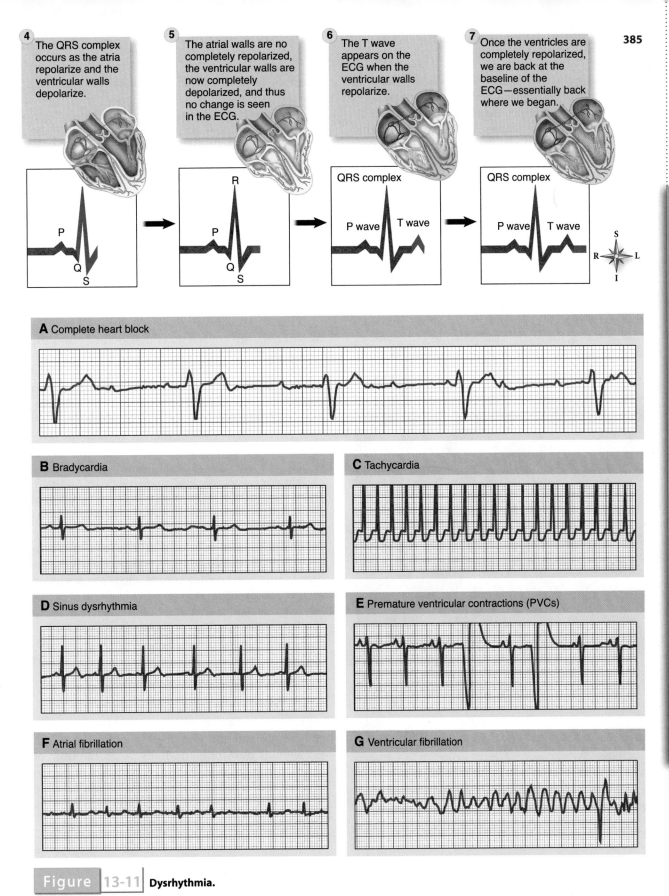

4 The QRS complex occurs as the atria repolarize and the ventricular walls depolarize.

5 The atrial walls are no completely repolarized, the ventricular walls are now completely depolarized, and thus no change is seen in the ECG.

6 The T wave appears on the ECG when the ventricular walls repolarize.

7 Once the ventricles are completely repolarized, we are back at the baseline of the ECG—essentially back where we began.

A Complete heart block

B Bradycardia

C Tachycardia

D Sinus dysrhythmia

E Premature ventricular contractions (PVCs)

F Atrial fibrillation

G Ventricular fibrillation

Figure 13-11 Dysrhythmia.

Examples of different types of dysrhythmia are shown as they would appear in an electrocardiogram (ECG strip recording).

physician may treat heart block by implanting in the heart an **artificial pacemaker,** a battery-operated device implanted under the skin and connected by thin wires to the myocardium (Figure 13-12). This device stimulates the myocardium with timed electrical impulses that cause ventricular contractions at a rate fast enough to maintain an adequate circulation of blood.

Bradycardia (bray-dee-KAR-dee-ah) is a slow heart rhythm—less than 60 beats per minute (Figure 13-11, *B*). Slight bradycardia is normal during sleep and in conditioned athletes while they are awake (but at rest). Abnormal bradycardia can result from improper autonomic nervous control of the heart or from a damaged SA node. If the problem is severe, artificial pacemakers can be used to increase the heart rate by taking the place of the SA node. For example, *demand pacemakers* take over SA node function only

when the heart rate falls below a level programmed into the pacemaker by the physician.

Tachycardia (tak-ee-KAR-dee-ah) is a rapid heart rhythm—more than 100 beats per minute (Figure 13-11, *C*). Tachycardia is normal during and after exercise and during the stress response. Abnormal tachycardia can result from improper autonomic control of the heart, blood loss or shock, the action of drugs and toxins, fever, and other factors.

Sinus dysrhythmia is a variation in heart rate during the breathing cycle (Figure 13-11, *D*). Typically, the rate increases during inspiration and decreases during expiration. The causes of sinus dysrhythmia are not clear. This phenomenon is common in young people and does not require treatment.

Premature contractions, or *extrasystoles* (eks-trah-SIS-tol-ees), are contractions that occur before the next expected contraction in a series of cardiac cycles. For example, *premature atrial contractions (PACs)* may occur shortly after the ventricles contract—an early P wave on the ECG. *Premature ventricular contractions (PVCs)* occur when the electrical signal begins in the ventricle rather than in the SA node (Figure 13-11, *E*). Premature contractions often occur with lack of sleep, anxiety, cold medications, too much caffeine or nicotine, alcoholism, or heart damage. PVCs can occur in otherwise healthy newborns, young children, and adult athletes following intense activity.

Frequent premature contractions can lead to **fibrillation** (fib-ril-AY-shun), a condition in which cardiac muscle fibers contract out of step with each other. This event can be seen in an ECG as the absence of regular P waves or abnormal QRS and T waves. In fibrillation, the affected heart chambers do not effectively pump blood. *Atrial fibrillation (AF or A-fib)* occurs commonly in mitral stenosis, rheumatic heart disease, and infarction of the atrial myocardium. Figure 13-11, *F*, shows an example of atrial fibrillation in an ECG strip.

Ventricular fibrillation (VF or V-fib) is an immediately life-threatening condition in which the lack of ventricular pumping suddenly stops the flow of blood to vital tissues. Unless ventricular fibrillation is corrected immediately by defibrillation or some other method, death may occur within minutes. Figure 13-11, *G*, shows an example of atrial fibrillation in an ECG strip.

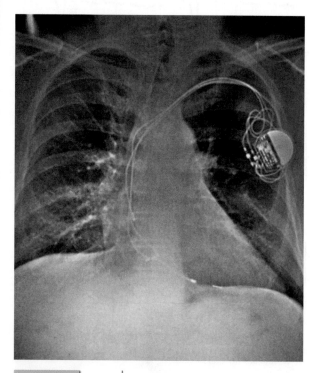

Figure 13-12 **Artificial pacemaker.**

This x-ray photograph shows the stimulus generator in the subcutaneous tissue of the chest wall. Thin, flexible wires extend through veins to the heart, where timed electrical impulses stimulate the myocardium.

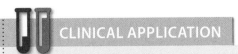

HEART MEDICATIONS

Numerous drugs are used in the treatment of heart disease both in the critical care unit and in home health care. Here are a few examples of the basic pharmacological tools of cardiac care.

Anticoagulants and antiplatelet agents—These drugs prevent clot formation in patients with valve damage or who have experienced a myocardial infarction. Warfarin (Coumadin), heparin, dalteparin, and danaparoid are examples of commonly used anticoagulants—agents that disrupt or block the blood clotting mechanism. Antiplatelet agents prevent platelets from sticking together to produce a blood clot. Examples of antiplatelet drugs are acetylsalicylic acid (aspirin), clopidogrel (Plavix), and ticlopidine (Ticlid).

Beta-adrenergic blockers—These drugs block norepinephrine receptors in cardiac muscle and thus reduce the rate and strength of the heartbeat. Such drugs can help correct certain dysrhythmias, as well as reduce the amount of oxygen required by the myocardium. Propranolol (Inderal) and related drugs are beta-adrenergic blockers.

Calcium-channel blockers—These drugs block the flow of calcium into cardiac muscle cells, thus reducing heart contractions. Calcium-channel blockers may be used in treating certain dysrhythmias and coronary heart disease. Some examples include diltiazem, verapamil, and nifedipine.

Digitalis—This drug slows and increases the strength of cardiac contractions. It plays an important part in the treatment of congestive heart failure and certain dysrhythmias. Digoxin is one of several commonly used digitalis preparations.

Nitroglycerin—This drug dilates (widens) coronary blood vessels, thus increasing the flow of oxygenated blood to the myocardium. Nitroglycerin is often used to prevent or relieve angina pectoris.

Tissue plasminogen activator (TPA)—Usually a synthetic version of a naturally occurring substance from the walls of blood vessels, TPA activates a substance in the blood called *plasminogen*, which dissolves clots that may be blocking coronary arteries. Another preparation called *streptokinase*, an enzyme produced by *Streptococcus* bacteria, has similar effects.

Fibrillation may be treated immediately by *defibrillation*—application of an electric shock to force cardiac muscle fibers to once again contract in rhythm. In atrial fibrillation, a drug such as digoxin (digitalis) may be used to prevent ventricular involvement. In ventricular fibrillation, epinephrine may be injected into the bloodstream to increase blood pressure (and blood flow) enough to make defibrillation successful. If initial defibrillation is unsuccessful, then drugs that help reduce dysrhythmia also may be injected into the bloodstream.

Automatic external defibrillators (AEDs) are becoming increasingly available in public places. AEDs are small, lightweight devices that detect a person's heart rhythm using small electrode pads placed on the torso. If ventricular fibrillation is detected, then a non-medical rescuer will be talked through some simple steps to defibrillate the victim.

Heart Failure

Heart failure is the inability of the heart to pump enough blood to sustain life. Heart failure can be the result of many different heart diseases. Valve disorders can reduce the pumping efficiency of the heart enough to cause heart failure. **Cardiomyopathy** (kar-dee-oh-my-OP-ath-ee), or disease of the myocardial tissue, may reduce pumping effectiveness. A specific event, such as myocardial infarction, can result in myocardial damage that causes heart failure. Dysrhythmias, such as complete heart block or ventricular fibrillation, also can impair the pumping effectiveness of the heart and thus cause heart failure.

Failure of the right side of the heart, or *right-sided heart failure,* accounts for about one fourth of all cases of heart failure. Right-sided heart failure often results from the progression of disease that begins in the left side of the heart. Failure of the left side of the heart results in reduced pumping of blood returning from the lungs. Blood backs up into the pulmonary circulation, then into the right heart—causing an increase in pressure that the right side of the heart simply cannot overcome. Right-sided heart failure also can be caused by lung disorders that obstruct normal pulmonary blood flow and thus overload the right side of the heart—a condition called **cor pulmonale** (kor pul-mon-AHL-ee) (Figure 13-13).

Congestive heart failure (CHF), or simply *left-sided heart failure,* is the inability of the left ventricle to pump blood effectively. Most often, such failure results from myocardial infarction caused by coronary artery disease. It is called *congestive heart failure* because it decreases pumping pressure in the systemic circulation, which in turn causes the body to retain fluids. Portions of the systemic circulation thus become congested with extra fluid. As stated above, left-sided heart failure also causes congestion of blood in the pulmonary circulation, termed *pulmonary edema*—possibly leading to right heart failure.

Patients in danger of death because of heart failure may be candidates for heart *transplants* or heart *implants.* Heart transplants are surgical procedures in which healthy hearts from recently deceased donors replace the hearts of patients with heart disease (Figure 13-14). Unfortunately, a continuing problem with this procedure is the tendency of the body's immune system to reject the new heart as a foreign tissue. More details about the rejection of transplanted tissues are found in Chapter 15. Heart implants are artificial hearts that are made of biologically inert synthetic materials. After decades of false starts and cumbersome implants with external pumps, the era of the "artificial heart" seems to have finally arrived. In July of 2001, the first artificial heart was successfully implanted into Robert Tools by University of Louisville researchers. The one-kilogram (2-pound) implant is the first to allow the patient to move around freely without external pumps.

> **QUICK CHECK**
>
> 1. What does the term *dysrhythmia* mean?
> 2. What is the difference between *tachycardia* and *bradycardia*?
> 3. How is *fibrillation* corrected?
> 4. How does *heart failure* occur?

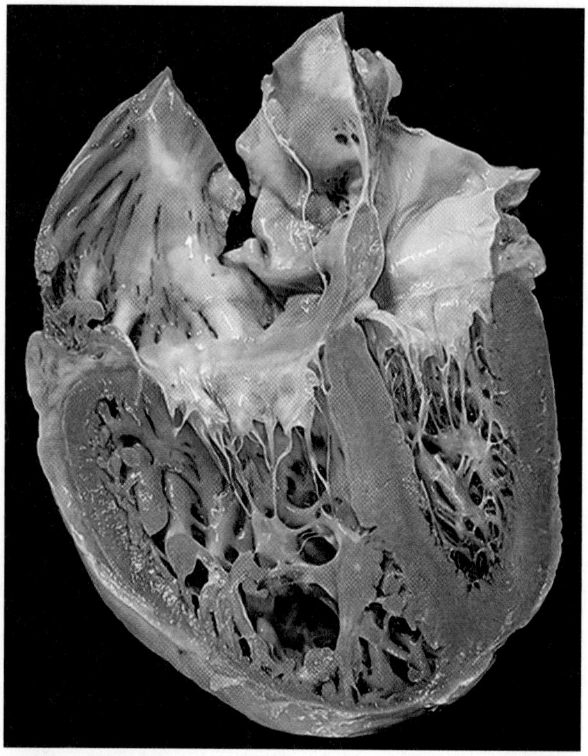

Figure 13-13 Cor pulmonale.

When pulmonary blood backs up into the right side of the heart during right-sided heart failure, it may stretch the right ventricle as seen in this photograph.

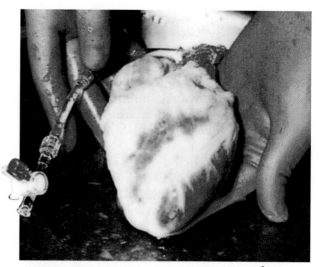

Figure 13-14 Heart transplant.

Human heart prepared for transplantation into a patient. I

SCIENCE APPLICATIONS

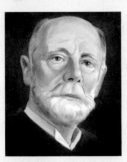

Willem Einthoven
(1860–1927)

CARDIOLOGY

Cardiology, the study and treatment of the heart, owes much to Dutch physiologist Willem Einthoven and his invention of the modern electrocardiograph in 1903. Einthoven's first major contribution was the invention of a machine that could record electrocardiograms (ECGs) with far greater sensitivity than the crude machines of the 19th century. Then, with the help of British physician Lewis Thomas, Einthoven demonstrated and named the P, Q, R, S, and T waves and proved that these waves precisely record the electrical activity of the heart (see Figure 13-10). In 1905, he even invented a way that ECG data could be sent from a patient over the telephone line to his laboratory where they could be recorded and analyzed—a technique now called *telemetry*. His detailed studies of ECG recordings changed the practice of heart medicine forever. In fact, his invention was later applied to the study of nerve impulses and led to breakthrough discoveries in the neurosciences.

Cardiologists today still use modern versions of Einthoven's machine to diagnose heart disorders. Of course, biomedical engineers continue to develop refinements to electrocardiograph equipment and to invent new machines to monitor heart function. In fact, engineers and designers have worked with cardiologists to develop artificial heart valves, artificial pacemakers, and even artificial hearts! With all of this medical equipment being used in cardiology, and in medicine in general, there are also many technicians working to keep it all in good repair.

Outline Summary

To download an MP3 version of the chapter summary for use with your iPod or portable media player, access the **Audio Chapter Summaries** on your CD.

Location, Size, and Position of the Heart

A. Triangular organ located in mediastinum with two thirds of the mass to the left of the body midline and one third to the right; the apex is on the diaphragm; shape and size of a closed fist (Figure 13-1)

B. Cardiopulmonary resuscitation (CPR)—heart lies between the sternum in front and the bodies of the thoracic vertebrae behind; rhythmic compression of the heart between the sternum and vertebrae can maintain blood flow during cardiac arrest; if combined with artificial respiration procedure, it can be lifesaving

Anatomy of the Heart

A. Heart chambers (Figure 13-2)
   1. Two upper chambers are called *atria* (receiving chambers)—right and left atria
   2. Two lower chambers are called *ventricles* (discharging chambers)—right and left ventricles

   3. Wall of each heart chamber is composed of cardiac muscle tissue called *myocardium*
   4. Endocardium—smooth lining of heart chambers
      a. Inflammation of endocardium is called *endocarditis*
      b. Inflamed endocardium can become rough and abrasive and thereby cause a thrombus

B. The pericardium and pericarditis
   1. Pericardium—a two-layered fibrous sac with a lubricated space between the two layers
      a. Inner layer is called *visceral pericardium,* or *epicardium*
      b. Outer layer is called *parietal pericardium*
   2. Pericarditis—inflammation of the pericardium
   3. Cardiac tamponade—compression of the heart caused by fluid building up between the visceral pericardium and parietal pericardium

C. Heart action
   1. Contraction of the heart is called *systole*
   2. Relaxation of the heart is called *diastole.*

D. Heart valves and valve disorders (Figure 13-3)
 1. Valves keep blood flowing through the heart; prevent backflow
 2. Atrioventricular (AV) valves
  a. Tricuspid—at the opening of the right atrium into the ventricle
  b. Bicuspid (mitral)—at the opening of the left atrium into the ventricle
 3. Semilunar (SL) valves
  a. Pulmonary semilunar—at the beginning of the pulmonary artery
  b. Aortic semilunar—at the beginning of the aorta
 4. Valve disorders
  a. Incompetent valves "leak," allowing some blood to flow backward into the chamber from which it came
  b. Stenosed valves are narrower than normal, reducing blood flow (Figure 13-4)
  c. Rheumatic heart disease—cardiac damage resulting from a delayed inflammatory response to streptococcal infection
  d. Mitral valve prolapse (MVP)—incompetence of mitral valve caused by its edges extending back into the left atrium when the left ventricle contracts (Figure 13-5)

Heart Sounds

A. Two distinct heart sounds in every heartbeat, or cycle—"lub-dup"
B. First sound (lub) is caused by the vibration and closure of AV valves during contraction of the ventricles
C. Second sound (dup) is caused by the closure of the semilunar valves during relaxation of the ventricles
D. Heart murmurs—abnormal heart sounds often caused by abnormal valves

Blood Flow Through the Heart

A. Heart acts as two separate pumps—the right atrium and ventricle performing different functions from the left atrium and ventricle (Figure 13-6)
B. Sequence of blood flow
 1. Venous blood enters the right atrium through the superior and inferior venae cavae—passes from the right atrium through the tricuspid valve to the right ventricle
 2. From the right ventricle through the pulmonary semilunar valve to the pulmonary artery to the lungs—blood from the lungs to

the left atrium, passing through the bicuspid (mitral) valve to left ventricle
 3. Blood in the left ventricle is pumped through the aortic semilunar valve into the aorta and is distributed to the body as a whole

Coronary Circulation and Coronary Heart Disease

A. Blood, which supplies oxygen and nutrients to the myocardium of the heart, flows through the right and left coronary arteries (Figure 13-7)
B. Blockage of blood flow through the coronary arteries can cause myocardial infarction (heart attack)
C. Atherosclerosis (type of "hardening of arteries" in which lipids build up on the inside wall of blood vessels) can partially or totally block coronary blood flow
D. Angina pectoris—chest pain caused by inadequate oxygen to the heart

Cardiac Cycle

A. Heartbeat is regular and rhythmic—each complete beat called a *cardiac cycle*—average is about 72 beats per minute
B. Each cycle, about 0.8 second long, subdivided into systole (contraction phase) and diastole (relaxation phase)
C. Stroke volume is the volume of blood ejected from one ventricle with each beat
D. Cardiac output is amount of blood that one ventricle can pump each minute—average is about 5 L per minute at rest

Conduction System of the Heart

A. Normal structure and function (Figure 13-9)
 1. SA (sinoatrial) node, the pacemaker—located in the wall of the right atrium near the opening of the superior vena cava
 2. AV (atrioventricular) node—located in the right atrium along the lower part of the interatrial septum
 3. AV bundle (bundle of His)—located in the septum of the ventricle
 4. Purkinje fibers—located in the walls of the ventricles
B. Electrocardiography (Figure 13-10)
 1. Specialized conduction system structures generate and transmit the electrical impulses that result in contraction of the heart

2. These tiny electrical impulses can be picked up on the surface of the body and transformed into visible tracings by a machine called an *electrocardiograph*
3. The visible tracing of these electrical signals is called an *electrocardiogram*, or ECG
4. The normal ECG has three deflections, or waves
   a. P wave—associated with depolarization of the atria
   b. QRS complex—associated with depolarization of the ventricles
   c. T wave—associated with repolarization of the ventricles
C. Cardiac dysrhythmia—abnormality of heart rhythm (Figure 13-11)
   1. Heart block—conduction of impulses is blocked
      a. Complete heart block—impaired AV node conduction, producing complete dissociation of P waves from QRS complexes
      b. Can be treated by implanting an artificial pacemaker (Figure 13-12)
   2. Bradycardia—slow heart rate (less than 60 beats/min)
   3. Tachycardia—rapid heart rate (more than 100 beats/min)
4. Sinus dysrhythmia—variation in heart rate during breathing cycle
5. Premature contraction (extrasystole)—contraction that occurs sooner than expected in a normal rhythm
6. Fibrillation—condition in which cardiac muscle fibers are "out of step," producing no effective pumping action

Heart Failure

A. Heart failure—inability to pump enough returned blood to sustain life—can be caused by many different heart diseases
B. Right-sided heart failure—failure of the right side of the heart to pump blood, usually because the left side of the heart is not pumping effectively (Figure 13-13)
C. Left-sided heart failure (congestive heart failure)—inability of the left ventricle to pump effectively, resulting in congestion of the systemic and pulmonary circulations
D. Diseased hearts can be replaced by donated living hearts (transplants) or by artificial hearts (implants), although both procedures have yet to be perfected (Figure 13-14)

New Words

aorta	myocardium	**Diseases and Other Clinical Terms**	echocardiography
aortic semilunar valve	P wave		electrocardiogram (ECG)
atrioventricular (AV) node	pacemaker		electrocardiograph
atrioventricular (AV) valve	parietal pericardium	angina pectoris	endocarditis
atrium (*pl.*, atria)	pericardium	artificial pacemaker	fibrillation
AV bundle (bundle of His)	pulmonary artery	atherosclerosis	heart block
bicuspid (mitral) valve	pulmonary circulation	automatic external defibrillator (AED)	heart disease
cardiac cycle	pulmonary semilunar valve	bradycardia	heart failure
cardiac output	pulmonary vein	cardiac tamponade	heart murmur
chordae tendineae	Purkinje fiber	cardiologist	incompetent valve
coronary artery	QRS complex	cardiomyopathy	mitral valve prolapse (MVP)
coronary circulation	semilunar (SL) valve	cardiopulmonary resuscitation (CPR)	myocardial infarction (MI)
coronary sinus	sinoatrial node	congestive heart failure (CHF)	pericarditis
diastole	stroke volume	cor pulmonale	premature contractions
endocardium	superior vena cava	coronary bypass surgery	rheumatic heart disease
epicardium (visceral pericardium)	systemic circulation	dysrhythmia	sinus dysrhythmia
inferior vena cava	systole		stenosed valve
mitral valve	T wave		tachycardia
	tricuspid valve		

Review Questions

1. Describe the heart and its position in the body.
2. Name the four chambers of the heart.
3. What is the *myocardium*? What is the *endocardium*?
4. Describe the two layers of the pericardium. What is the function of pericardial fluid?
5. Define or explain *pericarditis* and *pericardial effusion*.
6. What is *systole*? What is *diastole*?
7. Name and give the locations of the four heart valves.
8. Explain what is meant by a mitral valve prolapse.
9. Explain what occurs in a myocardial infarction.
10. Trace the flow of blood from the superior vena cava to the aorta.
11. What is angina pectoris?
12. Differentiate between stroke volume and cardiac output.
13. Trace the path and name the structures involved in the conduction system of the heart.
14. What is *heart block?* What is *bradycardia?* What is *tachycardia?*
15. What is *fibrillation?* Which is more dangerous, atrial fibrillation or ventricular fibrillation?

Critical Thinking

16. Explain how the tracings on an ECG relate to the electrical activity of the heart.
17. Explain how right-sided heart failure is usually caused by left-sided heart failure.

Chapter Test

1. _____ are the thicker chambers of the heart, sometimes called the discharging chambers.
2. _____ are the thinner chambers of the heart, sometimes called the receiving chambers.
3. Cardiac muscle tissue also may be called _____.
4. The ventricles of the heart are separated into right and left sides by a wall called the _____.
5. The thin layer of tissue lining the interior of each of the heart chambers is called the _____.
6. Another word for the visceral pericardium is the _____.
7. When the heart is contracting, it is said to be in _____.
8. When the heart is relaxing, it is said to be in _____.
9. The heart valve located between the right atrium and right ventricle is called the _____ valve.
10. The term _____ refers to the volume of blood ejected from the ventricle during each beat.

11. The _____ is the pacemaker of the heart and begins the contraction of the atria.
12. The _____ are extensions of the atrioventricular fibers and cause the contraction of the ventricles.
13. The ECG tracing that occurs when the ventricles are depolarizing is called _____.
14. The ECG tracing that occurs when the atria are depolarizing is called the _____.
15. Place the following structures in their proper order in relation to blood flow through the heart. Put a *1* in front of the first structure the blood would pass through and a *10* in front of the last structure the blood would pass through.
    _____ **a.** left atrium
    _____ **b.** tricuspid valve (right atrioventricular valve)
    _____ **c.** right ventricle
    _____ **d.** pulmonary vein
    _____ **e.** aortic semilunar valve
    _____ **f.** mitral valve (left atrioventricular valve)
    _____ **g.** left ventricle
    _____ **h.** pulmonary artery
    _____ **i.** right atrium
    _____ **j.** pulmonary semilunar valve

Match each heart disorder in Column A with its corresponding description or cause in Column B.

Column A

16. _____ pericarditis
17. _____ mitral valve prolapse
18. _____ myocardial infarction
19. _____ angina pectoris
20. _____ heart block
21. _____ bradycardia
22. _____ tachycardia
23. _____ fibrillation
24. _____ congestive heart failure

Column B

a. damage to the heart cells due to a lack of blood flow
b. slow heart rhythm
c. a condition in which the cardiac muscles contract out of step with each other
d. rapid heart rhythm
e. also called left-sided heart failure
f. inflammation of the pericardium
g. a condition in which contraction impulses are prevented from getting through to the ventricles
h. severe chest pain that occurs when the heart muscle is deprived of oxygen
i. a condition that allows blood to leak back into the left atrium when the left ventricle contracts

Study Tips

continued from page 373

but ventricles must contract from the bottom up so the contraction impulse must be carried to the bottom of the ventricles before they start contracting. The letters for the ECG waves do not stand for anything; they are arbitrary, but they do indicate a sequence of events (that is, the P tracing comes before the QRS complex).

4. Make a chart of the disorders of the heart. Organizing them based on their cause would be useful: the pericardium, the heart muscle, the heart valves, the conduction system, or general heart failure.

5. Bring photocopies of heart illustrations (for example, Figures 13-1, 13-2, and 13-9) to your study group. Blacken out the labels and use them as tools for learning the structures of the heart.

6. In your study group, discuss the flow of blood through the heart, the conduction system, the parts of the ECG, and the chart of the disorders of the heart. Go over the questions at the end of the chapter and discuss possible test questions.

Case Studies

1. You are visiting a friend in the hospital. Beside her bed is a video monitor that displays your friend's ECG. She asks you what the large spikes represent—can you tell her? Suddenly the ECG line becomes completely disorganized, with no discernible P, QRS, or T waves. What may have happened? What, if anything, should be done for her?

2. Your classmate Vivian told you during lunchtime today that she has been diagnosed as having mitral valve prolapse. Describe this structural abnormality and describe its possible effects on heart function.

3. Uncle John is about to undergo coronary bypass surgery. His surgeon carefully explained Uncle John's condition and the surgical procedure to correct it, but your uncle was too upset to pay close attention. Now that he has calmed a bit, he realizes that he has very little idea of what his "triple bypass surgery" is all about. Describe to your uncle the probable condition of his heart and explain the concept of the planned surgery.

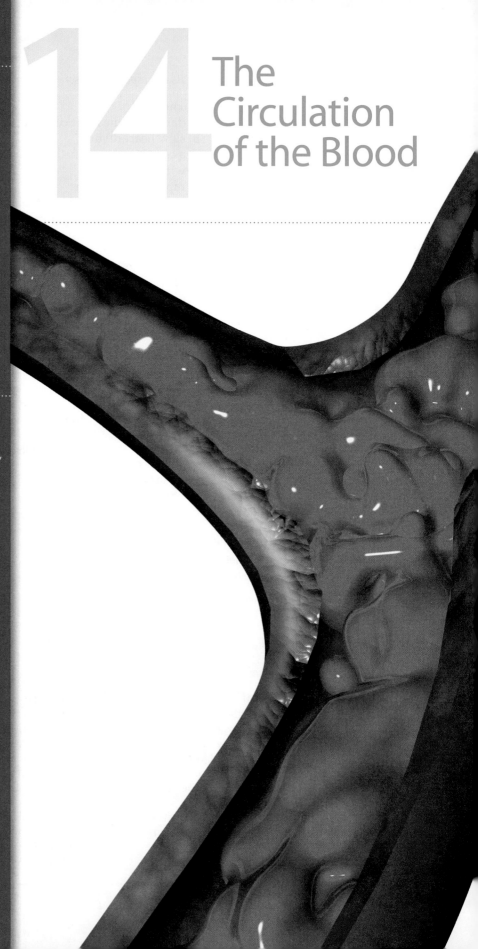

Outline

Objectives

After you have completed this chapter, you should be able to:

1. Describe the structure and function of each major type of blood vessel: artery, vein, and capillary.

2. List the major disorders of blood vessels and explain how they develop.

3. Trace the path of blood through the systemic, pulmonary, portal, and fetal circulations.

4. Identify and discuss the factors involved in the generation of blood pressure and how they relate to each other.

5. Define pulse and locate the major pulse points on the body.

6. Explain what is meant by the term *circulatory shock* and describe the major types.

14

The Circulation of the Blood

In the previous chapter we discussed the basic structure and function of the circulatory system's pump: the heart. In this chapter, we continue our explanation of how blood circulates through the internal environment of the body. First, the structure and function of blood vessels is discussed in some detail. Then how the vessels fit together into routes for the conduction of blood is explained. The last part of this chapter deals with blood pressure, the driving force of blood circulation. We, of course, also discuss major circulatory disorders as appropriate throughout the chapter.

STUDY TIPS

The arteries and veins are composed of three different tissue layers. There is a difference in thickness in these layers because arteries carry blood under higher pressure. Arteries and veins carry blood in opposite directions: arteries away from the heart and veins toward the heart. Capillaries are the most important blood vessels in the system. The exchange of substances (e.g., O_2, CO_2, glucose) between the blood and the tissues, the function of the cardiovascular system, occurs in the capillaries. Because of this, the walls of the capillaries must be very thin.

1. If you are asked to learn the names and locations of specific blood vessels, make flash cards and use the figures in this chapter as learning tools.
2. Systemic and pulmonary circulation is fairly self-explanatory. The hepatic portal system makes more sense if you see it as a homeostatic mechanism. The liver helps keep the blood leaving the digestive system from having too high a concentration of various nutrients, such as glucose. It also has a protective function: detoxifying the blood.
3. Fetal circulation will make sense to you if you consider the environment in which the fetus is living. The blood sent to the fetus is already oxygenated and full of digested food, so it doesn't have to go to the lungs or liver. Figure 14-9 provides a visual that will help you remember the circulation route.
4. A liquid always moves from a higher pressure to a lower pressure, so pressure would be highest leaving the heart and lowest in the vena cava. Make a chart with the disorders of the vessels. It helps to organize them by whether they are arterial disorders or venous disorders.

continued on page 419

Blood Vessels

Types

Arterial blood is pumped from the heart through a series of large distribution vessels—the **arteries.** The largest artery in the body is the aorta. Arteries subdivide into vessels that become progressively smaller and finally become tiny **arterioles** (ar-TEER-ee-ols) that control the flow into microscopic exchange vessels called **capillaries** (KAP-i-lair-ees). In the so-called *capillary beds,* the exchange of nutrients and respiratory gases occurs between the blood and tissue fluid around the cells. Blood exits, or is drained, from the capillary beds and then enters the small **venules** (VEN-yools), which join with other venules and increase in size, becoming **veins.** The largest veins are the superior vena cava and the inferior vena cava.

As noted in Chapter 13, arteries carry blood away from the heart and toward capillaries. Veins carry blood toward the heart and away from capillaries, and capillaries carry blood from the tiny arterioles into tiny venules. The aorta carries blood out of the left ventricle of the heart, and the venae cavae return blood to the right atrium after the blood has circulated through the body.

Structure

Arteries, veins, and capillaries differ in structure. Three coats or layers are found in both arteries and veins (Figure 14-1). The outermost layer is called the **tunica externa.** This outer layer is made of connective tissue fibers that reinforce the wall of the vessel so that it will not burst under pressure.

Figure 14-1 shows that smooth muscle tissue is found in the middle layer, or **tunica media,** of arteries and veins. This muscle layer is much thicker in arteries than it is in veins. Why is this important? Because the thicker muscle layer in the artery wall is able to resist great pressures generated by ventricular systole. In arteries, the tunica media plays a critical role in maintaining blood pressure and controlling blood distribution. This is a smooth muscle, so it is controlled by the autonomic nervous system.

An inner layer of endothelial cells called the **tunica intima** lines arteries and veins. The tunica intima is actually a single layer of squamous epithelial cells called **endothelium** (en-doh-THEE-lee-um) that lines the inner surface of the entire circulatory system. This single layer of cells provides a very smooth lining that prevents the accidental formation of blood clots. The tunica intima also sometimes includes a thin layer of elastic fibrous tissue.

As you can see in Figure 14-1, veins have a unique structural feature not present in arteries. They are equipped with one-way valves that prevent the backflow of blood.

When a surgeon cuts into the body, only arteries, arterioles, veins, and venules can be seen. Capillaries cannot be seen because they are microscopic. The most important structural feature of capillaries is their extreme thinness—only one layer of flat, endothelial cells composes the capillary membrane. Instead of three layers or coats, the capillary wall is composed of only one—the tunica intima. Substances such as glucose, oxygen, and wastes can quickly pass through it on their way to or from cells.

Smooth muscle cells called **precapillary sphincters** guard the entrances to the capillaries and determine how much blood will flow into each capillary bed.

Functions

Arteries, veins, and capillaries all have different functions.

Arteries and arterioles distribute blood from the heart to capillaries in all parts of the body. In addition, by constricting or dilating, arterioles help maintain arterial blood pressure at a normal level.

Venules and veins collect blood from capillaries and return it to the heart. They also serve as blood reservoirs because they carry blood under lower pressure (than arteries) and can expand to hold a larger volume of blood or constrict to hold a much smaller amount.

Capillaries function as exchange vessels. For example, glucose and oxygen move out of the blood in capillaries into interstitial fluid and then on into cells. Carbon dioxide and other substances move in the opposite direction (that is, into the capillary blood from the cells). Fluid is also exchanged between capillary blood and interstitial fluid (see Chapter 20).

Study Figure 14-2 and Table 14-1 to learn the names of the main arteries of the body and Figure 14-3 and Table 14-2 for the names of the main veins.

QUICK CHECK

1. What are the main types of blood vessel in the body? How are they different from each other?
2. Describe the three major layers of a large blood vessel.
3. What are capillaries?

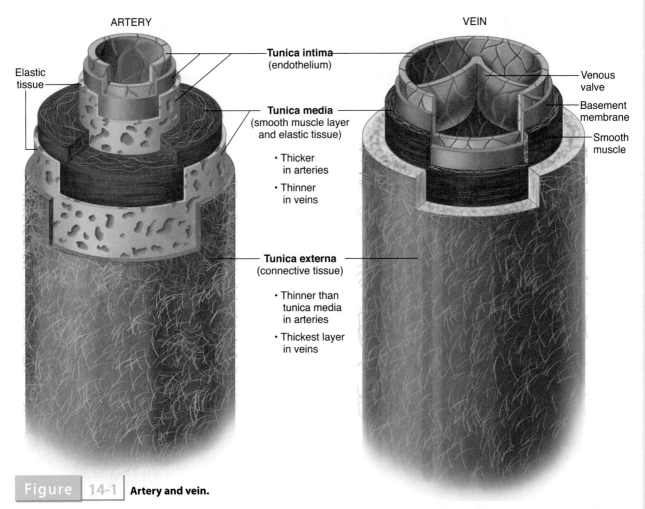

Figure 14-1 **Artery and vein.**

Schematic drawings of an artery and a vein show comparative thicknesses of the three layers: the outer layer or tunica externa, the muscle layer or tunica media, and the tunica intima made of endothelium. Note that the muscle and outer layers are much thinner in veins than in arteries and that veins have valves.

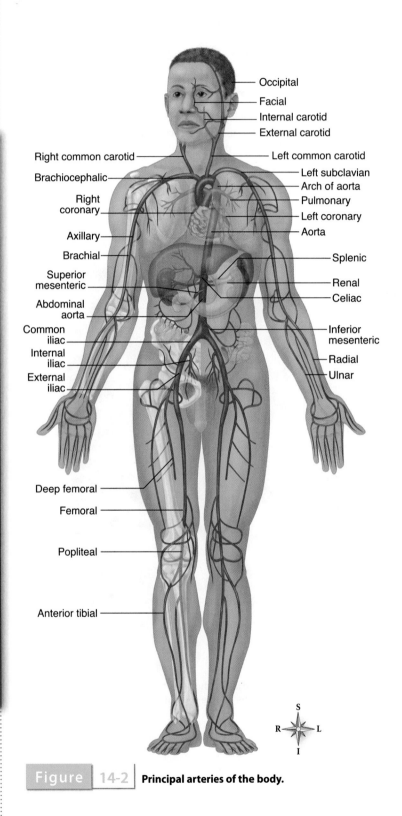

Occipital
Facial
Internal carotid
External carotid
Right common carotid
Left common carotid
Brachiocephalic
Left subclavian
Arch of aorta
Right coronary
Pulmonary
Left coronary
Axillary
Aorta
Brachial
Splenic
Superior mesenteric
Renal
Abdominal aorta
Celiac
Common iliac
Inferior mesenteric
Internal iliac
External iliac
Radial
Ulnar
Deep femoral
Femoral
Popliteal
Anterior tibial

S
R — L
I

Figure 14-2 | **Principal arteries of the body.**

Table 14-1	The Major Systemic Arteries	
ARTERY	**TISSUES SUPPLIED**	
HEAD AND NECK		
Occipital	Posterior head and neck	
Facial	Mouth, pharynx, and face	
Internal carotid	Anterior brain and meninges	
External carotid	Superficial neck, face, eyes, and larynx	
Common carotid	Head and neck	
Vertebral	Brain and meninges	
THORAX		
Left subclavian	Left upper extremity	
Brachiocephalic	Head and arm	
Arch of aorta	Branches to head, neck, and upper extremities	
Coronary	Heart muscle	
ABDOMEN		
Celiac	Stomach, spleen, and liver	
Splenic	Spleen	
Renal	Kidneys	
Superior mesenteric	Small intestine; upper half of the large intestine	
Inferior mesenteric	Lower half of the large intestine	
UPPER EXTREMITY		
Axillary	Axilla (armpit)	
Brachial	Arm	
Radial	Lateral side of the hand	
Ulnar	Medial side of the hand	
LOWER EXTREMITY		
Internal iliac	Pelvic viscera and rectum	
External iliac	Genitalia and lower trunk muscles	
Deep femoral	Deep thigh muscles	
Femoral	Thigh	
Popliteal	Leg and foot	
Anterior tibial and posterior tibial	Leg	

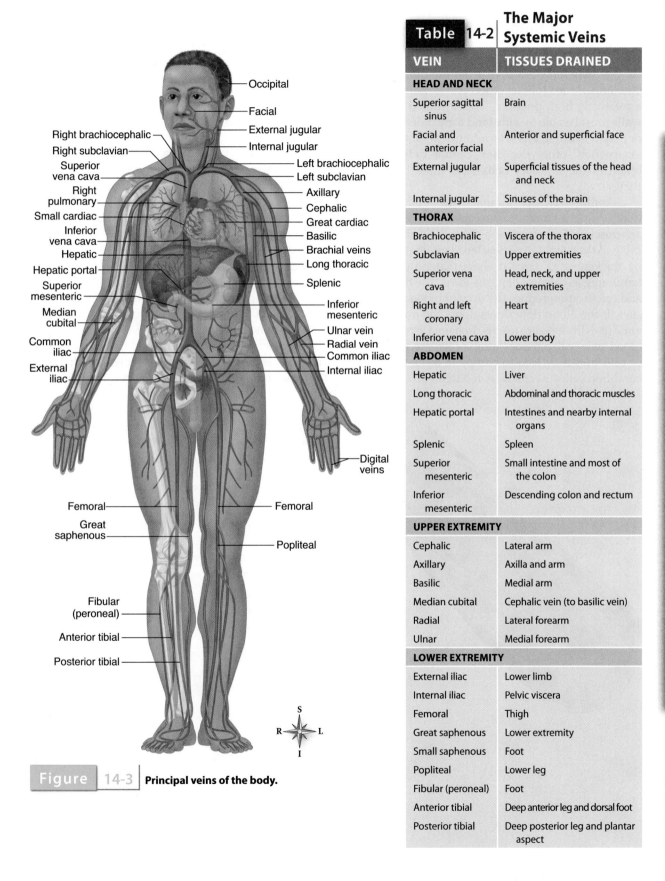

Occipital
Facial
External jugular
Internal jugular
Left brachiocephalic
Left subclavian
Axillary
Cephalic
Great cardiac
Basilic
Brachial veins
Long thoracic
Splenic
Inferior mesenteric
Ulnar vein
Radial vein
Common iliac
Internal iliac
Digital veins
Femoral
Popliteal

Right brachiocephalic
Right subclavian
Superior vena cava
Right pulmonary
Small cardiac
Inferior vena cava
Hepatic
Hepatic portal
Superior mesenteric
Median cubital
Common iliac
External iliac
Femoral
Great saphenous
Fibular (peroneal)
Anterior tibial
Posterior tibial

S
R — L
I

Figure 14-3 **Principal veins of the body.**

The Major Systemic Veins

Table 14-2	
VEIN	**TISSUES DRAINED**
HEAD AND NECK	
Superior sagittal sinus	Brain
Facial and anterior facial	Anterior and superficial face
External jugular	Superficial tissues of the head and neck
Internal jugular	Sinuses of the brain
THORAX	
Brachiocephalic	Viscera of the thorax
Subclavian	Upper extremities
Superior vena cava	Head, neck, and upper extremities
Right and left coronary	Heart
Inferior vena cava	Lower body
ABDOMEN	
Hepatic	Liver
Long thoracic	Abdominal and thoracic muscles
Hepatic portal	Intestines and nearby internal organs
Splenic	Spleen
Superior mesenteric	Small intestine and most of the colon
Inferior mesenteric	Descending colon and rectum
UPPER EXTREMITY	
Cephalic	Lateral arm
Axillary	Axilla and arm
Basilic	Medial arm
Median cubital	Cephalic vein (to basilic vein)
Radial	Lateral forearm
Ulnar	Medial forearm
LOWER EXTREMITY	
External iliac	Lower limb
Internal iliac	Pelvic viscera
Femoral	Thigh
Great saphenous	Lower extremity
Small saphenous	Foot
Popliteal	Lower leg
Fibular (peroneal)	Foot
Anterior tibial	Deep anterior leg and dorsal foot
Posterior tibial	Deep posterior leg and plantar aspect

Disorders of Blood Vessels

Disorders of Arteries

As you may have gathered from the previous discussion, arteries contain blood that is maintained at a relatively high pressure. This means the arterial walls must be able to withstand a great deal of force, or they will burst. The arteries must also stay free of obstruction; otherwise they cannot deliver their blood to the capillary beds (and thus the tissues they serve).

A common type of vascular disease that occludes (blocks) arteries and weakens arterial walls is called **arteriosclerosis** (ar-teer-ee-oh-skleh-ROH-sis), or *hardening of the arteries*. Arteriosclerosis is characterized by thickening of arterial walls that progresses to hardening as calcium deposits form. The thickening and calcification reduce the flow of blood to the tissues. If the blood flow slows down too much, **ischemia** (is-KEE-mee-ah) results. Ischemia, or decreased blood supply to a tissue, involves the gradual death of cells and may lead to complete tissue death—a condition called **necrosis** (neh-KROH-sis). If a large section of tissue becomes necrotic, it may begin to decay. Necrosis that has progressed this far is called **gangrene** (GANG-green).

Because of the potential tissue damage involved, arteriosclerosis may be not only painful—it may be life threatening as well. For example, ischemia of heart muscle can lead to *myocardial infarction* (see Chapter 13).

There are several types of arteriosclerosis, but perhaps the most well known is *atherosclerosis*, described in Chapter 13 as the blockage of arteries by lipids and other matter (Figure 14-4).

Eventually, the fatty deposits in the arterial walls become fibrous and perhaps calcified—resulting in sclerosis (hardening). High blood levels of triglycerides and cholesterol, which may be caused by a high-fat, high-cholesterol diet, smoking, and a genetic predisposition, are associated with atherosclerosis. (See Chapter 2 for a discussion of triglycerides and cholesterol.)

In general, arteriosclerosis develops with advanced age, diabetes, high-fat and high-cholesterol diets, hypertension (high blood pressure), and smoking. Arte-

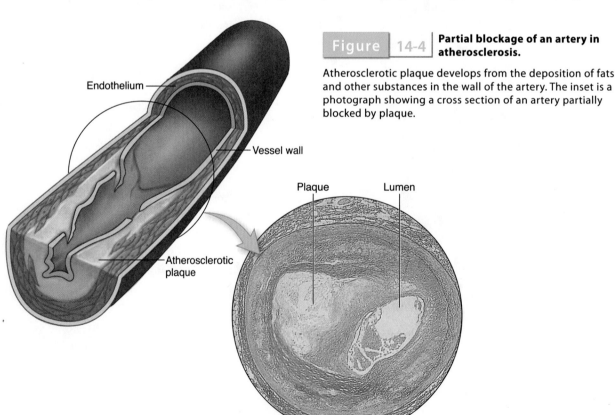

Figure 14-4 | **Partial blockage of an artery in atherosclerosis.**

Atherosclerotic plaque develops from the deposition of fats and other substances in the wall of the artery. The inset is a photograph showing a cross section of an artery partially blocked by plaque.

riosclerosis can be treated by drugs called *vasodilators* that trigger the smooth muscles of the arterial walls to relax, thus causing the arteries to dilate (widen).

Some cases of atherosclerosis are treated by mechanically opening the affected area of an artery, a type of procedure called **angioplasty** (AN-jee-oh-plas-tee). In one such procedure, a deflated balloon attached to a long tube called a *catheter* is inserted into a partially blocked artery and then inflated (Figure 14-5). As the balloon inflates, the *plaque* (fatty deposits and tissue) is pushed outward, and the artery widens to allow near-normal blood flow.

In a similar procedure, metal springs or mesh tubes called *stents* are inserted in affected arteries and hold them open. Other types of angioplasty use lasers, drills, or spinning loops of wire to clear the way for normal blood flow. Severely affected arteries also can be surgically bypassed or replaced, as discussed in Chapter 13.

Damage to arterial walls caused by arteriosclerosis or other factors may lead to the formation of an **aneurysm** (AN-yoor-iz-em). An aneurysm is a section of an artery that has become abnormally widened because of a weakening of the arterial wall. Aneurysms sometimes form a saclike extension of the arterial wall.

One reason aneurysms are dangerous is because they, like atherosclerotic plaques, promote the formation of thrombi (abnormal clots). A thrombus may cause an embolism (blockage) in the heart or some other vital tissue. Another reason aneurysms are dangerous is their tendency to burst, causing severe hemorrhaging that may result in death.

A brain aneurysm may lead to a *stroke,* or **cerebrovascular accident (CVA).** A stroke results from ischemia of brain tissue caused by an embolism or ruptured aneurysm. Depending on the amount of tissue affected and the place in the brain the CVA occurs, effects of a stroke may range from hardly noticeable to crippling to fatal.

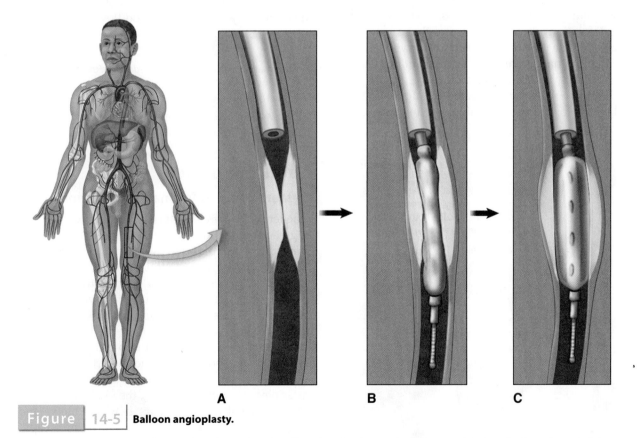

A   **B**   **C**

Figure 14-5 | **Balloon angioplasty.**

A, A catheter is inserted into the vessel until it reaches the affected region. **B,** A probe with a metal tip is pushed out the end of the catheter into the blocked region of the vessel. **C,** The balloon is inflated, pushing the walls of the vessel outward. Sometimes metal coils or tubes (stents) are inserted to keep the vessel open.

To learn more about angioplasty, go to **AnimationDirect** on your CD.

Disorders of Veins

Varicose veins are veins in which blood tends to pool rather than continue on toward the heart. Varicosities, also called **varices** (VAIR-i-seez) (singular, *varix*), most commonly occur in *superficial veins* near the surface of the body (Figure 14-6). The *great saphenous vein,* the largest superficial vein of the leg (see Figure 14-3), often becomes varicose in people who stand for long periods. The force of gravity slows the return of venous blood to the heart in such cases, causing blood-engorged veins to dilate. As the veins dilate, the distance between the flaps of venous valves widens, eventually making them incompetent (leaky). Incompetence of valves causes even more pooling in affected veins—a positive-feedback phenomenon.

Hemorrhoids (HEM-eh-royds), or *piles,* are varicose veins in the rectum. Excessive straining during defecation can create pressures that cause hemorrhoids. The unusual pressures of carrying a child during pregnancy predispose expectant mothers to hemorrhoids and other varicosities.

Varicose veins can be treated by supporting the dilated veins from the outside. For instance, support stockings can reduce blood pooling in the great saphenous vein. Surgical removal of varicose veins can be performed in severe cases. Advanced cases of hemorrhoids are often treated this way. Symptoms of milder cases can be relieved by removing the pressure that caused the condition.

A number of factors can cause **phlebitis** (fleh-BYE-tis), or vein inflammation. Irritation by an intravenous catheter, for example, is a common cause of vein inflammation. **Thrombophlebitis** (thromb-boh-fleh-BYE-tis) is acute phlebitis caused by clot (thrombus) formation. Veins are more likely sites of thrombus formation than arteries because venous blood moves more slowly and is under less pressure. Thrombophlebitis is characterized by pain and discoloration of the surrounding tissue. If a piece of a clot breaks free, it may cause an embolism when it blocks a blood vessel. **Pulmonary embolism,** for example, could result when an embolus lodges in the circulation of the lung (see Figure 12-17 on p. 362). Pulmonary embolism can lead to death quickly if too much blood flow is blocked.

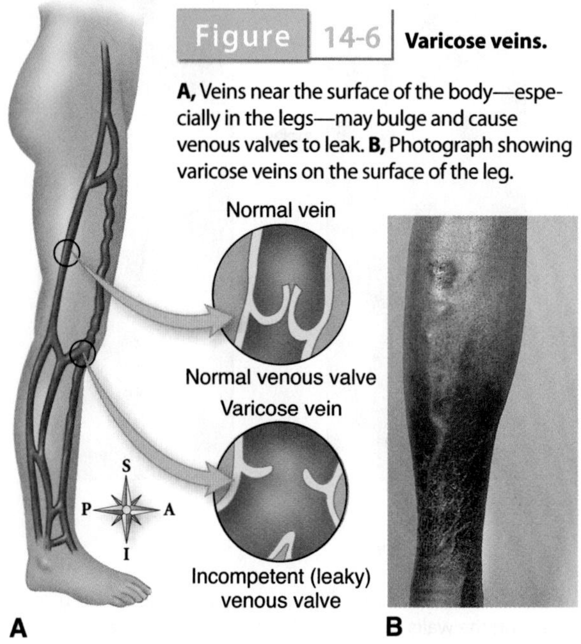

> **QUICK CHECK**
>
> 1. What is the medical term for *hardening of the arteries?* Describe this condition.
> 2. What is an *aneurysm?*
> 3. What causes *varicose veins?*

Circulation of Blood

Systemic and Pulmonary Circulation

The term *blood circulation* is self-explanatory, meaning that blood flows through vessels that are arranged in a complete circuit or circular pattern.

Blood flow from the left ventricle of the heart through blood vessels to all parts of the body and back to the right atrium of the heart was described in Chapter 13 as the **systemic circulation.** The left ventricle pumps blood into the aorta. From there, it flows into arteries that carry it into the tissues and organs of the body. As indicated in Figure 14-7, within each structure, blood moves from arteries to arterioles to capillaries. There, the vital two-way exchange of substances occurs between blood and cells. Next, blood flows out of each organ's capillary beds by way of its venules and then its veins to drain eventually into the inferior or superior vena

Figure 14-6 **Varicose veins.**

A, Veins near the surface of the body—especially in the legs—may bulge and cause venous valves to leak. **B,** Photograph showing varicose veins on the surface of the leg.

Normal vein

Normal venous valve

Varicose vein

Incompetent (leaky) venous valve

A

B

cava. These two great veins return venous blood to the right atrium of the heart.

At that point the blood is short of coming full circle back to its starting point in the left ventricle. To reach the left ventricle and start on its way again, it must first flow through another circuit, referred to in Chapter 13 as the **pulmonary circulation.** Observe in Figure 14-7 that venous blood moves from the right atrium to the right ventricle and then to the pulmonary artery to lung arterioles and capillaries. There, the exchange of gases between the blood and air takes place, converting the deep crimson color typical of venous blood to the scarlet color of arterial blood. This oxygenated blood then flows through lung venules into four pulmonary veins and returns to the left atrium of the heart. From the left

atrium, it enters the left ventricle, from which it will once again be pumped throughout the body in the systemic circulation.

 To learn more about pulmonary circulation and systemic circulation, go to **AnimationDirect** on your CD.

Hepatic Portal Circulation

The term **hepatic portal circulation** refers to the route of blood flow through the liver. Veins from the spleen, stomach, pancreas, gallbladder, and intestines do not pour their blood directly into the inferior vena cava as do the veins from other abdominal organs. Instead, blood flow from these organs

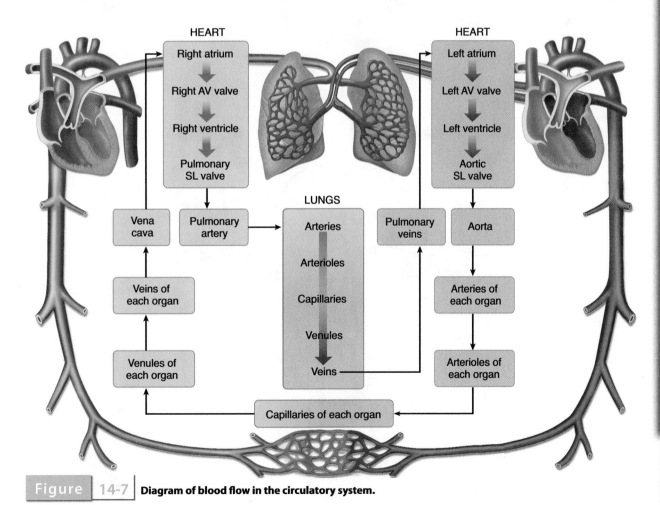

Figure 14-7 | **Diagram of blood flow in the circulatory system.**

Blood leaves the heart through arteries, then travels through arterioles, capillaries, venules, and veins before returning to the opposite side of the heart. *AV,* Atrioventricular; *SL,* semilunar.

is funneled to the liver by means of the hepatic portal vein (Figure 14-8). The blood then passes through the liver before it reenters the more direct venous return pathway to the heart. Blood leaves the liver by way of the hepatic veins, which drain into the inferior vena cava.

As noted in Figure 14-7, most of the blood flows from arteries to arterioles to capillaries to venules to veins and back to the heart. Blood flow that is diverted to the hepatic portal circulation, however, does not follow this direct route. The diverted venous blood, instead of return-

ing directly to the heart, is sent instead through a second capillary bed in the liver. The hepatic portal vein shown in Figure 14-8 is located between two capillary beds—one located in the digestive organs and the other in the liver. Once blood exits from the liver capillary beds, it returns to the systemic blood pathway, returning to the right atrium of the heart.

The detour of venous blood through a second capillary bed in the liver before its return to the heart serves some valuable purposes. For example, when a meal is being absorbed, the blood in the portal vein contains a higher-than-normal concentration of glu-

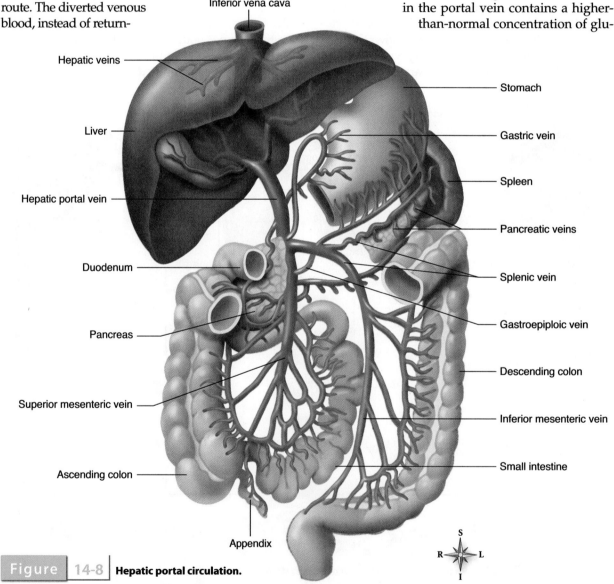

Figure 14-8 | **Hepatic portal circulation.**

In this very unusual circulation, a vein is located between two capillary beds. The hepatic portal vein collects blood from capillaries in visceral structures located in the abdomen and empties it into the liver. Hepatic veins return blood to the inferior vena cava. (Note that organs are not drawn to scale in this illustration and portion of pancreas has been removed to show veins.)

cose. Liver cells remove the excess glucose and store it as glycogen; therefore blood leaving the liver usually has a normal blood glucose concentration. Liver cells also remove and detoxify various poisonous substances that may be present in the blood. The hepatic portal system is an excellent example of how "structure follows function" in helping the body maintain homeostasis.

 To learn more about hepatic portal circulation, go to **AnimationDirect** on your CD.

Fetal Circulation

Circulation in the body before birth differs from circulation after birth because the fetus must secure oxygen and food from maternal blood instead of from its own lungs and digestive organs.

For the exchange of nutrients and oxygen to occur between fetal and maternal blood, specialized blood vessels must carry the fetal blood to the **placenta** (plah-SEN-tah), where the exchange occurs, and then return it to the fetal body. Three vessels (shown in Figure 14-9 as part of the **umbilical cord**) accomplish this purpose. They are the two small **umbilical arteries** and a single, much larger **umbilical vein.** The move-

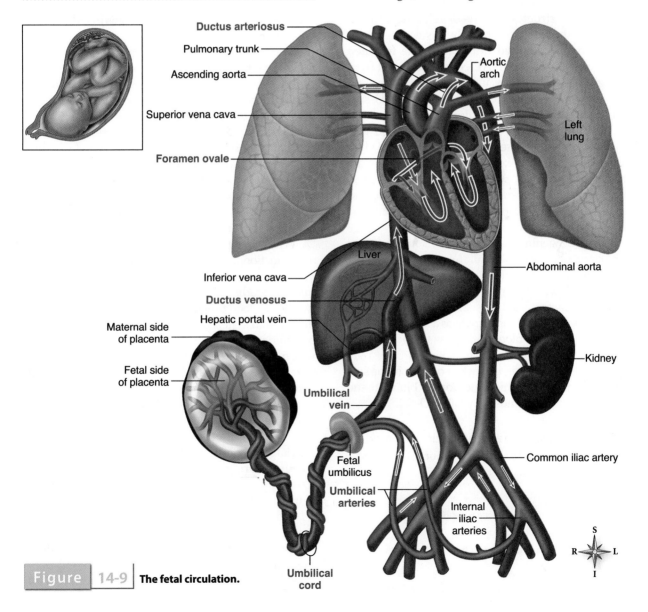

Figure 14-9 **The fetal circulation.**

ment of blood in the umbilical vessels may seem unusual at first in that the umbilical vein carries oxygenated blood, and the umbilical artery carries oxygen-poor blood. Remember that arteries are vessels that carry blood away from the heart, whereas veins carry blood toward the heart, regardless of the oxygen content these vessels may have.

Another structure unique to fetal circulation is called the **ductus venosus** (DUK-tus veh-NO-sus). As you can see in Figure 14-9, it is actually a continuation of the umbilical vein. It serves as a shunt, allowing most of the blood returning from the placenta to bypass the immature liver of the developing baby and empty directly into the inferior vena cava.

Two other structures in the developing fetus allow most of the blood to bypass the developing lungs, which remain collapsed until birth. The **foramen ovale** (foh-RAY-men oh-VAL-ee) shunts blood from the right atrium directly into the left atrium, and the **ductus arteriosus** (DUK-tus ar-teer-ee-OH-sus) connects the aorta and the pulmonary artery.

At birth, the baby's specialized fetal blood vessels and shunts must be rendered nonfunctional. When the newborn infant takes its first deep breaths, the circulatory system is subjected to increased pressure. The result is closure of the foramen ovale and rapid collapse of the umbilical blood vessels, the ductus venosus, and ductus arteriosus.

Several congenital disorders result from the failure of the circulatory system to shift from the fetal route of blood flow at the time of birth. The ductus arteriosus may fail to close, for example, and allow deoxygenated blood to bypass the lungs. Similarly, the foramen ovale may fail to close and remain as a so-called *hole in the heart* that allows blood to bypass the pulmonary circulation. In such cases, a light-skinned baby may appear bluish because of the lack of oxygen in the systemic arterial blood. This condition of bluish tissue coloration is called **cyanosis** (sye-ah-NO-sis).

 To learn more about fetal circulation, go to **AnimationDirect** on your CD.

QUICK CHECK

1. How do *systemic* and *pulmonary* circulations differ?
2. What is the *hepatic portal circulation*?
3. How is fetal circulation different from adult circulation?
4. What is *cyanosis*?

Blood Pressure

Defining Blood Pressure

A good way to explain blood pressure might be to first answer a few questions about it. What is blood pressure? Just what the words indicate—**blood pressure** is the pressure or "push" of blood as it flows through the circulatory system.

Where does blood pressure exist? It exists in all blood vessels, but it is highest in the arteries and lowest in the veins. In fact, if we list blood vessels in order according to the amount of blood pressure in them and draw a graph, as in Figure 14-10, the graph looks like a hill, with aortic blood pressure at the top and vena caval pressure at the bottom. This blood pressure "hill" is spoken of as the **blood pressure gradient.**

More precisely, the blood pressure gradient is the difference between two blood pressures. The blood pressure gradient for the entire systemic circulation is the difference between the average or mean blood pressure in the aorta and the blood pressure at the termination of the venae cavae where they join the right atrium of the heart. The mean blood pressure in the aorta, given in Figure 14-10, is 100 mm of mercury (mmHg), and the pressure at the termination of the venae cavae is 0. Therefore, with these typical normal figures, the systemic blood pressure gradient is 100 mmHg (100 minus 0).

Why is it important to understand how blood pressure functions? The blood pressure gradient is vitally involved in keeping the blood flowing. When a blood pressure gradient is present, blood circulates; conversely, when a blood pressure gradient is not present, blood does not circulate. For example, suppose that the blood pressure in the arteries were to decrease to a point at which it became equal to the average pressure in arterioles. The result would be no blood pressure gradient between arteries and arterioles, and therefore no force would be available to move blood out of arteries into arterioles. Circulation would stop, in other words, and very soon life itself would cease. That is why when arterial blood pressure is observed to be falling rapidly, whether during surgery or in some other circumstance, emergency measures must be started quickly to try to reverse this fatal trend.

What we have just said may start you wondering about why high blood pressure (meaning, of course, high arterial blood pressure) and low blood pressure are bad for circulation. High blood pressure, or **hypertension** (HI-per-TEN-shun) **(HTN),**

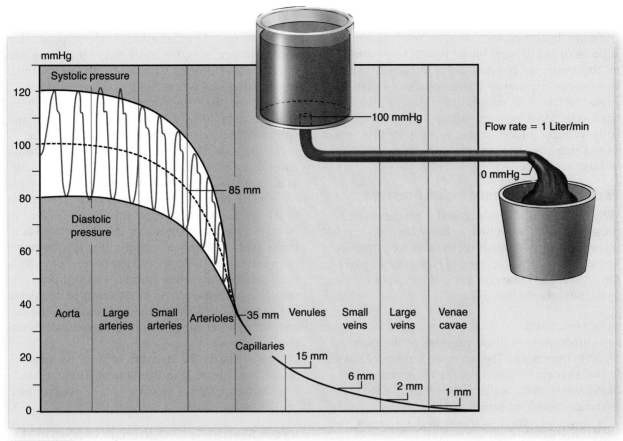

Figure 14-10 **Pressure gradients in blood flow.**

Blood flows down a "blood pressure hill" from arteries, where blood pressure is highest, into arterioles, where it is somewhat lower, into capillaries, where it is lower still, and so on. All numbers on the graph indicate blood pressure measured in millimeters of mercury. The broken line, starting at 100 mm, represents the average pressure in each part of the circulatory system.

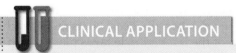

CLINICAL APPLICATION

REYNAUD PHENOMENON

A disorder characterized by sudden decreases in circulation in the digits (fingers or toes), often in response to stress or temperature change, is called *Reynaud* (ray-NO) *phenomenon*. The decreased blood flow often causes pale discoloration of the affected digits (see figure), followed by numbness and cyanosis (blue discoloration) as oxygen levels drop. As blood flow returns to the digits, they may become dark and redder—often swelling and throbbing with pain. Symptoms range from mild to severe. There is no known cause of Reynaud phenomenon, but some cases have been associ-

ated with inflammatory conditions such as scleroderma, rheumatoid arthritis, and lupus erythematosus.

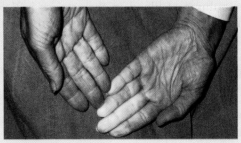

is bad for several reasons. For one thing, if blood pressure becomes too high, it may cause the rupture of one or more blood vessels (for example, in the brain, as happens in a stroke). But low blood pressure can be dangerous too. If arterial pressure falls low enough, circulation and thus life cease. Massive hemorrhage, which dramatically reduces blood pressure, kills in this way. Blood pressure problems are discussed further in later sections.

Factors That Influence Blood Pressure

What causes blood pressure, and what makes blood pressure change from time to time? Factors such as blood volume, the strength of each heart contraction, heart rate, and the thickness of blood are all part of the answers to these questions. We explain further in the paragraphs that follow.

BLOOD VOLUME

The direct cause of blood pressure is the *volume* of blood in the vessels. The larger the volume of blood in the arteries, for example, the more pressure the blood exerts on the walls of the arteries, or the higher the arterial blood pressure.

Conversely, the less blood in the arteries, the lower the blood pressure tends to be. Hemorrhage demonstrates this relationship between blood volume and blood pressure. Hemorrhage is a pronounced loss of blood, and this decrease in the volume of blood causes blood pressure to drop. In fact, the major sign of hemorrhage is a rapidly falling blood pressure. Another example is the fact that *diuretics*—drugs that promote water loss by increasing urine output—are often used to treat hypertension (high blood pressure). As water is lost from the body, blood volume decreases, and thus blood pressure decreases to a lower level.

The volume of blood in the arteries is determined by how much blood the heart pumps into the arteries and how much blood the arterioles drain out of them. The diameter of the arterioles plays an important role in determining how much blood drains out of arteries into arterioles.

STRENGTH OF HEART CONTRACTIONS

The strength and the rate of the heartbeat affect cardiac output and therefore blood pressure. Each time the left ventricle contracts, it squeezes a cer-

tain volume of blood (the stroke volume) into the aorta and on into other arteries. The stronger that each contraction is, the more blood it pumps into the aorta and arteries. Conversely, the weaker that each contraction is, the less blood it pumps.

Suppose that one contraction of the left ventricle pumps 70 ml of blood into the aorta, and suppose that the heart beats 70 times a minute; 70 ml × 70 equals 4900 ml. Almost 5 L of blood would enter the aorta and arteries every minute (the cardiac output). Now suppose that the heartbeat were to become weaker and that each contraction of the left ventricle pumps only 50 ml instead of 70 ml of blood into the aorta. If the heart still contracts just 70 times a minute, it will obviously pump much less blood into the aorta—only 3500 ml instead of the more normal 4900 ml per minute. This decrease in the heart's output decreases the volume of blood in the arteries, and the decreased arterial blood volume decreases arterial blood pressure.

In summary, the strength of the heartbeat affects blood pressure in this way: a stronger heartbeat increases blood pressure, and a weaker beat decreases it.

HEART RATE

The rate of the heartbeat also may affect arterial blood pressure. You might reason that when the heart beats faster, more blood enters the aorta, and therefore the arterial blood volume and blood pressure would increase.

This is true only if the stroke volume does not decrease sharply when the heart rate increases. Often, however, when the heart beats faster, each contraction of the left ventricle takes place so rapidly that it has little time to fill with blood and therefore squeezes out much less blood than usual into the aorta.

For example, suppose that the heart rate speeded up from 70 to 100 times per minute and that at the same time its stroke volume decreased from 70 ml to 40 ml. Instead of a cardiac output of 70 × 70 or 4900 ml per minute, the cardiac output would have changed to 100 × 40 or 4000 ml per minute. Arterial blood volume decreases under these conditions, and therefore blood pressure also decreases, even though the heart rate has increased.

What generalization, then, can we make? We can say only that an increase in the rate of the heartbeat increases blood pressure, and a decrease in the rate decreases blood pressure. But whether a change in the heart rate actually produces a similar change in blood pressure depends on whether the stroke volume also changes and in which direction.

BLOOD VISCOSITY

Another factor that needs to be mentioned in connection with blood pressure is the viscosity of blood, or in plainer language, its thickness. If blood becomes less viscous than normal, blood pressure decreases.

For example, if a person suffers a hemorrhage, fluid moves into the blood from the interstitial fluid. This dilutes the blood and decreases its viscosity, and blood pressure then falls because of the decreased viscosity. After hemorrhage, transfusion of whole blood or plasma is preferred to infusion of saline solution. The reason is that saline solution is not a viscous liquid and so cannot keep blood pressure at a normal level.

In a condition called **polycythemia** (pol-ee-sye-THEE-mee-ah), the number of red blood cells increases beyond normal and thus increases blood viscosity. This in turn increases blood pressure. Polycythemia can occur when oxygen levels in the air decrease and the body attempts to increase its ability to attract oxygen to the blood—as happens when working at high altitude.

RESISTANCE TO BLOOD FLOW

A factor that has a huge impact on local blood pressure gradients, and thus on blood flow, is any factor that changes the resistance to blood flow. The term **peripheral** (peh-RIF-er-al) **resistance** describes any force that acts against the flow of blood in a blood vessel. Viscosity of blood, for example, affects peripheral resistance by influencing the ease with which blood flows through blood vessels.

Another factor that affects peripheral resistance is the tension in muscles of the blood vessel wall (Figure 14-11). When these muscles are relaxed, resistance is low and therefore blood pressure is low—thus blood may flow easily down its pressure gradient and into the vessel. When vessel wall muscles are contracted, however, resistance increases and therefore so does the blood pressure—thus the pressure gradient is reduced and blood will not flow so easily into the vessel. Such adjustment of muscle tension in vessel walls to control blood pressure, and therefore blood flow, is often called the **vasomotor mechanism** (vay-so-MOH-tor MEK-ah-niz-em).

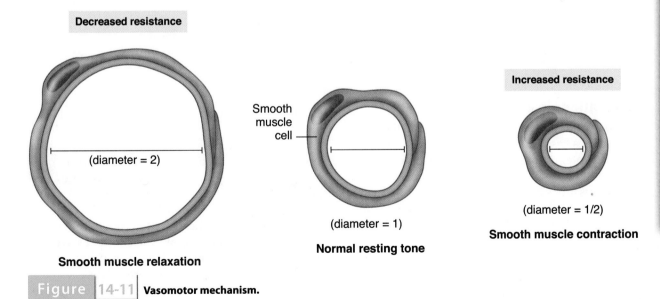

Decreased resistance

(diameter = 2)

Smooth muscle relaxation

Smooth muscle cell

(diameter = 1)

Normal resting tone

Increased resistance

(diameter = 1/2)

Smooth muscle contraction

Figure 14-11 **Vasomotor mechanism.**

Changes in smooth muscle tension in the wall of an arteriole influence the resistance of the vessel to blood flow. Relaxation of muscle results in decreased resistance; contraction of muscle results in increased resistance.

HEALTH & WELL-BEING

CHANGES IN BLOOD FLOW DURING EXERCISE

Not only does the overall rate of blood flow increase during exercise, but also the relative blood flow through the different organs of the body changes. During exercise, blood is routed away from the kidneys and digestive organs and toward the skeletal muscles, cardiac muscle, and skin. Rerouting of blood is accomplished by contracting precapillary sphincters in some tissues (thus reducing blood flow) while relaxing precapillary sphincters in other tissues (thus increasing blood

flow). How can homeostasis be better maintained as a result of these changes? One reason is that glucose and oxygen levels drop rapidly in muscles as they use up these substances to produce energy for exercising. Increased blood flow restores normal levels of glucose and oxygen more rapidly. Blood that has been warmed up in active muscles flows to the skin for cooling. This helps keep the body temperature from getting too high. Can you think of other ways this change in blood flow helps maintain homeostasis?

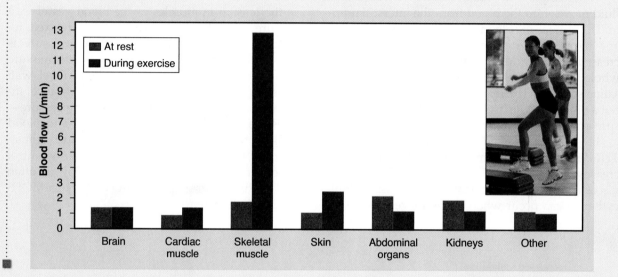

Fluctuations in Blood Pressure

No one's blood pressure stays the same all the time. It fluctuates, even in a perfectly healthy individual. For example, it goes up when a person exercises strenuously. Not only is this normal, but the increased blood pressure serves a good purpose. It increases circulation to bring more blood to muscles each minute and thus supplies them with more oxygen and food for more energy.

A normal arterial blood pressure is below 120/80, or 120 mmHg systolic pressure (as the ventricles contract) and 80 mmHg diastolic pressure (as the ventricles relax). Remember, however, that what is "normal" varies somewhat among individuals and also varies with age.

The venous blood pressure, as you can see in Figure 14-10, is very low in the large veins and falls almost to 0 by the time blood leaves the venae cavae and enters the right atrium. The venous blood pressure within the right atrium is called the **central venous pressure.** This pressure level is important because it influences the pressure that exists in the large peripheral veins. If the heart beats strongly, the central venous pressure is low as blood enters and leaves the heart chambers efficiently. However, if the heart is weakened, central venous pressure increases, and the flow of blood into the right atrium is slowed. As a result, a person suffering heart failure, who is sitting at rest in a chair, often has distended external jugular veins as blood "backs up" in the venous network.

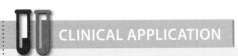

BLOOD PRESSURE READINGS

A device called a **sphygmomanometer** (sfig-moh-mah-NAH-meh-ter) is often used to measure blood pressures in both clinical and home health care situations. The traditional sphygmomanometer is an inverted tube of mercury (Hg) with a balloonlike air cuff attached via an air hose. The air cuff is placed around a limb, usually the subject's upper arm as shown in the figure. A stethoscope sensor is placed over a major artery (the brachial artery in the figure) to listen for the arterial pulse. A hand-operated pump fills the air cuff, increasing the air pressure and pushing the column of mercury higher. While listening through the stethoscope, the operator opens the air cuff's outlet valve and slowly reduces the air pressure around the limb. Loud, tapping Korotkoff sounds suddenly begin when the cuff pressure measured by the mercury column equals the systolic pressure—often below 120 mm. As the air pressure surrounding the arm continues to decrease, the Korotkoff sounds disappear. The pressure measurement at which the sounds disappear is equal to the diastolic pressure—often 70 to 80 mm. The subject's blood pressure is then expressed as systolic pressure (the maximum arterial pressure during each cardiac cycle) over the diastolic pressure (the minimum arterial pressure), such as 120/80 (read "one-twenty over eighty"). The final reading can

then be compared to the expected value, patient's age, and various other individual factors. Mercury sphygmomanometers have been replaced in many clinical settings by nonmercury devices that similarly measure the maximum and minimum arterial blood pressures. In home health care settings, patients can often learn to monitor their own blood pressure.

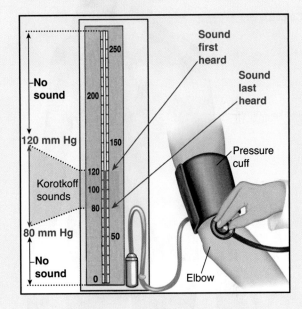

Five mechanisms help to keep venous blood moving back through the circulatory system and into the right atrium. They include the following:

1. Continued beating of the heart, which pumps blood through the entire circulatory system

2. Adequate blood pressure in the arteries, to push blood to and through the veins

3. Semilunar valves in the veins that ensure continued blood flow in one direction (toward the heart)

4. Contraction of skeletal muscles, which squeeze veins, producing a kind of pumping action

5. Changing pressures in the chest cavity during breathing that produce a kind of pumping action in the veins in the thorax

QUICK CHECK

1. How does the blood pressure gradient explain what makes blood flow?

2. Name four factors that influence blood pressure.

3. Does a person's blood pressure stay the same all the time? Explain why this is so.

Pulse

What you feel when you take a **pulse** is an artery expanding and then recoiling alternately. To feel a pulse, you must place your fingertips over an artery that lies near the surface of the body and over a bone or other firm base. The pulse is a valuable clinical sign. It can provide information, for example, about the rate, strength, and rhythmicity of the heartbeat. It is also easily determined with little or no danger or discomfort. The nine major "pulse points" are named after

Superficial temporal artery

Facial artery

Carotid artery

Brachial artery

Radial artery

Femoral artery

Popliteal (posterior to knee)

Posterior tibial

Dorsalis pedis

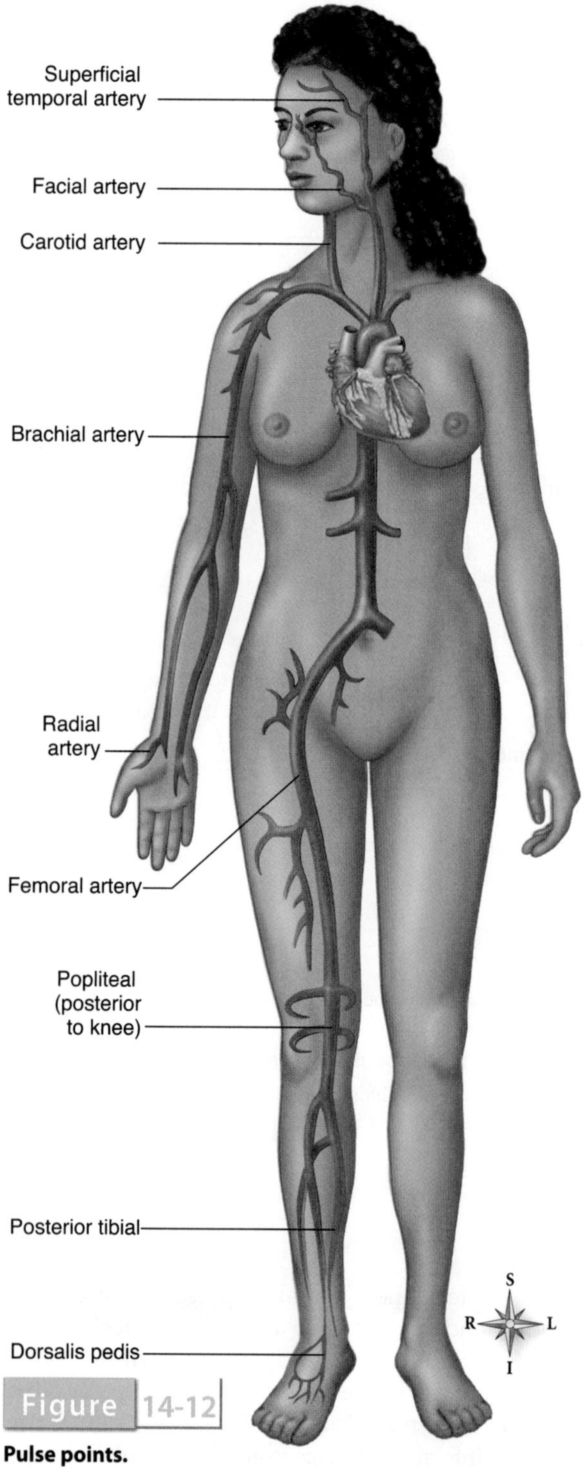

Figure 14-12

Pulse points.
Each pulse point is named after the artery with which it is associated.

the arteries over which they are felt. Locate each pulse point on Figure 14-12 and on your own body.

Three pulse points are located on each side of the head and neck: (1) over the superficial temporal artery in front of the ear, (2) the common carotid artery in the neck along the front edge of the sternocleidomastoid muscle, and (3) over the facial artery at the lower margin of the mandible at a point below the corner of the mouth.

A pulse is also detected at three points in the upper limb: (1) in the axilla over the axillary artery, (2) over the brachial artery at the bend of the elbow along the inner or medial margin of the biceps brachii muscle, and (3) at the radial artery at the wrist. The so-called *radial pulse* is the most frequently monitored and easily accessible pulse in the body.

The pulse also can be felt at three locations in the lower extremity: (1) over the femoral artery in the groin, (2) at the popliteal artery behind and just proximal to the knee, and (3) at the dorsalis pedis artery on the front surface of the foot, just below the bend of the ankle joint.

Hypertension

More visits to a physician's office are related to **hypertension (HTN),** or high blood pressure, than any other factor. More than 60 million cases of HTN have been diagnosed in the United States. This condition occurs when the force of blood exerted by the arterial blood vessel exceeds a blood pressure of 140/90 mmHg. Ninety percent of HTN cases are classified as *primary-essential,* or idiopathic, with no single known causative etiology. Another classification, secondary HTN, is caused by kidney disease or hormonal problems or induced by oral contraceptives, pregnancy, or other causes.

Another way of classifying hypertension is illustrated in the accompanying chart adapted from the National High Blood Pressure Education Program (Figure 14-13). This system uses systolic and diastolic blood pressure values to classify hypertension into stages according to severity. The guidelines that accompany this scheme emphasize the belief that there is no precise distinction between normal and abnormal values—thus even those in the high-normal range or the *prehypertension* range may be treated as having HTN.

Many risk factors have been identified in the development of HTN. Genetic factors play a large role. There is an increased susceptibility or predisposition with a family history of HTN. Men experience higher rates of HTN at an earlier age than women, and HTN in African Americans far exceeds that of Caucasians in the United States. There is also a direct relationship between age and high blood pressure. This is because as age advances, the blood vessels become less compliant and there is a higher incidence of atherosclerotic plaque buildup. HTN can also be fatal if undetected in women taking oral contraceptives. Risk factors include high stress levels, obesity, calcium deficiencies, high levels of alcohol and caffeine intake, smoking, and lack of exercise.

Untreated HTN has many potential complications including ischemic heart disease and heart failure, kidney failure, and stroke. As many as 400,000 people per year experience a stroke. Because HTN manifests minimal or no overt signs, it is known as the "silent killer." Headaches, dizziness, and fainting have been reported but are not always symptomatic of HTN. Regular screenings at the worksite and screening booths in malls and in hospitals often help to identify asymptomatic HTN.

Circulatory Shock

The term **circulatory shock** refers to the failure of the circulatory system to adequately deliver oxygen to the tissues, resulting in the impairment of cell function throughout the body. If left untreated, circulatory shock may lead to death. Circulatory failure has a variety of causes, all of which in some way reduce the flow of blood through the blood vessels of the body. Because of the variety of causes, circulatory shock is often classified as follows:

1. **Cardiogenic** (kar-dee-oh-JEN-ik) **shock** results from any type of heart failure, such as that after severe myocardial infarction (heart attack), heart infections, and other heart conditions. Because the heart can no longer pump blood effectively, blood flow to the tissues of the body decreases or stops.

2. **Hypovolemic** (hye-poh-voh-LEE-mik) **shock** results from the loss of blood volume in the blood vessels (*hypovolemia* means "low blood volume"). Reduced blood volume results in low blood pressure and reduced flow of blood to tissues. Hemorrhage is a common cause of blood volume loss leading to hypovolemic shock. Hypovolemia also can be caused by loss of interstitial fluid, causing blood plasma to drain out of the vessels and into the tissue spaces. Loss of interstitial fluid is common in chronic diarrhea or vomiting, dehydration, intestinal blockage, severe or extensive burns, and some other conditions.

3. **Neurogenic** (noo-roh-JEN-ik) **shock** results from widespread dilation of blood vessels caused by an imbalance in autonomic stimulation of smooth muscles in vessel walls. You may recall from Chapter 9 that autonomic effectors such as smooth muscle tissues are controlled by a balance of stimulation from the sympathetic and parasympathetic divisions of the autonomic nervous system. Normally, sympathetic stimulation maintains the muscle tone that keeps blood vessels at their usual diameter. If sympathetic stimulation is disrupted by an injury to the spinal cord or medulla, depressive drugs, emotional stress, or some other factor, blood vessels dilate significantly. Widespread vasodilation reduces blood pressure, thus reducing blood flow.

4. **Anaphylactic** (an-ah-fi-LAK-tik) **shock** results from an acute allergic reaction called *anaphylaxis*. Anaphylaxis causes the same kind of blood vessel dilation characteristic of neurogenic shock.

Blood Pressure (BP) Classification

Classification	Systolic BP		Diastolic BP
Normal	less than 120	and	less than 80
Prehypertension	120-139	or	80-89

High blood pressure

Stage 1 hypertension	140-159	or	90-99
Stage 2 hypertension	greater than or equal to 160	or	greater than or equal to 100

Figure 14-13 | **Classification of hypertension.**

This chart is adapted from the National High Blood Pressure Education Program. After age 50, the systolic pressure becomes more significant than diastolic pressure in assessing high blood pressure and associated risk of cardiovascular and renal disease.

5. **Septic shock** results from complications of *septicemia,* a condition in which infectious agents release toxins into the blood. The toxins often dilate blood vessels, thereby causing shock. The situation is usually made worse by the damaging effects of the toxins on tissues combined with the increased cell activity caused by the accompanying fever. One type of septic shock is *toxic shock syndrome (TSS),* which usually results from staphylococcal infections that begin in the vagina of menstruating women and spread to the blood (see Appendix A on page A-1 of your book).

The body has a number of mechanisms that compensate for the changes that occur during shock. However, these mechanisms may fail to compensate for changes that occur in severe cases, perhaps resulting in death.

> **QUICK CHECK**
>
> 1. Where are the places on your body that you can likely feel your pulse?
> 2. What general condition is called *circulatory shock?*
> 3. Describe four different causes of circulatory failure.

SCIENCE APPLICATIONS

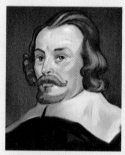

William Harvey (1578–1657)

CIRCULATION OF THE BLOOD

The English physician William Harvey was the first to prove that blood circulates. Until Harvey's time, scientists believed that the blood of the arteries was separate from the blood of the veins—each having different functions in the body. However, Harvey's observations of the body led him to discover that blood moves in a complete circle. Although he did not directly observe the capillaries (even though microscopes became available in his day), Harvey proved that they must exist by means of a series of clever experiments. Harvey not only completely changed the way we think of the body, he also proved his point with logical experiments.

William Harvey's work provides the conceptual basis for a variety of modern ideas and methods. For example, toxicologists (scientists who study the effects of poisons) know that the rapid spread of poisons in the body is explained by Harvey's model of circulation. Phlebotomists, technicians who draw blood for medical tests, know which vessels will work best for drawing blood. Nurses and technicians specializing in IV (intravenous) therapy must know how the blood circulates in order to effectively add therapeutic fluids to their patients' bloodstream. Radiologists and radiological technicians must know which way blood flows in different vessels so that contrast dyes can be added to the bloodstream to help visualize structures of the body in an x-ray film. Many different health professionals rely on their familiarity with the body's blood flow circuit when they measure blood pressure, inject intravenous drugs, perform surgeries, take pulses, attempt to stop bleeding after trauma to the body, and in many other medical procedures.

Outline Summary

 To download an MP3 version of the chapter summary for use with your iPod or portable media player, access the **Audio Chapter Summaries** on your CD.

Blood Vessels

A. Types
   1. Arteries—carry blood away from the heart and toward capillaries
   2. Veins—carry blood toward the heart and away from capillaries
   3. Capillaries—carry blood from the arterioles to the venules

B. Structure (Figure 14-1)
   1. Arteries
      a. Tunica intima—inner layer of endothelial cells
      b. Tunica media—smooth muscle, thick in arteries; some elastic tissue; important in blood pressure regulation
      c. Tunica externa—outer layer of fibrous connective elastic tissue
   2. Capillaries—microscopic vessels
      a. Only one layer thick—the tunica intima
      b. Precapillary sphincters determine how much blood will flow into each bed of capillaries
   3. Veins
      a. Tunica intima—inner layer; valves prevent retrograde movement of blood
      b. Tunica media—smooth muscle; thin in veins
      c. Tunica externa—heavy layer of fibrous connective tissue in many veins

C. Functions
   1. Arteries—distribute nutrients, gases, etc., carried in the blood by way of high pressure; assist in maintaining the arterial blood pressure; serve as blood reservoirs
   2. Capillaries—serve as exchange vessels for nutrients, wastes, and fluids

   3. Veins—collect blood for return to the heart; low pressure flow of blood (compared to arteries)

D. Names of main arteries—see Figure 14-2 and Table 14-1

E. Names of main veins—see Figure 14-3 and Table 14-2

Disorders of Blood Vessels

A. Disorders of arteries—arteries must withstand high pressure and remain free of blockage
   1. Arteriosclerosis—hardening of arteries caused by calcification of fatty deposits on arterial walls (Figure 14-4)
      a. Thickening and calcification of arterial walls reduce flow of blood, possibly causing ischemia
      b. Ischemia may progress to necrosis (tissue death) and then gangrene
      c. High blood levels of triglycerides and cholesterol, smoking, hypertension, advanced age, and genetic predisposition are associated factors
      d. May be corrected by vasodilators (vessel-relaxing drugs) or angioplasty (mechanical widening of vessels, see Figure 14-5) or surgical replacement
   2. Aneurysm—abnormal widening of arterial wall
      a. Promotes formation of thrombi that may obstruct blood flow to vital tissues
      b. Arterial walls may burst, resulting in life-threatening hemorrhaging
      c. Cerebrovascular accident (CVA), or stroke—ischemia of brain tissue caused by embolism or hemorrhage

B. Disorders of veins—low-pressure vessels
  1. Varicose veins (varices)—enlarged veins in which blood pools (Figure 14-6)
    a. Hemorrhoids—varicose veins in the rectum
    b. Treatments include supporting affected veins or surgical removal of veins
  2. Thrombophlebitis—vein inflammation (phlebitis) accompanied by clot (thrombus) formation; may result in fatal pulmonary embolism

Circulation of Blood

A. Systemic and pulmonary circulation
  1. Blood circulation—refers to the flow of blood through all the vessels, which are arranged in a complete circuit or circular pattern (Figure 14-7)
  2. Systemic circulation
    a. Carries blood throughout the body
    b. Path goes from left ventricle through aorta, smaller arteries, arterioles, capillaries, venules, venae cavae, to right atrium
  3. Pulmonary circulation
    a. Carries blood to and from the lungs
    b. Arteries deliver deoxygenated blood to the lungs for gas exchange
    c. Path goes from right ventricle through pulmonary arteries, lungs, pulmonary veins, to left atrium
B. Hepatic portal circulation (Figure 14-8)
  1. Unique blood route through the liver
  2. Vein (hepatic portal vein) exists between two capillary beds
  3. Assists with homeostasis of blood glucose levels
C. Fetal circulation (Figure 14-9)
  1. Refers to circulation before birth
  2. Modifications required for fetus to efficiently secure oxygen and nutrients from the maternal blood

  3. Unique structures include the placenta, umbilical arteries and vein, ductus venosus, ductus arteriosus, and foramen ovale
  4. Failure of fetal circulation to shift to usual post-birth circulation may result in cyanosis caused by lack of oxygen

Blood Pressure

A. Defining blood pressure
  1. "Push" or force of blood in the blood vessels
  2. Exists in all blood vessels—highest in arteries, lowest in veins (Figure 14-10)
  3. Blood pressure gradient—causes blood to circulate; liquids can flow only from areas of high pressure to areas of low pressure
    a. Low or nonexistent blood pressure gradient is fatal if not reversed
    b. Hypertension (high blood pressure) can cause a blood vessel to rupture
B. Factors that influence blood pressure
  1. Blood volume—the larger the volume, the more pressure is exerted on vessel walls
  2. Strength of heart contractions—affect cardiac output; stronger heartbeat increases pressure; weaker beat decreases it
  3. Heart rate—increased rate increases pressure; decreased rate decreases pressure
  4. Blood viscosity (thickness)—less than normal viscosity decreases pressure, more than normal viscosity increases pressure
  5. Resistance to blood flow (peripheral resistance)—affected by many factors, including the vasomotor mechanism (vessel muscle contraction/relaxation) (Figure 14-11)
C. Fluctuations in blood pressure
  1. Blood pressure varies within normal range from time to time

2. Central venous pressure—influences pressure in large peripheral veins
3. Venous return of blood to the heart depends on five mechanisms
   a. A strongly beating heart
   b. An adequate arterial blood pressure
   c. Valves in the veins
   d. Pumping action of skeletal muscles as they contract
   e. Changing pressures in the chest cavity caused by breathing

Pulse

A. Definition—alternate expansion and recoil of the blood vessel wall
B. Nine major pulse points named after arteries over which they are felt (Figure 14-12)

Hypertension (HTN)

A. Occurs when blood pressure exceeds 140/90 mm Hg (Figure 14-13)
B. 90% of HTN cases are primary-essential (idiopathic); secondary HTN can be caused by kidney disease or other causes
C. Many risk factors for HTN, including genetics, age, stress, obesity, and more
D. Untreated HTN may contribute to heart disease, kidney failure, and stroke

Circulatory Shock

A. Circulatory shock—failure of the circulatory system to deliver oxygen to the tissues adequately, resulting in cell impairment
B. When the cause is known, shock can be classified as follows:
   1. Cardiogenic shock—caused by heart failure
   2. Hypovolemic shock—caused by a drop in blood volume that causes blood pressure (and blood flow) to drop
   3. Neurogenic shock—caused by nerve condition that relaxes (dilates) blood vessels and thus reduces blood flow
   4. Anaphylactic shock—caused by a severe allergic reaction characterized by blood vessel dilation
   5. Septic shock—results from complications of septicemia (toxins in blood resulting from infection)

New Words

arteriole	placenta	**Diseases and Other**	hypovolemic shock
artery	precapillary sphincter	**Clinical Terms**	ischemia
blood pressure	pulse	anaphylactic shock	necrosis
blood pressure gradient	tunica externa	aneurysm	neurogenic shock
capillary	tunica intima	angioplasty	phlebitis
central venous pressure	tunica media	arteriosclerosis	pulmonary embolism
ductus arteriosus	umbilical	cardiogenic shock	septic shock
ductus venosus	vasomotor mechanism	circulatory shock	sphygmomanometer
endothelium	vein	cyanosis	thrombophlebitis
foramen ovale	venule	gangrene	varices (*sing.,* varix)
hepatic portal circulation		hemorrhoid	varicose vein
peripheral resistance		hypertension (HTN)	

Review Questions

1. Name and describe the main types of blood vessels in the body.
2. Name the three tissue layers that make up arteries and veins.
3. What is arteriosclerosis?
4. What is ischemia? What is gangrene?
5. What is an aneurysm?
6. What is phlebitis?
7. Describe both systemic and pulmonary circulation.
8. Name and briefly explain the four factors that influence blood pressure.
9. List five mechanisms that keep venous blood moving toward the right atrium.
10. What is circulatory shock? List the five types of circulatory shock.
11. Name four locations on the body where the pulse can be felt.

Critical Thinking

12. Explain how the formation of varicose veins is an example of a positive feedback mechanism.
13. Explain hepatic portal circulation. How is it different from normal circulation, and what advantages are gained from this type of circulation?
14. Explain the differences between normal postnatal circulation and fetal circulation. Based on the environment of the fetus, explain how these differences make fetal circulation more efficient.

Chapter Test

1. The _____ are blood vessels that carry blood back to the heart.
2. The _____ are blood vessels that carry blood away from the heart.
3. The _____ are microscopic blood vessels where substances are exchanged between the blood and the tissues.
4. The innermost tissue layer in an artery is called the _____.
5. The outermost tissue layer in an artery is called the _____.
6. Systemic circulation involves moving blood throughout the body; _____ circulation involves moving blood to the lungs and back.
7. The two structures in the fetus that allow most of the blood to bypass the lungs are the _____ and the _____.
8. The strength of the heart contraction and blood volume are two factors that influence blood pressure. Two other factors are _____ and _____.

Match each disorder in Column A with its corresponding description or cause in Column B.

Column A
9. _____ arteriosclerosis
10. _____ necrosis
11. _____ aneurysm
12. _____ varicose veins
13. _____ phlebitis
14. _____ cardiogenic shock
15. _____ hypovolemic shock
16. _____ septic shock
17. _____ anaphylactic shock
18. _____ neurogenic shock

Column B
a. cell death caused by ischemia
b. dilated, blood-engorged veins, usually found in the legs
c. circulatory shock caused by heart failure
d. circulatory shock that is a complication of septicemia
e. circulatory shock caused by an acute allergic reaction
f. also called "hardening of the arteries"
g. circulatory shock caused by autonomic stimulation of the smooth muscles in the blood vessels
h. circulatory shock due to loss of blood volume
i. inflammation of a vein
j. a section of an artery that has widened due to a weakening of the arterial wall

Study Tips

continued from page 395

5. The types of circulatory shock are fairly self-explanatory. Review the descriptions found in the chapter.
6. In your study group, review the structure of the blood vessels and try to relate it to its function. Discuss hepatic portal circulation and fetal circulation in terms of their advantages or efficiencies. Go over the factors influencing blood pressure and the location of places where a pulse can be taken. Review the chart of disorders and the types of shock. Review the questions at the end of the chapter and discuss possible test questions.

Case Studies

1. Kevin has just learned that he has hypercholesterolemia (high blood cholesterol). On the advice of his physician, he is starting a regular exercise program. How might this affect Kevin's cholesterol problem? (HINT: See Appendix A on page A-1 of your book.) What vascular disorder might Kevin develop if he is not able to correct his hypercholesterolemia?
2. Leo is a middle-age man who has recently been experiencing pain in his legs, especially when he walks for even moderate distances. His physician tells him that he has atherosclerosis in a major artery in the affected leg. Why does this cause pain when Leo walks? What treatments might Leo's physician recommend to correct this problem? Explain how each will improve Leo's condition.
3. If balloon angioplasty is used to correct mitral valve stenosis (see Chapter 13), what route must the catheter travel if it enters at the femoral artery?

15 The Lymphatic System and Immunity

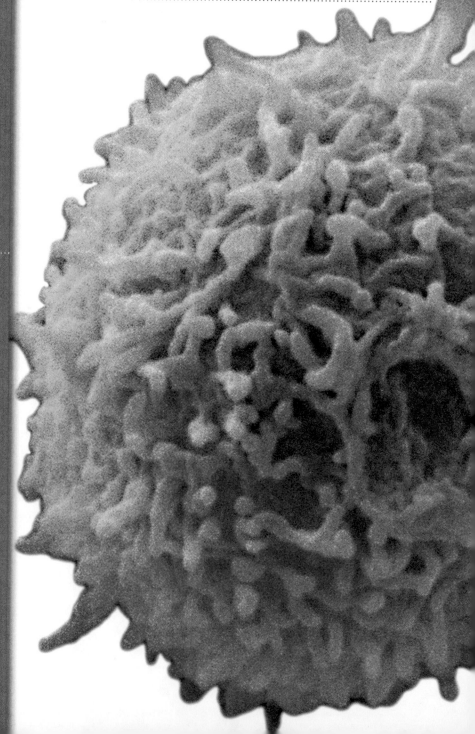

Objectives

After you have completed this chapter, you should be able to:

1. Describe general functions of the lymphatic system and list the main lymphatic structures.

2. Compare nonspecific and specific, inherited and acquired, and active and passive immunity.

3. Name the major disorders associated with the lymphatic system.

4. Discuss the major types of immune system molecules and indicate how antibodies and complement proteins function.

5. Discuss and contrast the development and functions of B and T cells.

6. Compare and contrast humoral and cell-mediated immunity.

7. Describe the mechanisms of allergy, autoimmunity, and isoimmunity.

8. List the major types of immune deficiencies and explain their causes.

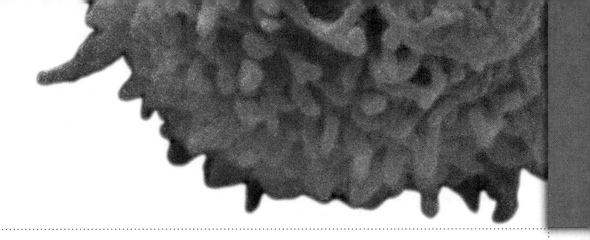

All of us live in a hostile and dangerous environment. Each day we are faced with potentially harmful toxins, disease-causing bacteria, viruses, and even cells from our own bodies that have been transformed into cancerous invaders. Fortunately, we are protected from this staggering variety of differing biological enemies by a remarkable set of defense mechanisms. We refer to this protective "safety net" as the **immune system.**

This system is characterized by structural components, the lymphatic organs, and by a functional group of defensive cells and molecules that protect us from infection and disease. This chapter begins with an overview of the lymphatic system, discussing vessels that help maintain fluid balance and lymphoid tissues that help defend the internal environment. We then discuss the basic principles of immunity and the ways that highly specialized cells and molecules provide us with effective and very specific resistance to disease.

STUDY TIPS

Before beginning your study of Chapter 15, review the synopsis of the lymphatic system in Chapter 4. The lymphatic system is partly a "sewer" system of the body. Plasma is pushed out of the capillaries and washes over the tissue cells. The interstitial fluid (IF) carries bacteria and other cellular debris, along with proteins and lipids, into open-ended capillaries in the lymphatic system. The fluid is then called *lymph*. It is carried to the lymph node, where it is filtered, cleaned, and then carried by ducts back to the blood. Keep this process in mind when you study the structures of the lymphatic system.

1. There are several specific organs in the lymphatic system. Flash cards that include their names, locations, and functions will help you learn them.
2. The immune system is divided into nonspecific and specific immunity. Most of the nonspecific immunity is fairly simple; the most complex part is the inflammation response, so study that well.
3. Specific immunity can be classified as natural or artificial depending on how the body was exposed to the specific antigen, and active or passive

continued on page 450

The Lymphatic System

Lymph and Lymphatic Vessels

Maintaining the constancy of the fluid around each body cell is possible only if numerous homeostatic mechanisms function effectively together in a controlled and integrated response to changing conditions. know from Chapter 12 that the cardiovascu plays a key role in bringing many needed es to cells and then removing the waste prod accumulate as a result of metabolism. This e of substances between blood and tissue fluid capillary beds. Many additional substances that cannot enter or return through the capillary walls, including excess fluid and protein molecules, are returned to the blood as **lymph.** Lymph is a fluid formed in the tissue spaces that is transported by way of **lymphatic vessels** to eventually reenter the circulatory system. In addition to lymph and the lymphatic vessels, the lymphatic system includes lymph nodes and lymphatic organs such as the thymus and spleen (Figure 15-1).

Lymph forms in this way: blood plasma filters out of the capillaries into the microscopic spaces between tissue cells because of the pressure generated by the pumping action of the heart. There, the liquid is called **interstitial fluid (IF),** or tissue fluid. Much of the interstitial fluid goes back into the blood by the same route it came out (that is, through the capillary membrane). The remainder of the interstitial fluid enters the lymphatic system before it returns to the blood. The fluid, called *lymph* at this point, enters a network of tiny blind-ended tubes distributed in the tissue spaces. These tiny vessels, called *lymphatic capillaries,* permit excess tissue fluid and some other substances such as dissolved protein molecules to leave the tissue spaces. Figure 15-2 shows the role of the lymphatic system in fluid homeostasis.

Lymphatic and blood capillaries are similar in many ways. Both types of vessels are microscopic and both are formed from sheets consisting of a cell layer of simple squamous epithelium called *endothelium* (en-doh-THEE-lee-um). The flattened endothelial cells that form blood capillaries, however, fit tightly together so that large molecules cannot enter or exit from the vessel. The "fit" between endothelial cells forming the lymphatic capillaries is not as tight. As a

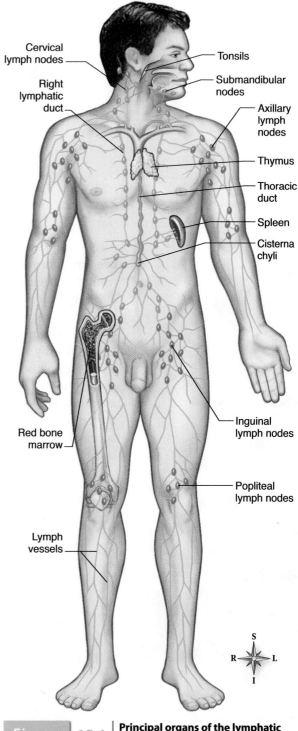

Cervical lymph nodes

Right lymphatic duct

Red bone marrow

Lymph vessels

Tonsils

Submandibular nodes

Axillary lymph nodes

Thymus

Thoracic duct

Spleen

Cisterna chyli

Inguinal lymph nodes

Popliteal lymph nodes

Figure **15-1** **Principal organs of the lymphatic system.**

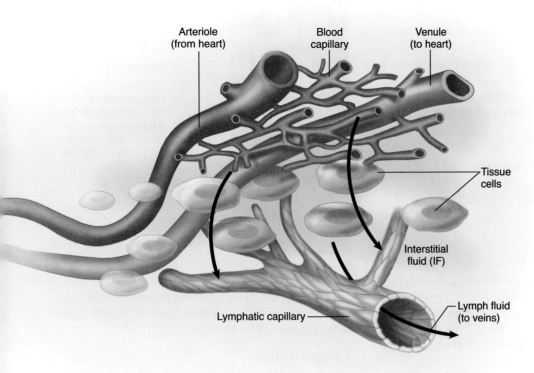

Figure 15-2

Role of lymphatic system in fluid homeostasis.

Fluid from blood plasma that is not reabsorbed by blood vessels drains into lymphatic vessels. Lymphatic drainage prevents accumulation of too much tissue fluid.

result, they are more porous and allow larger molecules, including proteins and other substances, as well as the fluid itself, to enter the vessel and eventually return to the general circulation.

The movement of lymph in the lymphatic vessels is one way. Unlike blood, lymph does not flow over and over again through vessels that form a circular route.

Lymph flowing through the lymphatic capillaries next moves into successively larger and larger vessels called *lymphatic venules* and veins and eventually empties into two terminal vessels called the **right lymphatic duct** and the **thoracic duct,** which empty their lymph into the blood in veins in the neck region.

Lymph from about three fourths of the body eventually drains into the thoracic duct, which is the largest lymphatic vessel in the body. Lymph from the right upper extremity and from the right side of the head, neck, and upper torso flows into the right lymphatic duct (Figure 15-3).

The lymphatic vessels often have a "beaded" appearance caused by the presence of valves that assist in maintaining a one-way flow of lymph. Note in Figure 15-1 that the thoracic duct in the abdomen has an enlarged pouchlike structure called the **cisterna chyli** (sis-TER-nah KYE-lee) that serves as a

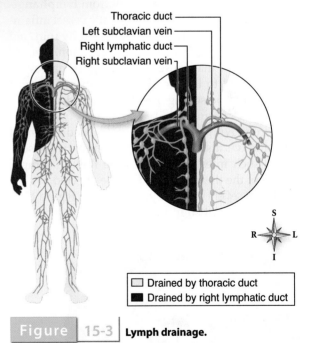

Figure 15-3   **Lymph drainage.**

The right lymphatic duct drains lymph from the upper right quarter of the body into the right subclavian vein. The thoracic duct drains lymph from the rest of the body into the left subclavian vein.

storage area for lymph moving toward its point of entry into the venous system.

Lymphatic capillaries in the wall of the small intestine are given the special name of **lacteals** (LAK-tee-als). They transport fats obtained from food to the bloodstream and are discussed further in Chapter 17.

 To learn more about lymph and lymphatic vessels, go to **AnimationDirect** on your CD.

Lymphedema

Lymphedema (lim-feh-DEE-mah) is an abnormal condition in which tissues exhibit swelling (edema) because of the accumulation of lymph. Lymph may accumulate in tissue when the lymphatic vessels are partially blocked (Figure 15-4). This may result from a congenital abnormality or a specific injury or blockage of lymphatic drainage.

Lymphedema may also result from **lymphangitis** (lim-fan-JYE-tis), that is, lymphatic vessel inflammation. Lymphangitis is characterized by thin, red streaks extending from an infected region. The infectious agent that causes lymphangitis may eventually spread to the bloodstream, causing septicemia ("blood poisoning") and possibly death from septic shock (Figure 15-5).

Rarely, lymphedema may be caused by small parasitic worms that infest the lymphatic vessels. When such infestation blocks the flow of lymph, edema of the tissues drained by the affected vessels occurs. In severe cases, as you can see in Figure 15-6, the tissues swell so much that the limbs look as if

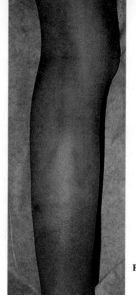

Figure 15-5

Lymphangitis.

This condition is characterized by inflamed lymphatic vessels that appear as red streaks radiating from the source of infection.

they belong to an elephant! For this reason, the condition is often called **elephantiasis**—literally "condition of being like an elephant."

Lymph Nodes

As lymph moves from its origin in the tissue spaces toward the thoracic or right lymphatic ducts and then into the venous blood, it is filtered by way of moving through **lymph nodes,** which are

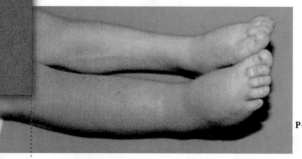

Figure 15-4 **Lymphedema.**

Notice the significant swelling in the subject's right leg and foot.

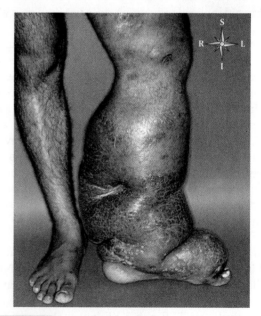

Figure 15-6 **Elephantiasis.**

Lymphedema caused by prolonged infestation by *Filaria* worms produces elephant-like limbs.

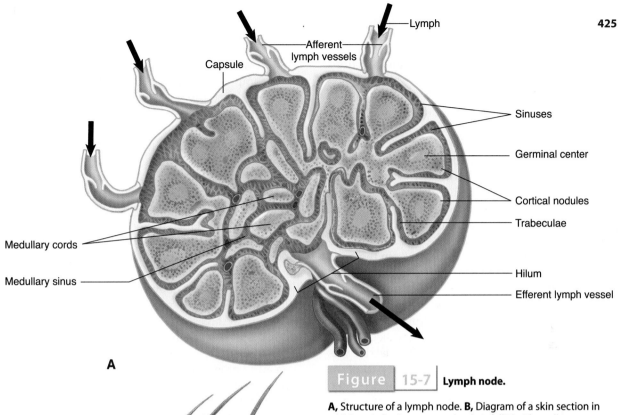

Lymph

Afferent
lymph vessels

Capsule

Sinuses

Germinal center

Cortical nodules

Trabeculae

Medullary cords

Medullary sinus

Hilum

Efferent lymph vessel

A

 Figure 15-7 **Lymph node.**

A, Structure of a lymph node. **B,** Diagram of a skin section in
which an infection surrounds a hair follicle. The yellow areas
represent dead and dying cells (pus). The black dots around the
yellow areas represent bacteria. Bacteria entering the lymph
node via the afferent lymphatics are filtered out.

Dead and dying
cells (pus)

Bacteria

Afferent lymph
vessel

Lymph node

Efferent lymph
vessel

B

immune functions: defense and white blood cell
formation.

Lymph nodes are *lymphoid organs* because they
contain *lymphoid tissue,* which is a mass of developing lymphocytes and related cells. Lymphoid organs such as lymph nodes, tonsils, thymus, and
spleen are important structural components of the
immune system because they provide immune defense and development of immune cells.

To learn more about lymph nodes, go to
AnimationDirect on your CD.

DEFENSE FUNCTION: BIOLOGICAL FILTRATION
Figure 15-7 shows the structure of a typical lymph
node. In this example, a small node located next to
an infected hair follicle is shown filtering bacteria
from lymph. Lymph nodes perform biological filtration, a process in which cells (phagocytic cells
in this case) alter the contents of the filtered fluid.
Biological filtration of bacteria and other abnormal

located in clusters along the pathway of lymphatic
vessels. Some of these nodes may be as small as
a pinhead, and others may be as large as a lima
bean. With the exception of a comparatively few
single nodes, most lymph nodes occur in groups
or clusters in certain areas. Figure 15-1 shows the
locations of the clusters of greatest clinical importance. The structure of the lymph nodes makes
it possible for them to perform two important

cells by phagocytosis prevents local infections from spreading.

Figure 15-7 shows that lymph enters the node through four **afferent** (Latin "to carry toward") **lymphatic vessels.** These vessels deliver lymph to the node. Once lymph enters the node, it "percolates" slowly through spaces called *sinuses* that surround *nodules* found in the outer (cortex) and inner (medullary) areas of the node (Figure 15-7). In passing through the node, lymph is filtered so that bacteria, cancer cells, and damaged tissue cells are removed and prevented from entering the blood and circulating all over the body. Lymph exits from the node through a single **efferent** (Latin "to carry away from") **lymphatic vessel.**

Clusters of lymph nodes allow a very effective biological filtration of lymph flowing from specific body areas. Figure 15-8 shows an x-ray image called a *lymphangiogram* (lym-FAN-jee-oh-gram). A special dye was injected into the soft tissues that drain the part of the lymphatic network that appears in the image. You can see that the dyed lymph appears in the vessels and nodes of the inguinal and pelvic regions.

Knowledge of lymph node location and function is important in clinical medicine. For example, a school nurse monitoring the progress of a child with an infected finger will watch the elbow and axillary regions for swelling and tenderness of the lymph nodes—a condition called **lymphadenitis** (limf-ad-en-EYE-tis).

These nodes filter lymph returning from the hand and may become infected by the bacteria they trap. As mentioned in the Clinical Application box (Lymphedema After Breast Surgery), a surgeon uses knowledge of lymph node function when removing lymph nodes under the arms (axillary nodes) and in other nearby areas during an operation for breast cancer (Figure 15-9). These nodes may contain cancer cells filtered out of the lymph drained from the breast. Cancer of the breast is one of the most common forms of this disease in women. Unfortunately, cancer cells from a single tumorous growth in the breast often spread to other areas of the body through the lymphatic system. Figure 15-10 shows a cluster of cancer cells moving through a lymphatic vessel during the process of *metastasis* (spread of a cancer).

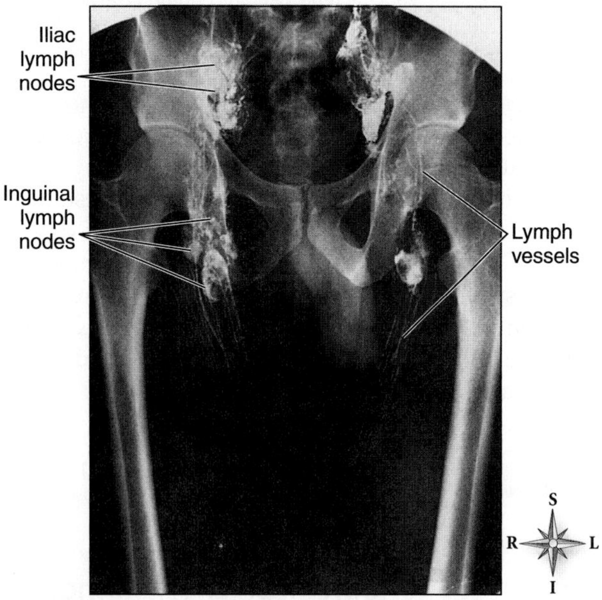

Figure 15-8 **Lymphangiogram.**

A special dye that is opaque to x-rays is injected into the tissue fluids that drain into the inguinal and pelvic lymphatic pathways. Thus the outlines of the lymphatic vessels and lymph nodes can be visualized.

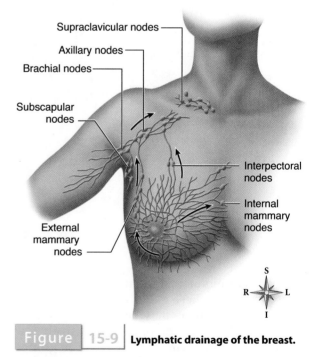

Figure 15-9 **Lymphatic drainage of the breast.**

Note the extensive network of nodes that receive lymph from the breast.

Tumor cells   Lymphatic vessel

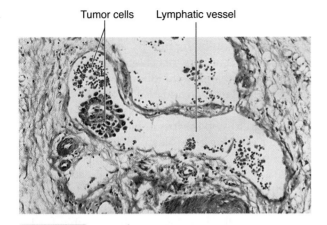

Figure 15-10 **Lymphatic metastasis.**

This cluster of cancer cells moving through a lymphatic vessel may eventually start another cancerous tumor in another part of the body.

Lymphoma

As you may recall from Chapter 5, *lymphoma* is a term that refers to lymphatic tumors. Lymphomas are most often malignant but in rare cases can be benign. The two principal categories of lymphoma are **Hodgkin disease** and **non-Hodgkin lymphoma.** All types of lymphoma characteristically cause painless

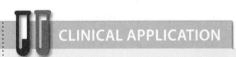

CLINICAL APPLICATION

LYMPHEDEMA AFTER BREAST SURGERY

Surgical procedures called *mastectomies,* in which some or all of the breast tissues are removed, are sometimes done to treat breast cancer. Because cancer cells can spread so easily through the extensive network of lymphatic vessels associated with the breast (see Figure 15-9), the lymphatic vessels and their nodes are sometimes also removed. Occasionally, such procedures interfere with the normal flow of lymph fluid from the arm. When this happens, tissue fluid may accumulate in the arm—resulting in lymphedema.

In home health care situations, the affected arm may be exercised and massaged to reduce swelling and encourage the growth of new lymphatic vessels. Some women wear an elastic sleeve that has a similar effect.

enlargements of the lymph nodes in the neck and other regions. This sign is followed by anemia, weight loss, weakness, fever, and spread to other lymphatic tissues. In later stages, the lymphoma spreads to many other areas of the body. When discovered early, lymphoma can be successfully treated with intensive radiation and chemotherapy. Lymphoma occurs more often in men than in women.

> **QUICK CHECK**
>
> 1. How does the lymphatic system return fluid to the blood?
> 2. What is the role of *lymph nodes* in the body?

Thymus

As you can see in Figure 15-1, the **thymus** (THYE-mus) is a small lymphoid tissue organ located in the mediastinum, extending upward in the midline of the neck. It is composed of lymphocytes in a meshlike framework. The thymus, also called the *thymus gland*, is largest at puberty and even then weighs only about 35 or 40 g—a little more than an ounce.

Although small in size, the thymus plays a central and critical role in the body's vital immunity mechanism. First, it is a source of lymphocytes before birth and is then especially important in the "maturation" or development of a type of lymphocytes that then leave the thymus and circulate to the spleen, tonsils, lymph nodes, and other lymphoid tissues. These **T lymphocytes,** or **T cells,** are critical to the functioning of the immune system and are discussed later. They develop under the influence of a hormone secreted by the thymus, **thymosin** (THYE-moh-sin).

The thymus appears to complete much of its work early in childhood, reaching its maximum size at puberty. The thymus tissue is then gradually replaced by fat and connective tissue, a process called *involution*. By age 60, the thymus is about half its maximum size and is virtually gone by age 80 or so.

Tonsils

Masses of lymphoid tissue called *tonsils* are located in a protective ring under the mucous membranes in the mouth and back of the throat (Figure 15-11). They help protect us against bacteria that may invade tissues in the area around the openings between the nasal and oral cavities. The **palatine tonsils** are located on each side of the throat. The **pharyngeal tonsils,** known as **adenoids** (AD-eh-noyds) when they become swollen, are near the posterior opening of the nasal cavity. A third type of tonsil, the **lingual tonsils,** are near the base of the tongue. The tonsils serve as the first line of defense from the exterior and as such are subject to chronic infection, or **tonsillitis** (tahn-sil-LYE-tis). They may have to be removed surgically if antibiotic therapy is not successful at treating the chronic infection or if swelling impairs breathing.

Spleen

The spleen is the largest lymphoid organ in the body. As you can see in Figure 15-1, it is located high in the upper left quadrant of the abdomen lateral to the stomach. Although the spleen is protected by the lower ribs, it can be injured by abdominal trauma. The spleen has a very rich blood supply and may contain more than 500 ml (about 1 pint) of blood. If the spleen is damaged and bleeding, surgical removal, called a **splenectomy** (splen-NEK-toh-mee), may be required to stop the loss of blood.

After entering the spleen, blood flows through dense, pulplike accumulations of lymphocytes. As blood flows through the pulp, the spleen removes by filtration and phagocytosis many bacteria and other foreign substances, destroys worn-out RBCs and salvages the iron found in hemoglobin for future use, and serves as a reservoir for blood that can be returned to the circulatory system when needed.

Splenomegaly (spleh-no-MEG-ah-lee), or abnormal spleen enlargement, is observed in a variety of disorders. For example, infectious conditions such as scarlet fever, syphilis, and typhoid fever are characterized by splenomegaly. Spleen enlargement sometimes accompanies hypertension. Splenomegaly also accompanies some forms of hemolytic anemia in which red blood cells appear to be broken apart at an abnormally fast rate. Surgical removal of the spleen often cures such cases.

To learn more about the spleen, go to **AnimationDirect** on your CD.

QUICK CHECK

1. Why is the *thymus* important for immunity?
2. What are *tonsils?* What is their function?
3. What is the role of the *spleen?*

The Immune System

Function of the Immune System

The body's defense mechanisms protect us from disease-causing microorganisms that invade our bodies, from foreign tissue cells that may have been transplanted into our bodies, and from our own cells when they have turned malignant or cancerous. The body's overall defense system is called the *im-*

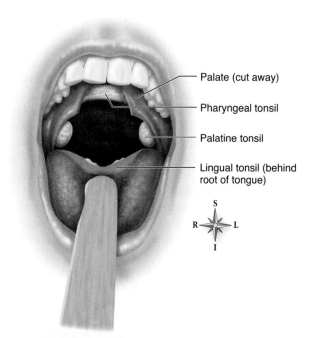

Palate (cut away)

Pharyngeal tonsil

Palatine tonsil

Lingual tonsil (behind root of tongue)

Figure 15-11 **Location of the tonsils.**

Small segments of the roof and floor of the mouth have been removed to show the protective ring of tonsils (lymphoid tissue) around the internal opening of the nose and throat.

mune system. The immune system makes us immune—that is, able to resist these threats to our health and survival.

In the lymphatic system, we have seen many organs that provide defense: lymph nodes, tonsils, thymus, and spleen. The immune system is not simply a small group of organs working together. Instead, it is an interactive network of many organs and billions of freely moving cells and trillions of free-floating molecules in many different areas of the body.

Nonspecific Immunity

Nonspecific immunity is maintained by mechanisms that attack any irritant or abnormal substance that threatens the internal environment. In other words, nonspecific immunity confers general protection rather than protection from certain kinds of threatening cells or chemicals. Because we are born with nonspecific defenses that do not require prior exposure to a harmful substance or threatening cell, nonspecific immunity is often called *innate immunity.*

There are many types of nonspecific immune defenses in the body. The skin and mucous membranes, for example, are mechanical barriers that prevent entry into the body by bacteria and many other substances such as toxins and harmful chemicals. Tears and mucus also contribute to nonspecific immunity. Tears wash harmful substances from the eyes, and mucus traps foreign material that may enter through the respiratory tract. Phagocytosis of bacteria by white blood cells (WBCs) is a nonspecific form of immunity.

The **inflammatory response** is a set of nonspecific responses that often occurs in the body. In the example shown in Figure 15-12, bacteria cause tissue damage that, in turn, triggers the release of mediators from any of a variety of immune cells. Some of the mediators attract WBCs to the area. Many of these factors produce the characteristic signs of inflammation: heat, redness, pain, and swelling. These signs are caused by increased blood flow (resulting in heat and redness) and vascular permeability (resulting in tissue swelling and the pain that it causes) in the affected region. Such changes help phagocytic WBCs reach the general area and enter the affected tissue.

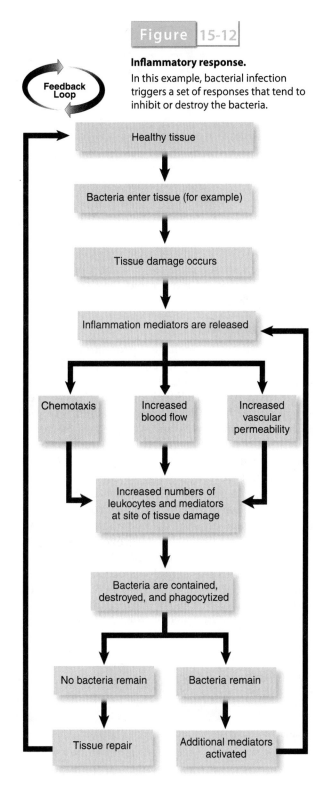

Figure 15-12

Inflammatory response. In this example, bacterial infection triggers a set of responses that tend to inhibit or destroy the bacteria.

Table 15-1	Nonspecific and Specific Immunity	
	NONSPECIFIC IMMUNITY	**SPECIFIC IMMUNITY**
Synonyms	Innate immunity, native immunity, genetic immunity	Adaptive immunity, acquired immunity
Specificity	Not specific—recognizes variety of nonself or abnormal cells and particles	Specific—recognizes certain antigens on certain cells or particles
Speed of reaction	Rapid—immediate up to several hours	Slower—several hours to several days
Memory	None—same response to repeated exposures to same antigen	Yes—enhanced response to repeated exposures to same antigen
Chemicals	Complement proteins, interferons, others	Antibodies, various signaling chemicals
Cells	Phagocytes (neutrophils, macrophages, dendritic cells)	Lymphocytes (B cells and T cells)

As you can see in Table 15-1, nonspecific immune responses are more rapid than specific immune responses.

Specific Immunity

Specific immunity includes protective mechanisms that confer very specific protection against certain types of threatening microorganisms or other toxic materials. Specific immunity involves memory and the ability to recognize and respond to certain harmful substances or bacteria. Because it is able to adapt to newly encountered "enemies," specific immunity is often called *adaptive immunity*.

In specific immunity, when the body is first attacked by particular bacteria or viruses, disease symptoms may occur as the body fights to destroy the threatening organism. However, if the body is exposed a second time to the same threatening organism, no serious symptoms occur because the organism is destroyed quickly—the person is said to be *immune* to that particular organism. Immunity to one type of disease-causing bacteria or virus does not protect the body against others. Immunity can be very selective.

As Table 15-1 shows, specific immune responses are slow compared to nonspecific immune responses. However, specific immune responses have memory—the ability to produce a stronger, faster response to repeated exposure to the same antigen. Table 15-1 summarizes other important features of both types of immunity, some of which will be discussed later in this chapter.

Specific immunity may be classified as either "natural" or "artificial" depending on how the body is exposed to the harmful agent (Table 15-2). Natural exposure is not deliberate and occurs in the course of everyday living. We are naturally exposed to many disease-causing agents on a regular basis. Artificial exposure is called *immunization* and is the deliberate exposure of the body to a potentially harmful agent.

Natural and artificial immunity may be "active" or "passive." Active immunity occurs when an individual's own immune system responds to a harmful agent, regardless of whether that

Table 15-2	Types of Specific Immunity
TYPE	**EXAMPLE**
Natural immunity	Exposure to the causative agent is not deliberate
Active (exposure)	A child develops measles and acquires an immunity to a subsequent infection
Passive (exposure)	A fetus receives protection from the mother through the placenta, or an infant receives protection via the mother's milk
Artificial immunity	Exposure to the causative agent is deliberate
Active (exposure)	Intentional exposure to the causative agent, such as a vaccination against polio, confers immunity
Passive (exposure)	Injection of protective material (antibodies) that was developed by another individual's immune system is given

agent was naturally or artificially encountered. Passive immunity results when immunity to a disease that has developed in another individual or animal is transferred to an individual who was not previously immune. For example, antibodies in a mother's milk confer passive immunity to her nursing infant. Active immunity generally lasts longer than passive immunity. Passive immunity, although temporary, provides immediate protection. Table 15-1 lists the various forms of specific immunity and gives examples of each.

QUICK CHECK

1. What is the difference between specific immunity and nonspecific immunity?
2. Outline the changes that occur in the body's inflammatory response?

HEALTH & WELL-BEING

EFFECTS OF EXERCISE ON IMMUNITY

Exercise physiologists have found that moderate exercise increases the number of white blood cells (WBCs), specifically granular leukocytes and lymphocytes. Not only is the number of circulating immune cells higher after exercise, but the activity of activated T cells is also increased. But at the same time, research also shows that strenuous exercise may actually inhibit immune function. Nevertheless, moderate exercise such as walking, when engaged in immediately after a trauma such as surgery, is often encouraged because of its immunity-strengthening effects.

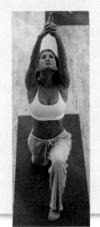

RESEARCH, ISSUES, AND TRENDS

MONOCLONAL ANTIBODIES

Techniques that have permitted biologists to produce large quantities of pure and very specific antibodies have resulted in dramatic advances in medicine. As a new medical technology, the development of **monoclonal antibodies** has been compared in importance with advances in recombinant DNA or genetic engineering.

Monoclonal antibodies are specific antibodies produced or derived from a population or culture of identical, or *monoclonal,* cells. In the past, antibodies produced by the immune system against a specific antigen had to be "harvested" from serum containing literally hundreds of other antibodies. The total amount of a specific antibody that could be recovered was very limited, so the cost of recovery was high. Monoclonal antibody techniques are based on the ability of immune system cells to produce individual antibodies that bind to and react with very specific antigens. We know, for example, that if the body is exposed to the varicella virus of chickenpox, WBCs will produce an antibody that will react very specifically with that virus and no other. With monoclonal antibody techniques, lymphocytes that are produced by the body after the injection of a specific antigen are "harvested" and then "fused" with other cells that have been transformed to grow and divide indefinitely in a tissue culture medium. These fused or hybrid cells, called **hybridomas** (hye-brid-OH-mahs), continue to produce the

same antibody produced by the original lymphocyte (see the figure). The result is a rapidly growing population of identical or monoclonal cells that produce large quantities of a very specific antibody. Monoclonal antibodies have now been produced against a wide array of different antigens, including disease-producing organisms and various types of cancer cells.

The availability of very pure antibodies against specific disease-producing agents is the first step in the commercial preparation of diagnostic tests that can be used to identify viruses, bacteria, and even specific cancer cells in the blood or other body fluids. The use of monoclonal antibodies may serve as the basis for specific treatment of many human diseases.

Monoclonal antibodies are also used in over-the-counter early pregnancy test kits. The antibodies in such kits bind to the hormone *human chorionic gonadotropin (hCG)* found in the urine of women in the early stages of pregnancy. When the antibodies in the kit bind to hCG molecules, they trigger a chemical reaction that produces a color change.

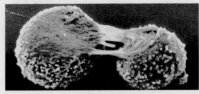

Hybridoma dividing

Immune System Molecules

The immune system functions because of adequate amounts of defensive protein molecules and protective cells. The protein molecules critical to immune system functioning are called **antibodies** (AN-ti-bod-ees) and **complement** (KOM-pleh-ment) proteins.

Antibodies

DEFINITION

Antibodies are protein compounds that are normally present in the body. A defining characteristic of an antibody molecule is the uniquely shaped concave regions called **combining sites** on its surface. Another defining characteristic is the ability of an antibody molecule to combine with a specific compound called an **antigen** (AN-ti-jen). All antigens are compounds whose molecules have small regions on their surfaces that are uniquely shaped to fit into the combining sites of a specific antibody molecule

as precisely as a key fits into a specific lock. Antigens are often protein molecules imbedded in the surface membranes of threatening or diseased cells such as microorganisms or cancer cells.

FUNCTIONS

In general, antibodies produce **humoral,** or **antibody-mediated, immunity** by changing the antigens in a way that prevents them from harming the body (Figure 15-13). To do this, an antibody must first bind to its specific antigen. This forms an *antigen-antibody complex.* The antigen-antibody complex then acts in one or more ways to make the antigen, or the cell on which it is present, harmless. For example, if the antigen is a toxin, a substance poisonous to body cells, the toxin is neutralized or made nonpoisonous by becoming part of an antigen-antibody complex. Or if antigens are molecules in the surface membranes of threatening cells, when antibodies combine with them, the resulting antigen-antibody complexes may **agglutinate** the

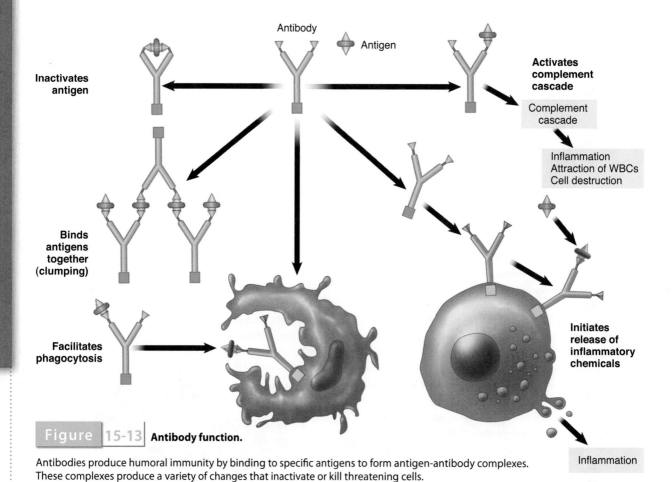

Figure 15-13 **Antibody function.**
Antibodies produce humoral immunity by binding to specific antigens to form antigen-antibody complexes. These complexes produce a variety of changes that inactivate or kill threatening cells.

enemy cells (that is, make them stick together in clumps). Then macrophages or the other phagocytes can rapidly destroy them by ingesting and digesting large numbers of them at one time.

Another important function of antibodies is promotion and enhancement of phagocytosis. Certain antibody fractions help promote the attachment of phagocytic cells to the object they will engulf. As a result, the contact between the phagocytic cell and its victim is enhanced, and the object is more easily ingested. This process contributes to the efficiency of immune system phagocytic cells, which is described below and on p. 434.

Probably the most important way in which antibodies act is a process called the **complement cascade.** Often, when antigens that are molecules on an antigenic or foreign cell's surface combine with antibody molecules, they change the shape of the antibody molecule slightly, just enough to expose two previously hidden regions. These are called **complement-binding sites.** Their exposure initiates a series of events that eventually kill the cell. The next section describes these events.

Complement Proteins

Complement is the name used to describe a group of protein enzymes normally present in an inactive state in blood. These proteins may be activated by exposure of complement-binding sites on antibodies when they attach to antigens. The result is formation of highly specialized protein molecules that target foreign cells for destruction. Recall that this process is a rapid-fire cascade or sequence of events collectively called the **complement cascade.** The end result of this process is that doughnut-shaped protein rings (complete with a hole in the middle) are formed and literally bore holes in the foreign cell!

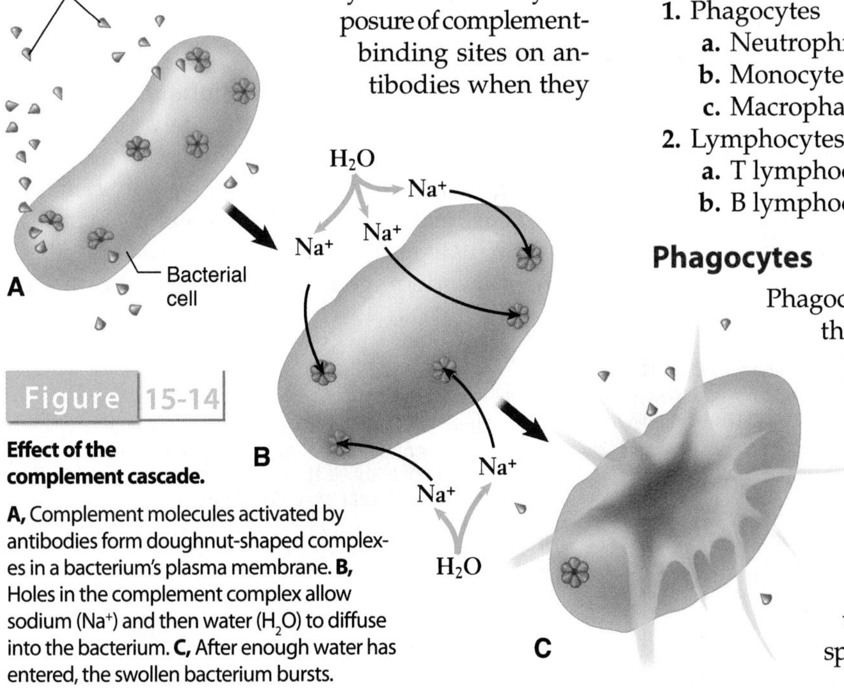

The tiny holes allow sodium to rapidly diffuse into the cell; then water follows through the process of osmosis. The cell literally bursts as the internal osmotic pressure increases (Figure 15-14).

Complement proteins also serve other roles in the immune system, such as attracting immune cells to a site of infection, activating immune cells, marking foreign cells for destruction, and increasing permeability of blood vessels. Complement proteins also play a vital role in producing the inflammatory response.

> **QUICK CHECK**
>
> 1. What are *antibodies?* How do they work?
> 2. What are *complement proteins?* How do they work?

Immune System Cells

The primary cells of the immune system include the following:

1. Phagocytes
   a. Neutrophils
   b. Monocytes
   c. Macrophages
2. Lymphocytes
   a. T lymphocytes
   b. B lymphocytes

Phagocytes

Phagocytic WBCs are an important part of the immune system. In Chapter 12, phagocytes were described as cells derived from the bone marrow that carry on phagocytosis, or ingestion and digestion, of foreign cells or particles. Two important phagocytes are neutrophils and monocytes (see Figure 12-9, p. 356). These blood phagocytes migrate out of the blood and into the tissues in response to an infection. The neutrophils

Figure 15-14

Effect of the complement cascade.

A, Complement molecules activated by antibodies form doughnut-shaped complexes in a bacterium's plasma membrane. **B,** Holes in the complement complex allow sodium (Na^+) and then water (H_2O) to diffuse into the bacterium. **C,** After enough water has entered, the swollen bacterium bursts.

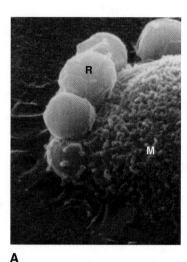

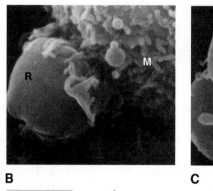

B

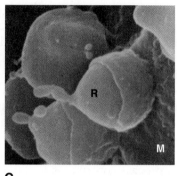

C

A

Figure 15-15 **Phagocytosis.**

This series of scanning electron micrographs shows the progressive steps in phagocytosis of damaged red blood cells (RBCs) by a macrophage. **A,** RBCs *(R)* attach to the macrophage *(M)*. **B,** Plasma membrane of the macrophage begins to enclose the RBC. **C,** The RBCs are almost totally ingested by the macrophage.

are functional but short-lived in the tissues. The pus found at some infection sites is mostly dead neutrophils. Once in the tissues, monocytes develop into phagocytic cells called **macrophages** (MAK-roh-fay-jes). Most macrophages then "wander" throughout the tissues to engulf bacteria wherever they find them.

Another type of phagocytic cell is called the **dendritic cell (DC).** These highly branched (*dendrite* "branch") cells are produced in bone marrow and are released into the bloodstream. Some remain in the blood but many migrate to tissues in contact with the external environment—the skin, respiratory lining, digestive lining, and so on.

Antibody molecules that bind to and coat certain foreign particles help macrophages function effectively. They serve as "flags" that alert the macrophage to the presence of foreign material, infectious bacteria, or cellular debris. They also help bind the phagocyte to the foreign material so that it can be engulfed more effectively (Figure 15-15).

Macrophages and DCs perform another important immune function besides destruction of threatening cells and particles. They also act as **antigen-presenting cells (APCs).** Macrophages and DCs ingest a cell or particle, remove its antigens, and display some of them on their cell surfaces. The displayed antigens can then be presented to other immune cells to trigger additional, specific immune responses.

Lymphocytes

The most numerous cells of the immune system are the lymphocytes; they are ultimately responsible for antibody production. Several million strong, lymphocytes continually patrol the body, searching out any enemy cells that may have entered. Lymphocytes circulate in the body's fluids. Huge numbers of them wander vigilantly through most of its tis-

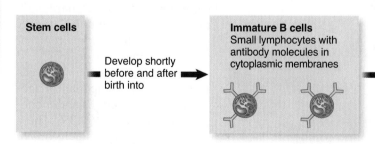

Stem cells

Develop shortly before and after birth into

Immature B cells
Small lymphocytes with antibody molecules in cytoplasmic membranes

Mature B cells migrate to lymph nodes, liver, and spleen; binding of antigen to antibody on surfaces of inactive B cells and chemical signal from T cells changes them into

sues. Lymphocytes densely populate the body's widely scattered lymph nodes and its other lymphatic tissues, especially the thymus gland in the chest and the spleen and the liver in the abdomen.

There are two major types of lymphocytes, sometimes designated as *B* and *T lymphocytes,* but usually called **B cells** and **T cells.** Each type of lymphocyte has a different set of roles to play in immunity.

DEVELOPMENT OF B CELLS

All lymphocytes that circulate in the tissues arise from primitive cells in the bone marrow called *stem cells* and go through two stages of development. The first stage of B-cell development, transformation of stem cells into immature B cells, occurs in the liver and bone marrow before birth but only in the bone marrow in adults. Because this process was first discovered in a bird organ called the *bursa,* these cells were named B cells.

Immature B cells are small lymphocytes that have each synthesized and inserted into their cytoplasmic membranes numerous molecules of one specific kind of antibody (Figure 15-16). After they mature, B cells eventually leave the tissue where they were formed. Each mature, but inactive, B cell carries a different type of antibody. The various B cells then enter the blood and are transported to their new place of residence, chiefly the lymph nodes.

The second stage of B-cell development changes a mature, inactive B cell into an activated B cell. Not all B cells undergo this change. They do so only if an inactive B cell comes into contact with certain nonself or abnormal molecules—antigens—whose shape fits the shape of the B cell's surface antibody molecules. If this happens, the antigens lock onto the antibodies and by so doing change the inactive B cell into an activated B cell. B-cell activation also requires a chemical signal from another immune cell—a type of T cell. Then the activated B cell, by dividing rapidly and repeatedly, develops into clones of many identical cells—all having the same type of antibody. A **clone** is a family of many identical cells, all descended from one cell.

Each clone of B cells is made up of two kinds of cells, **plasma cells** (also called **effector cells**) and **memory cells,** as you can see in Figure 15-16. Plasma cells secrete huge amounts of antibody into the blood—reportedly 2000 antibody molecules per second by each plasma cell for every second of the few days that it lives. Antibodies circulating in the blood constitute an enormous, mobile, ever-on-duty army.

Memory cells can secrete antibodies but do not immediately do so. They remain in reserve in the lymph nodes until they are contacted by the same antigen that led to their formation. Then, very quickly, the memory cells develop into plasma cells and secrete large amounts of antibody. Memory cells, in effect, seem to remember their ancestor activated B cell's encounter with its appropriate antigen. They stand ready, at a moment's notice, to produce antibody that will combine with this antigen.

FUNCTION OF B CELLS

B cells function indirectly to produce humoral immunity. Recall that **humoral immunity** is resistance

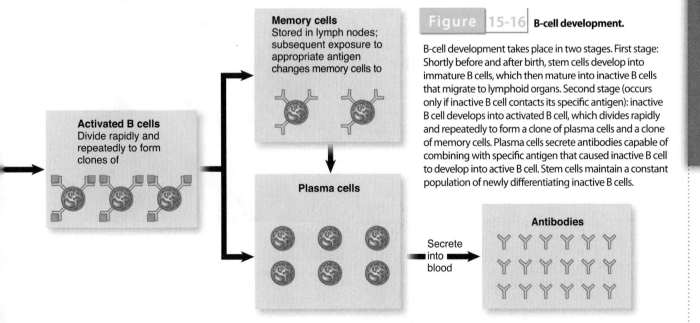

Figure 15-16 B-cell development.

B-cell development takes place in two stages. First stage: Shortly before and after birth, stem cells develop into immature B cells, which then mature into inactive B cells that migrate to lymphoid organs. Second stage (occurs only if inactive B cell contacts its specific antigen): inactive B cell develops into activated B cell, which divides rapidly and repeatedly to form a clone of plasma cells and a clone of memory cells. Plasma cells secrete antibodies capable of combining with specific antigen that caused inactive B cell to develop into active B cell. Stem cells maintain a constant population of newly differentiating inactive B cells.

Memory cells
Stored in lymph nodes; subsequent exposure to appropriate antigen changes memory cells to

Activated B cells
Divide rapidly and repeatedly to form clones of

Plasma cells

Antibodies

Secrete into blood

Figure 15-17 **T-cell development.**

The first stage takes place in the thymus gland shortly before and after birth. Stem cells maintain a constant population of newly differentiating cells as they are needed. The second stage occurs only if a T cell contacts antigen, which combines with certain proteins on the T cell's surface.

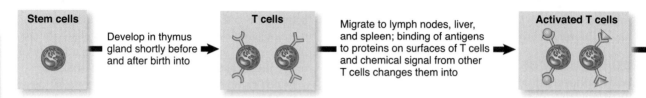

Stem cells → Develop in thymus gland shortly before and after birth into → **T cells** → Migrate to lymph nodes, liver, and spleen; binding of antigens to proteins on surfaces of T cells and chemical signal from other T cells changes them into → **Activated T cells**

to disease organisms produced by the actions of antibodies binding to specific antigens while circulating in body fluids. Activated B cells develop into plasma cells. Plasma cells secrete antibodies into the blood; they are the "antibody factories" of the body. These antibodies, like other proteins manufactured for extracellular use, are formed on the endoplasmic reticulum of the cell.

DEVELOPMENT OF T CELLS

T cells are lymphocytes that have undergone their first stage of development in the thymus gland. Stem cells from the bone marrow seed the thymus, and shortly before and after birth, they develop into T cells. The newly formed T cells stream out of the thymus into the blood and migrate chiefly to the lymph nodes, where they take up residence. Embedded in each T cell's cytoplasmic membrane are protein molecules shaped to fit only one specific kind of antigen molecule.

The second stage of T-cell development takes place when and if a T cell comes into contact with its specific antigen. If this happens, the antigen binds to the protein on the T cell's surface, thereby changing the T cell into an activated T cell (Figure 15-17). As with B cells, T cells must also receive a chemical signal from another T cell to become activated. Likewise, T cells also produce a clone of identical cells, all able to react with the same antigen. And as with B cells, T cells form a group of *effector cells* along with *memory cells*. The effector T cells actively engage in immune responses, whereas the memory T cells do not. Later, if more effector T cells are needed, the memory T cells can produce additional clones that include more effector T cells.

FUNCTIONS OF T CELLS

Activated T cells produce cell-mediated immunity. As the name suggests, **cell-mediated immunity** is

resistance to disease organisms resulting from the actions of cells—chiefly activated T cells. Some activated T cells kill infected cells and tumor cells directly (Figure 15-18). When bound to antigens, these *cytotoxic* (sye-toh-TOK-sik) *T cells* release a substance that acts as a specific and lethal poison against the abnormal cell.

Activated T cells called *helper T cells* produce their deadly effects indirectly by means of compounds that they release into the area around enemy cells. Among these is a substance that attracts macrophages into the neighborhood of the enemy cells. The as-

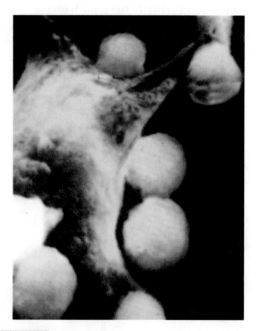

Figure 15-18 **T cells.**

The blue spheres seen in this scanning electron microscope view are T cells attacking a much larger cancer cell. The cells are a significant part of our defense against cancer and other types of foreign cells.

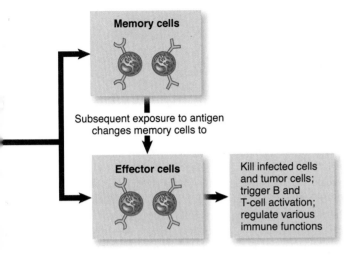

sembled macrophages then destroy the cells by phagocytosing (ingesting and digesting) them (Figure 15-19). Helper T cells also release the chemicals needed to help trigger the activation of B cells. Activated *regulatory T cells* help shut down an immune reaction after the antigens have been destroyed and also help prevent inappropriate immune reactions.

QUICK CHECK

1. What are *phagocytes?* How do they work?
2. What is the role of *B cells* in immunity?
3. What is the role of *T cells* in immunity?
4. What are memory cells?

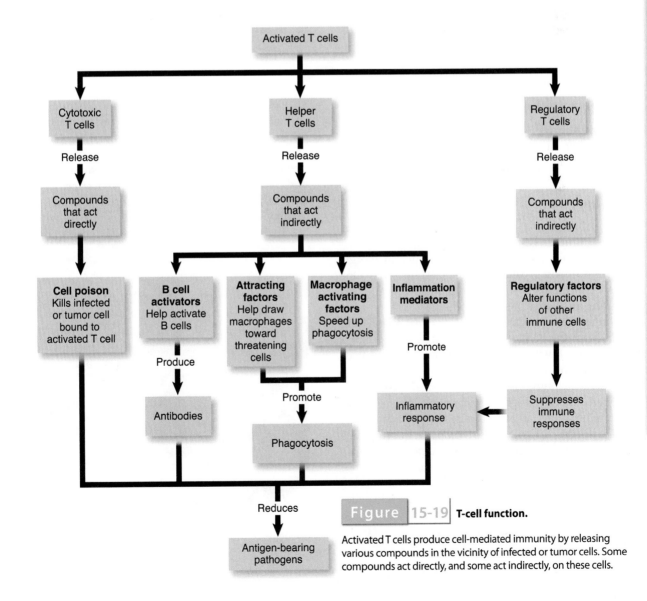

Figure 15-19 **T-cell function.**

Activated T cells produce cell-mediated immunity by releasing various compounds in the vicinity of infected or tumor cells. Some compounds act directly, and some act indirectly, on these cells.

RESEARCH, ISSUES, AND TRENDS

MUCOSAL IMMUNITY

The mucosal immune system is a complex system of defense distinct from the systemic (internal) immune system that we have been discussing in most of this chapter. It is an innate (nonspecific) and adaptive (specific) system that is found within the mucous barriers of the body: digestive tract, urinary/reproductive tracts, respiratory tract, exocrine ducts, conjunctiva (eye covering), middle ear, and so on. The immune cells that make up the mucosal immune system are located mainly in or near mucosal-associated lymphoid tissue (MALT).

The main functions of the mucosal immune system involve preventing pathogens from colonizing the mucous surfaces of the body, preventing the accidental absorption of antigens from outside the body, and preventing inappro-

priate or intense responses of the systemic immune system to these external antigens.

Understanding the mucosal immune system and its cooperation with the systemic (internal) immune system promises to reveal new strategies of immunization. For example, researchers have found that immunizing through the bloodstream activates only the internal (systemic) B cells and T cells. Thus a pathogen would have to actually enter the internal environment before this type of specific immunity could protect us. Immunization of the mucosal lymphocytes, however, can activate both mucosal and systemic lymphocytes—providing a more thorough type of protection. Another advantage of mucosal immunization is that it is easier to administer to patients than immunizations injected under the skin or into the bloodstream. For example, immunization can be delivered by nasal sprays or drops instead of "shots."

Hypersensitivity of the Immune System

Hypersensitivity (hye-per-sen-si-TIV-i-tee) is an inappropriate or excessive response of the immune system. There are three types: allergy, autoimmunity, and isoimmunity.

Allergy

The term **allergy** is used to describe hypersensitivity of the immune system to relatively harmless environmental antigens. Antigens that trigger an allergic response are often called **allergens** (AL-ler-jenz). One in six Americans has a genetic predisposition to exhibiting an allergy of some kind.

Immediate allergic responses involve antigen-antibody reactions. Before such a reaction occurs, a susceptible person must be exposed to an allergen repeatedly—triggering the production of antibodies. After a person is thus *sensitized,* exposure to an allergen causes antigen-antibody reactions that trigger the release of histamine, kinins, and other inflammatory substances. These responses usually cause typical allergy symptoms such as runny nose, conjunctivitis, and *urticaria* (hives). In some cases, however, these substances may cause constriction of the airways, relaxation of blood vessels, and irregular heart rhythms that can progress to a life-threatening condition called *anaphylactic shock* (see Chapter 14). Drugs called *antihistamines* are sometimes used to relieve the symptoms of this type of allergy.

Delayed allergic responses, on the other hand, involve cell-mediated immunity. In **contact dermatitis,** for example, T cells trigger events that lead to local skin inflammation a few hours or days after initial exposure to an antigen. Exposure to poison ivy, soaps, and certain cosmetics may cause contact dermatitis in this manner (Figure 15-20). Hypersensitive individuals may use *hypoallergenic* products (products without common allergens) to avoid such allergic reactions.

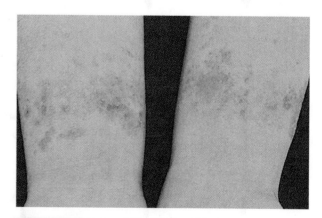

Figure 15-20 | **Contact dermatitis.**

Dermatitis, or skin inflammation, can result from contact with allergens—substances that trigger allergic responses in hypersensitive individuals.

To learn more about allergic response, go to **AnimationDirect** on your CD.

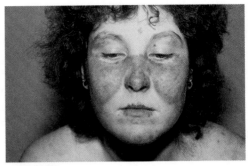

Figure 15-21 **Lupus erythematosus.**

A red "butterfly" rash on the face is sometimes seen in cases of systemic lupus erythematosus (SLE).

Autoimmunity

Autoimmunity (aw-toh-im-YOO-ni-tee) is an inappropriate and excessive response to self-antigens. Disorders that result from autoimmune responses are called *autoimmune diseases.* Examples of autoimmune diseases are given in Appendix B on the CD that accompanies your book. Self-antigens are molecules that are native to a person's body and that are used by the immune system to identify components of "self." Self-antigens can also be segments of a person's genetic material (DNA or RNA) or certain proteins or other chemicals made in the body. In autoimmunity, the immune system inappropriately attacks these antigens.

A common autoimmune disease is **systemic lupus erythematosus (SLE),** or simply *lupus.* Lupus is a chronic inflammatory disease that affects many tissues in the body: joints, blood vessels, kidneys, nervous system, and skin. The name *lupus erythematosus* refers to the red rash that often develops on the face of those afflicted with SLE (Figure 15-21). The "systemic" part of the name comes from the fact that the disease affects many systems throughout the body. The systemic nature of SLE results from the production of antibodies against many different self-antigens.

Isoimmunity

Isoimmunity (eye-so-im-YOO-ni-tee) is excessive reaction of the immune system to antigens from a different individual of the same species. It is important in relation to pregnancy and tissue transplants.

During pregnancy, antigens from the fetus may enter the mother's blood supply and sensitize her immune system. Antibodies that are formed as a result of this sensitization may enter the fetal circulation and cause an inappropriate immune reaction. One example, erythroblastosis fetalis, was discussed in Chapter 12. Other pathological conditions also may be caused by damage to developing fetal tissues resulting from attack by the mother's immune system. Examples include congenital heart defects, Graves disease, and myasthenia gravis.

Tissue or organ **transplants** are medical procedures in which tissue from a donor is surgically *grafted* into the body. For example, skin grafts are often done to repair damage caused by burns. Donated whole blood tissue is often transfused into a recipi-

ent after massive hemorrhaging. A kidney is sometimes removed from a living donor and grafted into a person suffering from kidney failure. Unfortunately, the immune system sometimes reacts against foreign antigens present in the grafted tissue, causing what is often called a *rejection syndrome.* The antigens most commonly involved in transplant rejection are called **human lymphocyte antigens (HLAs).**

Rejection of grafted tissues can occur in two ways. One is called *host-versus-graft rejection* because the recipient's immune system recognizes foreign HLAs and attacks them, destroying the donated tissue. The other is *graft-versus-host rejection* because the donated tissue (for example, bone marrow) attacks the recipient's HLAs, destroying tissue throughout the recipient's body. Graft-versus-host rejection may lead to death.

There are two ways to prevent rejection syndrome. One strategy is called *tissue typing,* in which HLAs and other antigens of a potential donor and recipient are identified. If they match, tissue rejection is unlikely to occur. Another strategy is the use of **immunosuppressive** (im-yoo-no-su-PRES-iv) **drugs** in the recipient. Immunosuppressive drugs such as *cyclosporine* and *prednisone* suppress the immune system's ability to attack the foreign antigens in the donated tissue.

QUICK CHECK

1. What is an *allergen?* How does it affect the immune system?
2. Why is *lupus* called an "autoimmune disorder"?
3. Why are immunosuppressive drugs given to organ transplant recipients?

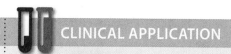

CLINICAL APPLICATION

INTERFERON

Interferons (in-ter-FEER-onz) **(IFs)** are small proteins produced most often by body cells in response to viral infections. IFs play a significant role in producing nonspecific (innate) immunity to many viruses. Groups of IFs designated as alphas, betas, and omegas all have unique biological activity and are being used more and more often in clinical medicine. One IF is produced by T cells within hours after they have been infected by a virus. This IF, when released from the T cells, protects other cells by interfering with the ability of the virus to reproduce as it moves from cell to cell. In the past, thousands of pints of blood had to be processed to harvest tiny quantities of leukocyte (T cell) IF for study.

Currently, different synthetic types of both human and non-naturally occurring IFs are being "manufactured" in bacteria as a result of gene-splicing techniques and are available in quantities sufficient for clinical use. Synthetic IF decreases the severity of many virus-related diseases including chickenpox, measles, and hepatitis. IF also shows promise as an anticancer agent. It has been shown to be effective in treating breast, skin, and other forms of cancer.

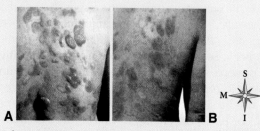

Interferon treatment. **A,** Cancerous skin tumors of Kaposi sarcoma (KS). **B,** After treatment with alpha interferon, the KS tumors have been reduced.

CLINICAL APPLICATION

IMMUNIZATION

Active immunity can be established artificially by using a technique called *vaccination*. The original vaccine was a live cowpox virus that was injected into healthy people to cause a mild cowpox infection. The term **vaccine** literally means "cow substance." Because the cowpox virus is similar to the deadly *smallpox* virus, vaccinated individuals developed antibodies that imparted immunity against both cowpox and smallpox viruses.

Modern vaccines work on a similar principle; substances that trigger the formation of antibodies against specific pathogens are introduced orally or by injection. Some of these vaccines are killed pathogens; some are live, attenuated (weakened) pathogens. Such pathogens still have their specific antigens intact, so they can trigger formation of the proper antibodies, but they are no longer *virulent* (able to cause disease). Although it is rare, these vaccines sometimes backfire and actually cause an infection. Many of the newer vaccines get around this potential problem by using only the part of the pathogen that contains antigens. Because the disease-causing portion is missing, such vaccines cannot cause infection.

The amount of antibodies in a person's blood produced in response to vaccination or an actual infection is called the *antibody titer*. As you can see in the graph, the initial injection of vaccine triggers a rise in the antibody titer that gradually diminishes. Often, a *booster shot,* or second injection, is given to keep the antibody titer high or to raise it to a level that is more likely to prevent infection. The secondary response is more intense than the primary response because memory B cells are standing ready to produce a large number of antibodies at a moment's notice. A later accidental exposure to the pathogen will trigger an even more intense response—thus preventing infection.

Toxoids are similar to vaccines but use an altered form of a bacterial toxin (poisonous chemical) to stimulate production of antibodies. Injection of toxoids imparts protection against toxins, whereas administration of vaccines imparts protection against pathogenic organisms and viruses.

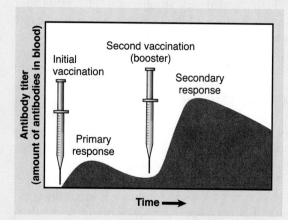

Immune System Deficiency

Immune deficiency, or *immunodeficiency,* is the failure of immune system mechanisms in defending against pathogens. Immune system failure usually results from disruption of lymphocyte (B or T cell) function. The chief characteristic of immune deficiency is the development of unusual or recurring severe infections or cancer. Although immune deficiency by itself does not cause death, the resulting infections or cancer can. There are two broad categories of immune deficiencies, based on the mechanism of lymphocyte dysfunction: *congenital* and *acquired.*

Congenital Immune Deficiency

Congenital immune deficiency, which is rare, results from improper lymphocyte development before birth. Depending on the stage of development of stem cells (B or T cells) during which the defect occurs, different diseases can result. For example, improper B-cell development can cause insufficiency or absence of antibodies in the blood. If stem cells are disrupted, a condition called **severe combined immune deficiency (SCID)** results. In most forms of SCID, humoral immunity and cell-mediated immunity are defective. Temporary immunity can be imparted to children with SCID by injecting them with a preparation of antibodies (gamma globulin). Bone marrow transplants, which replace the defective stem cells with healthy donor cells, have proved effective in treating some cases of SCID. Advances in using gene therapy also have been made in treating SCID patients (see discussion of gene therapy on pp. 678-681 in Chapter 24).

Acquired Immune Deficiency

Acquired immune deficiency develops after birth and is not related to genetic defects. A number of factors can contribute to acquired immune deficiency: nutritional deficiencies, immunosuppressive drugs or other medical treatments, trauma, stress, and viral infection.

One of the best known examples of acquired immune deficiency is **acquired immunodeficiency syndrome (AIDS).** AIDS was first recognized as a disease by the Centers for Disease Control and Prevention (CDC) in 1981. This syndrome (collection of symptoms) is caused by the human immunodeficiency virus, or HIV. HIV, a retrovirus, contains RNA that undergoes reverse transcription inside affected cells to form its own DNA. The viral DNA often becomes part of the cell's DNA. When the viral DNA is activated, it directs the synthesis of its own RNA and protein coat, thus "stealing" raw materials from the cell. When this occurs in certain T cells, the cell is destroyed and immunity is impaired. As the T cell dies, it releases new retroviruses that can spread the HIV infection.

Although HIV can invade several types of cells, it has its most obvious effects in a certain type of T cell called a CD4+ T cell. When T-cell function is impaired, infectious organisms and cancer cells can grow and spread much more easily than normal. Unusual conditions, such as *pneumocystosis* (a protozoan infection) and *Kaposi sarcoma,* or *KS* (a type of skin cancer), may also appear. Because their immune systems are deficient, AIDS patients usually die from one of these infections or cancers.

After infection with HIV, a person may not show signs of AIDS for months or years. This is because the immune system can hold the infection at bay for a long time before finally succumbing to it.

There are several strategies for controlling AIDS. Many agencies are trying to slow the spread of AIDS by educating people about how to avoid contact with the HIV retrovirus. HIV is spread by means of direct contact of body fluids, so preventing such contact reduces HIV transmission. Sexual relations, contaminated blood transfusions, and intravenous use of contaminated needles are common modes of HIV transmission. HIV can also be a **perinatal infection,** that is, an infection passing from mother to infant during birth. Many researchers are working on HIV vaccines. Like many viruses, such as those that cause the common cold, HIV changes rapidly enough to make development of a vaccine difficult at best.

Another way to inhibit the disease is by means of chemicals such as azidothymidine (AZT) and ritonavir (Norvir) that block HIV's ability to reproduce within infected cells. A breakthrough in the treatment of HIV came a few years ago when it was discovered that a "cocktail" of several antiviral drugs working together greatly reduced the number of virus particles in a patient's blood. More than a hundred such compounds in various combinations are being evaluated for use in halting the progress of HIV infections.

QUICK CHECK

1. What is the difference between *congenital* and *acquired* immune deficiency?
2. What causes AIDS?

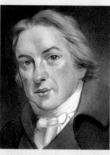

Edward Jenner (1749–1823).

VACCINES

English surgeon Edward Jenner changed the world forever in 1789 when he inoculated his young son and two others against the terrible viral disease, smallpox. Using material from the blisters of a patient with the milder disease swinepox, he was able to trigger immunity to smallpox—the world's first vaccination. Later, in 1796, he found that vaccination with material from cowpox blisters worked even better in protecting people from smallpox. A disease that had formerly killed millions upon millions of people worldwide even-

tually disappeared from the human population in the 20th century because of Jenner's pioneering efforts.

In this century, interest in smallpox vaccinations has resurfaced because of the threat of smallpox as a weapon. Immunologists are at work improving on this important vaccine to protect people against such weapons; they also continue to work on vaccines for other infectious diseases such as AIDS and even disorders such as heart disease and cancer. Many health professionals use vaccines in their practice, of course, to boost the immune systems of their clients. Many physicians also treat disorders of the immune system itself. For example, immune deficiencies such as AIDS, allergies such as "hay fever," and autoimmune disorders such as lupus and rheumatoid arthritis, are treated every day by physicians and other health professionals..

Outline Summary

To download an MP3 version of the chapter summary for use with your iPod or portable media player, access the **Audio Chapter Summaries** on your CD.

The Lymphatic System

A. Lymph—fluid in the tissue spaces that carries protein molecules and other substances back to the blood
B. Lymphatic vessels—permit only one-way movement of lymph (Figure 15-1)
  1. Lymphatic capillaries—tiny blind-ended tubes distributed in tissue spaces (Figure 15-2)
    a. Microscopic in size
    b. Sheets consisting of one cell layer of simple squamous epithelium
    c. Poor "fit" between adjacent cells results in porous walls
    d. Called *lacteals* in the intestinal wall (fat transportation from food to bloodstream)

2. Right lymphatic duct
  a. Drains lymph from the right upper extremity and right side of head, neck, and upper torso
3. Thoracic duct
  a. Largest lymphatic vessel
  b. Has an enlarged pouch along its course, called *cisterna chyli*
  c. Drains lymph from about three fourths of the body (Figure 15-3)
C. Lymphedema—swelling (edema) of tissues caused by blockage of lymphatic vessels (Figure 15-4)
  1. Lymphangitis—inflammation of lymphatic vessels, may progress to septicemia (blood infection) (Figure 15-5)

2. Elephantiasis—severe lymphedema of limbs resulting from parasite infestation of lymphatic vessels (Figure 15-6)
D. Lymph nodes
1. Filter lymph (Figure 15-7)
2. Located in clusters along the pathway of lymphatic vessels (Figure 15-8 and 15-9)
3. Lymphoid tissue—mass of lymphocytes and related cells inside a lymphoid organ; provides immune function and development of immune cells
4. Lymph nodes and other lymphoid organs have functions that include defense and WBC formation
5. Flow of lymph: to node via several afferent lymphatic vessels and drained from node by a single efferent lymphatic vessel
6. Lymphadenitis—swelling and tenderness of lymph nodes
7. Cancer cells can easily move through lymphatic vessels to other parts of the body in a process called metastasis (Figure 15-10)
E. Lymphoma—malignant tumor of lymph nodes
1. Two principal types: Hodgkin disease and non-Hodgkin lymphoma
2. All types cause painless enlargement of lymph nodes
3. Can spread to many other areas of the body
F. Thymus
1. Lymphoid tissue organ located in mediastinum
2. Total weight of about 35-40 g—a little more than an ounce
3. Plays a vital and central role in immunity
4. Produces T lymphocytes, or T cells
5. Secretes hormone called *thymosin*
6. Lymphoid tissue is largely replaced by fat in the process called *involution*
G. Tonsils (Figure 15-11)
1. Composed of three masses of lymphoid tissue around the openings of the mouth and throat
   a. Palatine tonsils ("the tonsils")
   b. Pharyngeal tonsils (also known as *adenoids*)
   c. Lingual tonsils
2. Subject to chronic infection
3. Enlargement of pharyngeal tonsils may impair breathing
H. Spleen
1. Largest lymphoid organ in body
2. Located in upper left quadrant of abdomen
3. Often injured by trauma to abdomen
4. Surgical removal called *splenectomy*
5. Functions include phagocytosis of bacteria and old RBCs; acts as a blood reservoir
6. Splenomegaly—enlargement of the spleen

The Immune System

A. Protects body from pathological bacteria, foreign tissue cells, and cancerous cells
B. Made up of defensive cells and molecules (Table 15-1)
C. Nonspecific immunity
1. Skin—mechanical barrier to bacteria and other harmful agents
2. Tears and mucus—wash eyes and trap and kill bacteria
3. Inflammation attracts immune cells to site of injury, increases local blood flow, increases vascular permeability; promotes movement of WBCs to site of injury or infection (Figure 15-12)
D. Specific immunity—ability of body to recognize, respond to, and remember harmful substances or bacteria (Table 15-2)
1. Inherited, or inborn immunity—inherited immunity to certain diseases from birth
2. Acquired immunity
   a. Natural immunity—exposure to causative agent is not deliberate
      (1) Active—active disease produces immunity
      (2) Passive—immunity passes from mother to fetus through placenta or

from mother to child through mother's milk
   b. Artificial immunity—exposure to causative agent is deliberate
      (1) Active—vaccination results in immunity
      (2) Passive—protective material developed in another individual's immune system and given to previously nonimmune individual

Immune System Molecules

A. Antibodies (Figure 15-13)
   1. Protein compounds with specific combining sites
   2. Combining sites attach antibodies to specific antigens (foreign proteins), forming an antigen-antibody complex—called *humoral,* or *antibody-mediated, immunity*
   3. Antigen-antibody complexes may:
      a. Neutralize toxins
      b. Clump or agglutinate enemy cells
      c. Promote phagocytosis
B. Complement proteins
   1. Group of proteins normally present in blood in inactive state
   2. Complement cascade
      a. Important mechanism of action for antibodies
         (1) Complement-binding sites on antibody are exposed after attaching to antigen
         (2) Complement triggers a series (cascade) of reactions that produce

tiny protein rings that create holes in the surface of a foreign cell
      b. Ultimately causes cell lysis by permitting entry of water through a defect created in the plasma membrane of the foreign cell (Figure 15-14)
   3. Complement proteins play many other roles in immunity, including the inflammatory response

Immune System Cells

A. **Phagocytes**
   1. Types
      a. Neutrophils—short-lived phagocytic cells
      b. Monocytes—develop into phagocytic macrophages and migrate to tissues (Figure 15-15)
      c. Dendritic cells (DCs)—often found at or near external surfaces
   2. Ingest and destroy foreign cells or other harmful substances via phagocytosis
   3. Macrophages and DCs act as antigen-presenting cells (APCs) by displaying ingested antigens on their outer surface to trigger specific immune cells
B. Lymphocytes
   1. Most numerous of immune system cells
   2. Development of B cells—primitive stem cells migrate from bone marrow and go through two stages of development (Figure 15-16)
      a. First stage—stem cells develop into immature B cells

(1) Takes place in the liver and bone marrow before birth and in the bone marrow only in adults

(2) B cells are small lymphocytes with antibody molecules (which they have synthesized) in their plasma membranes

(3) After they mature, inactive B cells migrate chiefly to lymph nodes

  b. Second stage—inactive B cell develops into activated B cell

(1) Initiated by inactive B cell's contact with antigens, which bind to its surface antibodies, plus signal chemicals from T cells

(2) Activated B cell, by dividing repeatedly, forms two clones of cells—plasma (effector) cells and memory cells

(3) Plasma cells secrete antibodies into blood; memory cells are stored in lymph nodes

(4) If subsequent exposure to antigen that activated B cell occurs, memory cells become plasma cells and secrete antibodies

3. Function of B cells—indirectly, B cells produce humoral immunity

  a. Activated B cells develop into plasma cells

  b. Plasma cells secrete antibodies into the blood

  c. Circulating antibodies produce humoral immunity (Figure 15-16)

4. Development of T cells—stem cells from bone marrow migrate to thymus gland (Figure 15-17)

  a. First stage—stem cells develop into T cells

(1) Occurs in thymus during few months before and after birth

(2) T cells migrate chiefly to lymph nodes

  b. Second stage—T cells develop into activated T cells

(1) Occurs when, and if, antigen binds to T cell's surface proteins and a chemical signal is received from another T cell

(2) As with B cells, clones made up of effector cells and memory cells are formed

5. Functions of T cells—produce cell-mediated immunity (Figures 15-18 and 15-19)

  a. Cytotoxic T cells—kill infected or tumor cells by releasing a substance that poisons infe cted or tumor cells

  b. Helper T cells—release chemicals that attract and activate macrophages to kill cells by phagocytosis; produce chemicals that help activate B cells

  c. Regulatory T cells—release chemicals to suppress immune responses

Hypersensitivity of the Immune System

A. Hypersensitivity—inappropriate or excessive immune response (Figure 15-20)

B. Allergy—hypersensitivity to harmless environmental antigens (allergens)
   1. Immediate allergic responses usually involve humoral immunity
   2. Delayed allergic responses usually involve cell-mediated immunity
C. Autoimmunity—inappropriate, excessive response to self-antigens
   1. Causes autoimmune diseases
   2. Systemic lupus erythematosus (SLE)—chronic inflammatory disease caused by numerous antibodies attacking a variety of tissues (Figure 15-21)
D. Isoimmunity—excessive reaction to antigens from another human
   1. May occur between mother and fetus during pregnancy
   2. May occur in tissue transplants (causing rejection syndrome)

Immune System Deficiency

A. Congenital immune deficiency, or immunodeficiency (rare)
   1. Results from improper lymphocyte development before birth
   2. Severe combined immune deficiency (SCID)—caused by disruption of stem cell development
B. Acquired immune deficiency
   1. Develops after birth
   2. Acquired immunodeficiency syndrome (AIDS)—caused by HIV infection of T cells

New Words

afferent	humoral immunity	autoimmunity	lymphedema
antibody-mediated (humoral) immunity	interferon (IF)	contact dermatitis	monoclonal antibody
	lymph	elephantiasis	non-Hodgkin lymphoma
antigen-presenting cell (APC)	macrophage	Hodgkin disease	perinatal infection
B cell (B lymphocyte)	memory cell	human lymphocyte antigen (HLA)	severe combined immune deficiency (SCID)
cell-mediated immunity	plasma cell (effector B cell)	hybridoma	splenectomy
cisterna chyli	T cell (T lymphocyte)	hypersensitivity	splenomegaly
clone		immune deficiency	systemic lupus erythematosus (SLE)
combining site	**Diseases and Other Clinical Terms**	immunosuppressive drug	tonsillitis
complement		inflammatory response	transplant
complement-binding site	acquired immunodeficiency syndrome (AIDS)	isoimmunity	vaccine
complement cascade	allergen	lymphadenitis	
dendritic cell (DC)	allergy	lymphangitis	
efferent			

Review Questions

1. Define *lymph* and explain its function.
2. Name the two major lymphatic ducts and the areas of the body each of them drains.
3. Describe the structure of a lymph node.
4. What is lymphedema? What is the cause of elephantiasis?
5. Explain the defense function of the lymph node.
6. Where is the thymus gland? What are its functions?
7. Name the three pairs of tonsils and give the location of each.
8. Give the location and function of the spleen.
9. Explain the types of nonspecific immunity.
10. Name and differentiate the four types of specific immunity.
11. What are antibodies? What are antigens?
12. Explain the role of complement in the immune system.
13. Explain the role of the macrophage in the immune system.
14. Explain the development and functioning of B cells.
15. Explain the development and functioning of T cells.
16. What is an allergy?
17. What is autoimmunity? Give an example of an autoimmune disease.
18. What is isoimmunity? Give an example of an isoimmunity disorder.
19. What are HLAs? How are they related to tissue typing?
20. What is SCID? What is its cause?
21. List three causes of acquired immunodeficiency syndrome.

Critical Thinking

22. Differentiate between lymphatic capillaries and blood capillaries. Explain how the different structures relate to their function.
23. Explain the role of the lymph node in the spread of cancer.
24. Explain the difference in mechanisms in the development of the allergic reaction of runny nose and hives, and the allergic reaction to poison ivy.

Chapter Test

1. _____ is the fluid that leaves the blood capillaries and is not directly returned to the blood.
2. Lymph from about three fourths of the body drains into the _____.
3. Lymph from the right upper extremity and the right side of the head drains into the _____.
4. An abnormal condition in which tissue swells because of accumulation of lymph is called _____.
5. The enlarged, pouchlike structure in the abdomen that serves as a storage area for lymph is called the _____.
6. The function of the _____ is to filter and clean the lymph.
7. The many lymphatic vessels that enter the lymph node are called _____ vessels; the single vessel leaving the lymph node is called the _____ vessel.
8. The _____ are white blood cells that mature in the thymus. The thymus also produces a hormone called _____.
9. The three pairs of tonsils are the _____, _____, and _____.
10. The largest lymphoid organ is the _____.
11. The signs of _____ are heat, redness, pain, and swelling.
12. _____ kills target cells by drilling holes in their plasma membrane, which disrupts the sodium and water balance.
13. Macrophages were originally _____ that migrated into the tissues.
14. A hypersensitivity of the immune system to a harmless environmental antigen is called an _____.
15. An extreme allergic reaction causing life-threatening symptoms is called _____.
16. An inappropriate and excessive response to self-antigen is called _____.
17. Erythroblastosis is an example of what excessive immune reaction? _____
18. An attempt to identify and match HLAs between the organ donor and the recipient is called _____.
19. A congenital immune deficiency in which both humoral and cellular immunity are defective is called _____.
20. The cause of AIDS is _____.

21. The immunity that develops against polio after receiving a polio vaccination is an example of:
    a. active natural immunity
    b. passive natural immunity
    c. active artificial immunity
    d. passive artificial immunity

22. The immunity that is given to the fetus or newborn by the immune system of the mother is an example of:
    a. active natural immunity
    b. passive natural immunity
    c. active artificial immunity
    d. passive artificial immunity

23. The immunity that comes from the injection of antibodies made by another individual's immune system is an example of:
    a. active natural immunity
    b. passive natural immunity
    c. active artificial immunity
    d. passive artificial immunity

24. The immunity that develops after a person has had a disease is an example of:
    a. active natural immunity
    b. passive natural immunity
    c. active artificial immunity
    d. passive artificial immunity

For each of the following phrases, write a *B* in front of it if it describes the development or functioning of a B cell or write a *T* in front of it if it describes the development or functioning of a T cell.

25. _____ produces antibodies
26. _____ some develop into plasma cells
27. _____ the main cell involved in cell-mediated immunity
28. _____ the main cell involved in humoral immunity
29. _____ develops in the thymus gland
30. _____ moves to the site of the antigen and releases cell poison
31. _____ divides rapidly into clones once it is activated
32. _____ releases a substance that attracts macrophages
33. _____ some differentiate into memory cells
34. _____ mediates the contact dermatitis allergic response

Study Tips

continued from page 421

depending on how involved the body's immune system was in developing the response.

4. The natural, active immune response is divided into humoral immunity and cell-mediated immunity. Humoral immunity is mediated by the B lymphocytes or B cells. They stay in the lymph node and secrete antibodies into the blood (*humor* means "body fluid"). They also form memory cells, which give lifelong immunity. T lymphocytes or T cells provide cell-mediated immunity. They leave the lymph node and actively engage the antigen.

5. The best way to learn the disorders of the immune system is to make a chart organized by the mechanism or cause of the disorder: allergic reaction, autoimmunity, isoimmunity, and immune deficiencies.

6. In your study group, use flash cards to quiz each other on the terms and structures of the lymphatic and immune systems. Discuss the process of how lymph is formed, filtered, and returned to the blood. Discuss nonspecific immunity, especially the inflammation response. Discuss the different types of specific immunity. Discuss the steps in humoral and cell-mediated immunity. Go over the disorder chart and the questions at the end of the chapter and discuss possible test questions.

Case Studies

1. After having an infection in the groin, a young boy complains of painful swelling in his leg. On examination, you see that the entire leg is swollen, but the opposite leg is fine. The attending physician explains that this is a complication of the recent groin infection, which involved the lymph nodes in that area. Can you explain how this may have caused the boy's leg to swell? Why isn't the other leg affected?

2. Keith was sledding in the snow with his friends when he accidentally hit a tree. After examining Keith, the emergency room physician concluded that he had ruptured his spleen in the accident. How might a ruptured spleen be treated? What might happen if Keith's family or physician delays this treatment? Does Keith need his spleen to survive?

3. Many years ago there was a famous case of a boy born with severe combined immune deficiency (SCID). His physicians placed him in a pathogen-free chamber that resembled a giant glass bubble. What purpose was served by doing this? What treatments are available today that might have helped this boy?

Outline

Objectives

After you have completed this chapter, you should be able to:

1. Discuss the generalized functions of the respiratory system.

2. List the major organs of the respiratory system and describe the function of each.

3. Compare, contrast, and explain the mechanism responsible for the exchange of gases that occurs during internal and external respiration.

4. List and discuss the volumes of air exchanged during pulmonary ventilation.

5. Identify and discuss the mechanisms that regulate respiration.

6. Identify and describe the major disorders of the upper respiratory tract.

7. Identify and describe the major disorders of the lower respiratory tract.

16 The Respiratory System

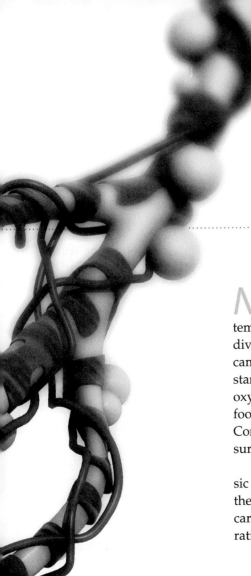
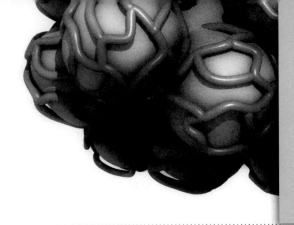

No one needs to be told how important the **respiratory system** is. The respiratory system serves the body much as a lifeline to an oxygen tank serves a scuba diver. Think how panicked you would feel if suddenly your lifeline became blocked—if you could not breathe for a few seconds! Of all the substances that cells and therefore the body as a whole must have to survive, oxygen is by far the most crucial. A person can live a few weeks without food, a few days without water, but only a few minutes without oxygen. Constant removal of carbon dioxide from the body is just as important for survival as a constant supply of oxygen.

The organs of the respiratory system are designed to perform two basic functions; they serve as an *air distributor* and as a *gas exchanger* for the body. The respiratory system ensures that oxygen is supplied to and carbon dioxide is removed from the body's cells. The process of respiration therefore is an important **homeostatic mechanism.** By constantly

STUDY TIPS

Before beginning your study of Chapter 16, review the synopsis of the respiratory system in Chapter 3. The structures of the respiratory system can be described as tubes and bags. All the structures except the alveoli are tubes. Their job is to get air to and from the alveoli, where oxygen and carbon dioxide are exchanged in the blood.

1. Flash cards can be used to learn the names, locations, and functions of the structures of the respiratory system.

2. Lungs are passive organs. Remember that in order for air to be moved in and out of the lung, the pressure of the chest cavity must be raised or lowered. To lower the pressure, the volume must increase (Boyle's law); this is done by contracting the diaphragm, which causes air to enter the lung. When the diaphragm relaxes, the volume of the chest cavity decreases, the pressure goes up, and the air is pushed out of the lung.

3. When oxygen gets to the lung, it forms a weak bond with hemoglobin in the blood. When the blood gets to the tissue, it gives up the oxygen and takes on carbon dioxide. The blood carries carbon dioxide as bicarbonate ion or by

continued on page 485

supplying adequate oxygen and by removing carbon dioxide as it forms, the respiratory system helps maintain a constant environment that enables our body cells to function effectively.

In addition to air distribution and gas exchange, the respiratory system effectively *filters, warms,* and *humidifies* the air we breathe. Respiratory organs or organs closely associated with the respiratory system, such as the **sinuses,** also help produce speech or other sounds and make possible the sense of smell, or **olfaction** (ol-FAK-shun). In this chapter the structural plan of the respiratory system is considered first, then the respiratory organs are discussed individually, followed by some facts about gas exchange and the nervous system's control of respiration. Further discussion

that relates to disorders of the upper and lower respiratory tracts emphasizes how disruptions in respiratory system homeostasis lead to both anatomical and physiological manifestations of disease.

Structural Plan

Respiratory organs include the **nose, pharynx** (FAIR-inks), **larynx** (LAIR-inks), **trachea** (TRAY-kee-ah), **bronchi** (BRONG-ki), and **lungs.** The basic structural design of this organ system is that of a tube with many branches ending in millions of extremely tiny, very thin-walled sacs called **alveoli** (al-VEE-oh-lye). Figure 16-1 shows the extensive branching of the "respiratory tree" in both lungs. Think of this air distribution system as an "upside-down tree." The trachea

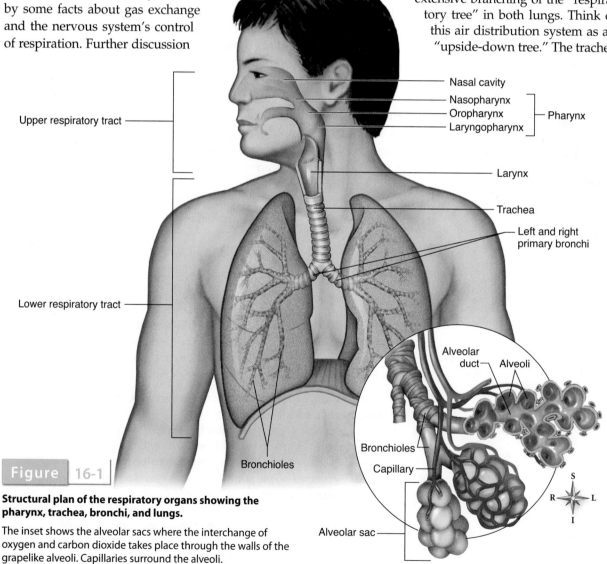

Upper respiratory tract

Nasal cavity
Nasopharynx
Oropharynx — Pharynx
Laryngopharynx

Larynx

Trachea

Left and right primary bronchi

Lower respiratory tract

Alveolar duct — Alveoli

Bronchioles

Capillary

Bronchioles

Alveolar sac

Figure 16-1

Structural plan of the respiratory organs showing the pharynx, trachea, bronchi, and lungs.

The inset shows the alveolar sacs where the interchange of oxygen and carbon dioxide takes place through the walls of the grapelike alveoli. Capillaries surround the alveoli.

or windpipe then becomes the trunk and the bronchial tubes the branches. This idea will be developed further when the types of bronchi and the alveoli are studied in more detail later in the chapter.

A network of capillaries fits like a hairnet around each microscopic alveolus. Incidentally, this is a good place for us to think again about a principle already mentioned several times, namely, that structure and function are intimately related. The function of alveoli—in fact, the function of the entire respiratory system—is to distribute air close enough to blood for a gas exchange to take place between air and blood. The passive transport process of **diffusion,** which was described in Chapter 3, is the mode for the exchange of gases that occurs in the respiratory system. You may want to review the discussion of diffusion on p. 49 before you study the mechanism of gas exchange that occurs in the lungs and body tissues.

Two characteristics about the structure of alveoli assist in diffusion and make them able to perform this function admirably. First, the wall of each alveolus is made up of a single layer of cells and so are the walls of the capillaries around it. This means that between the blood in the capillaries and the air in the alveolus, there is a barrier probably less than 1 micron thick. This extremely thin barrier is called the **respiratory membrane** (Figure 16-2). Second, there are millions of alveoli. This means that together they make an

Figure 16-2 The gas-exchange structures of the lung.

Each alveolus is continually ventilated with fresh air. The inset shows a magnified view of the respiratory membrane composed of the alveolar wall (surfactant, epithelial cells, and basement membrane), interstitial fluid, and the wall of a pulmonary capillary (basement membrane and endothelial cells). The gases, CO_2 (carbon dioxide) and O_2 (oxygen), diffuse across the respiratory membrane.

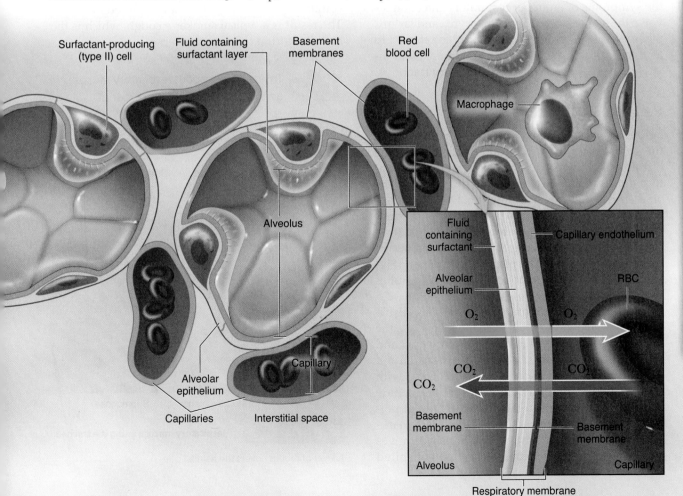

enormous surface (approximately 100 square meters, an area many times larger than the surface of the entire body) where large amounts of oxygen and carbon dioxide can rapidly be exchanged.

Respiratory Tracts

The respiratory system is often divided into upper and lower tracts, or divisions, to assist in the description of symptoms associated with common respiratory problems such as a cold. The organs of the upper respiratory tract are located outside of the thorax or chest cavity, whereas those in the lower tract, or division, are located almost entirely within it. The *upper respiratory tract* is composed of the nose, pharynx, and larynx. The *lower respiratory tract*, or division, consists of the trachea, all segments of the bronchial tree, and the lungs.

The designation *upper respiratory infection,* or URI, is often used by medical professionals to describe what many of us call a "head cold." Typically the symptoms of an upper respiratory infection involve the sinuses, nasal cavity, pharynx, and larynx, whereas the symptoms of what is often referred to as a "chest cold" are similar to pneumonia and involve the organs of the lower respiratory tract.

Respiratory Mucosa

Before beginning the study of individual organs in the respiratory system, it is important to review the histology, or microscopic anatomy, of the **respiratory mucosa**—the membrane that lines most of the air distribution tubes in the system. Do not confuse the respiratory membrane with the respiratory mucosa! The **respiratory membrane** (see Figure 16-2) separates the air in the alveoli from the blood in surrounding capillaries. The respiratory mucosa (Figure 16-3) is covered with mucus and lines the tubes of the respiratory tree.

Recall that in addition to serving as air distribution passageways or gas exchange surfaces, the anatomical components of the respiratory tract and lungs cleanse, warm, and humidify inspired air. Air entering the nose is generally contaminated with one or more common irritants; examples include some types of chemical air pollutants, dust, pollen, bacterial organisms, and even insects. A remarkably effective air purification mechanism removes almost every form of contaminant before inspired

air reaches the alveoli, or terminal air sacs, in the lungs.

A layer of protective mucus, called a *mucous blanket,* covers nearly the entire ciliated pseudo-stratified epithelial lining of the air distribution tubes in the respiratory tree (see Figure 16-3). It serves as the most important air purification mechanism. Air is purified when contaminants such as dust, pollen, and smoke particles stick to the mucus and become trapped. Only the vocal cords, which are covered by stratified squamous epithelium, are free of this mucous coating.

Normally, the cleansing layer of mucus containing inhaled contaminants moves upward to the pharynx from the lower portions of the bronchial tree on the millions of hairlike cilia that beat or move only in one direction. More than 125 ml of respiratory mucus is produced daily. Cigarette smoke and other chronic irritants both increase production of mucus and paralyze cilia, thus causing accumulations of contaminated mucus to build up and remain in the respiratory passageways for longer periods of time. The result is a typical smoker's cough, which is the body's effort to clear the secretions.

 To learn more about respiratory mucosa, go to **AnimationDirect** on your CD.

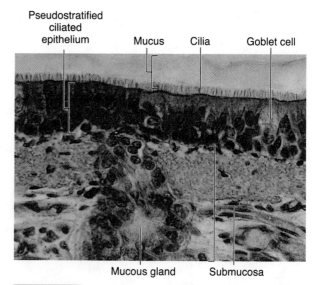

Pseudostratified ciliated epithelium   Mucus   Cilia   Goblet cell

Mucous gland   Submucosa

Figure 16-3 **Respiratory mucosa lining the trachea.**

A layer of mucus covers the hairlike cilia.

Nose

Air enters the respiratory tract through the **external nares** (NA-rees), or nostrils. It then flows into the right and left **nasal cavities,** which are lined by respiratory mucosa. A partition called the **nasal septum** separates these two cavities. **Nasal polyps** (POL-ips) are painless, noncancerous tissue growths that may project from the nasal mucosa. They are frequently associated with chronic hay fever. Over time, nasal polyps may grow in size, partially obstruct the nasal passage, and impair breathing. In severe cases, surgical removal may be required.

The surface of the nasal cavities is moist from mucus and warm from blood flowing just under it. Nerve endings responsible for the sense of smell (olfactory receptors) are located in the nasal mucosa.

Four **paranasal sinuses**—frontal, maxillary, sphenoidal, and ethmoidal—drain into the nasal cavities (Figure 16-4). The paranasal sinuses are lined with a mucous membrane that assists in the production of mucus for the respiratory tract. In addition, these hollow spaces help to lighten the skull bones and serve as resonant chambers that enhance the production of sound.

Because the mucosa that lines the sinuses is continuous with the mucosa that lines the nose, sinus infections, called **sinusitis** (sye-nyoo-SYE-tis), often develop from colds in which the nasal mucosa is inflamed. Symptoms of sinusitis include pressure, pain, headache, and often external tenderness, swelling, and redness. In chronic cases, infection may spread to adjacent bone or into the cranial cavity inflaming meninges or brain tissue. Treatment includes decongestants, analgesics, antibiotics, and in some cases surgery to improve drainage.

Two ducts from the *lacrimal* (LAK-rim-al) *sacs* also drain into the nasal cavity, as Figure 16-4 shows. The lacrimal sacs collect tears from the corner of each eyelid and drain them into the nasal cavity.

Note in Figure 16-4 that three shelflike structures called **conchae** (KONG-kee) protrude into the nasal cavity on each side. The nasal conchae are sometimes called *turbinates.* The mucosa-covered conchae greatly increase the surface over which air must flow as it passes through the naval cavity. As air moves over the conchae and through the nasal cavities, it is warmed and humidified. This helps explain why breathing through the nose is more effective in humidifying inspired air than is breathing through the mouth.

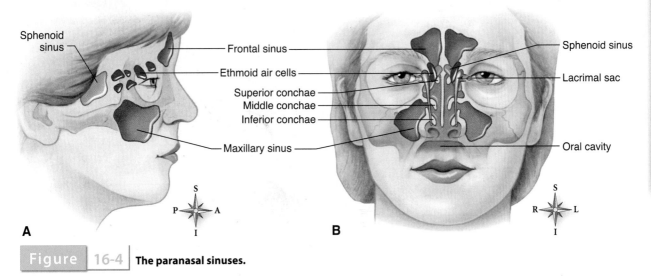

A, Lateral view of the position of the sinuses. **B,** The anterior view shows the anatomical relationship of the paranasal sinuses to each other and to the nasal cavity.

Figure 16-4 | **The paranasal sinuses.**

Pharynx

The **pharynx** is the structure that many of us call the throat. It is about 12.5 cm (5 inches) long and can be divided into three portions (Figure 16-5). The uppermost part of the tube just behind the nasal cavities is called the **nasopharynx** (nay-zoh-FAIR-inks). The portion behind the mouth is called the **oropharynx** (o-ro-FAIR-inks). The last or lowest segment is called the **laryngopharynx** (lah-ring-go-FAIR-inks).

The pharynx as a whole serves the same purpose for the respiratory and digestive tracts as a hallway serves for a house. Air and food pass through the pharynx on their way to the lungs and the stomach, respectively. Air enters the pharynx from the two nasal cavities and leaves it by way of the larynx; food enters it from the mouth and leaves it by way of the esophagus.

The right and left **auditory,** or *eustachian* (yoo-STAY-she-an), **tubes** open into the nasopharynx; they connect the middle ears with the nasopharynx (see Figure 16-5). This connection permits equalization of air pressure between the middle ear and the exterior ear. The lining of the auditory tubes is continuous with the lining of the nasopharynx and middle ear. Thus just as sinus infections can develop from colds in which the nasal mucosa is inflamed, middle ear infections can develop from inflammation of the nasopharynx.

Masses of lymphatic tissue called **tonsils** are embedded in the mucous membrane of the pharynx. Recall the location of the tonsils from the previous chapter (see pp. 427-428). The *palatine tonsils* are located in the oropharynx and the *pharyngeal* (fah-RIN-jee-al) *tonsils,* also called the *adenoids* (AD-eh-noyds), are located in the nasopharynx.

As you read in Chapter 15, these tonsils form a ring of lymphoid tissue in the throat that pro-

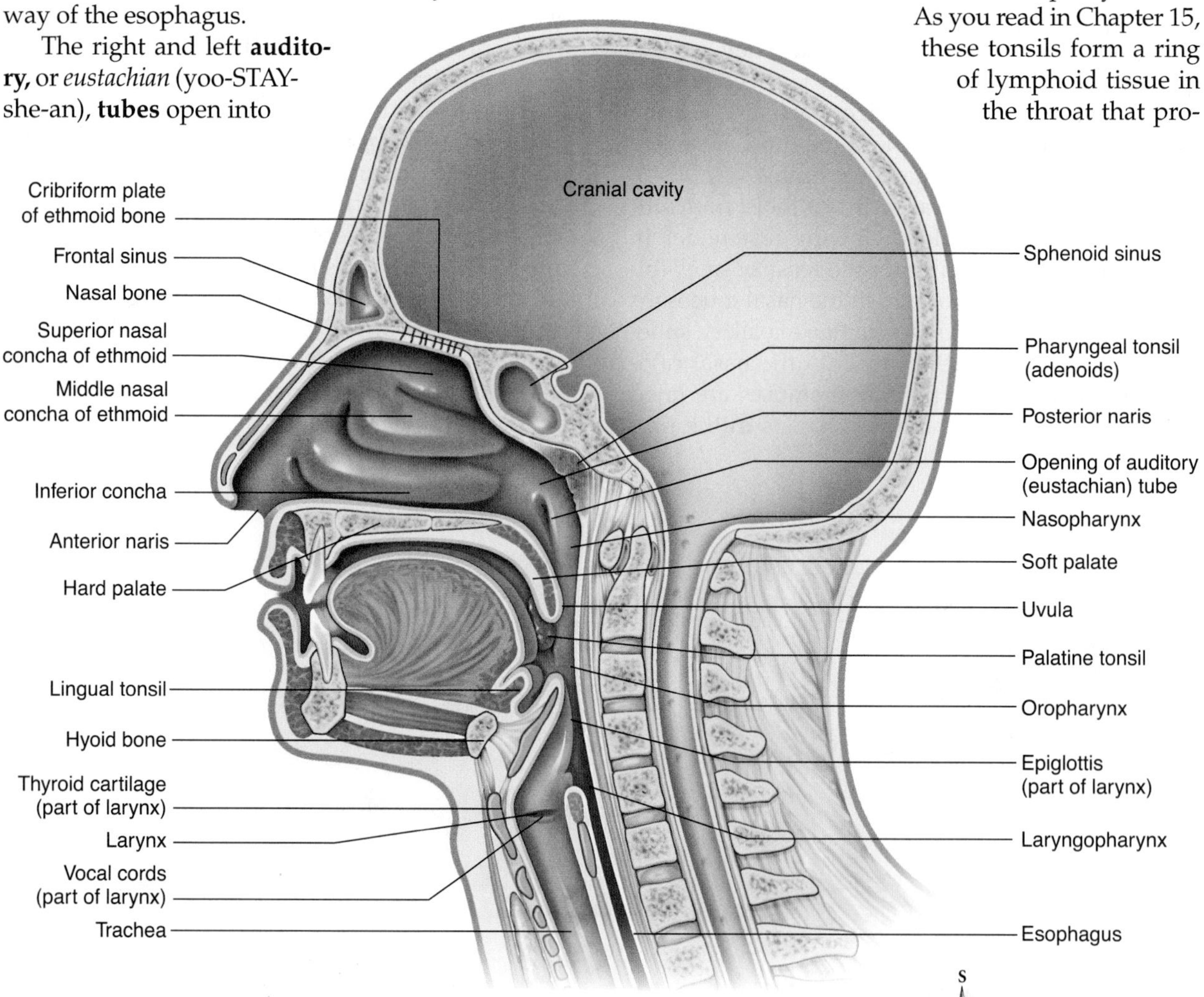

Cribriform plate of ethmoid bone
Frontal sinus
Nasal bone
Superior nasal concha of ethmoid
Middle nasal concha of ethmoid
Inferior concha
Anterior naris
Hard palate
Lingual tonsil
Hyoid bone
Thyroid cartilage (part of larynx)
Larynx
Vocal cords (part of larynx)
Trachea

Cranial cavity

Sphenoid sinus
Pharyngeal tonsil (adenoids)
Posterior naris
Opening of auditory (eustachian) tube
Nasopharynx
Soft palate
Uvula
Palatine tonsil
Oropharynx
Epiglottis (part of larynx)
Laryngopharynx
Esophagus

Figure 16-5 | **Sagittal section of the head and neck.**

The nasal septum has been removed, exposing the right lateral wall of the nasal cavity so that the nasal conchae can be seen. Note also the divisions of the pharynx and the position of the tonsils.

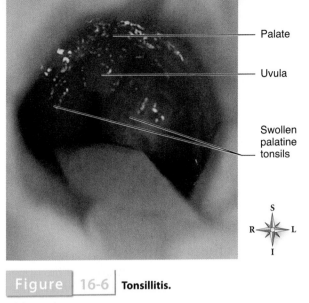

Figure 16-6 **Tonsillitis.**

Enlarged palatine tonsils can be seen nearly meeting at the midline of the pharynx.

vides immune protection at a critical boundary with the external environment. Although the tonsils usually protect us, they can also become infected and inflamed themselves—a condition called **tonsillitis** (Figure 16-6). Swelling of the pharyngeal tonsils caused by infections may make it difficult or im-

possible for air to travel from the nose into the throat. In these cases the individual is forced to breathe through the mouth.

In a **tonsillectomy** (ton-si-LEK-toh-mee) both tonsils are generally removed by a surgeon. Once a very common surgical procedure, tonsillectomy, with its potentially serious complications—including severe hemorrhage—is now performed only after other options have been exhausted. Physicians now recognize the value of lymphatic tissue in the body's defense mechanism and delay removal of the tonsils—even in cases of inflammation (tonsillitis). Although surgical removal may eventually be necessary in cases of repeated infections or when nonsurgical treatments such as intensive antibiotic therapy prove ineffective, the number of tonsillectomies performed each year continues to decrease.

Larynx

The **larynx,** or voice box, is located just below the pharynx. It is composed of several pieces of cartilage. You know the largest of these (the *thyroid cartilage*) as the "Adam's apple" (Figure 16-7).

Figure 16-7

The larynx.
A, Sagittal section of the larynx. **B,** Superior view of the larynx. **C,** Photograph of the larynx taken with an endoscope (optical device) inserted through the mouth and pharynx to the epiglottis.

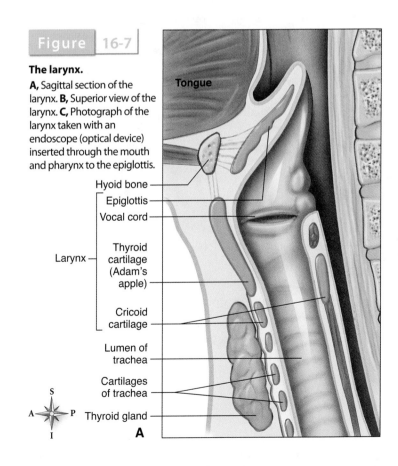

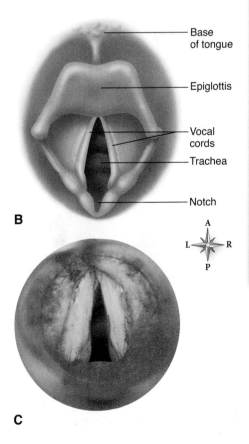

Two short fibrous bands, the **vocal cords,** stretch across the interior of the larynx. Muscles that attach to the larynx cartilages can pull on these cords in such a way that they become tense or relaxed. When they are tense, the voice is high pitched; when they are relaxed, it is low pitched. The space between the vocal cords is the **glottis.** Another piece of cartilage, the **epiglottis** (ep-i-GLOT-is), partially covers the opening of the larynx (see Figure 16-7). The epiglottis acts like a trapdoor, closing off the larynx during swallowing and preventing food from entering the trachea.

The risk of *laryngeal cancer* increases with smoking and alcohol abuse. It occurs most often in men over age 50 and is often diagnosed because of persistent hoarseness and difficulty in swallowing. A number of therapeutic treatments including surgery, radiation, and chemotherapy can be curative but about one third of those affected will die of the disease. If treatment involves surgical removal of the larynx, the individual must learn "esophageal speech" or use an electric artificial larynx to speak.

Disorders of the Upper Respiratory Tract

Upper Respiratory Infection

Any infection localized in the mucosa of the upper respiratory tract (nose, pharynx, and larynx) can be called an *upper respiratory infection (URI).* Although

CLINICAL APPLICATION

KEEPING THE TRACHEA OPEN

Often a tube is placed through the mouth, pharynx, and larynx into the trachea before patients leave the operating room, especially if they have been given a muscle relaxant. This procedure is called **endotracheal intubation** (en-doh-TRAY-kee-al in-too-BAY-shun). The purpose of the tube is to ensure an open airway (see parts A and B of the figure). To ensure that the tube enters the trachea rather than the nearby esophagus (which leads to the stomach), anatomical landmarks such as the vocal folds are used. Likewise, the dis-tinct feel of the V-shaped posterior groove called the *interarytenoid notch* (in-ter-AIR-ih-ten-oyd) (see Figure 16-7, *B*) can help guide the proper insertion of the tube.

Another procedure done frequently in today's modern hospitals is a **tracheostomy** (tray-kee-OS-toh-mee). This procedure involves the cutting of an opening into the trachea (part C of the figure). A surgeon may perform this procedure so that a suction device can be inserted to remove secretions from the bronchial tree or so that an *intermittent positive-pressure breathing (IPPB)* machine can be used to improve ventilation of the lungs.

ENDOTRACHEAL INTUBATION

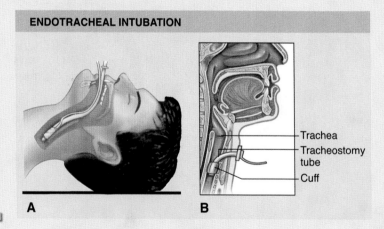

— Trachea
— Tracheostomy tube
— Cuff

A B

TRACHEOSTOMY

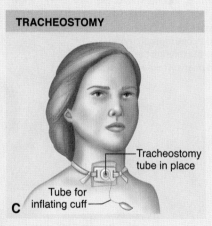

— Tracheostomy tube in place

Tube for inflating cuff —

C

the general designation URI is often used, such infections are sometimes named for the specific structure involved.

Rhinitis (rye-NYE-tis), from the Greek *rhinos,* "nose," is inflammation and swelling of the nasal mucosa. A red, itchy, "runny nose" and partially obstructed breathing are universally recognized as symptoms of *infectious rhinitis.* Most cases of infectious rhinitis are caused by viruses responsible for the common cold (rhinoviruses) or the flu (influenza viruses). Although potentially serious in susceptible individuals, most cases of infectious rhinitis resolve with (or without!) supportive treatment after about 7 to 10 days of misery. The term *allergic rhinitis,* or "hay fever," is used to describe sensitivity-type reactions to many types of nasal irritants and airborne allergens including animal dander and plant pollens. Symptoms similar to infectious rhinitis may become chronic and result in formation of nasal polyps and secondary infections.

Pharyngitis (fair-in-JYE-tis), or *sore throat,* is inflammation or infection of the pharynx (throat). Pain, redness, and difficulty in swallowing are characteristic of pharyngitis. Pharyngitis may be caused by any of several pathogens, including the streptococcal bacteria that cause "strep throat" (see Appendix A on page A-1 of your book).

Laryngitis (lair-in-JYE-tis) is inflammation of the mucous lining of the larynx. The inflammation is accompanied by edema of the laryngeal structures. If swelling of the vocal cords occurs, hoarseness or loss of voice results. The condition may be caused by bacteria, viruses, exposure to allergens, or by overuse of the voice, smoking, and other factors. Even a moderate amount of laryngeal swelling or edema, especially in a young child, can obstruct air flow and result in asphyxiation.

Epiglottitis is a life-threatening condition caused by *Haemophilus influenzae* type B (Hib) infection. Hib often struck children between 3 and 7 years of age a generation ago. However, introduction of Hib vaccines at the end of the twentieth century produced a 99% drop in the incidence of this infection, making this type of epiglottitis rare in our day.

The term **croup** is used to describe a non–life-threatening type of laryngitis generally seen in children younger than age 3. It is caused by the parainfluenza viruses. Symptoms include a harsh bark-like cough and labored inspiration. Affected children often develop symptoms after going to sleep and awaken frightened and coughing but without a fever.

URIs are rather common, occurring several times a year in most individuals, because the upper respiratory tract is easily accessible to common airborne pathogens. Because the upper respiratory mucosa is continuous with the mucous lining of the sinuses, the eustachian tube and middle ear, and lower respiratory tract, URIs have the unfortunate tendency to spread. It is not unusual therefore to see a common cold progress to become sinusitis or *otitis media* (middle ear infection).

Anatomical Disorders

Deviated septum is a condition in which the nasal septum strays from the midline of the nasal cavity. Nobody's nasal septum is *exactly* on the midsagittal plane, but most are fairly close. Some people, however, are born with a congenital defect of the septum that results in some degree of blockage to one or both sides of the nasal cavity. Others acquire a deviated septum after birth as a result of damage from an injury or infection. In either case, surgical correction of the anatomical abnormality often results in normal breathing through the nose.

Injury to the nose occurs relatively often because the nose projects some distance from the front of the head. Usually, common bumps and other injuries cause little if any serious damage. Occasionally, **epistaxis** (ep-i-STAKS-is), or nosebleed, occurs. The most common cause of nosebleed is a strong bump or blow, but it can result from severe inflammation or rubbing (as in rhinitis), hypertension, or even brain injury. Because of the rich blood supply close to the inside surface of the nasal cavity, even minor nosebleeds can produce a great deal of blood—causing them to appear more serious than they are.

CLINICAL APPLICATION

ABDOMINAL THRUST MANEUVER

The **abdominal thrust maneuver** is an effective and often lifesaving technique that can be used to open a windpipe that has suddenly been obstructed. It was originally named after the physician who helped develop it for general use, Henry Heimlich (see box on p. 479). More recently, the *eponym* (term that includes a person's name), that is, *Heimlich maneuver,* is being dropped and the technique is now often called simply **abdominal thrusts**.

Choking often occurs when something becomes lodged in the larynx and cannot be dislodged by normal coughing. Many experts recommend that a person who is choking should receive back slaps to help dislodge foreign material from the larynx. If back slaps are not effective, then abdominal thrusts may be applied.

The maneuver (see the figures) uses air already present in the lungs to expel the object obstructing the airway. Most accidental airway obstructions result from pieces of food aspirated during a meal—the condition is sometimes referred to as "cafe coronary." Other objects such as chewing gum or balloons are frequently the cause of obstructions in children. Individuals trained in emergency procedures must be able to tell the difference between airway obstruction and other conditions that produce similar symptoms, such as heart attacks. The key question they must ask the person who appears to be choking is, "Can you talk?" A person with an obstructed airway will not be able to speak, even while conscious.

The abdominal thrust maneuver, if the victim is standing, consists of the rescuer grasping the victim with both arms around the victim's waist just below the rib cage and above the navel. The rescuer makes a fist with one hand, grasps it with the other, and then delivers an upward thrust against the diaphragm just below the xiphoid process of the sternum. Air trapped in the lungs is pressurized, forcing the object that is choking the victim out of the airway.

Technique if Victim Can Be Lifted (see Figure A)

1. The rescuer stands behind the victim and wraps both arms around the victim's chest slightly below the rib cage and above the navel. The victim is allowed to fall forward with the head, arms, and chest over the rescuer's arms.
2. The rescuer makes a fist with one hand and grasps it with the other hand, pressing the thumb side of the fist against the victim's abdomen below the end of the xiphoid process and above the navel.
3. The hands only are used to deliver the upward subdiaphragmatic thrusts. Each thrust is performed with sharp flexion of the elbows, in an upward rather than inward direction, and is usually repeated 4 times. It is very important that neither the rib cage nor sternum be compressed during the abdominal thrust maneuver.

Technique if Victim Has Collapsed or Cannot Be Lifted (see Figure B)

1. Rescuer places victim on floor face up.
2. Facing victim, rescuer straddles the hips.
3. Rescuer places one hand on top of the other, with the bottom hand on the victim's abdomen slightly above the navel and below the rib cage.
4. Rescuer performs a forceful upward thrust with the heel of the bottom hand, repeating several times if necessary.

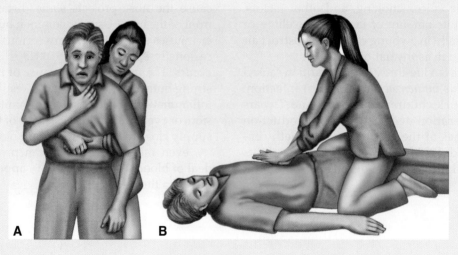

A   **B**

Trachea

The **trachea** or windpipe is a tube about 11 cm (4.5 inches) long that extends from the larynx in the neck to the bronchi in the chest cavity (Figures 16-1 and 16-8). The trachea performs a simple but vital function: it provides part of the open passageway through which air can reach the lungs from the outside.

By pushing with your fingers against your throat about an inch above the sternum, you can feel the shape of the trachea or windpipe. Nature has taken precautions to keep this lifeline open. Its framework is made of an almost noncollapsible material—15 to 20 **C-shaped rings of cartilage** placed one above the other with only a little soft tissue between them (see Figure 16-8). The trachea is lined by the typical respiratory mucosa. Glands below the ciliated epithelium help produce the blanket of mucus that continually moves upward toward the pharynx.

Despite the structural safeguard of cartilage rings, closing of the trachea sometimes occurs. A tumor or an infection may enlarge the lymph nodes of the neck so much that they squeeze the trachea shut, or a person may aspirate (breathe in) a piece of food or something else that blocks the windpipe. Because air has no other way to get to the lungs, complete tracheal obstruction causes death in a matter of minutes.

Choking on food and other substances caught in the trachea kills more than 4000 people each year and is the fifth major cause of accidental deaths in the United States. A lifesaving technique developed by Dr. Henry Heimlich (see box on p. 479) is now widely used to free the trachea of ingested food or other foreign objects that would otherwise block the airway and cause death in choking victims.

> **QUICK CHECK**
>
> 1. Name the paranasal sinuses and the three divisions of the pharynx.
> 2. What is the common name for infectious rhinitis?
> 3. What disorder of the upper respiratory tract is considered life threatening?
> 4. What keeps the trachea from collapsing?

Bronchi, Bronchioles, and Alveoli

Recall that one way to picture the thousands of air tubes that make up the lungs is to think of an upside-down tree. The trachea is the main trunk of this tree; the right bronchus (the tube leading into the right lung) and the left bronchus (the tube leading into the left lung) are the trachea's first branches or **primary bronchi.** The right primary bronchus is more vertical and "in line" with the

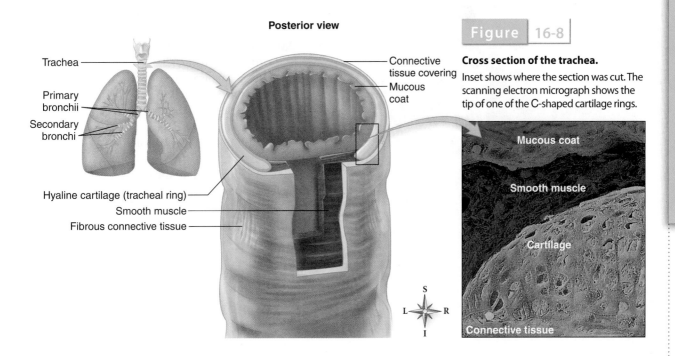

Posterior view

Trachea
Primary bronchii
Secondary bronchi
Hyaline cartilage (tracheal ring)
Smooth muscle
Fibrous connective tissue

Connective tissue covering
Mucous coat

Mucous coat
Smooth muscle
Cartilage
Connective tissue

Figure 16-8

Cross section of the trachea.
Inset shows where the section was cut. The scanning electron micrograph shows the tip of one of the C-shaped cartilage rings.

terminal trachea than is the left. As a result, aspirated objects that enter the trachea tend to enter and lodge in the right primary bronchus or lung more often than the left.

In each lung, the primary bronchi branch into smaller, or **secondary, bronchi** whose walls, like those of the trachea and bronchi, are kept open by rings of cartilage for air passage. These secondary bronchi divide into smaller and smaller tubes, ultimately branching into tiny tubes whose walls contain only smooth muscle. These very small passageways are called **bronchioles.**

The bronchioles subdivide into microscopic tubes called **alveolar ducts,** which resemble the main stem of a bunch of grapes (Figure 16-9). Each alveolar duct ends in several **alveolar sacs,** each of which resembles a cluster of grapes, and the wall of each alveolar sac is made up of numerous **alveoli,** each of which resembles a single grape.

Alveoli are very effective in exchanging gas, mainly because they are extremely thin walled; each alveolus lies in contact with a blood capillary, and there are millions of alveoli in each lung. The surface of the respiratory membrane inside the alveolus is covered by a substance called **surfactant** (sur-FAK-tant). This important substance helps reduce surface tension in the alveoli and keeps them from collapsing as air moves in and out during respiration.

 To learn more about respiratory membrane, go to **AnimationDirect** on your CD.

Respiratory Distress

Respiratory distress results from the body's relative inability to inflate the alveoli of the lungs normally. **Respiratory distress syndrome (RDS)** is a condition most often caused by absence or impairment of the surfactant in the fluid that lines the alveoli.

Infant respiratory distress syndrome, or **IRDS,** is a very serious, life-threatening condition that often affects prematurely born infants of less than 37 weeks' gestation or those who weigh less than 2.2 kg (5 lb) at birth. IRDS is the leading cause of death among premature infants in the United States, claiming more than 5000 premature babies each year. The disease, characterized by a lack of **surfactant** in the alveolar air sacs, affects 50,000 babies annually.

Surfactant is manufactured by *type II cells* in the walls of the alveoli. Surfactant reduces the surface tension of the fluid on the free surface of the alveolar walls and permits easy movement of air into and out of the lungs. The ability of the body to manufacture this important substance is not fully developed until shortly before birth—normally about 40 weeks after conception.

In newborn infants who are unable to manufacture surfactant, many air sacs collapse during expiration because of the increased surface tension. The effort required to reinflate these collapsed alveoli is much greater than that needed to reinflate normal alveoli with adequate surfactant. The baby soon develops labored breathing, and symptoms of respiratory distress appear shortly after birth.

In the past, treatment of IRDS was limited to keeping the alveoli open so that delivery and exchange of oxygen and carbon dioxide could occur. To accomplish this, a tube was inserted

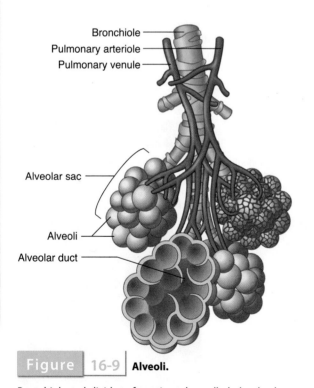

Bronchiole
Pulmonary arteriole
Pulmonary venule

Alveolar sac

Alveoli

Alveolar duct

Figure 16-9 | **Alveoli.**

Bronchioles subdivide to form tiny tubes called *alveolar ducts,* which end in clusters of alveoli called *alveolar sacs.*

into the respiratory tract, and oxygen-rich air was delivered under sufficient pressure to keep the alveoli from collapsing at the end of expiration. A newer treatment involves delivering air under pressure and applying prepared surfactant directly into the baby's airways by means of a tube.

Adult respiratory distress syndrome (ARDS) is caused by impairment or removal of surfactant in the alveoli. For example, accidental inhalation of foreign substances such as water, vomit, smoke, or chemical fumes can cause ARDS. Edema of the alveolar tissue can impair surfactant and reduce the alveoli's ability to stretch, causing respiratory distress.

Lungs and Pleura

The **lungs** are fairly large organs. Note in Figure 16-10 that the right lung has three lobes and the left lung has two. Figure 16-10 shows the relationship of the lungs to the rib cage at the end of a normal expiration. The narrow, superior position of each lung, up under the collarbone, is the apex; the broad, inferior portion resting on the diaphragm is the base.

The **pleura** covers the outer surface of the lungs and lines the inner surface of the rib cage. The pleura resembles other serous membranes in relation to its structure and function. Like the peritoneum or pericardium, the pleura is an extensive, thin, moist, slippery membrane. It lines a large, closed cavity of the

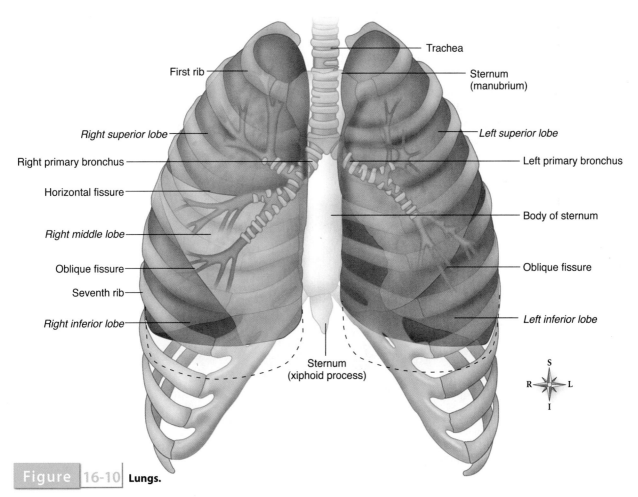

Figure 16-10 **Lungs.**

The trachea is an airway that branches to form a treelike formation of bronchi and bronchioles. Note that the right lung has three lobes and the left lung has two lobes.

body and covers the organs located within it. The parietal pleura lines the walls of the thoracic cavity; the visceral pleura covers the lungs, and the intrapleural space lies between the two pleural membranes (Figure 16-11).

Pleurisy (PLOOR-i-see) is an inflammation of the parietal pleura, characterized by difficulty in breathing and stabbing pain. The discomfort and restriction of normal breathing associated with pleurisy are caused by the constant rubbing back and forth of the visceral and parietal pleurae during breathing. Pleurisy can be caused by tumors, infections (such as pneumonia and tuberculosis), and other factors.

Normally the intrapleural space contains just enough fluid to make both portions of the pleura moist and slippery and able to glide easily against each other as the lungs expand and deflate with each breath.

However, the pleural space sometimes fills with other substances, which increases the pressure on the lung from the outside—causing it to collapse. Incomplete expansion or collapse of the lung for any reason is called **atelectasis** (at-eh-LEK-tah-sis). While collapsed, the lung cannot be ventilated,

making the affected lung useless in breathing. For example, a puncture wound to the chest wall or a rupture of the visceral pleura may cause **pneumothorax** (noo-moh-THOR-aks) (Figure 16-12). Pneumothorax (literally "air in the thorax") is the presence of air in the pleural space on one side of the chest. An injury or disease also may cause **hemothorax** (hee-moh-THOR-aks), the presence of blood in the pleural space. Both conditions are potentially life threatening unless medical treatment is received.

> **QUICK CHECK**
>
> 1. What lung structures serve to distribute air and which structures serve as gas exchangers?
> 2. Infant respiratory distress syndrome (IRDS) is caused by a lack of what substance?
> 3. What causes pleurisy?

Respiration

Respiration means exchange of gases (oxygen and carbon dioxide) between a living organism and its environment. If the organism consists of only

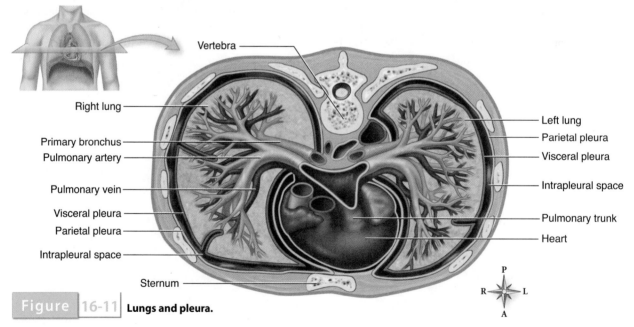

Figure 16-11 **Lungs and pleura.**

The inset shows where the body was cut to show this transverse section of the thorax. A serous membrane lines the thoracic wall (parietal pleura) and then folds inward near the bronchi to cover the lung (visceral pleura). The intrapleural space contains a small amount of serous pleural fluid.

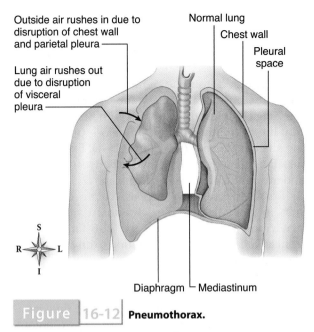

Outside air rushes in due to disruption of chest wall and parietal pleura

Normal lung

Chest wall

Pleural space

Lung air rushes out due to disruption of visceral pleura

S

R   L

I

Diaphragm — Mediastinum

Figure 16-12 Pneumothorax.

Air in the pleural space may accumulate when the visceral pleura ruptures and air from the lung rushes out or when atmospheric air rushes in through a wound in the chest wall and parietal pleura. In either case, the lung collapses and normal respiration is impaired. If blood accumulates in the pleural space, the condition is called *hemothorax.*

one cell, gases can move directly between it and the environment. If, however, the organism consists of billions of cells, as do our bodies, most of its cells are too far removed from the air source for a direct exchange of gases to occur. To overcome this difficulty, a pair of organs—the lungs—provides a place where air and a circulating fluid (blood) can come close enough to each other for oxygen to move out of the air into the blood while carbon dioxide moves out of the blood into the air.

Breathing, or **pulmonary ventilation,** is the process that moves air into and out of the lungs. It makes possible the exchange of gases between air in the lungs and in the blood. This exchange is often called **external respiration.** In addition, exchange of gases occurs between the blood and the cells of the body—a process called **internal respiration.** *Cellular respiration* refers to the actual use of oxygen by cells in the process of metabolism, which is discussed in Chapter 18.

Mechanics of Breathing

Pulmonary ventilation, or breathing, has two phases. **Inspiration,** or *inhalation,* moves air into the lungs, and **expiration,** or *exhalation,* moves air out of the lungs. The lungs are enclosed within the thoracic cavity. Thus changes in the shape and size of the thoracic cavity result in changes in the air pressure within that cavity and in the lungs. This difference in air pressure causes the movement of air into and out of the lungs. Air moves from an area where pressure is high to an area where pressure is lower. Respiratory muscles are responsible for the changes in the shape of the thoracic cavity that cause the air movements involved in breathing.

INSPIRATION

Inspiration occurs when the chest cavity enlarges. As the thorax enlarges, the lungs expand along with it, and air rushes into them and down into the alveoli. This happens because of a very important law of physics: the volume and pressure of a gas are inversely proportional. That means that when volume of a gas goes up, as lung volume goes up as we expand the thorax, then the pressure goes down. Thus air pressure in the lungs decreases during inspiration. When air pressure in the lungs is less than atmospheric air pressure, air rushes into the lungs.

Muscles that increase the volume of the thorax are classified as **inspiratory muscles.** These include the *diaphragm* (DYE-ah-fram) and the external intercostals.

The diaphragm is the dome-shaped muscle separating the abdominal cavity from the thoracic cavity. The diaphragm flattens out when it contracts during inspiration. Instead of protruding up into the chest cavity, it moves down toward the abdominal cavity. Thus the contraction or flattening of the diaphragm makes the chest cavity longer from top to bottom. The diaphragm is the most important muscle of inspiration. Nerve impulses passing through the *phrenic nerve* stimulate the diaphragm to contract.

The external intercostal muscles are located between the ribs. When they contract, they enlarge the thorax by increasing the size of the cavity from front to back and from side to side. Contraction of the inspiratory muscles increases the volume of the thoracic cavity and reduces lung air pressure below atmospheric air pressure, drawing air into the lungs (Figure 16-13).

EXPIRATION

Quiet, resting expiration is ordinarily a passive process that begins when the inspiratory muscles relax and contract to their resting length. The thoracic cavity then returns to its smaller size. The elastic nature of thoracic and lung tissue also causes these organs to "recoil" and decrease in size. Because volume and pressure are inversely proportional (one goes up as the other goes down), as lung volume decreases the lung air pressure increases. As the lung air pressure rises above atmospheric air pressure, air flows down its pressure gradient and outward through the respiratory passageways.

When we speak, sing, or do heavy work, we may need more forceful expiration to increase the rate and depth of ventilation. During more forceful expiration, the **expiratory muscles** (internal intercostals and abdominal muscles) contract.

When contracted, the internal intercostal muscles pull the rib cage inward and decrease the front-to-back size of the thorax. Contraction of the abdominal muscles pushes the abdominal organs against the underside of the diaphragm, pushing it farther upward into the thoracic cavity. As the thoracic cavity decreases in size, the air pressure within it increases above atmospheric air pressure and air flows out of the lungs (see Figure 16-13).

Exchange of Gases in Lungs

Blood pumped from the right ventricle of the heart enters the pulmonary artery and eventually enters the lungs. It then flows through the thousands of tiny lung capillaries that are in close proximity to the air-filled alveoli (see Figure 16-1). External respiration or the exchange of gases between the blood and alveolar air occurs by diffusion.

Recall that diffusion is a passive process that results in movement of particles down a concentration gradient. During diffusion, substances move from an area of high concentration to an area of low concentration.

Blood flowing into lung capillaries is low in oxygen. Oxygen is continually removed from the blood and used by the cells of the body. By the time it enters the lung capillaries, it is low in oxygen content. Because alveolar air is rich in oxygen, diffusion causes movement of oxygen from the area of high concentration (alveolar air) to the area of low concentration (capillary blood). Note in Figure 16-14 that most of the oxygen (O_2) entering the blood combines with hemoglobin (Hb) in the red blood cells (RBCs) to form **oxyhemoglobin** (ahk-see-HEE-moh-glo-bin) (HbO_2) so that it can be carried to the tissues and used by the body cells.

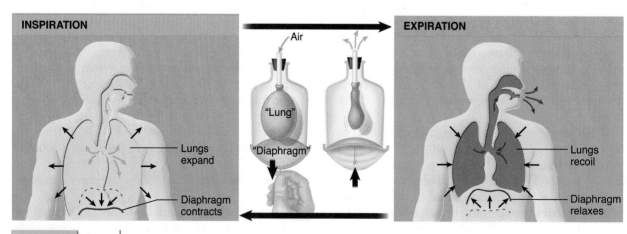

Figure 16-13 **Mechanics of breathing.**

During *inspiration,* the diaphragm contracts, increasing the volume of the thoracic cavity. This increase in volume results in a decrease in pressure, which causes air to rush into the lungs. During *expiration,* the diaphragm returns to an upward position, reducing the volume in the thoracic cavity. Air pressure increases then, forcing air out of the lungs. The inserts show the classic model in which a jar represents the rib cage, a rubber sheet represents the diaphragm, and a balloon represents the lungs.

Diffusion of carbon dioxide (CO_2) also occurs between blood in lung capillaries and alveolar air. Blood flowing through the lung capillaries is high in carbon dioxide. As cells remove oxygen from circulating blood, they add the waste product *carbon dioxide* to it. As a result, the blood flowing toward pulmonary cap-

illaries eventually becomes low in oxygen and high in carbon dioxide. Diffusion of carbon dioxide results in its movement from an area of high concentration in the pulmonary capillaries to an area of low concentration in alveolar air. Then from the alveoli, carbon dioxide leaves the body in expired air.

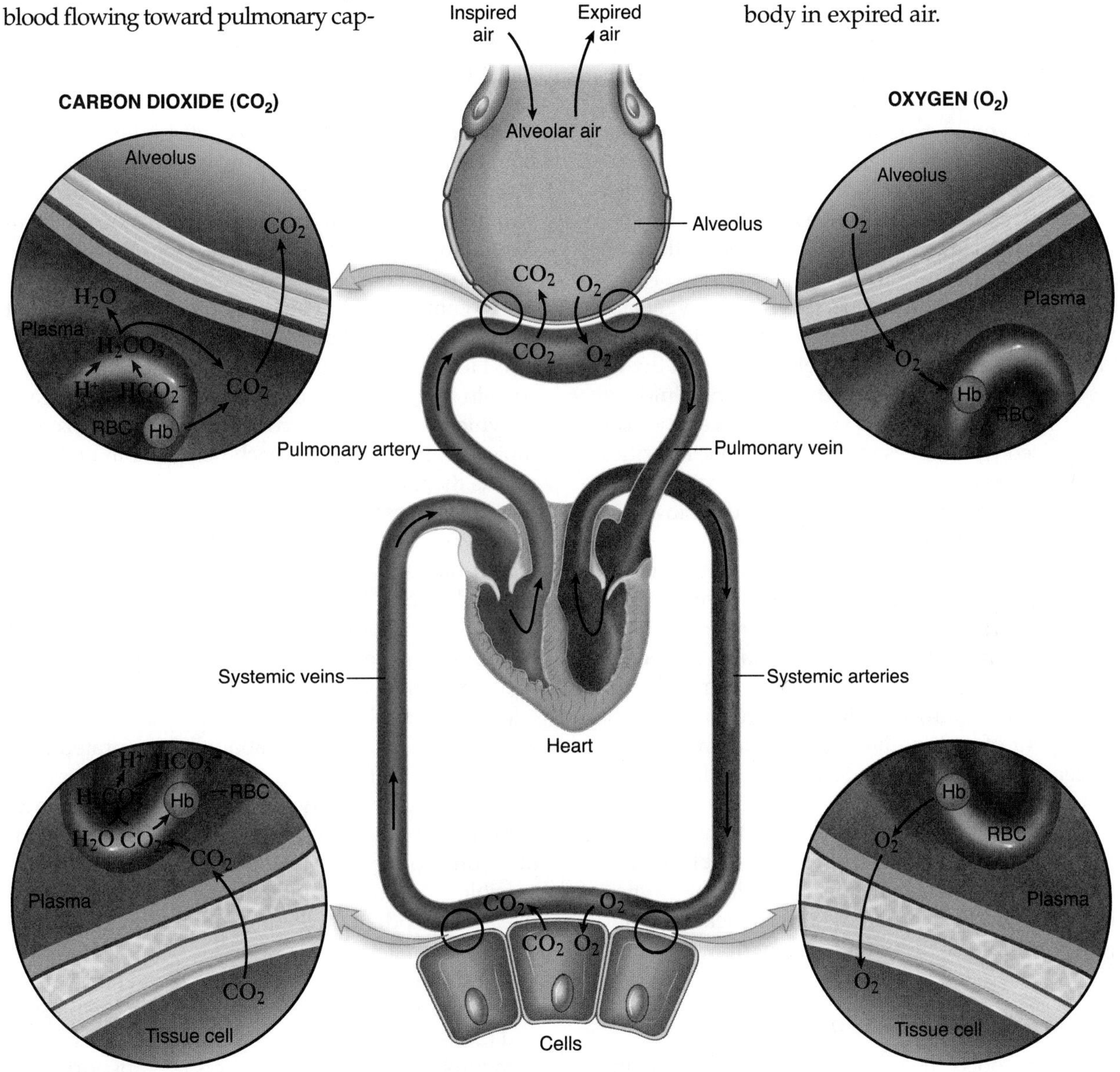

Figure 16-14 **Exchange of gases in lung and tissue capillaries.**

The right insets show O_2 diffusing out of alveolar air into blood and associating with hemoglobin (Hb) in lung capillaries to form oxyhemoglobin. In tissue capillaries, oxyhemoglobin dissociates, releasing O_2, which diffuses from the RBC and then crosses the capillary wall to reach the tissue cells. As the left insets show, CO_2 diffuses in the opposite direction (into RBCs) and some of it associates with Hb to form carbaminohemoglobin. However, most CO_2 combines with water to form carbonic acid (H_2CO_3), which dissociates to form H^+ and HCO_3^- (bicarbonate) ions. Back in the lung capillaries CO_2 dissociates from the bicarbonate and carbamino-hemoglobin molecules and diffuses out of blood into alveolar air.

Most carbon dioxide is carried as bicarbonate ion (HCO_3^-) in the blood. Some, as depicted in Figure 16-14, combines with the hemoglobin in RBCs to form **carbaminohemoglobin** (kar-bam-i-no-HEE-moh-glo-bin) ($HbCO_2$).

Exchange of Gases in Tissues

The exchange of gases that occurs between blood in tissue capillaries and the body cells is called *internal respiration.*

As you would expect, the direction of movement of oxygen and carbon dioxide during internal respiration is just the opposite of that noted in the exchange that occurs during external respiration when gases are exchanged between the blood in the lung capillaries and the air in alveoli. As shown in Figure 16-14, oxyhemoglobin breaks down into oxygen and hemoglobin in the tissue capillaries. Oxygen molecules move rapidly out of the blood through the tissue capillary membrane into the interstitial fluid and on into the cells that compose the tissues. The oxygen is used by the cells in their metabolic activities. Diffusion results in the movement of oxygen from an area of high concentration to an area of low concentration in the cells where it is needed.

While oxygen is moving down its concentration gradient, carbon dioxide molecules leave the cells, entering the tissue capillaries where bicarbonate ions are formed and where hemoglobin molecules unite with carbon dioxide to form carbaminohemoglobin. Once again, diffusion is responsible for the movement of carbon dioxide from an area of high concentration in the cells to an area of lower concentration in the capillary blood.

In brief, oxygenated blood enters tissue capillaries and is changed into deoxygenated blood as it flows through them. In the process of losing oxygen, the waste product carbon dioxide is picked up and transported to the lungs for removal from the body.

Blood Transportation of Gases

Blood transports the respiratory gases, oxygen and carbon dioxide, in a dissolved state, either as a single substance or combined with other chemicals. Immediately upon entering the blood, both oxygen and carbon dioxide dissolve in the plasma, but because fluids can hold only small amounts of gas in solution, most of the oxygen and carbon dioxide rapidly form a chemical union with some other molecule—such as hemoglobin—another plasma protein found in the blood—or water. Once gas molecules are bound to another molecule, their plasma concentration (partial pressure) decreases and more gas can diffuse into the plasma. In this way, comparatively large volumes of the gases can be transported.

Transport of Oxygen

Only very limited amounts of oxygen can be dissolved in the blood. Of the total amount of oxygen that blood can transport, about 20.4 ml in 100 ml of blood, only about 1.5% or 0.3 ml is actually dissolved. Many times that amount, about 21.1 ml, combines with the hemoglobin (Hb) in 100 ml of blood to form **oxyhemoglobin** (HbO_2) so that it can be carried to the tissues and used by the body cells.

To combine with hemoglobin, oxygen must first diffuse into the red blood cells to form oxyhemoglobin. Hemoglobin molecules are large proteins that contain four iron-containing **heme** components, each of which is capable of combining with an oxygen molecule. In many ways each hemoglobin molecule acts as the ultimate "oxygen sponge."

Oxygen associates with hemoglobin rapidly—so rapidly, in fact, that about 97% of the blood's hemoglobin has united with oxygen, and become "oxygenated blood," by the time it leaves the lung capillaries to return to the heart. Oxygenated blood is found in the systemic arteries and pulmonary veins. Normally, oxygenated blood is 97% "saturated." So-called "deoxygenated blood," found in the systemic veins and pulmonary arteries, is about 70% saturated with oxygen. The difference in oxygen saturation results from the release of oxygen from oxyhemoglobin to supply the body cells. Therefore, the chemical combination of oxygen and hemoglobin is said to be "reversible" with oxyhemoglobin formation or oxygen release dependent on the partial pressure of oxygen driving the reaction.

Summing up, we can say that oxygen travels in two forms: (1) as simply dissolved O_2 in the plasma and (2) as a combination of O_2 and hemoglobin (oxyhemoglobin). Of these two forms of transport, oxyhemoglobin is the carrier of the vast majority of the total oxygen transported by the blood.

Transport of Carbon Dioxide

Carbon dioxide is a by-product of cellular metabolism and plays an important and necessary role in regulating the pH of body fluids. However, if it accumulates in the body beyond normal limits (40 to

50 mmHg in venous blood), it can quickly become toxic. Elimination of excess CO_2 from the body occurs when it enters the alveoli and is expelled during expiration. For this to occur, CO_2 must be transported in the blood to the lungs in one of three forms:

1. **As dissolved carbon dioxide (CO_2).** About 10% of the total amount of carbon dioxide is carried in the dissolved form. It is this dissolved CO_2 that produces the PCO_2 of blood plasma.

2. **As carbaminohemoglobin** (kahr-bam-i-no-hee-moh-GLOH-bin). About 20% of the total CO_2 transported in the blood is in the form of carbaminohemoglobin. It is formed by the union of carbon dioxide, hemoglobin, and certain other plasma proteins. The formation of this compound is accelerated by an increase in PCO_2 and slowed by a decrease in PCO_2.

3. **As bicarbonate ions** (HCO_3^-). About 70% of the total CO_2 transported in the blood is carried in the form of bicarbonate ions. When CO_2 dissolves in water (as in blood plasma), some of the CO_2 molecules associate with water (H_2O) to form carbonic acid (H_2CO_3). Once formed, some of the H_2CO_3 molecules dissociated to form hydrogen (H^+) and bicarbonate (HCO_3^-) ions. The speed of this process is quite slow when it occurs in the plasma, but the rate of reaction increases dramatically within red blood cells (RBCs) because of the presence of an enzyme called *carbonic anhydrase* (kar-BON-ik an-HYE-drays). The reaction is summarized by the following chemical equation:

$$CO_2 + H_2O \rightleftharpoons H_2CO_3 \rightleftharpoons$$

Carbon   Water   Carbonic
dioxide   acid

$$H^+ + HCO_3^-$$

Hydrogen   Bicarbonate
ion   ion

Note that the arrows go in both directions. This indicates that the reaction is *reversible*—it can go in either direction. If bicarbonate is being formed, CO_2 molecules entering into plasma can continually be removed from the blood and transported to the lungs. And, when the process is reversed in the lungs, CO_2 can be released to enter the alveolar air and then be exhaled.

 To learn more about gas exchange, go to **AnimationDirect** on your CD.

Volumes of Air Exchanged in Pulmonary Ventilation

A special device called a **spirometer** is used to measure the amount of air exchanged in breathing. Figure 16-15 illustrates the various pulmonary volumes that can be measured as a subject breathes into a spirometer. We take 500 ml (about a pint) of air into our lungs with each normal inspiration and expel it

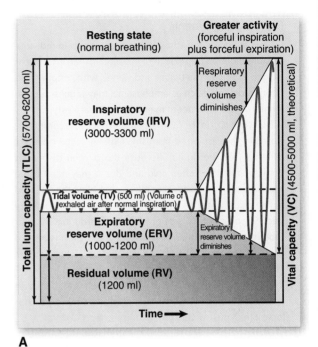

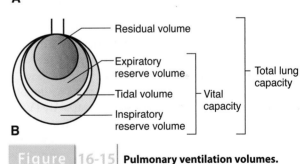

Figure 16-15 **Pulmonary ventilation volumes.**

The chart in **A** shows a tracing like that produced with a spirometer. The diagram in **B** shows the pulmonary volumes as relative proportions of an inflated balloon (see Figure 16-13). During normal, quiet breathing, about 500 ml of air is moved into and out of the respiratory tract, an amount called the *tidal volume*. During forceful breathing (like that during and after heavy exercise), an extra 3300 ml can be inspired (the *inspiratory reserve volume*), and an extra 1000 ml or so can be expired (the *expiratory reserve volume*). The largest volume of air that can be moved in and out during ventilation is called the *vital capacity*. Air that remains in the respiratory tract after a forceful expiration is called the *residual volume*.

MAXIMUM OXYGEN CONSUMPTION

Exercise physiologists use maximum oxygen consumption ($VO_{2\,max}$) as a predictor of a person's capacity to do aerobic exercise. An individual's $VO_{2\,max}$ represents the amount of oxygen taken up by the lungs, transported to the tissues, and used to do work. $VO_{2\,max}$ is determined largely by hereditary factors, but aerobic (endurance) training can increase it by as much as 35%. Many endurance athletes are now using $VO_{2\,max}$ measurements to help them determine and then maintain their peak condition.

Oxygen Supplements

Oxygen therapy is the administration of oxygen to individuals suffering from **hypoxia** (hy-POK-see-ah)—an insufficient oxygen supply to the tissues. Individuals with certain respiratory problems, such as emphysema, may require supplemental oxygen in order to maintain a normal lifestyle.

Oxygen (O_2) in the form of compressed gas is commonly stored in and dispensed from small, green, metal cylinders or tanks (see the figure). Because the oxygen dispensed from such tanks is often cold and dry, it may need to be warmed and moistened, generally by bubbling the released gas through water, to prevent damage to the respiratory tract. Supplemental oxygen is delivered through a mask or tubes that lead into the nasal passage (nasal prongs).

Supplemental (and generally very expensive) oxygen is now being dispensed for recreational purposes at trendy "oxygen bars." Delivery is at low flow levels and, although considered safe for healthy individuals, has more psychological than measurable physiological effects.

Breathing supplemental oxygen for short periods after strenuous exercise is another nonmedical application of oxygen therapy. Although it may shorten recovery times for some athletes, it seldom provides more than transitory benefits. Some endurance athletes, such as cyclists and long-distance runners who perform at high altitudes, have used "oxygen tents" or "bags" to provide lower O_2 levels over longer periods of sleep or rest to improve performance or reduce the need for high altitude training prior to competition. Most sport sanctioning groups have now questioned the ethics of this longer-term use of supplemental oxygen or have banned the practice outright as a form of "doping" (see box p. 350).

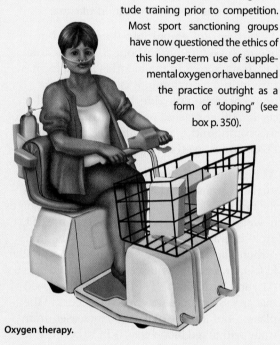

Oxygen therapy.

---

with each normal expiration. Because this amount comes and goes regularly like the tides of the sea, it is referred to as the **tidal volume (TV).**

The largest amount of air that we can breathe out in one expiration is known as the **vital capacity (VC).** In normal young adults, this is about 4800 ml. Tidal volume and vital capacity are frequently measured in patients with lung or heart disease, conditions that often lead to abnormal volumes of air being moved in and out of the lungs.

Observe the area in Figure 16-15 that represents the **expiratory reserve volume (ERV).** This is the amount of air that can be forcibly exhaled after expiring the tidal volume. Compare this with the area in Figure 16-15 that represents the **inspiratory reserve volume (IRV).** The IRV is the amount of air that can be forcibly inspired over and above a normal inspiration. As the tidal volume increases, the ERV and IRV decrease.

Note in Figure 16-15 that vital capacity (VC) is the total of tidal volume, inspiratory reserve volume,

and expiratory reserve volume—or expressed in another way: VC = TV + IRV + ERV. **Residual volume (RV)** is simply the air that remains in the lungs after the most forceful expiration.

> **QUICK CHECK**
>
> 1. How does the diaphragm operate during inspiration? During expiration?
> 2. In what form does oxygen travel in the blood? What form of carbon dioxide?
> 3. What is the vital capacity? How is it measured?

Regulation of Respiration

We know that the body uses oxygen to obtain energy for the work it has to do. The more work the body does, the more oxygen that must be delivered to its millions of cells. One way this is accomplished is by increasing the rate and depth of respirations. Although we may take only 12 to 18 breaths a minute when we are not moving about, we take considerably more than this when we are exercising. Not only do we take more breaths, but our tidal volume also increases.

To help supply cells with more oxygen when they are doing more work, automatic adjustments occur not only in respirations but also in circulation. Most notably, the heart beats faster and harder and therefore pumps more blood through the body each minute. This means that the millions of RBCs make more round trips between the lungs and tissues each minute and so deliver more oxygen per minute to tissue cells.

Working cells not only require more oxygen but also produce more waste products, such as carbon dioxide and certain metabolic acids. The increase in respirations during exercise shows us how the body automatically regulates its vital functions. By increasing the rate and depth of respiration, we can adjust to the varying demands for increased oxygen while increasing the elimination of metabolic waste products in expired air to maintain homeostasis.

Normal respiration depends on proper functioning of the muscles of respiration. These muscles are stimulated by nervous impulses that originate in **respiratory control centers** located in the brainstem. The brainstem centers are influenced by input from a number of sensory receptors located in different areas of the body. These receptors can sense the need for changing the rate or depth of respirations to maintain homeostasis. Certain receptors sense carbon dioxide or oxygen levels, whereas others sense blood acid levels or the amount of stretch in lung tissues.

A group of control centers in the medulla—the *medullary rhythmicity area*—seem to produce the basic rhythm of breathing. A normal resting breathing rate is about 12 to 18 breaths a minute. The two most important control centers in the medulla for regulating breathing rhythm are called the *ventral respiratory group (VRG)* and the *dorsal respiratory group (DRG)*. The VRG provides the basic rhythm generator for breathing. DRG adjusts the breathing rhythm when blood pH or carbon dioxide levels change—as they would during exercise.

Several control centers in the pons—the *pontine respiratory group (PRG)*—seem to provide input to the DRG and thus help to modulate the basic rhythm as needed under a variety of changing conditions in the body.

The depth and rate of respiration can be influenced by many "inputs" to the respiratory control centers from other areas of the brain or from sensory receptors located outside of the central nervous system (Figure 16-16).

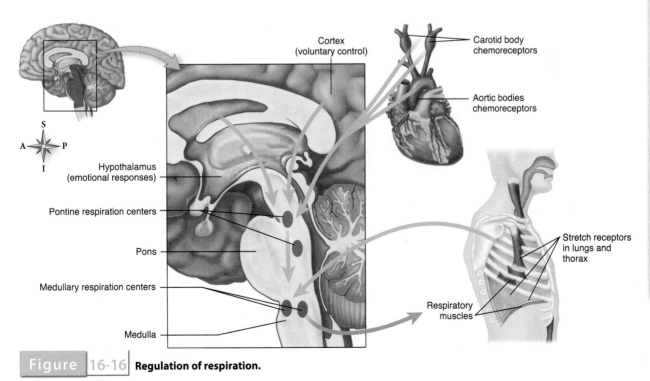

Figure 16-16 | Regulation of respiration.

Respiratory control centers in the brainstem control the basic rate and depth of breathing. The brainstem also receives input from other parts of the body; information from chemoreceptors and stretch receptors can alter the basic breathing pattern, as can emotional and sensory input. Despite these controls, the cerebral cortex can override the "automatic" control of breathing to some extent to accomplish activities such as singing or blowing up a balloon. Green arrows show the flow of regulatory information as it flows into the respiratory control centers. The purple arrow shows the flow of regulatory information from the control centers to the respiratory muscles that provide the power needed for breathing.

Cerebral Cortex

The cerebral cortex can influence respiration by sending nerve signals that affect the function of the respiratory centers of the brainstem. In other words, an individual may voluntarily override the "automatic" brainstem rhythm of breathing and speed up or slow down the breathing rate—or greatly change the pattern of respiration during activities. This ability permits us to change respiratory patterns and even to hold our breath for short periods to accommodate activities such as speaking, eating, or swimming under water.

This voluntary control of respiration, however, has limits. As indicated in a later section, other factors such as blood carbon dioxide levels are much more powerful in controlling respiration than conscious control. Regardless of cerebral intent to the contrary, we resume breathing when our bodies sense the need for more oxygen or if carbon dioxide levels increase to certain levels.

Receptors Influencing Respiration

CHEMORECEPTORS

Chemoreceptors (KEE-moh-ree-SEP-tors) located in the **carotid** and **aortic bodies** are sensory receptors that are sensitive to increases in blood carbon dioxide level and decreases in blood oxygen level. They also can sense and respond to increasing blood acid levels.

The carotid body receptors are found at the point where the common carotid arteries divide, and the aortic bodies are small clusters of chemosensitive cells that lie adjacent to the aortic arch near the heart (see Figure 16-16). When stimulated by increasing levels of blood carbon dioxide, decreasing oxygen levels, or increasing blood acidity, these receptors send nerve impulses to the respiratory regulatory centers that in turn modify respiratory rates.

PULMONARY STRETCH RECEPTORS

Sensory stretch receptors in the lungs are located throughout the pulmonary airways and in the alveoli (see Figure 16-16). Nerve impulses generated by these receptors influence the normal pattern of breathing and protect the respiratory system from excess stretching caused by harmful overinflation.

When the tidal volume of air has been inspired, the lungs are expanded enough to stimulate stretch receptors that then send inhibitory impulses to the inspiratory center. Relaxation of inspiratory muscles occurs, and expiration follows. After expiration, the lungs are sufficiently deflated to inhibit the stretch receptors, and inspiration is then allowed to start again.

Breathing Patterns

A number of terms are used to describe breathing patterns. **Eupnea** (YOOP-nee-ah), for example, refers to a normal respiratory rate. During eupnea, the need for oxygen and carbon dioxide exchange is being met, and the individual is usually not aware of the breathing pattern.

The terms **hyperventilation** and **hypoventilation** describe very rapid and deep or slow and shallow respirations, respectively. Hyperventilation sometimes results from a conscious voluntary effort preceding exertion or from psychological factors—"hysterical hyperventilation."

Dyspnea (DISP-nee-ah) refers to labored or difficult breathing and is often associated with hypoventilation. Dyspnea that is relieved by moving into an upright or sitting position is called **orthopnea** (or-THOP-nee-ah).

If breathing stops completely for a brief period, regardless of cause, it is called **apnea** (AP-nee-ah). A series of cycles of alternating apnea and hyperventilation is called **Cheyne-Stokes** (chain-stokes) **respiration (CSR).** CSR occurs in critical diseases such as congestive heart failure, brain injuries, or brain tumors. CSR also may occur in the case of a drug overdose. Failure to resume breathing after a period of apnea is called **respiratory arrest.**

Examples of breathing patterns are summarized in Table 16-1.

 To learn more about normal and abnormal breathing patterns, go to **AnimationDirect** on your CD.

QUICK CHECK

1. Where are the respiratory control centers located?
2. What is a chemoreceptor? How does it influence breathing?
3. What is hyperventilation? Hypoventilation?

Disorders of the Lower Respiratory Tract

Lower Respiratory Infection

Acute **bronchitis** (brahn-KYE-tis) is a common condition characterized by acute inflammation of the bronchi, most commonly caused by infection. Because the trachea is often also involved, the condition may be called *tracheobronchitis*. This condition is often pre-

Table 16-1	Examples of Breathing Patterns and Spirograms
NAME OF PATTERN	**DESCRIPTION**
Eupnea	Normal breathing
Hyperventilation	Rapid, deep respirations
Hypoventilation	Slow, shallow respirations
Apnea	Cessation of respirations
Cheyne-Stokes respiration	Alternating apnea and hyperventilation

ceded by a URI that seems to move down into the trachea and bronchi after several days. Acute bronchitis often starts with a nonproductive cough that progresses to a deep cough that produces *sputum* (SPYOO-tum) containing mucus and pus.

Pneumonia (noo-MOH-nee-ah) is an acute inflammation of the lungs in which the alveoli and bronchi become plugged with thick fluid (exudate). The vast majority of pneumonia cases result from infection by *Streptococcus pneumoniae* bacteria, but can be caused by several other bacteria, viruses, and fungi (see Appendix A on page A-1 of your book). Pneumonia is characterized by a high fever, severe chills, headache, cough, and chest pain. The fact that each day more than 10,000 liters of potentially contaminated air enters the respiratory system helps explain why pneumonia is such a common illness—especially in individuals with lowered resistance or impaired immune systems.

Types of pneumonia include *lobar pneumonia,* which typically affects an entire lobe of the lung, and *bronchopneumonia* in which patches of infection are scattered along portions of the bronchial tree (see Figure 16-17). The term *aspiration pneumonia* describes lung infections caused by inhalation of vomit or other infective material. It is common in acute alcohol intoxication and as a result of anesthesia.

Tuberculosis (too-ber-kyoo-LO-sis) **(TB)** is a chronic bacillus infection caused by *Mycobacterium tuberculosis* (see Appendix A on page A-1 of your book). TB is a highly contagious disease transmitted through inhalation or swallowing of droplets contaminated with the TB bacillus. It usually affects the lungs and sur-

rounding tissues but can invade any other tissue or organ as well. Early stages of TB are characterized by fatigue, chest pain, pleurisy, weight loss, and fever. As the disease progresses, lung hemorrhage and dyspnea may develop.

The name *tuberculosis* literally means "condition of having tubercles," which describes the protective capsules the body forms around colonies of TB bacilli. Successful treatment requires a combination of drugs and other therapies for an extended period—usually longer than a year. TB is still a major cause of death in many poor, densely populated regions of the world. It has recently reemerged as a serious health problem in some major U.S. cities.

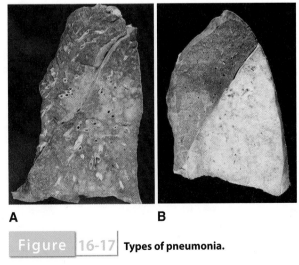

A   B

Figure 16-17 **Types of pneumonia.**

A, Bronchopneumonia. **B,** Lobar pneumonia.

Restrictive Pulmonary Disorders

Restrictive pulmonary disorders involve restriction (reduced stretch) of the alveoli, as the name implies. Because they inhibit inspiration, restrictive disorders reduce pulmonary volumes and capacities such as inspiratory reserve volume and vital capacity. Some restrictive disorders arise in connective tissue of the lung itself. For example, inflammation or fibrosis (scarring) of lung tissue caused by exposure to asbestos, coal, or silicon dust can restrict alveoli. Restriction of breathing also can be caused by the pain that accompanies pleurisy or mechanical injuries.

Obstructive Pulmonary Disorders

A number of different conditions may cause obstruction of the airways. For example, exposure to cigarette smoke and other common air pollutants can trigger a reflexive constriction of bronchial airways. Obstructive disorders may obstruct *inspiration* and *expiration*, whereas restrictive disorders mainly restrict *inspiration*. In obstructive disorders, the total lung capacity may be normal, or even high, but the time it takes to inhale or exhale maximally is significantly increased. Some major obstructive disorders are summarized here and in Figure 16-18.

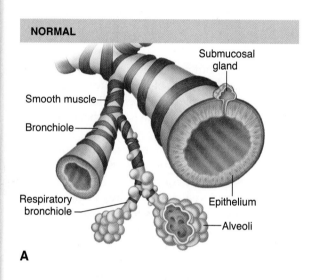

NORMAL

Submucosal gland

Smooth muscle

Bronchiole

Respiratory bronchiole

Epithelium

Alveoli

A

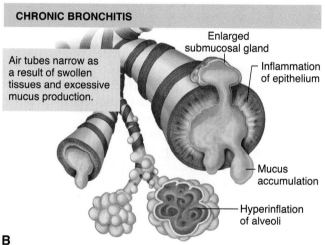

CHRONIC BRONCHITIS

Air tubes narrow as a result of swollen tissues and excessive mucus production.

Enlarged submucosal gland

Inflammation of epithelium

Mucus accumulation

Hyperinflation of alveoli

B

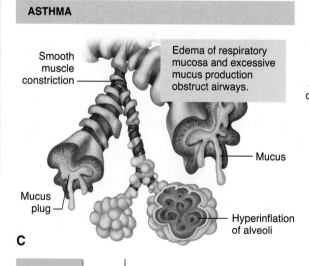

ASTHMA

Smooth muscle constriction

Edema of respiratory mucosa and excessive mucus production obstruct airways.

Mucus

Mucus plug

Hyperinflation of alveoli

C

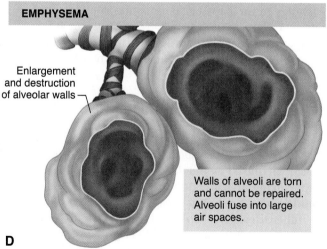

EMPHYSEMA

Enlargement and destruction of alveolar walls

Walls of alveoli are torn and cannot be repaired. Alveoli fuse into large air spaces.

D

Figure 16-18 **Major obstructive pulmonary disorders.**

Chronic obstructive pulmonary disease (COPD) is a broad term used to describe conditions of progressive irreversible obstruction of expiratory air flow. People with COPD have chronic difficulties with breathing, mainly emptying their lungs, and have visibly hyperinflated chests. Those with COPD often have a productive cough and intolerance of activity. The major disorders observed in people with COPD are chronic bronchitis and emphysema.

In North America, tobacco use is the primary cause of COPD, but air pollution, asthma, and respiratory infections also play a role. COPD is a leading cause of death and the death rate from COPD is *increasing!* Until a few years ago, more men had COPD than women. However, the increase of smoking among women is thought to account for the fact that the rate for female COPD is growing rapidly.

Acute respiratory failure can occur when any of the disorders that produce COPD become intense. Heart failure resulting from the pulmonary disease and the vascular resistance that develops with COPD is another possible outcome. Although there is no cure for chronic obstructive respiratory conditions, limiting symptoms can improve quality of life. Bronchodilators and corticosteroids have been used to relieve some of the airway obstruction involved in COPD.

Acute obstruction of the airways, as when a piece of food blocks air flow, requires immediate action to avoid death from suffocation (see the box on p. 462).

Chronic bronchitis is a chronic inflammation of the bronchi and bronchioles. It is characterized by edema and excessive mucus production, which block air passages. People with chronic bronchitis have

RESEARCH, ISSUES, AND TRENDS

LUNG VOLUME REDUCTION SURGERY

Lung volume reduction surgery (LVRS) is a "treatment of last resort" for severe cases of emphysema. It involves the removal of 20% to 30% of each lung. Diseased tissue is generally removed from the upper or apical areas of the superior lobes. Evidence from a number of large clinical trials has shown that the LVRS procedure may benefit or at least help stabilize selected emphysema patients whose lung function continues to decline despite aggressive pulmonary rehabilitation efforts and other more conservative forms of treatment.

More than 2 million Americans, most of whom are older than age 50 and are current or former smokers, have emphysema—a major cause of disability and death in the United States. Emphysema is one of a number of conditions discussed in Chapter 24 and classified as a **chronic obstructive pulmonary disease,** or **COPD**. Although lung damage caused by emphysema is irreversible, in some cases the disease may be halted or its progression slowed by LVRS. In the end stages of this chronic disease, breathing becomes labored as the lungs fill with large irregular spaces resulting from the enlargement and rupture of many alveoli (see illustration). The LVRS procedure removes part of the diseased lung tissue and increases available space in the pleural cavities. As a result, the diaphragm and other respiratory muscles can more effectively move air into and out of the remaining lung tissue, thereby improving pulmonary function and making breathing easier.

LVRS may reduce the need for lung transplantation procedures and augment the effectiveness of such supporting medical treatments as nutritional supplementation and exercise training in the treatment of selected late-stage emphysema patients. Newer and less invasive techniques involving smaller incisions and tiny video equipment inserted into the thoracic cavity (video-assisted thoracic surgery) are now being used for many LVRS procedures. As a result, the relatively long hospital stays and home recovery periods previously required after more traditional open-chest surgery have been shortened.

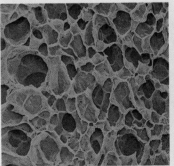 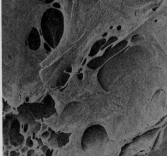

A **B**

Emphysema.
The effects of emphysema can be seen in these scanning electron micrographs of lung tissue. **A,** Normal lung with many small alveoli. **B,** Lung tissue affected by emphysema. Notice that the alveoli have merged into larger air spaces, reducing the surface area for gas exchange.

difficulty with exhaling and often cough deeply as they try to dislodge the accumulating mucus. The major cause of chronic bronchitis is cigarette smoking or exposure to cigarette smoke. Exposure to other air pollutants also may cause chronic bronchitis.

Emphysema (em-fi-SEE-mah) may result from the progression of chronic bronchitis or other conditions as air becomes trapped within alveoli and causes them to enlarge. As the alveoli enlarge, their walls rupture and then fuse into large irregular spaces. The rupture of alveoli reduces the total surface area of the lung, making breathing difficult. Emphysema victims often develop *hypoxia,* or oxygen deficiency, in the internal environment.

Asthma (AZ-mah) is an obstructive disorder characterized by recurring spasms of the smooth muscle in the walls of the bronchial air passages. The muscle contractions narrow the airways, making breathing difficult. Inflammation (edema and excessive mucus production) usually accompanies the spasms, further obstructing the airways. Asthma can be triggered by stress, heavy exercise, infection, or inhaling allergens or other irritants.

Lung Cancer

Lung cancer is a malignancy of pulmonary tissue that not only destroys the vital gas-exchange tissues of the lungs but, like other cancers, also may invade other parts of the body (metastasis). Lung cancer most often develops in damaged or diseased lungs. The most common predisposing condition associated with lung cancer is cigarette smoking (accounting for about 75% of lung cancer cases). Other factors thought to cause lung cancer include exposure to "second-hand" cigarette smoke, asbestos, chromium, coal products, petroleum products, rust, and ionizing radiation (as in radon gas).

Lung cancer may be arrested if detected early with routine chest x-ray films or other diagnostic procedures. Depending on the exact type of malignancy involved and the extent of lung involvement, a number of strategies are available for treatment. Chemotherapy can cause a cure or remission in selected cases, as can radiation therapies. Surgery is the most effective treatment known, but only half of the persons diagnosed as having lung cancer are good candidates for surgery because of extensive spread of the disease (metastasis) at the time of diagnosis. In a **lobectomy** (lo-BEK-toh-mee), only the affected lobe of a lung is removed. **Pneumonectomy** (noo-moh-NEK-toh-mee) is the surgical removal of an entire lung.

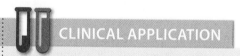

QUICK CHECK

1. What is the difference between bronchopneumonia and lobar pneumonia?

2. Do restrictive pulmonary disorders restrict mainly inspiration or expiration?

3. Give two examples of chronic obstructive pulmonary disease (COPD).

CLINICAL APPLICATION

SUDDEN INFANT DEATH SYNDROME

Sudden infant death syndrome (SIDS) is the third-ranking cause of infant death and accounts for about 1 in 9 of the nearly 30,000 infant deaths reported each year in the United States. Sometimes called "crib death," SIDS occurs most frequently in babies with no obvious medical problems who are younger than 3 months of age. The exact cause of death can seldom be determined even after extensive testing and autopsy.

SIDS occurs at a higher rate in African-American and Native-American babies than in white, Hispanic, or Asian infants, although the reasons remain a mystery. Regardless of infant ethnicity, recent data suggest that certain precautions, such as having babies sleep only on their backs and keeping cribs free of pillows or plush toys that might partially cover the nose or mouth, may reduce the incidence of SIDS. Also important is the elimination of smoking during pregnancy and protecting infants from exposure to "second-hand" cigarette smoke after birth.

Although the exact cause of SIDS remains unknown, abnormalities in the regulatory centers of the brainstem that control breathing may play a role in this tragic problem.

SCIENCE APPLICATIONS

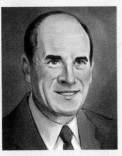

Henry Heimlich, born 1920

RESPIRATORY MEDICINE
The name of American physician Henry Heimlich is known to many people around the world because of the abdominal thrust maneuver that he developed in 1974 to save the lives of people who are choking (see box on p. 462). What many do not know is that Heimlich has made remarkable breakthroughs throughout his life. For example, after witnessing a soldier die after being shot in the chest in 1945 he went on to develop the Heimlich chest drain valve that drains blood and air out of the chest. In 1980, he developed a tiny tube called the *Heimlich MicroTrach* that can be inserted into the trachea under local anesthesia and used in oxygen therapy. Later, he developed a method for teaching stroke victims who were fed through a tube to once again swallow.

Even today, Heimlich's first-aid techniques are being used by countless emergency medical technicians, paramedics, police and firefighters trained in first aid, and even ordinary citizens who have been trained in these lifesaving procedures. Physicians, respiratory therapists, and many other health professionals continue to use Heimlich's medical procedures along with many other respiratory treatments to save the lives of their patients.

Outline Summary

To download an MP3 version of the chapter summary for use with your iPod or portable media player, access the **Audio Chapter Summaries** on your CD.

Structural Plan

A. Basic plan of respiratory system would be similar to an inverted tree if it were hollow (Figure 16-1); leaves of the tree would be comparable to alveoli, with the microscopic sacs enclosed by networks of capillaries (Figure 16-2)
B. Diffusion is the mode for gas exchange that occurs in the respiratory mechanism

Respiratory Tracts

A. Upper respiratory tract—nose, pharynx, and larynx
B. Lower respiratory tract—trachea, bronchial tree, and lungs

Respiratory Mucosa

A. Mucous membrane that lines the air distribution tubes in the respiratory tree (Figure 16-3)
B. More than 125 ml of mucus produced each day forms a "mucus blanket" over much of the respiratory mucosa
C. Mucus serves as an air purification mechanism by trapping inspired irritants such as dust and pollen

D. Cilia on mucosal cells beat in only one direction, moving mucus upward to pharynx for removal

Nose

A. Structure
  1. Nasal septum separates interior of nose into two cavities
  2. Mucous membrane lines nose
  3. Nasal polyps—noncancerous growths that project from nasal mucosa (associated with chronic hay fever)
  4. Frontal, maxillary, sphenoidal, and ethmoidal sinuses drain into nose (Figure 16-4)
B. Functions
  1. Warms and moistens inhaled air
  2. Contains sense organs of smell

Pharynx

A. Structure (Figure 16-5)
  1. Pharynx (throat) about 12.5 cm (5 inches) long
  2. Divided into nasopharynx, oropharynx, and laryngopharynx

3. Two nasal cavities, mouth, esophagus, larynx, and auditory tubes all have openings into pharynx
4. Pharyngeal tonsils and openings of auditory tubes open into nasopharynx; other tonsils found in oropharynx
5. Mucous membrane lines pharynx

B. Functions
1. Passageway for food and liquids
2. Air distribution; passageway for air
3. Tonsils—masses of lymphoid tissue embedded in pharynx provide immune protection

Larynx

A. Structure (Figure 16-7)
1. Located just below pharynx; also referred to as the voice box
2. Several pieces of cartilage form framework
   a. Thyroid cartilage (Adam's apple) is largest
   b. Epiglottis partially covers opening into larynx
3. Mucous lining
4. Vocal cords stretch across interior of larynx; space between cords is the glottis

B. Functions
1. Air distribution; passageway for air to move to and from lungs
2. Voice production

C. Laryngeal cancer
1. Incidence increases with age and alcohol abuse
2. Occurs most often in men over age 50
3. If larynx removed, "esophageal speech" or electric artificial larynx needed for speech

Disorders of the Upper Respiratory Tract

A. Upper respiratory infection (URI)
1. Rhinitis—nasal inflammation, as in a cold, influenza, or allergy
   a. Infectious rhinitis—common cold
   b. Allergic rhinitis—hay fever
2. Pharyngitis (sore throat)—inflammation or infection of the pharynx
3. Laryngitis—inflammation of the larynx resulting from infection or irritation
   a. Epiglottitis—life threatening
   b. Croup—non-life threatening

B. Anatomical disorders

1. Deviated septum—septum that is abnormally far from the midsagittal plane (congenital or acquired)
2. Epistaxis (bloody nose) can result from mechanical injuries to the nose, hypertension, or other factors

Trachea

A. Structure (Figure 16-8)
1. Tube (windpipe) about 11 cm (4.5 inches) long that extends from larynx into the thoracic cavity
2. Mucous lining
3. C-shaped rings of cartilage hold trachea open

B. Function—passageway for air to move to and from lungs

C. Obstruction
1. Blockage of trachea occludes the airway and if complete causes death in minutes
2. Tracheal obstruction causes more than 4000 deaths annually in the United States
3. Abdominal thrust maneuver (p. 462) is a lifesaving technique used to free the trachea of obstructions; also called *abdominal thrusts*
4. Tracheostomy—surgical procedure in which a tube is inserted into an incision in the trachea so that a person with a blocked airway can breathe

Bronchi, Bronchioles, and Alveoli

A. Structure
1. Trachea branches into right and left bronchi
   a. Right primary bronchus more vertical than left
   b. Aspirated objects most often lodge in right primary bronchus or right lung
2. Each bronchus branches into smaller and smaller tubes (secondary bronchi), eventually leading to bronchioles
3. Bronchioles end in clusters of microscopic alveolar sacs, the walls of which are made up of alveoli (Figure 16-9)

B. Function
1. Bronchi and bronchioles—air distribution; passageway for air to move to and from alveoli
2. Alveoli—exchange of gases between air and blood

C. Respiratory distress—relative inability to inflate the alveoli

1. Infant respiratory distress syndrome (IRDS)—leading cause of death in premature infants, resulting from lack of surfactant production in alveoli
2. Adult respiratory distress syndrome (ARDS)—impairment of surfactant by inhalation of foreign substances or other conditions

Lungs and Pleura

A. Structure (Figure 16-10)
   1. Size—large enough to fill the chest cavity, except for middle space occupied by heart and large blood vessels
   2. Apex—narrow upper part of each lung, under collarbone
   3. Base—broad lower part of each lung; rests on diaphragm
   4. Pleura—moist, smooth, slippery membrane that lines chest cavity and covers outer surface of lungs; reduces friction between the lungs and chest wall during breathing (Figure 16-11)
B. Function—breathing (pulmonary ventilation)
C. Pleurisy—inflammation of the pleura
D. Atelectasis—incomplete expansion or collapse of the lung (alveoli) (Figure 16-12); can be caused by:
   1. Pneumothorax—presence of air in the pleural space
   2. Hemothorax—presence of blood in the pleural space

Respiration

A. Mechanics of breathing (Figure 16-13)
   1. Pulmonary ventilation includes two phases called *inspiration* (movement of air into lungs) and *expiration* (movement of air out of lungs)
   2. Changes in size and shape of thorax cause changes in air pressure within that cavity and in the lungs because as volume changes, pressure changes in the opposite direction
   3. Air moves into or out of lungs because of pressure differences (pressure gradient); air moves from high air pressure toward low air pressure
B. Inspiration
   1. Active process—muscles increase volume of thorax, decreasing lung pressure, which causes air to move from atmosphere into lungs (down the pressure gradient)
   2. Inspiratory muscles include diaphragm and external intercostals
      a. Diaphragm flattens during inspiration—increases top-to-bottom length of thorax
      b. External intercostals—contraction elevates the ribs and increases the size of the thorax from front to back and from side to side
C. Expiration
   1. Reduction in the size of the thoracic cavity decreases its volume and thus increases its pressure, so air moves down the pressure gradient and leaves the lungs
   2. Quiet expiration is ordinarily a passive process
   3. During expiration, thorax returns to its resting size and shape
   4. Elastic recoil of lung tissues aids in expiration
   5. Expiratory muscles used in forceful expiration are internal intercostals and abdominal muscles
      a. Internal intercostals—contraction depresses the rib cage and decreases the size of the thorax from front to back
      b. Contraction of abdominal muscles elevates the diaphragm, thus decreasing size of the thoracic cavity from top to bottom
D. Exchange of gases in lungs (Figure 16-14)
   1. Carbaminohemoglobin breaks down into carbon dioxide and hemoglobin
   2. Carbon dioxide moves out of lung capillary blood into alveolar air and out of body in expired air
   3. Oxygen moves from alveoli into lung capillaries
   4. Hemoglobin combines with oxygen, producing oxyhemoglobin
E. Exchange of gases in tissues
   1. Oxyhemoglobin breaks down into oxygen and hemoglobin
   2. Oxygen moves out of tissue capillary blood into tissue cells
   3. Carbon dioxide moves from tissue cells into tissue capillary blood
   4. Hemoglobin combines with carbon dioxide, forming carbaminohemoglobin

Blood Transportation of Gases

A. Transport of oxygen
   1. Only small amounts of oxygen can be dissolved in blood
   2. Most oxygen combines with hemoglobin to form oxyhemoglobin to be carried in blood
B. Transport of carbon dioxide
   1. Dissolved carbon dioxide—10%

2. Carbaminohemoglobin—20%
3. Bicarbonate ions—70%
C. Volumes of air exchanged in pulmonary ventilation (Figure 16-15)
   1. Volumes of air exchanged in breathing can be measured with a spirometer
   2. Tidal volume (TV)—amount normally breathed in or out with each breath
   3. Vital capacity (VC)—largest amount of air that one can breathe out in one expiration
   4. Expiratory reserve volume (ERV)—amount of air that can be forcibly exhaled after expiring the tidal volume
   5. Inspiratory reserve volume (IRV)—amount of air that can be forcibly inhaled after a normal inspiration
   6. Residual volume (RV)—air that remains in the lungs after the most forceful expiration

Regulation of Respiration

A. Regulation of respiration permits the body to adjust to varying demands for oxygen supply and carbon dioxide removal
B. Central regulatory centers in the brainstem are called *respiratory control centers* (Figure 16-16)
   1. Medullary centers—under resting conditions the medullary rhythmicity area produces a normal rate and depth of respirations (12 to 18 per minute)
   2. Pontine centers—as conditions in the body vary, these centers in the pons can alter the activity of the medullary rhythmicity area, thus adjusting breathing rhythm
   3. Brainstem centers are influenced by information from other parts of the brain and from sensory receptors located in other body areas
C. Cerebral cortex—voluntary (but limited) control of respiratory activity
D. Receptors influencing respiration
   1. Chemoreceptors—respond to changes in carbon dioxide, oxygen, and blood acid levels—located in carotid and aortic bodies
   2. Pulmonary stretch receptors—respond to the stretch in lungs, thus protecting respiratory organs from overinflation

Breathing Patterns

A. Eupnea—normal breathing
B. Hyperventilation—rapid and deep respirations

C. Hypoventilation—slow and shallow respirations
D. Dyspnea—labored or difficult respirations
E. Orthopnea—dyspnea relieved by moving into an upright or sitting position
F. Apnea—stopped respiration
G. Cheyne-Stokes respiration (CSR)—cycles of alternating apnea and hyperventilation associated with critical conditions
H. Respiratory arrest—failure to resume breathing after a period of apnea

Disorders of the Lower Respiratory Tract

A. Lower respiratory infection
   1. Acute bronchitis, or tracheobronchitis—inflammation of the bronchi or bronchi and trachea caused by infection (usually resulting from the spread of a URI)
   2. Pneumonia (Figure 16-17)—acute inflammation (infection) in which lung airways become blocked with thick exudates
      a. Lobar pneumonia—affects entire lobe of lung
      b. Bronchopneumonia—infection scattered along bronchial tree
   3. Tuberculosis (TB)—chronic, highly contagious lung infection characterized by tubercles in the lung; can progress to involve tissues outside the lungs and pleura
B. Restrictive pulmonary disorders reduce the ability of lung tissues to stretch (as during inspiration)
   1. Factors inside the lungs, such as fibrosis (scarring) or inflammation, may restrict breathing
   2. Factors outside the lungs, such as pain from injury or pleurisy, may restrict breathing
C. Obstructive pulmonary disorders
   1. Obstruct breathing
   2. Chronic obstructive pulmonary disease (COPD) can develop from preexisting obstructive conditions (Figure 16-18)
   3. Chronic bronchitis—chronic inflammation of the bronchial tree
   4. Emphysema—reduced surface area of lungs caused by rupture or other damage to alveoli
   5. Asthma—recurring spasms of the airways accompanied by edema and mucus production
D. Lung cancer—malignant tumor of the lungs, occasionally treatable with surgery, chemotherapy, radiation, photodynamic therapy

New Words

alveolar duct	nasopharynx	adult respiratory distress	laryngitis
alveolar sac	olfaction	syndrome (ARDS)	lobectomy
alveoli (*sing.*, alveolus)	oropharynx	apnea	nasal polyp
aortic body	oxyhemoglobin	asthma	orthopnea
bronchi (*sing.*, bronchus)	paranasal sinus	atelectasis	pharyngitis
bronchiole	pharynx	bronchitis	photodynamic therapy
carbaminohemoglobin	pleura	Cheyne-Stokes respiration (CSR)	pleurisy
carotid body	pulmonary ventilation	chronic obstructive pulmo-	pneumonectomy
conchae	residual volume (RV)	nary disease (COPD)	pneumonia
epiglottis	respiration	croup	pneumothorax
expiration (exhalation)	respiratory control center	deviated septum	primary bronchi
expiratory reserve volume (ERV)	respiratory membrane	dyspnea	respiratory arrest
external nares	respiratory mucosa	emphysema	respiratory distress syndrome
external respiration	spirometer	endotracheal intubation	rhinitis
glottis	surfactant	epiglottitis	secondary bronchi
heme	tidal volume (TV)	epistaxis	sinusitis
homeostatic mechanism	trachea	eupnea	spirometer
inspiration (inhalation)	vital capacity (VC)	hemothorax	sudden infant death
inspiratory reserve volume (IRV)	vocal cords	hyperventilation	syndrome (SIDS)
internal respiration		hypoventilation	tracheostomy
laryngopharynx	**Diseases and Other**	hypoxia	tuberculosis (TB)
larynx	**Clinical Terms**	infant respiratory distress	
nasal cavity	abdominal thrusts (abdomi-	syndrome (IRDS)	
nasal septum	nal thrust maneuver)		

Review Questions

1. Differentiate between the respiratory membrane and the respiratory mucosa.
2. List the functions of the paranasal sinuses.
3. What is the function of the auditory tube?
4. What is the function of the epiglottis?
5. Describe, in decreasing order of size, the air tubes of the lung.
6. What constitutes an upper respiratory infection?
7. Describe rhinitis, pharyngitis, and laryngitis.
8. What is IRDS? What substance is missing from the lung that causes IRDS?
9. Describe the pleura. What is the function of pleural fluid?
10. What is atelectasis?
11. Describe Cheyne-Stokes respiration.
12. Differentiate between external, internal, and cellular respiration.
13. Explain the mechanical process of inspiration.
14. Explain the mechanical process of expiration.
15. Explain how gas is exchanged between the lung and the blood, and the blood and the tissues.
16. How is oxygen carried in the blood? How is carbon dioxide carried in the blood?
17. Name and explain the volumes that make up vital capacity.
18. Explain the function of chemoreceptors in regulating breathing.
19. Explain the function of stretch receptors in regulating breathing.
20. What is bronchitis?

21. Distinguish between lobar pneumonia, bronchopneumonia, and aspiration pneumonia.
22. How is tuberculosis transmitted from person to person? What is the pathogen that causes tuberculosis?
23. What process in emphysema causes the reduction in lung surface area?
24. What occurs to restrict breathing in asthma?

Critical Thinking

25. Explain the effect smoking has on the body's ability to move material trapped in the respiratory mucosa.
26. Explain the role of other systems in the regulation of respiration.

Chapter Test

1. The organs of the respiratory system are designed to perform two basic functions: _____ and _____.
2. The upper respiratory tract consists of the _____, the _____, and the _____.
3. The lower respiratory tract consists of the _____, the _____, and the _____.
4. The membrane that separates the air in the alveoli from the blood in the surrounding capillaries is called the _____.
5. The membrane that lines most of the air distribution tubes of the respiratory system is called the _____.
6. The frontal, maxillary, sphenoidal, and ethmoidal cavities make up the _____.
7. The _____ sacs drain tears into the nasal cavity.
8. The _____ protrude into the nasal cavities and function to warm and humidify the air.
9. The _____ is the structure that can also be called the *throat*.
10. The _____ is also called the *voice box*.
11. The _____ is the large air tube in the neck.
12. The four progressively smaller air tubes that connect the trachea and the alveoli are the _____, _____, _____, and _____.
13. A _____ is a substance made by the lung to reduce the surface tension of water in the alveoli.
14. The right lung is made up of _____ lobes, and the left lung is made up of _____ lobes.

15. A collapse of the lung for any reason is called _____.
16. Air in the pleural space is called a _____.
17. Blood in the pleural space is called a _____.
18. A series of cycles of alternating apnea and hyperventilation is called _____ respiration.
19. The exchange of gases between the blood and the tissues is called _____.
20. The exchange of gases between the blood and the air in the lungs is called _____.
21. The _____ is the most important muscle in respiration.
22. Oxygen is carried in the blood as _____.
23. Carbon dioxide is carried in the blood as the _____ ion or combines with hemoglobin as _____.
24. The basic respiratory rhythm centers are located in what part of the brain? _____.
25. _____ are the sensory receptors that help keep the lung from overexpanding.
26. _____ are the sensory receptors that help modify respiratory rates by detecting the amount of carbon dioxide, oxygen, or acid levels in the blood.
27. The amount of air that is moved in and out of the lung during normal, quiet breathing is called _____ volume.
28. The three volumes that make up vital capacity are _____, _____, and _____.
29. The volume included in total lung capacity, but not vital capacity, is _____ volume.

Match each disorder in Column A with its description or cause in Column B.

Column A
30. _____ rhinitis
31. _____ pharyngitis
32. _____ laryngitis
33. _____ deviated septum
34. _____ epistaxis
35. _____ IRDS
36. _____ pneumonia
37. _____ tuberculosis
38. _____ emphysema
39. _____ asthma

Column B
a. nosebleed
b. a condition in which the nasal septum strays from the midline of the nasal cavity
c. a chronic bacillus infection that usually affects the lung, caused by a mycobacterium
d. an inflammation of the mucous lining of the larynx
e. a condition in which ruptured alveoli reduce the surface area of the lung, making breathing difficult
f. an inflammation of the nasal mucosa
g. an obstructive disorder characterized by recurring spasms of the smooth muscles of the bronchi
h. an acute inflammation of the lungs
i. an inflammation or infection of the pharynx
j. a disease characterized by a lack of surfactant in the alveoli; usually occurs in premature infants

Study Tips

continued from page 453

combining it with hemoglobin. When the blood gets to the lung, the carbon dioxide dissociates and is exhaled. Figure 16-2 shows CO_2 leaving the blood.
4. The different lung volumes can be learned by using flash cards.
5. The disorders of the respiratory system can be learned by making a chart of the various disorders. Organize the chart by mechanism or cause: upper

respiratory infections, lower respiratory infections, restrictive disorders, and obstructive disorders.
6. In your study group, go over the flash cards of the structures of the respiratory system and pulmonary volumes. Discuss the processes of inspiration, expiration, and regulation of respiration. Discuss external and internal respiration. Go over the respiratory disorders chart and the questions at the end of the chapter, and discuss possible test questions.

Case Studies

1. Curtis was having fun alongside a neighborhood swimming pool when he was accidentally pushed into the pool. Although he is a good swimmer, the suddenness of the fall caught him off guard and he inhaled some water before he was able to gain control of the situation. Luckily, a nearby swimmer assisted Curtis to the edge of the pool, but Curtis continued to have great difficulty in breathing. Can you name the syndrome that Curtis must be exhibiting? Explain what has happened to Curtis's lungs to cause his breathing difficulty.
2. Walter has aspergillosis in his lungs. This disease has caused a partial blockage of both of his bronchi. Does

Walter have a restrictive or obstructive condition? What signs would you look for to confirm your diagnosis if Walter uses a spirometer to test his breathing? What type of pathogenic organism caused Walter's problem? (HINT: see Appendix A on page A-1 of your book.)
3. While you are chatting with your friend at an expensive restaurant, she suddenly stops in midswallow and looks panicked. When you ask what is wrong, she indicates that she can't speak and runs toward the restroom. What should you do? Assume that your first aid does not work—what procedure might emergency medical personnel use to help your friend?

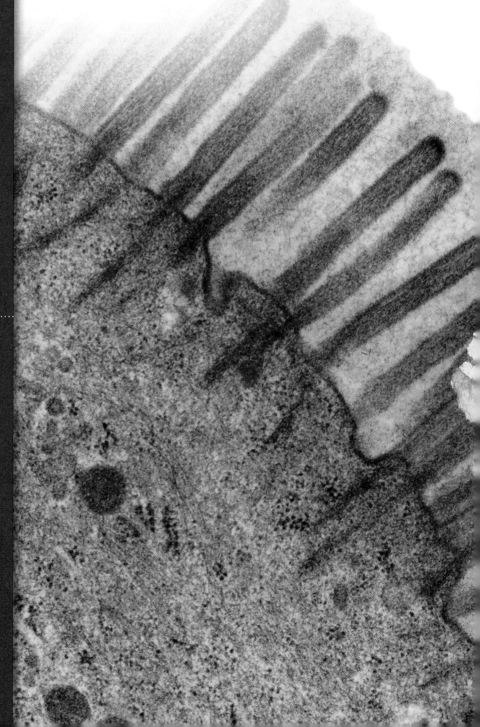

17 The Digestive System

Outline

Objectives

After you have completed this chapter, you should be able to:

1. List in sequence each of the component parts or segments of the alimentary canal from the mouth to the anus and identify the accessory organs of digestion.

2. List and describe the four layers of the wall of the alimentary canal. Compare the lining layer in the esophagus, stomach, small intestine, and large intestine.

3. List and describe the major disorders of the digestive organs.

4. Discuss the basics of protein, fat, and carbohydrate digestion and give the end-products of each process.

5. Define and contrast mechanical and chemical digestion.

6. Define *peristalsis, bolus, chyme, jaundice, ulcer,* and *diarrhea*.

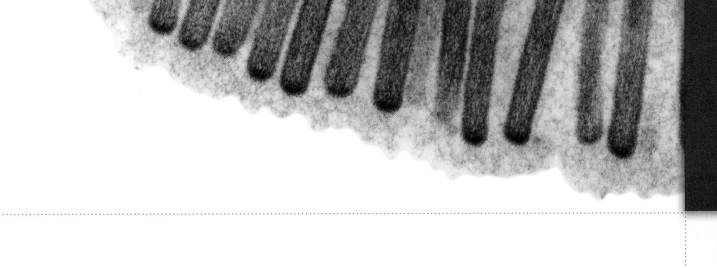

The principal structure of the **digestive system** is an irregular tube, open at both ends, called the **alimentary** (al-i-MEN-tar-ee) **canal,** or the **gastrointestinal** (gas-tro-in-TES-ti-nal) **(GI) tract** (Figure 17-1). In the adult, this hollow tube is about 9 m (29 feet) long.

Although this may seem strange, food or other material that enters the digestive tube is not really *inside* the body. Most parents of young children quickly learn that a button or pebble swallowed by their child will almost always pass unchanged and with little difficulty through the tract. Think of the tube as a passageway that extends through the body like a hallway through a building.

Food must be broken down, or *digested,* and then absorbed through the walls of the digestive tube before it can actually enter the body and be used by cells. The breakdown or digestion of food material is both mechanical and chemical in nature. The teeth are used to physically break down food material before it is swallowed. The churning of food in the stomach then continues the mechanical breakdown process. Chemical breakdown results from the action of

STUDY TIPS

Before studying Chapter 17, review the synopsis of the digestive system in Chapter 3. The structures of the digestive system can be divided into two parts: the tube called the *gastrointestinal tract* and the accessory organs (organs that are not part of the tube). In most cases, the accessory organs produce substances that are released into the tube. The tube is composed of four layers of tissue. The actual process of digestion occurs in this tube.

1. Make flash cards to help you learn the name, location, and function of the organs of the gastrointestinal tract and the accessory organs.
2. Make a chart of the disorders of the digestive system. Group them by the organ that is affected and the mechanism or cause of the disorder.
3. The two processes of the digestive system are digestion and absorption. Digestion is what happens physically and chemically to the food. Absorption is the process of moving digested food into the blood.
4. The process of digestion is explained in terms of what type of food is being digested: carbohydrates, fats, or proteins. The chemical process of digestion uses

continued on page 523

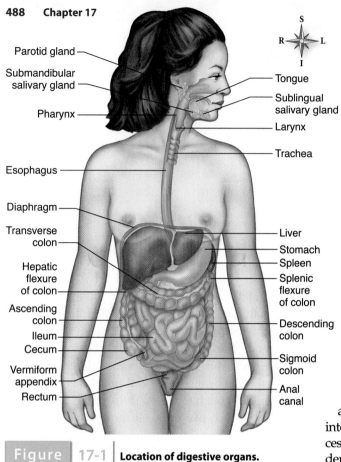

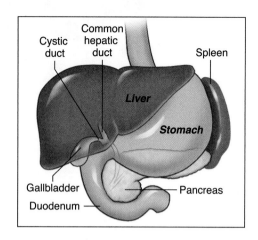

Figure 17-1 | Location of digestive organs.

digestive enzymes and other chemicals acting on food as it passes through the GI tract. In chemical digestion, large food molecules are reduced to smaller molecules that can be absorbed through the lining of the intestinal wall and then distributed to body cells for use. This process of altering the chemical and physical composition of food so that it can be absorbed and used by body cells is known as **digestion,** and it is the function of the gastrointestinal system.

Part of the digestive system, the large intestine, serves also as an organ of elimination, ridding the body of the waste material or **feces** (FEE-seez) resulting from the digestive process. The large intestine also supports the growth of bacteria that add to the amount of the feces; vitamin K is produced in the large intestine as well. Table 17-1 lists both main and accessory digestive organs, which include the teeth, tongue, gallbladder, and appendix, as well as a number of glands that secrete their products into the digestive tube.

Foods undergo three forms of processing in the body: **digestion, absorption,** and **metabolism.** Digestion and absorption are performed by the organs of the digestive system (Figure 17-1). Metabolism, on the other hand, is performed by all body cells. This chapter describes digestive organs, associated disease states, and the processes of digestion and absorption. The metabolism of food after it has been absorbed is discussed in Chapter 18.

Mouth

The *mouth,* or **oral cavity,** is a hollow chamber with a roof, a floor, and walls. Food enters, or is ingested, into the digestive tract through the mouth, and the process of digestion begins immediately. Like the remainder of the digestive tract, the mouth is lined with mucous membrane. Typically, mucous membranes line

Table 17-1 | Organs of the Digestive System

MAIN ORGAN	ACCESSORY ORGAN
Mouth	Teeth and tongue
Pharynx (throat)	Salivary glands
Esophagus (food pipe)	Parotid
Stomach	Submandibular
Small intestine	Sublingual
Duodenum	Liver
Jejunum	Gallbladder
Ileum	Pancreas
Large intestine	Vermiform appendix
Cecum	
Colon	
Ascending colon	
Transverse colon	
Descending colon	
Sigmoid colon	
Rectum	
Anal canal	

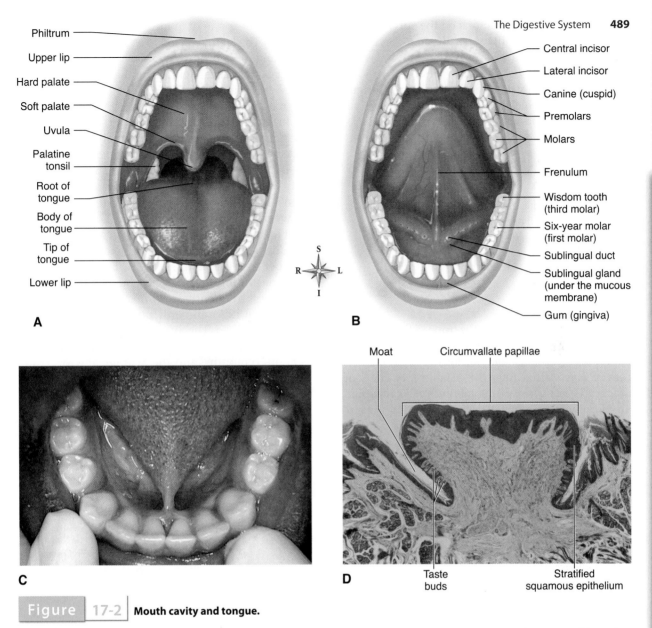

Philtrum
Upper lip
Hard palate
Soft palate
Uvula
Palatine tonsil
Root of tongue
Body of tongue
Tip of tongue
Lower lip

A

Central incisor
Lateral incisor
Canine (cuspid)
Premolars
Molars
Frenulum
Wisdom tooth (third molar)
Six-year molar (first molar)
Sublingual duct
Sublingual gland (under the mucous membrane)
Gum (gingiva)

B

Moat   Circumvallate papillae

Taste buds   Stratified squamous epithelium

C   **D**

Figure 17-2 | Mouth cavity and tongue.

A, Mouth cavity showing hard and soft palates, tongue surface, and uvula. **B,** Undersurface of tongue showing frenulum, sublingual gland, and opening of sublingual duct. **C,** Photograph shows an abnormally short lingual frenulum, which may result in faulty speech. **D,** Papillae with taste buds located on the lateral surfaces.

hollow organs, such as the digestive tube, that open to the exterior of the body. Mucus produced by the lining of the GI tract protects the epithelium from digestive juices and lubricates food passing through the lumen.

The roof of the mouth is formed by the *hard* and *soft* **palates** (Figure 17-2). The hard palate is a bony structure in the anterior or front portion of the mouth, formed by parts of the palatine and maxillary bones. The soft palate is located above the posterior or rear portion of the mouth. It is soft because it consists chiefly of muscle. Hanging down from the center of the soft palate is an elongated process called the **uvula** (YOO-vyoo-lah). The uvula and the soft palate prevent any

food and liquid from entering the nasal cavities above the mouth and also assist in speech and swallowing, also known as **deglutition** (dee-glu-TISH-un).

The floor of the mouth consists of the tongue and its muscles. The tongue is made of skeletal muscle covered with mucous membrane. It is anchored to bones in the skull and to the hyoid bone in the neck. A thin membrane called the **frenulum** (FREN-yoo-lum) attaches the tongue to the floor of the mouth. Occasionally the frenulum is too short to allow free movements of the tongue. Individuals with this condition cannot enunciate words normally and are said to be tongue-tied (Figure 17-2, *C*).

The many small elevations on the surface of the tongue are called **papillae** (pa-PIL-ee.). The largest are the *circumvallate* (ser-kum-VAL-ate) type, which form an inverted V-shaped row of about 10 to 12 mushroom-like elevations at the back of the tongue. The taste buds, which contain sensory receptors, are located on the sides of the papillae (Figure 17-2, *D*).

Teeth

Types of Teeth

The shape and placement of the teeth assist them in their functions and are classified as one of four types:

1. Incisors
2. Canines
3. Premolars
4. Molars

The **incisors** are considered the front teeth; they have a sharp cutting edge (Figure 17-3) used to bite off or cut food into manageable portions to begin the process of **mastication** (mas-ti-KAY-shun), or chewing of food. The **canine teeth,** sometimes called **cuspids,** are usually more elongated and pointed in appearance and function to pierce or tear the food that is being eaten into smaller shreds. This tooth type is particularly apparent in meat-eating mammals such as dogs. The teeth referred to as premolars, or **bicuspids,** and molars, or **tricuspids,** have comparatively larger surface areas with several grinding or crushing sharp points (cuspids) on the surface. The chewing made possible by the teeth begins the mechanical breakdown of food for digestion. After food has been chewed, it is formed into a small rounded mass called a **bolus** (BO-lus) so that it can be swallowed.

By the time a baby is 2 years old, he or she probably has a full set of 20 baby (primary or deciduous) teeth. By the time a young adult is somewhere between 17 and 24 years old, a full set of 32 permanent teeth is generally present. If an individual does not form wisdom teeth (third molars), then the number of adult teeth will be 28. This is considered a normal variation and occurs most often in Asians (30%), less frequently in whites and Native Americans (about 12%), and only rarely in African-Americans (1% to 2%). The average age for "cutting" the first tooth (eruption of tooth through gum tissue) is about 6 months, and the average age for losing the first baby tooth and starting to cut the permanent teeth is about 6 years. Figure 17-3 gives the names of the teeth and shows which ones are lacking in the deciduous (dee-SID-yu-us), or baby, set of teeth.

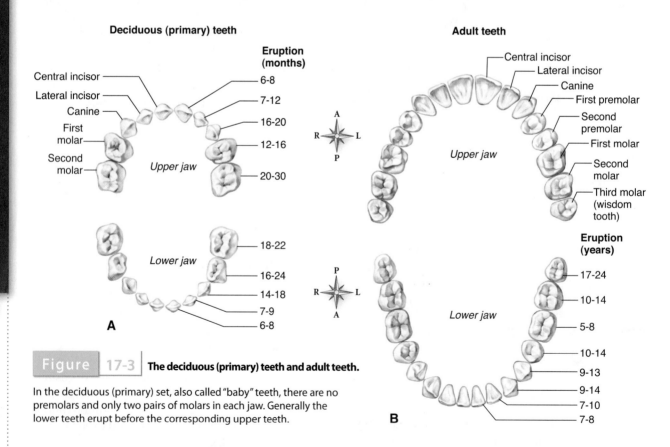

Figure 17-3 | **The deciduous (primary) teeth and adult teeth.**

In the deciduous (primary) set, also called "baby" teeth, there are no premolars and only two pairs of molars in each jaw. Generally the lower teeth erupt before the corresponding upper teeth.

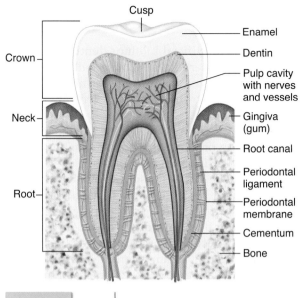

Figure 17-4 | **Longitudinal section of a tooth.**

A molar is sectioned here to show its bony socket and details of its three main parts: crown, neck, and root. Enamel (over the crown) and cementum (over the neck and root) surround the dentin layer. The pulp contains nerves and blood vessels.

Typical Tooth

A typical tooth can be divided into three main parts: crown, neck, and root (Figure 17-4). The **crown** is the portion that is exposed and visible in the mouth. It is largely made of a bony material called **dentin** that

is covered by enamel. Enamel is the hardest material made by the body and is ideally suited to withstand the grinding that occurs during the chewing of hard and brittle foods. The root and neck of each tooth are covered by **cementum** (see-MEN-tum). The center of the tooth contains a pulp cavity consisting of connective tissue, blood and lymphatic vessels, and sensory nerves.

The *neck* of a tooth is the narrow portion surrounded by the pink gingival (JIN-ji-val) or gum tissue. The neck joins the crown of the tooth to the root. The *root* fits into the socket of the upper or lower jaw and is supported by a fibrous **periodontal membrane** that lines each tooth socket.

Disorders of the Mouth and Teeth

Infections, cancer, congenital defects, and other disorders of the mouth and teeth can result in a variety of serious complications. Such conditions may cause pain or even damage to the mouth and teeth that makes chewing and swallowing difficult—perhaps causing a person to reduce the intake of food, thereby resulting in malnutrition. Mouth infections or cancer may spread to nearby tissues: the nasal cavity (then on to the sinuses, middle ear, and brain) or **pharynx** (FAIR-inx), also called the throat, (and on to the esophagus, larynx, and thoracic organs).

Cancer of the mouth may result from exposure to carcinogens found in tobacco smoke or in so-called smokeless tobacco (chewing tobacco), especially in combination with heavy alcohol consumption. Smokers may develop white patches, or **leukoplakia** (loo-koh-PLAK-ee-ah), which may develop into malignant tumors. Leukoplakia often develops in the fold between "cheek and gum" in users of smokeless tobacco (Figure 17-5, *A*). The condition, called **snuff dipper's**

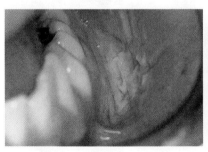

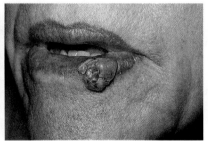

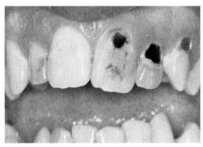

A   **B**   **C**

Figure 17-5 | **Disorders of the mouth and teeth.**

A, Snuff dipper's pouch. This individual has developed leukoplakia in the area between cheek and gum used for placement of chewing tobacco. **B,** Squamous cell carcinoma of lip. Excessive long-term exposure to ultraviolet light (UV) such as in sunlight increases the risk of skin cancer. **C,** Dental caries. These permanent defects, or cavities, are filled with decayed dental tissues.

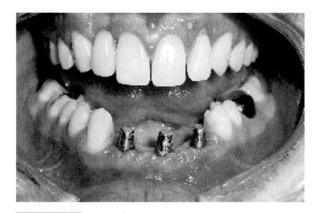

Figure 17-6 | **Dental implant.**

A permanent dental prosthesis will be affixed to the anchor after bone grows and healing has occurred.

pouch, may lead to tooth and gum diseases and oral cancer. Lip cancer may result from the carcinogenic effects of sunlight, which can be avoided by the use of lip balms containing sunscreen. The most common form of mouth cancer is squamous cell carcinoma (Figure 17-5, *B*).

Tooth decay, or dental **caries** (KAIR-ees), is one of the most common diseases in the developed world. It is a disease of the enamel, dentin, and cementum of teeth that results in the formation of a permanent defect called a **cavity** (Figure 17-5, *C*). Many people living in the United States, Canada, and Europe are affected by the disease. Decay occurs on tooth surfaces where food debris, acid-secreting bacteria, and plaque accumulate. Sugar is the main ingredient in food that allows bacteria to produce the acid that damages the protective tooth enamel.

If the disease goes untreated, tooth decay results in infection, loss of teeth, and inflammation of the soft tissues in the mouth. Bacteria also may invade the paranasal sinuses or extend to the surface of the face and neck or enter the bloodstream, causing serious complications.

Dental caries are treated by removal of the decayed portion of the tooth followed by repair and filling of the defect using a variety of restorative materials including porcelain and metal alloys. If lost because of disease or trauma, teeth can be replaced with *dental appliances,* which include removable dentures and permanently fixed or implanted teeth. So called "dental implants" are anchors screwed into holes that have been drilled into the jawbone

to support an artificial tooth or denture. About 6 months after insertion, new bone will have fused with and stabilized the anchor, permitting the attachment of the artificial tooth or dental appliance (Figure 17-6).

Gingivitis (jin-ji-VYE-tis) is the general term for inflammation or infection of the gums. Most cases of gingivitis result from poor oral hygiene—inadequate brushing and no flossing. Gingivitis also may be a complication of other conditions such as diabetes mellitus, vitamin deficiency, or pregnancy.

Thrush, or **oral candidiasis** (KAN-di-DI-a-sis), is a mouth infection caused by a yeastlike fungal organism. It causes cream-colored "cheesy" patches of exudate to appear on an inflamed tongue and oral mucosa (Figure 17-7). Thrush is sometimes observed in otherwise healthy children but is most often seen in adults who are immunosuppressed, such as AIDS patients, or in individuals who have been on antibiotic therapy. The healthy bacteria that normally inhabit the mouth usually prevent the yeast from growing.

Periodontitis (pair-ee-oh-don-TYE-tis) is the inflammation of the periodontal membrane, or *periodontal ligament,* which anchors the tooth to the bone of the jaw. Periodontitis is often a complication of advanced or untreated gingivitis, and may spread to the surrounding bony tissue. Destruction of periodontal membrane and bone results in loosening and eventually complete loss of teeth. Periodontitis is the leading cause of tooth loss among adults.

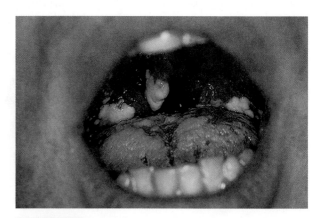

Figure 17-7 | **Oral thrush *(Candida albicans).***

Inflamed mucous membrane is covered with patches of creamy-white exudates.

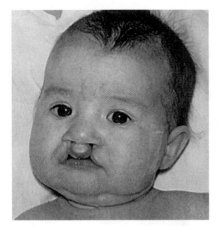

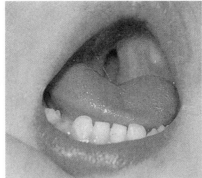

Figure 17-8

Congenital defects of the mouth.
A, Bilateral cleft lip in an infant.
B, Cleft palate.

A   **B**

Cleft lip and **cleft palate** (Figure 17-8) represent the most common forms of congenital defect affecting the mouth. They may occur alone or together and are caused by a failure of structures in the upper lip or palate to fuse or close properly during embryonic development. The condition may be inherited or be a spontaneous abnormality. Cleft lip, which may occur on one or both sides, is generally repaired soon after birth. Surgical repair of cleft palate is usually done later in the first year of life. Modern reconstructive surgery techniques help minimize possible long-term complications that could include scarring, speech impairment, dental problems, and potential emotional maladjustment.

QUICK CHECK

1. What are the three main parts of a typical tooth?
2. What is snuff dipper's pouch?
3. Distinguish between dental caries, gingivitis, and periodontitis.
4. Name the two most common forms of congenital defect affecting the mouth.

CLINICAL APPLICATION

MALOCCLUSION

Malocclusion of the teeth occurs when missing teeth create wide spaces in the dentition, when teeth overlap, or when malposition of one or more teeth prevents correct alignment of the maxillary and mandibular dental arches (Figures *A* and *B*). Malocclusion that results in protrusion of the upper front teeth causing them to hang over the lower front teeth is called *overbite* (Figure *A*), whereas the positioning of the lower front teeth outside the upper front teeth is called *underbite* (Figure *B*).

Dental malocclusion may cause significant problems and chronic pain in the functioning of the temporomandibular joint, contribute to the generation of headaches, or complicate routine mastication of food. Fortunately, even severe malocclusion problems can be corrected by the use of braces and other dental appliances. **Orthodontics** (or-thoh-DON-tiks) is that branch of dentistry that deals with the prevention and correction of positioning irregularities of the teeth and malocclusion.

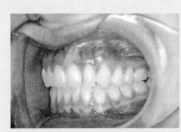

A

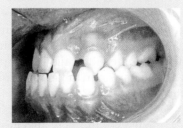

B

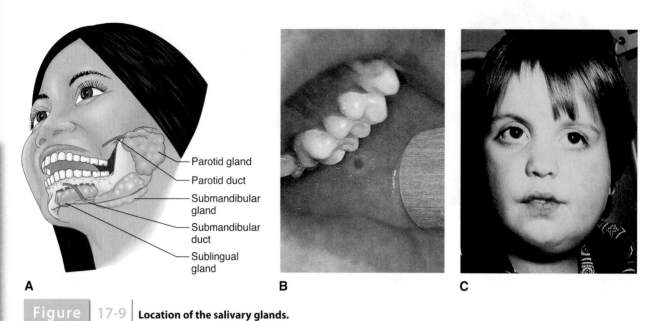

Parotid gland
Parotid duct
Submandibular gland
Submandibular duct
Sublingual gland

A   **B**   **C**

Figure | 17-9 | **Location of the salivary glands.**

A, The salivary glands and their associated ducts. **B,** Photo shows the inflamed opening of the parotid duct into the mouth of a patient with mumps. **C,** Mumps (paramyxovirus) inflammation and swelling of the parotid gland in a child.

Salivary Glands

Three pairs of salivary glands—the parotids, submandibulars, and sublinguals—secrete most (about 1 L) of the saliva produced each day in the adult. The salivary glands (Figure 17-9) are typical of the accessory glands associated with the digestive system because they are located outside the digestive tube itself and must convey their secretions by way of ducts into the tract.

The **parotid glands,** largest of the salivary glands, lie just below and in front of each ear at the angle of the jaw. The parotid gland secretes a solution rich in bicarbonate that helps neutralize bacterial acids and provides moisture to form dry foods into a bolus for swallowing. The openings of the parotid ducts are found by looking in a mirror at the insides of the cheeks and next to the second molar tooth on either side of the upper jaw. Photo insert in Figure 17-9, *B* shows a red and inflamed parotid duct papilla opening into the mouth of a patient with a viral infection called mumps. This disease is now uncommon in developed countries because of the mumps vaccination given to most children. The virus causes the parotid gland to swell and become tender and may also infect other organs such as the testis of older boys (Figure 17-9, *C*).

The ducts of the **submandibular glands** open into the mouth on either side of the lingual frenulum (Figure 17-2, *B*). The ducts of the **sublingual glands** open into the floor of the mouth.

Saliva contains mucus and a digestive enzyme called **salivary amylase** (AM-i-lays). Mucus moistens the food and allows it to pass with less friction through the esophagus and on into the stomach. Salivary amylase begins the chemical digestion of carbohydrates.

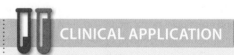

CLINICAL APPLICATION

MUMPS

Mumps is an acute viral disease characterized by swelling of the parotid salivary glands. Most of us think of mumps as a childhood disease because it most often affects children between the ages of 5 and 15 years of age. However, it can occur in adults—often producing a more severe infection. The mumps infection can affect other tissues in addition to the parotid gland, including the joints, pancreas, myocardium, and kidneys. In about 25% of infected men, mumps causes inflammation of the testes, or *orchitis*. Orchitis resulting from mumps very rarely causes enough damage to render a man sterile.

To learn more about the mouth and associated structures in mechanical digestion, go to **AnimationDirect** on your CD.

To learn more about the pharynx, go to **AnimationDirect** on your CD.

and food must pass through it on its way to the stomach.

Pharynx

The **pharynx,** or throat, is a tubelike structure made of muscle and lined with mucous membrane (Figure 17-10). Because of its location behind the nasal cavities and mouth, it functions as part of both the respiratory and digestive systems. Air must pass through the pharynx on its way to the lungs,

Wall of the Digestive Tract

The digestive tract has been described as a tube that extends from the mouth to the anus. However, it is only when food leaves the pharynx and enters the esophagus that the true tubular nature of the GI tract becomes apparent. The wall

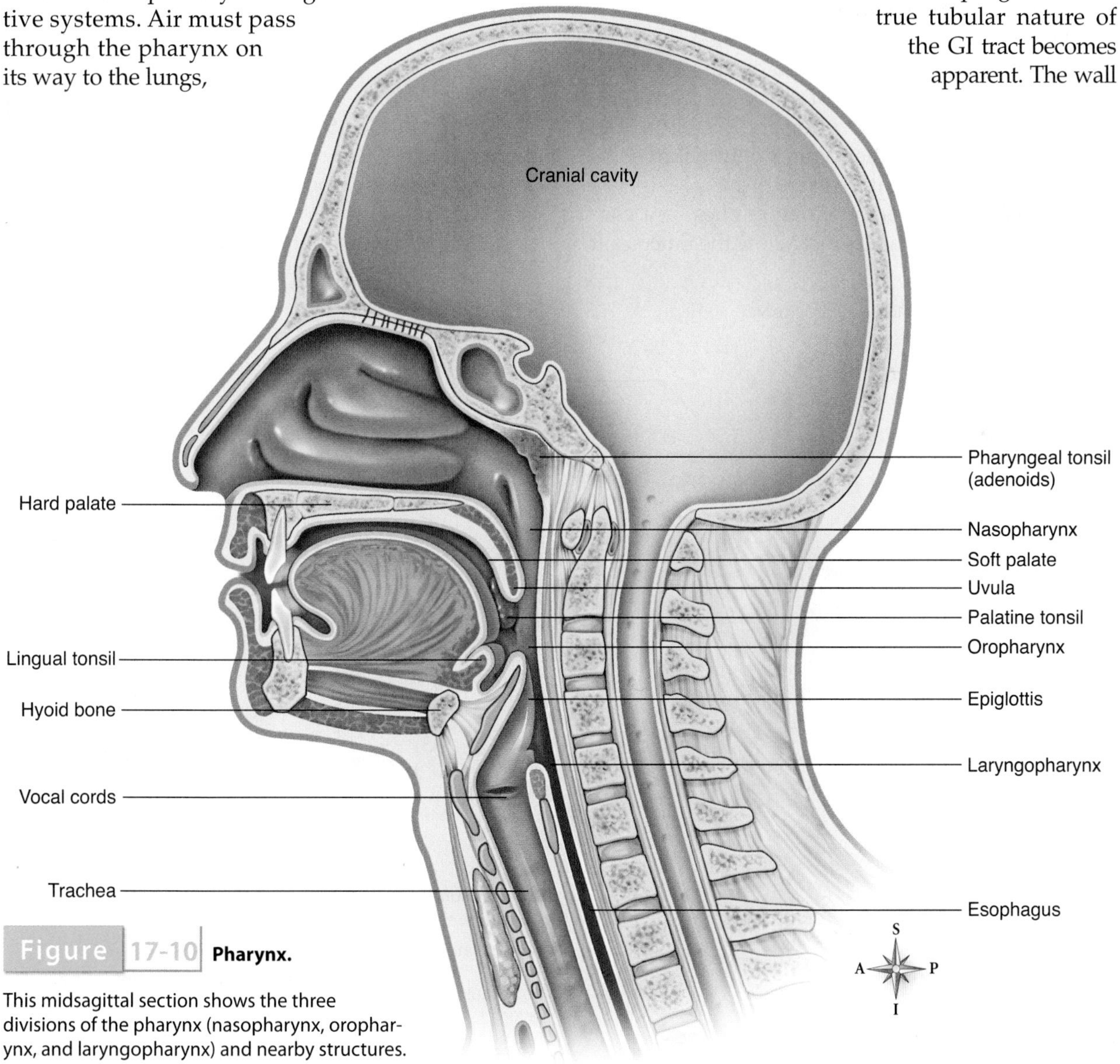

Cranial cavity

Hard palate

Lingual tonsil

Hyoid bone

Vocal cords

Trachea

Pharyngeal tonsil (adenoids)

Nasopharynx

Soft palate

Uvula

Palatine tonsil

Oropharynx

Epiglottis

Laryngopharynx

Esophagus

Figure 17-10 **Pharynx.**

This midsagittal section shows the three divisions of the pharynx (nasopharynx, oropharynx, and laryngopharynx) and nearby structures.

of this digestive tube is composed of four layers of tissue. Figure 17-11 shows the four layers as they appear in a section of the small intestine. The inside or hollow space within the tube is called the **lumen.** The four layers, named from the inside coat to the outside of the tube, are as follows:

1. Mucosa, or mucous membrane
2. Submucosa
3. Muscularis
4. Serosa

Although the same four tissue coats form the organs of the alimentary tract, their structures vary in different organs. The **mucosa** of the esophagus, for example, is composed of tough and stratified abrasion-resistant epithelium. The mucosa of the remainder of the tract is a delicate layer of simple columnar epithelium designed for absorption and secretion. The mucus produced by either type of epithelium coats the lining of the alimentary canal.

The **submucosa,** as the name implies, is a connective tissue layer that lies just below the mucosa. It contains many blood vessels and nerves. The layers of muscle tissue called the **muscularis** have an important function in the digestive process. By a wave-like, rhythmic contraction of the muscular coat, called **peristalsis** (pair-i-STAL-sis), food material is moved through the digestive tube. In addition, the contraction of the muscularis also assists in the mixing of food with digestive juice and in the further mechanical breakdown of larger food particles.

The **serosa** is the outermost covering or coat of the digestive tube. In the abdominal cavity it is composed of the visceral peritoneum. The loops of the digestive tract are anchored to the posterior wall of the abdominal cavity by a large double fold of peritoneal tissue called the **mesentery** (MEZ-en-tair-ee).

Esophagus

The **esophagus** (eh-SOF-ah-gus) is a collapsible, muscular, mucus-lined tube about 25 cm (10 inches) long that extends from the pharynx to the stomach. It is the first segment of the digestive tube proper, and the four layers that form the wall of the GI tract

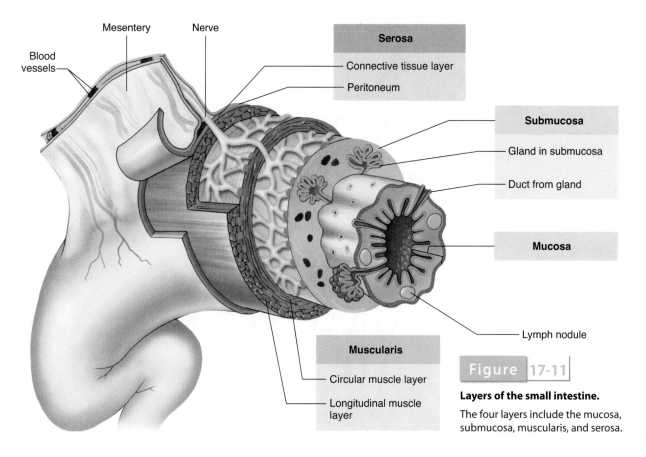

Mesentery

Nerve

Blood vessels

Serosa

Connective tissue layer

Peritoneum

Submucosa

Gland in submucosa

Duct from gland

Mucosa

Lymph nodule

Muscularis

Circular muscle layer

Longitudinal muscle layer

Figure 17-11

Layers of the small intestine.

The four layers include the mucosa, submucosa, muscularis, and serosa.

can be identified when it is sectioned. Its muscular walls make it a dynamic passageway able to push food toward the stomach.

Each end of the esophagus is guarded by a muscular *sphincter* (SFINK-ter). Sphincters are valvelike rings of muscle tissue that often surround tubular structures or body openings. In the GI tract they normally act to keep ingested material moving in one direction down the tube. The **upper esophageal sphincter (UES)** helps prevent air from entering the tube during respiration, and the **lower esophageal sphincter (LES)** normally prevents backflow of acidic stomach contents.

The terms *heartburn* and *acid indigestion* are often used to describe a number of unpleasant symptoms experienced by more than 60 million Americans each month. Backward flow of stomach acid up into the esophagus causes these symptoms (Figure 17-12), which typically include burning and pressure behind the breastbone. The term **gastroesophageal reflux disease (GERD)** is used to better describe this very common and sometimes serious medical condition.

In its simplest form, GERD symptoms are mild and occur only infrequently (twice a week or less). In these cases, avoiding problem foods or beverages, stopping smoking, or losing weight if needed may

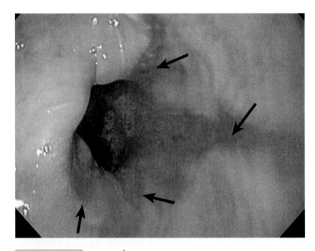

Figure 17-13 **Esophageal inflammation.**

Chronic inflammation of the esophagus is characteristic of GERD (gastroesophageal reflux disease). Arrows show reddened, inflamed areas about midway along esophagus. This damage is caused by the frequent "splashing back" of acids from the stomach.

solve the problem. Additional treatment with over-the-counter antacids or non-prescription-strength acid-blocking medications also may be helpful. More severe and frequent episodes of GERD can trigger asthma attacks, cause severe chest pain, result in bleeding, or promote a narrowing (stricture) or chronic irritation of the esophagus (Figure 17-13). In these cases, more powerful inhibitors of stomach acid production may be prescribed. Other drugs that strengthen the LES and thus reduce backflow of stomach acid are also used in moderate to severe cases of GERD.

Several minimally invasive surgical procedures for treating serious cases of GERD are also available. In such procedures, which are done on an outpatient basis, a flexible tube called an *endoscope* is used to insert and then remove the necessary medical devices required for treatment. If GERD is left untreated, serious pathological (precancerous) changes in the esophageal lining may develop—a condition called **Barrett esophagus**.

A sign of Barrett esophagus is evident when the esophagus is viewed with an endoscope. The color of the esophageal mucosa changes from a pink to a reddish salmon color, indicating cellular changes that are caused by continual exposure of the esophagus to stomach acid. A sample of the lining of the esophagus is removed and viewed under the microscope to make the diagnosis of Barrett esophagus.

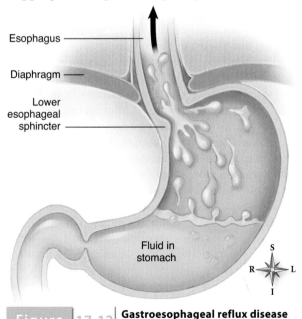

Esophagus

Diaphragm

Lower esophageal sphincter

Fluid in stomach

Figure 17-12 **Gastroesophageal reflux disease (GERD).**

Reflux of gastric acid up into the esophagus, causing irritation of the lining of the esophagus.

Other than heartburn, symptoms of Barrett may include trouble swallowing, vomiting blood, and weight loss that results because eating is painful. Treatment may include medications that reduce stomach acid production and lifestyle changes aimed at preventing the reflux of acid into the esophagus. These changes include eating smaller and more frequent meals; not lying down until 3 hours after eating; elevating the head of the bed to prevent reflux during sleep; avoiding foods that trigger heartburn, which includes caffeine, nicotine, and alcohol; and maintaining a healthy weight to decrease pressure on the stomach.

GERD is a common symptom of **hiatal hernia** (hye-AY-tal HER-nee-ah). A hernia results from an organ being pushed through a wall that normally acts as a barrier. In hiatal hernia, the stomach pushes through the gap, or hiatus, in the diaphragm that allows the esophagus to pass through it (Figure 17-14). Often the lower esophagus becomes enlarged, allowing acidic stomach contents to bypass the LES and flow upward into the esophagus.

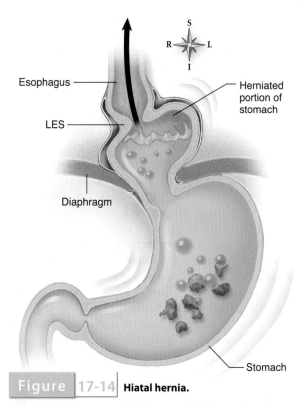

Figure 17-14 **Hiatal hernia.**

Note herniated portion of stomach pushed through diaphragm. *LES,* Lower esophageal sphincter.

 To learn more about the esophagus, go to **AnimationDirect** on your CD.

Stomach

The **stomach** (Figure 17-15) lies in the upper part of the abdominal cavity just under the diaphragm. It serves as a pouch that food enters after it has been chewed, swallowed, and passed through the esophagus. The stomach looks small after it is emptied, not much bigger than a large sausage, but it expands considerably after a large meal. Have you ever felt so uncomfortably full after eating that you could not take a deep breath? If so, it probably meant that your stomach was so full of food that it occupied more space than usual and was pushed up against the diaphragm. This made it hard for the diaphragm to contract and move downward as much as necessary for you to take a deep breath.

After food has entered the stomach by passing through the muscular LES at the distal end of the esophagus, the digestive process continues. Contraction of the stomach's muscular walls mixes the food thoroughly with the gastric juice and breaks it down into a semisolid mixture called **chyme** (KIME). Gastric juice contains hydrochloric acid and enzymes that function in the digestive process. Chyme formation is a continuation of the mechanical digestive process that begins in the mouth.

There are three layers of smooth muscle in the stomach wall (Figure 17-15). The muscle fibers that run lengthwise, around, and obliquely make the stomach one of the strongest internal organs—well able to break up food into tiny particles and to mix them thoroughly with gastric juice to form chyme. Stomach muscle contractions result in peristalsis, which propels food down the digestive tract. Mucous membrane lines the stomach; it contains thousands of microscopic **gastric glands** that secrete gastric juice and hydrochloric acid into the stomach. Cells in the stomach also secrete a chemical called *intrinsic factor* that protects vitamin B$_{12}$ and saves it for its later absorption in the distal small intestine. Some individuals may require vitamin B$_{12}$ injections after some stomach surgeries. When the stomach is empty, its lining lies in folds called **rugae.**

The three divisions of the stomach shown in Figure 17-15 are the **fundus, body,** and **pylorus** (pye-

Figure 17-15 | Stomach.

A portion of the anterior wall has been cut away to reveal the three muscle layers of the stomach wall. Notice that the mucosa lining the stomach forms folds called *rugae*.

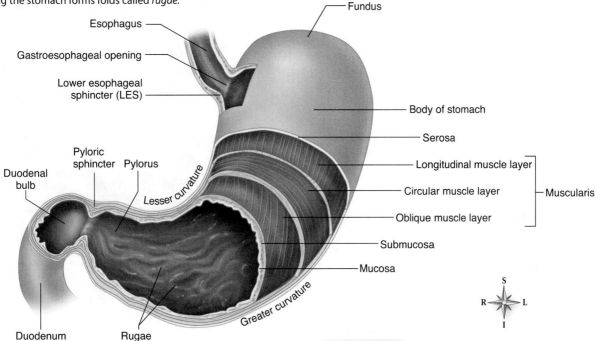

LOR-us). The fundus is the enlarged portion to the left of and above the opening of the esophagus into the stomach. The body is the central part of the stomach, and the pylorus is its lower narrow section, which joins the first part of the small intestine. Partial digestion occurs after food is held in the stomach by the **pyloric** (pi-LOR-ik) **sphincter** muscle. The smooth muscle fibers of the sphincter stay contracted most of the time and thereby close off the opening of the pylorus into the small intestine. The upper right border of the stomach is known as the *lesser curvature*, and the lower left border is called the *greater curvature*. After food has been mixed in the stomach, chyme begins its passage through the pyloric sphincter into the first part of the small intestine.

 To learn more about the stomach, go to **AnimationDirect** on your CD.

QUICK CHECK

1. Name the three pairs of salivary glands. Which salivary gland is inflamed in mumps?
2. Identify the four layers of the stomach.
3. What is GERD?
4. Name the three divisions of the stomach.

Disorders of the Stomach

Gastroenterology (gas-tro-en-ter-AHL-o-jee) is the study of the stomach (*gastro-*) and intestines (*entero-*) and their diseases. The stomach is the potential site of numerous diseases and conditions, some of which are briefly described in this section. Many of these disorders are characterized by one or more of these signs and symptoms:

1. **Gastritis** (gas-TRY-tis)—stomach inflammation
2. **Anorexia** (an-or-EKS-ee-ah)—chronic loss of appetite
3. **Nausea** (NAW-zee-ah)—unpleasant feeling that often leads to vomiting
4. **Emesis** (EM-e-sis)—vomiting

UPPER GASTROINTESTINAL X-RAY STUDY

The upper GI (UGI) study consists of a series of x-rays of the lower esophagus, stomach, and duodenum, produced with the aid of a contrast medium, usually barium sulfate. The test is used to detect ulcerations, tumors, inflammations, or anatomical malpositions such as *hiatal hernia* (distention of the diaphragm that allows the stomach to protrude). Obstruction of the upper GI tract is also easily detected with the UGI series.

First the patient drinks a flavored liquid containing barium sulfate. Then x-rays are taken periodically as the contrast medium travels through the system—the lower esophagus, gastric wall, pyloric channel, and duodenum; each structure is evaluated for defects.

Benign peptic ulcer is a common pathological condition that may affect these GI areas. Tumors, cysts, or enlarged organs near the stomach also can be identified by an anatomical distortion of the outline of the upper GI tract. Compare the x-ray image shown here with the stomach structures depicted in Figure 17-15. Identify as many of these structures as you can in the x-ray. Can you locate the greater and lesser curvatures? Fundus, body, and pyloric areas? Area of the pyloric sphincter? Note that although a majority of the barium contrast material has pooled in the stomach, some has passed through the pyloric sphincter, thereby outlining the duodenum.

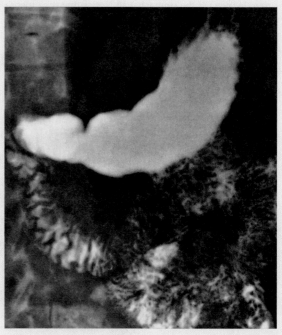

The pyloric sphincter is of clinical importance because **pylorospasm** (pie-LO-ro-spasm) is a fairly common condition in infants. The pyloric muscle fibers do not relax normally in infants with this condition. As a result, food is not able to leave the stomach, and the infant vomits food instead of digesting and absorbing it. The condition is relieved by the administration of a drug that relaxes smooth muscles. Another abnormality of the pyloric sphincter is called **pyloric stenosis** (pie-LO-rik ste-NO-sis); an obstructive narrowing of its opening can be corrected surgically in infancy.

An **ulcer** is a craterlike wound or sore in a membrane caused by tissue destruction. Current statistics show that about 1 in 10 individuals in the United States will suffer from either a gastric (stomach) or duodenal ulcer in his or her lifetime (Figure 17-16, *A*).

Ulcers cause disintegration, loss, and death of tissue as they erode the layers of the wall of the stomach or duodenum. These craterlike lesions cause gnawing or burning pain and may ultimately result in hemorrhage, perforation, widespread inflammation, scarring, and other very serious medical complications. Usually perforation does not occur, but small, repeated hemorrhages over long periods can cause anemia.

Excessive acid secretion was thought for many years to be the primary cause of ulcers. It is now known that most gastric and duodenal ulcers result from infection with the *Helicobacter pylori* (hel-i-ko-BAK-ter PIL-o-ri) *(H. pylori)* bacterium (Figure 17-16, *B*). This is especially so if the infected individual has a genetic predisposition to ulcer development. The bacterium burrows through the protective mucus lining the GI tract and impairs the lining's ability to produce protective mucus. *H. pylori* infection is diagnosed by biopsy, breath, or blood antibody tests.

Long-term use of certain pain medications such as aspirin and ibuprofen, called *nonsteroidal antiinflammatory drugs (NSAIDs)* can also cause ulcers because they too decrease the secretion of mucus. NSAID-induced ulcers can be treated by stopping NSAID use and taking acid-reducing drugs until the ulcer heals.

The discovery that most ulcers are caused by a bacterial organism led to development of a number of treatment programs. These treatments were designed to eradicate the bacteria by use of antibiotics while simultaneously blocking or reducing stomach acid secretion. Currently, the standard antibiotic-based treatment used most often to both heal ulcers and prevent recurrences is called **triple therapy.** It requires that three medications be taken concurrently for about 2 weeks. More than one cycle may be required. Triple therapy combines a stomach-lining protector such as bismuth subsalicylate (Pepto-Bismol) and/or an acid reducer with two different antibiotics.

Stomach cancer has been linked to excessive alcohol consumption, use of chewing tobacco, eating smoked or heavily preserved food, and to *H. pylori* infection. Unfortunately, there is no practical way to screen the general population for stomach cancer in its earliest stages. Most stomach cancers, usually adenocarcinomas, have already metastasized before they are found because patients treat themselves for the early warning signs of heartburn, belching, and nausea. Later warning signs of stomach cancer include chronic indigestion, vomiting, anorexia, stomach pain, and blood in the feces. Surgical removal of the malignant tumors has been the most successful method of treating stomach cancer.

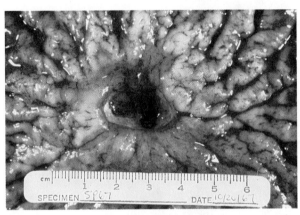

A

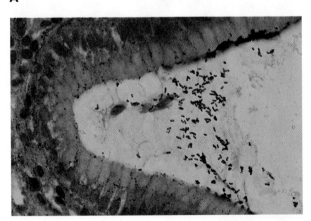

B

Figure 17-16 | **Disorders of the stomach.**

A, Gastric ulcer. **B,** *H. pylori* (black particles) infecting the stomach mucosa.

Small Intestine

The **small intestine** is roughly 7 meters (20 feet) long. However, it is noticeably smaller in diameter than the large intestine, so in this respect its name is appropriate. Different names identify three different sections of the small intestine, which include the **duodenum** (doo-oh-DEE-num), **jejunum**, (jeh-JOO-num), and **ileum** (IL-ee-um).

The mucous lining of the small intestine, like that of the stomach, contains thousands of microscopic glands. These **intestinal glands** secrete the intestinal digestive juice that is rich in a variety of enzymes as well as water and ions. The pancreas excretes bicarbonate into the lumen (hollow interior) of the duodenum to neutralize the stomach acid and also adds enzymes to digest fats, proteins, and carbohydrates that are absorbed in the intestine. A structural feature of the lining of the small intestine that makes it especially well suited to absorption of food and water is multiple circular folds called

plicae (PLYE-kee) (Figure 17-17). These folds are themselves covered with thousands of tiny fingers called **villi** (VILL-eye). Under the microscope, the villi can be seen projecting into the lumen of the intestine. Inside each villus lies a rich network of blood capillaries that absorb the products of carbohydrate and protein digestion (sugars and amino acids) and lymph capillaries (lacteals) that absorb

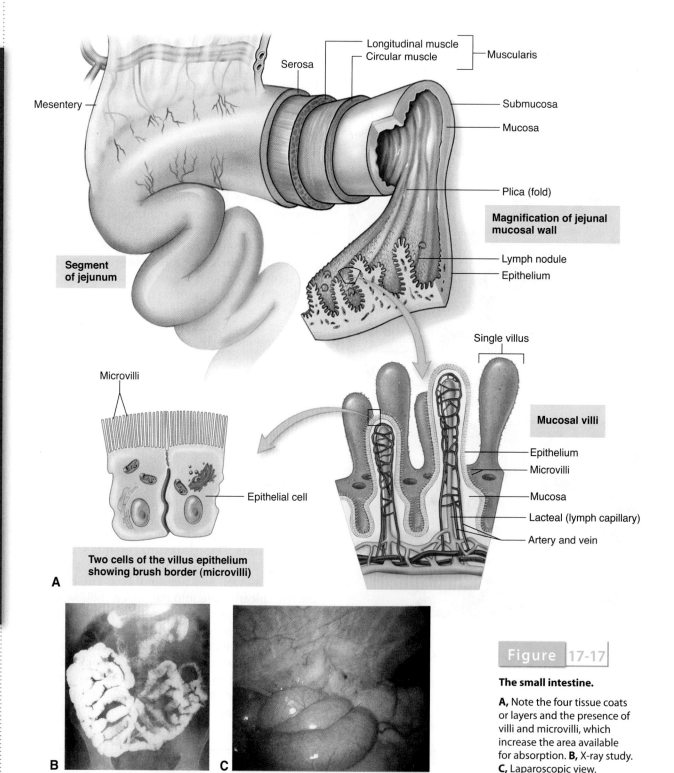

Figure 17-17

The small intestine.

A, Note the four tissue coats or layers and the presence of villi and microvilli, which increase the area available for absorption. **B,** X-ray study. **C,** Laparoscopic view.

fats. Millions and millions of villi jut inward from the mucous lining. This large contact area offers faster absorption of food from the intestine into the blood and lymph.

In addition to the thousands of villi that increase surface area in the small intestine, each villus is itself covered by epithelial cells, which have a brushlike border composed of **microvilli.** The microvilli further increase the surface area of each villus for absorption of nutrients.

Most of the chemical digestion occurs in the first subdivision of the small intestine, known as the *duodenum.* The duodenum is C shaped (Figure 17-18) and curves around the head of the pancreas. The acid chyme enters the duodenum from the stomach. This area is the site of frequent ulceration (duodenal ulcers.) The middle third of the duodenum contains the openings of ducts that empty pancreatic digestive juice and bile from the liver into the small intestine. The two openings are located at two bumps called the *greater* and *lesser duodenal papillae* (Figure 17-18).

Occasionally a gallstone blocks the ducts that drain through the major duodenal papilla, causing symptoms such as severe pain, jaundice, and digestive problems. The inset in Figure 17-18 shows an x-ray study taken during a specialized procedure called *retrograde endoscopic cholangiography* (KOLAN-jee-OG-rafee). During the procedure, x-rays images are made that allow visualization of the gallbladder and ducts that carry bile. The process begins with passage of a flexible endoscope tube surrounding a hollow catheter and other laparoscopic instruments through the mouth, esophagus, and stomach into the duodenum. Once in the duodenum, the catheter is threaded into the major duodenal papilla and contrast material is injected into the biliary tract. This procedure also can be used to fill the pancreatic duct and its branches with contrast material to obtain very high-quality x-ray images.

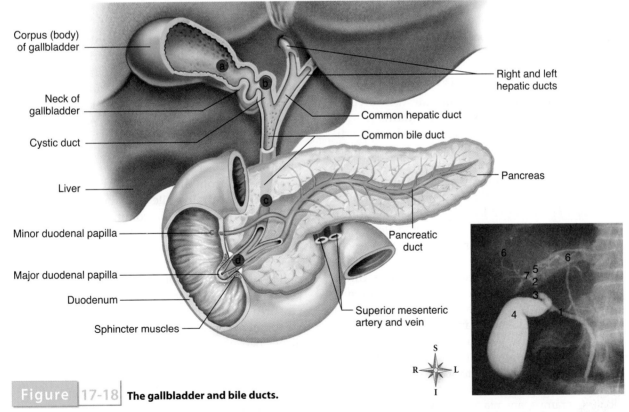

Figure 17-18 **The gallbladder and bile ducts.**

Obstruction of the hepatic or common bile duct by stone or spasm blocks the exit of bile from the liver, where it is formed, and prevents bile from being ejected into the duodenum. The drawing shows gallstone locations: in the gallbladder (a), blocking the cystic duct (b), in the common bile duct (c), and blocking both the pancreatic duct and the common bile duct (d). Inset shows an x-ray of the gallbladder and the ducts that carry bile taken during a specialized procedure called an *endoscopic cholangiography*. See text for explanation. *Inset: 1,* Common bile duct; *2,* common hepatic duct; *3,* cystic duct; *4,* gallbladder; *5,* left hepatic duct; *6,* liver shadow with tributaries of hepatic ducts; *7,* right hepatic duct.

EXERCISE AND FLUID UPTAKE

Replacement of fluids lost during exercise, primarily through sweating, is essential for maintaining homeostasis. Nearly everyone increases his or her intake of fluids during and after exercise. The main limitation to efficient fluid replacement is how quickly fluid can be absorbed, rather than how much a person drinks. Very little water is absorbed until it reaches the intestines, where it is absorbed almost immediately. Thus the rate of *gastric emptying* into the intestine is critical.

Large volumes of fluid leave the stomach and enter the intestines more rapidly than small volumes. How-

ever, large volumes may create an uncomfortable feeling during exercise. Cool fluids (8° C to 13° C) empty more quickly than warm fluids. Fluids with a high solute concentration empty slowly and may cause nausea or stomach cramps. Thus large amounts of cool, dilute, or isotonic fluids are best for replacing fluids quickly during exercise.

The duration of exercise does not affect gastric emptying, but the intensity can. Strenuous exercise practically shuts down gastric emptying. Thus the harder you work, the harder it is to replace lost fluids.

Smooth muscle in the wall of the small intestine contracts to produce peristalsis, the wavelike contraction that moves food through the GI tract and to the large intestine.

 To learn more about the small intestine, go to **AnimationDirect** on your CD.

Disorders of the Small Intestine

Many disorders of the small intestine involve inflammation, a condition termed **enteritis** (en-ter-EYE-tis). If the stomach is also inflamed, the condition is termed **gastroenteritis** (gas-troh-en-ter-EYE-tis). Bacterial toxins or other irritants in the chyme, including stomach acid, can cause enteritis. Irritation or inflammation in the duodenum can produce a feeling of nausea that leads to emesis (vomiting). Because the duodenum may be emptied along with the stomach during vomiting, it is common to observe yellowish or brownish bile in the vomit. X-ray studies of the small intestine, as well as direct viewing of either the inside lumen or exterior surface using an endoscope, are useful tools in both diagnosis and treatment of intestinal disease.

Malabsorption syndrome is a general term referring to a group of symptoms resulting from the failure of the small intestine to absorb nutrients properly. These symptoms include anorexia, abdominal bloating, cramps, anemia, and fatigue. A number of underlying conditions can cause malabsorption syndrome such as mucosal changes due to surgery, blood

flow changes, or disease. Another disorder called **maldigestion** involves a deficit of digestive enzymes or bile salts that reduce the amount of material that can be absorbed by the intestine.

Liver and Gallbladder

The liver is so large that it fills the entire upper right section of the abdominal cavity and even extends partway into the left side. Because its cells secrete a substance called **bile** into ducts, the liver is classified as an exocrine gland; in fact, it is the largest gland in the body. The liver also has a wide variety of metabolic functions that are discussed in Chapter 18.

The hepatic ducts (Figure 17-18) drain bile out of the liver, a fact suggested by the name hepatic, which comes from the Greek word for liver *(hepar)*. The duct that drains bile into the small intestine (duodenum) is called the common bile duct. This duct is formed by the union of the common hepatic duct with the cystic duct that exits the bile storage sack called the gallbladder.

Fats form large globules, and these must be broken down into smaller particles to increase the surface area for digestion. The function of bile is similar to how soap helps break up fat when washing dishes because it mechanically breaks up or **emulsifies** (e-MUL-seh-fyz) fats. When chyme containing lipid or fat enters the duodenum, it initiates a mechanism that contracts the gallbladder and forces bile into the small intestine.

Fats in chyme stimulate or trigger the secretion of the hormone **cholecystokinin** (koh-leh-sis-toh-KYE-nin), or **CCK,** from the intestinal mucosa of the duodenum. This hormone then stimulates the contraction of the gallbladder and the relaxation of smooth muscles that control the opening of the duodenal papilla, allowing the bile to flow into the duodenum. Between meals, when the opening of the duodenal papilla is closed, bile moves up the cystic duct into the gallbladder. The gallbladder thus concentrates and stores bile that is produced in the liver.

QUICK CHECK

1. What bacterium is associated with ulcers?
2. Identify the different sections of the small intestine in the order in which food passes through them.
3. What is gastroenteritis?
4. Where is bile formed and what is its function?

Disorders of the Liver and Gallbladder

Gallstones are solid clumps of material (mostly cholesterol) that form in the gallbladder in 1 in 10 Americans. Some gallstones never cause problems and are called *silent gallstones,* whereas others produce painful symptoms or other medical complications and are called *symptomatic gallstones.* Gallstones often form when the cholesterol concentration in bile becomes excessive, causing crystallization or precipitation to occur (Figure 17-19). Stone formation is much more likely to occur if the gallbladder does not empty regularly and chemically imbalanced or cholesterol-laden bile remains in the gallbladder for long periods of time. **Cholelithiasis** (koh-leh-li- THEE-ah-sis) literally means condition of having bile (gall) stones and often occurs in the presence of gallbladder inflammation, or **cholecystitis** (koh-leh-sis-TYE-tis).

When a gallstone blocks the common bile duct (choledocholithiasis) (Figure 17-18), bile is not able to drain into the duodenum. In such a case, feces then appear gray-white because the pigments from bile that normally give feces its characteristic color are absent. Furthermore, excessive amounts of bile pigments are absorbed into the blood. A yellowish skin discoloration called **jaundice** (JAWN-dis) results. Often, pain accompanies this condition. The pain is called *biliary colic.* Obstruction of the common hepatic duct also leads to jaundice because when bile cannot drain out of the liver, it is absorbed into the blood. Bile is not absorbed from the gallbladder so no jaundice occurs if only the cystic duct is blocked.

The relationship of dieting and weight loss to gallstone formation is under intense scrutiny. Physicians have known for years that in severely obese individuals (body mass index [BMI] over 40) the liver produces higher levels of cholesterol and the risk of developing gallstones is increased. However, only recently have scientists established with certainty that significant and rapid weight loss greatly increases the risk of symptomatic gallstone formation that may require surgery—a procedure called **cholecystectomy** (KO-le-cys-TEK-to-my).

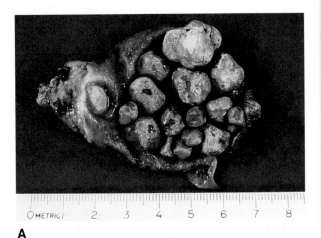

A

B

Figure 17-19 **Gallstones.**

A, Inflamed gallbladder filled with yellow cholesterol gallstones. **B,** Laparoscopic view of the gallbladder before removal.

Bariatrics (from Greek word *baros,* weight) is a specialized field of medicine that deals with treatment of obesity. So called *bariatric surgical procedures* used for producing weight loss, such as the Lap Band Adjustable Gastric Banding System, the more traditional restrictive gastric banding procedure (vertical-banded gastroplasty), or more extensive bypass operations (RGB, or Roux-en-Y gastric bypass), all reduce the size of the stomach and almost always result in rapid postsurgical weight loss, but more than one third of these patients develop gallstones. Unfortunately, individuals who choose nonsurgical approaches to achieve significant and rapid weight loss, such as very–low-calorie, ultra–low-fat or carbohydrate diets, also experience higher rates of gallstone formation. In these cases, stone formation is related to imbalances in bile chemistry and delayed emptying or incomplete gallbladder contractions.

If surgery is required for removal of symptomatic gallstones, laparoscopic techniques have made the need for open abdominal surgical procedures less common (Figure 17-19, *B*). Gallstones can sometimes be treated (dissolved) over time or prevented from developing in individuals experiencing rapid weight loss by oral administration of a naturally occurring bile constituent called *ursodeoxycholic acid* (Actigall).

Hepatitis (hep-ah-TYE-tis) is a general term referring to inflammation of the liver. Hepatitis is characterized by jaundice, liver enlargement, anorexia, abdominal discomfort, gray-white feces, and dark urine. A number of different conditions can produce hepati-tis. Alcohol, drugs, or other toxins may cause hepatitis. It also may be a complication of bacterial or viral infection or parasite infestation. *Hepatitis A,* for example, results from infection by a virus that may be found in contaminated food. Another viral hepatitis, *hepatitis B,* is more severe. It was historically called *serum hepatitis* because it is often transmitted by contaminated blood serum. Improperly sterilized tattooing needles contaminated with even trace amounts of hepatitis B–infected blood (0.004 ml), will cause disease. Hepatitis C is a form of viral liver inflammation most often associated with transfusion of contaminated blood or intravenous drug abuse. The disease may become chronic and result in cirrhosis (see below) or liver cancer many months or even years after exposure. There are vaccines to prevent infection with both hepatitis A and hepatitis B viruses.

Hepatitis, chronic alcohol abuse, malnutrition, or infection may lead to a degenerative liver condition known as **cirrhosis** (si-ROH-sis). The liver's ability to regenerate damaged tissue is well known, but it has its limits. For example, when the toxic effects of alcohol accumulate faster than the liver can regenerate itself, damaged tissue is replaced with a nodular, pebble-like fibrous or fatty tissue instead of normal tissue (Figure 17-20, *A*). No matter what the cause of liver cirrhosis, the symptoms are the same: nausea, anorexia, gray-white stools, weakness, and pain. If the cause of cirrhosis is removed and high-protein foods are eaten, the liver may be able to repair itself—given enough time. If the dam-

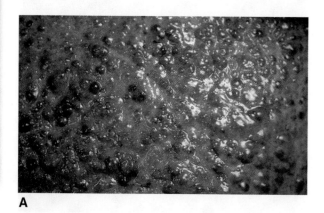

A

Figure 17-20 **Liver damage.**

A, Alcoholic cirrhosis where liver surface is hard and covered with nodules that look like pebbles. **B,** Varicose veins (varicies) of the esophagus caused by reduction of blood flow through liver with cirrhosis.

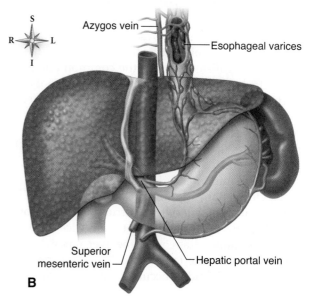

Azygos vein

Esophageal varices

Superior mesenteric vein

Hepatic portal vein

B

age is extensive, a liver transplant may be the only hope of saving someone with cirrhosis of the liver.

Acute or chronic liver disorders such as hepatitis or cirrhosis can block the flow of blood through the liver, thus causing it to back up into the *hepatic portal circulation* (Figure 17-20, *B*). As a result, the blood pressure in the hepatic circulation increases abnormally—a condition called *portal hypertension*. To relieve the pressure, new veins that connect to the systemic veins are formed. This often causes the veins lining the esophagus, stomach, and other organs to widen and become varicose. If these varicosities rupture after erosion by stomach acid, vomiting of blood occurs. This massive bleeding may result in death.

Pancreas

The pancreas lies behind the stomach in the concavity produced by the C shape of the duodenum. It is an exocrine gland that secretes pancreatic juice into ducts and also an endocrine gland that secretes hormones (insulin and glucagon) into the blood. The cells that secrete the blood glucose–regulating hormones are located between the duct cells in areas called

the *pancreatic islet (of Langerhans)*. Pancreatic juice secreted into the duodenum contains enzymes that digest all three major kinds of foods. It also contains sodium bicarbonate, an alkaline substance that neutralizes the hydrochloric acid in the gastric juice that enters the intestines. Pancreatic juice enters the duodenum of the small intestine at the same place that bile enters because both the common bile and pancreatic ducts open into the duodenum at the major duodenal papilla (Figure 17-18).

Between the cells that secrete pancreatic juice into ducts lie clusters of cells that have no contact with any ducts. These are the pancreatic islets (of Langerhans), which secrete the hormones of the pancreas described in Chapter 11. Locate the pancreas and nearby structures in Figure 17-21, which shows a transverse section of a human cadaver.

Disorders of the pancreas include diabetes mellitus (the inability of the islet cells to make insulin) and **pancreatitis** (pan-kree-ah-TYE-tis) (or inflammation of the pancreas). *Acute pancreatitis* may result from blockage of the common bile duct. The blockage causes pancreatic enzymes to "back up" into the pancreas and digest it. This is a very serious and potentially fa-

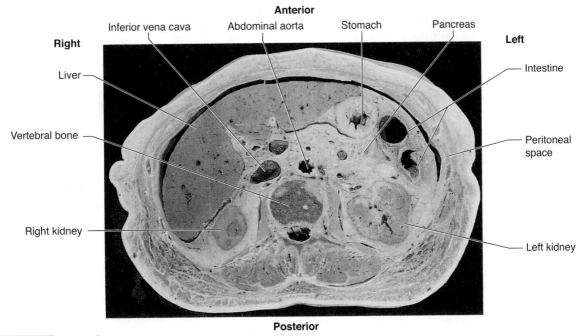

Figure 17-21 **Horizontal (transverse) section of the abdomen.**

The photograph of a cadaver section shows the relative position of some of the major digestive organs of the abdomen. Such a view is typical in newer imaging methods such as computed tomography (CT) scanning and magnetic resonance imaging (MRI).

tal condition. Another condition that blocks the flow of pancreatic enzymes is **cystic fibrosis (CF),** which is an inherited disorder that disrupts cell transport and causes exocrine glands to produce excessively thick secretions. Thick pancreatic secretions may build up and block pancreatic ducts, disrupting the flow of pancreatic enzymes and damaging the pancreas.

Another serious pancreatic disorder is pancreatic cancer. Usually a form of *adenocarcinoma,* pancreatic cancer claims the lives of nearly all its victims within 5 years after diagnosis.

Large Intestine

The **large intestine** is only about 1.5 meters (5 feet) in length. It has a much larger diameter than the small intestine and forms the lower or terminal portion of the digestive tract. Undigested and unabsorbed food material enters the large intestine after passing through a sphincter-like structure (Figure 17-22, *A*) called the **ileocecal** (il-ee-o-SEE-kal) **valve.**

The word *chyme* is no longer appropriate for describing food material once it enters the large intestine. Chyme, which has the consistency of soup and is found in the small intestine, changes to the consistency of fecal matter as water and salts are reabsorbed during its passage through the large intestine.

During its movement through the large intestine, material that escaped digestion in the small intestine is acted upon by bacteria. As a result of this bacterial action, additional nutrients may be released from cellulose and other fibers and are then absorbed. In addition to their digestive role, bacteria in the large intestine have other important functions. They are responsible for the synthesis of vitamin K needed for normal blood clotting and for the production of some of the B-complex vitamins. Once formed, these vitamins are absorbed from the large intestine and then enter the blood.

Although some absorption of water, salts, and vitamins occurs in the large intestine, this segment of the digestive tube is not as well suited for absorption as is the small intestine. Salts, especially sodium, are absorbed by active transport, and water is moved into the blood by osmosis. No villi are present in the mucosa of the large intestine. As a result, much less surface area is available for absorption, and the efficiency and speed of movement of substances through the wall of the large intestine are lower than in the

small intestine. Normal passage of material through the large intestine takes about 3 to 5 days.

The subdivisions of the large intestine are listed below in the order in which fecal matter passes through them.

1. Cecum
2. Ascending colon
3. Transverse colon
4. Descending colon
5. Sigmoid colon
6. Rectum
7. Anal canal

These areas can be studied and identified by tracing the passage of material from its point of entry into the large intestine at the ileocecal valve to its elimination from the body through the external opening called the **anus.**

The ileocecal valve opens into a pouchlike area called the **cecum** (SEE-kum). The opening itself is about 5 or 6 cm (2 inches) above the beginning of the large intestine (Figure 17-22, *A*). Food residue in the cecum flows upward on the right side of the body in the *ascending colon.* The **hepatic,** or **right, colic flexure** is the bend between the ascending colon and the *transverse colon,* which extends across the front of the abdomen from right to left. The **splenic,** or **left, colic flexure** marks the point where the *descending colon* turns downward on the left side of the abdomen. The **sigmoid colon** is the S-shaped segment that terminates in the **rectum.** The terminal portion of the rectum is called the **anal canal,** which ends at the external opening or anus.

Two sphincter muscles stay contracted to keep the anus closed except during defecation. Smooth or involuntary muscle composes the *inner anal sphincter,* but striated, or voluntary, muscle composes the *outer sphincter.* This anatomical fact sometimes becomes highly important from a practical standpoint. For example, often after a person has had a stroke, the voluntary anal sphincter at first becomes paralyzed. This means, of course, that the individual has no control at that time over bowel movements.

 To learn more about the large intestine, go to **AnimationDirect** on your CD.

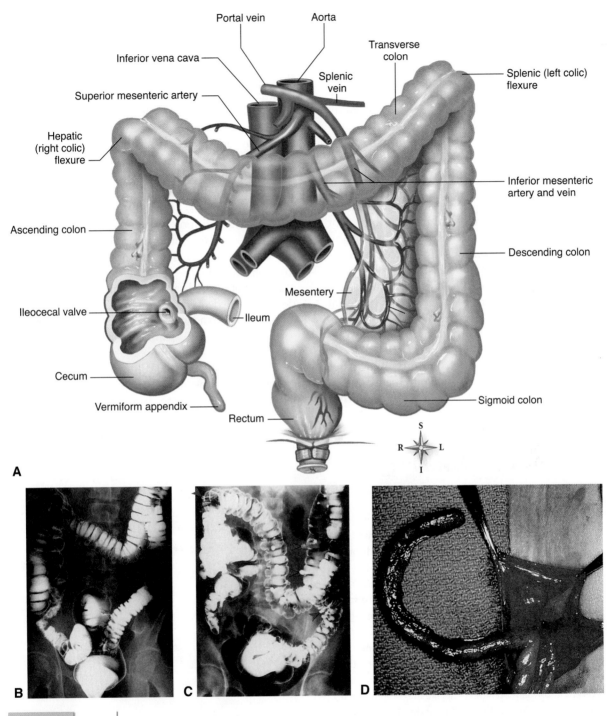

Figure 17-22 **Divisions of the large intestine.**

A, Artist's drawing of the large intestine. **B,** X-ray of large intestine and terminal ileum filled with barium contrast material (barium enema). **C,** X-ray of a barium enema showing diverticulosis *(arrowheads)*. **D,** Acute appendicitis. Appendix is gangrenous and showing signs of ischemia and putrefaction.

Disorders of the Large Intestine

Many of the more common disorders of the large intestine relate to *inflammation* or *abnormal motility*, or rate of movement of the intestinal contents. Abnormally rapid motility through the large intestine may result in *diarrhea*, and abnormally slow motility may result in *constipation*. These and other conditions are briefly described in this section.

Diarrhea (dye-ah-REE-ah) usually occurs when the intestinal contents move so quickly that the resulting feces are more fluid than normal. Diarrhea is characterized by frequent passing of watery feces. In inflammatory conditions such as **dysentery,** the watery feces also may contain mucus, blood, or pus. Diarrhea also may be accompanied by abdominal cramps—a symptom caused by excessive contractions of the intestinal muscles.

The increased intestinal motility that causes diarrhea often results from the presence of bacterial toxins, parasites, or other irritants. The intestines reflexively "speed up," a mechanism that quickly disposes of the irritant. The high water content of loose stools can be caused by high motility, which decreases the time the intestines have to reabsorb water from the feces. Watery stools also may result from the action of toxins that causes cells in the intestinal lining to move water into the GI tract rather than out of the tract. Because of the water loss involved, untreated diarrhea may quickly lead to dehydration—and possibly convulsions or death (see box on infant diarrhea, p. 511).

Constipation results from decreased intestinal motility. If passage of feces through the large intestine is prolonged beyond 5 days, the feces lose volume and become more solid because of excessive water reabsorption. This reduction in volume decreases stimulation of the bowel-emptying reflex, resulting in retention of feces—a positive-feedback affect that makes the condition even worse.

Acute constipation often results from intestinal blockage, low-fiber diets, tumors, or **diverticulitis** (dye-ver-tik-yoo-LYE-tis). Diverticulitis is an inflammation of abnormal saclike outpouchings of the intestinal wall called *diverticula* (Figure 17-22, C). Diverticula often develop in adults older than 50 years of age who eat low-fiber foods. Treatment of acute constipation usually involves treatment of the underlying cause.

Colitis (koh-LYE-tis) refers to any inflammatory condition of the large intestine. If present for prolonged periods of time, inflammatory bowel dis-

CLINICAL APPLICATION

COLOSTOMY

Colostomy (koh-LAH-stoh-mee) is a surgical procedure in which an artificial anus is created on the abdominal wall by cutting the colon and bringing the cut end or ends out to the surface to form an opening called a *stoma* (see figure). Home health care workers help patients learn to accept the change in body image, which may cause emotional discomfort. The patient or caregiver is also trained in the regular changing of the disposable bag, including how to clean the stoma and how to prevent irritation, chapping, or infection. Irrigation of the colon with isotonic solutions is sometimes necessary. Deodorants may be added to the fresh bag to prevent unpleasant odors. Patients are also taught to manage their diet to include low-residue food and to avoid foods that produce gas or cause diarrhea. Fluid intake after colostomy is also carefully managed.

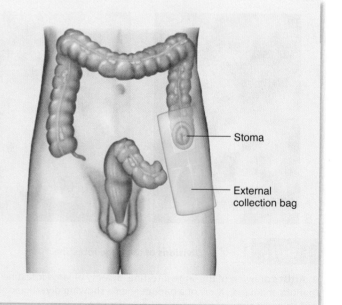

Stoma

External collection bag

ease becomes a significant risk factor for colorectal cancer. Symptoms of colitis include diarrhea and abdominal cramps or constipation. Some forms of colitis may also produce bleeding and intestinal ulcers. Colitis may be a result of emotional stress, as in *irritable bowel syndrome.* It also may result from an autoimmune disease, as in *ulcerative colitis.* Another type of autoimmune colitis is **Crohn disease,** which often also affects the small intestine. If more conservative treatments fail, colitis may be corrected by surgical removal of the affected portions of the colon.

Colorectal (kol-oh-REK-tal) **cancer** is a malignancy, usually *adenocarcinoma,* of the columnar epithelium that lines the lumen of the colon and/or rectum. Most colorectal cancers originate from nonmalignant *colonic polyps* that gradually undergo malignant transformation. Colorectal cancer occurs most often after age 50 and increases in incidence dramatically after age 75. The disease is slightly more common in men than in women and constitutes the second leading cause of death from cancer in the United States and the fourth most common type of cancer diagnosed after prostate, breast, and lung malignancy.

Diagnosis of colorectal cancer is made during a digital rectal examination or as a result of direct visualization of the rectum and lower colon during *sigmoidoscopy* (sig-moi-DOS-koh-pee) or of the entire colon during a *colonoscopy* (koh-lon-OS-koh-pee). Other diagnostic tools include the use of barium enemas, ultrasound, various x-ray–based techniques, and magnetic resonance imaging. Certain dietary habits, especially a high saturated fat intake, and genetic predisposition are known risk factors. The prognosis for recovery from colorectal cancer is based on a number of factors, including the degree of penetration (if any) of the tumor through the bowel wall, and the presence or absence of cancer cells in regional lymph nodes or distant body locations (metastases).

Early warning signs of this common type of cancer include changes in bowel habits (constipation or diarrhea), decreased stool diameter, rectal bleeding that may be obvious (gross or visible) or hidden (occult or microscopic), abdominal pain, unexplained anemia, weight loss, and fatigue. Large bowel obstruction is the most common complication of colon cancer.

Treatment requiring surgical removal of a tumor in the distal rectum also may require the creation of a **colostomy** (koh-LAH-stoh-mee) (see box on facing page). In addition to surgery, both rectal and colon cancer are often treated by use of chemotherapy. Radiation therapy is seldom used in treatment of colon cancer but has an important role in treatment of rectal malignancy.

CLINICAL APPLICATION

INFANT DIARRHEA

Severe diarrhea caused by a *rotavirus,* an intestinal infection, kills more than 500,000 infants and young children worldwide each year. Death results from severe dehydration caused by 20 or more episodes of diarrhea in a single day. Currently, more than 3 million U.S. children suffer symptoms of rotavirus intestinal infection annually and 55,000 require hospitalization. Good medical care has limited the number of U.S. infant deaths caused by the disease each year to just a few. In developed countries, relatively new and promising vaccines provide good protection against the virus. Unfortunately, in developing countries, rotavirus-induced diarrhea remains one of the leading causes of infant mortality. Until rotavirus vaccines can be more widely distributed and administered, one of the best treatment options available in many areas of the world involves oral administration of liberal doses of a simple, easily prepared solution containing sugar and salt. The salt-sugar solution used in this *oral rehydration therapy* replaces nutrients and electrolytes lost in diarrheal fluid. Because the replacement fluid can be prepared from readily available and inexpensive ingredients, it is particularly valuable in the treatment of infant diarrhea in developing countries.

Appendix and Appendicitis

The **vermiform appendix** (Latin *vermiformis* from *vermins* or worm and *forma* or shape) is, as the name implies, a wormlike, tubular structure that is attached directly to the cecum (Figure 17-22, *A*). Although it serves no important digestive function in humans, it does contain lymphatic tissue and may play a minor role in the immunologic defense mechanisms of the body. The appendix contains a blind, tubelike interior lumen that communicates with the lumen of the large intestine 3 cm (1 inch) below the opening of the ileocecal valve into the cecum. If the mucous lining of the appendix becomes inflamed, the resulting condition is the well-known affliction **appendicitis** (Figure 17-22, *D*).

The opening between the lumen of the appendix and the cecum is quite large in children and young adults—a fact of great clinical significance because food or fecal material trapped in the appendix will irritate and inflame its mucous lining, causing appendicitis. The opening between the appendix and the cecum is often completely obliterated in elderly persons, which explains the low incidence of appendicitis in this population.

If infectious material becomes trapped in an inflamed appendix, the appendix may rupture and release the material into the abdominal cavity. Infection of the peritoneum and other abdominal organs can be life threatening. Appendicitis is the most common of the acute abdominal conditions requiring surgery. It affects 7% to 12% of the population, generally before age 30.

QUICK CHECK

1. What is cholelithiasis? Cirrhosis?
2. What is the role of the gallbladder?
3. Name the seven subdivisions of the large intestine.
4. What is the most common acute abdominal condition requiring surgery?

Peritoneum

The **peritoneum** is a large, moist, slippery sheet of serous membrane that lines the abdominal cavity and covers the organs located in it, including most of the digestive organs. The parietal layer of the peritoneum lines the abdominal cavity. The visceral layer of the peritoneum forms the outer, or covering, layer of each abdominal organ. The small space between the parietal and visceral layers is called the *peritoneal space*. It contains just enough peritoneal fluid to keep both layers of the peritoneum moist and able to slide freely against

each other during breathing and digestive movements (Figure 17-23, *A*). Organs outside the peritoneum (such as the kidneys) are said to be retroperitoneal.

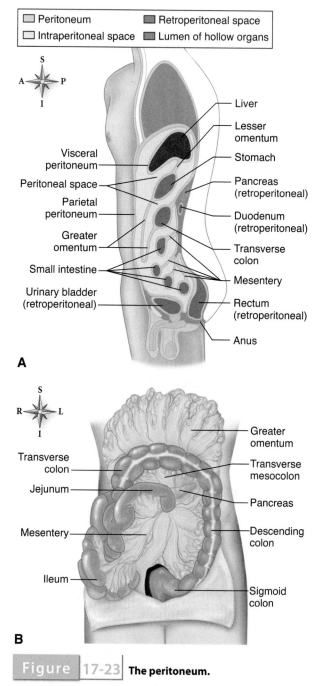

A, The parietal layer of the peritoneum lines the abdominopelvic cavity and then extends as a series of mesenteries to form the visceral layer that covers abdominal organs. **B,** The transverse colon and greater omentum are raised and the small intestine is pulled to the side to show the mesentery.

Figure 17-23 **The peritoneum.**

Extensions

The two most prominent extensions of the peritoneum are the mesentery and the greater omentum. The **mesentery** (Figure 17-23, *B*), an extension between the parietal and visceral layers of the peritoneum, is shaped like a giant, pleated fan. Its smaller edge attaches to the lumbar region of the posterior abdominal wall, and its long, loose outer edge encloses most of the small intestine, anchoring it to the posterior abdominal wall. The **greater omentum** is a pouchlike extension of the visceral peritoneum from the lower edge of the stomach, part of the duodenum, and the transverse colon. Shaped like a large apron, it hangs down over the intestines, and because spotty deposits of fat give it a lacy appearance, it has been nicknamed the *lace apron*. It may envelop a badly inflamed appendix, walling it off from the rest of the abdominal organs.

Peritonitis

Peritonitis (pair-i-toh-NYE-tis) is the inflammation of the peritoneum resulting from a bacterial infection or another irritating condition. Peritonitis most commonly results from an infection that occurs after the rupture of the appendix or other abdominopelvic organ. It is characterized by abdominal distention, pain, nausea, vomiting, tachycardia (rapid heart rate), fever, dehydration, and other signs and symptoms. Circulatory shock progressing to heart failure may result.

Ascites

Ascites (ah-SYE-teez) is the abnormal accumulation of fluid in the peritoneal space (Figure 17-24). Fluid enters the peritoneal space from the blood because of local hypertension (high blood pressure) or an osmotic imbalance in the plasma (low plasma protein). This condition may be accompanied by abdominal swelling and decreased urinary output. It commonly occurs as a complication of cirrhosis, congestive heart failure, kidney disease, peritonitis, cancer, or malnutrition .

Digestion

Digestion, a complex process that occurs in the alimentary canal, consists of physical and chemical changes that prepare food for absorption. *Mechanical digestion* breaks food into tiny particles, mixes them with digestive juices, moves them along the alimentary canal, and finally eliminates the digestive wastes from the body. Chewing or mastication, swallowing or **deglutition** (deg-loo-TISH-un), peristalsis, and defecation are the main processes of mechanical digestion. *Chemical digestion* breaks down

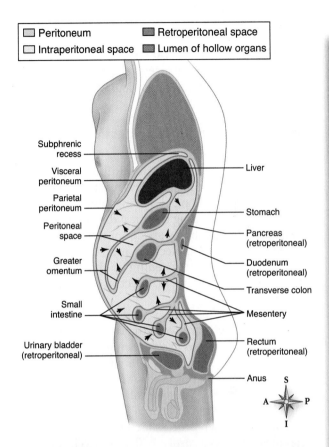

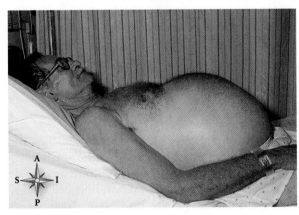

Figure 17-24 **Ascites.**

Ascites results from an accumulation of fluid in the peritoneal space. The arrows indicate water filtering out of the peritoneal blood vessels, resulting from hypertension, or diffusing out of the vessels because of an osmotic imbalance in the blood.

large, nonabsorbable food molecules into smaller, absorbable molecules—molecules that are able to pass through the intestinal mucosa into blood and lymph. Chemical digestion consists of numerous chemical reactions catalyzed by enzymes in saliva, gastric juice, pancreatic juice, and intestinal juice.

 To learn more about the initiation of mechanical digestion, go to **AnimationDirect** on your CD.

Enzymes and Chemical Digestion

Enzymes (EN-zymes) are specialized protein molecules that act as *catalysts* (KAT-ah-lists). That is, they speed up specific chemical reactions without themselves being changed or consumed during the reaction process. During chemical digestion, certain enzymes very selectively speed up the breakdown of specific nutrient molecules and no others. Enzymes responsible for speeding up the breakdown of fats, for example, have no effect on carbohydrates or proteins.

The names of many enzymes end with the suffix *-ase* combined with the word that describes the type of substance involved in the chemical reaction. Li*pase* (LYE-payse), for example, is a fat-digesting enzyme that acts on lipids (fats) and prote*ase* (PROH-tee-ayz) enzymes serve to break down protein nutrients into smaller molecules.

The breakdown process facilitated by digestive enzymes is called **hydrolysis** (hye-DROHL-i-sis)—an important type of chemical reaction first discussed in Chapter 2. Recall that during hydrolysis, enzymes speed up reactions that add water *(hydro)* to chemically break up or split *(lysis)* larger molecules into smaller molecules (see Figure 2-4 on p. 28).

Carbohydrate Digestion

Very little digestion of carbohydrates (starches and sugars) occurs before food reaches the small intestine. Salivary amylase usually has little time to do its work because so many of us swallow our food so fast. Gastric juice contains no carbohydrate-digesting enzymes. But after the food reaches the small intestine, pancreatic and intestinal juice enzymes digest the starches and sugars. A pancreatic enzyme (amylase) starts the process by changing starches

into a double sugar, namely, maltose. Three intestinal enzymes—maltase, sucrase, and lactase—digest double sugars by changing them into simple sugars, chiefly glucose (dextrose). Maltase digests maltose (malt sugar), sucrase digests sucrose (ordinary cane sugar), and lactase digests lactose (milk sugar).

The end products of carbohydrate digestion are the so-called *simple sugars*; the most abundant is glucose.

Protein Digestion

Protein digestion starts in the stomach with the secretion of pepsinogen. Pepsinogen is a component of gastric juice and is converted into the active enzyme pepsin by hydrochloric acid (also in gastric juice). Pepsin causes the large protein molecules to break up into simpler compounds. In the intestine, other enzymes (trypsin in the pancreatic juice and peptidases in the intestinal juice) finish the job of protein digestion.

Every protein molecule is made up of many amino acids joined together. When enzymes have split up the large protein molecule into its separate amino acids, protein digestion is completed. The end product of protein digestion is amino acids, which are also referred to as *protein building blocks*.

Fat Digestion

Just as with carbohydrates, very little fat digestion occurs before food reaches the small intestine. Most fats are undigested until after being emulsification by bile in the duodenum (where fat droplets are broken into very small droplets). After this action takes place, pancreatic lipase splits the fat molecules further into fatty acids and glycerol (glycerin), the end products of fat digestion.

Table 17-2 summarizes the main facts about chemical digestion. Enzyme names indicate the type of food digested by the enzyme. For example, the name **amylose** indicates that the enzyme digests the carbohydrate amylase or starch, **protease** indicates a protein-digesting enzyme, and **lipase** means a lipid or fat-digesting enzyme. When carbohydrate digestion has been completed, starches (polysaccharides) and double sugars (disaccharides) have been changed mainly to glucose, a simple sugar (monosaccharide). The end products of protein digestion, on the other hand, are amino acids. Fatty acid and glycerol are the end products of fat digestion.

Table 17-2 | Chemical Digestion

DIGESTIVE JUICES AND ENZYMES		SUBSTANCE DIGESTED (OR HYDROLYZED)	RESULTING PRODUCT*
SALIVA			
Salivary amylase		Starch (polysaccharide)	Maltose (a double sugar, or disaccharide)
GASTRIC JUICE			
Protease (pepsin) plus hydrochloric acid		Proteins	Partially digested proteins
PANCREATIC JUICE			
Proteases (e.g., trypsin)†		Proteins (intact or partially digested)	Peptides and **amino acids**
Lipases		Fats emulsified by bile	**Fatty acids, monoglycerides,** and **glycerol**
Amylase		Starch	Maltose
INTESTINAL ENZYMES‡			
Peptidases		Peptides	**Amino acids**
Sucrase		Sucrose (cane sugar)	**Glucose** and **fructose**§ (simple sugars, or monosaccharides)
Lactase		Lactose (milk sugar)	**Glucose** and **galactose** (simple sugars)
Maltase		Maltose (malt sugar)	**Glucose**

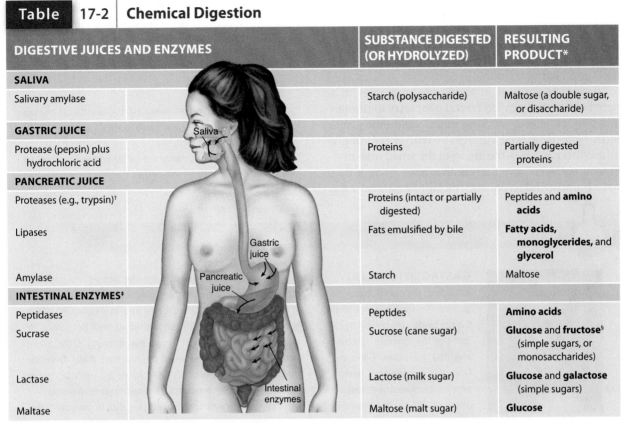

Saliva

Gastric juice

Pancreatic juice

Intestinal enzymes

*Substances in boldface type are end products of digestion (that is, completely digested nutrients ready for absorption).
†Secreted in inactive form (trypsinogen); activated by enterokinase, an enzyme in the intestinal brush border.
‡Brush-border enzymes.
§Glucose is also called *dextrose;* fructose is also called *levulose.*

Absorption

After food is digested, it is absorbed; that is, it moves through the mucous membrane lining of the small intestine into the blood and lymph. In other words, food absorption is the process by which molecules of amino acids, glucose, fatty acids, and glycerol move from the inside of the intestine into the circulating fluids of the body. Absorption of foods is just as essential as digestion of foods. The reason is fairly obvious. As long as food stays in the intestines, it cannot nourish the millions of cells that compose all other parts of the body. Their lives depend on the absorption of digested food and its transportation to them by the circulating blood.

Many important minerals, such as sodium, are actively transported through the intestinal mucosa. Water follows by osmosis. Other nutrients such as monosaccharides and amino acids are also actively transported through the intestinal mucosa and diffuse into the blood of capillaries in the intestinal villi. Fatty acids and glycerol diffuse into the absorptive cells of the GI tract and then are secreted into the lymphatic vessels or lacteals found in intestinal villi.

The so called "water-soluble vitamins" (vitamin C and the B vitamins) are dissolved in water and absorbed primarily from the small intestine. The "fat-soluble vitamins" (vitamins A, D, E, and K) are absorbed along with the end products of fat digestion in the small intestine and then pass into the lacteals. Bacterial action in the colon also produces some vitamin K that is absorbed through the lining of the large intestine.

Surface Area and Absorption

Structural adaptations of the digestive tube, including folds in the lining mucosa, villi, and microvilli, increase the absorptive surface and the efficiency and speed of transfer of materials from the intestinal lumen to body fluids.

Biologists are now applying the principles of a new field of study called **fractal geometry** to human anatomy. Scientists working in this field study surfaces—called "fractal surfaces"—with a seemingly infinite area, such as the lining of the small intestine. Fractal surfaces have bumps that have bumps that have bumps, and so on. The fractal-like nature of the

intestinal lining is represented in Figure 15-9. The plicae (folds) have villi, the villi have microvilli, and even the microvilli have bumps that cannot be seen in the figure. Thus the absorptive surface area of the small intestine is almost limitless.

> **QUICK CHECK**
>
> 1. Name the two most prominent extensions of the peritoneum.
> 2. What is the difference between mechanical digestion and chemical digestion?
> 3. What are the end products of carbohydrate digestion? fat digestion? protein digestion?

SCIENCE APPLICATIONS

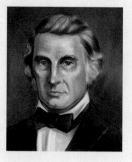

William Beaumont
(1785–1853)

GASTROENTEROLOGY

Analyzing the word parts of gastroenterology tells you that it is the study (-ology) and treatment of the stomach (gastro-) and the intestines (-entero-). One of the pioneering gastroenterologists was the American physician William Beaumont. In 1822, the young Québécois trapper Alexis St. Martin was shot with a musket near the Army hospital in Michigan where Beaumont was working. Beaumont treated his wound—although expecting St. Martin would die from the injury. However, St. Martin recovered and lived a long life even though the wound did not heal properly. For his entire life thereafter, an open hole remained in his abdomen that led directly into the stomach. Being grateful for his spared life, St. Martin allowed Beaumont to study gastric secretion through the opening. Over many years, Beaumont made careful observations about how the stomach works. Many of his conclusions are still valid today and serve as the foundation for modern gastroenterology.

Many physicians and nurses specialize in gastroenterology today; however, many other health care providers, such as health care technicians and nursing assistants, need a basic knowledge of digestive structure and function in order to care for patients effectively. Even workers in the fields of dietetics, nutrition, and food service benefit from knowledge of the principles of digestion.

Outline Summary

To download an MP3 version of the chapter summary for use with your iPod or portable media player, access the **Audio Chapter Summaries** on your CD.

Structures of the Digestive System (Figure 17-1)

A. Alimentary canal, or GI tract
   1. Extends from mouth to anus—9 m (29 feet) in length
   2. Involved in digestion, absorption, and metabolism of nutrients
B. Main organs and accessory organs (Table 17-1)
   1. Main organs: mouth; pharynx; esophagus; stomach; small intestine; large intestine; rectum; anal canal

   2. Accessory organs: teeth and tongue, salivary glands; liver; gallbladder; pancreas; vermiform appendix

Mouth

A. Also known as *oral cavity*—hollow chamber with a roof, floor, and walls
   1. Roof—formed by hard palate (parts of maxillary and palatine bones) and soft palate (an arch-shaped muscle separating mouth from pharynx)

2. Uvula—a downward projection of the soft palate (Figure 17-2, *A*)
   a. Uvula and soft palate prevent food and liquid from entering nasal cavities
   b. Assists in speech and swallowing (deglutition)
3. Floor—formed by tongue and its muscles
   a. Lingual frenulum—fold of mucous membrane that helps anchor the tongue to the floor of the mouth (Figure 17-2, *B*)
   b. Papillae—small elevations on mucosa of tongue; taste buds, found in many papillae

Teeth

A. Types of teeth—incisors, cuspids, bicuspids, and tricuspids
   1. Deciduous (also known as baby or primary) teeth—full set equals 20 teeth
      a. First tooth erupts at about 6 months
      b. Complete set in place at about 2 years of age
   2. Permanent teeth—full set equals 32 in most; 28 teeth is a normal variation in others
      a. First permanent tooth erupts at about 6 years of age
      b. Set complete usually between ages of 17 and 24 years (Figure 17-3)
B. Structures of a typical tooth—crown, neck, and root (Figure 17-4)

Disorders of the Mouth and Teeth

A. Infections, cancer, congenital defects, and other disorders can cause serious complications including malnutrition
B. Infections and cancer of the mouth may spread to other parts of the body
   1. Leukoplakia—precancerous condition of mouth tissue
      a. Snuff dipper's pouch—caused by use of chewing tobacco (Figure 17-5, *A*)
      b. Squamous cell carcinoma—most common form of mouth cancer (Figure 17-5, *B*)
   2. Dental caries (Figure 17-5, *C*)
      a. Tooth disease resulting in permanent defect called a "cavity"
      b. Infection may spread to other adjacent tissues or to blood
      c. Lost or diseased teeth may be replaced by dentures or implants (Figure 17-6)
   3. Gingivitis—gum inflammation or infection
      a. Most cases result from poor oral hygiene

      b. Can be a complication of diabetes, vitamin deficiency, or pregnancy
   4. Thrush, or oral candidiasis—caused by yeastlike fungal organism (Figure 17-7)
      a. Patches of "cheesy"-looking exudate form over an inflamed tongue and oral mucosa, which itches and bleeds easily
      b. Common in immunosuppressed individuals (with AIDS) or after antibiotic therapy
   5. Periodontitis—inflammation of periodontal membrane
      a. Often a complication of advanced or untreated gingivitis
      b. Leading cause of tooth loss among adults
   6. Cleft lip and cleft palate—most common congenital defects of the mouth (Figure 17-8)
      a. May occur alone or together
      b. Caused by failure of mouth structures to fuse during embryonic development

Salivary Glands (Figure 17-7)

A. Three pairs of salivary glands
   1. Secrete about 1 liter of saliva/day
   2. Located outside of GI tract
   3. Convey secretions via ducts into tract lumen (Figure 17-9)
B. Parotid glands—largest of salivary glands
   1. Located in front of ear at angle of jaw
   2. Ducts open into mouth opposite second molars
   3. Inflamed in mumps
C. Submandibular glands—ducts open on either side of lingual frenulum
D. Sublingual glands—ducts open into floor of mouth
E. Saliva contains salivary amylase—begins digestion of carbohydrates

Pharynx

A. Muscular tube (throat) lined with mucous membrane
B. Functions as part of both respiratory and digestive systems
C. Subdivided into three anatomical segments (Figure 17-10)

Wall of the Digestive Tract (Figure 17-11)

A. Lumen—hollow space within the "tube" of the digestive tract
B. Tissue layers of the wall of the digestive tube from inside to outside
   1. Mucosa—mucous epithelium

2. Submucosa—connective tissue
3. Muscularis—two layers of smooth muscle that move food through the tube by rhythmic muscular waves known as *peristalsis*
4. Serosa—serous membrane that covers the outside of abdominal organs
   a. Composed of visceral peritoneum in abdominal cavity
   b. It attaches the digestive tract to the wall of the abdominopelvic cavity by forming folds called *mesenteries* (Figure 17-23)

Esophagus

A. Muscular, mucus-lined tube about 25 cm (10 inches) long
B. Connects pharynx to stomach
C. Muscular walls help push food toward stomach
D. Sphincters at each end of esophagus help keep ingested material moving in one direction down the tube
   1. Upper esophageal sphincter (UES)
   2. Lower esophageal sphincter (LES)
E. GERD—gastroesophageal reflux disease
   1. Backflow of acidic stomach contents into esophagus causes symptoms of heartburn and indigestion
   2. Mild symptoms treated by nonsurgical measures include dietary changes, weight loss, acid blocking or buffering medications, and drugs that strengthen LES
   3. Severe and frequent episodes of GERD can trigger asthma attacks, cause severe chest pain, bleeding, or narrowing and chronic irritation of esophagus (Figure 17-12)
   4. Untreated GERD may result in a precancerous condition called Barrett esophagus.
   5. Common symptom of hiatal hernia (Figure 17-14)

Stomach (Figure 17-15)

A. Pouch for food that lies in upper part of abdominal cavity just under diaphragm
   1. About the size of a large sausage when empty
   2. Expands considerably after a large meal
B. Contraction of muscular walls of stomach mixes food with gastric juice and breaks it down into chyme
C. Mucous membrane lines the stomach
   1. Membrane lies in folds (rugae) when stomach is empty

2. Many microscopic glands secrete gastric juice and hydrochloric acid into stomach
D. Divisions of stomach—fundus, body, and pylorus
E. Pyloric sphincter muscle closes opening of pylorus (lower part of stomach) to retain food to facilitate partial digestion
F. Disorders of the stomach
   1. Gastroenterology—study of stomach and intestines and their diseases
      a. Stomach is potential site of numerous diseases and conditions
      b. Gastric diseases often exhibit these signs or symptoms: gastritis (inflammation), anorexia (appetite loss), nausea (upset stomach), and emesis (vomiting)
   2. Pylorospasm—abnormal spasms of the pyloric sphincter
      a. Common condition in infants
      b. Pyloric stenosis is similar abnormality—obstructive narrowing of the pyloric opening
   3. Ulcer—open wound caused by acid in gastric juice
      a. Often occurs in duodenum or stomach
      b. Associated with infection by the bacterium *Helicobacter pylori* and use of NSAIDs
      c. Current treatment involves triple therapy
   4. Stomach cancer
      a. Associated with consumption of alcohol or preserved food, use of chewing tobacco, and infection by *H. pylori*
      b. No practical way to screen for early stages

Small Intestine (Figure 17-17)

A. Size—about 7 meters (20 feet) long but only 2 cm or so in diameter
B. Divisions
   1. Duodenum
   2. Jejunum
   3. Ileum
C. Lining—mucous membrane
   1. Many microscopic glands (intestinal glands) secrete intestinal juice
   2. Arranged into multiple circular folds—plicae
   3. Folds covered with villi (microscopic finger-shaped projections from surface of mucosa into intestinal cavity)—contain blood and lymph capillaries
D. Disorders of the small intestine
   1. Enteritis—intestinal inflammation

2. Gastroenteritis—inflammation of stomach and intestines
3. Malabsorption syndrome—group of symptoms resulting from failure to absorb nutrients properly (e.g., anorexia, abdominal bloating, cramps, anemia, and fatigue)

Liver and Gallbladder (Figure 17-18)

A. Liver
   1. Size and location
      a. Liver is largest gland
      b. Fills upper right section of abdominal cavity and extends over into left side
   2. Classified as exocrine gland
      a. Secretes bile
      b. Has a variety of metabolic functions
   3. Ducts (Figure 17-18)
      a Hepatic—drains bile from liver
      b. Cystic—duct by which bile enters and leaves gallbladder
      c. Common bile—formed by union of hepatic and cystic ducts and drains bile from hepatic or cystic ducts into duodenum
B. Gallbladder
   1. Location—undersurface of the liver
   2. Function—concentrates and stores bile produced in the liver
C. Disorders of the liver and gallbladder
   1. Gallstones—hard clumps made of cholesterol crystallized bile pigments and calcium salts
      a. Cholelithiasis—condition of having gallstones (Figure 17-19)
      b. Cholecystitis—inflammation of the gallbladder; may accompany cholelithiasis
      c. Stones can obstruct bile canals, causing jaundice
   2. Hepatitis—liver inflammation
      a. Characterized by liver enlargement, jaundice, anorexia, discomfort, gray-white feces, and dark urine
      b. Caused by a variety of factors: toxins, bacteria, viruses, hepatitis A, B, and C, and parasites
   3. Cirrhosis—degeneration of liver tissue involving replacement of normal (but damaged) tissue with fibrous and fatty tissue (Figure 17-20, *A*)
   4. Portal hypertension—high blood pressure in the hepatic portal veins caused by obstruction of blood flow in a diseased liver; may cause varicosities of surrounding systemic veins (Figure 17-20, *B*)

Pancreas (Figure 17-18)

A. Location—behind stomach
B. Functions
   1. Pancreatic cells secrete pancreatic juice into pancreatic ducts; main duct empties into duodenum
   2. Pancreatic islets (of Langerhans)—cells not connected with pancreatic ducts; secrete hormones glucagon and insulin into the blood
C. Pancreatic disorders
   1. Pancreatitis—inflammation of pancreas
      a. Acute pancreatitis results from blocked ducts that force pancreatic juice to backflow
      b. Pancreatic enzymes digest the gland
   2. Cystic fibrosis—thick secretions block flow of pancreatic juice
   3. Pancreatic cancer—very serious; fatal in the majority of cases

Large Intestine (Figure 17-22)

A. Size and location—1.5 meters long; forms lower, or terminal, portion of digestive tract
B. Divisions
   1. Cecum
   2. Colon—ascending, transverse, descending, and sigmoid
   3. Rectum
   4. Anal canal
C. Opening to exterior—anus
D. Disorders of the large intestine often relate to abnormal motility (rate of movement of contents)
   1. Diarrhea—results from abnormally increased intestinal motility; may result in dehydration or convulsions
   2. Constipation—results from decreased intestinal motility
   3. Diverticulitis (inflammation of abnormal outpouchings called *diverticula*)—may cause constipation (Figure 17-22, *C*)
   4. Colitis—general name for any inflammatory condition of the large intestine
   5. Colorectal cancer—a common malignancy of the colon and rectum associated with colonic polyps; advanced age; low-fiber, high-fat diets; and genetic predisposition

Appendix and Appendicitis

A. Vermiform appendix is blind tube attached directly to cecum; no important digestive function in humans
B. Appendicitis—inflammation or infection of appendix
  1. If appendix ruptures, infectious material may spread to other organs (Figure 17-22, *D*)
  2. Most common acute abdominal condition requiring surgery
  3. Affects 7% to 12% of population younger than 30 years

Peritoneum (Figure 17-23)

A. Description—large sheet of serous membrane
  1. Parietal layer of peritoneum lines abdominal cavity
  2. Visceral layer of peritoneum covers abdominal organs
  3. Peritoneal space lies between parietal and visceral layers
B. Extensions of peritoneum—largest are the mesentery and greater omentum (Figure 17-23, *B*)
  1. Mesentery—extension of parietal peritoneum, which attaches most of small intestine to posterior abdominal wall
  2. Greater omentum, or "lace apron"—hangs down from lower edge of stomach and transverse colon over intestines
C. Peritonitis—inflammation of peritoneum resulting from infection or other irritant; often a complication of ruptured appendix
D. Ascites—abnormal accumulation of fluid in peritoneal space; often causes bloating of abdomen (Figure 17-24)

Digestion (Table 17-2)

A. Definition—process that transforms food into a form that can be absorbed and used by cells
  1. Mechanical digestion—chewing, swallowing, and peristalsis break food into tiny particles, mix them well with digestive juices, and move them along the digestive tract
  2. Chemical digestion—breaks up large food molecules into compounds having smaller molecules; brought about by digestive enzymes
B. Enzymes and chemical digestion
  1. Enzymes—protein molecules that act as catalysts, speeding up chemical reactions
  2. Chemical digestion—specific enzymes speed up breakdown of specific molecules and no others
  3. Hydrolysis—enzymes speed up reactions that add water to break large moleucles into smaller molecules
C. Carbohydrate digestion—mainly in small intestine
  1. Pancreatic amylase—changes starches to maltose
  2. Intestinal juice enzymes
    a. Maltase—changes maltose to glucose
    b. Sucrase—changes sucrose to glucose
    c. Lactase—changes lactose to glucose
D. Protein digestion—starts in stomach; completed in small intestine
  1. Gastric juice enzymes, rennin (in infants) and pepsin, partially digest proteins
  2. Pancreatic enzyme trypsin completes digestion of proteins to amino acids
  3. Intestinal enzymes, peptidases, complete digestion of partially digested proteins to amino acids
E. Fat digestion
  1. Bile contains no enzymes but emulsifies fats (breaks fat droplets into very small droplets)
  2. Pancreatic lipase changes emulsified fats to fatty acids and glycerol in small intestine

Absorption

A. Definition—digested food moves from intestine into blood or lymph
B. Absorption site—foods and most water are absorbed from small intestine; some water also absorbed from large intestine
  1. Minerals and other nutrients are actively transported through the intestinal mucosa; water absorbed by osmosis
  2. Fatty acids and glycerol diffuse into absorptive cells in GI tract
  3. "Water-soluble vitamins" are dissolved in water and absorbed, "fat-soluble vitamins" are absorbed with the end products of fat digestion
C. Surface area and absorption—large surface area of GI tract composed of mucosal folds, vili, and microvilli that increase efficiency and speed of absorption

New Words

absorption	intestinal gland	tricuspid (molar)	dysentery
alimentary canal	jejunum	upper esophageal sphincter	emesis
amylase	large intestine	(UES)	enteritis
anal canal	lipase	uvula	gallstone
anus	lower esophageal sphincter	vermiform appendix	gastritis
bicuspid (premolar)	(LES)	villus (*pl.,* villi)	gastroenteritis
bile	lumen		gastroenterology
bolus	mastication	**Diseases and Other**	gastroesophageal reflux
canine tooth (cuspid)	mesentery	**Clinical Terms**	disease (GERD)
cecum	oral cavity	anorexia	gingivitis
cementum	palate	appendicitis	heartburn
cholecystokinin (CCK)	papilla (*pl.,* papillae)	ascites	hepatitis
chyme	parotid gland	Bard endoscopic suturing	hiatal hernia
crown (of tooth)	periodontal membrane	system	jaundice
deglutition	peristalsis	Barrett esophagus	leukoplakia
dentin	peritoneum	caries (cavity)	malabsorption syndrome
digestion	plica (*pl.,* plicae)	cholecystectomy	maldigestion
duodenum	protease	cholecystitis	malocclusion
emulsify	pyloric sphincter	cholelithiasis	nausea
enzymes	pylorus	cirrhosis	orthodontics
fractal geometry	rectum	cleft lip	pancreatitis
frenulum	rugae	cleft palate	periodontitis
fundus (of stomach)	salivary amylase	colitis	peritonitis
gastric gland	serosa	colorectal cancer	pyloric stenosis
gastrointestinal (GI) tract	sigmoid colon	colostomy	pylorospasm
greater omentum	small intestine	constipation	snuff dipper's pouch
hepatic colic (right) flexure	splenic colic (left) flexure	Crohn disease	thrush (oral candidiasis)
ileocecal valve	sublingual gland	diarrhea	triple therapy
ileum	submandibular gland	diverticulitis	ulcer

Review Questions

1. Name and describe the four layers of the wall of the gastrointestinal tract.
2. What is the function of the uvula and soft palate?
3. Explain the function of the different types of teeth.
4. Describe the three main parts of the tooth.
5. What is leukoplakia? What could possibly develop from it?
6. Distinguish between gingivitis and periodontitis.
7. Name the three pairs of salivary glands and describe where the duct from each enters the mouth.
8. What is the function of the upper and lower esophageal sphincter muscles?
9. Define peristalsis.
10. What are the three parts of the triple therapy used to treat ulcers?
11. Explain how bile from the liver and gallbladder reaches the small intestine. What is the function of cholecystokinin?
12. What is the relationship between body weight and the formation of gallstones?
13. What is hepatitis? What are the signs and symptoms of hepatitis?
14. What is contained in pancreatic juice?
15. What do the bacteria in the large intestine contribute to the body?
16. List the seven subdivisions of the large intestine.

17. Describe the mesentery and the greater omentum.
18. What is peritonitis? What is ascites?
19. Differentiate between mechanical digestion and chemical digestion.
20. Briefly describe the process of carbohydrate digestion.
21. Briefly describe the process of fat digestion.
22. Briefly describe the process of protein digestion.
23. Explain the process of absorption. What function do the lacteals have in absorption?

Chapter Test

1. Food undergoes three kinds of processing in the body. All cells perform metabolism, but _____ and _____ are performed by the digestive system.
2. The _____ layer of the wall of the gastrointestinal tract produces peristalsis.
3. The _____ layer of the wall of the gastro-intestinal tract contains blood vessels and nerves.
4. _____ is the innermost layer of the wall of the gastrointestinal tract.
5. _____ is the outermost layer of the wall of the gastrointestinal tract.
6. The _____ and _____ prevent food and liquids from entering the nasal cavity above the mouth when food is swallowed.
7. The three main parts of the tooth are _____, _____, and _____.
8. The three salivary glands are the _____, _____, and _____.
9. The tube connecting the mouth and stomach is the _____.
10. The three divisions of the stomach are the _____, _____, and _____.

Critical Thinking

24. What structures in the small intestine increase the internal surface area? What advantage is gained by this increase in surface area?
25. Bile does not cause a chemical change; what is the effect of bile on fat, and why does this make fat digestion more efficient?
26. Some people are lactose intolerant. This means they are less able to fully digest lactose sugar. What enzyme is probably not functioning properly and what type of food should these people try to avoid?

11. The three divisions of the small intestines are the _____, _____, and _____.
12. The tiny finger-like projections covering the plicae of the small intestines are called _____.
13. The lymphatic vessels in the villi are called the _____.
14. The common bile duct is formed by the union of the _____ from the liver and the _____ from the gallbladder.
15. The part of the large intestine between the ascending and descending colon is the _____.
16. The part of the large intestine between the descending colon and the rectum is called the _____.
17. The two most prominent extensions of the peritoneum are the _____ and the _____.
18. The process by which digested food is moved from the digestive system to the circulating fluids is called _____.

Case Studies

1. Give the sequence of events in which a failure to brush and floss the teeth would lead to loss of teeth.
2. You have been diagnosed as having a duodenal ulcer. Your physician prescribed the drug famotidine (Pepcid). This drug has an action similar to cimetidine, but it is much more potent. How will famotidine help your ulcer? Your brother also has an ulcer, but his physician has prescribed sucralfate (Carafate), a medication that has an antipepsin action and tends to adhere to membrane injuries. Explain how sucralfate might help your brother's ulcer.

3. Fred has been experiencing recurring episodes of heartburn, especially when he bends over to lace his shoes or when he lies down in bed. His physician believes Fred may have a hiatal hernia. To confirm this diagnosis, she has scheduled Fred for a "barium swallow." In this test, a barium-containing fluid that blocks x-rays is swallowed so that the stomach appears as a bright mass in a radiograph. If Fred has a hiatal hernia, what should the radiologist see on the radiograph? Can you explain what caused the symptoms that brought Fred in to see his physician?

Match each term in Column A with its corresponding statement in Column B.

Column A
19. _____ emulsification
20. _____ amylase
21. _____ pepsin
22. _____ cholecystokinin
23. _____ peptidase
24. _____ cystic
25. _____ trypsin
26. _____ simple sugars
27. _____ amino acid
28. _____ liver
29. _____ lipase
30. _____ glycerol

Column B
a. enzyme that is made in the pancreas and digests fat
b. enzyme that is made in the small intestine and digests protein
c. gland that produces bile
d. the final end product of protein digestion
e. effect bile has on fat droplets
f. enzyme that is made in the pancreas and digests protein
g. the final end product of carbohydrate digestion
h. one of the final end products of fat digestion
i. enzyme that is made in both the salivary glands and the pancreas and digests starch
j. enzyme that is made in the stomach and digests protein
k. hormone that stimulates the contraction of the gallbladder
l. duct that connects the gallbladder to the common bile duct

Match each disorder in Column A with its cause or description in Column B.

Column A
31. _____ gingivitis
32. _____ periodontitis
33. _____ gastroenteritis
34. _____ ulcer
35. _____ cholecystitis
36. _____ hepatitis
37. _____ diverticulitis
38. _____ colitis
39. _____ peritonitis
40. _____ ascites

Column B
a. inflammation of the stomach and intestines
b. a liver inflammation; B type is more serious than A type
c. inflammation of abnormal outpouchings in the large intestine
d. inflammation of the periodontal membrane
e. abnormal accumulation of fluid in the peritoneal space
f. a general term for the inflammation of the large intestine
g. a general term for gum inflammation or infection
h. inflammation of the peritoneum
i. inflammation of the gallbladder
j. open wounds caused by gastric acid, often associated with *Helicobacter pylori*

Study Tips

continued from page 487

some suffixes that can make the processes easier to learn. The suffix *-ose* indicates that the substance is a carbohydrate. The suffix *-ase* indicates the substance is an enzyme. In many cases, the first part of the enzyme's name tells you what substance is being digested. Malt*ose* is digested by the enzyme malt*ase*. If you know this general rule, remembering what digests what becomes easier. The protein enzymes pepsin and trypsin do not fit this rule.

5. Absorption usually occurs by diffusion of nutrients into the cells of the small intestine and then into the blood. Villi on the interior of the small intestine greatly increase its surface area. This makes the process of absorption much more efficient.

6. In your study group, review your flash cards of the structures of the digestive system and your chart of the disorders of the digestive system. Use Table 17-2 to quiz each other on the enzymes, the substances they digest, and the end products they produce. Discuss the process of absorption, go over the questions at the back of the chapter, and discuss possible test questions.

18 Nutrition and Metabolism

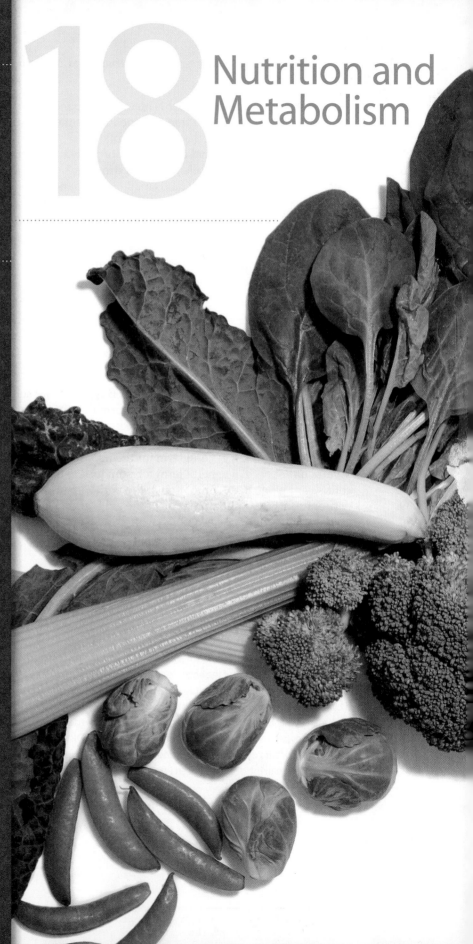

Objectives

After you have completed this chapter, you should be able to:

1. Define and contrast catabolism and anabolism.

2. Describe the metabolic roles of carbohydrates, fats, proteins, vitamins, and minerals.

3. Define basal metabolic rate and list some factors that affect it.

4. Describe three disorders associated with eating or metabolism.

5. Discuss the physiological mechanisms that regulate body temperature.

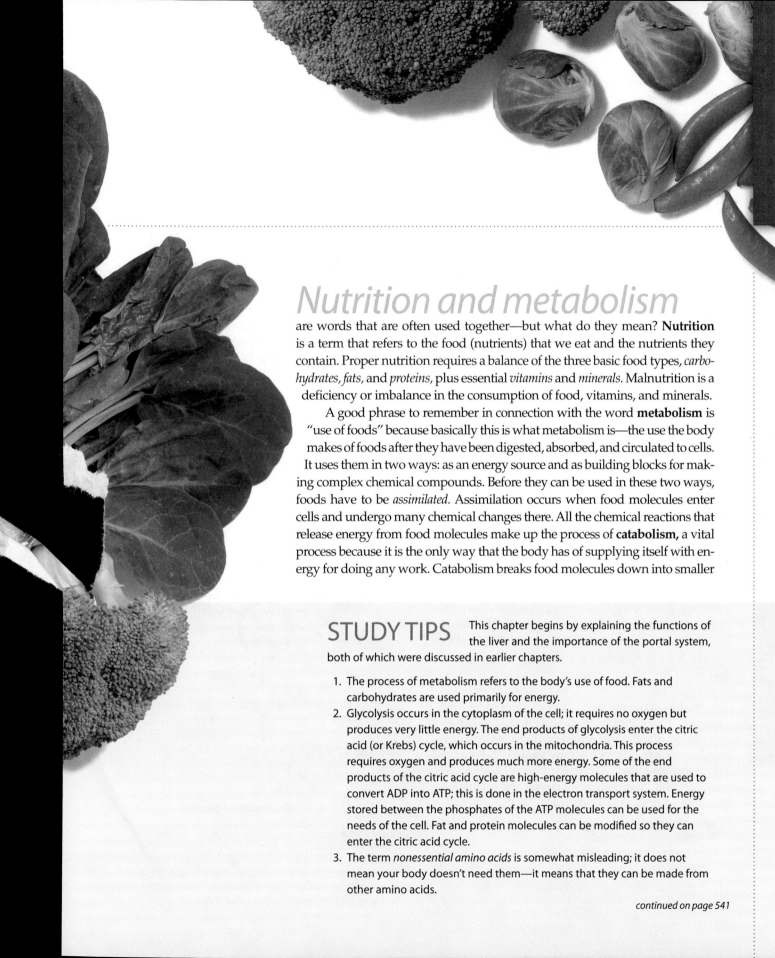

Nutrition and metabolism

are words that are often used together—but what do they mean? **Nutrition** is a term that refers to the food (nutrients) that we eat and the nutrients they contain. Proper nutrition requires a balance of the three basic food types, *carbohydrates, fats,* and *proteins,* plus essential *vitamins* and *minerals.* Malnutrition is a deficiency or imbalance in the consumption of food, vitamins, and minerals.

A good phrase to remember in connection with the word **metabolism** is "use of foods" because basically this is what metabolism is—the use the body makes of foods after they have been digested, absorbed, and circulated to cells. It uses them in two ways: as an energy source and as building blocks for making complex chemical compounds. Before they can be used in these two ways, foods have to be *assimilated.* Assimilation occurs when food molecules enter cells and undergo many chemical changes there. All the chemical reactions that release energy from food molecules make up the process of **catabolism,** a vital process because it is the only way that the body has of supplying itself with energy for doing any work. Catabolism breaks food molecules down into smaller

STUDY TIPS

This chapter begins by explaining the functions of the liver and the importance of the portal system, both of which were discussed in earlier chapters.

1. The process of metabolism refers to the body's use of food. Fats and carbohydrates are used primarily for energy.
2. Glycolysis occurs in the cytoplasm of the cell; it requires no oxygen but produces very little energy. The end products of glycolysis enter the citric acid (or Krebs) cycle, which occurs in the mitochondria. This process requires oxygen and produces much more energy. Some of the end products of the citric acid cycle are high-energy molecules that are used to convert ADP into ATP; this is done in the electron transport system. Energy stored between the phosphates of the ATP molecules can be used for the needs of the cell. Fat and protein molecules can be modified so they can enter the citric acid cycle.
3. The term *nonessential amino acids* is somewhat misleading; it does not mean your body doesn't need them—it means that they can be made from other amino acids.

continued on page 541

molecules and releases energy in the process. The many chemical reactions that build these smaller food molecules into more complex chemical compounds constitute the process of **anabolism.** Catabolism and anabolism make up the process of metabolism. An easy way to remember these terms is to imagine two small children with a set of blocks. Anna (anabolism) built a tower and Carter (catabolism) knocked it down.

This chapter explores many of the basic ideas about why certain nutrients are necessary for survival, how they are used by the body, and what can go wrong in metabolic and eating disorders.

Metabolic Functions of the Liver

As we discussed in Chapter 17, the liver plays an important role in mechanical digestion of lipids because it secretes *bile.* As you recall, bile breaks large fat globules into smaller droplets of fat that are more easily broken down. In addition, liver cells perform other functions necessary for healthy survival. They play a major role in the metabolism of all three kinds of foods. They help maintain a normal blood glucose concentration by carrying on complex and essential chemical reactions. Liver cells also carry out the first steps of protein and fat metabolism and synthesize several kinds of protein compounds. These proteins when released into blood are called the *blood proteins,* or *plasma proteins.* Prothrombin and fibrinogen, plasma proteins formed by liver cells, play essential parts in blood clotting (see pp. 360-362). Another protein made by liver cells, albumin, helps maintain normal blood volume. Liver cells detoxify the body of various poisonous substances such as bacterial products and certain drugs. They also store several substances, notably iron and vitamins A and D.

The liver is assisted by an interesting structural feature of the blood vessels that supply it. As you may recall from Chapter 14, the hepatic portal vein delivers blood directly from the gastrointestinal tract to the liver (see Figure 14-9). This arrangement allows blood that has just absorbed nutrients and other substances to be processed by the liver before being distributed throughout the body. Thus excess nutrients and vitamins can be stored and toxins can be removed from the bloodstream.

QUICK CHECK

1. What are the three basic food types?
2. What is metabolism?
3. Describe at least three functions of the liver.

Nutrient Metabolism

Carbohydrate Metabolism

Carbohydrates are the preferred energy food of the body. The larger carbohydrate molecules are composed of smaller "building blocks," primarily *glucose* (see Chapter 2). Human cells catabolize (break down) glu-

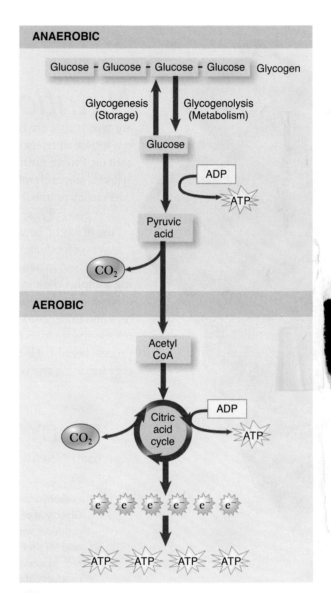

Figure 18-1 | **Metabolism of glucose.**

Glucose is liberated from glycogen stores in the body and is converted into pyruvic acid. Acetyl CoA is formed from the pyruvic acid generated during glycolysis and enters the citric acid cycle where high-energy electrons are released. These high-energy electrons enter the electron transport system where they are transferred to molecules of ATP.

cose rather than other substances as long as enough glucose enters them to supply their energy needs.

Three series of chemical reactions, **glycolysis** (glye-KOL-i-sis), **citric acid cycle**, and **electron transport system** occur in a precise sequence and make up the process of glucose catabolism.

Glycolysis takes place in the cytoplasm of a cell, whereas the citric acid cycle and electron transport system occur in the mitochondria, the cell's miniature power plants. Glycolysis is an **anaerobic** (an-er-OH-bik) process, meaning that it will take place with or without oxygen. Glycolysis doesn't *need* oxygen to occur. The citric acid cycle, in contrast, is an oxygen-using or **aerobic** (air-OH-bik) process. Glycolysis, as Figure 18-1 shows, changes glucose to pyruvic acid, which is then converted into acetyl CoA before it enters the citric acid cycle.

Acetyl CoA then moves into the citric acid cycle, also known as the *Krebs cycle* after its discoverer Hans Krebs. The citric acid cycle changes the acetyl CoA to carbon dioxide, and along the way a little bit of energy is produced. However, most of the energy leaving the citric acid cycle is in the form of high-energy electrons that enter the electron transport system to yield even more energy.

While the chemical reactions of glycolysis and the citric acid cycle occur, energy stored in the glucose molecule is being released. More than half of the released energy is in the form of high-energy electrons that enter a chain of carrier molecules embedded in the inner membrane of mitochondria. This chain of carrier molecules is known as the electron transport system, and it almost immediately transfers the energy to molecules of adenosine triphosphate (ATP). The rest of the energy originally stored in the glucose molecule is released as heat, which we can't use to do work but which contributes to a person's body temperature.

ATP serves as the direct source of energy for doing cellular work in all kinds of living organisms from one-cell plants to trillion-cell animals, including humans. Among biological compounds, therefore, ATP ranks as one of the most important. The energy transferred to ATP molecules differs in two ways from the energy stored in food molecules: (1) the energy in ATP molecules is not stored but is released almost instantaneously and (2) it can be used directly to do cellular work. Release of energy from food molecules occurs much more slowly because catabolism of food must occur first. Energy released from food molecules cannot be used directly for doing cellular work. It must first be transferred to ATP molecules and then be explosively released from them.

As Figure 18-2 shows, ATP is made up of an adenosine group and three phosphate groups. The capacity of ATP to store large amounts of energy is found in the high-energy bonds that hold the phosphate groups together, illustrated as curvy lines. When a phosphate group breaks off of the molecule, an adenosine diphosphate (ADP) molecule and free phosphate group result. Energy that had been holding the phosphate bond together is freed to do cellular work (muscle fiber contractions, for example).

As you can see in Figure 18-2, the ADP and phosphate are reunited by the energy produced by carbohydrate catabolism, making ATP a reusable energy-storage molecule. Only enough ATP for immediate cellular requirements is made at any one time, but new ATP is constantly being made to meet cellular demands. Glucose that is not needed is built up (by anabolic processes) into larger molecules that are stored for later use.

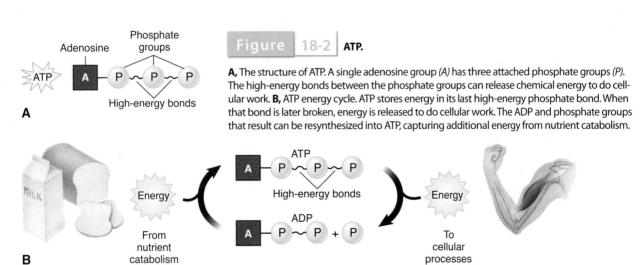

Figure 18-2 **ATP.**

A, The structure of ATP. A single adenosine group *(A)* has three attached phosphate groups *(P)*. The high-energy bonds between the phosphate groups can release chemical energy to do cellular work. **B,** ATP energy cycle. ATP stores energy in its last high-energy phosphate bond. When that bond is later broken, energy is released to do cellular work. The ADP and phosphate groups that result can be resynthesized into ATP, capturing additional energy from nutrient catabolism.

Glucose anabolism is called **glycogenesis** (glye-koh-JEN-eh-sis). Carried on chiefly by liver and muscle cells, glycogenesis consists of a series of reactions that join glucose molecules together, like many beads in a necklace, to form *glycogen*, a compound sometimes called *animal starch.*

Something worth noting is that the amount of nutrients in the blood normally does not change very much, not even when we go without food for many hours, when we exercise and use a lot of food for energy, or when we sleep and use little food for energy. The amount of glucose in our blood, for example, usually stays at about 80 to 110 mg in 100 ml of blood when we are "fasting" between meals.

Several hormones help regulate carbohydrate metabolism to keep blood glucose at a normal level. **Insulin** is one of the most important of these. Although the exact details of its mechanism of action are still being worked out, insulin is known to accelerate glucose transport through cell membranes. As insulin secretion increases, more glucose leaves the blood and enters the cells. The amount of glucose in the blood therefore decreases as the rate of glucose metabolism in cells increases (see p. 328).

Too little insulin secretion, which occurs in people with type 1 diabetes mellitus, or ineffective insulin secretion, which occurs in people with type 2 diabetes mellitus, produces the opposite effects. Less glucose leaves the blood and enters the cells; more glucose therefore remains in the blood, and less glucose is metabolized by cells. In other words, high blood glucose (hyperglycemia) and a low rate of glucose metabolism characterize insulin deficiency.

Insulin is the only hormone that significantly lowers the blood glucose level. Several other hormones, on the other hand, can increase it. Growth hormone secreted by the anterior pituitary gland, hydrocortisone secreted by the adrenal cortex, epinephrine secreted by the adrenal medulla, and glucagon secreted by the pancreatic islets are four of the most important hormones that increase blood glucose. More information about these hormones can be found in Chapter 11.

 To learn more about glycolysis and the citric acid cycle, go to **AnimationDirect** on your CD.

Fat Metabolism

Fats, like carbohydrates, are primarily energy foods. If cells have inadequate amounts of glucose to catabolize, they immediately shift to the catabolism of fats for energy. Fats are simply converted into a form of glucose that can enter the citric acid cycle. This happens normally when a person goes without food for many hours and forms the basis for low carbohydrate diets (see Health and Well-Being box). This conversion of glucose happens abnormally in those with an untreated diabetic condition. Because of an insulin deficiency, too little glucose enters the cells of a diabetic person to supply all energy needs. The result is that the cells catabolize fats to make up the difference (Figure 18-3). In all persons, fats not needed for catabolism are instead anabolized (built up) to form triglycerides and then are stored in adipose tissue, which contributes to weight gain.

HEALTH & WELL-BEING

LOW-CARB DIETS

Low-carbohydrate diets have become increasingly popular among those attempting weight loss. When carbohydrate catabolism equals energy needs, fats are not taken out of storage and catabolized. Low-carbohydrate diets are based on the rationale that when the body is not supplied with adequate amounts of carbohydrates to meet its energy needs, it will switch to fat metabolism. This will reduce triglyceride stores in the body, and as a result, the person loses weight. In addition, some research studies on these diets have demonstrated an improved plasma lipid profile. However, there is still controversy over the many types of low-carbohydrate diets and which are safe and effective for those struggling with obesity, diabetes, and other disorders. Ultimately, the most successful weight-reducing diet may be the one that each person can stick to for the longest duration.

HEALTH & WELL-BEING

CARBOHYDRATE LOADING

A number of athletes and others who must occasionally sustain endurance exercise for a significant period practice **carbohydrate loading,** or **glycogen loading.** As with liver cells, some skeletal muscle fibers can take up and store glucose in the form of glycogen. By ceasing intense exercise and switching to a diet high in carbohydrates 2 or 3 days before an endurance event, an athlete can cause the skeletal muscles to store almost twice as much glycogen as usual. This allows the muscles to sustain aerobic exercise for up to 50% longer than usual. The concept of carbohydrate loading has been used to promote the use of "energy bar" sport snacks.

Figure 18-3

Catabolism of nutrients.

Fats, carbohydrates, and proteins can be converted to products that enter the citric acid cycle to yield energy.

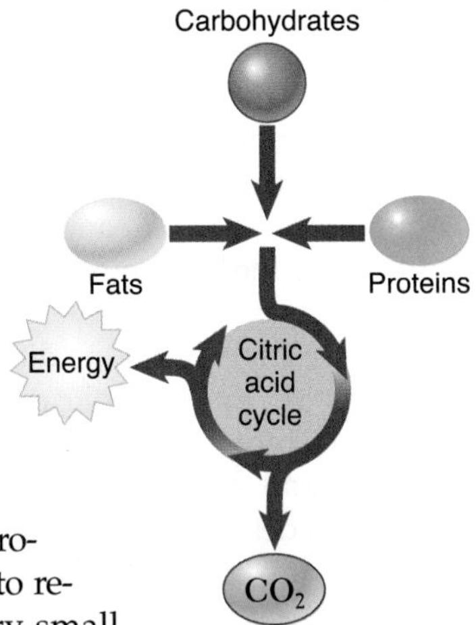

Carbohydrates

Fats   Proteins

Energy   Citric acid cycle

CO_2

Protein Metabolism

In a healthy person, proteins are catabolized to release energy to a very small extent. When fat reserves are low, as they are in the starvation that accompanies certain eating disorders such as anorexia nervosa, the body can start to use its protein molecules as an energy source. Specifically, the amino acids that make up proteins are each broken apart to yield an amine group that is converted to a form of glucose that can enter the citric acid cycle. This process is known as gluconeogenesis, and as discussed in Chapter 11, is a process that is performed mainly by liver cells. After a shift to reliance on protein catabolism as a major energy source occurs, death may quickly follow because vital proteins in the muscles and nerves are catabolized (see Figure 18-3).

A more common situation in normal bodies is protein anabolism, the process by which the body builds amino acids into complex protein compounds (for example, enzymes and proteins that form the structure of the cell). Proteins are assembled from a pool of 20 different kinds of amino acids. If any one type of amino acid is deficient, vital proteins cannot be synthesized—a serious health threat. One way your body maintains a constant supply of amino acids is by making them from other compounds already present in the body. Only about half of the required 20 types of amino acids can be made by the body, however. The remaining types of amino acids must be supplied in the diet. *Essential amino acids* are those that must be in the diet. *Nonessential amino acids* can be missing from the diet because they can be made by the body (Table 18-1).

QUICK CHECK

1. How are aerobic and anaerobic respiration different? How are they alike?
2. How is energy transferred from glucose to ATP?
3. How are proteins used once they are absorbed into the body?
4. What are essential amino acids?

CLINICAL APPLICATION

CHOLESTEROL

Cholesterol is a type of lipid that has many uses in the body (see Chapter 2). The body derives steroid hormones from cholesterol (see Chapter 11) and uses cholesterol to stabilize the phospholipid bilayer that forms the plasma membrane and membranous organelles of the cells. So why does such a useful substance have such a bad reputation? The reason lies in the fact that an *excess* of cholesterol in the blood, a condition called **hypercholesterolemia** (hye-per-kol-es-ter-ol-EE-mee-ah), increases the risk of developing atherosclerosis. You may recall from Chapter 14 that *atherosclerosis* develops into a type of arteriosclerosis, or "hardening of the arteries," that can lead to heart disease, stroke, and other problems. Hypercholesterolemia occurs most often in people with a genetic predisposition but is certainly also affected by other factors such as diet and exercise. People with hypercholesterolemia are encouraged to switch to diets low in cholesterol and saturated fats and to participate in aerobic exercise, both of which tend to lower blood cholesterol levels. Chapter 2 discusses different types of cholesterol and their roles in health and disease.

Table 18-1 | Amino Acids

ESSENTIAL (INDISPENSABLE)	NONESSENTIAL (DISPENSABLE)
Histidine*	Alanine
Isoleucine	Arginine
Leucine	Asparagine
Lysine	Aspartic acid
Methionine	Cysteine
Phenylalanine	Glutamic acid
Threonine	Glutamine
Tryptophan	Glycine
Valine	Proline
	Serine
	Tyrosine†

*Essential in infants and, perhaps, adult males.
†Can be synthesized from phenylalanine; therefore is nonessential as long as phenylalanine is in the diet.

Vitamins and Minerals

One glance at the label of any packaged food product reveals the importance we place on vitamins and minerals. We know that carbohydrates, fats, and proteins are used by our bodies to build important molecules and to provide energy. So why do we need vitamins and minerals?

First, let's discuss the importance of vitamins. **Vitamins** are organic molecules needed in small quantities for normal metabolism throughout the body. Most vitamin molecules attach to enzymes or *coenzymes* (molecules that assist enzymes) and help them work properly. Many enzymes are totally useless without the appropriate vitamins to activate them. Some vitamins play other important roles in the body. For example, a form of vitamin A plays an important role in detecting light in the sensory cells of the retina. Vitamin D can be converted to a hormone that helps regulate calcium homeostasis in the body, and vitamin E acts as an **antioxidant** that prevents highly re-

active molecules called **free radicals** from damaging DNA and molecules in cell membranes.

Most vitamins cannot be made by the body, so we must eat them in our food. The body can store fat-soluble vitamins—A, D, E, and K—in the liver for later use. Because the body cannot store water-soluble vitamins such as B vitamins and vitamin C, they must be continually supplied in the diet. Vitamin deficiencies can lead to severe metabolic problems. Table 18-2 lists some of the more well-known vitamins, their sources, functions, and symptoms of deficiency.

Vitamin deficiency, or **avitaminosis** (a-vye-tah-min-OS-is), can lead to severe metabolic problems. For example, *avitaminosis C* (vitamin C deficiency) can lead to **scurvy** (SKER-vee) (Figure 18-4). Scurvy results from the inability of the body to manufacture and maintain collagen fibers. As you may have gathered from your studies thus far, collagen fibers compose the connective tissues that hold most of the body together. In scurvy, the body falls apart in the same way that a ne-

Table 18-2	**Major Vitamins**		
VITAMIN	**DIETARY SOURCE**	**FUNCTIONS**	**SYMPTOMS OF DEFICIENCY**
Vitamin A	Green and yellow vegetables, dairy products, and liver	Maintains epithelial tissue and produces visual pigments	Night blindness and flaking skin
B-complex vitamins			
B_1 (thiamine)	Grains, meat, and legumes	Helps enzymes in the citric acid cycle	Nerve problems (beriberi), heart muscle weakness, and edema
B_2 (riboflavin)	Green vegetables, organ meat, eggs, and dairy products	Aids enzymes in the citric acid cycle	Inflammation of skin and eyes
B_3 (niacin)	Meat and grains	Helps enzymes in the citric acid cycle	Pellagra (scaly dermatitis and mental disturbances) and nervous disorders
B_5 (pantothenic acid)	Organ meat, eggs, and liver	Aids enzymes that connect fat and carbohydrate metabolism	Loss of coordination (rare); decreased gut motility
B_6 (pyridoxine)	Vegetables, meat, and grains	zHelps enzymes that catabolize amino acids	Convulsions, irritability, and anemia
B_{12} (cyanocobalamin)	Meat and dairy products	Involved in blood production and other processes	Pernicious anemia
Biotin	Vegetables, meat, and eggs	Helps enzymes in amino acid catabolism and fat and glycogen synthesis	Mental and muscle problems (rare)
Folic acid	Vegetables	Aids enzymes in amino acid catabolism and blood	Digestive disorders and anemia; neural defects in embryo or fetus
Vitamin C (ascorbic acid)	Fruits and green vegetables	Helps in manufacture of collagen fibers	Scurvy and degeneration of skin, bone, and blood vessels
Vitamin D (calciferol)	Dairy products and fish liver oil	Aids in calcium absorption	Rickets and skeletal deformity
Vitamin E (tocopherol)	Green vegetables and seeds	Protects cell membranes from oxydation damage	Muscle and reproductive disorders (rare)

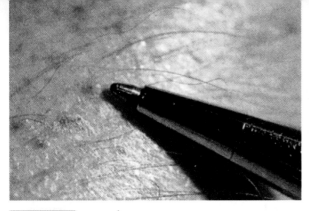

Figure 18-4 | **Scurvy.**

In scurvy, lack of vitamin C impairs the normal maintenance of collagen-containing connective tissues, causing bleeding and ulceration of the skin, gums, and other tissues, as these lesions on the skin show.

glected house eventually falls apart. More details about scurvy and other types of avitaminosis are given in Appendix C on the CD that accompanies your book.

Some forms of **hypervitaminosis** (hye-per-vye-tah-min-OS-is)—or vitamin excess—can be just as serious as a deficiency of vitamins. For example, chronic *hypervitaminosis A* can occur if very large amounts of vita-

min A are consumed daily over a period of 3 months or more. This condition first manifests itself with dry skin, hair loss, anorexia (appetite loss), and vomiting, but may progress to severe headaches and mental disturbances, liver enlargement, and occasionally cirrhosis. Acute hypervitaminosis A, characterized by vomiting, abdominal pain, and headache, can occur if a massive overdose is ingested. Excesses of the fat-soluble vitamins (A, D, E, and K) are generally more serious than excesses of the water-soluble vitamins (B complex and C) because fat-soluble vitamins are stored, whereas water-soluble vitamins can be excreted.

Minerals are just as important as vitamins. Minerals are inorganic elements or salts found naturally in the earth. As with vitamins, mineral ions can attach to enzymes and help them work. Minerals also function in a variety of other vital chemical reactions. For example, sodium, calcium, and other minerals are required for nerve conduction and for contraction in muscle fibers. Without these minerals, the brain, heart, and respiratory tract would cease to function. Information about some of the more important minerals is summarized in Table 18-3.

Table 18-3 | **Major Minerals**

MINERAL	DIETARY SOURCE	FUNCTIONS	SYMPTOMS OF DEFICIENCY
Calcium (Ca)	Dairy products, legumes, and vegetables	Helps blood clotting, bone formation, and nerve and muscle function	Bone degeneration and nerve and muscle malfunction
Chlorine (Cl)	Salty foods	Aids in stomach acid production and acid-base balance	Acid-base imbalance
Cobalt (Co)	Meat	Helps vitamin B_{12} in blood cell production	Pernicious anemia
Copper (Cu)	Seafood, organ meats, and legumes	Involved in extracting energy from the citric acid cycle and in blood production	Fatigue and anemia
Iodine (I)	Seafood and iodized salt	Aids in thyroid hormone synthesis	Goiter (thyroid enlargement) and decrease of metabolic rate
Iron (Fe)	Meat, eggs, vegetables, and legumes	Involved in extracting energy from the citric acid cycle and in blood production	Fatigue and anemia
Magnesium (Mg)	Vegetables and grains	Helps many enzymes	Nerve disorders, blood vessel dilation, and heart rhythm problems
Manganese (Mn)	Vegetables, legumes, and grains	Helps many enzymes	Muscle and nerve disorders
Phosphorus (P)	Dairy products and meat	Aids in bone formation and is used to make ATP, DNA, RNA, and phospholipids	Bone degeneration and metabolic problems
Potassium (K)	Seafood, milk, fruit, and meat	Helps muscle and nerve function	Muscle weakness, heart problems, and nerve problems
Sodium (Na)	Salty foods	Aids in muscle and nerve function and fluid balance	Weakness and digestive upset
Zinc (Zn)	Many foods	Helps many enzymes	Metabolic problems

Like vitamins, minerals are beneficial only when taken in the proper amounts. Many of the minerals listed in Table 18-3 are required in trace amounts. Any intake of such minerals beyond the recommended trace amount may become toxic—perhaps even life threatening.

Metabolic Rates

The **basal metabolic rate (BMR)** is the rate at which food is catabolized under basal conditions (that is, when the individual is resting but awake, is not digesting food, and is not adjusting to a cold external temperature). Or, stated differently, the BMR is the number of calories of heat that must be produced per hour by catabolism just to keep the body alive, awake, and comfortably warm. To provide energy for muscular work and digestion and absorption of food, an additional amount of food must be catabolized. The amount of additional food depends mainly on how much work the individual does. The more active he or she is, the more food the body must catabolize and the higher the total metabolic rate will be. The **total metabolic rate (TMR)** is the total amount of energy used by the body per day (Figure 18-5).

When the number of calories in your food intake equals your TMR, your weight remains constant (except for possible variations resulting from water retention or water loss). When your food intake provides more calories than your TMR, you gain weight; when your food intake provides fewer calories than your TMR, you lose weight. Nature does not forget to count calories. Reducing diets make use of this knowledge. They contain fewer calories than the TMR of the individual eating the diet.

 To learn more about the factors that influence metabolic rate, go to **AnimationDirect** on your CD.

Metabolic and Eating Disorders

Disorders characterized by a disruption or imbalance of normal metabolism can be caused by several different factors. For example, *inborn errors of metabolism* are a group of genetic conditions involving a deficiency or absence of a particular enzyme. Specific enzymes are required by cells to carry out each step of every metabolic reaction. Although an abnormal genetic code may affect the production of only a single enzyme, the resulting abnormal metabolism may have widespread effects. Specific diseases resulting from inborn errors of metabolism, such as *phenylketonuria (PKU)*, are discussed in Chapter 24.

A number of metabolic disorders are complications of other conditions. For example, you may recall from Chapter 11 that both hyperthyroidism and hypothyroidism have profound effects on the basal metabolic rate (BMR). Diabetes mellitus affects metabolism throughout the body when an insulin deficiency limits the amount of glucose available for use by the cells.

Some metabolic disorders result from normal mechanisms in the body that maintain homeostasis. For example, the body has several mechanisms that maintain a relatively constant level of glucose in the blood—glucose required by cells for life-sustaining catabolism. As mentioned earlier in this chapter, during *starvation* or in certain *eating disorders*, these mechanisms are taken to the extreme as they attempt to maintain blood glucose homeostasis. A few of the more well-known eating and nutrition disorders are briefly described here:

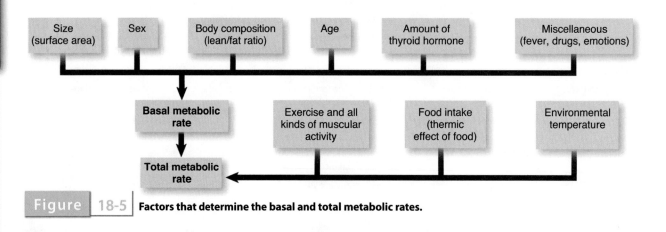

Figure 18-5 **Factors that determine the basal and total metabolic rates.**

1. **Anorexia nervosa** is a behavioral disorder characterized by chronic refusal to eat, often because of an abnormal fear of becoming obese. This condition is most commonly seen in teenage girls and young adult women and is often linked to emotional stress. Treatment is usually directed at solving the resulting nutritional deficit first, then dealing with the underlying behavioral problem.

2. **Bulimia** (boo-LEE-mee-ah) is a behavioral disorder characterized by insatiable craving for food alternating with periods of self-deprivation. The self-deprivation that follows a "food binge" is often accompanied by depression. People with a form of this disorder called **bulimarexia** (boo-lee-mah-REK-see-ah) purposely induce the vomiting reflex to purge themselves of food they just ate. Excessive vomiting in this way can have a variety of consequences, including damage to the esophagus, pharynx, mouth, and teeth by stomach acid.

3. **Obesity** is not an eating disorder itself but may be a result of chronic overeating behavior. Like anorexia nervosa and bulimia, eating disorders characterized by chronic overeating usually have an underlying emotional cause. Obesity is defined as an abnormal increase in the proportion of fat in the body. Most of the excess fat is stored in the subcutaneous tissue and around the viscera. Obesity is a risk factor for a variety of life-threatening diseases, including diabetes mellitus, many forms of cancer, and heart disease.

4. **Protein-calorie malnutrition (PCM)** is an abnormal condition resulting from a deficiency of calories in general and protein in particular. PCM is likely to result from reduced intake of food but may also be caused by increased nutrient loss or increased use of nutrients by the body. Table 18-4 summarizes a few of the many conditions that may lead to PCM. Mild cases occur frequently in illness; as many as one in five patients admitted to the hospital are significantly malnourished. More severe cases of PCM are likely to occur in parts of the world where food, especially protein-rich food, is relatively unavailable. There are two forms of advanced PCM: *marasmus* (mah-RAZ-mus) and

Table 18-4 | Some Causes of Protein-Calorie Malnutrition

CONDITION	IMPACT ON NUTRIENTS
CONDITIONS THAT REDUCE NUTRIENT INTAKE	
Anorexia	Absence of appetite; reduced motivation to eat
Dysphagia	Difficulty in swallowing; inhibition of normal eating
Gastrointestinal obstruction	Inability of food to be digested or absorbed
Nausea	Upset stomach; discomfort, which inhibits appetite
Pain	Discomfort, which discourages eating
Poverty	Inability to acquire proper nutrients
Social isolation	Absence of social cues or motivation for eating
Substance abuse	Reduction or replacement of the motivation to eat
Tooth problems	Difficulty in chewing, which discourages or prevents eating
CONDITIONS THAT INCREASE LOSS OF NUTRIENTS	
Diarrhea	Increased intestinal motility, which reduces absorption of nutrients
Glycosuria	Loss of glucose in the urine
Hemorrhage	Loss of blood and the nutrients it contains
Malabsorption	Failure to properly absorb nutrients, which causes nutrients to pass through the body unabsorbed
CONDITIONS THAT INCREASE THE USE OF NUTRIENTS BY THE BODY	
Burns	Loss of nutrients from damaged tissues
Fever	Increased temperature and metabolic rate, which increase rate of nutrient catabolism
Infection	Increased immune activity and tissue repair, which increase the rate of nutrient use
Trauma and surgery	Increased immune activity, tissue repair, and homeostatic-compensating mechanisms, which increase the rate of nutrient use
Tumors	Increased tissue growth, which increases the rate of nutrient use

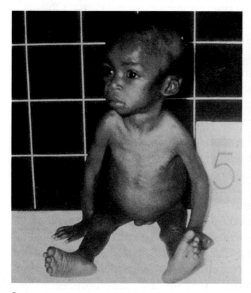

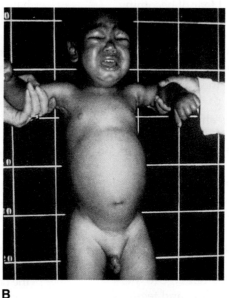

A   **B**

Figure 18-6

Protein-calorie malnutrition (PCM).

A, Marasmus results from starvation. **B,** Kwashiorkor results from a diet sufficient in calories but deficient in protein. Note the abdominal bloating typical in kwashiorkor.

kwashiorkor (kwah-shee-OR-kor) (Figure 18-6). Marasmus results from an overall lack of calories and proteins, such as when sufficient quantities of food are not available. Marasmus is characterized by progressive wasting of muscle and subcutaneous tissue accompanied by fluid and electrolyte imbalances. Kwashiorkor results from a protein deficiency in the presence of sufficient calories, as when a child is weaned from milk to low-protein foods. Kwashiorkor also causes wasting of tissues, but unlike marasmus, it also causes pronounced ascites (abdominal bloating) and flaking dermatitis. The ascites results from a deficiency of plasma proteins, which changes the osmotic balance of the blood and thus promotes osmosis of water from the blood into the peritoneal space (see Figure 17-23).

Nutrition disorders, including many specific deficiency diseases, are summarized in Appendix B on the CD that accompanies your book.

QUICK CHECK

1. How do *anorexia nervosa* and *bulimia* differ? How are these conditions alike?
2. Name at least eight causes of *protein-calorie malnutrition.*

Body Temperature

Considering that more than 60% of the energy released from food molecules during catabolism is converted to heat rather than being transferred to ATP, it is no wonder that maintaining a constant body temperature is a challenge. Maintaining homeostasis of body temperature, or **thermoregulation,** is the function of the hypothalamus. The hypothalamus operates a variety of negative-feedback mechanisms that keep body temperature in its normal range (36.2° to 37.6° C, or 97° to 100° F).

The skin is often involved in negative-feedback loops that maintain body temperature. When the body is overheated, blood flow to the skin increases

RESEARCH, ISSUES, AND TRENDS

MEASURING ENERGY

Physiologists studying metabolism must be able to express a quantity of energy in mathematical terms. The unit of energy measurement most often used is the calorie (cal). A **calorie** is the amount of energy needed to raise the temperature of 1 g of water 1 degree C. Because physiologists often deal with very large amounts of energy, the larger unit, **kilocalorie** (kcal) or **Calorie** (notice the uppercase C), is used. There are 1000 cal in 1 kcal or Calorie. Nutritionists prefer to use *Calorie* when they express the amount of energy stored in a food.

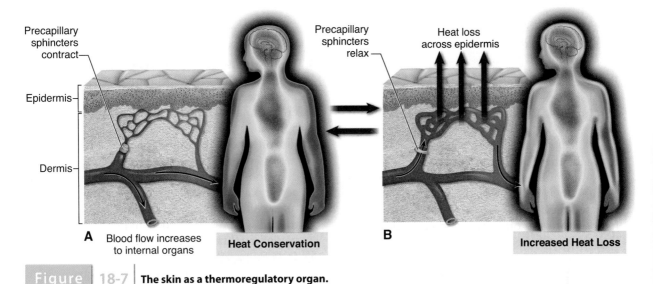

Precapillary sphincters contract

Epidermis

Dermis

A Blood flow increases to internal organs

Heat Conservation

Precapillary sphincters relax

Heat loss across epidermis

B

Increased Heat Loss

Figure 18-7 | **The skin as a thermoregulatory organ.**

When homeostasis requires that the body conserve heat, blood flow in the warm organs of the body's core increases *(left)*. When heat must be lost to maintain the stability of the internal environment, flow of warm blood to the skin increases *(right)*. Heat can be lost from the blood and skin by means of radiation, conduction, convection, and evaporation.

(Figure 18-7). Warm blood from the body's core can then be cooled by the skin, which acts as a radiator. At the skin, heat can be lost from blood by the following mechanisms:

1. Radiation—flow of heat waves away from the blood
2. Conduction—transfer of heat energy to the skin and then the external environment
3. Convection—transfer of heat energy to air that is continually flowing away from the skin
4. Evaporation—absorption of heat by water (sweat) vaporization

When necessary, heat can be conserved by reducing blood flow in the skin, as you can see in Figure 18-7.

A number of other mechanisms can be called on to help maintain the homeostasis of body temperature. Heat-generating muscle activity such as shivering and secretion of metabolism-regulating hormones are two of the body's processes that can be altered to adjust the body's temperature. The concept of using feedback control loops in homeostatic mechanisms was introduced in Chapter 1.

Abnormal Body Temperature

Maintenance of a body temperature within a narrow range is necessary for normal functioning of the body. As Figure 18-8 shows, straying too far out of the normal range of body temperatures can have

Figure 18-8 | **Body temperature.**

This diagram, modeled after a thermometer, shows some of the physiological consequences of abnormal body temperature. The normal range of body temperature under a variety of conditions is shown in the inset.

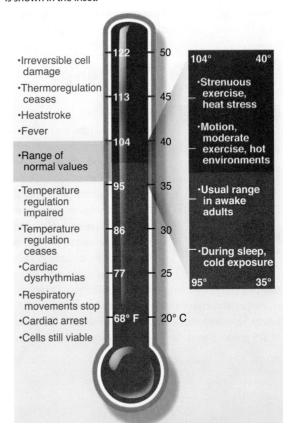

- Irreversible cell damage
- Thermoregulation ceases
- Heatstroke
- Fever
- Range of normal values
- Temperature regulation impaired
- Temperature regulation ceases
- Cardiac dysrhythmias
- Respiratory movements stop
- Cardiac arrest
- Cells still viable

122 — 50
113 — 45
104 — 40
95 — 35
86 — 30
77 — 25
68° F — 20° C

104° 40°

- Strenuous exercise, heat stress
- Motion, moderate exercise, hot environments
- Usual range in awake adults
- During sleep, cold exposure

95° 35°

very serious physiological consequences. A few important conditions related to body temperature are listed below and on p. 537.

1. **Fever**—As explained in Chapter 5, a fever or febrile state is an unusually high body temperature associated with a systemic inflammation response. In the case of infections, chemicals called *pyrogens* (literally, "fire-makers") cause the thermostatic control centers of the hypothalamus to produce a fever. Because the body's "thermostat" is reset to a higher setting, a person feels a need to warm up to this new temperature and often experiences "chills" as the febrile state begins. The high body temperature associated with infectious fever is thought to enhance the body's immune responses, eliminating the pathogen. Strategies aimed at reducing the temperature of a febrile person are normally counteracted by the body's heat-generating mechanisms and have the effect of further weakening the infected person. Under ordinary circumstances, it is best to let the fever "break" on its own after the pathogen is destroyed.

2. **Malignant hyperthermia (MH)** is an inherited condition characterized by an abnormally increased body temperature (hyperthermia) and muscle rigidity when exposed to certain anesthetics. The drug *dantrolene (Dantrium)*, which inhibits heat-producing muscle contractions, has been used to prevent or relieve effects of this condition.

3. **Heat exhaustion** occurs when the body loses a large amount of fluid resulting from heat-loss mechanisms. This usually happens when environmental temperatures are high. Although a normal body temperature is maintained, the loss of water and electrolytes can cause weakness, vertigo, nausea, and possibly loss of consciousness. Heat exhaustion also may be accompanied by skeletal muscle cramps that are often called *heat cramps.* Heat exhaustion is treated with rest (in a cool environment) accompanied by fluid replacement.

4. **Heatstroke,** or *sunstroke,* is a severe, sometimes fatal condition resulting from the inability of the body to maintain a normal temperature in an extremely warm environment. Such thermoregulatory failure may result from factors such as old age, disease, drugs that impair thermoregulation, or simply overwhelming elevated environmental temperatures. Heatstroke is characterized by body temperatures of 41° C (105° F) or higher, tachycardia, headache, and hot, dry skin. Confusion, convulsions, or loss of consciousness may occur. Unless the body is cooled and body fluids replaced immediately, death may result.

5. **Hypothermia** (hye-poh-THER-mee-ah) is the inability to maintain a normal body temperature

SCIENCE APPLICATIONS

FOOD SCIENCE

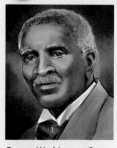

George Washington Carver (1864–1943)

At the dawn of the twentieth century, one figure loomed large in the world of food science—George Washington Carver. Born a slave on a Missouri plantation during the Civil War, Carver overcame great obstacles to become one of the most admired American scientists in history. Although talented in music and art, it was his knack for agriculture that led him to a long and successful career as a professor, researcher, and inventor in the agriculture department of Alabama's Tuskegee Institute. There, his work resulted in the creation of 325 products made from peanuts, nearly 200 products from yams (sweet potatoes), and hundreds more from other plants native to the southern United States. Development of these new products helped poor farmers survive by allowing them to make money from a variety of crops that thrived on their land.

Today, breakthroughs continue to be made in the world of agriculture and food science. Farmers and ranchers work closely with agricultural scientists and technicians to improve the end product of food crops and livestock they grow—and also to improve methods of raising them. As did Carver, they strive to work in ways that benefit the land as well as the people. Of course, nutritionists, dietitians, chefs, and food preparers all play a role in getting these crops to our table in a healthy and appetizing way. Food scientists and other industrial scientists work to develop technologies and methods for preparing, preserving, storing, and packaging foods.

in extremely cold environments. Hypothermia is characterized by body temperatures lower than 35° C (95° F), shallow and slow respirations, and a faint, slow pulse. Hypothermia is usually treated by slowly warming the affected person's body.

6. **Frostbite** is local damage to tissues caused by extremely low temperatures. Damage to tissues results from formation of ice crystals accompanied by a reduction in local blood flow. Necro-

sis (tissue death) and even gangrene (decay of dead tissue) can result from frostbite.

QUICK CHECK

1. Describe the four main ways that heat leaves the body.
2. Is *fever* a normal or abnormal response to injury or infection?
3. What can happen to the body with excessive exposure to heat?

Outline Summary

To download an MP3 version of the chapter summary for use with your iPod or portable media player, access the **Audio Chapter Summaries** on your CD.

Definitions

A. Nutrition—food, vitamins, and minerals that are ingested and assimilated into the body
B. Metabolism—process of using food molecules as energy sources and as building blocks for our own molecules
C. Catabolism—process that breaks food molecules down, releasing their stored energy; oxygen used in catabolism
D. Anabolism—process that builds food molecules into complex chemical compounds

Metabolic Functions of the Liver

A. Secretes bile to help mechanically digest lipids
B. Processes blood immediately after it leaves the gastrointestinal tract
   1. Helps maintain normal blood glucose concentration
   2. Site of protein, carbohydrate, and fat metabolism
   3. Removes toxins from the blood
   4. Synthesizes several kinds of protein compounds, such as albumins, fibrinogen, clotting factors, etc.
   5. Stores some vitamins

Nutrient Metabolism

A. Carbohydrate metabolism
   1. Carbohydrates are the preferred energy food of the body

2. Three series of chemical reactions that occur in a precise sequence make up the process of glucose metabolism
   a. Glycolysis—occurs in cytoplasm of the cell
      (1) Anaerobic process (uses no oxygen)
      (2) Changes glucose to pyruvic acid, which is then converted into acetyl CoA
      (3) Yields small amount of energy (transferred to ATP)
   b. Citric acid (Krebs) cycle—occurs in the mitochondria
      (1) Aerobic process (requires oxygen)
      (2) Changes acetyl CoA to carbon dioxide
      (3) Yields small amount of energy
      (4) Most energy leaving the citric acid cycle is in the form of high-energy electrons
   c. Electron transport system—occurs in the mitochondria
      (1) Transfers energy from high-energy electrons (from citric acid cycle) to ATP molecules
      (2) ATP serves as direct source of energy for cells (Figure 18-2)
3. Energy transferred to ATP differs from energy in food molecules
   a. Not stored; released almost instantly
   b. Can be used directly to do cellular work
4. Carbohydrates are primarily catabolized for energy (Figure 18-1), but small amounts are anabolized by glycogenesis (a series of chemical reactions that changes glucose to glycogen—occurs mainly in liver cells where glycogen is stored)

5. Blood glucose (imprecisely, blood sugar)—amount of glucose in blood
   a. Normally stays between about 80 and 110 mg per 100 ml of blood during fasting
   b. Insulin accelerates the movement of glucose out of the blood into cells, therefore decreases blood glucose and increases glucose catabolism
B. Fat metabolism
   1. Fats are primarily an energy food
   2. Converted to glucose by catabolism
   3. Excess fat is anabolized to form adipose tissue (Figure 18-3)
C. Protein metabolism
   1. Proteins are catabolized for energy only after carbohydrate and fat stores are depleted
   2. Gluconeogenesis breaks apart amino acids to convert them to glucose

Vitamins and Minerals

A. Vitamins—organic molecules that are needed in small amounts for normal metabolism (Table 18-2)
   1. Avitaminosis—deficiency of a vitamin
      a. Can lead to severe metabolic problems
      b. Avitaminosis C can lead to scurvy
   2. Hypervitaminosis—excess of a vitamin
      a. Can be just as serious as avitaminosis
      b. May be chronic or acute
B. Minerals—inorganic molecules found naturally in the earth
   1. Required by the body for normal function, including nerve conduction (Table 18-3)
   2. Can attach to enzymes to facilitate their work

Metabolic Rates

A. Basal metabolic rate (BMR)—rate of metabolism when a person is lying down but awake and not digesting food and when the environment is comfortably warm
B. Total metabolic rate (TMR)—the total amounts of energy, expressed in calories, used by the body per day (Figure 18-5)

Metabolic and Eating Disorders

A. Disruption or imbalance of normal metabolism can be caused by several different factors
   1. Inborn errors of metabolism—genetic conditions involving deficient or abnormal metabolic enzymes

2. Some metabolic disorders are complications of other conditions
   a. Hormonal imbalances
   b. Eating disorders
      (1) Anorexia nervosa—characterized by chronic refusal to eat
      (2) Bulimia—an alternating pattern of craving of food followed by a period of self-denial; in bulimarexia, the self-denial triggers self-induced vomiting
      (3) Obesity—abnormally high proportion of fat in the body; may be a symptom of an eating disorder
      (4) Protein-calorie malnutrition (PCM)—results from a deficiency of calories in general and proteins in particular (Figure 18-6)

Body Temperature

A. Hypothalamus—regulates the homeostasis of body temperature (thermoregulation) through a variety of processes
   1. Blood flow to the skin increases when body is overheated
   2. Heat is lost through the skin by radiation, conduction, convection, evaporation (Figure 18-7)
B. Abnormal body temperature can have serious physiological consequences
   1. Fever (febrile state)—unusually high body temperature associated with systemic inflammation response
   2. Malignant hyperthermia (MH)—inherited condition that causes increased body temperature (hyperthermia) and muscle rigidity when exposed to certain anesthetics
   3. Heat exhaustion—results from loss of fluid as the body tries to cool itself; may be accompanied by heat cramps
   4. Heatstroke (sunstroke)—overheating of body resulting from failure of thermoregulatory mechanisms in a warm environment
   5. Hypothermia—reduced body temperature resulting from failure of thermoregulatory mechanisms in a cold environment
   6. Frostbite—local tissue damage caused by extreme cold; may result in necrosis or gangrene

New Words

aerobic	electron transport system	**Diseases and Other Clinical Terms**	hypercholesterolemia
anabolism	free radical		hypervitaminosis
anaerobic	glycogenesis	anorexia nervosa	hypothermia
antioxidant	glycolysis	avitaminosis	malignant hyperthermia (MH)
basal metabolic rate (BMR)	kilocalorie (kcal; *also* Calorie)	bulimarexia	obesity
calorie		bulimia	protein-calorie malnutrition (PCM)
carbohydrate (glycogen) loading	nutrition	frostbite	scurvy
catabolism	thermoregulation	heat exhaustion	
citric acid (Krebs) cycle	total metabolic rate (TMR)	heatstroke	
	vitamin		

Review Questions

1. Define anabolism and catabolism.
2. Explain the function of the liver.
3. Briefly explain the process of glycolysis.
4. Briefly explain the citric acid cycle.
5. What is the function of the electron transport system?
6. Explain the ways in which energy stored in ATP is different from energy stored in food molecules.
7. List the hormones that tend to increase the amount of sugar in the blood.
8. When does fat catabolism usually occur?
9. When does protein catabolism usually occur?
10. Explain what is meant by a nonessential amino acid.
11. Name three water-soluble and three fat-soluble vitamins.
12. What is avitaminosis? Name a disorder caused by avitaminosis. What vitamin deficiency causes this disorder?
13. What are the signs and symptoms of vitamin A hypervitaminosis?
14. Name three minerals needed by the body.
15. What is the function of vitamins and minerals in the body?
16. Differentiate between basal and total metabolic rate.
17. Distinguish between marasmus and kwashiorkor.
18. Name and explain three ways heat can be lost through the skin.
19. What is the cause of malignant hyperthermia?
20. Distinguish between heat exhaustion and heatstroke in terms of a person's body temperature.

Critical Thinking

21. Differentiate between absorption and assimilation.
22. Explain the advantage the body gains by having the blood go through the hepatic portal system.
23. Diagram the ATP-ADP cycle. Include where the energy is added and where the energy is released.
24. A man went on a 10-day vacation. His total metabolic rate was 2600 calories a day. His total calorie intake was 3300 calories a day. He began the trip weighing 178 pounds. What did he weigh when he got back from vacation? (3500 excess calories = 1 pound)
25. Why is trying to lower a moderate fever counterproductive to the body's attempt to fight off an infection?

Chapter Test

1. The process of _____ occurs when food molecules enter the cell and undergo chemical change.

2. _____ is the term used to describe all the chemical processes that release energy from food.

3. _____ is the term used to describe all the chemical processes that build food molecules into larger compounds.

4. The plasma proteins _____ and _____ are made in the liver and are important in blood clot formation.

5. The vitamins _____ and _____ can be stored in the liver.

6. The B vitamins are _____ soluble, whereas vitamins K and E are _____ soluble.

7. _____ is the total amount of energy used by the body per day.

8. _____ is the number of calories that must be used just to keep the body alive, awake, and comfortably warm.

9. In order to lose weight, your total caloric intake must be less than your _____ .

10. One way heat can be lost by the skin is _____ , which is the transfer of heat to the air that is continually flowing away from the skin.

11. One way heat can be lost by the skin is _____ , which is the absorption of heat by water (sweat) vaporization.

12. _____ is the process used by the body as the second choice of energy metabolism.

13. In the healthy body, _____ is used almost exclusively for anabolism rather than catabolism.

14. _____t are amino acids needed by the body, but they can be made from other amino acids if they are not supplied directly by the diet.

Match each term in Column A with its corresponding description in Column B.

Column A
15. _____ glycolysis
16. _____ citric acid cycle
17. _____ electron transport system
18. _____ mitochondria
19. _____ cytoplasm
20. _____ ATP
21. _____ glycogenesis
22. _____ ADP

Column B
a. part of the cell in which glycolysis occurs
b. the part of carbohydrate metabolism that does not require oxygen
c. process that converts high-energy molecules from the citric acid cycle into ATP
d. the part of carbohydrate metabolism that requires oxygen
e. the body's direct source of energy
f. molecule that results when adenine triphosphate loses a phosphate group
g. the part of the cell in which the citric acid cycle takes place
h. glucose anabolism

Match each disorder in Column A with its corresponding description or cause in Column B.

Column A
23. _____ avitaminosis
24. _____ hypervitaminosis
25. _____ anorexia nervosa
26. _____ bulimia
27. _____ marasmus
28. _____ kwashiorkor
29. _____ malignant hyperthermia
30. _____ heat exhaustion
31. _____ heatstroke
32. _____ hypothermia
33. _____ frostbite

Column B
a. behavioral disorder characterized by a chronic refusal to eat
b. increased body temperature caused by exposure to anesthetics
c. type of malnutrition that results from an overall lack of calories
d. an overheating problem in which the body is dehydrated but the body temperature is normal
e. local tissue damage caused by ice crystals forming in the cells
f. condition that results in the development of scurvy
g. behavioral disorder characterized by insatiable craving for food alternating with self-deprivation; may include food binges
h. a body temperature lower than 95° F
i. overheating problem in which the body temperature can be as high as 105° F; potentially life-threatening
j. type of malnutrition that results from a lack of protein with sufficient total calories
k. a vitamin excess, usually involving fat-soluble vitamins

Study Tips

continued from page 525

4. Vitamins and minerals assist in enzyme function. You can learn the names and functions of the vitamins and minerals from the tables in the text or by making flash cards.
5. Metabolic rates describe how quickly your body is using food. The basal metabolic rate is the amount of food you burn just to stay alive and awake. Your total metabolic rate depends on how active you are.
6. Make a chart to help you learn the metabolic disorders. Organize the chart based on the mecha-nism or cause of each disorder: deficiency or excess of vitamins, nutrition disorders, and disorders of temperature regulation.
7. In your study group, review the flash cards for the vitamins and minerals or Tables 18-2 and 18-3. Discuss the processes of carbohydrate, protein, and fat metabolism. Discuss what constitutes basal and total metabolic rates and the ways heat can be lost from the body. Review the metabolic disorders chart and the questions at the end of the chapter, and discuss possible test questions.

Case Studies

1. A friend of yours is helping you chop firewood on a hot day. She complains of muscle cramps and nausea but has a normal body temperature. What has happened to her? How would you help your friend?
2. While looking through an old family album, you can't help but notice that your great-great-great-grandfather's smile reveals that he has no teeth. When asked why this ancestor lost his teeth at an early age, your grandmother replies that he suffered from scurvy as a merchant marine and lost all his teeth as a result. Is this possible? Can you explain how scurvy can cause the loss of teeth?
3. Andrea is planning to adopt a totally vegetarian diet—a diet that includes no meats or animal products. Her friends have voiced some concern that her new diet may not contain certain essential amino acids. What is an essential amino acid? Why must her diet contain these nutrients?

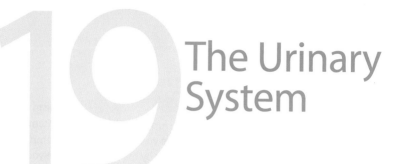

19 The Urinary System

Outline

Objectives

After you have completed this chapter, you should be able to:

1. Identify the major organs of the urinary system and give the generalized function of each.

2. Name the parts of a nephron and describe the role each component plays in the formation of urine.

3. Explain the importance of filtration, tubular reabsorption, and tubular secretion in urine formation.

4. Discuss the mechanisms that control urine volume.

5. Explain how the kidneys act as vital organs in maintaining homeostasis.

6. List the major renal and urinary disorders and explain the mechanism of each.

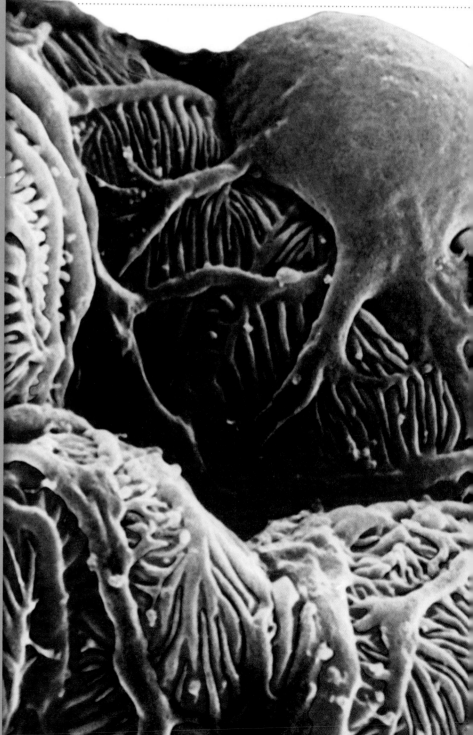

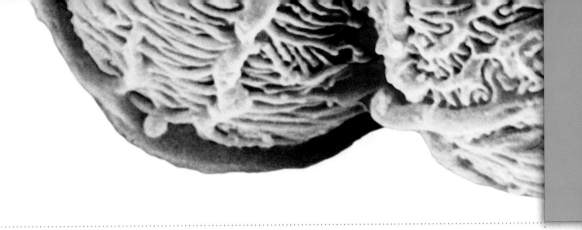

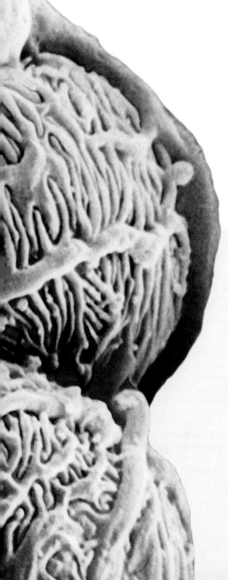

As you might guess from its name, the urinary system performs the functions of producing and excreting urine from the body. What you might not guess so easily is how essential these functions are for the maintenance of homeostasis and healthy survival. The constancy of body fluid volumes and the levels of many important chemicals depend on normal urinary system function. Unless the urinary system operates normally, the normal composition of blood cannot be maintained for long, and serious consequences soon follow.

The urinary system is composed of two kidneys, two ureters, one bladder, and one urethra (Figure 19-1). We begin our discussion with the kidneys. The kidneys "clear" or clean the blood of the many waste products continually produced as a result of metabolism of nutrients in the body cells. As nutrients are burned for energy, the waste products produced must be removed from the blood, or they quickly accumulate to toxic levels—a condition called **uremia** (yoo-REE-mee-ah) or **uremic poisoning.**

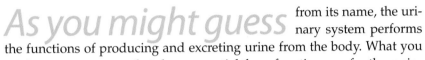

STUDY TIPS   Before studying Chapter 19, review the synopsis of the urinary system in Chapter 3. The function of the urinary system is to maintain the homeostasis of the blood plasma.

1. The names, locations, and functions of the organs of the urinary system, the internal structure of the kidney, and the microscopic structures of the nephron all can be learned using flash cards.
2. The formation of urine involves three processes: filtration, resorption, and secretion. Filtration was discussed in Chapter 2. Resorption is the process of taking material out of the urine and returning it to the blood. Secretion is the process of taking material out of the blood and putting it into the urine.
3. Urine volume is controlled by three hormones, each produced by a different organ. Remember that the body cannot directly move water; it must first move solute and then pull the water after it by way of diffusion. Make flash cards for each of the three hormones; include the name of the hormone, where it is made, its mechanism of action, and its effect on urine volume.

continued on page 567

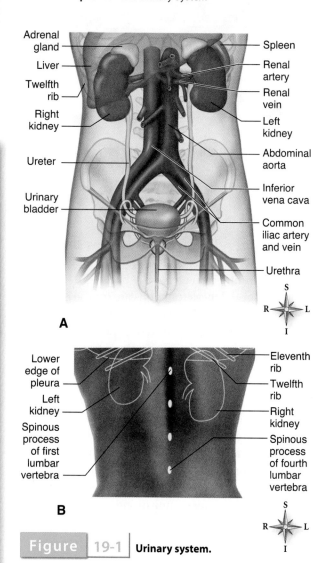

A, Anterior view of urinary organs. **B,** Surface markings of the kidneys, eleventh and twelfth ribs, spinous processes of L1 to L4, and lower edge of pleura viewed from behind.

The kidneys also play a vital role in maintaining electrolyte, water, and acid-base balances in the body. In this chapter, we discuss the structure and function of each organ of the urinary system. We also discuss disease conditions produced by abnormal functioning of the urinary system.

 To learn more about the urinary system, go to **AnimationDirect** on your CD.

KIDNEYS

Location

To locate the kidneys in your own body, stand erect and put your hands on your hips with your thumbs meeting over your backbone. When you are in this position, your kidneys lie above your thumbs on either side of your spinal column, but their placement is higher than you might think. Note in Figure 19-1 that the right kidney, which touches the liver, is slightly lower than the left.

Both kidneys are protected a bit by the lower rib cage and are located under the muscles of the back and behind the parietal peritoneum (the membrane that lines the abdominal cavity). Because of this **retroperitoneal** (RET-roh-pair-i-toh-NEE-all) location, a surgeon can operate on a kidney without cutting through the peritoneum. Once the peritoneum has been cut or opened, the potential for spread of infection throughout the entire abdominal cavity increases. The prefix "retro" (from the Latin meaning "back of") appropriately describes the placement of both kidneys behind this important membrane. The anatomical relationship of the upper portions of both kidneys to the lower edge of the thoracic parietal pleura (the membrane that lines the thoracic cavity) is shown in Figure 19-1, *B*. The close relationship between these structures also has important clinical implications (see Box on Kidney Biopsy). A heavy cushion of fat normally encases each kidney and helps hold it in place.

Note the relatively large diameter of the renal arteries in Figure 19-1. Normally, a little more than 20% of the total blood pumped by the heart each minute enters the kidneys. The rate of blood flow through this organ is among the highest in the body. This is understandable because one of the main functions of the kidney is to remove waste products from the blood. Maintenance of a high rate of blood flow and normal blood pressure in the kidneys is essential for the formation of urine.

Internal Structure

If you were to slice through a kidney from side to side and open it like the pages of a book (called a coronal section), you would see the structures shown in Figure 19-2. Identify each of the following parts:

1. **Renal cortex** (KOR-teks)—the outer part of the kidney (the word *cortex* comes from the Latin

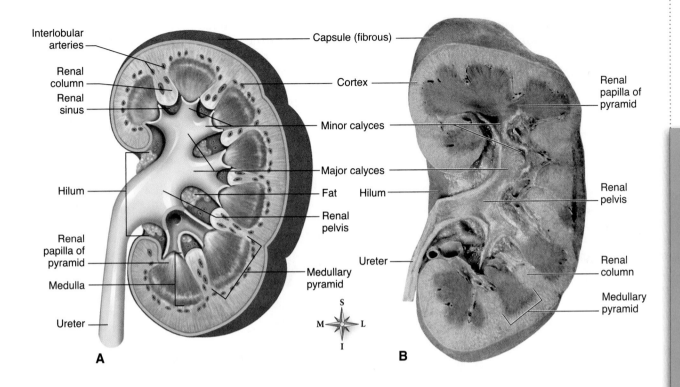

Figure 19-2 | **Internal structure of the kidney.**

A, Coronal section of the kidney in an artist's rendering. **B,** Photo of coronal section of a preserved human kidney.

word for "bark" or "rind," so the cortex of an organ is its outer layer; each kidney and adrenal gland, as well as the brain, has a cortex)

2. **Renal medulla** (meh-DUL-ah)—the inner portion of the kidney

3. **Renal pyramids** (PIR-ah-mids)—the triangular divisions of the medulla of the kidney. Extensions of cortical tissue that dip down into the medulla between the renal pyramids are called **renal columns**

4. **Renal papilla** (pah-PIL-ah) (*pl.,* papillae)—narrow, innermost end of a pyramid

5. **Renal pelvis**—(the kidney or renal pelvis) an expansion of the upper end of a ureter (the tube that drains urine into the bladder)

6. **Calyx** (KAY-liks) (*pl.,* calyces)—a division of the renal pelvis (the papilla of a pyramid opens into each calyx)

Microscopic Structure

More than a million microscopic units called **nephrons** (NEF-rons) make up each kidney's interior. The shape of a nephron is unique, unmis-

CLINICAL APPLICATION

KIDNEY BIOPSY

Suspected disease of the kidney, such as renal cancer, often requires a needle **biopsy** to confirm the diagnosis. In this procedure, a hollow (biopsy) needle is inserted through the skin surface and then guided into the diseased organ to withdraw a tissue sample for analysis. In a renal biopsy, tissue is removed from the lower rather than the upper or superior pole of the diseased kidney. This avoids the possibility of damage to the pleura that could be caused by the biopsy needle and a resulting pneumothorax.

takable, and admirably suited to its function of producing urine. It looks a little like a tiny funnel with a very long stem, but it is an unusual stem in that it is highly convoluted (that is, it has many bends in it). The nephron is composed of two principal components: the **renal corpuscle** and the **renal tubule.** The renal corpuscle can be subdivided still further into two parts and the renal tubule into four regions or segments. Identify each part of the renal corpuscle and renal tubule described below and on pp. 547 and 548 in Figures 19-3 and 19-4.

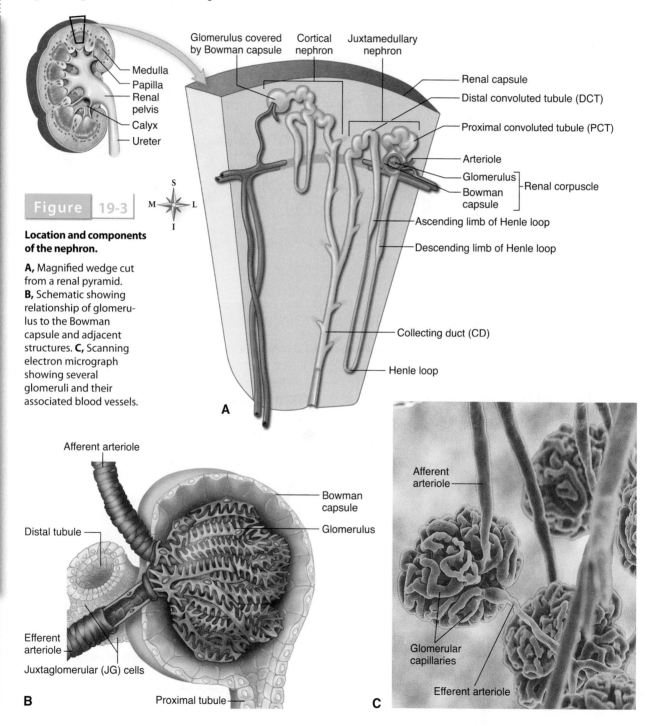

Figure 19-3

Location and components of the nephron.

A, Magnified wedge cut from a renal pyramid. **B,** Schematic showing relationship of glomerulus to the Bowman capsule and adjacent structures. **C,** Scanning electron micrograph showing several glomeruli and their associated blood vessels.

1. **Renal corpuscle**
   a. **Bowman capsule**—the cup-shaped top of a nephron. The hollow, saclike Bowman capsule surrounds the glomerulus.
   b. **Glomerulus** (glo-MAIR-yoo-lus) (*pl.*, glomeruli)—a network of blood capillaries tucked into the Bowman capsule. Note in Figure 19-3 that the small artery (afferent arteriole) that delivers blood to the glomerulus is larger in diameter than the blood vessel (efferent arteriole) that drains blood from it and that it is relatively short. This explains the high blood pressure that exists in the glomerular capillaries. This high pressure is required to filter wastes from the blood.

2. **Renal tubule**
   a. **Proximal convoluted tubule** (PCT)—the first segment of a renal tubule. The PCT is called *proximal* because it lies nearest the tubule's origin from the Bowman capsule, and it is called *convoluted* because it has several bends.
   b. **Henle loop** (HEN-lee)—the extension of the proximal tubule. Observe that the

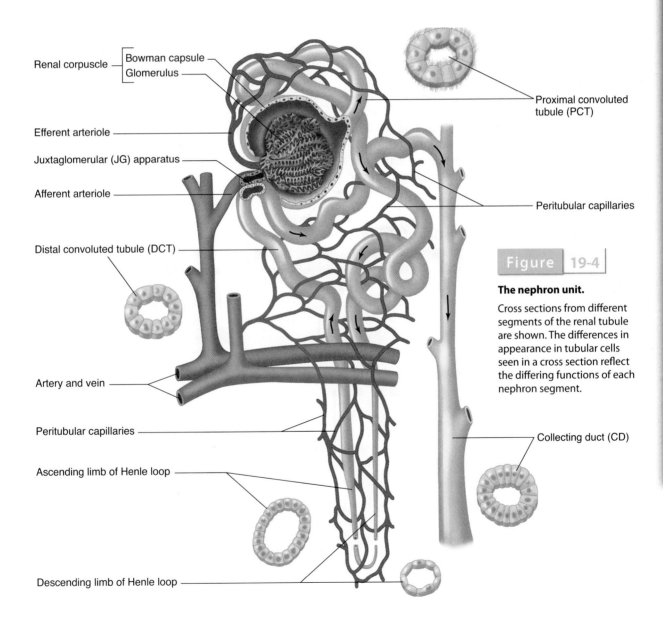

Renal corpuscle — Bowman capsule
Glomerulus

Efferent arteriole

Juxtaglomerular (JG) apparatus

Afferent arteriole

Distal convoluted tubule (DCT)

Artery and vein

Peritubular capillaries

Ascending limb of Henle loop

Descending limb of Henle loop

Proximal convoluted tubule (PCT)

Peritubular capillaries

Collecting duct (CD)

Figure 19-4

The nephron unit.

Cross sections from different segments of the renal tubule are shown. The differences in appearance in tubular cells seen in a cross section reflect the differing functions of each nephron segment.

Henle loop consists of a straight descending limb, a hairpin loop, and a straight ascending limb. It is also called *loop of Henle* or *nephron loop.*

    c. **Distal convoluted tubule** (DCT)—the part of the tubule distal to the ascending limb of the Henle loop. The DCT is the extension of the ascending limb.

    d. **Collecting duct** (CD)—a straight (that is, not convoluted) part of a renal tubule. Distal tubules of several nephrons join to form a single collecting duct or tubule.

Look again at Figure 19-3. Notice the differing locations of the two nephrons in the illustration. One is located high in the cortex and is typical of about 85% of all nephrons. Nephrons in this group are located almost entirely in the renal cortex and are called **cortical nephrons.** The remainder, called **juxtamedullary nephrons,** have their renal corpuscles near the junction (juxta) between cortex and medullary layers. These nephrons have Henle loops that dip far into the medulla. Juxtamedullary nephrons have an important role in concentrating urine. Urine from the collecting ducts

exits from the pyramid through the papilla and enters the calyx and renal pelvis before flowing into the ureter.

 To learn more about the nephron, go to **AnimationDirect** on your CD.

Function

The kidneys are vital organs. The function they perform, that of forming urine, is essential for homeostasis and maintenance of life. Early in the process of urine formation, fluid, electrolytes, and wastes from metabolism are filtered from the blood and enter the nephron. Additional wastes may be secreted into the tubules of the nephron as substances useful to the body are reabsorbed into the blood. Table 19-1 lists the components of normal versus abnormal urine.

Normally the kidneys balance the amount of many substances entering and leaving the blood over time so that normal concentrations can be maintained. In short, the kidneys adjust their output to equal the intake of the body. By eliminat-

Table 19-1 | Characteristics of Urine

NORMAL CHARACTERISTICS	ABNORMAL CHARACTERISTICS
COLOR	
Transparent yellow, amber, or straw colored	Abnormal colors or cloudiness, which may indicate presence of blood, bile, bacteria, drugs, food pigments, or high-solute concentration
COMPOUNDS	
Mineral ions (e.g., Na$^+$, Cl$^-$, K$^+$)	Acetone
Nitrogenous wastes: ammonia, creatinine, urea, uric acid	Albumin
Suspended solids, (sediment)*: bacteria, blood cells, casts	Bile (solid matter)
Urine pigments	Glucose
ODOR	
Slight odor	Acetone odor, which is common in diabetes mellitus
pH	
4.6-8.0	High in alkalosis; low in acidosis
SPECIFIC GRAVITY	
1.001-1.035	High specific gravity can cause precipitation of solutes and formation of kidney stones

*Occasional trace amounts.

ing wastes and adjusting fluid balance, the kidneys play an essential part in maintaining homeostasis. Homeostasis cannot be maintained—nor can life itself—if the kidneys fail and the condition is not soon corrected. Nitrogenous waste products accumulate as a result of protein breakdown and quickly reach toxic levels if not excreted. If kidney function ceases because of injury or disease, life can be maintained by using an artificial kidney to cleanse the blood of wastes (see box below).

Excretion of toxins and of waste products containing nitrogen such as urea and ammonia represents only one of the important responsibilities of the kidney. The kidney also plays a key role in regulating the levels of many chemical substances in the blood such as chloride, sodium, potassium, and bicarbonate. The kidneys also regulate the proper balance between body water content and salt by selectively retaining or excreting both substances as requirements demand.

In addition, the cells of the **juxtaglomerular** (jucks-tah-gloh-MER-u-lar) **(JG) apparatus** (see Figures 19-3, *B*, and 19-4) also function in blood volume and blood pressure regulation. When blood pressure is low, which often occurs when blood plasma volume is low, these JG cells secrete an enzyme that triggers a system (discussed later in this chapter) to restore normal blood volume and pressure.

Yet another important function of the kidney is the secretion of the hormone **erythropoietin** (eh-RITH-roh-POY-eh-tin) **(EPO)**. During *hypoxia*, a deficiency of oxygen in the body, the erythropoietin is released into the bloodstream and travels to the red bone marrow and stimulates the production of additional erythrocytes (red blood cells). The additional erythrocytes increase the ability of the blood to absorb and transport oxygen to oxygen-starved tissues. EPO is sometimes used as a drug (one brand is Procrit) to treat anemia caused by critical illness such as cancer. As you probably guessed, kidney disease can cause anemia by reducing the body's ability to produce EPO when needed.

With all these vital functions, it is easy to understand why the kidneys are often considered to be the most important homeostatic organs in the body.

To learn more about the kidney, go to **AnimationDirect** on your CD.

QUICK CHECK
1. What are the two main regions of the kidney?
2. Describe the structure of a nephron.
3. What is the role of filtration in the kidney?

HEALTH & WELL-BEING

THE AGING KIDNEY

As with other body organs, the kidneys undergo both age-related structural changes and decreasing functional capacity. Adults over 35 years of age gradually lose functional nephron units, and kidney weight actually decreases. By approximately 80 to 85 years of age, most individuals will have experienced a 30% reduction in total kidney mass.

In spite of a numerical reduction in actual kidney nephron units and a decrease in the metabolic activity of remaining tubular cells, most individuals continue to exhibit normal kidney function as they age. This is pos-

sible because older persons generally have a lower overall lean body mass and therefore a reduced production of waste products that must be excreted from the body. However, the "margin of safety" is reduced and any stress on the remaining functional nephrons, such as a systemic infection or a reduction in kidney blood flow, can produce almost immediate symptoms of kidney failure.

Marginal kidney function in old age may make it difficult to excrete drugs that are easily cleared from the blood of younger persons, and dosages of many medications have to be adjusted accordingly for older patients.

Formation of Urine

The kidney's 2 million or more nephrons form urine by way of a series of three processes: (1) filtration, (2) reabsorption, and (3) secretion (Figure 19-5).

Filtration

Urine formation begins with the process of **filtration,** which goes on continually in the renal corpuscles (Bowman capsules plus their encased glomeruli). Blood flowing through the glomeruli exerts pressure, and this glomerular blood pressure is high enough to push water and dissolved substances out of the glomeruli into the Bowman capsule. Briefly, glomerular blood pressure causes filtration through the glomerular-capsular membrane. If the glomerular blood pressure drops below a certain level, filtration and urine formation cease. Hemorrhage, for example, may cause a precipitous drop in blood pressure followed by kidney failure.

Glomerular filtration normally occurs at the rate of 125 ml per minute. As a result, about 180 liters (al-most 190 quarts) of **glomerular filtrate** is produced by the kidneys every day.

Obviously no one ever excretes anywhere near 180 liters of urine per day. Why? Because most of the fluid that leaves the blood by glomerular filtration, the first process in urine formation, returns to the blood by the second process—reabsorption.

Reabsorption

Reabsorption is the movement of substances out of the renal tubules into the blood capillaries located around the tubules (peritubular capillaries). Water, glucose and other nutrients, and sodium and other ions are substances that are reabsorbed. Reabsorption begins in the proximal convoluted tubules and continues in the Henle loop, distal convoluted tubules, and collecting ducts.

Large amounts of water—approximately 178 L per day—are reabsorbed by osmosis from the proximal tubules. In other words, nearly 99% of the 180 L of water that leaves the blood each day by glomerular filtration returns to the blood by proximal tubule reabsorption. Smaller amounts of water are also reabsorbed in the Henle loops, distal tubules, and collecting ducts.

The nutrient glucose is reabsorbed from the proximal tubules into peritubular capillary blood. None of this valuable nutrient is wasted by being lost in the urine. However, exceptions to this do occur. For example, in *diabetes mellitus,* if blood glucose concentration increases above a certain level, called the **renal threshold,** the tubular filtrate then contains more glucose than kidney tubule cells can reabsorb. Some of the glucose therefore remains behind in the urine. Glucose in the urine—**glycosuria** (glye-koh-SOO-ree-ah)—is a well-known sign of diabetes mellitus.

Common table salt (NaCl) consumed in the diet or introduced by intravenous (IV) infusion of normal saline (0.9% NaCl) or other NaCl-containing fluids, provides the body with sodium ions (Na$^+$) and chloride ions (Cl$^-$). For the most part, sodium ions are actively transported back into blood from the tubular urine, the amount reabsorbed depending largely on intake. In general the greater the amount of sodium intake, the less the amount reabsorbed and the greater the amount excreted in the urine. Also, the less sodium intake, the greater the reabsorption from kidney tubules and the less excreted in the urine.

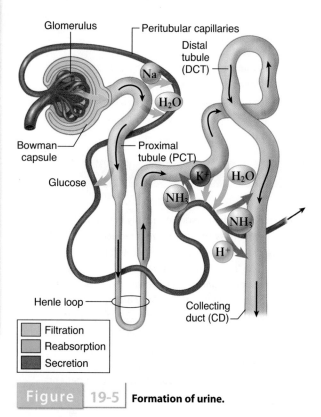

Glomerulus
Peritubular capillaries
Distal tubule (DCT)
Na$^+$
H$_2$O
Bowman capsule
Proximal tubule (PCT)
Glucose
K$^+$
H$_2$O
NH$_3$
NH$_3$
H$^+$
Henle loop
Collecting duct (CD)

☐ Filtration
☐ Reabsorption
☐ Secretion

Figure 19-5 | Formation of urine.

Diagram shows the steps in urine formation in successive parts of a nephron: filtration, reabsorption, and secretion.

Rather than being actively reabsorbed from renal tubules as are sodium ions (Na^+), chloride ions (Cl^-) passively move into blood because they carry a negative electrical charge. The positively charged sodium ions that have been reabsorbed and moved into the blood "attract" the negatively charged chloride ions from the tubule fluid into the peritubular capillaries.

The kidneys cannot *reabsorb* potassium ions (K^+) from the renal tubules. Therefore, urine values of this important mineral ion will vary greatly with diet. Some *diuretic* (dye-yoo-RET-ik) *drugs,* which stimulate the production of urine (see the box on p. 578), are said to be "potassium wasting" because they increase *secretion* of potassium into tubular fluid and, ultimately, its excretion in the urine.

Secretion

Secretion is the process by which substances move into urine in the distal and collecting ducts from blood in the capillaries around these tubules. In this respect, secretion is reabsorption in reverse. Whereas reabsorption moves substances out of the urine into the blood, secretion moves substances out of the blood into the urine. Substances secreted are hydrogen ions, potassium ions, ammonia, and certain drugs. Hydrogen ions, potassium ions, and some drugs are secreted by being actively transported out of the blood into tubular urine. Ammonia is secreted by diffusion. Kidney tubule secretion plays a crucial role in maintaining the body's acid-base balance (see Chapter 21).

In summary, the following processes occurring in successive portions of the nephron accomplish the function of urine formation (Table 19-2):

1. **Filtration**—of water and dissolved substances out of the blood in the glomeruli into the Bowman capsule

2. **Reabsorption**—of water and dissolved substances out of kidney tubules back into blood (This prevents substances needed by the body from being lost in urine. Usually, 97% to 99% of water filtered out of glomerular blood is retrieved from tubules.)

3. **Secretion**—of hydrogen ions, potassium ions, and certain drugs

Control of Urine Volume

The body has ways to control the amount and composition of the urine that it excretes. It does this mainly by controlling the amount of water and dissolved substances that are reabsorbed by the convoluted tubules.

An example of regulating water reabsorption in kidney tubules involves a hormone called *antidiuretic hormone (ADH)* secreted from the posterior pituitary gland. ADH decreases the amount of urine by making collecting ducts permeable to water. If no ADH is present, the tubules are practically impermeable to water, so little or no water is reabsorbed from them. When ADH is present in the blood, collecting ducts are permeable to water and water is reabsorbed from them. As a result, less water is lost from the body as urine, or more water is retained from the tubules—whichever way you wish to say it. At any rate, for this reason ADH is accurately described as the "water-retaining hormone." You might also think of it as the "urine-decreasing hormone."

The hormone aldosterone, secreted by the adrenal cortex, plays an important part in controlling the kidney tubules' reabsorption of salt. Primarily it stimulates the tubules to reabsorb sodium salts at a faster rate. Secondarily, aldosterone also increases tubular water reabsorption. The term *salt- and wa-*

Table 19-2	Functions of the Parts of the Nephron in Urine Formation	
PARTS OF NEPHRON	**PROCESS IN URINE FORMATION**	**SUBSTANCES MOVED**
Glomerulus	Filtration	Water and solutes (e.g., sodium and other ions, glucose and other nutrients filtering out of glomeruli into the Bowman capsules)
Proximal tubule	Reabsorption	Water and solutes
Henle loop	Reabsorption	Sodium and chloride ions
Distal and collecting ducts	Reabsorption	Water, sodium, and chloride ions
	Secretion	Ammonia, potassium ions, hydrogen ions, and some drugs

ter-retaining hormone therefore is a descriptive nickname for aldosterone. Like ADH, aldosterone reduces urine volume.

The kidney itself is responsible for triggering aldosterone secretion, a fact that illustrates the importance of the kidney in regulating overall fluid volume and blood pressure in the body. When blood volume and pressure drop below normal, this is sensed by cells in the juxtaglomerular (JG) apparatus. JG cells then release an enzyme called **renin** (REE-nin) that initiates the **renin-angiotensin-aldosterone** (REE-nin-an-jee-oh-TEN-sin-al-DAH-stair-ohn) **system (RAAS).** The RAAS eventually produces constriction of blood vessels and thus raises blood pressure. The RAAS also triggers adrenal gland secretion of aldosterone, which promotes water retention and thus increases total blood volume—also contributing to a rise in blood pressure. Figure 19-6 illustrates the main events of the RAAS and how it acts to restore normal plasma volume and blood pressure. Aldosterone mechanisms are also discussed in the next chapter.

Another hormone, **atrial natriuretic hormone (ANH)** secreted from the heart's atrial wall, has the opposite effect of aldosterone. ANH is the primary *atrial natriuretic peptide (ANP)* hormone in humans. ANH stimulates kidney tubules to secrete more sodium and thus lose more water. ANH is a *salt- and water-losing hormone.* Thus ANH increases urine volume.

The body secretes ADH, aldosterone, and ANH in different amounts, depending on the homeostatic balance of body fluids at any particular moment.

Sometimes the kidneys do not excrete normal amounts of urine as a result of kidney disease, endocrine imbalances, cardiovascular disease, stress, or a variety of other conditions. Here are some terms associated with abnormal amounts of urine:

1. **Anuria** (ah-NOO-ree-ah)—absence of urine
2. **Oliguria** (ol-i-GOO-ree-ah)—scanty amounts of urine
3. **Polyuria** (pol-ee-YOO-ree-ah)—an unusually large amount of urine

QUICK CHECK

1. What are the three basic processes that occur in the nephron?
2. How do ADH and aldosterone affect urine output?
3. What is anuria? polyuria?

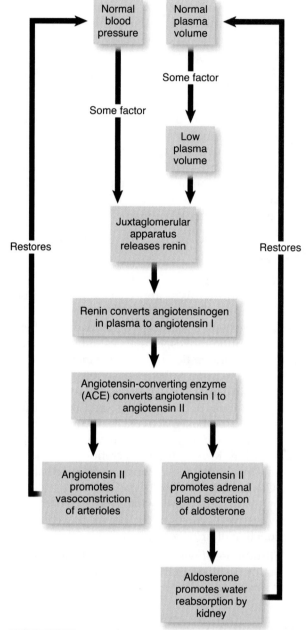

Figure 19-6 Renin-angiotensin-aldosterone system (RAAS).

Low plasma volume reduces blood pressure below normal, which is detected by juxtaglomerular (JG) cells in the juxtaglomerular apparatus of the kidney. This triggers the release of renin, which converts angiotensinogen into angiotensin I. The enzyme ACE then converts angiotensin I to angiotension II. Angiotensin II stimulates constriction of arteriolar smooth muscles and thus increases blood pressure back toward normal. Angiotensin II also triggers adrenal gland secretion of aldosterone, which promotes water retention by the kidney and thus restoration of normal blood volume and pressure.

Ureters

Urine drains out of the collecting ducts of each kidney into the renal pelvis and down the ureter into the urinary bladder (see Figure 19-1). The **renal pelvis** is the basin-like upper end of the ureter located inside the kidney. Ureters are narrow tubes less than 6 mm (¼ inch) wide and 25 to 30 cm (10 to 12 inches) long. Mucous membranes line both ureters and each renal pelvis. Note in Figure 19-7 that the ureter has a thick, muscular wall. Contraction of the muscular coat produces peristaltic-type movements that assist in moving urine down the ureters into the bladder. The lining membrane of the ureters is richly supplied with sensory nerve endings.

Attacks of **renal colic**—pain caused by the passage of a kidney stone—have been described in medical writings since antiquity. Kidney stones cause intense pain if they have sharp edges or are large enough to distend the walls or cut the lining of the renal pelvis, ureters, bladder, or urethra as they pass from the kidneys to the exterior of the body.

Urinalysis

The physical, chemical, and microscopic examination of urine is termed *urinalysis.* Like blood, urine is a fluid that reveals much about the function of the body. Changes in the normal characteristics of urine or the appearance of abnormal urine characteristics may be a sign of disease. Table 19-1 lists the characteristics of urine.

Physical characteristics of urine such as color, turbidity (cloudiness), odor, and specific gravity (density) are general indicators of the composition of urine and may serve as unique and useful "diagnostic clues" in clinical medicine. For example, an abnormally dark or amber color may indicate the presence of excess bile pigments or the presence of hemoglobin—possible signs of liver disease or bleeding somewhere in the urinary system. A turbid, milky appearing urine suggests the abnormal presence of fatty components and a mousy, musty smelling urine in infants is suggestive of an "inborn error of metabolism" called **phenylketonuria** (feen-il-kee-toh-NOO-ree-ah), or **PKU** (see Chapter 24). Changes in specific gravity of urine may indicate disease or simply result from insufficient fluid intake.

Although a change in any particular physical characteristic of urine may be a useful diagnostic tool, such changes do not provide the detailed information that a chemical analysis provides.

Chemical analysis of urine usually provides information about pH, urea concentration, or the presence of abnormal chemicals such as glucose, acetone, albumin (protein), or bile. As mentioned previously, the presence of a significant amount of glucose in the urine (glycosuria) is a well-known sign of diabetes mellitus.

Urine specimens are often spun in a *centrifuge* to force suspended particles to the bottom of a test tube. The sediment that forms is then examined with a microscope to detect the presence of abnormal cells or other particles. Blood cells may indicate bleeding or infection somewhere along the urinary tract. An abnormal urine sample may contain numerous *casts,* small particles formed by deposits of minerals or cells on the walls of renal tubules that break off into the urine. A large number of casts may indicate any of several kidney disorders, depending on the composition of the casts.

In clinical and laboratory situations, a standard urinalysis is often referred to as a "routine and microscopic" urinalysis, or simply an "R and M." The "routine" portion is a series of physical and chemical tests, whereas the "microscopic" part refers to the study of urine sediment with a microscope. This series of laboratory tests provides the variety of information often necessary for a physician to make a diagnosis. Tests included in typical routine and microscopic urinalysis studies are listed in Appendix C on the CD that accompanies your book.

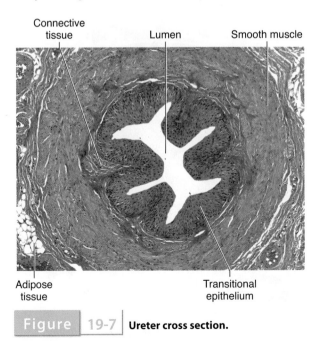

Connective tissue   Lumen   Smooth muscle

Adipose tissue   Transitional epithelium

Figure 19-7 | **Ureter cross section.**

Note the thick layer of muscle around the tube.

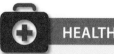

PROTEINURIA AFTER EXERCISE

Proteinuria is the presence of abnormally large amounts of plasma proteins in the urine. Proteinuria usually indicates kidney disease (**nephropathy**) because only damaged nephrons consistently allow many plasma protein molecules to leave the blood. However, intense exercise causes temporary proteinuria in many individuals. Some exercise physiologists believed that intense athletic activities cause kidney damage, but subsequent research has ruled out that explanation. One current hypothesis is that hormonal changes during strenuous exercise increase the permeability of the nephron's filtration membrane, allowing more plasma proteins to enter the filtrate. Some post-exercise proteinuria is usually considered normal.

Urinary Bladder

The empty urinary bladder lies in the pelvis just behind the pubic symphysis. When full of urine, it projects upward into the lower portion of the abdominal cavity.

Elastic fibers and involuntary muscle fibers in the wall of the urinary bladder make it well suited for expanding to hold variable amounts of urine and then contracting to empty itself. Mucous membrane containing transitional epithelium lines the urinary bladder (see Chapter 3). The lining is loosely attached to the deeper muscular layer so that the bladder is very wrinkled and lies in folds called *rugae* when it is empty. When the bladder is filled, its inner surface is smooth. Note in Figure 19-8 that one triangular area on the back or posterior surface of the bladder is free of rugae. This area, called the **trigone,** is always smooth. There, the lining membrane is tightly fixed to the deeper muscle coat. The trigone extends between the openings of the two ureters above and the point of exit of the urethra below.

Urethra

To leave the body, urine passes from the bladder, down the urethra, and out of its external opening, the **urinary meatus.** In other words, the urethra is the lowest part of the urinary tract. The same sheet of mucous membrane that lines each renal pelvis, the ureters, and the bladder extends down into the urethra, too. It is worth noting the continuity of the urinary mucous lining because it accounts for the fact that an infection of the urethra may spread upward through the urinary tract.

The urethra is a narrow tube of varying length. It is only about 4 cm (1½ inches) long in a woman, but it is about 20 cm (8 inches) long in a man. In a man, the urethra has two functions: (1) it is the terminal portion of the urinary tract, and (2) it is the passageway for transport of the reproductive fluid (semen) from the body. In a woman, the urethra is a part of the urinary tract only.

Micturition

The terms **micturition** (mik-too-RISH-un), **urination** (yoor-i-NAY-shun), and **voiding** all refer to the passage of urine from the body or the emptying of the bladder.

Micturition is an involuntary reflex action in infants or very young children. Although there is considerable variation among individuals, most children between 2 and 3 years of age learn to urinate voluntarily and also to inhibit voiding if the urge comes at an inconvenient time. **Enuresis** (EN-yoo-REE-sis) refers to involuntary urination, generally bed wetting at night (*nocturnal en-*

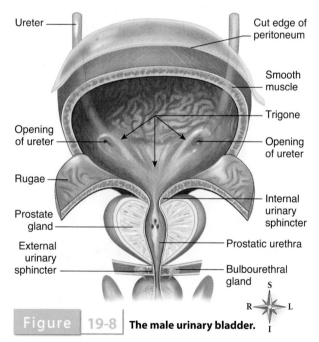

Figure 19-8 | **The male urinary bladder.**

This view (with bladder cut to show the interior) shows how the prostate gland surrounds the urethra as it exits from the bladder. The glands associated with the male reproductive system are further discussed in Chapter 22.

uresis), in a child who is beyond the age when voluntary bladder control is expected. Incidence is higher in boys than in girls and is often due to maturational delay.

Two **sphincters** (SFINGK-ters), or rings of muscle tissue, guard the pathway leading from the bladder. The *internal urethral sphincter* is located at the bladder exit, and the *external urethral sphincter* circles the urethra just below the neck of the bladder (see Figure 19-8). When contracted, both sphincters seal off the bladder and allow urine to accumulate without leaking to the exterior. The internal urethral sphincter is involuntary, and the external urethral sphincter is composed of striated muscle and is under voluntary control.

The muscular wall of the bladder permits this organ to accommodate a considerable volume of urine with very little increase in pressure until a volume of 300 to 400 ml is reached. As the volume of urine in-

creases, the need to void may be noticed at volumes of 150 ml, but micturition in adults does not normally occur much below volumes of 350 ml.

As the bladder wall stretches, nerve impulses are transmitted to the second, third, and fourth sacral segments of the spinal cord, and an **emptying reflex** is initiated. The reflex causes contraction of the muscle of the bladder wall and relaxation of the internal sphincter. Urine then enters the urethra. If the external sphincter, which is under voluntary control, is relaxed, micturition occurs. Voluntary contraction of the external sphincter suppresses the emptying reflex until the bladder is filled to capacity with urine and loss of control occurs. Contraction of this powerful sphincter also abruptly terminates urination voluntarily.

Higher centers in the brain also function in micturition by integrating bladder contraction and internal

CLINICAL APPLICATION

URINARY CATHETERIZATION

Urinary **catheterization** is the passage or insertion of a hollow tube or catheter through the urethra into the bladder for the withdrawal of urine (see figure). It is a medical procedure commonly performed on many patients who undergo prolonged surgical or diagnostic procedures or who experience problems with urinary retention.

Correct catheterization procedures require aseptic techniques to prevent the introduction of infectious bacteria

into the urinary system. Clinical studies have proved that improper catheterization techniques cause bladder infections—a condition called cystitis—and point out the need for extensive training of health professionals who perform catheterizations. To minimize the risk of infection, some facilities now use ultrasound imaging of the bladder to determine whether urine is being involuntarily retained in the bladder—replacing the former practice of catheterizing a patient.

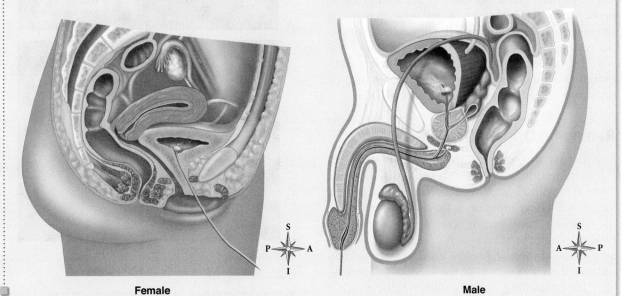

Female   **Male**

and external sphincter relaxation, with the cooperative contraction of pelvic and abdominal muscles. **Urinary retention** is a condition in which no urine is voided. The kidneys produce urine, but the bladder, for one reason or another, cannot empty itself. In **urinary suppression** the opposite is true. The kidneys do not produce any urine, but the bladder retains the ability to empty itself.

Micturition is a complex body function. It requires control and integration of both voluntary and involuntary nervous system components acting on a variety of anatomic structures. Unfortunately, homeostatic control problems occur quite frequently in this complex system. In addition to the 15% to 20% of children who experience some degree of enuresis, voiding dysfunction affects nearly 15 million adult Americans. People over 60 are especially at risk, with elderly women affected almost twice as often as men.

Urinary **incontinence** (in-KON-ti-nens) refers to involuntary voiding or loss of urine in an older child or adult. *Urge incontinence* is associated with detrusor overactivity or involuntary detrusor muscle contractions. The term *stress incontinence* is often used to describe the type of urine loss associated with laughing, coughing, or heavy lifting. It is a common problem in women with weakened pelvic floor muscles following pregnancy. So-called *overflow incontinence* is characterized by intermittent dribbling of urine. It results from urinary retention and an overdistended bladder—a common problem in men with an enlarged prostate gland (see Chapter 22). *Reflex incontinence* occurs in the absence of any sensory warning or awareness. It is common following a stroke or spinal cord injury. If totally cut off from spinal innervation, the bladder musculature acquires some automatic action, and periodic but unpredictable voiding occurs—a condition called **neurogenic bladder.**

Renal and Urinary Disorders

You may have experienced the discomfort and painful, burning urination, called **dysuria** (dis-UR-e-ah), associated with a bladder infection or know someone who has. Bladder infection is the most common urinary disorder, but it usually is not serious if promptly treated. A number of renal and urinary disorders are very serious, however. Any disorder that significantly reduces the effectiveness of the kidneys is immediately life threatening. In this section, we discuss some life-threatening kidney diseases, as well as a few of the less serious but more common disorders.

Obstructive Disorders

Obstructive urinary disorders are abnormalities that interfere with normal urine flow anywhere in the urinary tract. The severity of obstructive disorders depends on the location of the interference and the degree to which the flow of urine is impaired. Obstruction of urine flow usually results in "backing up" of the urine, perhaps all the way to the kidney itself.

The term **hydronephrosis** (hye-droh-nef-ROH-sis) is used to describe pathological swelling or enlargement of the renal pelvis and calyces caused by blockage of urine outflow. The condition may be the result of congenital problems or be caused by blockage caused by stones, tumors, or inflammation. Regardless of cause, if left untreated, much of the internal structure of the kidney is lost as the cortex thins and medullary tissue is destroyed (Figure 19-9, *A*).

Some of the more important obstructive conditions are summarized in the following paragraphs.

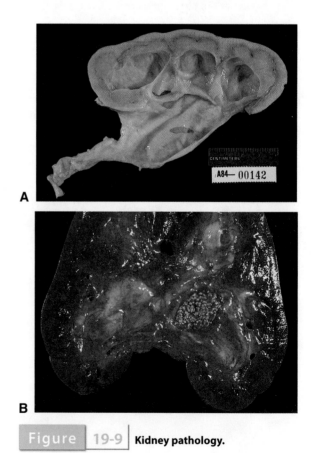

A

B

Figure 19-9 **Kidney pathology.**

A, Hydronephrosis. Note the dramatic enlargement of the renal pelvis and calyces with loss of kidney tissue. **B,** Renal calculi. Coronal section of kidney showing a large stone in the renal pelvis.

RENAL CALCULI

Renal calculi, or *kidney stones,* are crystallized mineral chunks that develop in the renal pelvis or calyces. Calculi develop when calcium and other minerals, such as uric acid, crystallize on the renal papillae, then break off into the urine. *Staghorn calculi* are large, branched stones that form in the pelvis and branched calyces.

If the stones are small enough, they will simply flow through the ureters and eventually be voided with the urine. Larger stones may obstruct the ureters, causing an intense pain called **renal colic** as rhythmic muscle contractions of the ureter attempt to dislodge the stones (Figure 19-9, *B*). Hydronephrosis may occur if the stone does not move from its obstructing position.

TUMORS

Tumors of the urinary system typically obstruct urine flow, possibly causing hydronephrosis in one or both kidneys. Most kidney tumors are malignant neoplasms called *renal cell carcinomas.* They usually occur only in one kidney. Renal cell carcinoma metastasizes most often to the lungs and bone tissue. *Bladder cancer* occurs about as frequently as renal cancer (each accounts for about two in every hundred cancer cases) and is often found in association with bladder stones.

Renal and bladder cancer have few symptoms early in their development, other than traces of blood in the urine, or **hematuria** (hem-ah-TOO-ree-ah). As the cancer develops, pelvic pain and symptoms of urinary obstruction may occur. Insertion of a **cystoscope** (SIS-toh-skohp) through the urethra and into the bladder permits direct inspection, biopsy, and surgical removal or treatment of bladder and other urinary tract lesions (Figure 19-10, *A*). The

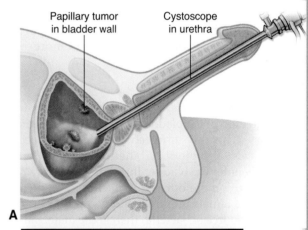

Papillary tumor in bladder wall   Cystoscope in urethra

A

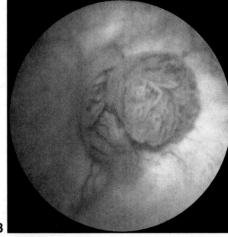

B

Figure 19-10 **Cystoscopic view of bladder cancer.**

A, Cystoscope in male bladder. **B,** Cystoscopic view of a cancerous growth (a transitional cell carcinoma) on the bladder wall.

CLINICAL APPLICATION

REMOVAL OF KIDNEY STONES USING ULTRASOUND

Statistics suggest that approximately 1 in every 1000 adults in the United States suffers from kidney stones, or **renal calculi** (KAL-kyoo-lye), at some point in his or her life. Although symptoms of excruciating pain are common, many kidney stones are small enough to pass spontaneously out of the urinary system. If this is possible, no therapy is required other than treatment for pain and antibiotics if the calculi are associated with infection. Larger stones, however, may obstruct the flow of urine and therefore are much more serious and difficult to treat.

Formerly, only traditional surgical procedures were effective in removing relatively large stones that formed in the calyces and renal pelvis of the kidney. In addition to the risks that always accompany major medical procedures, surgical removal of stones from the kidneys frequently requires rather extensive hospital and home recovery periods, lasting 6 weeks or more.

A technique that uses ultrasound to pulverize the stones so that they can be flushed out of the urinary tract without surgery is now used in hospitals across the United States. The specially designed ultrasound generator required for the procedure is called a **lithotriptor** (li-thoh-TRIP-ter). Using a lithotriptor, physicians break up the stones with ultrasound waves—in a process called *lithotripsy*—without making an incision. Recovery time is minimal, and both patient risk and costs are reduced.

hollow tube allows passage of light, a viewing lens, and various catheters and operative devices. Figure 19-10, *B* shows the appearance of a malignant tumor on the bladder wall before its removal during a surgical cystoscopic procedure.

Urinary Tract Infections

Most *urinary tract infections (UTIs)* are caused by bacteria, most often gram-negative types. UTIs can involve the urethra, bladder, ureter, and kidneys. Common types of urinary tract infections are summarized in the following paragraphs.

URETHRITIS

Urethritis (yoo-reth-RYE-tis) is inflammation of the urethra that commonly results from bacterial infection, often *gonorrhea* (Appendix A on page A-1 of your book). Nongonococcal urethritis is usually caused by *chlamydial* infection (Appendix A on page A-1 of your book). Males (particularly infants) suffer from urethritis more often than do females.

CYSTITIS

Cystitis (sis-TYE-tis) is a term that refers to an inflammation of the bladder. Cystitis most commonly occurs as a result of infection but also can accompany calculi, tumors, or other conditions. Bacteria usually enter the bladder through the urethra. Cystitis occurs more often in women than in men because the female urethra is shorter and closer to the anus (a source of bacteria) than in the male. Bladder infections are characterized by pelvic pain, an urge to urinate frequently, painful urination (dysuria), and hematuria.

If cystitis caused by bacterial infection becomes severe and chronic, the bladder epithelium may become ulcerated and covered with exudate. Extension of the infection may then inflame the ureters, renal pelvis, and kidney tissues. One common form of "nonbacterial" cystitis is *urethral syndrome.* Urethral syndrome, which occurs most commonly in young women, has unknown causes but often develops into a bacterial infection.

The term **overactive bladder** refers to the need for frequent urination. The amounts voided are generally small, and feelings of extreme urgency and pain (dysuria) are common. The condition is called *interstitial* (IN-tur-STISH-ul) *cystitis* and is treated with drugs to decrease nervous stimulation and with physical distention of the bladder with fluid to increase capacity. The condition is another type of "nonbacterial" cystitis because symptoms occur without evidence of bacterial infection. Some clinicians believe it is autoimmune in origin because it is often associated with lupus (see Chapter 15).

PYELONEPHRITIS

Nephritis (nef-RYE-tis) is a general term referring to kidney disease, especially inflammatory conditions. **Pyelonephritis** (pie-el-o-nef-RYE-tis) is literally "pelvis nephritis" and refers to inflammation of the renal pelvis and connective tissues of the kidney. As with cystitis, pyelonephritis is usually caused by bacterial infection but also can result from viral infection, mycosis, calculi, tumors, pregnancy, and other conditions.

Acute pyelonephritis develops rapidly and is characterized by fever, chills, pain in the sides (flank), nausea, and an urge to urinate frequently. It often results from the spread of infection from the lower urinary tract or through the blood from other organs. *Chronic pyelonephritis* may be an autoimmune disease but is often preceded by a bacterial infection or urinary blockage.

Glomerular Disorders

Glomerular disorders, collectively called **glomerulonephritis** (gloh-mair-yoo-lo-nef-RYE-tis), result from damage to the glomerular-capsular membrane. This damage can be caused by immune mechanisms, heredity, or bacterial infections. Without successful treatment, glomerular disorders can progress to kidney failure.

NEPHROTIC SYNDROME

Nephrotic (nef-ROT-ik) **syndrome** is a collection of signs and symptoms that accompany various glomerular disorders. This syndrome is characterized by the following:

1. **Proteinuria** (pro-teen-YOO-ree-ah)—presence of proteins (especially *albumin*) in the urine. Protein, normally absent from urine, filters through damaged glomerular-capsular

membranes and is not reabsorbed by the kidney tubules.

2. **Hypoalbuminemia** (hye-poh-al-byoo-min-EE-mee-ah)—low albumin concentration in the blood, resulting from the loss of albumin from the blood through holes in the damaged glomeruli. Albumin is the most abundant plasma protein. Because it normally cannot leave the blood vessels, it usually remains as a "permanent" solute in the plasma. This keeps plasma water concentration low and thus prevents osmosis of large amounts of water out of the blood and into tissue spaces. (You may wish to review the discussion of osmosis in Chapter 3 to help you understand this process.) In hypoalbuminemia, this function is lost and fluid leaks out of the blood vessels and into tissue spaces, causing widespread edema.

3. **Edema**—general tissue swelling caused by accumulation of fluids in the tissue spaces. Edema associated with nephrotic syndrome is caused by loss of plasma protein (albumin) and the resulting osmosis of fluid from the blood.

Note that hematuria (blood in the urine) is not a feature of nephrotic syndrome.

ACUTE GLOMERULONEPHRITIS

Acute glomerulonephritis is the most common form of kidney disease. It is caused by a delayed immune response to streptococcal infection—the same mechanism that causes valve damage in rheumatic heart disease (see Chapter 13). For this reason, it is sometimes called *postinfectious glomerulonephritis.* Occurring 1 to 6 weeks after a streptococcal infection, this disorder is characterized by hematuria, oliguria, proteinuria, and edema.

Antibiotic therapy and bed rest are the usual treatments for acute glomerulonephritis. Recovery is often complete but may progress to a chronic form of glomerulonephritis.

CHRONIC GLOMERULONEPHRITIS

Chronic glomerulonephritis is the general name for a variety of noninfectious glomerular disorders characterized by progressive kidney damage that leads to renal failure. Early stages of chronic glomerulonephritis are asymptomatic. As this disorder progresses, hematuria, proteinuria, oliguria, and edema develop. Immune mechanisms are believed to be the major causes of chronic glomerulonephritis.

Kidney Failure

Kidney failure, or **renal failure,** is simply the failure of the kidney to properly process blood and form urine. Renal failure can be classified as either *acute* or *chronic.*

ACUTE RENAL FAILURE

Acute renal failure is an abrupt reduction in kidney function characterized by oliguria and a sharp rise in nitrogenous compounds in the blood. The concentration of nitrogenous wastes in the blood is often assessed by the *blood urea nitrogen (BUN)* test. A high BUN result indicates failure of the kidneys to remove urea from the blood. Acute renal failure can be caused by a variety of factors that alter blood pressure or otherwise affect glomerular filtration. For example, hemorrhage, severe burns, acute glomerulonephritis or pyelonephritis, or obstruction of the lower urinary tract may progress to kidney failure. If the underlying cause of acute renal failure is successfully treated, recovery is usually rapid and complete.

CHRONIC RENAL FAILURE

Chronic renal failure is a slow, progressive condition resulting from the gradual loss of nephrons. There are dozens of diseases that may result in the gradual loss of nephron function, including infections, glomerulonephritis, tumors, systemic autoimmune disorders, and obstructive disorders.

Polycystic kidney disease (PKD) is one of the most common genetic disorders in humans. In PKD, large fluid-filled pockets (cysts) develop in the epithelium of the kidney tubules. In this condition, *primary cilia* (nonmoving cilia) on the epithelial cells that form kidney tubules fail to do their normal job of regulating cell growth. The epithelial cells then overpopulate and obstruct the kidney tubules. The obstructions result in pockets of backed-up urine called *cysts.* Eventually, the kidney fails.

One of the most common forms of PKD is called *adult polycystic kidney disease.* It is hereditary and

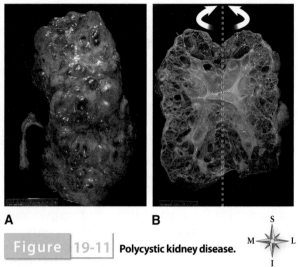

A, External view shows characteristic cysts. **B,** Lateral view of a kidney partially cut along a frontal plane and then opened like a book to view the cysts inside the kidney.

Figure 19-11 Polycystic kidney disease.

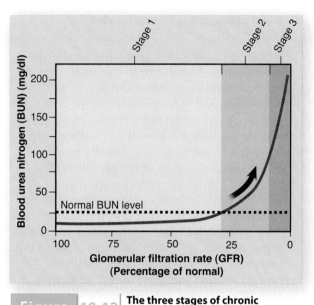

Figure 19-12 The three stages of chronic renal failure.

Stage 1: As nephrons are lost (indicated by decreasing GFR), the remaining healthy nephrons compensate—keeping BUN values within the normal range. *Stage 2:* As more than 75% of kidney function is lost, BUN levels begin to climb. *Stage 3:* Uremia (elevated BUN) results from massive loss of kidney function.

appears in 1 in 500 to 1000 persons. Symptoms of the disease, which include flank pain and hematuria, generally appear after age 40 and progress slowly. Eventually, the kidneys achieve enormous size as they fill with growing numbers of cysts (Figure 19-11). Destruction of tissue results in progressive renal failure.

As kidney function is lost, the glomerular filtration rate (GFR) decreases, causing the blood urea nitrogen (BUN) and creatinine levels to climb. Chronic renal failure can be described as progressing through the three stages shown in Figure 19-12 and described here:

1. **Stage 1**—During the first stage, some nephrons are lost but the remaining healthy nephrons compensate by enlarging and taking over the function of the lost nephrons. This stage is often asymptomatic and may last for years, depending on the underlying cause.

2. **Stage 2**—The second stage is often called *renal insufficiency*. During this stage, the kidney can no longer adapt to the loss of nephrons. The remaining healthy nephrons cannot handle the urea load, and BUN levels climb dramatically. Because the kidney's ability to concentrate urine is impaired, polyuria and dehydration may occur.

3. **Stage 3**—The final stage of chronic renal failure is called *uremia* or *uremic syndrome.* Uremia literally means "high blood urea" and is characterized by a very high BUN value caused by loss of kidney function. During this stage, low GFR causes low urine production and oliguria. Because fluids are retained by the body rather than being eliminated by the kidneys, edema and hypertension often occur. The uremic syndrome includes a long list of other symptoms caused directly or indirectly by the loss of kidney function. Unless an artificial kidney is used or a new kidney is transplanted, the progressive loss of kidney function eventually causes death.

QUICK CHECK

1. Through what tube does urine leave the kidney?
2. What structural characteristics of the bladder allow it to expand to hold urine?
3. Through what structure does urine pass from the bladder to the outside of the body?
4. What is incontinence?

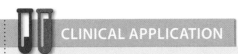

CLINICAL APPLICATION

ARTIFICIAL KIDNEY

The artificial kidney is a mechanical device that uses the principle of dialysis to remove or separate waste products from the blood. In the event of kidney failure, the process, appropriately called **hemodialysis** (Greek *haima* "blood" and *lysis* "separate"), is implemented as a reprieve from death for the patient.

During a hemodialysis treatment, a semipermeable membrane is used to separate large (nondiffusible) particles such as blood cells from small (diffusible) ones such as urea and other wastes. Figure *A* shows blood from the radial artery passing through a porous (semipermeable) cellophane tube that is housed in a tanklike container. The tube is surrounded by a bath or dialyzing solution containing varying concentrations of electrolytes and other chemicals. The pores in the membrane are small and allow only very small molecules, such as urea, to escape into the surrounding fluid. Larger molecules and blood cells cannot escape and are returned through the tube to reenter the patient via a wrist vein. By constantly replacing the bath solution in the dialysis tank with freshly mixed solution, waste materials can be kept at low levels. As a result, wastes such as urea in the blood rapidly pass into the surrounding wash solution.

For a patient with complete kidney failure, two or three hemodialysis treatments a week are required. These dialysis treatments are now being monitored and controlled by sophisticated computer components and software that have been integrated into the most current hemodialysis equipment. New and dramatic advances in both treatment techniques and equipment are expected in the future. Although most hemodialysis treatments are administered in hospital or clinical settings, equipment designed for use in the home is available and is appropriate for many individuals. Patients and their families using this equipment are initially instructed in its use and then monitored and supported on an ongoing basis by home health care professionals.

Another technique used in the treatment of renal failure is called **continuous ambulatory peritoneal dialysis (CAPD).** In this procedure, 1 to 3 L of sterile dialysis fluid is introduced directly into the peritoneal cavity through an opening in the abdominal wall (Figure *B*). Peritoneal membranes in the abdominal cavity transfer waste products from the blood into the dialysis fluid, which is then drained back into a plastic container after about 2 hours. This technique is less expensive than hemodialysis and does not require the use of complex equipment. CAPD is the more frequently used home-based dialysis treatment for patients with chronic renal failure. Successful long-term treatment is greatly enhanced by support from professionals trained in home health care services.

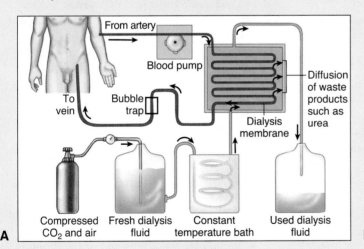

A

From artery

Blood pump

To vein

Bubble trap

Dialysis membrane

Diffusion of waste products such as urea

Compressed CO_2 and air   Fresh dialysis fluid   Constant temperature bath   Used dialysis fluid

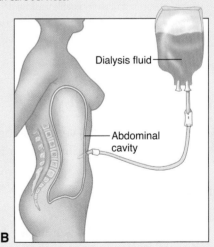

B

Dialysis fluid

Abdominal cavity

 To learn more about hemodialysis, go to **AnimationDirect** on your CD.

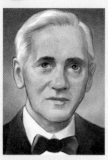

Alexander Fleming
(1881–1955)

FIGHTING INFECTION

Unfortunately, the structure of the urinary tract puts it at risk for infection by bacteria and other microorganisms. Because it is open to the external environment, bacteria can enter easily. In women, the short length of the urethra and its location close to the anus may further increase the risk of bacteria getting to the urinary bladder. Another risk factor is poor technique by health care workers when they insert catheters (tubes) into the urethras of patients who need help voiding their bladders of urine.

A breakthrough in the treatment of urinary tract infections (UTIs) came in 1928 in the laboratory of Scots researcher Alexander Fleming. Some mold spores accidentally contaminated one of the dishes in which Fleming was growing bacteria. He marveled at the fact that no bacteria could grow near the colony of mold. He isolated a substance from the mold that was responsible for this antibacterial effect and named it *penicillin*. Earlier Fleming had discovered another natural antibiotic (lysozyme) that effectively attacked bacteria that did not often cause disease so this concept was not totally new to him. However, through further experiments, Fleming showed that penicillin was effective against a variety of bacteria that do cause serious infections in humans, which made it an invaluable treatment tool.

Penicillin was touted as the first "miracle drug" and rapidly became the tool of choice in fighting bacteria. In 1943

another breakthrough came when laboratory worker Mary Hunt brought a moldy cantaloupe to work and researchers found that the new type of mold produced enough penicillin to make commercial production of the antibiotic possible.

Although forms of penicillin and other antibiotics derived from natural sources are still the weapon of choice in battling many infections, the infectious bacteria are evolving into strains that resist common antibiotics. UTIs and other types of infections now require more powerful antibiotics and other special techniques to stop them. Some scientists fear that the era of simple antibiotic therapy may be nearing an end.

Many professions are involved in the fight against infection. Medical supply technicians ensure that devices such as urethral catheters are sterile (free of microorganisms) before they are packaged and sent to hospitals and clinics. Physicians, nurses, and others who deal directly with patients learn proper "sterile technique" to ensure that infections are not introduced by medical procedures. To help in this effort, most organizations designate an infection control manager—a health professional with the responsibility of preventing **nosocomial** (no-zoh-KOAM-ee-al) **infections** (infections that begin in the hospital). Community health experts including epidemiologists and health service officers from the U.S. government's Centers for Disease Control and Prevention (CDC) also help prevent the spread of infection in local communities and worldwide. Of course, pharmacology researchers and others continue in the quest to find newer and better treatments for UTIs and other infections that threaten human health.

Outline Summary

To download an MP3 version of the chapter summary for use with your iPod or portable media player, access the **Audio Chapter Summaries** on your CD.

Kidneys

A. Location
   1. Kidneys lie under back muscles, behind parietal peritoneum, just above waistline
   2. Right kidney is usually a little lower than left (Figure 19-1)
B. Internal structure (Figure 19-2)
   1. Renal cortex—outer layer of kidney
   2. Renal medulla—inner portion of kidney
   3. Renal pyramids—triangular divisions of medulla
      a. Renal columns—cortical tissue that dips down between renal pyramids

   4. Renal papilla—narrow, innermost end of pyramid
   5. Renal pelvis—expansion of upper end of ureter; lies inside kidney
   6. Renal calyces—divisions of renal pelvis
C. Microscopic structure
   1. Interior of kidney composed of more than 1 million microscopic nephron units (Figures 19-3 and 19-4)
      a. Unique shape of nephron well suited to function
      b. Principal components are renal corpuscle and renal tubule
   2. Renal corpuscle

a. Bowman capsule—cup-shaped top of nephron

b. Glomerulus—network of blood capillaries surrounded by Bowman capsule

c. Cortical nephrons—85% of total; located mostly in renal cortex

d. Juxtamedullary nephrons—have important role in concentrating urine; located near junction between cortex and medullary layers

3. Renal tubule

a. Proximal convoluted tubule (PCT)—first segment

b. Henle loop—extension of proximal tubule; consists of descending limb, loop, and ascending limb

c. Distal convoluted tubule (DCT)—extension of ascending limb of Henle loop

d. Collecting duct (CD)—straight extension of distal tubule

4. Location of nephrons

a. Cortical nephrons—85% of total; located mostly in renal cortex

b. Juxtamedullary nephrons—have important role in concentrating urine; located near junction between cortex and medullary layers

D. Function

1. Excrete toxins and nitrogenous wastes

2. Regulate levels of many chemicals in blood

3. Maintain water balance

4. Help regulate blood pressure and volume

5. Regulate red blood cell production by secreting erythropoietin (EPO)

Formation of Urine (Figure 19-5)

A. Filtration

1. Goes on continually in renal corpuscles

2. Glomerular blood pressure causes water and dissolved substances to filter out of glomeruli into the Bowman capsule

3. Normal glomerular filtration rate 125 ml per minute

B. Reabsorption

1. Movement of substances out of renal tubules into blood in peritubular capillaries

2. Water, nutrients, and ions are reabsorbed

3. Water is reabsorbed by osmosis from proximal tubules

C. Secretion

1. Movement of substances into urine in the distal and collecting ducts from blood in peritubular capillaries

2. Hydrogen ions, potassium ions, and certain drugs are secreted by active transport

3. Ammonia is secreted by diffusion

D. Control of urine volume

1. ADH—secreted by posterior pituitary; promotes water reabsorption by collecting ducts; reduces urine volume

2. Aldosterone—secreted by adrenal gland, triggered by RAAS process; promotes sodium and water reabsorption in nephron; reduces urine volume (Figure 19-6)

3. ANH—one of the peptide hormones (ANPs) secreted by atrial cells in heart; promotes loss of sodium and water into kidney tubules; increases urine volume

Ureters

A. Structure

1. Narrow long tubes with expanded upper end (renal pelvis) located inside kidney

2. Lined with mucous membrane and muscular layer (Figure 19-7)

B. Function—drain urine from renal pelvis to urinary bladder

C. Urinalysis

1. Examination of the physical, chemical, and microscopic characteristics of urine

2. May help determine the presence and nature of a pathologic condition

Urinary Bladder

A. Structure (Figure 19-8)

1. Elastic muscular organ, capable of great expansion

2. Lined with mucous membrane arranged in rugae, like stomach mucosa

B. Function

1. Storage of urine before voiding

2. Voiding

Urethra

A. Structure

1. Narrow tube from urinary bladder to exterior

2. Lined with mucous membrane

3. Opening of urethra to the exterior called *urinary meatus*

B. Function

1. Passage of urine from bladder to exterior of the body
2. Passage of male reproductive fluid (semen) from the body

Micturition

A. Passage of urine from body (also called *urination* or *voiding*)
B. Regulatory sphincters
   1. Internal urethral sphincter (involuntary)
   2. External urethral sphincter (voluntary)
C. Bladder wall permits storage of urine with little increase in pressure
D. Emptying reflex
   1. Initiated by stretch reflex in bladder wall
   2. Bladder wall contracts
   3. Internal sphincter relaxes
   4. External sphincter relaxes and urination occurs
   5. Enuresis—involuntary urination in young child; nighttime bed wetting called *nocturnal enuresis*
E. Urinary retention—urine produced but not voided
F. Urinary suppression—no urine produced but bladder is normal
G. Incontinence—urine is voided involuntarily
   1. Urge incontinence—associated with detrusor overactivity or involuntary detrusor muscle contractions
   2. Stress incontinence—associated with weakened pelvic floor muscles
   3. Overflow incontinence—associated with urinary retention and overdistended bladder
   4. Reflex incontinence occurs in absence of any sensory warning or awareness—common following a stroke or spinal cord injury
   5. Neurogenic bladder— periodic but unpredictable voiding; related to paralysis or abnormal function of the bladder

Renal and Urinary Disorders

A. Obstructive disorders interfere with normal urine flow, possibly causing urine to back up and cause hydronephrosis or other kidney damage
   1. Renal calculi (kidney stones)—crystallized mineral chunks in renal pelvis or calyces; may block ureters, causing intense pain called *renal colic*
   2. Tumors—renal cell carcinoma (kidney cancer) and bladder cancer (Figure 19-10); often characterized by hematuria (blood in the urine)

3. Hydronephrosis—enlargement of renal pelvis and calyces caused by blockage of urine flow (Figure 19-9, *A*)
B. Urinary tract infections (UTIs) are often caused by gram-negative bacteria
   1. Urethritis—inflammation of the urethra
   2. Cystitis—inflammation or infection of the urinary bladder
   3. Pyelonephritis—inflammation of the renal pelvis and connective tissues of the kidney; may be acute (infectious) or chronic (autoimmune)
C. Glomerular disorders result from damage to the glomerular-capsular membrane of the renal corpuscles
   1. Nephrotic syndrome accompanies many glomerular disorders
      a. Proteinuria—protein in the urine
      b. Hypoalbuminemia—low plasma protein (albumin) level; caused by loss of proteins to urine
      c. Edema—tissue swelling caused by loss of water from plasma as a result of hypoalbuminemia
   2. Acute glomerulonephritis is caused by delayed immune response to a streptococcal infection
   3. Chronic glomerulonephritis is a slow inflammatory condition caused by immune mechanisms and often leads to renal failure
D. Kidney failure, or renal failure, occurs when the kidney fails to function
   1. Acute renal failure—abrupt reduction in kidney function that is usually reversible
   2. Chronic renal failure—slow, progressive loss of nephrons caused by a variety of underlying diseases
      a. Polycystic kidney disease (PKD)—numerous fluid-filled cysts destroy kidney tissue as they grow; hereditary (Figure 19-11)
      b. Progression of kidney failure (Figure 19-12)
         (1) Stage 1—early in this disorder, healthy nephrons often compensate for the loss of damaged nephrons
         (2) Stage 2—often called *renal insufficiency;* loss of kidney function ultimately results in uremia (high BUN levels) and its life-threatening consequences
         (3) Stage 3—called *uremia* or *uremic syndrome;* complete kidney failure results in death unless a new kidney is transplanted or an artificial kidney substitute is used

New Words

atrial natriuretic hormone (ANH)	renal columns	**Diseases and Other Clinical Terms**	nephritis
Bowman capsule	renal corpuscle		nephropathy
calyx	renal cortex	anuria	nephrotic syndrome
collecting duct (CD)	renal medulla	catheterization	neurogenic bladder
cortical nephron	renal papilla	continuous ambulatory	nosocomial infection
distal convoluted tubule (DCT)	renal pelvis	peritoneal dialysis (CAPD)	oliguria
	renal pyramid	cystitis	overactive bladder
emptying reflex	renal threshold	cystoscope	phenylketonuria (PKU)
erythropoietin (EPO)	renal tubule	dysuria	polycystic kidney disease (PKD)
glomerular filtrate	renin-angiotensin-	edema	polyuria
glomerulus	aldosterone system (RAAS)	enuresis	proteinuria
juxtaglomerular (JG) apparatus	retroperitoneal	glomerulonephritis	pyelonephritis
juxtamedullary nephron	secretion	glycosuria	renal calculi
Henle loop	sphincter	hematuria	renal colic
micturition	trigone	hemodialysis	renal failure
nephron	urinary meatus	hydronephrosis	uremia (uremic poisoning)
proximal convoluted tubule (PCT)	urination	hypoalbuminemia	urethritis
	voiding	incontinence	urinary retention
		lithotriptor	urinary suppression

Review Questions

1. Describe the location of the kidneys.
2. Name and describe the internal structures of the kidneys.
3. Define filtration, reabsorption, and secretion as they apply to kidney function.
4. Briefly explain the formation of urine.
5. Name several substances eliminated or regulated by the kidney.
6. Explain the function of the juxtaglomerular apparatus.
7. Describe the structure of the ureters.
8. Chemical urinalysis provides information about what substances in the urine?
9. Casts are sometimes found in a urine sample; what are casts?
10. Describe the structure of the bladder. What is the trigone?
11. Describe the structure of the urethra.
12. Briefly explain the process of micturition.
13. Differentiate between retention and suppression of urine.
14. What is incontinence? What can cause incontinence?
15. What is the most common urinary disorder?
16. What is hydronephrosis?
17. What is another term for renal calculi? What are they usually made of?
18. Briefly explain the following disorders: urethritis, cystitis, and pyelonephritis.
19. What is proteinuria? What is hypoalbuminemia?
20. Briefly describe the three stages of chronic renal failure.

Critical Thinking Questions

21. Explain the salt and water balance maintained by aldosterone and ADH.
22. Why is proper blood pressure necessary for proper kidney function?
23. If a person were doing strenuous work on a hot day and perspiring heavily, would there be a great deal of ADH in the blood or very little? Explain your answer.

Chapter Test

1. The kidneys receive about _____ % of the total amount of blood pumped by the heart each minute.

2. The renal corpuscle is made up of two structures, the _____ and the _____.

3. The two parts of the renal tubules that extend into the medulla of the kidney are the _____ and the _____.

4. The two parts of the renal tubules that are in the cortex of the kidney are the _____ and the _____.

5. The process of _____ is the movement of substances out of the renal tubules and into the blood capillaries.

6. The process of _____ causes substances in the glomerulus to be pushed into the Bowman capsule as a result of blood pressure.

7. The process of _____ is the movement of substances from the blood into the distal tubule or collecting tube.

8. The hormone _____ is released from the posterior pituitary gland and reduces the amount of water lost in the urine.

9. The hormone _____ is produced in the heart and stimulates the tubules to secrete sodium.

10. The hormone _____ is made in the adrenal cortex and causes the tubules to absorb sodium.

11. A physical, chemical, and microscopic examination of the urine is called a _____.

12. Small mineral deposits or cells found in a urine sample are called _____.

13. The involuntary muscle, _____, is at the exit of the bladder.

14. _____ is a condition in which the bladder is able to empty itself but no urine is being produced by the kidneys.

15. _____ is a condition in which a person voids urine involuntarily.

16. _____ is a condition in which the bladder is full and the kidney is producing urine but the bladder is unable to empty itself.

Match each term in Column A with its corresponding description in Column B.

Column A

17. _____ cortex
18. _____ medulla
19. _____ pyramid
20. _____ pelvis
21. _____ urethra
22. _____ bladder
23. _____ ureter
24. _____ trigone
25. _____ Bowman capsule
26. _____ glomerulus
27. _____ Henle loop

Column B

a. inner layer of the kidney
b. expansion of the ureter in the kidney
c. cup-shaped part of the nephron that catches filtrate
d. tube leading from the bladder to outside of the body
e. network of capillaries nestled within the Bowman capsule
f. saclike structure used to hold urine until it is voided
g. outer part of the kidney
h. an area of the bladder that has openings for the two ureters and the urethra
i. the part of the renal tubules that is located between the proximal and distal convoluted tubules
j. tube connecting the kidney and bladder
k. triangular division in the medulla of the kidney

Match each disorder in Column A with its corresponding description or cause in Column B.

Column A

28. _____ hydronephrosis
29. _____ renal calculi
30. _____ urethritis
31. _____ cystitis
32. _____ pyelonephritis
33. _____ hypoalbuminemia
34. _____ proteinuria

Column B

a. an inflammation of the urethra that commonly results from a bacterial infection
b. another term for a kidney stone
c. protein, especially albumin, in the urine
d. condition caused by urine backing up into the kidney, causing swelling of the renal pelvis and calyces
e. an inflammation of the bladder
f. low albumin in the blood due to loss of albumin through damaged glomeruli
g. inflammation of the renal pelvis and connective tissue of the kidney

Study Tips

continued from page 543

4. Make a chart of the disorders of the urinary system. Organize it based on the mechanism or cause of each disorder: obstructive disorders, urinary tract infections, glomerular disorders, and kidney failure.
5. Be sure you can differentiate the three stages of kidney failure.
6. In your study group, review the material in this chapter using the flash cards and photocopies of the figures of the organs of the urinary system, the internal structure of the kidney, and the microscopic structure of the nephron. Discuss how the kidney forms urine and the hormones involved in regulating urine volume. Make sure you know whether each of the hormones will increase or decrease urine volume. Go over the process of micturition, the chart of disorders of the urinary system, and the questions at the end of the chapter; discuss possible test questions.

Case Studies

1. Sue has *anorexia nervosa* (see Chapter 17). Her body fat content has decreased to a level that is far below normal. How might the changing structure of the body affect the position of Sue's kidneys? How can a change in the position of one or both kidneys lead to kidney failure?
2. Drugs called *thiazide diuretics* are sometimes prescribed to control hypertension (high blood pressure). These drugs act on kidney tubules in a way that inhibits reabsorption of water. How does inhibition of water reabsorption by the kidney reduce high blood pressure? What effects would such drugs have on the volume of urine output?
3. Harriet is receiving *continuous ambulatory peritoneal dialysis (CAPD)*. As you may recall from the boxed essay earlier in this chapter, fluid is introduced into the peritoneal cavity and later withdrawn. Do you think that this dialysis fluid is hypertonic, isotonic, or hypotonic to normal blood plasma? Give reasons for your answer.

Outline

Objectives

**After you have completed this chapter,
you should be able to:**

1. List, describe, and compare the
   body fluid compartments and their
   subdivisions.

2. Discuss avenues by which water
   enters and leaves the body and the
   mechanisms that maintain fluid
   balance.

3. Discuss the nature and importance
   of electrolytes in body fluids and
   explain the aldosterone mechanism of
   extracellular fluid volume control.

4. Explain the interaction between
   capillary blood pressure and blood
   proteins.

5. Give examples of common fluid
   imbalances.

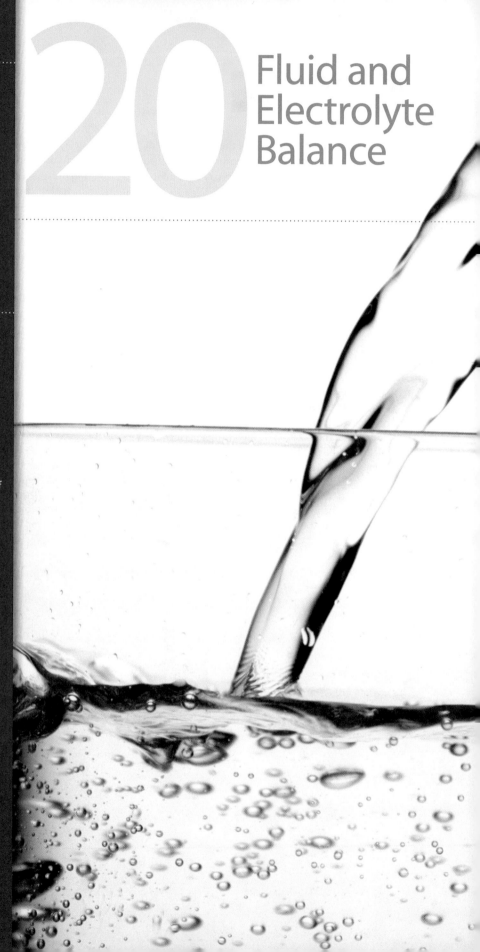

20 Fluid and Electrolyte Balance

Have you ever wondered why you sometimes excrete great volumes of urine and at other times excrete almost none at all? Why sometimes you feel so thirsty that you can hardly get enough to drink and other times you want no liquids at all? These conditions and many more relate to one of the body's most important functions—that of maintaining its **fluid and electrolyte balance.**

The phrase *fluid balance* implies homeostasis, or relative constancy of body fluid levels—a condition required for healthy survival. It means that both the total volume and distribution of water in the body remain normal and relatively constant. Body "input" of water must be balanced by "output." If water in excess of requirements enters the body, it must be eliminated, and, if excess losses occur, prompt replacement is critical. Because fluid balance refers to normal homeostasis, fluid imbalance means that the total volume of water in the body or the amounts in one or more of its fluid compartments have increased or decreased beyond normal limits.

STUDY TIPS

Chapter 20 expands on some of the material from Chapter 19. A quick review of Chapter 19 will better prepare you for this chapter.

1. Make flash cards to help you learn the terms in this chapter.
2. Remember that plasma and interstitial fluid make up the extracellular fluid.
3. Electrolytes are charged particles or ions. One of the functions of ions is to control water movement. The body cannot directly control water movement so it must move electrolytes and water will then follow.
4. The capillary pressure and blood protein mechanism regulates the movement of water between the blood and interstitial fluid. Blood pressure determines the amount of plasma that is pushed out into the interstitial fluid, and plasma proteins determine the amount of water that gets pulled back into the blood.
5. In your study group, review the flash cards with the terms. Discuss how electrolytes function in regulating water movement. Go over the aldosterone mechanism (Figure 20-7). Discuss the plasma protein and capillary

continued on page 585

Electrolytes are substances such as salts that dissolve or break apart in water solution. *Electrolyte balance* refers to homeostasis or relative constancy of normal electrolyte levels in the body fluids. The various types of body fluids serve differing functions in different areas of the body. To do so, each type of body fluid must maintain differing levels and types of electrolytes within a very narrow range of normal. For example, blood, lymph, intracellular fluid, interstitial fluid, cerebrospinal fluid, and joint and eye fluids all depend on complex homeostatic mechanisms to adjust and maintain normal levels of appropriate electrolytes required for that particular type of body fluid to function as it should.

The widespread and differing functions of body water and electrolytes can result in the development of many unique diseases and clinical problems if homeostasis of fluid and/or electrolyte balance is not maintained. Health and sometimes even survival itself depend on maintaining the proper volume and distribution of body water and the appropriate levels and types of electrolytes within it.

In this chapter you will find a discussion of body fluids and electrolytes, their normal values, the mechanisms that operate to keep them normal, and some of the more common types of fluid and electrolyte imbalances.

Body Fluids

Of the hundreds of compounds present in your body, the most abundant is water. Medical reference tables often refer to "average" fluid volumes based on healthy nonobese young adults. In such tables, males weighing 70 kg (154 pounds) will have on average about 60% of their body weight, nearly 40 L, as water (Figure 20-1); females about 50%.

The reason fluid volume values in reference tables are based on nonobese individuals is that adipose or fat tissue contains the least amount of water of any body tissue. The more fat present in the body, the less the total water content per kilogram of body weight. Therefore, regardless of age, obese individuals, with their high body fat content, have less body water per kilogram of weight than slender people. Although a nonobese male body typically consists of about 60% water, an obese male may consist of only 50% water or even less. The female body contains slightly less water per kilogram of

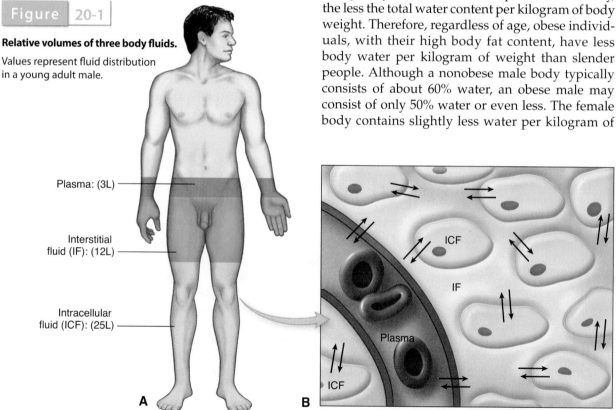

Figure 20-1

Relative volumes of three body fluids.
Values represent fluid distribution in a young adult male.

Plasma: (3L)

Interstitial fluid (IF): (12L)

Intracellular fluid (ICF): (25L)

ICF

IF

Plasma

ICF

A   **B**

weight because it contains slightly more fat than the male body.

Note in Figure 20-2 that age as well as gender influences the amount of water in the body.

Infants have more water as compared with body weight than adults of either sex. In a newborn, water may account for up to 80% of total body weight. The percentage of water is even higher in premature infants. The need for a high water content in the early stages of life is the reason fluid imbalances in infants caused by diarrhea, for example, can be so serious.

The percentage of body water decreases rapidly during the first 10 years of life and by adolescence, adult values are reached and gender differences, which account for about a 10% variation in body fluid volumes between the sexes, have developed.

In elderly individuals, the amount of water per kilogram of body weight decreases. One reason is that old age is often accompanied by a decrease in muscle mass (65% water) and an increase in fat (20% water). Certain drugs or toxins may have more potent effects in the elderly because they become more concentrated in the smaller volume of water present in the bodies of some elderly people. Of course, such drugs or toxins may have a reduced effect when diluted in the larger relative amount of water in a young person's body. In both cases, the key factor is the percentage of body weight represented by water.

Body Fluid Compartments

For the sake of discussion, the fluids of the body are thought of as being contained in theoretical "compartments." Each of these **fluid compartments** is actually a group of separated spaces in the body that in many ways function as if they are all in one compartment. Using this concept, total body fluid can be subdivided into two major fluid compartments called the *extracellular* and the *intracellular* fluid compartments.

Extracellular fluid (ECF) consists mainly of the liquid part of whole blood called the *plasma,* found in the blood vessels, and the *interstitial fluid* (IF) that surrounds the cells. In addition, the lymph, cerebrospinal fluid, humors of the eye, and the synovial joint fluids are also considered as extracellular fluid.

The term **intracellular fluid (ICF)** refers to the largest volume of body fluid by far. It is located inside all the cells of the body. Water has many func-

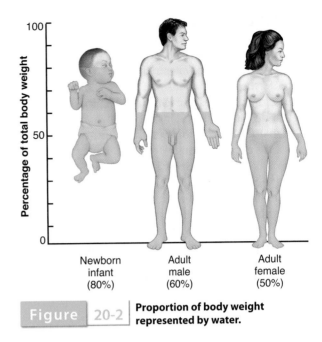

Figure 20-2 Proportion of body weight represented by water.

tions inside the cell but mainly serves as a solvent in which important chemical reactions of the cell can occur.

Figure 20-2 illustrates the typical proportion of body weight represented by water in the newborn and in adults by gender. Remember that body fluids are not all in a single, continuous space in the body—but often function as if they are.

> **QUICK CHECK**
>
> 1. What are the two main fluid compartments of the body?
> 2. What is meant by the term *fluid balance?*

Mechanisms That Maintain Fluid Balance

Under normal conditions, homeostasis of the total volume of water in the body is maintained or restored primarily by devices that adjust output (urine volume) to intake and secondarily by mechanisms that adjust fluid intake. There is no question about which of the two mechanisms is more important; the body's chief mechanism, by far, for maintaining fluid balance is that of adjusting its fluid output so that it equals its fluid intake.

Obviously, as long as output and intake are equal, the total amount of water in the body does not change. Figure 20-3 shows the three sources of fluid intake: the liquids we drink, the water in the foods we eat, and the water formed by catabolism of foods. Table 20-1 gives the normal volumes of each. However, these can vary a great deal and still be considered normal.

Table 20-1 also indicates that fluid output from the body occurs through four organs: the kidneys, lungs, skin, and intestines. The fluid output that fluctuates the most is that excreted from the kidneys. The body maintains fluid balance mainly by changing the volume of urine excreted to match changes in the volume of fluid intake. Everyone knows this from experience. The more liquid one drinks, the more urine one excretes. Conversely, the less the fluid intake, the less the urine volume. How changes in urine volume come about was discussed on pp. 551-552. This would be a good time to review those paragraphs.

It is important to remember from your study of the urinary system that the rate of water and salt resorption by the renal tubules is the most important factor in determining urine volume. Urine volume is regulated chiefly by hormones that affect kidney tubule function. Recall that *antidiuretic hormone (ADH)* from the posterior pituitary and *aldosterone* from the adrenal cortex both reduce urine volume by promoting water reabsorption from the kidney tubule back into the blood. Thus they are water-conserving hormones. *Atrial natriuretic hormone (ANH)* from the atrial wall of the heart, on the other hand, increases urine volume. Therefore, ANH is a water-loss hormone— or *diuretic* hormone. Please review hormonal control of urine volume in Chapter 19 (p. 551-552).

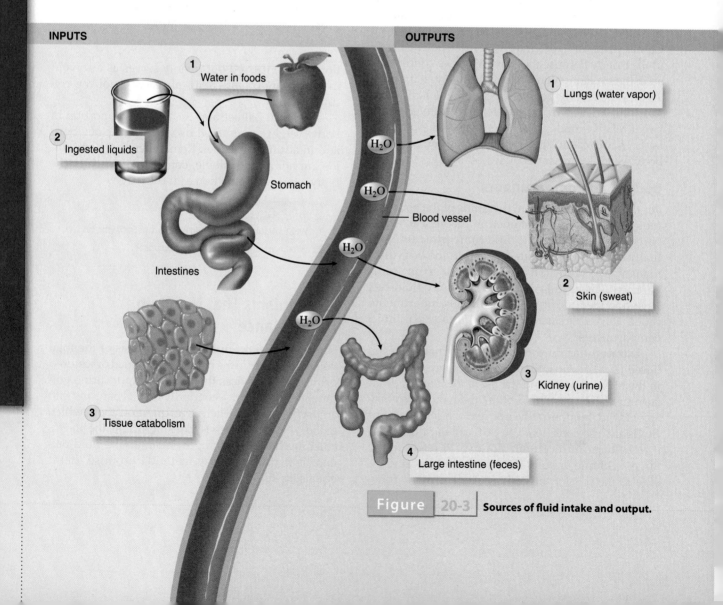

INPUTS

1 Water in foods
2 Ingested liquids
Stomach
Intestines
3 Tissue catabolism

OUTPUTS

H_2O
H_2O
H_2O
H_2O

1 Lungs (water vapor)
Blood vessel
2 Skin (sweat)
3 Kidney (urine)
4 Large intestine (feces)

Figure 20-3 **Sources of fluid intake and output.**

Table 20-1	**Typical Normal Values for Each Portal of Water Entry and Exit (in 24 Hours)**		
INTAKE	**AMOUNT***	**OUTPUT**	**AMOUNT***
Water in foods	700 ml	Lungs (water in expired air)	350 ml
Ingested liquids	1500 ml	Skin	
Water formed by catabolism	200 ml	By diffusion	350 ml
		By sweat	100 ml
		Kidneys (urine)	1400 ml
		Intestines (in feces)	200 ml
TOTALS	2400 ml		2400 ml

*Amounts vary widely among individuals and within the same individual depending on many factors.

A number of factors act as mechanisms for controlling plasma, IF, and ICF volumes. We shall limit our discussion to naming only three of these factors, stating their effects on fluid volumes and giving some specific examples of them. Those three main factors are as follows:

1. Concentration of electrolytes in ECF
2. Capillary blood pressure
3. Concentration of proteins in blood

Regulation of Fluid Intake

Physiologists disagree about the details of the mechanism for controlling and regulating fluid intake to compensate for factors that would lead to dehydration.

In general the mechanism for regulating fluid intake appears to operate in the following ways. When dehydration starts to develop—that is, when fluid loss from the body exceeds fluid intake—changes occur in the extracellular fluid. The extracellular fluid volume decreases and the solute concentration (osmotic pressure) of the extracellular fluid increases. Sensory receptors in the brain and elsewhere in the body also detect a change in the volume and concentration of extracellular fluids and relay this information to the thirst centers of hypothalamus. Signals from the hypothalamus cause salivary secretion to decrease, producing a "dry-mouth feeling" and the sensation of thirst. The dry mouth causes a person to "feel thirsty" and to drink water. Drinking water increases fluid intake and thereby compensates for previous fluid losses. This tends to restore fluid balance (Figure 20-4).

If an individual takes nothing by mouth for days, can his fluid output decrease to zero? The answer—no—becomes obvious after reviewing the information in Table 20-1. Despite every effort of homeostatic mechanisms to compensate for zero intake, some output (loss) of fluid occurs as long as life continues.

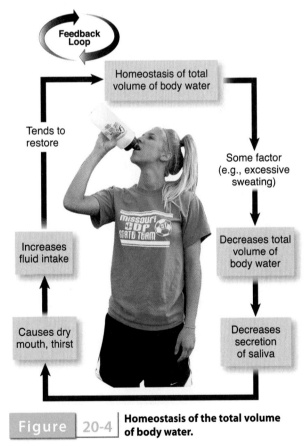

| Figure 20-4 | **Homeostasis of the total volume of body water.** |

A basic mechanism for adjusting intake to compensate for excess output of body fluid is diagrammed here.

Water is continually lost from the body through expired air and diffusion through skin.

Although the body adjusts fluid intake, factors that adjust fluid output, such as electrolytes and blood proteins, are far more important.

QUICK CHECK

1. Which does the body primarily adjust, fluid *intake* or fluid *output*?
2. What are the chief ways that fluid leaves the body?

Importance of Electrolytes in Body Fluids

The bonds that hold together the molecules of certain organic substances such as glucose are such that they do not permit the compound to break up, or **dissociate,** in water solution. Such compounds are called **nonelectrolytes.** Compounds such as ordinary table salt, or sodium chloride (NaCl), that have molecular bonds that permit them to break up, or dissociate, in water solution into separate particles (Na$^+$ and Cl$^-$) are **electrolytes.** The dissociated particles of an electrolyte are **ions** and carry an electrical charge. Sometimes the dissociated ions are themselves called *electrolytes.*

Important positively charged ions include sodium (Na$^+$), calcium (Ca^{++}), potassium (K$^+$), and magnesium (Mg^{++}). Important negatively charged ions include chloride (Cl$^-$), bicarbonate (HCO$_3^-$), phosphate (HPO$_4^-$), and many proteins. Figure 20-5 shows that although blood plasma contains a number of important ions, by far the most abundant are sodium (positive) and chloride (negative).

A variety of electrolytes have important nutrient or regulatory roles in the body. Many ions are major or important "trace" elements in the body (see Appendix C on the CD that accompanies your book). Iron, for example, is required for hemoglobin production, and iodine must be available for synthesis of thyroid hormones. Electrolytes are also required for many cellular activities such as nerve conduction and muscle contraction.

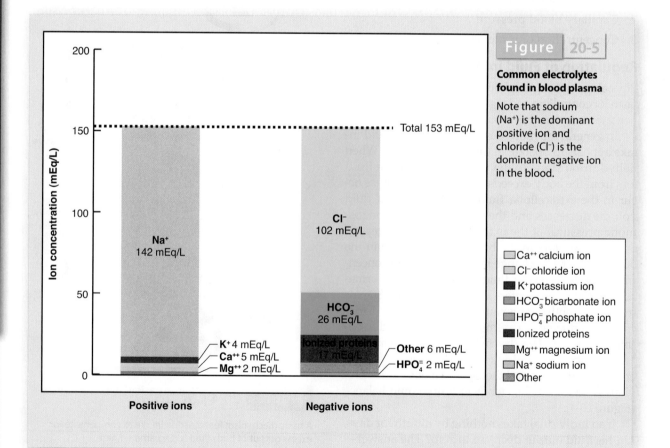

Figure 20-5

Common electrolytes found in blood plasma

Note that sodium (Na$^+$) is the dominant positive ion and chloride (Cl$^-$) is the dominant negative ion in the blood.

Legend:
- ☐ Ca^{++} calcium ion
- ☐ Cl$^-$ chloride ion
- ■ K$^+$ potassium ion
- ☐ HCO$_3^-$ bicarbonate ion
- ☐ HPO$_4^=$ phosphate ion
- ■ Ionized proteins
- ☐ Mg^{++} magnesium ion
- ☐ Na$^+$ sodium ion
- ☐ Other

Total 153 mEq/L

Na$^+$ 142 mEq/L

Cl$^-$ 102 mEq/L

HCO$_3^-$ 26 mEq/L

Ionized proteins 17 mEq/L

K$^+$ 4 mEq/L
Ca^{++} 5 mEq/L
Mg^{++} 2 mEq/L

Other 6 mEq/L
HPO$_4^=$ 2 mEq/L

Ion concentration (mEq/L)

Positive ions   Negative ions

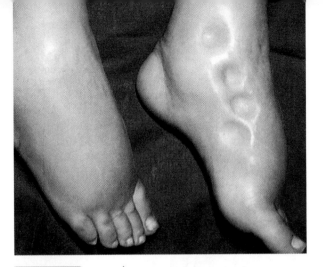

Figure 20-6 | **Pitting edema.**

Note the fingertip-shaped depressions that do not rapidly refill after an examiner has exerted pressure.

example, the concentration of sodium in interstitial fluid spaces rises above normal, the volume of IF soon reaches abnormal levels, too—a condition called **edema,** which results in tissue swelling (see box on p. 576). Edema may occur in any organ or tissue of the body. However, the lungs, brain, and dependent body areas such as the legs and lower back are affected most often. One of the most common areas for swelling to occur is in the subcutaneous tissues of the ankle and foot.

The term **pitting edema** is used to describe depressions in swollen subcutaneous tissue that do not rapidly refill after an examiner has exerted finger pressure (Figure 20-6). This type of edema is often a symptom in those with congestive heart failure.

Figure 20-7 traces one mechanism that tends to maintain fluid homeostasis. Aldosterone, secreted by the adrenal cortex, increases Na^+ reabsorption by the kidney tubules. Water reabsorption also increases, causing an increase in ECF volume. Begin in the upper right of the diagram and follow, in sequence, each of the informational steps. In summary they are as follows:

In addition, electrolytes influence the movement of water among the three fluid compartments of the body. To remember how ECF electrolyte concentration affects fluid volumes, remember this one short sentence: *Where sodium goes, water soon follows.* If, for

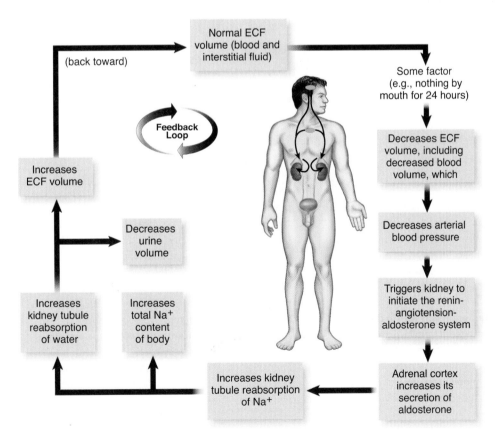

Figure 20-7

Aldosterone mechanism.

Aldosterone restores normal extracellular fluid (ECF) volume when such levels decrease below normal. Excess aldosterone, however, leads to excess ECF volume—that is, excess blood volume (hypervolemia) and excess interstitial fluid volume (edema)—and also leads to an excess of the total Na^+ content of the body.

1. Overall fluid balance requires that fluid output equal fluid intake.
2. The type of fluid output that changes most is urine volume.
3. Renal tubule regulation of salt and water is the most important factor in determining urine volume.
4. Aldosterone controls sodium reabsorption in the kidney.
5. The presence of sodium forces water to move (where sodium goes, water soon follows).

The flow chart diagram in Figure 20-7 explains, in a very brief way, the aldosterone mechanism that helps to restore normal ECF volume when it decreases below normal.

Although wide variations are possible, the average daily diet contains about 100 milliequivalents of sodium. The *milliequivalent (mEq)* (see Figure 20-5) is a unit of measurement related to ion reactivity. In a healthy individual, sodium excretion from the body by the kidney is about the same as intake. The kidney acts as the chief regulator of sodium levels in body fluids. It is important to know that many electrolytes such as sodium not only pass into and out of the body but also move back and forth between a number of body fluids during each 24-hour period.

Figure 20-8 shows the large volumes of sodium-containing internal secretions produced each day.

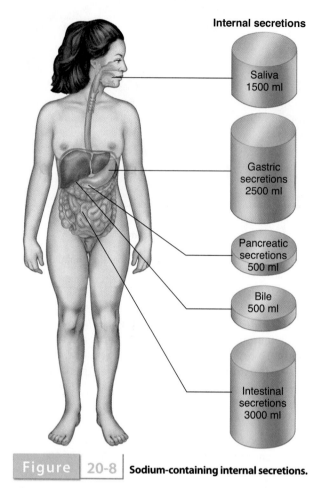

Internal secretions

Saliva
1500 ml

Gastric
secretions
2500 ml

Pancreatic
secretions
500 ml

Bile
500 ml

Intestinal
secretions
3000 ml

Figure 20-8 | **Sodium-containing internal secretions.**
The total volume of these secretions may reach 8000 ml or more in 24 hours.

CLINICAL APPLICATION

EDEMA

Edema may be defined as the presence of abnormally large amounts of fluid in the intercellular tissue spaces of the body. The condition is a classic example of fluid imbalance and may be caused by disturbances in any factor that governs the interchange between blood plasma and IF compartments. Examples include the following:

1. **Retention of electrolytes (especially Na⁺) in the extracellular fluid**. This can result from increased aldosterone secretion or can occur after serious kidney disease.
2. **An increase in capillary blood pressure.** Normally, fluid is drawn from the tissue spaces into the venous end of a tissue capillary because of the low venous pressure and the relatively high water-pulling force of the plasma proteins. This balance is upset by anything that increases the capillary hydrostatic pressure. The generalized venous congestion of heart failure is the most common cause of widespread edema. In patients with this condition, blood cannot flow freely through the capillary beds, and therefore the pressure will increase until venous return of blood improves.
3. **A decrease in the concentration of plasma proteins.** This decrease can be caused by "leakage" into the interstitial spaces of proteins normally retained in the blood. This may occur as a result of increased capillary permeability caused by infection, burns, or shock.

During a 24-hour period, more than 8 liters of fluid containing 1000 to 1300 mEq of sodium are poured into the digestive system as part of saliva, gastric secretions, bile, pancreatic juice, and IF secretions. This sodium, along with most of that contained in the diet, is almost completely reabsorbed in the large intestine. Very little sodium is lost in the feces. Precise regulation and control of sodium levels are required for survival.

 To learn more about the aldosterone regulation mechanism, go to **AnimationDirect** on your CD.

QUICK CHECK

1. What is the difference between an *electrolyte* and a *nonelectrolyte*?
2. What are some of the major roles of ions in the body?
3. What hormones regulate ions in the body?

Capillary Blood Pressure and Blood Proteins

Capillary blood pressure is a "water-pushing" force. It pushes fluid out of the blood in capillaries into the IF. Therefore if capillary blood pressure increases, more fluid is pushed—filtered—out of blood into the IF. The effect of an increase in capillary blood pressure, then, is to transfer fluid from blood to IF. In turn, this *fluid shift,* as it is called, changes blood and IF volumes. It decreases blood volume by increasing IF volume. If, on the other hand, capillary blood pressure decreases, less fluid filters out of blood into IF.

Water continually moves in both directions through the membranous walls of capillaries (see Figure 20-1). The amount that moves out of capillary blood into IF depends largely on capillary blood pressure, a water-pushing force. The amount that moves in the opposite direction (that is, into blood from IF) depends largely on the concentration of proteins in blood plasma.

Plasma proteins contribute to osmotic pressure and thereby act as a water-pulling or water-holding force. They hold water in the blood and pull it into the blood from IF. If, for example, the concentration of proteins in blood decreases appreciably—as it does in some abnormal conditions such as dietary deficiency—less water moves into blood from IF. As a result, blood volume decreases and IF volume increases.

Of the three main body fluids, IF volume varies the most. Plasma volume usually fluctuates only slightly and briefly. If a pronounced change in its volume occurs, adequate circulation cannot be maintained.

 To learn more about fluid shift, go to **AnimationDirect** on your CD.

Fluid Imbalances

Fluid imbalances are common ailments. They take several forms and stem from a variety of causes, but they all share a common characteristic—that of abnormally low or abnormally high volumes of one or more body fluids.

Dehydration is the fluid imbalance seen most often. In this potentially dangerous condition, IF volume decreases first, but eventually, if treatment has not been given, ICF and plasma volumes also decrease below normal levels. Either too small a fluid intake or too large a fluid output causes dehydration. Prolonged diarrhea or vomiting may result in dehydration due to the loss of body fluids. This is particularly true in infants where the total fluid volume is much smaller than it is in adults. Loss of skin elasticity is a clinical sign of dehydration (Figure 20-9).

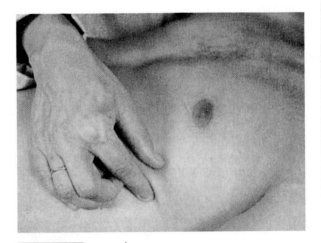

Figure 20-9 **Testing for dehydration.**

Loss of skin elasticity is a sign of dehydration. Skin that does not return quickly to its normal shape after being pinched (or tented) indicates interstitial water loss.

CLINICAL APPLICATION

DIURETICS

The word **diuretic** is from the Greek word *diouretikos* meaning "causing urine." By definition a *diuretic drug* is a substance that promotes or stimulates the production of urine. Recall that an increase in urine volume represents a loss of water from the body.

As a group, diuretics are among the most commonly used drugs in medicine. They are used because of their role in influencing water and electrolyte balance, especially sodium, in the body. Diuretics have their effect on tubular function in the nephron, and the differing types of diuretics are often classified according to their major site of action. Examples would include (1) *proximal tubule diuretics* such as acetazolamide (Diamox), (2) *Henle loop diuretics* such as ethacrynic acid (Edecrin) or furosemide (Lasix), and (3) *distal tubule diuretics* such as chlorothiazide (Diuril). Caffeine produces its mildly diuretic effects by inhibiting water reabsorption in the proximal tubules of the kidney.

Classification of diuretic drugs also can be made according to the effect the drug has on the level or concentration of sodium (Na^+), chloride (Cl^-), potassium (K^+), and bicarbonate (HCO_3^-) ions in the tubular fluid.

Alcohol is also a diuretic. It reduces secretion of ADH, which is a water-conserving hormone. Thus water that would have otherwise been conserved by the body is lost under the influence of alcohol.

Diuretics are sometimes used by athletes to quickly reduce their weight just prior to an event or "weigh-in." Loss of water from the body does in fact reduce a person's weight, but it also reduces his or her athletic ability by creating the condition of dehydration. Diuretics (except for legitimate therapeutic use) are included on the Prohibited List by the World Anti-Doping Agency.

Nursing implications for caregivers monitoring patients receiving diuretics both in hospitals and in home health care environments include (1) keeping a careful record of fluid intake and output and (2) assessing the patient for signs and symptoms of electrolyte and water imbalance. For example, diuretic-induced dehydration resulting in a loss of only 6% of initial body weight will cause tingling in the extremities, stumbling gait, headache, fever, and an increase in both pulse and respiratory rates.

Overhydration also can occur but is much less common than dehydration. One grave danger of giving intravenous fluids too rapidly or in too large of an amount is overhydration, which can put too heavy a burden on the heart by increasing the volume of blood to be pumped.

Water intoxication may result from rapidly drinking large volumes of water or giving hypotonic solutions to persons unable to dilute and excrete urine normally. This may occur in patients with kidney insufficiency or abnormal "thirst" mechanisms resulting from neurological disorders. Water content is elevated, and plasma sodium levels are diluted. Development of subtle mental changes such as confusion and lethargy occur. If intoxication is severe, stupor, seizures, and coma may result. Correction of the neurological impairment along with water restriction can reverse the symptoms.

Water intoxication can happen in normal individuals if water intake is so rapid that the urinary mechanisms of water loss cannot keep up. Although this is unusual, it can happen—as witnessed by millions a few years ago when a radio station held a "water drinking race" on the air and a contestant died from the effects of severe water intoxication.

Electrolyte Imbalances

Electrolyte balance, like fluid balance, is related to "intake" and "output" of specific electrolytes. Also important is the absorption of electrolytes once ingested, their final distribution in the body fluids, and their "availability" for use by the body cells. Extracellular fluid normally contains differing levels of some electrolytes than do intracellular fluid. In order to maintain different concentrations of electrolytes in the different body fluids, differing homeostatic mechanisms that influence intake, absorption, distribution, and excretion of these electrolytes are needed.

Any disruption in a homeostatic mechanism controlling the level or normal chemical activity of a particular electrolyte in any of the different body fluids produces an *electrolyte imbalance*. Such imbalances are widespread and often very serious and sometimes fatal manifestations of disease.

Appendix C (found on the CD that accompanies your book) lists the normal values of many important electrolytes and identifies disease states that may result in variations above or below normal levels. Electrolyte imbalances involving sodium, potassium, and calcium are common in clinical medicine and are described below.

Sodium Imbalance

The term *Natrium* is the Latin word for sodium. The prefixes *hyper-* and *hypo-* refer to "above" and "below," respectively. Knowing this makes the terms *hypernatremia* (hye-per-nah-TREE-mee-ah) and *hyponatremia* (hye-poh-nah-TREE-mee-ah) easier to understand and remember. **Hypernatremia** is used to describe a blood sodium level of more than 145 mEq/L. **Hyponatremia** occurs when blood sodium level is below 136 mEq/L (Appendix C on the CD that accompanies your book).

Hypernatremia may result from overuse of salt tablets, dehydration, or prolonged diarrhea. Regardless of cause, the condition is characterized by a relative deficit of water to salt in the extracellular fluid. Hyponatremia occurs when there is relatively too much water in the extracellular fluid compartment for the amount of sodium present. This can occur if excessive antidiuretic hormone is produced or after massive infusion of IV fluids, such as 5% dextrose in water, that do not contain sodium.

Hyponatremia also may be caused by excessive salt loss resulting from burns or certain diuretics. Both of these conditions affect central nervous system functioning and are characterized by headache, confusion, seizures, and, in the most severe cases, coma and death.

Potassium Imbalance

The normal range for potassium in blood is 3.8 to 5.1 mEq/L (Appendix C on the CD that accompanies your book). Although most of the total body potassium is inside the cells, fluctuations or imbalance in the relatively small amounts present in the extracellular fluid will cause serious illness.

Hyperkalemia (hye-per-kal-EE-mee-ah) is the clinical term used to describe blood potassium levels of more than 5.1 mEq/L. (*Kalium* is the Latin term for potassium.) Elevation of potassium may be related to increased intake, a shift from the intracellular fluid into the blood—caused by tissue trauma or burns, or in cases of renal failure, by an in-

ability of the kidneys to excrete excess potassium. Many of the clinical manifestations of hyperkalemia are related to muscle malfunction. As potassium levels increase, skeletal muscles weaken and paralysis develops. Severe hyperkalemia results in cardiac arrest.

Hypokalemia refers to a low blood potassium level (below 3.8 mEq/L); it may be caused by fasting, fad diets low in dietary potassium, abuse of laxatives and certain diuretics in extreme weight loss programs, or by loss of potassium because of diarrhea, vomiting, or gastric suction. As with hyperkalemia, low potassium levels cause skeletal muscle weakness and cardiac problems. In addition, smooth muscle in the gastrointestinal tract does not contract properly, causing abdominal distention and diminished rate of passage of intestinal contents.

Calcium Imbalance

Calcium is the most abundant mineral in the body. It serves as a basic structural building block in bone and teeth. In addition, it is essential for the maintenance of a normal heartbeat, for functioning of nerves and muscles, and for the role it plays in metabolism, blood coagulation, and in many other enzymatic reactions. Failure of homeostatic mechanisms that regulate levels of this important electrolyte can result in catastrophic illness.

The normal range for serum calcium is 8.4 to 10.5 mg/dl (Appendix C on the CD that accompanies your book). **Hypercalcemia** (hye-per-kal-SEE-mee-ah) occurs when blood calcium levels rise above normal limits. The condition may be caused by excessive input or by increased absorption that may occur following an overdose of vitamin D. Elevated levels can also result from shifts of calcium from bone into the extracellular fluid caused by Paget disease (see p. 192-193), other bone tumors, or hyperparathyroidism blood levels that will also increase if the kidney cannot normally excrete excess calcium in the urine—a side effect of certain diuretics. Regardless of cause, hypercalcemia decreases neuromuscular irritability resulting in fatigue, muscle weakness, diminished reflexes, and delayed atrioventricular conduction in the heart.

Hypocalcemia may result from dietary calcium deficiency, decreased absorption or availability, and as a result of increased calcium excretion. Diseases such as pancreatitis, hypoparathyroidism, rickets, and osteomalacia and chronic renal insufficiency all lower blood calcium levels. Clinical signs of hypocalcemia involve *increased* neuromuscular irritability, cramping and twitching of muscles, hyperactive reflexes, and abnormal cardiac rhythms characterized by impairment of myocardial contractility.

SCIENCE APPLICATIONS

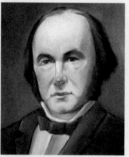

Claude Bernard (1813–1877)

THE CONSTANCY OF THE BODY

In 1834, a young Claude Bernard left what he thought of at the time as his "boring job" as an apprentice apothecary (druggist) in Lyon, France, to make his fortune as a playwright in Paris. His plays were not appreciated in Paris, but he took a medical course while there and found that many of the doctors appreciated his research skills. Bernard went on to become one of the most important figures in the study of human physiology.

Bernard made groundbreaking discoveries in the functions of the pancreas and the liver, discovered the existence of muscles that control blood vessel dilation, and wrote a manual on experimental medicine that set the standard in research practice for a century. However, one of the most fundamental contributions he made to human physiology is the idea that the body is made up of cells living in an internal fluid environment.

Bernard stated that the internal fluid environment of the body is maintained in a relatively constant state—and that's what ensures the survival of the cells and therefore also ensures the survival of the whole body. Recall from Chapter 1 that we now call this concept *homeostasis* (see pp. 13–15). It was Bernard who showed that the actions of hormones and other control mechanisms maintain constant conditions in the body's internal fluid environment. And it was Bernard who showed that nearly every function of the body somehow relates to the success of keeping body fluids constant.

Today, nearly every health care professional uses concepts based on Bernard's original idea to help keep patients alive and healthy. Those who use these ideas most directly are the nurses, health technicians, IV (intravenous) therapists, and others who care for patients on an hour by hour basis. It is these professionals who must constantly assess the fluid balance of patients and possibly administer therapies to bring their fluids back into balance. Maintaining a healthy fluid and electrolyte balance is one of the key elements of successful patient care in the modern hospital and clinic.

Outline Summary

 To download an MP3 version of the chapter summary for use with your iPod or portable media player, access the **Audio Chapter Summaries** on your CD.

Body Fluids

A. Water is most abundant body compound
   1. References to "average" body water volume in reference tables are based on a healthy, nonobese, 70-kg male
   2. Volume averages 40 L in a 70-kg male (Figure 20-1)
     a. Plasma (3 L)
     b. Interstitial fluid (12 L)
     c. Intracellular fluid (25 L)
   3. Water is 80% of body weight in newborn infants; 60% in adult males; 50% in adult females (Figure 20-2)
   4. Variation in total body water is related to:
     a. Total body weight of individual
     b. Fat content of body—the more fat in the body the less the total water content per kilogram of body weight (adipose tissue is low in water content)
     c. Gender—female body has about 10% less than male body (Figure 20-2)
     d. Age—in a newborn infant, water may account for 80% of total body weight. In the elderly, water per kilogram of weight decreases (muscle tissue—high in water—replaced by fat which is lower in water)
B. Body fluid compartments
   1. Extracellular fluid (ECF)—called internal environment of body; surround cells and transports substances to and from them
     a. Plasma—liquid part of whole blood
     b. Interstitial fluid (IF)—surrounds the cells
     c. Miscellaneous—lymph; joint fluids; cerebrospinal fluid; eye humors
   2. Intracellular fluid (ICF)—largest fluid compartment
     a. Located inside cells
     b. Serves as solvent to facilitate intracellular chemical reactions

Mechanisms That Maintain Fluid Balance

A. Sources of fluid intake (Figure 20-3)
   1. Liquids we drink
   2. Water in food we eat
   3. Water formed by catabolism of food
B. Organs responsible for fluid output—lungs, skin, kidneys, and large intestine
   1. Fluid output, mainly urine volume, adjusts to fluid intake
   2. ADH from posterior pituitary gland and aldosterone from adrenal cortex act to increase kidney tubule reabsorption of sodium and water from tubular urine into blood, thereby tending to increase ECF (and total body fluid) by decreasing urine volume (Figure 20-7)
   3. Three main factors affect plasma, IF, and ICF volumes
C. Regulation of fluid intake (Figure 20-4)
   1. Sensory receptors detect change in volume and EDF concentration and send signals to the hypothalamus
   2. Signals from hypothalamus cause sensation of thirst, which triggers drinking of fluids to restore balance
D. Importance of electrolytes in body fluids
   1. Nonelectrolytes—organic substances that do not break up or dissociate when placed in water solution (e.g., glucose)
   2. Electrolytes—compounds that break up or dissociate in water solution into separate particles called ions (e.g., ordinary table salt or sodium chloride)
   3. Ions—the dissociated particles of an electrolyte that carry an electrical charge
     a. Positively charged ions (e.g., potassium [K^+] and sodium [Na^+])

   b. Negatively charged particles (ions) (e.g., chloride [Cl^-] and bicarbonate [HCO_3^-])
   4. Electrolyte composition of blood plasma (Figure 20-5)
   5. Edema—swelling caused by high IF volume; pitting edema occurs when depressions in skin do not rapidly refill (Figure 20-6)
   6. Aldosterone mechanism restores normal ECF volume (Figure 20-7)
   7. Sodium-containing internal secretions (Figure 20-8)
E. Capillary blood pressure and blood proteins
   1. Increased capillary blood pressure transfers fluid from blood to IF—a fluid shift
   2. Blood plasma protein concentration contributes to osmotic pressure

Fluid Imbalances

A. Dehydration—total volume of body fluids smaller than normal
   1. IF volume shrinks first, and then if treatment is not given, ICF volume and plasma volume decrease
   2. Dehydration occurs when fluid output exceeds intake for an extended period (Figure 20-9)
B. Overhydration—total volume of body fluids larger than normal
   1. Fluid intake exceeds output
   2. Excess volume burdens pumping action of heart
C. Water intoxication—possibly life-threatening neurological impairment caused by severe overhydration and accompanying electrolyte imbalance

Electrolyte Imbalance

A. Related to "intake" and "output" of electrolytes and also absorption and distribution of electrolytes in body fluids and availability for use by body cells
B. Sodium imbalance
   1. Hypernatremia—blood sodium more than145 mEq/L
      a. Characterized by relative deficit of water to salt in extracellular fluid
      b. Causes include overuse of salt tablets; dehydration; and prolonged diarrhea
   2. Hyponatremia—blood sodium less than 136 mEq/L
      a. Results when there is relatively too much water in the extracellular fluid for the amount of sodium present
      b. Causes include excessive secretion of antidiuretic hormone; massive infusion of sodium-free IV solution; burns; and prolonged use of certain diuretics
      c. Symptoms of both hyper- and hyponatremia are related to CNS malfunction and include headache, confusion, seizures, and coma
C. Potassium imbalance
   1. Hyperkalemia—blood potassium more than 5.1 mEq/L
      a. Causes include increased intake; shift potassium from ICF to blood caused by tissue trauma and burns; renal failure
      b. Clinical signs of hyperkalemia are related to muscle malfunction and include skeletal muscle weakness, paralysis, and cardiac arrest
   2. Hypokalemia—blood potassium less than 3.8 mEq/L
      a. Causes include fasting; diets low in potassium; abuse of laxatives and certain diuretics; diarrhea; vomiting; gastric suction
      b. Clinical signs include skeletal muscle and cardiac problems; smooth muscle weakness causing abdominal distention; and slow rate of passage of GI contents
D. Calcium imbalance
   1. Hypercalcemia—blood calcium levels more than 10.5 mg/dl
      a. Caused by excessive input; increased absorption; shifts of calcium

from bone to ECF; Paget disease
and other bone tumors; hyperparathyroidism
  b. Clinical signs related to decreased
neuromuscular activity—fatigue;
muscle weakness; diminished reflexes;
cardiac problems
  2. Hypocalcemia—blood calcium levels less
than 8.4 mg/dl

  a. Caused by dietary deficiency; dcreased
absorption or availability; increased
excretion; pancreatitis; hypoparathyroidism; rickets and osteomalacia; and
renal insufficiency
  b. Clinical signs related to increased
neuromuscular irritability—cramping
muscle twitching; hyperactive reflexes;
and abnormal cardiac rhythms

New Words

dissociate	fluid compartment	**Diseases and Other Clinical Terms**	hypernatremia
electrolyte	interstitial fluid (IF)		hypocalcemia
electrolyte balance	intracellular fluid (ICF)	dehydration	hypokalemia
extracellular fluid (ECF)	ion	diuretic	hyponatremia
fluid balance	nonelectrolyte	hypercalcemia	overhydration
		hyperkalemia	pitting edema
			water intoxication

Review Questions

1. Name and give the location of the three main fluid compartments of the body. Which of these make up extracellular fluid?
2. What factors influence the percentage of water in the body? Explain the effect of each factor.
3. List the three sources of water for the body.
4. List the four organs from which fluid output occurs.
5. Differentiate between an electrolyte and a nonelectrolyte.
6. Name three important negative ions.
7. Name three important positive ions.
8. Explain why the body is unable to reduce its fluid output to zero no matter how dehydrated it is.
9. Explain how aldosterone influences water movement between the kidney tubules and the blood.
10. Explain the role of capillary blood pressure in water movement between the plasma and interstitial fluid.
11. Explain the role of plasma proteins in water movement between the plasma and interstitial fluid.
12. Define dehydration and give a possible cause.
13. Define overhydration and give a possible cause.

Critical Thinking

14. Name the three hormones that regulate urine volume. State where each is made and the specific effect each has on urine volume.
15. Atrial natriuretic hormone has the opposite effect of aldosterone. Explain its effect on water movement between the kidney tubules and the blood.

Chapter Test

1. The extracellular fluid compartment is composed of _____ and _____.
2. The largest volume of water in the human body is contained in which fluid compartment? _____
3. The body's chief mechanism for maintaining fluid balance is to adjust its _____.
4. The body has three sources of fluid intake; the liquids we drink, the foods we eat, and _____.
5. The four organs from which fluid output occurs are the _____, _____, _____, and _____.
6. Urine volume is regulated by three hormones: ADH released from the pituitary gland, _____ released from the adrenal cortex, and _____ released from the heart.
7. When electrolytes dissociate in water, they form charged particles called _____.
8. The most abundant negatively charged particle in the blood is _____.
9. The most abundant positively charged particle in the blood is _____.

Indicate whether each of the next three questions is *true* or *false:*

10. _____ In general, an obese person has more water per pound of body weight than a slim person.
11. _____ In general, a man has less water per pound of body weight than a woman.
12. _____ In general, an infant has less water per pound of body weight than an adult.
13. When the blood level of aldosterone increases:
    a. sodium is moved from the blood to the kidney tubules
    b. sodium is moved from the kidney tubules to the blood
    c. more urine is formed
    d. ANH is released
14. Aldosterone causes:
    a. an increase in intracellular fluid
    b. a decrease in intracellular fluid
    c. an increase in extracellular fluid
    d. a decrease in extracellular fluid
15. Increased capillary pressure:
    a. moves fluid from the intracellular compartment to the extracellular compartment
    b. moves fluid from the plasma to the interstitial fluid
    c. moves fluid from the interstitial fluid to the plasma
    d. has no effect on fluid movement
16. Blood plasma proteins act to:
    a. move interstitial fluid into the plasma
    b. move plasma into the interstitial fluid
    c. move extracellular fluid into the intracellular space
    d. move interstitial fluid into the extracellular space

Study Tips

continued from page 569

blood pressure mechanism for regulating the balance between blood plasma and interstitial fluid. Review the questions at the end of the chapter and discuss possible test questions.

Case Studies

1. Like most people in the United States, Tom ingests 20 to 30 times more sodium each day than he needs for survival. How does Tom's body compensate for this imbalance to restore homeostasis?
2. Jo has not eaten anything all day but has consumed an excessive amount of distilled water. Will this affect her urine output? What unusual characteristics are likely to appear in a urinalysis of Jo's urine?
3. Jo is overhydrated (see Case study number 2). This chapter states that *overhydration* can place a dangerously heavy burden on the heart. Explain how overhydration can tax the heart.

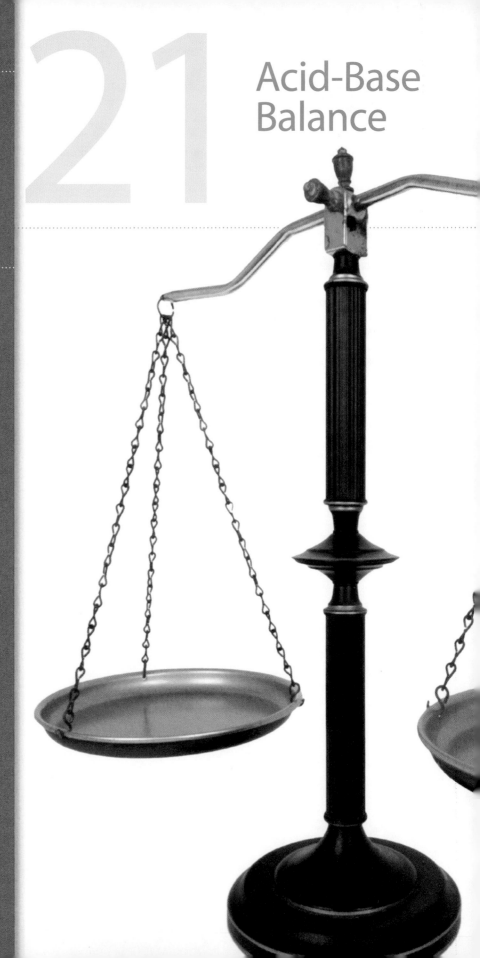

21

Acid-Base Balance

Outline

Objectives

After you have completed this chapter, you should be able to:

1. Discuss the concept of pH and define the term *acid-base balance*.

2. Define the terms *buffer* and *buffer pair* and contrast strong and weak acids and bases.

3. Contrast the respiratory and urinary mechanisms of pH control.

4. Discuss compensatory mechanisms that may help return blood pH to near-normal levels in cases of pH imbalances.

5. Compare and contrast metabolic and respiratory types of pH imbalances.

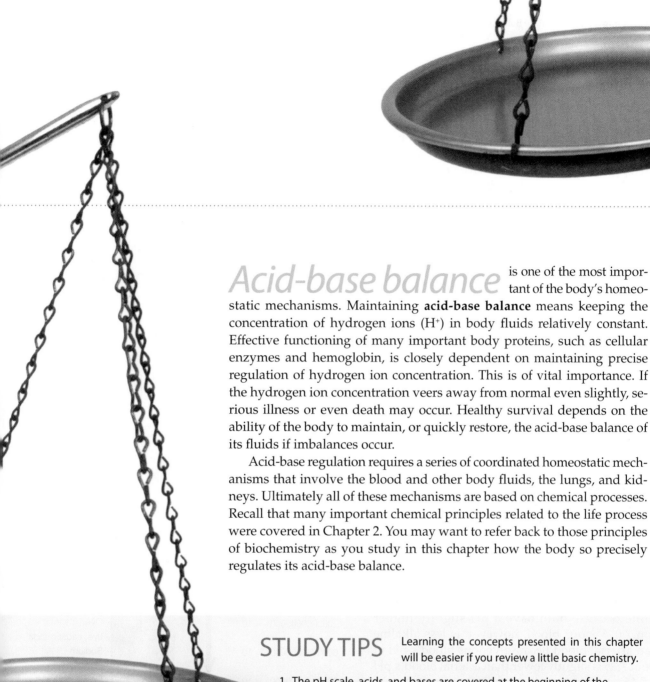

Acid-base balance is one of the most important of the body's homeostatic mechanisms. Maintaining **acid-base balance** means keeping the concentration of hydrogen ions (H⁺) in body fluids relatively constant. Effective functioning of many important body proteins, such as cellular enzymes and hemoglobin, is closely dependent on maintaining precise regulation of hydrogen ion concentration. This is of vital importance. If the hydrogen ion concentration veers away from normal even slightly, serious illness or even death may occur. Healthy survival depends on the ability of the body to maintain, or quickly restore, the acid-base balance of its fluids if imbalances occur.

Acid-base regulation requires a series of coordinated homeostatic mechanisms that involve the blood and other body fluids, the lungs, and kidneys. Ultimately all of these mechanisms are based on chemical processes. Recall that many important chemical principles related to the life process were covered in Chapter 2. You may want to refer back to those principles of biochemistry as you study in this chapter how the body so precisely regulates its acid-base balance.

STUDY TIPS
Learning the concepts presented in this chapter will be easier if you review a little basic chemistry.

1. The pH scale, acids, and bases are covered at the beginning of the chapter. If you need more of an explanation than that presented here, review Chapter 2.

2. Buffer systems can be thought of as hydrogen or hydroxide ion sponges. They remove those ions so they will have less of an effect on the pH of a solution, in this case, the blood. In the $NaHCO_3$–H_2CO_3 buffer system, the sodium bicarbonate can absorb hydrogen ions by having the hydrogen replace the sodium. The carbonic acid can give up one of its hydrogen atoms that then can react with a hydroxide ion to form water. In both cases the pH of the solution will change very little.

3. Blood carries carbon dioxide as carbonic acid. When the lungs exhale carbon dioxide, there is less carbonic acid in the blood and so the pH of the

continued on page 601

pH of Body Fluids

Water and all water solutions contain **hydrogen ions (H⁺)** and **hydroxide ions (OH⁻).** pH is an acronym for "power of H⁺." The term **pH** followed by a number indicates a solution's relative hydrogen ion concentration compared to hydroxide concentration.

At pH 7.0 a solution contains an equal concentration of hydrogen and hydroxide ions. Therefore pH 7.0 also indicates that a fluid is neutral in reaction (that is, neither acid nor alkaline) (Figure 21-1). The pH of pure water, for example, is 7.0.

A pH higher than 7.0 indicates an alkaline, or basic, solution (that is, one with a lower concentration of hydrogen than hydroxide ions). The more alkaline a solution, the higher is its pH value.

A pH lower than 7.0 indicates an acid solution (that is, one with a higher hydrogen ion concentration than hydroxide ion concentration). The higher the hydrogen ion concentration, the lower the pH and the more acid a solution is.

With a pH of about 1.6, gastric juice is the most acid substance in the body. Saliva has a pH of 7.7, on the alkaline side. Normally, the pH of arterial blood is about 7.45, and the pH of venous blood is about 7.35.

By applying the information given in the previous paragraph, you can deduce the answers to the following questions. Is arterial blood slightly acid or slightly alkaline? Is venous blood slightly acid or slightly alkaline? Which is a more accurate statement—venous blood is more acid than arterial blood or venous blood is less alkaline than arterial blood?

Arterial and venous blood are both slightly alkaline because both have a pH slightly higher than 7.0. Venous blood, however, is less alkaline than arterial blood because venous blood's pH of about 7.35 is slightly lower than arterial blood's pH of 7.45.

The pH unit is based on exponents of 10 from one unit to the next. That means that on the pH scale moving from one unit to the next multiplies the relative H⁺ concentration by 10 times. Thus the difference between pH 7 and pH 6 is a *tenfold* increase in H⁺. Moving from pH 7 to pH 5 is a *hundredfold* decrease in H⁺ concentration. This fact is important to remember when we look at the normal pH range of blood—what may seem like a small change in acidity at first glance is really 10 times bigger than it looks!

Mechanisms That Control pH of Body Fluids

The body has three mechanisms for regulating the pH of its fluids. They are (1) the buffer mechanism, (2) the respiratory mechanism, and (3) the urinary

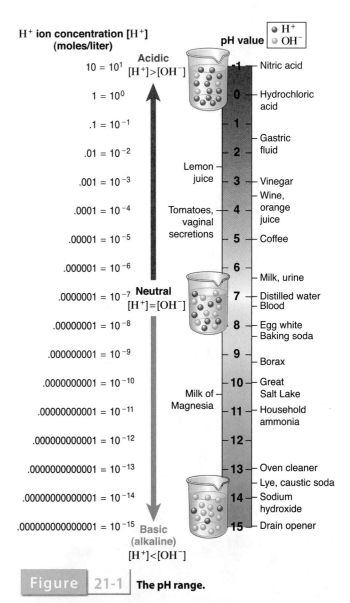

Figure 21-1 The pH range.

The overall pH range is expressed numerically on what is called a *logarithmic scale* of 1 to 14. This means that a change of 1 pH unit represents a tenfold difference in actual concentration of hydrogen ions. Note that as the concentration of H⁺ ions increases, the solution becomes increasingly acidic and the pH value decreases. As OH⁻ concentration increases, the pH value also increases, and the solution becomes more and more basic, or alkaline. A pH of 7 is neutral; a pH of 1 is very acidic, and a pH of 13 is very basic.

mechanism. Together, they constitute the complex pH homeostatic mechanism—the machinery that normally keeps blood slightly alkaline with a pH that stays remarkably constant. Its usual limits are very narrow, about 7.35 to 7.45.

The slightly lower pH of venous blood compared with arterial blood results primarily from carbon dioxide (CO_2) entering venous blood as a waste product of cellular metabolism. As carbon dioxide enters the blood, some of it combines with water (H_2O) and is converted into carbonic acid by **carbonic anhydrase (CA),** an enzyme found in red blood cells. The following chemical equation represents this reaction. If you need to review chemical formulas and equations, please refer to Chapter 2.

$$CO_2 + H_2O \xrightarrow{\text{carbonic anhydrase}} H_2CO$$

The lungs remove the equivalent of over 30 L of carbonic acid each day from the venous blood by elimination of CO_2. This almost unbelievable quantity of acid is so well buffered that a liter of venous blood contains only about $1/100,000,000$ g more H^+ than does 1 L of arterial blood. What incredible constancy! The pH homeostatic mechanism does indeed control effectively—astonishingly so.

Integration of the three homeostatic mechanisms that act to maintain the pH of body fluids is illustrated in Figure 21-2. Think of the circulating blood and RBCs as providing a *chemical pH control mechanism,* which is based on buffers (discussed below), and which acts immediately to help prevent harmful swings in pH when added acids or bases enter body fluids. If this immediate-acting chemical control mechanism is unable to stabilize the pH, the lungs and kidneys can both provide a *physiological pH control mechanism* to halt and reverse harmful pH shifts. The lungs respond in 1 to 2 minutes when the brainstem adjusts the respiratory rate (see Figure 16-16) and thus the elimination of CO_2 is accomplished. If the respiratory mechanism is unable to stop the pH shift, powerful but slower-acting renal mechanisms will be initiated within 24 hours. Details of each mechanism are discussed in the paragraphs that follow.

Buffers

Buffers are chemical substances that prevent a sharp change in the pH of a fluid when an acid or base is added to it. Strong acids and bases, if added to blood, would "dissociate" almost completely and release large quantities of H^+ or OH^- ions. The result would be drastic changes in blood pH. Survival itself depends on protecting the body from such drastic pH changes.

More acids than bases are usually added to body fluids. This is because catabolism, a process that goes on continually in every cell of the body, produces acids that enter blood as it flows through tissue capillaries. Almost immediately, one of the salts present in blood—a buffer, that is—reacts with these relatively strong acids to change them into weaker acids. The weaker acids decrease blood pH only slightly, whereas the stronger acids formed by catabolism would have decreased it greatly if they were not buffered.

Buffers consist of two kinds of substances and are therefore often called **buffer pairs.** One of the main blood buffer pairs is ordinary baking soda (sodium bicarbonate, or $NaHCO_3$) and carbonic acid (H_2CO_3).

Let us consider, as a specific example of buffer action, how the $NaHCO_3$–H_2CO_3 system works with a strong acid or base.

If, on the other hand, a strong base, such as sodium hydroxide (NaOH), were added to the same buffer system, the reaction shown in Figure 21-4 would take place. The H^+ of H_2CO_3 (H • HCO_3), the weak

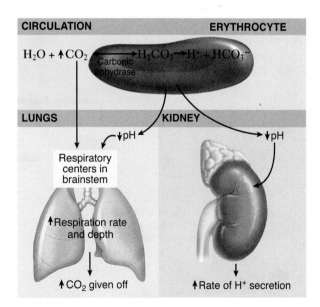

Figure 21-2 | **Integration of pH control mechanisms.**

Elevated CO_2 levels result in increased formation of carbonic acid in red blood cells. The resulting increase in hydrogen ions, coupled with elevated CO_2 levels, results in an increase in respiratory rate and secretion of hydrogen ions by the kidneys, thus helping to regulate the pH of body fluids.

acid of the buffer pair, combines with the OH⁻ of the strong base NaOH to form H_2O. Note what this accomplishes. It decreases the number of OH⁻ ions added to the solution, and this in turn prevents the drastic rise in pH that would occur without buffering.

Figure 21-3 shows how a buffer system works with a strong acid. Although useful in demonstrating the principles of buffer action, HCl or similar strong acids are never introduced directly into body fluids under normal circumstances. Instead, the $NaHCO_3$ buffer system is most often called on to buffer a number of weaker acids produced during catabolism. Lactic acid is a good example. As a weak acid, it does not "dissociate" as completely as HCl. Incomplete dissociation of lactic acid results in fewer hydrogen ions being added to the blood and a less drastic lowering of blood pH than would occur if HCl were added in an equal amount.

Without buffering, however, lactic acid buildup results in significant H⁺ accumulation over time. The resulting decrease of pH can produce serious acidosis. Ordinary baking soda (sodium bicarbonate, or $NaHCO_3$) is one of the main buffers of the normally occurring "fixed" acids in blood. Lactic acid is one of the most abundant of the "fixed" acids (acids that do not break down to form a gas).

Figure 21-5 shows the compounds formed by buffering of lactic acid (a "fixed" acid), produced by normal catabolism. The following changes

in blood result from buffering of fixed acids in tissue capillaries:

1. The amount of H_2CO_3 in blood increases slightly because an acid (such as lactic acid) is converted to H_2CO_3.

2. The amount of bicarbonate in blood (mainly $NaHCO_3$) decreases because bicarbonate ions become part of the newly formed H_2CO_3. Normal arterial blood with a pH of 7.45 contains 20 times more $NaHCO_3$ than H_2CO_3. If this ratio decreases, blood pH decreases below 7.45.

3. The H⁺ concentration of blood increases slightly. H_2CO_3 adds hydrogen ions to blood, but it adds fewer of them than lactic acid would have because it is a weaker acid than lactic acid. In other words, the buffering mechanisms do not totally prevent blood hydrogen ion concen-tration from increasing. It simply minimizes the increase.

4. Blood pH decreases slightly because of the small increase in blood H⁺ concentration.

H_2CO_3 is the most abundant acid in body fluids because it is formed by the buffering of fixed acids and also because CO_2 forms it by combining with H_2O. Large amounts of CO_2, an end product of catabolism, continually pour into tissue capillary blood from cells. Much of the H_2CO_3 formed in blood diffuses into red blood cells where it is buffered by the potassi-

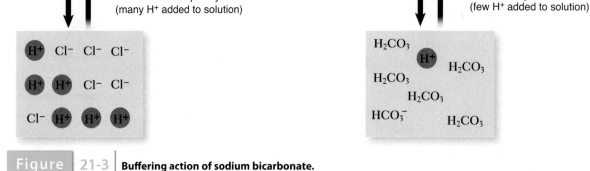

Figure 21-3 | **Buffering action of sodium bicarbonate.**

Buffering of acid HCl by $NaHCO_3$. As a result of the buffer action, the strong acid (HCl) is replaced by a weaker acid (H · HCO_3). Note that HCl, being a strong acid, "dissociates" almost completely and releases more H⁺ than H_2CO_3. Buffering decreases the number of H⁺ ions in the system.

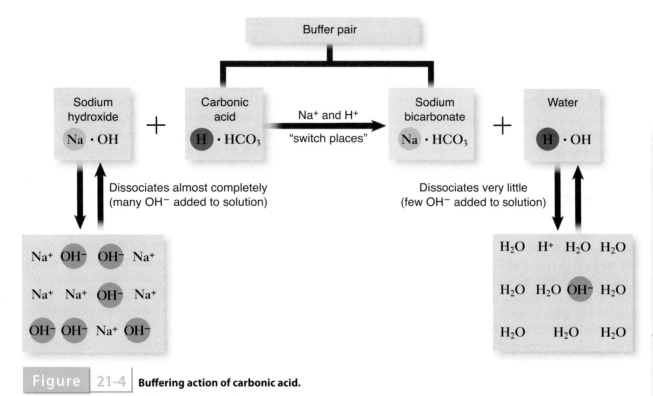

Figure 21-4 **Buffering action of carbonic acid.**

Buffering of base NaOH by H_2CO_3. As a result of buffer action, the strong base (NaOH) is replaced by $NaHCO_3$ and H_2O. As a strong base, NaOH "dissociates" almost completely and releases large quantities of OH^-. Dissociation of H_2O is minimal. Buffering decreases the number of OH^- ions in the system.

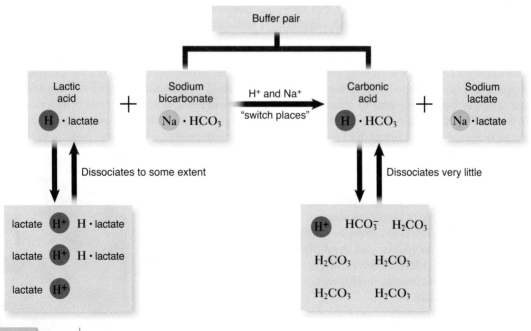

Figure 21-5 **Lactic acid buffered by sodium bicarbonate.**

Lactic acid (H · lactate) and other "fixed" acids are buffered by $NaHCO_3$ in the blood. Carbonic acid (H · HCO_3, or H_2CO_3, a weaker acid than lactic acid) replaces lactic acid. As a result, fewer H^+ ions are added to blood than would be added if lactic acid were not buffered.

um salt of hemoglobin. H_2CO_3 breaks down to form the gas CO_2 and water (H_2O). This takes place in the blood as it moves through the lung capillaries. The next several paragraphs explain how this affects blood pH.

> ## QUICK CHECK
>
> 1. What three mechanisms does the body have for regulating pH of body fluids?
> 2. What are buffers?

Respiratory Mechanism of pH Control

Respirations play a vital part in controlling pH. With every expiration, CO_2 and H_2O leave the body in the expired air. The CO_2 has diffused out of the venous blood as it moves through the lung capillaries. Less CO_2 therefore remains in the arterial blood leaving the lung capillaries, so less of it is available for combining with water to form H_2CO_3. Hence after expiration the arterial blood contains less H_2CO_3 and fewer hydrogen ions and has a higher pH (7.45) than does the venous blood (pH 7.35).

Let us consider now how a change in respirations can change blood pH. Suppose you were to pinch your nose shut and hold your breath for a full minute or a little longer. Obviously, no CO_2 would leave your body by way of expired air during that time, and the blood's CO_2 content would consequently increase. This would increase the amount of H_2CO_3 and the hydrogen-ion concentration of blood, which in turn would decrease blood pH.

However, this situation would not last for long. The respiratory control centers in your brainstem detect the dropping pH and rising CO_2 in your blood and respond strongly by forcing you to inhale (see Chapter 16, p. 468-470). This survival mechanism explains why a person cannot hold his or her breath indefinitely. It also explains why during exercise, a drop in pH caused by increased muscle production of CO_2 triggers an increase in breathing rate. Of course, the opposite is true as well—when blood pH increases to or above normal, then the rate of breathing slows.

Here then are two useful facts to remember. Anything that causes an appreciable decrease in respirations will in time produce **acidosis.** Conversely, anything that causes an excessive increase in respirations will in time produce **alkalosis.**

Urinary Mechanism of pH Control

Most people know that the kidneys are vital organs and that life soon ebbs away if they stop functioning. One reason is that the kidneys are the body's most effective regulators of blood pH. They can eliminate much larger amounts of acid than can the lungs and, if it becomes necessary, they can also excrete excess base. The lungs cannot. In short, the kidneys are the body's last and best defense against wide variations in blood pH. If they fail, homeostasis of pH—acid-base balance—fails.

Because more acids than bases usually enter blood, more acids than bases are usually excreted by the kidneys. In other words, most of the time the kidneys acidify urine; that is, they excrete enough acid to give urine an acid pH, frequently as low as 4.8. (How does this compare with normal blood pH?)

The distal tubules of the kidneys rid the blood of excess acid and at the same time conserve the base present in it by the two mechanisms illustrated by Figures 21-6 and 21-7. To understand these figures fully, you need to have some grasp of basic chemistry. If necessary, refer to Chapter 2 before proceeding.

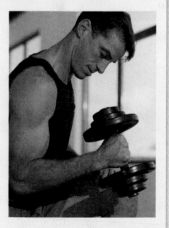

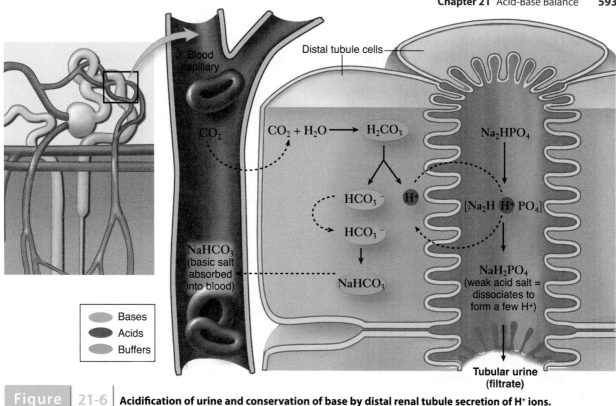

Bases
Acids
Buffers

Figure 21-6 | **Acidification of urine and conservation of base by distal renal tubule secretion of H⁺ ions.**

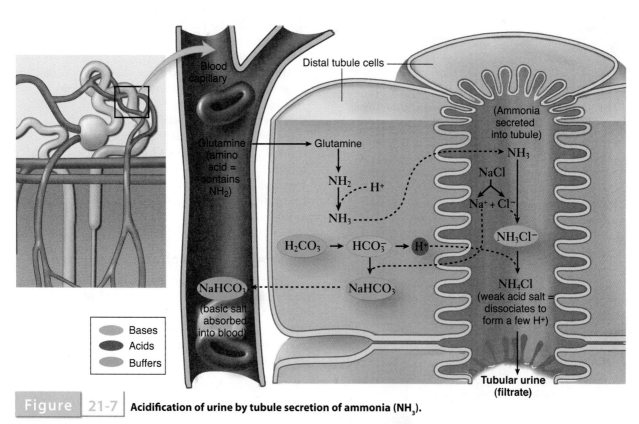

Figure 21-7 | **Acidification of urine by tubule secretion of ammonia (NH₃).**

An amino acid (glutamine) moves into the tubule cell and loses an amino group (NH₂) to form ammonia, which is secreted into urine. In exchange, the tubule cell reabsorbs a basic salt (mainly NaHCO₃) into blood from urine.

Now look at Figure 21-6 and find the CO_2 leaving the blood (as it flows through a kidney capillary) and entering one of the cells that helps form the wall of a distal kidney tubule. Note that in this cell the CO_2 combines with water to form H_2CO_3. This occurs rapidly because the cell contains carbonic anhydrase, an enzyme that accelerates this reaction. As soon as H_2CO_3 forms, some of it dissociates to yield hydrogen ions and bicarbonate ions. Note what happens to these ions. Hydrogen ions diffuse out of the tubule cell into the urine trickling down the tubule. There, it replaces one of the sodium ions (Na^+) in a salt (Na_2HPO_4) to form another salt (NaH_2PO_4), which leaves the body in the urine. Notice next that the Na^+ displaced from Na_2HPO_4 by the H^+ moves out of the tubular urine into a tubular cell. Here it combines with a bicarbonate (HCO_3^-) ion to form sodium bicarbonate, which then is resorbed into the blood.

What this complex of reactions has accomplished is to add hydrogen ions to the urine—that is, acidify it—and to conserve $NaHCO_3$ by reabsorbing it into the blood.

CLINICAL APPLICATION

DIABETIC KETOACIDOSIS

An important part of home care for diabetics involves monitoring the level of glucose in the blood and, especially for patients taking insulin, carefully watching for the appearance of **ketone bodies** in the urine.

Accumulation of these acidic substances in the blood results from the excessive metabolism of fats, most often in those people with uncontrolled type I diabetes. Some type II diabetics may also develop ketoacidosis under severe conditions. These individuals have trouble metabolizing carbohydrates and instead burn fat as a primary energy source. Ketone bodies are one way that the body transports the fatty acids from stored fat to other cells of the body.

The accumulation of ketone bodies results in a condition called **diabetic ketoacidosis** that causes the blood to become dangerously acidic. As blood levels of ketones increase, they "spill over" into the urine and can be detected by use of appropriate reagent strips. Ketones may also give a "fruity" odor to the breath and urine. As the body compensates for the acidosis, rapid breathing may occur.

Figure 21-7 illustrates another method of acidifying urine, as explained in the legend.

 To learn more about the urinary mechanism of pH control, go to **AnimationDirect** on your CD.

QUICK CHECK

1. How can breathing affect the pH of the blood?
2. By what mechanism can the kidney change the pH of the blood?

pH Imbalances

Acidosis and **alkalosis** are the two kinds of pH or acid-base imbalance. In acidosis the blood pH falls as H^+ ion concentration increases (or because of a loss of bases). Only rarely does it fall as low as 7.0 (neutrality) and almost never does it become even slightly acid, because death usually intervenes before the pH drops that much. In alkalosis, which develops less often than acidosis, the blood pH is higher than normal. Alkalosis results from a loss of acids or an accumulation of bases.

From a clinical standpoint, disturbances in acid-base balance can be considered dependent on the relative quantities (ratio) of H_2CO_3 and $NaHCO_3$ in the blood. Components of this important buffer pair must be maintained at the proper ratio (20 times more $NaHCO_3$ than H_2CO_3) if acid-base balance is to remain normal. It is fortunate that the body can regulate both chemicals in the $NaHCO_3$–H_2CO_3 buffer system. Blood levels of $NaHCO_3$ can be regulated by the kidneys and H_2CO_3 levels by the respiratory system (lungs).

Metabolic and Respiratory Disturbances

Two types of disturbances, metabolic and respiratory, can alter the proper ratio of these components. Metabolic disturbances affect the bicarbonate ($NaHCO_3$) element of the buffer pair, and respiratory disturbances affect the H_2CO_3 element, as follows:

1. Metabolic disturbances
   a. Metabolic acidosis (bicarbonate deficit).
      Patients that have metabolic acidosis with a

CLINICAL APPLICATION

VOMITING

Vomiting, sometimes referred to as *emesis* (EM-e-sis), is the forcible emptying or expulsion of gastric and occasionally intestinal contents through the mouth. It can occur as a result of many stimuli, including foul odors or tastes, irritation of the stomach or intestinal mucosa caused by food poisoning, certain bacterial or viral infections, and alcohol intoxication.

A "vomiting center" in the brainstem regulates the many coordinated, but primarily involuntary, steps involved (see illustration). The pernicious vomiting of pregnancy, the severe and repetitive (cyclic) vomiting that sometimes occurs in childhood, especially with pyloric obstruction in infants, can be life threatening because of the fluid, electrolyte, and acid-base imbalances that may result.

One of the most frequent and serious complications of repetitive vomiting that continues over time is **metabolic alkalosis.** The bicarbonate excess of metabolic alkalosis results indirectly because of the massive loss of chloride. The lost chloride, which is a component of hydrochloric acid (HCl) in gastric secretions, is replaced by bicarbonate in the extracellular fluid. The result is metabolic alkalosis (see illustration). The body "compensates" for the imbalance by suppressing respirations to increase blood CO_2 levels and, ultimately, levels of H_2CO_3 in the extracellular fluid. The kidneys also assist in the compensation process by conserving H^+ and eliminating additional HCO_3^- in an alkaline urine.

Therapy to actually *restore* the buffer pair (NaHCO$_3$ to H$_2$CO$_3$) ratio to normal includes intravenous administration of chloride-containing solutions such as **normal saline.** The chloride ions of the solution replace the bicarbonate ions and thus help relieve the bicarbonate excess that is responsible for the imbalance.

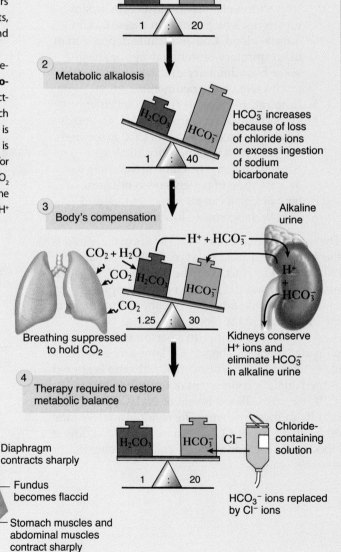

1 Metabolic balance before onset of alkalosis

H_2CO_3 HCO_3^-
1 : 20

2 Metabolic alkalosis

H_2CO_3 HCO_3^-
1 : 40

HCO_3^- increases because of loss of chloride ions or excess ingestion of sodium bicarbonate

3 Body's compensation

Alkaline urine

$CO_2 + H_2O$
CO_2 H_2CO_3 HCO_3^-
CO_2
$H^+ + HCO_3^-$
$H^+ + HCO_3^-$
1.25 : 30

Breathing suppressed to hold CO_2

Kidneys conserve H^+ ions and eliminate HCO_3^- in alkaline urine

4 Therapy required to restore metabolic balance

H_2CO_3 HCO_3^- Cl^-
1 : 20

Chloride-containing solution

HCO_3^- ions replaced by Cl^- ions

Hypersalivation occurs

Larynx and hyoid bone are drawn forward

Cardiac sphincter relaxes

Soft palate rises

Epiglottis closes

Diaphragm contracts sharply

Fundus becomes flaccid

Stomach muscles and abdominal muscles contract sharply

bicarbonate deficit often suffer from renal disease, uncontrolled diabetes, prolonged diarrhea, or have ingested toxic chemicals such as antifreeze (ethylene glycol) or wood alcohol (methanol).

   b. Metabolic alkalosis (bicarbonate excess). The bicarbonate excess in metabolic alkalosis can result from diuretic therapy, loss of acid-containing gastric fluid caused by vomiting or suction, or from certain diseases such as Cushing syndrome.

2. Respiratory disturbances

   a. Respiratory acidosis (H_2CO_3 excess). The increase in H_2CO_3 characteristic of respiratory acidosis is caused most often by slow breathing, which results in excess CO_2 in arterial blood. Causes include depression of the respiratory center by drugs or anesthesia or by pulmonary diseases such as emphysema and pneumonia.

   b. Respiratory alkalosis (H_2CO_3 deficit). Hyperventilation leads to an H_2CO_3 deficit caused by excessive loss of CO2 in expired air. The result is respiratory alkalosis. Anxiety (hyperventilation syndrome), overinflation of patients on ventilators, or hepatic coma can all reduce H_2CO_3 and CO2 to dangerously low levels.

The *ratio* of $NaHCO_3$ to H_2CO_3 levels in the blood is the key to acid-base balance. If the normal ratio ($20:1$ $NaHCO_3/H_2CO_3$) can be maintained, the acid-base balance and pH remain normal despite changes in the absolute amounts of either component of the buffer pair in the blood.

As a clinical example, in a person suffering from untreated diabetes, abnormally large amounts of acids enter the blood. The normal 20:1 ratio is altered as the $NaHCO_3$ component of the buffer pair reacts with the acids. Blood levels of $NaHCO_3$ decrease rapidly in these patients. The result is a lower *ratio* of $NaHCO_3$ to H_2CO_3 (perhaps 10:1) and lower blood pH. The condition is called *uncompensated metabolic acidosis*.

The body attempts to correct or *compensate* for the acidosis by altering the *ratio* of $NaHCO_3$ to H_2CO_3. Acidosis in a diabetic patient is often accompanied by rapid breathing or hyperventilation. This compensatory action of the respiratory system results in a "blow-off" of CO_2. Decreased blood levels of CO_2 result in lower H_2CO_3 levels. A new compensated ratio of $NaHCO_3$ to H_2CO_3 (perhaps 10:0.5) may result. In such individuals the blood pH returns to normal or near-normal levels. The condition is called *compensated metabolic acidosis*.

QUICK CHECK

1. What is acidosis? What is alkalosis?
2. What factors may cause a metabolic disturbance in pH?
3. What situations may cause a respiratory disturbance in pH?
4. How does vomiting sometimes create an acid-base imbalance?

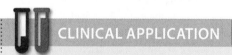

CLINICAL APPLICATION

LACTIC ACIDOSIS AND METFORMIN

Metformin hydrochloride (Glucophage) is one of the most widely used and effective of the oral antidiabetic drugs. It is used along with diet and exercise to lower blood glucose levels in those with type 2 diabetes mellitus. A rare but very serious complication of metformin therapy is *lactic acidosis*. It is characterized by elevated blood lactate levels, electrolyte disturbances, and decreased blood pH. It is reported in only about 1 in 33,000 patients taking metformin over the course of a year. However, when it does occur, it can be fatal in nearly 50% of cases.

Symptoms of this complication include a variety of gastrointestinal and respiratory complaints and feelings of weakness and muscle pain. Patients with kidney and liver disease are known to be at higher risk of developing lactic acidosis while taking the drug.

SCIENCE APPLICATIONS

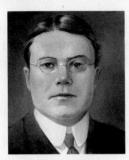

Walter Bradford Cannon
(1871–1945)

THE BODY IN BALANCE

Keeping the pH of the body stable is but one aspect of maintaining health. The American physiologist Walter Cannon gave us a name for the principle of balance, or constancy, of the internal fluid environment of the body—*homeostasis*. In 1932, his popular book *The Wisdom of the Body* finally gave a name to the concept first explained by Claude Bernard seven decades earlier (see p. 580). However, Cannon did more than name the concept. In his book, Cannon explained the incredibly complex set of mechanisms that allow our bodies to adjust to tremendous internal and external fluctuations that would otherwise kill us.

Much of Cannon's thought came from his groundbreaking discoveries in how the body copes with stress. In examining the fight-or-flight response, the effects of emotional stimuli, the mechanisms of cardiovascular shock, and in developing the "case study" approach to learning about human health and disease, Walter Cannon developed a clear understanding of the interactive nature of the organs of the body. It was Cannon who led scientists to look at their work in this new framework that explains the "big picture" of human body function.

Cannon's explanation of homeostasis revolutionized the way we look at the body—and how we look at patient care. As with fluid and electrolyte balance, knowledge of the mechanisms of acid-base balance is critical in providing direct patient care. Therefore, many physicians, nurses, IV therapists, first responders (e.g., emergency medical technicians and paramedics) and others need a basic knowledge of how the body maintains a constancy of pH in the blood.

Outline Summary

To download an MP3 version of the chapter summary for use with your iPod or portable media player, access the **Audio Chapter Summaries** on your CD.

pH of Body Fluids (Figure 21-1)

A. pH—a number that indicates the relative hydrogen ion (H^+) concentration (compared to OH^-) of a fluid
  1. pH 7.0 indicates neutrality (neutral solution)
  2. pH higher than 7.0 indicates alkalinity (alkaline or basic solution; base)
  3. pH less than 7.0 indicates acidity (acid solution)
B. Normal range of blood pH is approximately 7.35 to 7.45
  1. Arterial blood pH—about 7.45
  2. Venous blood pH—about 7.35
C. pH scale based on multiples of 10
  1. H+ concentration changes by 10 times for each pH unit
  2. Large pH fluctuations may appear small

Mechanisms that Control pH of Body Fluids (Figure 21-2)

A. pH homeostatic mechanism—three coordinated homeostatic mechanisms act to maintain the normal pH of body fluids and prevent pH swings when excess acids or bases are present

1. Chemical pH control mechanism—based on buffers in blood/RBCs/and body fluids—act immediately
2. Physiological pH control mechanisms
   a. Changes in pH regulated by changes in respiratory rate that result in changes in blood CO_2—act within minutes
   b. Changes in pH regulated by altered renal activity—act within hours

B. Buffers
1. Definition—chemical substances that prevent a sharp change in the pH of a fluid when an acid or base is added to it (Figures 21-3 and 21-4)
2. Buffers usually include two different chemicals—called a *buffer pair*
3. "Fixed" acids are buffered mainly by sodium bicarbonate ($NaHCO_3$)
4. Changes in blood produced by buffering of "fixed" acids in the tissue capillaries
   a. Amount of carbonic acid (H_2CO_3) in blood increases slightly
   b. Amount of $NaHCO_3$ in blood decreases; ratio of amount of $NaHCO_3$ to the amount of H_2CO_3 does not normally change; normal ratio is 20:1
   c. H^+ concentration of blood increases slightly
   d. Blood pH decreases slightly below arterial level

C. Respiratory mechanism of pH control
1. Respirations remove some CO_2 from blood as blood flows through lung capillaries
2. Amount of H_2CO_3 in blood is decreased and thereby its H^+ concentration is decreased; this in turn increases blood pH from its venous to its arterial level
3. Respiratory control centers in brainstem react to dropping pH and promote increased respirations; when pH increases, then breathing slows

D. Urinary mechanism of pH control
1. Kidneys are the body's most effective regulator of blood pH
2. Usually urine is acidified by way of the distal tubules secreting hydrogen ions and ammonia (NH_3) into the urine from blood in exchange for $NaHCO_3$ being reabsorbed into the blood

pH Imbalances

A. Acidosis and alkalosis are the two kinds of pH, or acid-base, imbalances
1. Disturbances in acid-base balance depend on relative quantities of $NaHCO_3$ and H_2CO_3 in the blood
2. Body can regulate both of the components of the $NaHCO_3$–H_2CO_3 buffer system
   a. Blood levels of $NaHCO_3$ are regulated by kidneys
   b. H_2CO_3 levels are regulated by lungs

B. Metabolic and respiratory disturbances—both can alter the normal 20:1 ratio of $NaHCO_3$ to H_2CO_3 in blood
1. Metabolic disturbances affect the $NaHCO_3$ levels in blood
   a. Metabolic acidosis—bicarbonate ($NaHCO_3$) deficit
   b. Metabolic alkalosis—bicarbonate ($NaHCO_3$) excess; complication of severe vomiting (see box, p. 595)
2. Respiratory disturbances affect the H_2CO_3 levels in blood
   a. Respiratory acidosis (H_2CO_3 excess)
   b. Respiratory alkalosis (H_2CO_3 deficit)
3. In *uncompensated metabolic acidosis*, the normal ratio of $NaHCO_3$ to H_2CO_3 is changed
4. In *compensated metabolic acidosis*, the ratio remains at 20:1, but the total amount of $NaHCO_3$ and H_2CO_3 changes

New Words

acid-base balance	hydroxide ion (HO⁻)	**Diseases and Other**	metabolic alkalosis
bicarbonate loading	ketone bodies	**Clinical Terms**	respiratory acidosis
buffer pairs	normal saline	diabetic ketoacidosis	respiratory alkalosis
carbonic anhydrase (CA)	pH	metabolic acidosis	
hydrogen ion (H⁺)			

Review Questions

1. Explain the relationship between pH and the relative concentration of hydrogen and hydroxide ions in a solution.
2. Write out the chemical reaction formula that converts carbon dioxide and water to carbonic acid. What enzyme catalyzes this reaction?
3. What is a buffer?
4. Explain how a buffer pair would react if more hydrogen ions were added to the blood.
5. Explain how a buffer pair would react if more hydroxide ions were added to the blood.
6. List the four changes that occur in the blood as the result of buffering fixed acids.
7. Explain the respiratory mechanism of pH control.
8. Describe how changes in the respiration rate can affect blood pH.
9. Explain how the chemical reaction that occurs in the distal tubule of the kidney using NaH_2PO_4 removes hydrogen ions from the blood.
10. Define *acidosis* and *alkalosis*.
11. Explain metabolic disturbances of the buffer pair.
12. Explain respiratory disturbances of the buffer pair.

Critical Thinking

13. Explain how excessive vomiting causes metabolic alkalosis and explain why normal saline can be used to correct it.
14. What is the proper ratio of $NaHCO_3$ and H_2CO_3 in a buffer pair? Explain how the body can use this ratio to correct uncompensated metabolic acidosis.

Chapter Test

1. The enzyme that converts carbon dioxide and water into carbonic acid is _____.
2. _____ are chemicals that prevent sharp changes in pH when an acid or base is added to a solution.
3. If a strong acid such as HCl were added to the buffer pair $NaHCO_3$ and H_2CO_3, the $NaHCO_3$ would become _____.
4. If a strong base such as NaOH were added to the buffer pair in question 3, the H_2CO_3 would become _____.
5. The part of the nephron that is important in regulation of blood pH is the _____.
6. When Na_2HPO_4 is used by the kidney to remove hydrogen ions from the blood, the end product that leaves the body in the urine is

   _____.
7. When ammonia is used by the kidney to remove hydrogen ions from the blood, the end product that leaves the body in the urine is

   _____.
8. The kidney is more effective in pH regulation than the lung because it can remove _____, which the lung cannot.
9. The condition in which the blood pH is higher than normal is called _____.
10. The condition in which the blood pH is lower than normal is called _____.
11. In order for the buffer pair to function correctly, the concentration of $NaHCO_3$ must be _____ times greater than the concentration of H_2CO_3.
12. Metabolic disturbances usually have an effect on the _____ part of the buffer pair.
13. Respiratory disturbances usually have an effect on the _____ part of the buffer pair.
14. Severe vomiting is a metabolic disturbance that can cause metabolic _____.
15. An acid solution has:
    a. a pH greater than 7.0
    b. a pH less than 7.0

    c. more hydroxide ions than hydrogen ions
    d. both b and c
16. An alkaline solution has:
    a. a pH greater than 7.0
    b. a pH less than 7.0
    c. more hydrogen ions than hydroxide ions
    d. both b and c
17. Which of the following statements is true?
    a. A solution with a pH of 5 has more hydrogen ions than a solution with a pH of 2.
    b. A solution with a pH of 9 is a base.
    c. The pH value increases as the number of hydrogen ions increases.
    d. Both a and c are true.
18. Arterial blood has a pH of 7.45, and venous blood has a pH of 7.35; therefore:
    a. arterial blood is slightly more acid than venous blood
    b. arterial blood is slightly more alkaline than venous blood
    c. venous blood is slightly more alkaline than arterial blood
    d. both a and c

For questions 19 through 24, fill in the blank with either *increases* or *decreases*, as appropriate.

19. When a fixed acid is buffered in the blood, the amount of $NaHCO_3$ in the blood _____.
20. When a fixed acid is buffered in the blood, the amount of hydrogen ions in the blood

    _____.
21. When a fixed acid is buffered in the blood, the amount of H_2CO_3 in the blood _____.
22. When a fixed acid is buffered in the blood, the pH of the blood _____.
23. Anything that causes an excessive increase in the respiration rate causes the pH of the blood to _____.
24. Anything that causes an appreciable decrease in the respiration rate causes the pH of the blood to _____.

Study Tips

continued from page 587

blood rises. The kidneys use a similar buffer system to secrete hydrogen ions.

4. The buffer system in the blood usually works well, but it can be overwhelmed. Acidosis is a condition in which the blood becomes too acidic, and alkalosis is a condition in which the blood becomes too basic.

5. If you have difficulty with the chemistry in this chapter, discuss it in your study group. Someone in the group may have a stronger chemistry background. Discuss the pH system. Carefully go over the diagrams of the blood and kidney buffer systems. Review the types of acidosis and alkalosis and what causes each of them. Go over the questions at the end of the chapter and discuss possible test questions.

Case Studies

1. Compensated respiratory acidosis is commonly found in persons with chronic bronchitis, an obstructive respiratory disorder discussed in Chapter 16. State what abnormal blood values a person should expect in such a case, and what factors produced them.

2. Larry is a diabetic who is suffering from metabolic acidosis. His breathing seems abnormally rapid. Is there a connection between Larry's acidosis and his rapid breathing? If so, explain the connection.

3. The hormone aldosterone affects kidney tubule function. One of its effects is to increase H^+ secretion by the kidney tubules. What effect does this action have on the pH of the internal environment (blood plasma)? What might occur if there is hypersecretion of aldosterone? Hyposecretion of aldosterone?

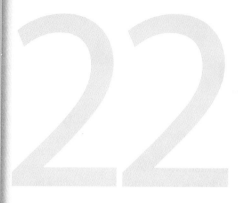

Outline

Objectives

After you have completed this chapter, you should be able to:

1. List the essential and accessory organs of the male and female reproductive systems and give the generalized function of each.

2. Describe the gross and microscopic structure of the gonads in both sexes and explain the developmental steps in spermatogenesis and oogenesis.

3. Discuss the primary functions of the sex hormones and identify the cell type or structure responsible for their secretion.

4. Identify and discuss the phases of the endometrial or menstrual cycle and correlate each phase with its occurrence in a typical 28-day cycle.

5. List the major disorders of the male and female reproductive systems and briefly describe each.

6. Define the term sexually transmitted disease and describe the major types.

22

The Reproductive Systems

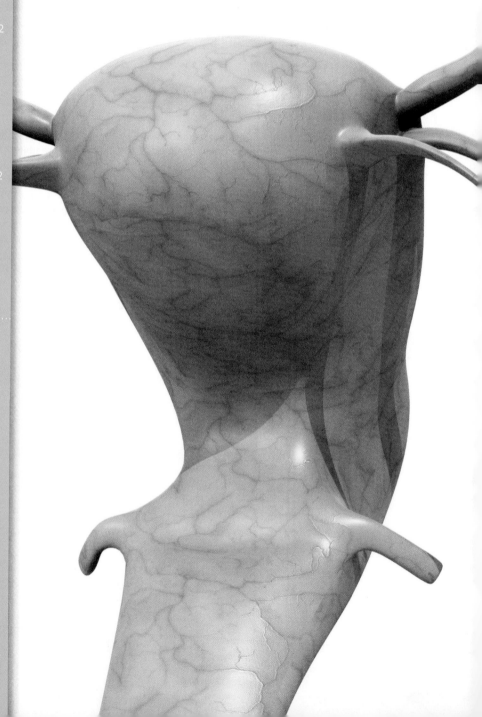

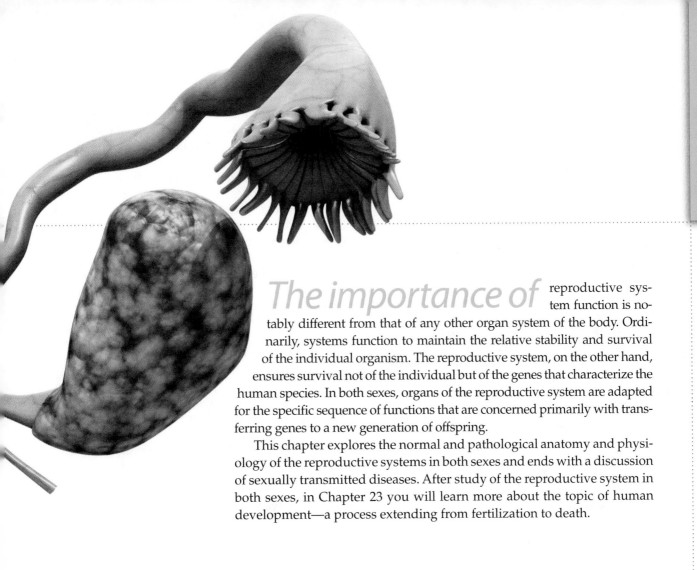

The importance of reproductive system function is notably different from that of any other organ system of the body. Ordinarily, systems function to maintain the relative stability and survival of the individual organism. The reproductive system, on the other hand, ensures survival not of the individual but of the genes that characterize the human species. In both sexes, organs of the reproductive system are adapted for the specific sequence of functions that are concerned primarily with transferring genes to a new generation of offspring.

This chapter explores the normal and pathological anatomy and physiology of the reproductive systems in both sexes and ends with a discussion of sexually transmitted diseases. After study of the reproductive system in both sexes, in Chapter 23 you will learn more about the topic of human development—a process extending from fertilization to death.

STUDY TIPS

Before studying Chapter 22, review the synopsis of the male and female reproductive systems in Chapter 4.

1. Much of Chapter 22 deals with the names, locations, and functions of the structures of the male and female reproductive systems. Make flash cards to help you learn this material.

2. Meiosis is the process of forming the male and female gametes. Gametes are reproductive cells with half the number of chromosomes of other body cells. Just before meiosis begins, the primary oocyte or spermatocyte doubles its chromosome number to 92. The first division produces cells with 46 chromosomes; the second division produces cells with 23 chromosomes.

3. The role of the male in reproduction is to produce as many sperm as possible, so four functional sperm are produced from meiosis. The female's role is the production of one egg containing 23 chromosomes; 69 of the original 92 chromosomes need to be "thrown away." This is the function of the polar bodies.

continued on page 637

Sexual Reproduction

Sexual reproduction requires two parent organisms, a male and female, each of which contributes half of the nuclear chromosomes needed to form the first cell of an offspring organism. *Asexual reproduction*, on the other hand, requires only one parent who produces an offspring genetically identical to itself. An advantage of sexual reproduction is that a new mixture of genes in each offspring increases the variety of genetic characteristics in the population. This variety of characteristics makes it more likely that in the case of environmental changes such as disease, natural disaster, or shifting climatic conditions, there will be at least some individuals likely to survive and carry on the reproductive line.

The reproductive system of each parent produces the sex or reproductive cells called **gametes** (GAM-eets) needed to form the offspring. These gametes, called an **ovum** (from the female parent) and a **sperm** (from the male parent), fuse during the process of fertilization. The new offspring cell that results is called the **zygote** (ZYE-gote). After many complicated and amazing developmental stages, the zygote ultimately develops into the new individual.

Each reproductive system also produces hormones that regulate development of the secondary sex characteristics that promote successful reproduction. For example, hormones create structural and behavioral differences in the sexes that permit adults to recognize and form sexual attractions with the opposite sex. Reproductive hormones and other regulatory mechanisms give us the urge to have sex, which is often reinforced with the pleasant sensations that sexual activity can produce. This sex drive is essential to success in producing offspring.

Sexual maturity and the ability to reproduce occur at puberty. The male reproductive system consists of organs whose functions are to produce, transfer, and ultimately introduce mature sperm into the female reproductive tract, where the nuclear chromosomes from each parent can unite to form a new offspring.

Common Structural and Functional Characteristics Between the Sexes

Although the organs and specific functions of the male and female reproductive systems will be discussed separately, it is important to understand that a common general structure and function can be identified between the systems in both sexes and that both sexes contribute in uniquely important ways to overall reproductive success.

In both men and women, the organs of the reproductive system are adapted for the specific sequence of functions that permit development of sperm or ova followed by successful fertilization and then the normal development and birth of a baby. In addition, production of hormones that permit development of secondary sex characteristics, such as breast development in women and beard growth in men, occurs as a result of normal reproductive system activity.

As you study the specifics of each system, keep in mind that the male organs function to produce, store, and ultimately introduce mature sperm into the female reproductive tract and that the female system is designed to produce ova, receive the sperm, and permit fertilization. In addition, the reproductive system in women permits the fertilized ovum to develop and mature until birth.

The complex and cyclic control of reproductive functions in both men and women are particularly crucial to overall reproductive success in humans. The production of sex hormones is required not only for development of the secondary sexual characteristics but also for normal reproductive functions in both sexes.

> **QUICK CHECK**
>
> 1. What are gametes?
> 2. What is the ultimate function of the reproductive systems?

Male Reproductive System

Structural Plan

So many organs make up the male reproductive system that we need to look first at the structural plan of the system as a whole. Reproductive organs can be classified as *essential* or *accessory.*

ESSENTIAL ORGANS

The essential organs of reproduction in men and women are called the **gonads.** The gonads of men consist of a pair of main sex glands called the **testes** (TES-teez). The testes produce the male sex cells, or **spermatozoa** (sper-mah-toh-ZOH-ah).

ACCESSORY ORGANS

The accessory organs of reproduction in men consist of the following structures:

Table 22-1	Male Reproductive Organs	
ESSENTIAL ORGANS	**ACCESSORY ORGANS**
Gonads: testes (right testis and left testis)	Ducts: epididymis (two), vas deferens (two), ejaculatory duct (two), and urethra
	Supportive sex glands: seminal vesicles (two), bulbourethral (Cowper) glands (two), and prostate gland
	External genitals: scrotum and penis

1. A series of passageways or ducts that carry the sperm from the testes to the exterior
2. Additional sex glands that provide secretions that protect and nurture sperm
3. The external reproductive organs called the *external genitals*

Table 22-1 lists the names of the essential and accessory organs of reproduction in men, and Figure 22-1 shows the location of most of them. The table and the illustration are included very early in the chapter to provide a preliminary but important overview. Refer back to this table and illustration frequently as you learn about each organ in the pages that follow.

Testes

STRUCTURE AND LOCATION

The paired **testes** are the gonads of men. They are located in the pouchlike **scrotum** (SKROH-tum), which is suspended outside of the body cavity behind the penis as you can see in Figure 22-1. This exposed location provides an environment about 1° to 3° C cooler than normal core body temperature, an important requirement for the normal production and survival of sperm.

Each testis is a small, oval gland about 3.8 cm (1.5 inches) long and 2.5 cm (1 inch) wide. The testis is shaped like an egg that has been flattened slight-

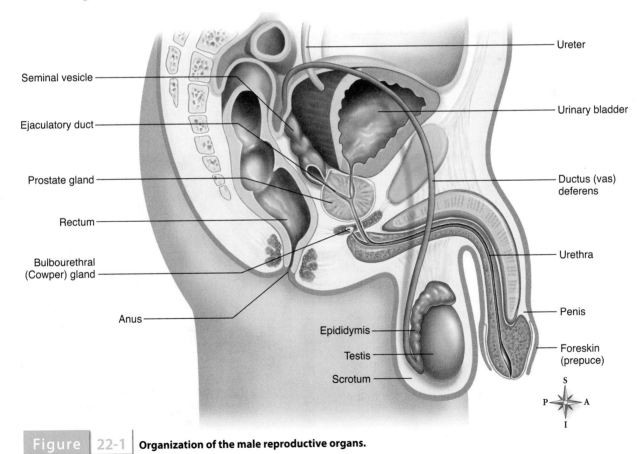

Figure 22-1 | **Organization of the male reproductive organs.**

Sagittal section of pelvis showing placement of male reproductive organs.

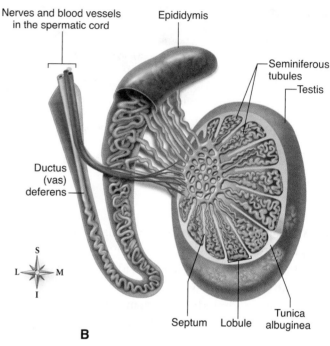

A

B

Figure 22-2 | Tubules of the testis and epididymis.

The ducts and tubules are exaggerated in size. In the photograph, the testis is the darker sphere in the center; note that the comma-shaped epididymis, seen on the left, is continuous with the ductus (vas) deferens.

ly from side to side. Note in Figure 22-2 that each testis is surrounded by a tough, whitish membrane called the **tunica** (TOO-ni-kah) **albuginea** (al-byoo-JIN-ee-ah). This membrane covers the testis and then enters the gland to form the many septa that divide it into sections or lobules.

As you can see in Figure 22-2, each lobule consists of a narrow but long and coiled **seminiferous** (seh-mi-NIF-er-us) **tubule.** These coiled structures form the bulk of the testicular tissue mass. Small endocrine cells lying near the septa that separate the lobules can be seen in Figure 22-3. These are the **interstitial cells** of the testes that secrete the male sex hormone **testosterone** (tes-TOS-teh-rone).

Each seminiferous tubule is a long duct with a central lumen or passageway (see Figure 22-3). Sperm develop in the walls of the tubule and are then released into the lumen and begin their journey to the exterior of the body.

TESTIS FUNCTIONS
Spermatogenesis
Sperm production is called **spermatogenesis** (sper-mah-toh-JEN-eh-sis). From puberty on, the seminifer-

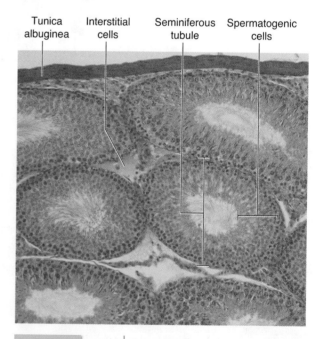

Figure 22-3 | Testis tissue.

Several seminiferous tubules surrounded by septa containing interstitial cells are shown.

ous tubules continuously form spermatozoa, or sperm. Although the number of sperm produced each day diminish with increasing age, most men continue to produce significant numbers throughout life.

The testes prepare for sperm production before puberty by increasing the numbers of sperm precursor (stem) cells called **spermatogonia** (sper-mah-toh-GO-nee-ah). These cells are located near the outer edge of each seminiferous tubule (Figure 22-4, *A*). Before puberty, spermatogonia increase in number by the process of mitotic cell division, which was described in Chapter 3. Recall that mitosis results in the division of a "parent" cell into two "daughter" cells, each identical to the parent and each containing a complete copy of the genetic material represented in the normal number of 46 chromosomes.

When a boy enters puberty, circulating levels of follicle-stimulating hormone (FSH) cause a spermatogonium to undergo a unique type of cell division. When the spermatogonium undergoes cell division and mitosis under the influence of FSH, it produces two daughter cells. One of these cells remains as a spermatogonium and the other forms another type of cell called a **primary spermatocyte** (sper-MAH-toh-cyte). These primary spermatocytes then undergo a type of cell division characterized by **meiosis** (my-OH-sis), which ultimately results in sperm formation.

Note in Figure 22-4, *B*, that in meiosis two cell divisions occur (not one as in mitosis) and that four daughter cells (not two as in mitosis) are formed. The daughter cells are called **spermatids** (SPER-mah-tids). Unlike the two daughter cells that result from mitosis, the four spermatids each have only half the genetic material in its nucleus and half of the nuclear chromosomes (23) of other body cells. These spermatids then develop into spermatozoa.

In women, meiosis results in a single ovum, which also has only 23 chromosomes. This will be discussed in more detail later in the chapter.

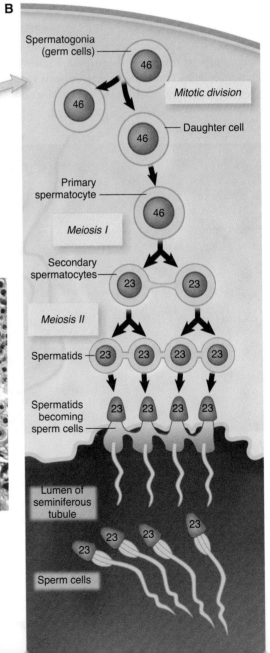

A, Cross section of tubule shows progressive meiotic cell types in the wall of a seminiferous tubule. **B,** Diagram of meiotic events and cell types leading to sperm formation.

A

Figure 22-4 | **Spermatogenesis.**

Look again at the diagram of meiosis in Figure 22-4, *B*. It shows that each primary spermatocyte ultimately produces four sperm cells. Note that, in the portion of a seminiferous tubule shown in Figure 22-4, spermatogonia are found at the outer surface of the tubule, primary and secondary spermatocytes lie deeper in the tubule wall, and mature but immotile sperm are seen about to enter the lumen of the tube and begin their journey through the reproductive ducts to the exterior of the body.

 To learn more about spermatogenesis, go to **AnimationDirect** on your CD.

Spermatozoa

Spermatozoa are among the smallest and most unusual cells in the body (Figure 22-5, *A*). All of the characteristics that a baby will inherit from its father at fertilization are contained in the condensed nuclear (genetic) material found in each sperm head. However, this genetic information from the father can fuse with genetic material contained in the mother's ovum only if successful fertilization occurs. The forceful ejection of fluid containing sperm, or **ejaculation**, into the female vagina during sexual intercourse is only one step in the long journey that these sex cells must make before they can meet and fertilize an ovum. To accomplish their task, these tiny packages of genetic information are equipped with tails for motility and are designed to penetrate the outer membrane of the ovum when contact occurs with it.

The structure of a mature sperm is diagrammed in Figure 22-5, *B*. Note the sperm head containing the nucleus with its genetic material from the father. The sperm head is covered by the **acrosome** (AK-roh-sohm)—a caplike structure containing enzymes that enable the sperm to break down the covering of the ovum and permit entry if contact occurs.

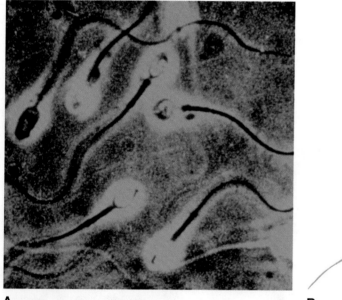

A

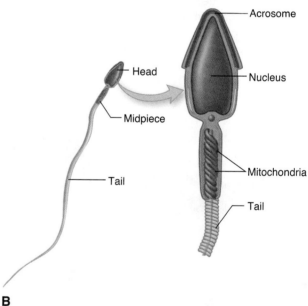

B

Figure 22-5 | **Human sperm.**

A, Micrograph shows the heads and long, slender tails of many spermatozoa. **B,** Illustration shows the components of a mature sperm cell and an enlargement of a sperm head and midpiece.

In addition to the head with its covering acrosome, each sperm has a midpiece and an elongated tail. Mitochondria in the midpiece break down adenosine triphosphate (ATP) to provide energy for the tail movements required to propel the sperm and allow them to "swim" for relatively long distances through the female reproductive ducts.

Production of testosterone

In addition to spermatogenesis, the other function of the testes is to secrete the male hormone testosterone. This function is carried on by the interstitial cells of the testes, not by their seminiferous tubules. Testosterone serves the following general functions:

1. It masculinizes. The various characteristics that we think of as "male" develop because of testosterone's influence. For instance, when a young boy's voice changes, it is testosterone that brings this about.

2. It promotes and maintains the development of the male accessory organs (prostate gland, seminal vesicles, and so on).

3. It has a stimulating effect on protein anabolism. Testosterone thus is responsible for the greater muscular development and strength of the male.

A good way to remember testosterone's functions is to think of it as "the masculinizing hormone" and the "anabolic hormone."

> **QUICK CHECK**
>
> 1. What is the name of the male gonads?
> 2. In what specific structures of the gonad are the sperm produced?
> 3. What hormone is produced in the male gonad?

Reproductive Ducts

The ducts through which sperm must pass after exiting from the testes until they reach the exterior of the body are important components of the accessory reproductive structures. The other two components included in the listing of accessory organs of reproduction in the male—the supportive sex glands and external genitals—are discussed separately here.

Sperm are formed within the walls of the seminiferous tubules of the testes. When they exit from these tubules within the testis, they enter and then pass, in sequence, through the epididymis, ductus (vas) deferens, ejaculatory duct, and the urethra on their journey out of the body.

EPIDIDYMIS

Each **epididymis** (ep-i-DID-i-mis) consists of a single and very tightly coiled tube about 6 m (20 feet) in length. It is a comma-shaped structure (see Figure 22-2) that lies along the top and behind the testes inside the scrotum. Sperm mature and develop their ability to move, or swim, as they pass through the epididymis.

Epididymitis is a painful inflammation (the suffix *-itis* signifies "inflammation of") of the epididymis. It often occurs in association with sexually transmitted diseases, or STDs (see Table 22-4). The onset of pain is coupled with redness and swelling of the overlying scrotum, fever, and the appearance of white blood cells (WBCs) in the urine.

DUCTUS (VAS) DEFERENS

The **ductus** (DUK-tus) **deferens** (DEF-er-enz), or **vas deferens** is the tube that permits sperm to exit from the epididymis and pass from the scrotal sac upward into the abdominal cavity (Figure 22-1). Each ductus deferens is a thick, smooth, very muscular, and movable tube that can easily be felt or "palpated" through the thin skin of the scrotal wall. It passes through the inguinal canal into the abdominal cavity as part of the *spermatic cord,* a connective tissue sheath that also encloses blood vessels and nerves.

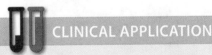
CLINICAL APPLICATION

VASECTOMY

Severing or clamping off the vas deferens—that is, a **vasectomy**, usually done through an incision in the scrotum—makes a man sterile. Why? Because it interrupts the route to the exterior from the epididymis. To leave the body, sperm must journey in succession through the epididymis, vas deferens, ejaculatory duct, and urethra.

EJACULATORY DUCT AND URETHRA

Once in the abdominal cavity, the ductus deferens extends over the top and down the posterior surface of the bladder, where it joins the duct from the seminal vesicle to form the **ejaculatory** (ee-JAK-yoo-lah-toe-ree) **duct.** Note in Figure 22-6 that the ejaculatory duct passes through the substance of the prostate gland and permits sperm to empty into the **urethra,** which eventually passes through the penis and opens to the exterior at the external urinary meatus.

 To learn more about male reproductive ducts, go to **AnimationDirect** on your CD.

Accessory or Supportive Sex Glands

The term **semen** (SEE-men), or **seminal fluid,** is used to describe the mixture of sex cells or sperm produced by the testes and the secretions of the accessory or supportive sex glands. The accessory glands, which contribute more than 95% of the secretions to the gelatinous fluid part of the semen, include the two seminal vesicles, one prostate gland, and two bulbourethral (Cowper) glands. In addition to the production of sperm, the seminiferous tubules of the testes contribute somewhat less than 5% of the seminal fluid volume.

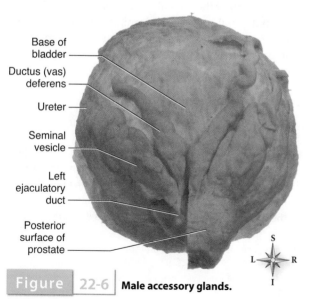

Base of bladder
Ductus (vas) deferens
Ureter
Seminal vesicle
Left ejaculatory duct
Posterior surface of prostate

Figure 22-6 | **Male accessory glands.**

Dissection photo showing bladder, prostate, ductus deferens, left ejaculatory duct, and seminal vesicles from behind.

Usually 3 to 5 ml (about 1 teaspoon) of semen is ejaculated at one time, and each milliliter normally contains about 100 million sperm. These numbers vary considerably in healthy men, even from day to day. Semen is slightly alkaline and protects sperm from the acidic environment of the female reproductive tract.

SEMINAL VESICLES

The paired **seminal vesicles** (Figure 22-1) are pouch-like glands that contribute about 60% of the seminal fluid volume. Their secretions are yellowish, thick, and rich in the sugar fructose. This fraction of the seminal fluid helps provide a source of energy for the highly motile sperm.

PROSTATE GLAND

The **prostate gland** lies just below the bladder and is shaped like a doughnut. The urethra passes through the center of the prostate before traversing the penis to end at the external urinary orifice.

The prostate secretes a thin, milk-colored fluid that constitutes about 30% of the total seminal fluid volume. This portion of the ejaculate helps to activate the sperm and maintain their motility.

BULBOURETHRAL GLANDS

Each of the two **bulbourethral** (BUL-bo-yoo-REE-thral) **glands** (also called *Cowper glands*) resemble peas in size and shape. They are located just below the prostate gland and empty their secretions into the penile portion of the urethra. The mucus-like secretions of these glands lubricate the terminal portion of the urethra to decrease friction damage to sperm at the time of ejaculation and contribute less than 5% of the seminal fluid volume.

External Genitals

The **penis** (PEE-nis) and **scrotum** constitute the external reproductive organs, or **genitalia** (jen-i-TAIL-yah) (or simply **genitals)** of men. The penis (Figure 22-7) is the organ that, when made stiff and erect by the filling of its spongy, or erectile, tissue components with blood during sexual arousal, can enter and deposit sperm in the vagina during intercourse. The penis has three separate columns of erectile tissue in its shaft: one **corpus** (KOR-pus) **spongiosum** (spun-jee-OH-sum), which surrounds the urethra, and two **corpora** (KOR-por-ah) **cavernosa** (kav-er-NO-sah), which lie above. The spongy nature of erectile tissue is apparent in Figure 22-7.

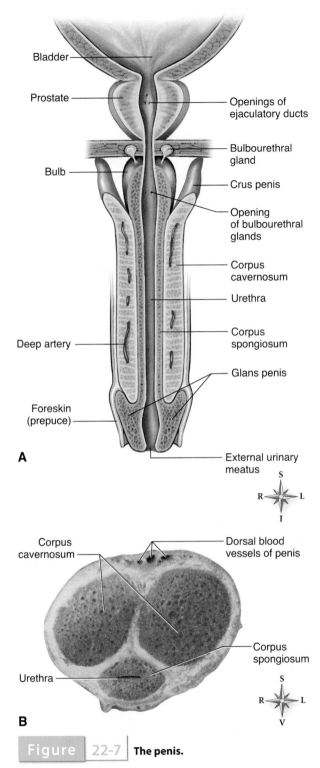

A, In this sagittal section of the penis viewed from above, the urethra is exposed throughout its length and can be seen exiting from the bladder and passing through the prostate gland before entering the penis to end at the external urinary meatus. **B,** Photograph of a cross section of the shaft of the penis showing the three columns of erectile or cavernous tissue. Note the urethra within the substance of the corpus spongiosum.

Figure 22-7 | The penis.

Labels (Part A):
- Bladder
- Prostate
- Bulb
- Deep artery
- Foreskin (prepuce)
- Openings of ejaculatory ducts
- Bulbourethral gland
- Crus penis
- Opening of bulbourethral glands
- Corpus cavernosum
- Urethra
- Corpus spongiosum
- Glans penis
- External urinary meatus

Labels (Part B):
- Corpus cavernosum
- Urethra
- Dorsal blood vessels of penis
- Corpus spongiosum

At the distal end of the shaft of the penis is the enlarged *glans penis,* or more simply **glans.** The external urinary meatus is the opening of the urethra at the tip of the glans.

The skin of the distal end of the penis is folded doubly to form a loose-fitting retractable collar around the glans called the **foreskin,** or **prepuce** (PRE-pus). Surgical removal of the foreskin is called **circumcision** (see Box).

The scrotum is a skin-covered pouch suspended from the groin. Internally, it is divided into two sacs by a septum; each sac contains a testis, epididymis, the lower part of the ductus deferens, and the beginning of the spermatic cords.

Disorders of the Male Reproductive System

Several disorders of the male reproductive system cause **infertility.** Infertility is an abnormally low ability to reproduce. If there is a complete inability to reproduce, the condition is called **sterility.** Infertility or sterility involves an abnormally reduced capacity to deliver healthy sperm to the female reproductive tract. Reduced reproductive capacity may result from factors such as a decrease in the testes' production of sperm, structural abnormalities in the sperm, or obstruction of the reproductive ducts.

Disorders of the Testes

Disruption of the sperm-producing function of the seminiferous tubules can result in decreased sperm production, a condition called **oligospermia** (ol-i-go-SPER-mee-ah). If the *sperm count* is too low, infertility may result. A large number of sperm is needed to ensure that many sperm will reach the ovum and dissolve its coating, allowing a single sperm to unite with the ovum. Oligospermia can result from factors such as infection, fever, radiation, malnutrition, and high temperature in the testes. In some cases, oligospermia is temporary—as in some acute infections. Oligospermia is a leading cause of infertility. Of course, total absence of sperm production results in sterility.

Early in fetal life the testes are located in the abdominal cavity near the kidneys but normally descend into the scrotum about 2 months before birth. Occasionally a baby is born with undescended testes, a condition called **cryptorchidism** (krip-TOR-ki-di-zem), which is readily observed by palpation of the scrotum at delivery. The word *cryptorchidism* is from the Greek words *kryptikos* (hidden) and *orchis* (testis). Failure of the testes to descend may be caused by hormonal imbalances in the developing fetus or by a physical deficiency or obstruction. Regardless of cause, in the cryptorchid infant, the testes remain "hidden" in the abdominal cavity. Because the higher temperature inside the body cavity inhibits spermatogenesis, measures must be taken to bring the testes down into the scrotum to prevent permanent sterility. Early treatment of this condition by injection of testosterone, which stimulates the testes to descend, may result in normal testicular and sexual development. The condition may also be corrected surgically.

Most *testicular tumors* are cancerous and arise from sperm-producing cells of the seminiferous tubules. Externally, they most often appear as a nontender mass fixed on the testis. Malignancies of the testes are most common among men 15 to 30 years old. In addition to age group, this type of cancer is associated with genetic predisposition, trauma or infection of the testis, and cryptorchidism.

Treatment of testicular cancer is most effective when the diagnosis is made early in the development of the tumor. Many physicians encourage male patients to perform monthly self-examination of their testes, especially if they are in a high-risk group. The self-examination involves palpating each testis—preferable after a warm shower when the scrotum is relaxed and the testes are descended and accessible. Each testis should be palpated through the scrotal wall between the thumb and the index and middle fingers. They should feel firm, smooth, and rubbery

but not hard. The examination may result in some tenderness but should not be painful. Any lump or change in texture should be reported to a physician for further assessment.

Disorders of the Prostate

A noncancerous condition called **benign** (bee-NINE) **prostatic hypertrophy** (hye-PER-troh-fee) **(BPH)** is a common problem in older men. The condition is characterized by an enlargement or hypertrophy of the prostate gland. The fact that the urethra passes through the center of the prostate after exiting from the bladder is a matter of considerable clinical significance in this condition. As the prostate enlarges, it squeezes the urethra, frequently closing it so completely that urination becomes very difficult or even impossible. In such cases, surgical removal of a part of or all of the gland, a procedure called **prostatectomy** (pross-tah-TEK-toh-mee), may become necessary. Other options, especially for treatment of cancerous prostatic growths, include systemic chemotherapy, cryotherapy (freezing) of prostatic tissue, microwave therapy, hormonal therapy, and various types of external beam x-ray radiation treatments.

A relatively recent treatment involves placing small radioactive "seeds" directly into the prostate tumor, where they give off very localized cancer-cell–destroying radiation for about a year. The treatment is called **brachytherapy** (BRAY-kee-ther-ah-pee)—from the Greek term "brachy"—meaning short distance. The radiation is limited to a short distance because the radioactive seeds are placed in or near the tumor itself, thus reducing any healthy tissue radiation exposure.

Disorders of the Penis and Scrotum

The penis is subject to *cancerous tumors* and is affected by numerous **sexually transmitted diseases,** or **STDs** (see Table 22-4). Development of herpes vesicles, genital warts, and various lesions of the foreskin, glans, and penile shaft are common. *Structural abnormalities* such as *phimosis* and *paraphimosis*, discussed in the box on p. 611), can obstruct the flow of urine or result in urinary tract infections.

The term **hypospadias** (hye-poh-SPAY-dee-us) describes a congenital condition that is characterized by the opening of the urethral meatus on the underside of the glans or penile shaft. Surgical correction is performed if the defect is likely to cause urological or reproductive problems. The term **epispadias** (ep-i-SPAY-dee-us) refers to a much less common congenital defect that involves the opening of the urethral meatus on the dorsal or top surface of the glans or penile shaft.

Failure to achieve an erection of the penis adequate enough to permit sexual intercourse is called **erectile dysfunction (ED)** or *impotence* (IM-poh-tense). ED affects men of all ages but is experienced most often after age 65. Impotence does not affect sperm production but infertility often results because normal intercourse may not be possible. In the past, psychological problems such as anxiety, depression, and stress were often cited as the most important causes of impotence in sexually active men. There is no doubt that such conditions contribute to ED. However, current research suggests that purely psychological problems probably account for far fewer cases of impotence than previously thought. We now know that ED is frequently caused by medical problems related to abnormal vascular or neural control of penile blood flow. Arteriosclerosis, diabetes, alcohol abuse, numerous medications, radiation therapy, tumors, spinal cord trauma, and surgery, especially if pelvic organs such as the prostate are involved, may all contribute to ED.

Treatment options for ED include use of drugs that increase blood flow to the spongy cavernous tissue of the penis causing it to stiffen and become erect. Oral medications such as Viagra (sildenafil), Levitra (vardenafil), Cialis (tadalafil), and Uprima (apomorphine) are generally preferred by men who do not have medical conditions that preclude their use. One drug called Muse (alprostadil) is available as a tiny soft pellet that is inserted into the urethra using a small applicator. A similar drug available in solution, Caverject, is injected directly into the penis. As a result of multiple options, even moderate to severe erectile dysfunction occurring in sexually active men can be treated with considerable success.

Swelling of the scrotum can be caused by a variety of conditions. One of the most common causes of scrotal swelling is an accumulation of fluid called a **hydrocele** (HYE-droh-seel). Hydroceles may be congenital, resulting from structural abnormalities present at birth. In adults, hydrocele often occurs when fluid produced by the serous membrane lining the scrotum is not absorbed properly. The cause of adult hydrocele is not always known, but in some cases, it can be linked to trauma or infection.

 CLINICAL APPLICATION

DETECTING PROSTATE CANCER

Many of the 32,000 men who die each year from *prostate cancer*—the most common non-skin form of cancer in American men and a leading cause of cancer deaths in men over 50—could be saved if the cancer was detected early enough to allow effective treatment. Several screening tests are now available for early detection of prostate cancer.

For example, physicians can sometimes detect prostate cancer early by palpating the prostate through the wall of the rectum using a gloved, lubricated finger. This is called a *digital rectal exam*.

Digital rectal examinations are sometimes performed in conjunction with a screening test called the *PSA test*. This test is a type of blood analysis that screens for **prostate-specific antigen (PSA)**, a substance sometimes found in the blood of men with prostate cancer.

Because of the prevalence of prostate cancer, adult men are encouraged to have regular prostate examinations and to report any urinary or sexual difficulty to their physicians.

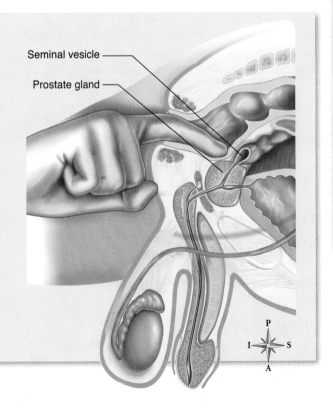

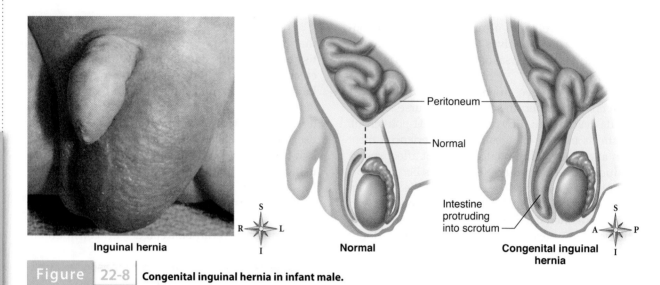

Inguinal hernia   Normal   Congenital inguinal hernia

Figure 22-8 | **Congenital inguinal hernia in infant male.**

Swelling of the scrotum may also occur when the intestines push through the weak area of the abdominal wall that separates the abdominopelvic cavity from the scrotum. This condition is a form of **inguinal** (IN-gwi-nal) **hernia.** If the intestines protrude too far into the scrotum, the digestive tract may become obstructed, resulting in death. In adults, inguinal hernia often occurs while lifting heavy objects, because of the high internal pressure generated by the contraction of abdominal muscles. Inguinal herniation also may be congenital (Figure 22-8). Small inguinal hernias may be treated with external supports that prevent organs from protruding into the scrotum; more serious hernias must be repaired surgically.

> **QUICK CHECK**
>
> 1. What duct leads from the epididymis?
> 2. Which organs produce the fluid in semen?
> 3. What is the function of erectile tissues?

Female Reproductive System

Structural Plan

The structural plan of the reproductive system in both sexes is similar in that organs are characterized as *essential* or *accessory.*

ESSENTIAL ORGANS

The essential organs of reproduction in women, the **gonads,** are the paired **ovaries.** The female sex cells, or **ova,** are produced in the ovaries.

ACCESSORY ORGANS

The accessory organs of reproduction in women consist of the following structures:

1. A series of ducts or modified duct structures that extend from near the ovaries to the exterior
2. Additional sex glands, including the mammary glands, which have an important reproductive function only in women
3. The external reproductive organs or external genitals

Table 22-2 lists the names of the essential and accessory organs of reproduction, and Figure 22-9 shows the location of most of them. Refer back to this table and illustration as you read about each structure in the pages that follow.

Ovaries

STRUCTURE AND LOCATION

The paired ovaries are the gonads of women. They have a puckered, uneven surface; each weighs about

Table 22-2	**Female Reproductive Organs**
ESSENTIAL ORGANS	**ACCESSORY ORGANS**
Gonads: ovaries (right ovary and left ovary)	Ducts: uterine tubes (two), uterus, vagina
	Accessory sex glands: vestibular glands (two pairs), breasts (two)
	External genitals: vulva

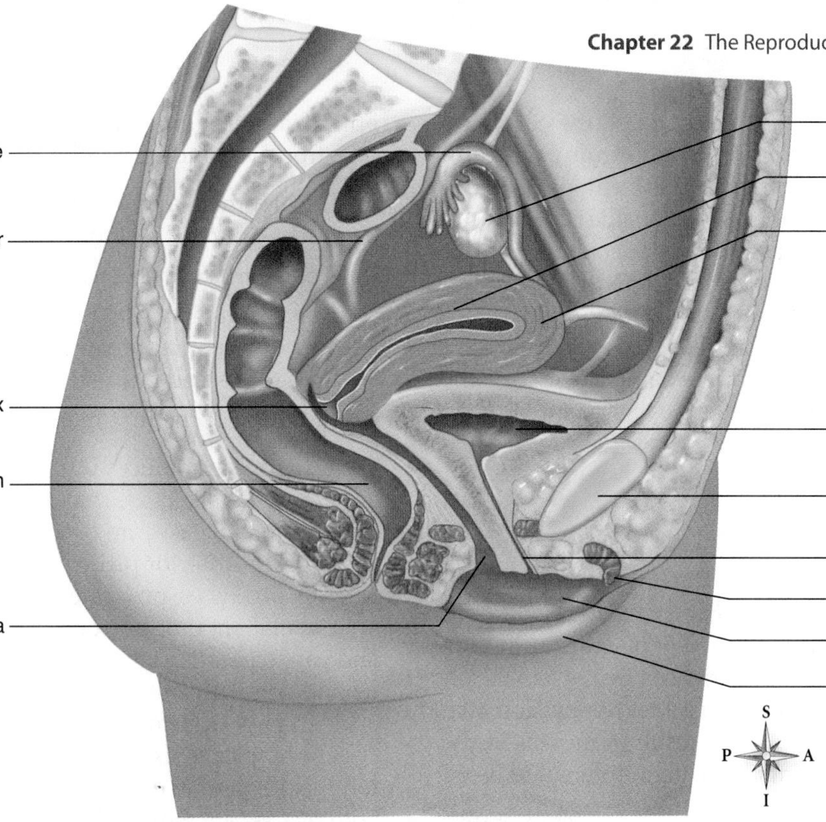

Uterine (fallopian) tube

Ureter

Cervix

Rectum

Vagina

Ovary

Body of uterus

Fundus of uterus

Urinary bladder

Symphysis pubis

Urethra

Clitoris

Labium minus

Labium majus

S
P — A
I

Figure 22-9 **Organization of the female reproductive organs.**

3 g. The ovaries resemble large almonds in size and shape and are attached to ligaments in the pelvic cavity on each side of the uterus.

Embedded in a connective tissue matrix just below the outer layer of each ovary in a newborn baby girl are about 1 million **ovarian follicles;** each contains an **oocyte,** an immature stage of the female sex cell. By the time a girl reaches puberty, however, further development has resulted in the formation of a reduced number (about 400,000) of what are then called **primary follicles.** Each primary follicle has a layer of **granulosa cells** around the oocyte. During the reproductive lifetime of most women, only about 350 to 500 of these primary follicles fully develop into *mature follicles.* It is the mature follicle that releases an ovum for potential fertilization—a process called **ovulation.** Follicles that do not mature degenerate and are reabsorbed into the ovarian tissue. The sac containing a mature ovum is sometimes called a **Graafian** (GRAHF-ee-an) **follicle,** in honor of the Dutch anatomist Regnier de Graaf who discovered them some 300 years ago.

The progression of development from primary follicle to ovulation is shown in Figure 22-10. As the thick-

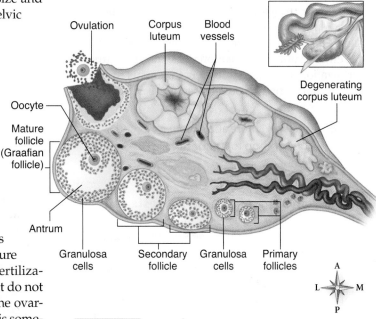

Ovulation Corpus luteum Blood vessels

Degenerating corpus luteum

Oocyte

Mature follicle (Graafian follicle)

Antrum

Granulosa cells

Secondary follicle

Granulosa cells

Primary follicles

A
L — M
P

Figure 22-10 **Diagram of ovary and oogenesis.**

Cross section of mammalian ovary shows successive stages of ovarian (Graafian) follicle and ovum development. Begin with the first stage (primary follicle) and follow around clockwise to the final state (degenerating corpus luteum).

ness of the granulosa cell layer around the oocyte increases, a hollow chamber called an **antrum** (AN-trum) appears, and a *secondary follicle* is formed. Development continues, and after ovulation, the ruptured follicle is transformed into a hormone-secreting glandular structure called the **corpus** (KOR-pus) **luteum** (LOO-tee-um), which is described later in this chapter. Corpus luteum is from the Latin word meaning "yellow body," an appropriate name to describe the yellow appearance of this glandular structure.

OVARY FUNCTIONS

Oogenesis
The production of female gametes, or sex cells, is called **oogenesis** (o-o-JEN-eh-sis). The unusual form of cell division that results in sperm formation, meiosis, is also responsible for development of ova. During the developmental phases experienced by the female sex cell from its earliest stage to just after fertilization, two meiotic divisions occur. As a result of meiosis in the female sex cell, the number of chromosomes is reduced equally in each daughter cell to half the number (23) found in other body cells (46). However, the amount of cytoplasm is divided unequally. The result is formation of one large ovum and small daughter cells called **polar bodies** that degenerate.

The ovum, with its large supply of cytoplasm, is one of the body's largest cells and is uniquely designed to provide nutrients for rapid development of the embryo until implantation in the uterus occurs. At fertilization, the sex cells from both parents fuse, and the normal chromosome number (46) is achieved.

 To learn more about oogenesis and meiosis, go to **AnimationDirect** on your CD.

Production of estrogen and progesterone
The second major function of the ovary, in addition to oogenesis, is secretion of the sex hormones, **estrogen** and **progesterone.** Hormone production in the ovary begins at puberty with the cyclic development and maturation of the ovum. The granulosa cells around the oocyte in the growing and mature follicle secrete estrogen. The corpus luteum, which develops after ovulation, chiefly secretes progesterone but also some estrogen.

Estrogen is the sex hormone that causes the development and maintenance of the female *secondary sex characteristics* and stimulates growth of the epithelial cells lining the uterus. Some of the actions of estrogen include the following:

1. Development and maturation of female reproductive organs, including the external genitals
2. Appearance of pubic hair and breast development
3. Development of female body contours by deposition of fat below the skin surface and in the breasts and hip region
4. Initiation of the first menstrual cycle

Progesterone is produced by the corpus luteum, which is a glandular structure that develops from a follicle that has just released an ovum. If stimulated by the appropriate anterior pituitary hormone, the corpus luteum produces progesterone for about 11 days after ovulation. Progesterone stimulates proliferation and vascularization of the epithelial lining of the uterus and acts with estrogen to initiate the menstrual cycle in girls entering puberty.

The surgical term **oophorectomy** (oh-off-eh-REK-toh-mee) is used to describe removal of the ovaries. If both ovaries are removed, sterility results and menopause follows.

QUICK CHECK

1. What is the name of the female gonads?
2. Where are the female glands located?
3. What is oogenesis?
4. What hormones are produced by the female gonads?

CLINICAL APPLICATION

HORMONE REPLACEMENT THERAPY
Hormone replacement therapy (HRT) using estrogen alone or in combination with progestin (synthetic progesterone) is sometimes used to reduce moderate to severe symptoms of menopause such as hot flashes. These symptoms result from the drop in estrogen that characterizes menopause. Although HRT may have some benefits in reducing or preventing chronic disorders such as osteoporosis, dementia, or heart disease, there are some health risks as well. Therefore HRT is used only for the more serious menopause cases and not to prevent chronic disease. To keep the risks low, HRT requires careful analysis of an individual's situation and determination of the lowest possible effective dose. Alternative drug therapies may be just as effective as HRT in some cases.

Reproductive Ducts

UTERINE TUBES

The two **uterine tubes,** also called **fallopian** (fal-LO-pee-an) **tubes** or **oviducts** (O-vi-dukts), serve as ducts for the ovaries, even though they are not attached to them. The outer end of each tube terminates in an expanded, funnel-shaped structure that has fringelike projections called **fimbriae** (FIM-bree-ee) along its edge. This part of the tube curves over the top of each ovary (Figure 22-11) and opens into the abdominal cavity. The inner end of each uterine tube attaches to the uterus, and the cavity inside the tube opens into the cavity in the uterus. Each tube is about 10 cm (4 inches) in length.

After ovulation the discharged ovum first enters the abdominal cavity and then enters the uterine tube assisted by the wavelike movement of the fimbriae and the beating of the cilia on their surface. Once in the tube, the ovum begins its journey to the uterus. Some ova never find their way into the oviduct and remain in the abdominal cavity where they are reabsorbed. In Chapter 23 the details of fertilization, which normally occurs in the outer one third of the uterine tube, are discussed.

The mucosal lining of the uterine tubes is directly continuous with the lining of the abdominal cavity on one end and with the lining of the uterus and vagina on the other. This is of great clinical significance because infections of the vagina or uterus such as gonorrhea may pass into the abdominal cavity, where they may become life threatening.

UTERUS

The **uterus** (YOO-ter-us) is a small organ—only about the size of a pear—but it is extremely strong. It is almost all muscle, or **myometrium** (my-oh-MEE-tree-um), with only a small cavity inside. During pregnancy the uterus grows many times larger so that it becomes big enough to hold a baby and a considerable amount of fluid.

The uterus is composed of several major regions. The upper portion of uterus is the **body.** Just above the level where the uterine tubes attach to the body of the uterus, it rounds out to form a bulging prominence called the **fundus** (see Figure 22-11). The lower, narrow neck section is called the **cervix.**

Except during pregnancy, the uterus lies in the pelvic cavity just behind the urinary bladder. By the end of pregnancy, it has become large enough to extend up to the top of the abdominal cavity. It then pushes the liver against the underside of the diaphragm—a fact that explains a comment such as "I can't seem to take a deep breath since I've gotten so big," made by many women late in their pregnancies.

Hysterectomy (hiss-teh-REK-toh-mee) is surgical removal of the uterus. It may be excised and removed through a typical incision in the abdomen (*abdominal hysterectomy*), through the vagina (*vaginal hysterectomy*), or laparoscopically (*laparoscopic hys-*

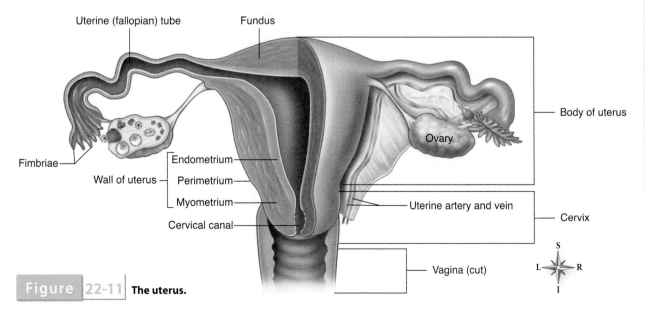

Figure 22-11 **The uterus.**

Sectioned view shows muscle layers of the uterus and its relationship to the ovaries and vagina.

terectomy). In *total hysterectomy* both the body and cervix are removed; in *subtotal hysterectomy* only the body of the uterus is removed, sparing the cervix.

The uterus functions in three processes—menstruation, pregnancy, and labor. The corpus luteum stops secreting progesterone and decreases its secretion of estrogens about 11 days after ovulation. About 3 days later, when the progesterone and estrogen concentrations in the blood are at their lowest, menstruation starts. Small pieces of the mucous membrane lining of the uterus, or the **endometrium** (en-doh-MEE-tree-um) pull loose, leaving torn blood vessels underneath. Blood and bits of endometrium trickle out of the uterus into the vagina and out of the body. Immediately after menstruation, the endometrium starts to repair itself. It again grows thick and becomes lavishly supplied with blood in preparation for pregnancy.

If fertilization does not take place, the uterus once more sheds the lining made ready for a pregnancy that did not occur. Because these changes in the uterine lining continue to repeat themselves, they are spoken of as the **menstrual cycle** (see pp. 620-622).

If fertilization occurs, pregnancy begins, and the endometrium remains intact. The events of pregnancy are discussed in Chapter 23.

Menstruation first occurs at puberty, often around the age of 12 to 13 years but sometimes even earlier. Normally it repeats itself about every 28 days or 13

times a year for some 30 to 40 years before it ceases at the time of **menopause** (MEN-o-pawz), when a woman is somewhere around the age of 50 years.

VAGINA

The **vagina** (vah-JYE-nah) is a distensible tube about 10 cm (4 inches) long made mainly of smooth muscle and lined with mucous membrane. It lies in the pelvic cavity between the urinary bladder and the rectum, as you can see in Figure 22-9. As the part of the female reproductive tract that opens to the exterior, the vagina is the organ that receives the penis during intercourse and through which sperm enter during their journey to meet an ovum. The vagina is also the organ from which a baby emerges to meet its new world, and so it is also called the *birth canal.*

 To learn more about female reproductive ducts, go to **AnimationDirect** on your CD.

Accessory or Supportive Sex Glands

VESTIBULAR GLANDS

Two pairs of exocrine glands lie imbedded in tissue to the left and right of the vaginal outlet and release mucus into the vestibule of the *vulva* (described later; Figure 22-13). One pair of these small glands are called the **greater vestibular** (ves-TIB-yoo-lar) **glands** and the other pair are called the **lesser vestibular glands**. The greater vestibular glands are also called **Bartholin** (BAR-toh-lin) **glands**. Mucus from these glands may contribute to lubrication during sexual intercourse.

The vestibular glands have clinical importance because they may become infected. For example, *Neisseria gonorrhoeae*—the bacteria that cause gonorrhea—are often hard to eliminate once they infect a vestibular gland (see Table 22-4).

BREASTS

The **breasts** lie over the pectoral muscles and are attached to them by connective tissue ligaments (of Cooper). Breast size is determined more by the amount of fat around the glandular (milk-secreting) tissue than by the amount of glandular tissue itself. Hence the size of the breast has little to do with its ability to secrete adequate amounts of milk after the birth of a baby.

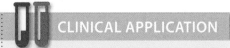

CLINICAL APPLICATION

ECTOPIC PREGNANCY

The term **ectopic** (ek-TOP-ic) **pregnancy** is used to describe a pregnancy resulting from the implantation of a fertilized ovum in any location other than the uterus. Occasionally, because the outer ends of the uterine tubes open into the pelvic cavity and are not actually connected to the ovaries, an ovum does not enter an oviduct but becomes fertilized and remains in the abdominal cavity. Although rare, if implantation occurs on the surface of an abdominal organ or on one of the mesenteries, development may continue to term. In such cases delivery by cesarean section is required. Most ectopic pregnancies involve implantation in the uterine tube and are therefore called *tubal pregnancies.* They result in fetal death and, if not treated, tubal rupture.

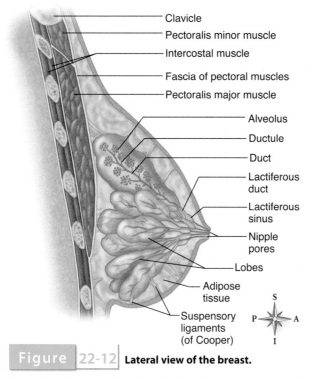

Clavicle
Pectoralis minor muscle
Intercostal muscle
Fascia of pectoral muscles
Pectoralis major muscle
Alveolus
Ductule
Duct
Lactiferous duct
Lactiferous sinus
Nipple pores
Lobes
Adipose tissue
Suspensory ligaments (of Cooper)

Figure 22-12 **Lateral view of the breast.**

Sagittal section shows the gland fixed to the overlying skin and the pectoral muscles by the suspensory ligaments of Cooper. Each lobule of secretory tissue is drained by a lactiferous duct that opens through the nipple.

Each breast consists of 15 to 20 divisions or lobes that are arranged radially (Figure 22-12). Each lobe consists of several lobules, and each lobule consists of milk-secreting glandular cells. The milk-secreting cells are arranged in grapelike clusters called *alveoli*. Small contractile cells surround the alveoli and push milk into ducts.

Small **lactiferous** (lak-TIF-er-us) **ducts** drain the alveoli and converge toward the nipple like the spokes of a wheel. Only one lactiferous duct leads from each lobe to an opening in the nipple. The colored surface area around the nipple is the **areola** (ah-REE-oh-lah).

Cancerous cells from breast tumors often spread to other areas of the body through the lymphatic system. This lymphatic drainage is discussed in Chapter 15 (see also Figure 15-9).

QUICK CHECK

1. What is another name for the uterine tubes?
2. What three major functions does the uterus perform?
3. What substance is conducted through lactiferous ducts?

External Genitals

The **external genitalia,** or **vulva** (VUL-vah), of women consist of the following:

1. Mons pubis
2. Clitoris
3. External urinary meatus
4. Labia minora (*sing.,* labium minus) (small lips)
5. Hymen
6. Opening of ducts of vestibular glands
7. Orifice (opening) of vagina
8. Labia majora (*sing.,* labium majus) (large lips)

The **mons pubis** is a skin-covered pad of fat over the symphysis pubis. Hair appears on this structure at puberty and persists throughout life. Extending downward from the elevated mons pubis are the **labia** (LAY-bee-ah) **majora** (mah-JOH-rah), or "large lips." These elongated folds, which are composed mainly of fat and numerous glands, are covered with pigmented skin and pubic hair on the outer surface and are smooth and free from hair on the inner surface. The **labia minora,** or "small lips," are located within the labia majora and are covered with modified skin. These two lips join anteriorly at the midline. The area between the labia minora is the **vesti-**

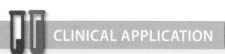

CLINICAL APPLICATION

FIBROCYSTIC DISEASE

The terms *fibrocystic disease* and *mammary dysplasia* are just two of the many names for a group of conditions characterized by benign lumps in one or both breasts. It is common in adult women before menopause, occurring in half of all women at some time, and is considered the most frequent breast lesion. The lumps that characterize fibrocystic disease are often painful, especially during the secretory phase of the reproductive cycle. Treatment is usually aimed at relieving pain or tenderness that may occur. Although it is commonly called a *disease,* most experts agree that fibrocystic disease is simply a collection of normal variations in breast tissue. Even though the lumps associated with fibrocystic disease are benign, any suspicious lump or other change in breast tissue should be regarded as possibly cancerous until determined otherwise by a physician.

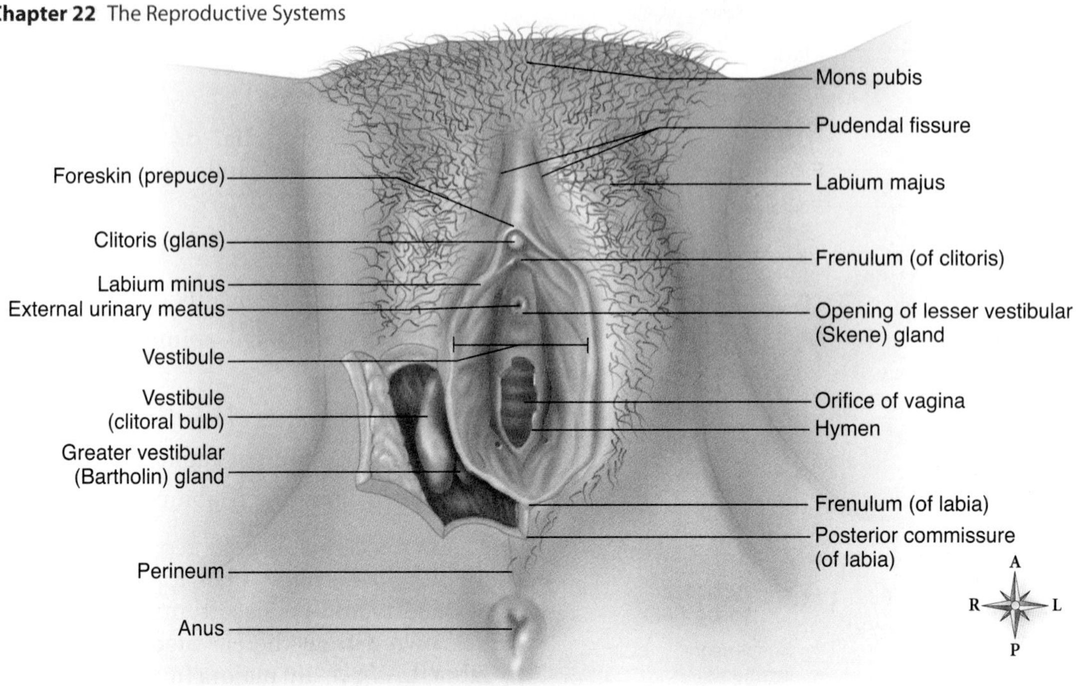

Foreskin (prepuce)

Clitoris (glans)

Labium minus

External urinary meatus

Vestibule

Vestibule
(clitoral bulb)

Greater vestibular
(Bartholin) gland

Perineum

Anus

Mons pubis

Pudendal fissure

Labium majus

Frenulum (of clitoris)

Opening of lesser vestibular
(Skene) gland

Orifice of vagina

Hymen

Frenulum (of labia)

Posterior commissure
(of labia)

Figure 22-13 **External genitals of the female.**

bule (Figure 22-13). Several genital structures are located in the vestibule.

The **clitoris** (KLIT-oh-ris), which is composed of erectile tissue, is located just behind the anterior junction of the labia minora. Situated between the clitoris above and the vaginal opening below is the orifice of the urethra. The vaginal orifice is sometimes partially closed by a membranous **hymen** (HYE-men). The ducts of vestibular glands open on either side of the vaginal orifice inside the labia minora.

The term **perineum** (pair-i-NEE-um) is used to describe the area between the vaginal opening and anus. This area is sometimes cut in a surgical procedure called an **episiotomy** (eh-piz-ee-OT-oh-mee) to prevent tearing of tissue during childbirth.

Menstrual Cycle

PHASES AND EVENTS

The menstrual cycle consists of many changes in the uterus, ovaries, vagina, and breasts and in the anterior pituitary gland's secretion of hormones (Figure 22-14). In the majority of women, these changes occur with almost precise regularity throughout their reproductive years. The first indication of changes comes with the first menstrual period. The first **menses** (MEN-seez) or menstrual flow is referred to as the **menarche** (meh-NAR-kee).

A typical menstrual cycle covers a period of about 28 days. However, the length of the cycle varies among women. Some women, for example, may have a regu-

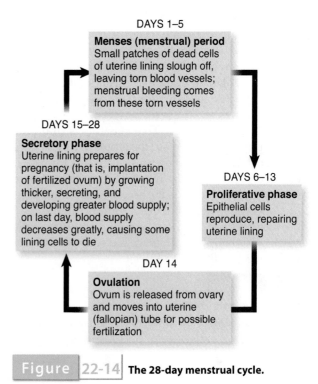

DAYS 1–5

Menses (menstrual) period
Small patches of dead cells of uterine lining slough off, leaving torn blood vessels; menstrual bleeding comes from these torn vessels

DAYS 15–28

Secretory phase
Uterine lining prepares for pregnancy (that is, implantation of fertilized ovum) by growing thicker, secreting, and developing greater blood supply; on last day, blood supply decreases greatly, causing some lining cells to die

DAYS 6–13

Proliferative phase
Epithelial cells reproduce, repairing uterine lining

DAY 14

Ovulation
Ovum is released from ovary and moves into uterine (fallopian) tube for possible fertilization

Figure 22-14 **The 28-day menstrual cycle.**

lar cycle that covers about 24 days. The length of the cycle also varies within one woman. Some women, for example, may have irregular cycles that range from 21 to 28 days, whereas others may be 2 to 3 months long.

Each cycle consists of three phases. The three periods of time in each cycle are called the **menses,** the **proliferative phase,** and the **secretory phase.** Re-

fer often to Figure 22-15 as you read about the events occurring during each phase of the cycle in the pituitary gland, the ovary, and in the uterus. Be sure that you do not overlook the event that occurs around day 14 of a 28-day cycle.

The menses is a period of 4 or 5 days characterized by menstrual

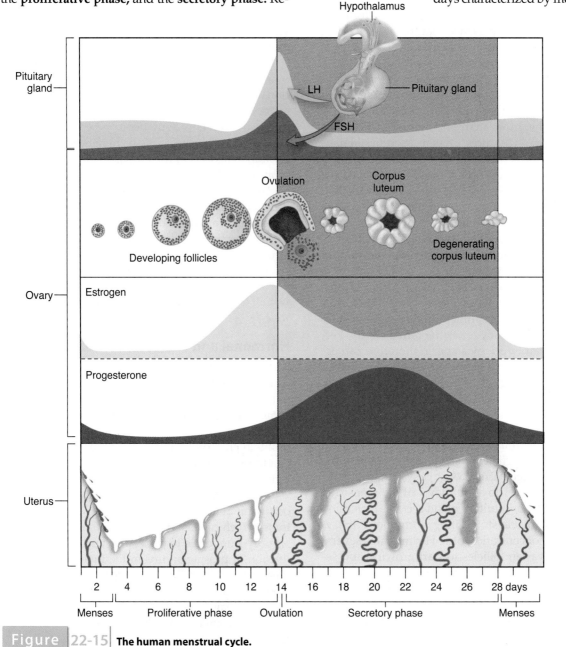

Figure 22-15 **The human menstrual cycle.**

Diagram illustrates the interrelationship of pituitary, ovarian, and uterine functions throughout a usual 28-day cycle. A sharp increase in luteinizing hormone (LH) levels causes ovulation, whereas menstruation (sloughing off of the endometrial lining) is initiated by lower levels of progesterone.

bleeding. The first day of menstrual flow is considered day 1 of the menstrual cycle. The proliferative phase begins after the menstrual flow ends and lasts until ovulation. During this period the follicles mature, the uterine lining thickens (proliferates), and estrogen secretion increases to its highest level. The secretory phase of the menstrual cycle begins at ovulation and lasts until the next menses begins. It is during this phase of the menstrual cycle that the uterine lining reaches its greatest thickness and the ovary secretes its highest levels of progesterone.

As a general rule, during the 30 or 40 years that a woman has periods, only one ovum matures each month. However, there are exceptions to this rule. Some months, more than one matures, and some months no ovum matures. Ovulation occurs 14 days before the next menses begins. In a 28-day cycle, this means that ovulation occurs around day 14 of the cycle, as shown in Figure 22-14. (Recall that the first day of the menses is considered the first day of the cycle.) In a 30-day cycle, however, ovulation would not occur on the fourteenth cycle day, but instead on the sixteenth. And in a 25-day cycle, ovulation would occur on the eleventh cycle day.

This matter of the time of ovulation has great practical importance. An ovum lives only a short time after it is ejected from its follicle, and sperm live only a short time after they enter the female body. Fertilization of an ovum by a sperm therefore can occur only around the time of ovulation. In other words, a woman's fertile period lasts only a few days each month.

CONTROL OF MENSTRUAL CYCLE CHANGES

The anterior pituitary gland plays a critical role in regulating the cyclic changes that characterize the functions of the female reproductive system (see Chapter 11). From day 1 to about day 7 of the menstrual cycle, the anterior pituitary gland secretes increasing amounts of follicle-stimulating hormone (FSH). A high blood concentration of FSH stimulates several immature ovarian follicles to start growing and secreting estrogens (see Figure 22-15).

As the estrogen content of blood increases, it stimulates the anterior pituitary gland to secrete another hormone, luteinizing hormone (LH). LH causes maturing of a follicle and its ovum, ovulation (rupturing of mature follicle with ejection of ovum), and luteinization (formation of a yellow body, the corpus luteum, from the ruptured follicle).

Which hormone—FSH or LH—would you call the "ovulating hormone"? Do you think ovulation could occur if the blood concentration of FSH remained low throughout the menstrual cycle? If you answered LH to the first question and no to the second, you answered both questions correctly. Ovulation cannot occur if the blood level of FSH stays low because a high concentration of this hormone is essential to stimulation of ovarian follicle growth and maturation. With a low level of FSH, no follicles start to grow, and therefore none become ripe enough to ovulate. Ovulation is caused by the combined actions of FSH and LH. Birth control pills that contain estrogen substances suppress FSH secretion. This indirectly prevents ovulation.

Ovulation occurs, as we have said, because of the combined actions of the two anterior pituitary hormones, FSH and LH. The next question is: what causes menstruation? A brief answer is this: a sudden, sharp decrease in estrogen and progesterone secretion toward the end of the secretory phase causes the uterine lining to break down and another menstrual period to begin.

Disorders of the Female Reproductive System

Hormonal and Menstrual Disorders

Menstrual cramps, or **dysmenorrhea** (dis-men-oh-REE-ah), are terms used to describe the cramping, painful periods that affect 75% to 80% of women at some time during their reproductive years. For significant numbers of those affected, severe lower abdominal cramping and back pain accompanied by headache, nausea, and vomiting will disrupt their school, work, athletic, or other activities.

Primary dysmenorrhea is the most common type occurring in adolescents and young women. Symptoms, which can last from hours to days and vary in severity from cycle to cycle, are caused by overproduction of prostaglandins in the inner lining of the uterus. Prostaglandins cause spasms that decrease blood flow and oxygen delivery to uterine muscle resulting in pain. Fortunately, primary dysmenorrhea is not associated with pelvic disease, such as an infection or tumor, and can generally be treated effectively with over-the-counter anti-inflammatory drugs such as ibuprofen and naproxen, which decrease prostaglandin production. In severe cases a physician may prescribe more powerful anti-inflammatory drugs or certain hormones, including oral contraceptives, to alter menstrual cycle activity.

Secondary dysmenorrhea refers to menstrual-related pain caused by some type of pelvic pathology. The problem is generally a gynecological problem affecting one or more reproductive organs. Treatment of secondary dysmenorrhea involves treating the underlying disorder.

Amenorrhea (ah-men-oh-REE-ah) is the absence of normal menstruation. *Primary amenorrhea* is the failure of menstrual cycles to begin and may be caused by a variety of factors, such as hormone imbalances, genetic disorders, brain lesions, or structural deformities of the reproductive organs.

Secondary amenorrhea occurs when a woman who has previously menstruated slows to three or fewer cycles per year. Secondary amenorrhea may occur with weight loss, pregnancy, lactation, menopause, or disease of the reproductive organs. Treatment involves treating the underlying disorder or condition. If amenorrhea occurs as a component of the "Sports Triad" (see Box), treatment may become part of extensive and long-term therapy needed to address a number of complex nutritional, hormonal, and self-image issues.

Dysfunctional uterine bleeding (DUB) is irregular or excessive uterine bleeding that most often results from either a hormonal imbalance or some type of structural problem that causes a disruption of blood supply. DUB is a significant medical problem affecting nearly 2 million women in the United States each year.

To diagnose the cause of DUB, a physician may employ x-ray or ultrasound studies to look at the contours of the uterine cavity, look directly inside the uterus using a telescope-like instrument inserted through the vagina and cervix or examine tissue obtained by biopsy to exclude cancer. If hormonal imbalance is the cause, it is the excessive growth and breakdown of delicate endometrial tissue that results in heavy bleeding. Structural problems, such as growth of a uterine malignancy, polyps, or fibroids (discussed on pp. 624-625), may also cause DUB by causing injury to the blood vessels of the uterine wall or lining. Excessive uterine bleeding over time can result in life-threatening anemia because of the chronic loss of blood.

Treatment of DUB generally begins with administration of nonsteroidal anti-inflammatory drugs and hormonal manipulation using low-dose birth control pills. If conservative treatment fails to stop the endometrial lining from hemorrhaging, hysterectomy remains one of the most effective curative options. Currently, about 20% of hysterectomies performed each year are for treatment of abnormal uterine bleeding. However, less invasive procedures, including **endometrial ablation** techniques, are now being used more frequently to destroy the endometrial lining and halt the bleeding. In *thermal ablation,* a balloon is inserted into the uterus and filled with fluid. A heat probe is then inserted into the balloon and the fluid is heated to a temperature that will destroy the endometrium. In *radiofrequency ablation,* a gold-plated mesh fabric is used to fill the uterine cavity and is then charged

CLINICAL APPLICATION

THE "SPORTS TRIAD" IN ELITE FEMALE ATHLETES
A disturbing trend among some elite female athletes involves development of a so-called "triad" of undesirable outcomes. In an attempt to improve performance, these athletes couple severe caloric restriction with over-training. The result is often a flawed sense of body image that equates thinness with athletic potential. The triad involves (1) low energy availability, (2) menstrual disorders, and (3) low bone mineral density.

Low energy availability often results from disordered eating and weight loss. *Amenorrhea* (failure to have a menstrual period) and other menstrual problems are caused by a drastic decrease in estrogen secretion as the body attempts to conserve energy by closing down the reproductive function. It is the decrease in estrogen levels that trigger early loss of bone density—perhaps

even *osteoporosis* and permanent skeletal damage. As it progresses, the *sports triad* may also be accompanied by development of other serious and potentially fatal outcomes.

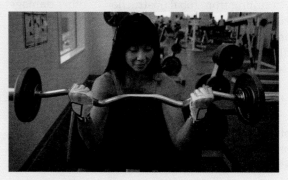

with radiofrequency energy that destroys the friable and bleeding endometrial cells. Both procedures carry less risk and have shorter recovery periods than does a hysterectomy.

Premenstrual syndrome (PMS) is a condition that involves a collection of symptoms that regularly occur in some women during the secretory phase of their reproductive cycles. Symptoms include irritability, fatigue, nervousness, depression, and other problems that are often distressing enough to affect personal relationships. Because the cause of PMS is still unclear, current treatments focus on relieving the symptoms.

Infection and Inflammation

Infections of the female reproductive tract are often classified as *exogenous* or *endogenous*. Exogenous infections result from pathogenic organisms transmitted from another person, such as **sexually transmitted diseases (STDs)**. Endogenous infections result from pathogens that normally inhabit the intestines, vulva, or vagina. You may recall from Chapter 5 that many areas of the body are normally inhabited by pathogenic microbes but that they cause infection only when there is a change in conditions or they are moved to a new area.

Pelvic inflammatory disease (PID) occurs as either an acute or chronic inflammatory condition that can be caused by several different pathogens, which usually spread upward from the vagina. PID is a major cause of infertility and sterility and affects more than 800,000 women each year in the United States. It is a common complication following infection by gonococcal *(Neisseria gonorrhoeae)* and chlamydial microorganisms (see Table 22-4).

In PID any inflammation involving the uterus, uterine tubes, ovaries, and other pelvic organs often results in development of scar tissue and adhesions. As a result, serious complications, including infertility resulting from tubal obstruction or other damage to the reproductive tract may occur. Uterine tube inflammation is termed **salpingitis** (sal-pin-JYE-tis) and inflammation of the ovaries is called **oophoritis** (oh-off-oh-RYE-tis).

Laparoscopic examination is often used to make a definitive diagnosis or to determine the severity of the infection and the reproductive organs involved. Although some chlamydial infections may not cause symptoms, most cases of PID are accompanied by fever, pelvic tenderness, and pain. Un-

fortunately, because of scarring and adhesions, pain may continue even after antibiotic therapy has eliminated the active infection. If left untreated, PID infections may spread to other tissues, including the blood, resulting in septic shock and death.

Vaginitis (vaj-in-EYE-tis) is inflammation or infection of the vaginal lining. Vaginitis most often results from STDs or from a "yeast infection." So-called yeast infections are usually opportunistic infections of the fungus *Candida albicans,* producing *candidiasis* (kan-did-EYE-as-is) (see Appendix A on page A-1 of your book). Candidiasis infections are characterized by a whitish discharge—a symptom known as **leukorrhea** (loo-koh-REE-ah).

Tumors and Related Conditions

The terms **fibroid, myoma** (my-OH-mah), and **fibromyoma** (fye-broh-my-OH-mah) are all words used to describe benign (non-cancerous) tumors of uterine fibrous or smooth muscle tissue. Individual fibroids may occur but multiple growths are not unusual. Fibroids are common in women during their reproductive years and develop most often in the myometrium of the uterine body and rarely in the cervix. The fact that they are seldom seen prior to puberty, increase in size during pregnancy, and tend to shrink in postmenopausal women suggests that age and estrogen levels may play a role in their development. Fibroids range in size from small asymptomatic nodules to massive tumors that may be painful and exert pressure on other pelvic organs. Growth during pregnancy may result in placental hemorrhage or malpresentation of the fetus complicating labor and delivery.

In addition to pain, symptoms of benign uterine tumors will vary depending on the size and location of the tumor. For example, if a large fibroid compresses the bladder and rectum, symptoms of urinary frequency and constipation may result. Even small tumors developing beneath the endometrium can cause severe hemorrhage (DUB).

Tumor size, location, and severity of symptoms will determine treatment options. A relatively new technique, similar to a heart catheterization, called *uterine artery embolization* involves snaking a small catheter through an artery in the groin into the arterial vessel supplying blood to a fibroid. Tiny inert pellets are then injected into the artery, blocking the flow of blood. The procedure results in dramatic shrinkage of the treated fibroid and a reduction in symptoms, including hemorrhage. Surgical removal of individual fibroids or, in more severe cases, hysterectomy may be indicated.

Polycystic ovary syndrome (PCOS) is a condition that affects 10% of reproductive-age women but can also affect girls as young as 11 years old. It is characterized by enlarged ovaries that usually are studded with fluid-filled cysts about 0.5 to 1.5 cm in diameter (Figure 22-16). The cysts are found on both ovaries and develop from mature follicles that fail to rupture completely. Corpora lutea are generally absent. Women with PCOS frequently have numerous endocrine abnormalities, including high levels of testosterone, infrequent menstrual cycles, and persistent anovulation. PCOS is the most common cause of female infertility.

Ovarian cysts are very common fluid-filled cysts that develop either from follicles that fail to rupture completely (*follicular cysts*) or from corpora lutea that fail to degenerate (*luteal cysts*). Most women develop a number of these cysts during their reproductive years and their presence does not represent a diagnosis of polycystic ovary syndrome. Although ovarian cysts are often multiple, they rarely become dangerous. However, on occasion they may become quite large and painful and be diagnosed by palpation or ultrasonography. Luteal cysts are less common than follicular cysts but tend to cause more symptoms, such as pelvic pain and menstrual irregularities. Rarely, rupture of a large luteal cyst will result in internal bleeding that requires surgical intervention. The vast majority of all ovarian cysts will disappear within a few months of their appearance, most within 60 days.

Endometriosis (en-doh-mee-tree-OH-sis) is the presence of functioning endometrial tissue outside the uterus. The displaced endometrial tissue can occur in many different places throughout the body but is most often found in or on pelvic and abdominal organs. The tissue reacts to ovarian hormones in the same way as the normal endometrium—exhibiting a cycle of growth and sloughing off. Symptoms of endometriosis may include unusual bleeding, dysmenorrhea, and pain during intercourse.

Malignancies of reproductive and related organs, especially the breasts, account for the majority of cancer cases among women. Some studies show that 1 in 10 women eventually get breast cancer, often a form of adenocarcinoma. Treatment of breast cancer is often successful if the cancerous tumor is detected ear-

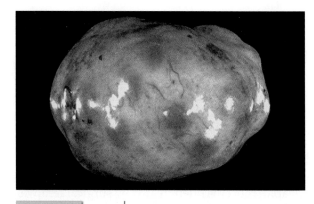

Figure 22-16 **Polycystic ovary syndrome (PCOS).** The ovary is studded with fluid-filled cysts developed from follicles that have failed to rupture.

ly. Because such tumors are often painless, most physicians recommend regular, frequent self-examination of breast tissue, as well as annual mammograms for women (see Chapter 5). Treatments often involve surgery, chemotherapy, and radiation therapy.

Breast surgeries can be very conservative, as in a simple lump removal or *lumpectomy*. If metastasis to surrounding tissue is suspected, a **radical mastectomy** (mas-TEK-toh-mee) may be performed. In this procedure the entire breast, with nearby muscle tissues and lymph nodes, is removed. Just as lumpectomy results in less trauma than radical mastectomy, so called *limited-field radiation* can provide effective treatment for clearly defined early-stage cancers that have not spread. It does so with shorter treatment cycles and fewer side effects than whole-breast radiation.

In the past, after women had completed their initial treatment for breast cancer they had few options available to lessen the possibility of recurrence. For a number of years the drug *tamoxifen* has been used extensively to prevent the recurrence of breast cancer fueled by estrogen. It does so by blocking the estrogen receptor sites on the cancer cell membrane. Unfortunately, tamoxifen effectiveness is limited to about 5 years. *Letrozole,* a relatively new drug, is classified as an "aromatase inhibitor." Instead of blocking estrogen receptor sites, it actually blocks estrogen production. It may replace tamoxifen or be prescribed for use after 5 years of tamoxifen therapy. Other "rational" drugs are being developed to alter or block crucial metabolic pathways in treating breast and other forms of cancer.

Ovarian cancer is another malignancy that affects 1 in 70 women in America. Usually a type of adeno-carcinoma, ovarian cancer is difficult to detect early and is often not easily apparent until it has grown into a large mass. Regular pelvic examinations that include palpation of the ovaries may result in earlier detection. Risk factors for ovarian cancer include age (over 40), infertility, childlessness or few children, a history of miscarriages, and endometriosis. Ovarian cancer is often treated by surgical removal of the ovaries combined with radiation therapy and chemotherapy.

Cancer of the uterus can affect the body of the uterus or the cervix. Cancers of the uterine body most often involve the endometrium *(endometrial cancer)* and mostly affect women beyond childbearing years; a common symptom is postmenopausal uterine bleeding. Risk factors for this type of cancer include obesity, prolonged estrogen therapy, and infertility. *Cervical cancer* occurs most often in women between the ages of 30 and 50.

Cervical cancer is often diagnosed early, through screening tests such as the **Papanicolaou** (pap-a-nik-oh-LAH-oo) **test,** or *Pap smear* (Figure 22-17). In this test, cells swabbed from the cervix are smeared on a glass slide, stained, and examined microscopically to determine whether any abnormalities exist. Current recommendations suggest two Pap smears 1 year apart beginning at age 21. If these two Pap smears are negative (that is, revealing no abnormalities), subsequent Pap smears should occur every 1 to 3 years thereafter. Because early or frequent intercourse is a risk factor for cervical cancer, sexually active young women should have their first Pap smear much earlier—and have follow-ups done more often.

Because screening tests and other early detection methods have been so successful, the death rates for uterine cancers have dropped dramatically over the last few decades. Because *human papillomavirus (HPV)* infections dramatically increase the risk of developing cervical cancer, widespread use of recently available HPV vaccines will likely further reduce the death rates from this type of cancer.

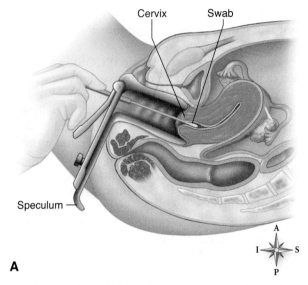

A

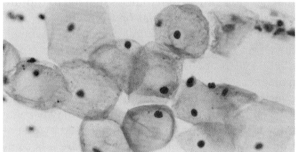

B

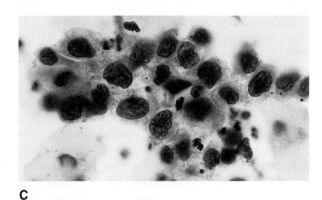

C

Figure 22-17 **Papanicolaou (Pap) smear.**

A, Obtaining a Pap smear. **B,** Appearance of normal cervical epithelial cells in Pap smear. **C,** Appearance of cervical cancer cells in Pap smear. Note the reduction in cytoplasm and increased prominence of the nuclei compared with normal epithelial cells.

Infertility

Like in the male reproductive system, various disorders can disrupt normal function of the female reproductive tract so that successful reproduction is unlikely (infertility) or impossible (sterility). Infections, tumors, hormonal imbalances, and other factors can contribute to infertility or sterility in women. For example, inflammation or infection of the uterine tubes can result in scarring that blocks sperm from reaching the ovum or prevents the ovum from traveling to the uterus. Infections, cancer, or hormonal imbalances may inhibit the female reproductive cycle, preventing the production and release of a healthy ovum each month. Such conditions also may interfere with the development of the uterine lining that is essential for successful pregnancy.

Because sexual reproduction requires normal function of both male and female systems, infertility of a couple may result from the infertility of either partner. A couple is considered infertile if a pregnancy does not occur after a year of reasonably frequent sexual intercourse (without contraception). When couples seek help for infertility problems, one of the first steps in diagnosis is to determine whether there is a problem in the male partner or the female partner—or both.

Summary of Male and Female Reproductive Systems

The reproductive systems in both sexes are centered around the production of reproductive cells, or gametes (sperm and ova), as well as mechanisms to ensure union of these two cells; the fusion of these cells enables transfer of parental genetic information to the next generation. Table 22-3 compares several analogous components of the reproductive systems in both sexes. You can see that men and women have similar structures to accomplish complementary functions. In addition, the female reproductive system permits development and birth of the offspring—the first subject of our next chapter.

Sexually Transmitted Diseases

Sexually transmitted diseases (STDs), formerly called *venereal diseases,* are infections caused by communicable pathogens such as viruses, bacteria, fungi, or protozoans (see Appendix A on page A-1 of your book). The term *sexually transmitted infection (STI)* is sometimes used in place of the term STD but does not have exactly the same meaning. An STI is an infection that may or may not cause symptoms. An STD occurs when an STI progresses to actually produce symptoms that make a person feel sick—making STI a broader term than STD.

The factor that links all these infections or diseases and gives this category its name is the fact that they are transmitted by sexual contact. The term *sexual contact* refers to normal intercourse in addition to any contact between the genitals of one person and the body of another person. Diseases classified as STDs can be transmitted sexually, but that is not the only way to transmit them. For example, *human immunodeficiency virus (HIV)* infection is a viral condition that can be spread through sexual contact but is also spread by transfusion of infected blood and use

Table 22-3	Analogous Features of the Reproductive Systems	
FEATURE	**FEMALE**	**MALE**
Essential organs	Ovaries	Testes
Sex cells	Ova (eggs)	Sperm
Hormones	Estrogen and progesterone	Testosterone
Hormone-producing cells	Granulosa cells and corpus luteum	Interstitial cells
Duct systems	Uterine (fallopian) tubes, uterus, and vagina	Epididymis, ductus (vas) deferens, and urethra
External genitals	Clitoris and vulva	Penis and scrotum

of contaminated medical instruments such as intravenous needles and syringes. Candidiasis, or yeast infection, is a common opportunistic infection, but it also can be transmitted through sexual contact. Sexually transmitted diseases are the most common of all communicable diseases. Table 22-4 summarizes a few of the principal STDs.

Table 22-4	Examples of Sexually Transmitted Diseases (STDs)	
DISEASE	**PATHOGEN**	**DESCRIPTION**
Acquired immunodeficiency syndrome (AIDS)	*Virus:* Human immunodeficiency virus (HIV)	HIV is transmitted by direct contact of body fluids, often during sexual contact. After a period that sometimes lasts many years, HIV infection produces the condition known as AIDS. AIDS is characterized by damage to lymphocytes (T cells), resulting in immune system impairment. Death results from secondary infections or tumors.
Candidiasis	*Fungus: Candida albicans*	This yeast infection is characterized by a white discharge (leukorrhea), peeling of skin, and bleeding. Although it can occur as an ordinary opportunistic infection, it may be transmitted sexually as well.
Chancroid	*Bacterium: Haemophilus ducreyi*	A highly contagious STI it is characterized by papules on the skin of the genitals that eventually ulcerate. About 90% of cases are reported by men.
Genital herpes	*Virus:* Herpes simplex virus (HSV)	HSV causes blisters on the skin of the genitals. The blisters may disappear temporarily but may reappear occasionally, especially as a result of stress.
Genital warts (cervical cancer)	*Virus:* Human papillomavirus (HPV-6, HPV-7)	Genital warts are nipple-like neoplasms of skin covering the genitals. (HPV is also involved in cervical cancer.)
Giardiasis	*Protozoan: Giardia lamblia*	This intestinal infection may be spread by sexual contact. Symptoms range from mild diarrhea to malabsorption syndrome, with about half of all cases being asymptomatic.
Gonorrhea	*Bacterium: Neisseria gonorrhoeae*	Gonorrhea primarily involves the genital and urinary tracts but can affect the throat, conjunctiva, or lower intestines. It may progress to PID.
Hepatitis	*Virus:* Hepatitis B virus (HBV)	This acute-onset liver inflammation may develop into a severe chronic disease, perhaps ending in death.
Lymphogranuloma venereum (LGV)	*Bacterium: Chlamydia trachomatis*	This chronic STD is characterized by genital ulcers, swollen lymph nodes, headache, fever, and muscle pain. *C. trachomatis* infection may cause a variety of other syndromes, including conjunctivitis, urogenital infections, and systemic infections. *C. trachomatis* infections constitute the most common STI in the United States (nongonorrheal urethritis) and often progress to PID.
Scabies	*Animal: Sarcoptes scabiei*	Scabies is caused by infestation by the *itch mite*, which burrows into the skin to lay eggs. About 2 to 4 months after initial contact, a hypersensitivity reaction occurs, causing a rash along each burrow that itches intensely. Secondary bacterial infection is possible.
Syphilis	*Bacterium: Treponema pallidum*	Although transmitted sexually, syphilis can affect any system. *Primary syphilis* is characterized by chancre sores on exposed areas of the skin. If the primary infection goes untreated, *secondary syphilis* may appear 2 months after chancres disappear. The secondary stage occurs when the spirochete has spread throughout the body, presenting a variety of symptoms, and it is still highly contagious—even through kissing. *Tertiary syphilis* may appear years later, possibly resulting in death.
Trichomoniasis	*Protozoan: Trichomonas vaginalis*	This urological infection is asymptomatic in most women and nearly all men. Vaginitis may occur, characterized by itching or burning, and a foul-smelling discharge.

SCIENCE APPLICATIONS

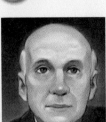

William Masters (1915–2001)

REPRODUCTIVE SCIENCES

The study of human reproduction, and especially sexual function, has many cultural implications. So it is no wonder that American researchers William Masters and Virginia Johnson encountered a great deal of controversy during their decades of pioneering work in the field of human sex and reproduction. After teaming up at Washington University in St. Louis in 1957, they were the first to study human sexual physiology in the laboratory. In 1966, their book *Human Sexual Response* clearly explained the physiology of sex for the first time. Besides making discoveries in the physiology of human sex and reproduction, they also developed therapies for treating sex-related conditions and trained therapists from around the world.

William Masters was a gynecologist (physician specializing in women's health) and Virginia Johnson was a psychologist. This partnership shows the importance of human reproduction in two major fields of study: medicine and psychology. Today, there are many opportunities to apply knowledge of reproductive science in a variety of professions. For example,

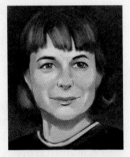

Virginia Johnson (born 1925)

many psychologists and counselors use biological principles in dealing with clients who seek help with reproductive or sexual issues. Social workers and legal professionals also find that such knowledge can be applied in their professions. Even politicians, religious leaders, social activists, and journalists must be aware of the latest findings in reproductive science in order to develop informed opinions and make reasonable judgments about applying such knowledge in our society.

Of course, the half-century since Masters and Johnson began their work has seen an increase in the number of health professionals working in fields related to human sex and reproduction. For example, urologists (who often deal with men's health issues) and gynecologists are physicians who directly apply reproductive science in their work. Many nurses, therapists, and health technicians join them in providing clients with the help they need. In addition, many community health workers find themselves dealing with their clients' issues related to sexual activity, pregnancy, and fertility.

Outline Summary

To download an MP3 version of the chapter summary for use with your iPod or portable media player, access the **Audio Chapter Summaries** on your CD.

Sexual Reproduction

A. Sexual reproduction involves two parents (unlike one-parent asexual reproduction); increases variation of genetic traits among offspring of same parents
B. Gametes—sex cells that fuse at fertilization to form a one-celled zygote, the first cell of the offspring
   1. Sperm—gamete from the male parent
   2. Ovum—gamete from the female parent
C. Reproductive hormones regulate sexual characteristics that promote successful reproduction
D. Ability to reproduce begins at puberty

Common Structural and Functional Characteristics Between the Sexes

A. Common general structure and function can be identified between the systems in both sexes
B. Systems adapted for development of sperm or ova followed by successful fertilization, development, and birth of offspring
C. Sex hormones in both sexes important in development of secondary sexual characteristics and normal reproductive system activity

Male Reproductive System

A. Structural plan—organs classified as essential or accessory (Figure 22-1; Table 22-1)
1. Essential organs of reproduction are the gonads (testes in men), which produce sex cells (spermatozoa)
2. Accessory organs of reproduction
   a. Ducts—passageways that carry sperm from testes to exterior
   b. Sex glands—produce protective and nutrient solution for sperm
   c. External genitals
B. Testes—the gonads of men
1. Structure and location (Figure 22-2)
   a. Testes in scrotum—temperature lower than inside body
   b. Covered by tunica albuginea, which divides testis into lobules containing seminiferous tubules
   c. Interstitial cells produce testosterone (Figure 22-3)
2. Testis functions
   a. Spermatogenesis is process of sperm production (Figure 22-4)
      (1) Sperm precursor cells called *spermatogonia*
      (2) Meiosis produces primary spermatocyte, which forms four spermatids with 23 chromosomes
      (3) Spermatozoa—male reproductive cell (Figure 22-5)
         (a) Ejaculation—forceful ejection (from the penis) of fluid containing sperm
         (b) Head contains genetic material
         (c) Acrosome contains enzymes to assist sperm in penetration of ovum
         (d) Mitochondria provide energy for movement
   b. Production of testosterone by interstitial cells
      (1) Testosterone "masculinizes" and promotes development of male accessory organs
      (2) Stimulates protein anabolism and development of muscle strength
C. Reproductive ducts—ducts through which sperm pass after exiting testes until they exit from the body

1. Epididymis—single, coiled tube about 6 m in length; lies along the top and behind the testis in the scrotum
   a. Sperm mature and develop the capacity for motility as they pass through the epididymis
   b. Epididymitis—painful inflammation
2. Ductus (vas) deferens—tube that receives sperm from the epididymis and transports them from scrotal sac through the abdominal cavity
   a. Passes through inguinal canal
   b. Joins duct of seminal vesicle to form the ejaculatory duct (Figure 22-6)
D. Accessory or supportive sex glands
1. Semen (seminal fluid): mixture of sperm and secretions of accessory sex glands
   a. Average of 3 to 5 ml per ejaculation
   b. Each milliliter contains about 100 million sperm
2. Seminal vesicles
   a. Pouchlike glands that produce about 60% of seminal fluid volume
   b. Secretion is yellowish, thick, and rich in fructose to provide energy needed by sperm for motility
3. Prostate gland
   a. Shaped like a doughnut and located below bladder
   b. Urethra passes through the gland
   c. Thin, milk-colored secretion that represents 30% of seminal fluid volume
   d. Activates sperm and is needed for ongoing sperm motility
4. Bulbourethral (Cowper) glands
   a. Resemble peas in size and shape
   b. Secrete mucus-like fluid (less than 5% of seminal fluid volume) that lubricates terminal portion of urethra
E. External genitals (Figure 22-7)
1. Penis and scrotum called *genitalia*
2. Penis has three columns of erectile tissue
   a. Two dorsal columns called *corpora cavernosa*
   b. One ventral column surrounding urethra called *corpus spongiosum*
3. Glans penis—distal end of penis
   a. Covered by foreskin (prepuce)
   b. Surgical removal of foreskin called *circumcision*

4. Scrotum—skin-covered pouch suspended from groin
 a. Divided into two sacs by a septum
 b. Each sac contains a testis, epididymis, part of ductus deferens, and beginning of spermatic cords

Disorders of the Male Reproductive System

A. May cause reduced reproductive ability (infertility) or total inability to reproduce (sterility)
B. Disorders of the testes
 1. Oligospermia—low sperm production
 2. Cryptorchidism—undescended testes
 3. Testicular cancer—most common in males ages 15 to 30
C. Disorders of the prostate
 1. Benign prostatic hypertrophy—enlargement of prostate common in older men
 2. Prostatectomy—surgical removal of part or all of the prostate
 3. Prostate cancer—malignancy of prostate tissue
 4. Brachytherapy—small radioactive "seeds" placed in prostate
D. Disorders of the penis and scrotum
 1. Phimosis—tight foreskin cannot be retracted over glans (Box, p. 611)
 2. Paraphimosis—foreskin cannot be replaced to usual position after it has been retracted behind the glans (Box, p. 611)
 3. Erectile dysfunction—failure to achieve erection of the penis
 4. Hydrocele—accumulation of watery fluid in the scrotum
 5. Inguinal hernia—protrusion of abdominopelvic organs, possibly into the scrotum (Figure 22-8)
 6. Hypospadias—urethra opens on underside of glans or shaft
 7. Epispadias—urethra opens on top of glans or shaft

Female Reproductive System

A. Structural plan—organs classified as essential or accessory (Figure 22-9; Table 22-2)
 1. Essential organs are gonads (ovaries), which produce sex cells (ova)
 2. Accessory organs of reproduction
 a. Ducts or modified ducts—including oviducts, uterus, and vagina
 b. Sex glands—including those in the breasts
 c. External genitals
B. Ovaries
 1. Structure and location
 a. Paired glands weighing about 3 g each
 b. Resemble large almonds
 c. Attached to ligaments in pelvic cavity on each side of uterus
 d. Microscopic structure (Figure 22-10)
 (1) Ovarian follicles—contain oocyte, which is immature sex cell (about 1 million at birth)
 (2) Primary follicles—about 400,000 at puberty are covered with granulosa cells
 (3) About 350 to 500 mature follicles ovulate during the reproductive lifetime of most women—sometimes called *graafian follicles*
 (4) Secondary follicles have hollow chamber called *antrum*
 (5) Corpus luteum forms after ovulation
 2. Ovary functions
 a. Oogenesis—this meiotic cell division produces daughter cells with equal chromosome numbers (23) but unequal cytoplasm
 (1) Resulting ovum is large
 (2) Polar bodies are small and degenerate
 b. Production of estrogen and progesterone
 (1) Granulosa cells surrounding the oocyte in the mature and growing follicles produce estrogen
 (2) Corpus luteum produces progesterone
 (3) Estrogen causes development and maintenance of secondary sex characteristics
 (4) Progesterone stimulates secretory activity of uterine epithelium and assists estrogen in initiating menses
 (5) Surgical removal of ovaries called *oophorectomy*
C. Reproductive ducts
 1. Uterine (fallopian) tubes (or oviducts)
 a. Extend about 10 cm from uterus into abdominal cavity

    b. Expanded distal end surrounded by fimbriae

    c. Mucosal lining of tube is directly continuous with lining of abdominal cavity

  2. Uterus—composed of body, fundus, and cervix (Figure 22-11)

    a. Lies in pelvic cavity just behind urinary bladder

    b. Myometrium is muscle layer

    c. Endometrium lost in menstruation

    d. Menopause—end of repetitive menstrual cycles (about 45–50 years of age)

    e. Surgical removal called *hysterectomy*

      (1) Removal may be abdominal, vaginal, or laparoscopic

      (2) Total hysterectomy—removal of both body and cervix of uterus

      (3) Subtotal hysterectomy—removal of body of uterus only (cervix remains)

  3. Vagina

    a. Distensible tube about 10 cm long

    b. Located between urinary bladder and rectum in the pelvis

    c. Receives penis during sexual intercourse and is birth canal for normal delivery of baby at end of pregnancy

D. Accessory or supportive sex glands

  1. Vestibular glands

    a. Greater (Bartholin) and lesser vestibular glands

    b. Secrete mucus into vestibule of vulva

    c. Clinically important when they become infected (e.g., *Neisseria gonorrhoeae* bacteria that cause gonorrhea)

  2. Breasts (Figure 22-12)

    a. Located over pectoral muscles of thorax

    b. Size determined by fat quantity more than amount of glandular (milk-secreting) tissue

    c. Lactiferous ducts drain at nipple, which is surrounded by pigmented areola

    d. Lymphatic drainage leads to spread of cancer cells to other body areas

E. External genitals (Figure 22-13)

  1. Include mons pubis, clitoris, external urinary meatus, openings of vestibular glands, orifice of vagina, labia minora and majora, and hymen

  2. Perineum—area between vaginal opening and anus

    a. Surgical cut during birth called episiotomy

F. Menstrual cycle—involves many changes in the uterus, ovaries, vagina, and breasts (Figures 22-14 and 22-15)

  1. Length—about 28 days, varies from month to month among individuals and in the same individual

  2. Phases

    a. Menses—about the first 4 or 5 days of the cycle, varies somewhat

      (1) Characterized by sloughing of bits of endometrium (uterine lining) with bleeding

      (2) First day of flow is day 1 of menstrual cycle

    b. Proliferative phase—days between the end of menses and ovulation; varies in length

      (1) The shorter the cycle, the shorter the proliferative phase; the longer the cycle, the longer the proliferative phase

      (2) Characterized by repair of endometrium

    c. Secretory phase—days between ovulation and beginning of next menses

      (1) Characterized by further thickening of endometrium and secretion by its glands in preparation for implantation of fertilized ovum

      (2) Combined actions of the anterior pituitary hormones FSH and LH cause ovulation

      (3) Sudden sharp decrease in estrogens and progesterone bring on menstruation if pregnancy does not occur

Disorders of the Female Reproductive System

A. Hormonal and menstrual disorders

  1. Menstrual cramps or dysmenorrhea—painful menstruation

  2. Amenorrhea—absence of normal menstruation

  3. Dysfunctional uterine bleeding (DUB)—irregular or excessive bleeding resulting from a hormonal imbalance or pathology

  4. Premenstrual syndrome (PMS)—collection of symptoms that occur in some women before menstruation

B. Infection and inflammation
1. Exogenous infections are often sexually transmitted; endogenous infections are caused by organisms already in or on the body
2. Pelvic inflammatory disease (PID)—acute inflammatory condition of the uterus, uterine tubes, or ovaries caused by infection
3. Vaginitis—infection of vaginal lining, it most often results from STDs or yeast infections

C. Tumors and related conditions
1. Myoma or fibroids—benign tumors of the uterus
2. Polycystic ovary syndrome (PCOS)—enlarged ovaries with many fluid-filled cysts
   a. Affects 10% of reproductive-age women
   b. Most common cause of female infertility (Figure 22-16)
3. Ovarian cysts—fluid-filled enlargements; usually benign
   a. Follicular cysts—most common
   b. Luteal cysts—most symptomatic
   c. Most resolve in 60 days
4. Endometriosis—presence of functioning endometrial tissue outside the uterus
5. Breast cancer is the most common type of cancer in women
6. Ovarian cancer can result from metastasis of breast cancer or can arise independently
7. Cervical cancer is often detected by a Papanicolaou test (Pap smear) (Figure 22-17)

D. Infertility can result from factors such as infection and inflammation, tumors, and hormonal imbalances

Summary of Male and Female Reproductive Systems

A. In men and women the organs of the reproductive system are adapted for the specific sequence of functions that permit development of sperm or ova followed by the successful fertilization and then the normal development and birth of offspring
B. The male organs produce, store, and ultimately introduce mature sperm into the female reproductive tract
C. The female system produces ova, receives the sperm, and permits fertilization followed by fetal development and birth, with lactation afterward
D. Production of sex hormones is required for development of secondary sex characteristics and for normal reproductive functions in both sexes

Sexually Transmitted Diseases

A. STDs are transmitted sexually but can also be transmitted in other ways
B. STDs are the most common of all communicable diseases
C. STDs are caused by a variety of organisms (Table 22-4)

New Words

acrosome	endometrium	graafian follicle	menopause
antrum	estrogen	greater vestibular	menses
areola	epididymis	(Bartholin) gland	menstrual cycle
bulbourethral (Cowper)	fimbriae	hymen	mons pubis
gland	foreskin (prepuce)	interstitial cells	myometrium
clitoris	fundus of uterus	labia majora	oocyte
corpora cavernosa	gametes	labia minora	oogenesis
corpus spongiosum	genitals (genitalia)	lactiferous duct	ovarian follicle
ductus (vas) deferens	glans	lesser vestibular gland	ovulation
ejaculation	gonads	meiosis	perineum
ejaculatory duct	granulosa cell	menarche	polar body

primary follicle
primary spermatocyte
progesterone
proliferative phase
scrotum
secretory phase
semen (seminal fluid)
seminal vesicle
seminiferous tubule
spermatid
spermatogenesis
spermatogonia
spermatozoa
testes
tunica albuginea
vestibule of the vulva
vulva
zygote

Diseases and Other Clinical Terms

amenorrhea
benign prostatic
   hypertrophy (BPH)
brachytherapy
circumcision
cryptorchidism
dysfunctional uterine
   bleeding (DUB)
dysmenorrhea (menstrual
   cramps)
ectopic pregnancy
endometrial ablation
endometriosis
epididymitis
episiotomy

epispadias
erectile dysfunction (ED)
fibroid
fibromyoma
hydrocele
hypospadias
hysterectomy
infertility
inguinal hernia
leukorrhea
myoma
oligospermia
oophoritis
oophorectomy
ovarian cyst
Papanicolaou test
paraphimosis

pelvic inflammatory
   disease (PID)
phimosis
polycystic ovary syndrome
   (PCOS)
premenstrual syndrome
   (PMS)
prostatectomy
prostatic-specific antigen
   (PSA)
radical mastectomy
salpingitis
sexually transmitted
   disease (STD)
sterility
vaginitis
vasectomy

Review Questions

1. Describe the structure and location of the testes.
2. Describe the structure of the spermatozoa.
3. List the functions of testosterone.
4. List and briefly describe the reproductive ducts of the male reproductive system.
5. List and briefly describe the glands of the male reproductive system. What does each gland contribute to the seminal fluid?
6. Distinguish between infertility, sterility, and impotence.
7. What is oligospermia? What is cryptorchidism?
8. Both a hydrocele and an inguinal hernia will produce swelling in the scrotum; explain the difference between the two.
9. Describe the structure and location of the ovaries.
10. Explain the development of an ovarian follicle from the primary follicle to the corpus luteum.
11. List the functions of estrogen.
12. List the functions of progesterone.
13. Describe the structure of the uterine tubes.
14. Describe the structure of the uterus.
15. Describe the structure of the vagina.
16. Describe the structure of the breast.
17. Explain what occurs during the proliferative phase of the reproductive cycle.
18. Explain what occurs during the secretory phase of the reproductive cycle.
19. Name the four hormones involved in the regulation of the reproductive cycle. Where is each made, and what is the function of each?
20. What is dysmenorrhea? What is amenorrhea?
21. Distinguish between salpingitis and oophoritis.
22. What is endometriosis?

Critical Thinking

23. Differentiate between spermatogenesis and oogenesis. How do these differences relate to the role of the male and female in reproduction?
24. Why are the testes located outside the body cavity in the scrotum?

Chapter Test

1. The essential organs of the male reproductive system are the _____.
2. The pouch-like sac where the male gonads are located is called the _____.
3. The membrane that covers the testis and also divides the interior into lobes is called the _____.
4. The _____ is a long duct in the testis where sperm develop.
5. The _____ are the cells in the testes that secrete testosterone.
6. The primary spermatocyte develops from a cell called the _____.
7. The primary spermatocyte forms sperm cells by undergoing a type of cell division called _____.
8. The sperm cell contains an _____, which contains an enzyme that can digest the covering of the ovum.
9. The _____ is a reproductive duct that consists of a tightly coiled tube that lies along the top and behind the testis.
10. The _____ is a reproductive duct that permits the sperm to move out of the scrotum upward into the abdominal cavity.
11. The _____ is a gland that secretes a thin, milk-colored fluid that makes up about 30% of the seminal fluid.
12. The _____ are a pair of glands that produce a thick, yellowish, fructose-rich fluid that makes up about 60% of the seminal fluid.
13. The penis is composed of three columns of erectile tissue: one is called the corpus spongiosum, and the other two are called the _____.
14. The essential organs of the female reproductive system are the _____.
15. Another name for a mature ovarian follicle is a _____ follicle.
16. The process that produces the female gamete is called _____.
17. Meiosis in the female produces one large ovum and three small daughter cells called _____, which degenerate.
18. The _____ are reproductive tubes connecting the ovary and the uterus.
19. The muscle layer of the uterus is called the _____.
20. The uterus is composed of two parts: the upper part, called the body, and the narrow lower part, called the _____.
21. The innermost layer of the uterus, which is shed during menstruation, is called the _____.
22. The _____ is the part of the female reproductive system that opens to the exterior.
23. The _____ glands are glands that secrete a mucus-like fluid into the vestibule.
24. The milk-secreting glandular cells of the breast are arranged in grape-like structures called _____. These drain into _____ ducts that converge toward the nipple.

Match each disorder in Column A with its description or cause in Column B.

Column A
25. _____ cryptorchidism
26. _____ benign prostatic
            hypertrophy
27. _____ hydrocele
28. _____ inguinal hernia
29. _____ dysmenorrhea
30. _____ amenorrhea
31. _____ salpingitis
32. _____ Pap smear
33. _____ myoma
34. _____ endometriosis
35. _____ syphilis
36. _____ genital herpes

Column B
a. a swelling of the scrotum caused by the overproduction of serous fluid
b. the lack of normal menstruation
c. used to screen for cervical cancer
d. the presence of functional endometrial tissue outside of the uterus
e. the inflammation of the uterine tubes
f. a sexually transmitted disease caused by a bacterium
g. condition that occurs when a testis fails to descend into the scrotum
h. painful menstruation syndrome
i. swelling of the scrotum caused by intestine pushing through a weak
    part of the abdominal wall
j. a sexually transmitted disease caused by a virus
k. a noncancerous condition characterized by enlargement of the prostate
l. benign fibroid tumor of the uterus

Match each term in Column A with its corresponding description in Column B.

Column A
37. _____ FSH
38. _____ menstruation
39. _____ corpus luteum
40. _____ estrogen
41. _____ secretory phase
42. _____ progesterone
43. _____ LH
44. _____ proliferative
            phase
45. _____ ovulation

Column B
a. term for the egg follicle after ovulation
b. ovarian hormone that reaches the highest concentration in the prolifera-
    tive phase
c. caused by a rapid drop in the blood levels of estrogen and progesterone
d. phase of the reproductive cycle that begins after ovulation
e. ovarian hormone that reaches its highest concentration during the
    secretory phase
f. term used to describe the egg being released from the ovary
g. phase of the reproductive cycle during which the uterine wall begins to
    thicken
h. pituitary hormone that stimulates the formation of an egg follicle
i. pituitary hormone that can be called the "ovulating hormone"

Study Tips

continued from page 603

4. The responsibility of the female reproductive system is to produce an egg and prepare the body for a possible pregnancy. The reproductive cycle assists in doing this.

5. The reproductive cycle is regulated by four hormones: two from the pituitary gland and two from the ovary. Follicle-stimulating hormone does exactly what its name implies. *Luteinizing* hormone helps stimulate ovulation that causes the egg follicle to become the corpus *luteum*. Estrogen begins the initial preparation of the uterus. Progesterone prepares the uterus to receive a fertilized egg. Think of progesterone as "pro" (in favor of) "gesterone" (gestation); this may help you remember what it does.

6. The disorders of the reproductive system can be put on a chart to help you learn them. Organize the disorders of the male reproductive system based on the specific structure of the male system that is affected. Disorders of the female system can be organized based on the specific structure of the female reproductive system or on menstruation disorders.

7. In your study group, go over the flash cards of the structures and photocopy figures to help you learn the locations. Discuss the process of meiosis and the differences between spermatogenesis and oogenesis. Discuss the reproductive cycle with emphasis on the function of the hormones. Go over the chart of the disorders and the questions at the end of the chapter, and discuss possible test questions.

Case Studies

1. As stated in the box on p. 613, one procedure that has been commonly used to screen for prostate cancer is palpation of the prostate through the wall of the rectum. Explain why digital (finger) palpation of the prostate is the only way to examine this gland from the outside without special equipment. What other prostate disorders might be detected this way?

2. Liz and Zeke have come to their physician with a problem: after 2 years of trying, they have not been able to conceive. According to the technical definition, is this couple infertile? On examination, Liz has been found to have pelvic inflammatory disease (PID). Could this condition have caused infertility?

3. Heather, age 22, briefly checks her breasts every few months and has never detected anything abnormal. However, a routine examination by her physician has revealed some small, tender lumps in both breasts. Does she have breast cancer? Can you think of any reason that Heather did not detect this condition herself?

Outline

Objectives

After you have completed this chapter, you should be able to:

1. Discuss the concept of development as a biological process characterized by continuous modification and change.

2. Discuss the major developmental changes characteristic of the prenatal stage of life from fertilization to birth.

3. Discuss the three stages of labor that characterize a normal vaginal birth.

4. Identify the three primary germ layers and several derivatives in the adult body that develop from each layer.

5. Identify and describe the major disorders associated with pregnancy.

6. List and discuss the major developmental changes characteristic of the four postnatal periods of life.

7. Discuss the effects of aging on the major body organ systems.

23 Growth and Development

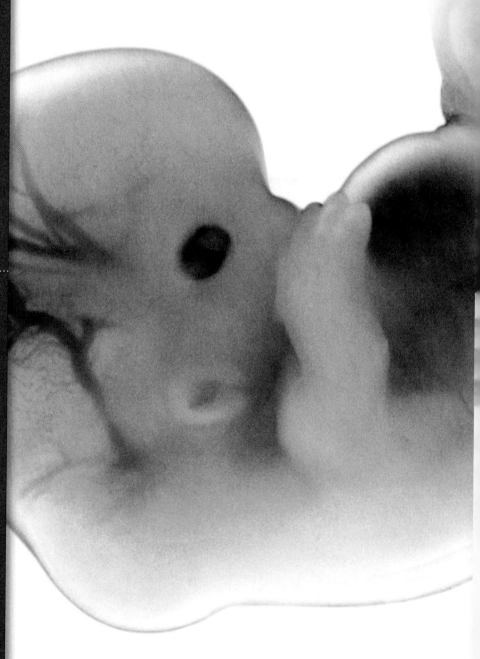

Many of your fondest and most vivid memories are probably associated with your birthdays. The day of birth is an important milestone of life. Most people continue to remember their birthday in some special way each year; birthdays serve as pleasant and convenient reference points to mark periods of transition or change in our lives. The actual day of birth marks the end of one phase of life called the **prenatal period** and the beginning of a second called the **postnatal period.** The prenatal period begins at conception and ends at birth; the postnatal period begins at birth and continues until death.

Although important periods in our lives such as childhood and adolescence are often remembered as a series of individual and isolated events, they are in reality part of an ongoing and continuous process. In reviewing the many changes that occur during the cycle of life from conception to death, it is often convenient to isolate

STUDY TIPS Before studying this chapter, quickly review the reproductive systems in Chapter 22. Also review the synopsis of all the organ systems found in Chapter 4.

1. Make flash cards to help you learn the early developmental stages. It would be helpful to include the order in which each developmental stage occurs. Remember to also include the functions of the amnion, chorion, and placenta.
2. The term *germ* in *primary germ layer* refers to "germinate." All of the structures of the body come from one of the primary germ layers. Each is named based on its location in the developing embryo. *Endoderm* means "inner skin," *mesoderm* means "middle skin," and *ectoderm* means "outer skin."
3. Make and use flash cards to help you learn to match up the primary germ layers and the structures that come from each. *Genesis* means to create, *histogenesis* means to create tissues, and *organogenesis* means to create organs.
4. Be sure you understand what distinguishes fraternal twins from identical twins.

continued on page 663

certain periods such as infancy or adulthood for study. It is important to remember, however, that life is not a series of stop-and-start events or individual and isolated periods of time. Instead, it is a biological process that is characterized by continuous modification and change.

This chapter discusses some of the events and changes that occur in the development of the individual from conception to death. Study of development during the prenatal period is followed by a discussion of the birth process and a review of changes occurring during infancy and adulthood. Finally some important changes that occur in the individual organ systems of the body as a result of aging are discussed.

Prenatal Period

The *prenatal stage of development* begins at the time of conception or fertilization (that is, at the moment the nuclei of the female ovum and the male sperm cells unite) (Figure 23-1). The period of prenatal development continues until the birth of the child about 39 weeks later. The science of the development of the individual before birth is called **embryology** (em-bree-OL-oh-jee). It is a story of biological marvels, describing the means by which a new human life is started and the steps by which a single microscopic cell is transformed into a complex human being.

Fertilization to Implantation

After ovulation the discharged ovum first enters the abdominal cavity and then finds its way into the uterine (fallopian) tubes. Sperm cells "swim" up the uterine tubes toward the ovum. Look at the relationship of the ovary, the two uterine tubes, and the uterus in Figure 23-2. Recall from Chapter 22 that each uterine tube extends outward from the uterus for about 10 cm. It then ends in the abdominal cavity near the ovary, as you can see in Figure 23-2, in an opening surrounded by fringelike processes, the *fimbriae*.

Sperm cells that are deposited in the vagina must enter and "swim" through the uterus and then move out of the uterine cavity and through the uterine tube to meet the ovum. **Fertilization** most often occurs in the outer one third of the oviduct as shown in Figure 23-2.

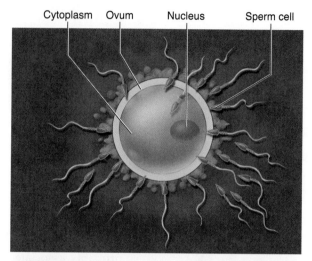

Cytoplasm   Ovum   Nucleus   Sperm cell

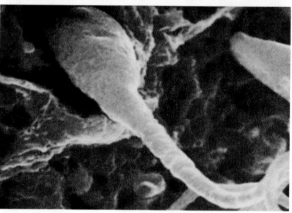

Figure 23-1 | **Fertilization.**

Fertilization is a specific biological event. It occurs when the male and female sex cells fuse. After union between a sperm cell and the ovum has occurred, the cycle of life begins. This scanning electron micrograph shows spermatozoa attaching themselves to the surface of an ovum. Only one will penetrate and fertilize the ovum.

The fertilized ovum or **zygote** (ZYE-gote) is genetically complete; it represents a new single-celled offspring. Time and nourishment are all that is needed for expression of characteristics such as sex, body build, and skin color that were determined at the time of fertilization. As you can see in the figure, the zygote immediately begins mitotic division, and in about 3 days a solid mass of cells called a **morula** (MOR-yoo-lah) is formed (see Figure 23-2). The cells of the morula continue to divide, and by the time the

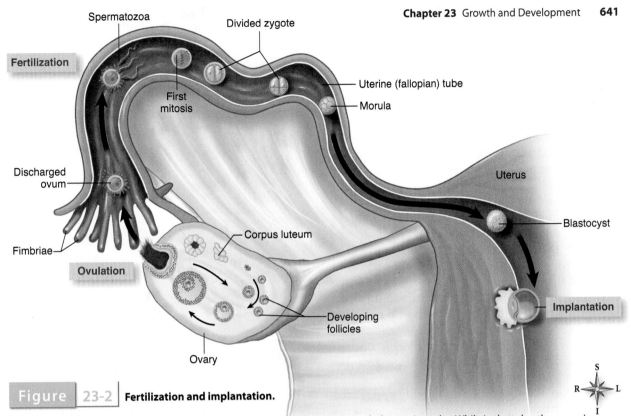

Figure 23-2 Fertilization and implantation.

At ovulation, an ovum is released from the ovary and begins its journey through the uterine tube. While in the tube, the ovum is fertilized by a sperm to form the single-celled zygote. After a few days of rapid mitotic division, a ball of cells called a *morula* is formed. After the morula develops into a hollow ball called a *blastocyst,* implantation occurs.

developing embryo reaches the uterus, it is a hollow ball of cells called a **blastocyst** (BLAS-toh-sist).

During the 10 days from the time of fertilization to the time when the blastocyst completes **implantation** in the uterine lining, no nutrients from the mother are available. The rapid cell division taking place up to the blastocyst stage occurs with no significant increase in total mass compared with the zygote (Figure 23-3). One of the specializations of the ovum is its incredible store of nutrients that help support this embryonic development until implantation has occurred.

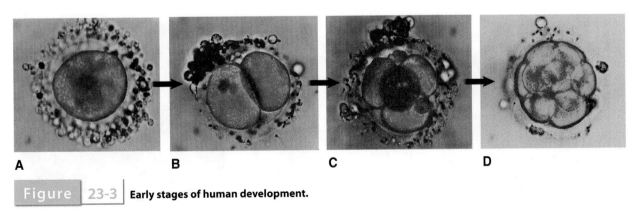

A **B** **C** **D**

Figure 23-3 Early stages of human development.

A, Fertilized ovum or zygote. **B** to **D,** Early cell divisions produce more and more cells. The solid mass of cells shown in **D** forms the morula—an early stage in embryonic development.

Note in Figure 23-4 that the blastocyst consists of an outer layer of cells and an inner cell mass. As the blastocyst develops, it forms a structure with two cavities, the **yolk sac** and **amniotic** (am-nee-OT-ik) **cavity.** The yolk sac is most important in animals, such as birds, that depend heavily on yolk as the sole source of nutrients for the developing embryo. In these animals the yolk sac digests the yolk and provides the resulting nutrients to the embryo. Because uterine fluids provide nutrients to the developing embryo in humans until the placenta develops, the function of the yolk sac is not a nutritive one. Instead, it has other functions, including production of blood cells.

The amniotic cavity becomes a fluid-filled, shock-absorbing sac, sometimes called the *bag of waters,* in which the embryo floats during development. The **chorion** (KO-ree-on), shown in Figures 23-4 and 23-5, develops into an important fetal membrane in the **placenta** (plah-SEN-tah). The *chorionic villi* shown in Figure 23-5 connect the blood vessels of the chorion to the placenta. The placenta (Figure 23-5) anchors the developing fetus to the uterus and provides a "bridge" for the exchange of nutrients and waste products between mother and baby.

The placenta is a unique and highly specialized structure that has a temporary but very important series of functions during pregnancy. It is composed of tissues from mother and child and functions not only as a structural "anchor" and nutritive bridge but also as an excretory, respiratory, and endocrine organ (Figure 23-5).

Placental tissue normally separates the maternal blood, which fills the lacunae of the placenta, from the fetal blood so that no intermixing occurs. The very thin layer of placental tissue that separates maternal and fetal blood also serves as an effective "barrier" that can protect the developing baby from many harmful

substances that may enter the mother's bloodstream. Unfortunately, toxic substances, such as alcohol and some infectious organisms, may penetrate this protective placental barrier and injure the developing baby. The *cytomegalovirus (CMV)* or the bacterium that causes syphilis, for example, can easily pass through the placenta and cause developmental defects in the fetus.

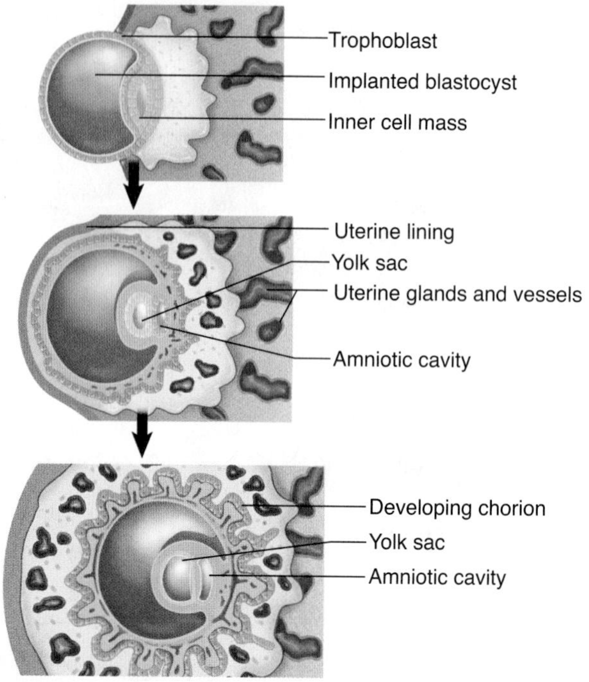

Figure 23-4 | **Implantation and early development.**

The hollow blastocyst implants itself in the uterine lining about 10 days after ovulation. Until the placenta is functional, nutrients are obtained by diffusion from uterine fluids. Notice the developing chorion and how the blastocyst eventually forms a yolk sac and amniotic cavity.

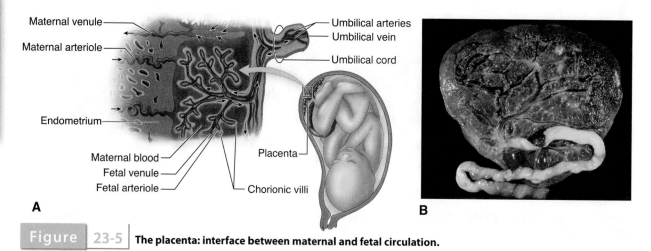

A

B

Figure 23-5 | **The placenta: interface between maternal and fetal circulation.**

The close placement of the fetal blood supply and the maternal blood in the lacunae of the placenta permits diffusion of nutrients and other substances. It also forms a thin barrier to prevent diffusion of most harmful substances. No mixing of fetal and maternal blood occurs. **A**, Diagram showing a cross section of the placental structure. **B**, Photograph of a normal, full-term placenta (fetal side) showing the branching of the placental blood vessels.

To learn more about fertilization and implantation, go to **AnimationDirect** on your CD.

Periods of Development

The length of pregnancy (about 39 weeks)—called the **gestation period**—is divided into three 3-month segments called *trimesters*. A number of terms are used to describe development during these periods known as the first, second, and third trimesters of pregnancy.

During the first trimester, or 3 months, of pregnancy, many terms are used. *Zygote* describes the ovum just after fertilization by a sperm cell. After about 3 days of constant cell division, the solid mass of cells, identified earlier as the *morula*, enters the uterus. Continued development transforms the morula into the hollow *blastocyst*, which then implants into the uterine wall.

The embryonic phase of development extends from the third week after fertilization until the end of week 8 of gestation. During this period in the first trimester, the term *embryo* is used to describe the developing individual. The fetal phase is used to indicate the period of development extending from week 9 to week 39. During this period, the term *embryo* is replaced by *fetus*.

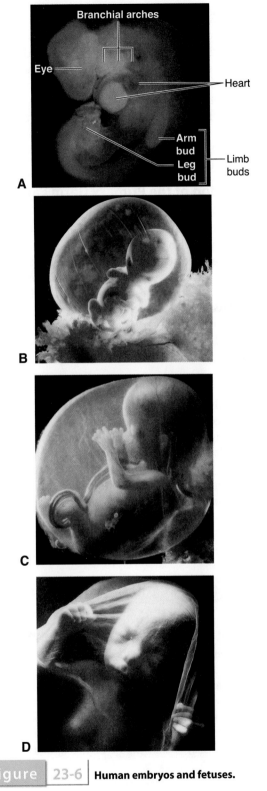

Figure 23-6 | **Human embryos and fetuses.**

A, At 35 days. **B,** At 49 days. **C,** At the end of the first trimester. **D,** At 4 months.

By day 35 of gestation (Figure 23-6, *A*), the heart is beating and, although the embryo is only 8 mm (about ⅜ inch) long, the eyes and so-called "limb buds," which ultimately form the arms and legs, are clearly visible. Figure 23-6, *C*, shows the stage of development of the fetus at the end of the first trimester of gestation. Body size is about 7 to 8 cm (3.2 inches) long. The facial features of the fetus are apparent, the limbs are complete, and gender can be identified. By month 4 (Figure 23-6, *D*) all organ systems are complete and in place.

Formation of the Primary Germ Layers

Early in the first trimester of pregnancy, three layers of unique cells develop that embryologists call the **primary germ layers** (Table 23-1). Each layer gives rise to definite structures such as the skin, nervous tissue, muscles, or digestive organs. Table 23-1 lists a number of structures derived from each primary germ layer called, respectively, **endoderm** (EN-doh-derm), or inside layer; **ectoderm** (EK-toh-derm), or outside layer; and **mesoderm** (MEZ-oh-derm), or middle layer.

Stem Cells

Stem cells are unspecialized cells that reproduce to form specific lines of specialized cells. At the very beginning of the embryonic stage, all the cells are stem cells. At this stage, they have their highest "stemness" or potency—that is, they are capable of producing many different kinds of cells in the body. Some stem cells remain throughout development and maturity such as the hematopoietic stem cells found in adult bone marrow. For example, adult stem cells

Table 23-1	Primary Germ Layer Derivatives	
ENDODERM	**ECTODERM**	**MESODERM**
Lining of gastrointestinal tract	Epidermis of skin	Dermis of skin
Lining of lungs	Tooth enamel	Cardiovascular system
Lining of hepatic and pancreatic ducts	Lens and cornea of eye	Many glands
Kidney ducts and bladder	Outer ear	Kidneys
Anterior pituitary gland (adenohypophysis)	Nasal cavity	Gonads
Thymus gland	Facial bones	Muscle
Thyroid gland	Skeletal muscles in head	Bones (except facial)
Parathyroid gland	Brain and spinal cord	
Tonsils	Sensory neurons	
	Adrenal medulla	

are found in the skin, many glands, muscles, nerve tissue, bone, and the gastrointestinal (GI) tract. Adult stem cells replace the specialized cells in a tissue and thus ensure stable, functional populations of the cell types needed for survival.

RESEARCH, ISSUES, AND TRENDS

HOW LONG DOES PREGNANCY LAST?

This seems like a silly question to most of us; the answer is 9 months, isn't it? Actually, the length of gestation (the amount of time one is pregnant) is defined in different ways in different situations and can vary from one pregnancy to another. The average gestation in humans is 266 days, starting at the day of conception. But physicians instead usually count from the beginning of the woman's last menstrual period, for an average of 280 days. But these are only averages. What is normal in one case can be different from what is normal in another case. In practice, any pregnancy of less than 37 weeks (259 days) is said to be premature, and any lasting more than 42 weeks (294 days) is said to be postmature. So as with many statistics regarding human function, what is "normal" can be spoken of only in generalities and averages.

Histogenesis and Organogenesis

The study of how the primary germ layers develop into many different kinds of tissues is called **histogenesis** (his-toh-JEN-eh-sis). The way that those tissues arrange themselves into organs is called **organogenesis** (or-gah-no-JEN-eh-sis).

The fascinating story of histogenesis and organogenesis in human development is long and complicated; its telling belongs to the science of embryology. But for the beginning student of anatomy and physiology, it seems sufficient to appreciate that human development begins when two sex cells unite to form a single-celled zygote and that the offspring's body evolves by a series of processes consisting of cell differentiation, multiplication, growth, and rearrangement, all of which take place in a definite, orderly sequence (Figure 23-7). Development of structure and function go hand in hand, and from 4 months of gestation, when every organ system is complete and in place, until term (about 280 days), fetal development is mainly a matter of growth. Figure 23-8, *A*, shows the normal intrauterine placement of a fetus just before birth in a full-term pregnancy.

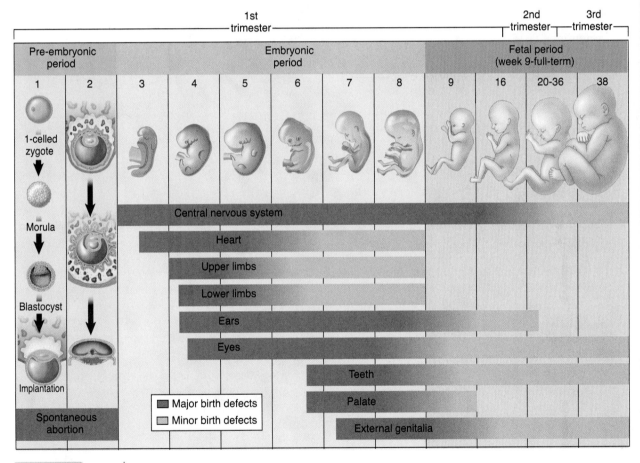

Figure 23-7 | **Critical periods of neonatal development.**

The red areas show when teratogens are most likely to cause major birth defects, and the yellow areas show when minor defects are more likely to arise.

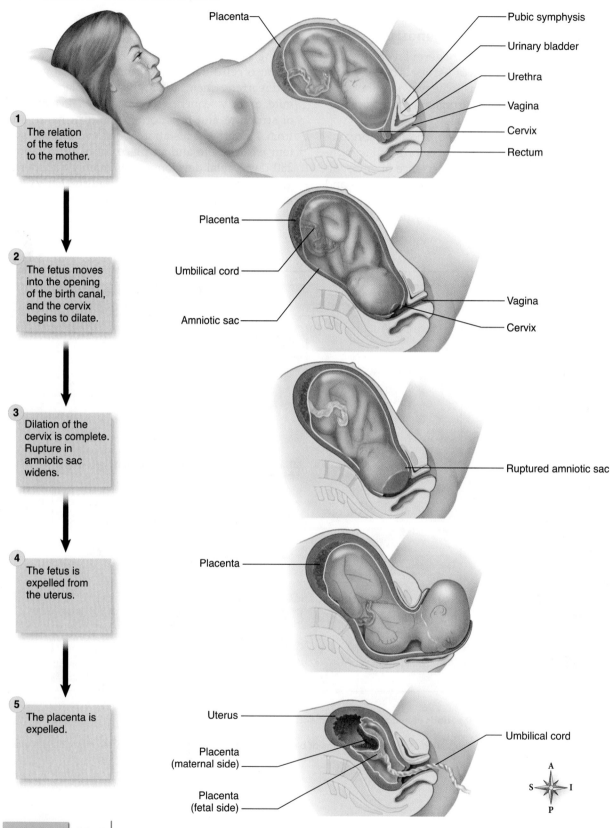

1. The relation of the fetus to the mother.

2. The fetus moves into the opening of the birth canal, and the cervix begins to dilate.

3. Dilation of the cervix is complete. Rupture in amniotic sac widens.

4. The fetus is expelled from the uterus.

5. The placenta is expelled.

Placenta

Pubic symphysis

Urinary bladder

Urethra

Vagina

Cervix

Rectum

Placenta

Umbilical cord

Amniotic sac

Vagina

Cervix

Ruptured amniotic sac

Placenta

Uterus

Placenta (maternal side)

Placenta (fetal side)

Umbilical cord

Figure 23-8 **Parturition.**

Birth or Parturition

The process of birth, or **parturition** (par-too-RISH-un), is the point of transition between the prenatal and postnatal periods of life. As pregnancy draws to a close, the uterus becomes "irritable" and, ultimately, muscular contractions begin and cause the cervix to dilate or open, thus permitting the fetus to move from the uterus through the vagina, or "birth canal," to the exterior. When contractions occur, the amniotic sac or "bag of waters" ruptures, and labor begins

The process normally begins with the fetus taking a head-down position against the cervix (Figure 23-8, *A*). A breech birth is one in which the fetus fails to turn head downward and consequently the feet are born first. This condition usually requires the baby to be born by **cesarean** (seh-ZAIR-ee-an) **section.** Often called simply a *C-section*, it is a surgical procedure in which the newborn is delivered through an incision in the abdomen and uterine wall. The procedure may be done when abnormal conditions of the mother or fetus (or both) make normal vaginal delivery hazardous or impossible.

Stages of Labor

Labor is the process that results in the birth of a baby. It has three stages (Figure 23-8, *B* to *E*):

1. Stage one—period from onset of uterine contractions until dilation of the cervix is complete.
2. Stage two—period from the time of maximal cervical dilation until the baby exits through the vagina.
3. Stage three—process of expulsion of the placenta through the vagina.

The time required for normal vaginal birth varies widely and may be influenced by many variables, including whether the woman has previously had a child. In most cases, stage one of labor lasts from 6 to 24 hours, and stage two lasts from a few minutes to an hour. Delivery of the placenta (stage three) normally occurs within 15 minutes after the birth of the baby.

To assess the general condition of a newborn, a system that scores five health criteria is often used. The criteria are heart rate (HR), respiration, muscle tone, skin color, and response to stimuli. Each aspect is scored as 0, 1, or 2—depending on the condition of the infant. The resulting total score is called the **Apgar score.** The Apgar score in a completely healthy newborn is 10.

 To learn more about the three stages of birth, go to **AnimationDirect** on your CD.

Multiple Births

The term *multiple birth* refers to the birth of two or more infants from the same pregnancy. The birth of twins is more common than the birth of triplets, quadruplets, or quintuplets. Multiple-birth babies are often born prematurely, so they are at a greater than normal risk of complications in infancy. However, premature infants that have modern medical care available have a much lower risk of complications than without such care.

Twinning, or double births, can result from at least two different natural processes:

1. **Identical (monozygotic) twins** result from the splitting of embryonic tissue from the same zygote early in development. As Figure 23-9, *A,*

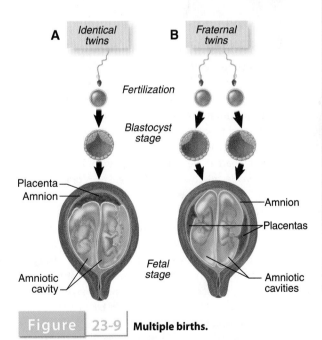

Figure 23-9 **Multiple births.**

A, Identical twins develop when embryonic tissue from a single zygote splits to form two individuals. Notice that the placenta and the part of the amnion separating the amniotic cavities are shared by the twins. **B,** Fraternal twins develop when two ova are fertilized at about the same time, producing two separate zygotes. Notice that each fraternal twin has its own placenta and amnion.

shows, identical, or monozygotic, twins usually share the same placenta but have separate umbilical cords. Because they develop from the same fertilized egg, identical twins have the same genetic code. Despite this, identical twins are not absolutely identical in terms of structure and function. Different environmental factors and personal experiences lead to individuality even in genetically identical twins.

2. **Fraternal (dizygotic) twins** result from the fertilization of two different ova by two different spermatozoa (Figure 23-9, *B*). Fraternal or dizygotic twinning requires the production of more than one mature ovum during a single menstrual cycle, a trait that is often inherited. Multiple ovulations may also occur in response to certain fertility drugs, especially the gonadotropin preparations. Fraternal twins are no more closely related genetically than any other brother-sister relationship. Because two separate fertilizations must occur, it is even possible for fraternal twins to have different biological fathers. Triplets, quadruplets, and other multiple births may be identical, fraternal, or any combination.

More and more often, multiple births result from medical treatments. For example, fertility-enhancing drugs sometimes increase the number of eggs released at ovulation and thus increase the likelihood of multiple births. *In vitro* fertilization (see the Research, Issues, and Trends box below) and other reproductive medical procedures often involve implantation of multiple embryos—increasing the odds of successful reproduction while also increasing the odds of multiple births.

> **QUICK CHECK**
>
> 1. What is meant by the term *parturition?*
> 2. What are the three stages of *labor?*
> 3. How do *multiple births* occur?

RESEARCH, ISSUES, AND TRENDS

FREEZING UMBILICAL CORD BLOOD

The concept of development of blood cells from red bone marrow, a process called *hemopoiesis,* was introduced in Chapter 12. Ultimately, the presence of **stem cells** is required for bone marrow to produce blood cells. The fact that umbilical cord blood is rich in these stem cells has great clinical significance.

In the past, if the stem cells in the bone marrow of a child were destroyed as a result of leukemia or by chemotherapy, death would result unless a bone marrow transplant was possible to provide replacement stem cells. "Matching" a child in need of stem cells with a suitable bone marrow donor occurs in only about 40% to 50% of cases, and the search for a match may take 3 or more months. The stem cells obtained from cord blood are as effective as those obtained from traditional bone marrow and are easier to match to the recipient. More than 2000 cord blood transfusions have been performed worldwide to provide stem cells for treatment of numerous genetic diseases, leukemia, sickle-cell anemia, lymphoma, and other types of cancer. As cord blood donations increase and supplies become more readily available, cord blood transfusions may eliminate or reduce the need for obtaining bone marrow as a source of stem cells, particularly for use in treating children.

After the umbilical cord is cut after birth, the blood that remains in the cord is simply drained into a sterile bag (see illustration), frozen, and then stored in liquid nitrogen in one of the numerous cord-blood centers in the United States.

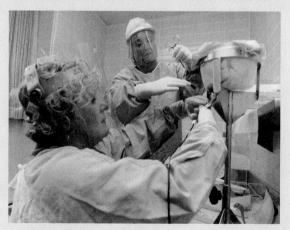

Disorders of Pregnancy

Implantation Disorders

A pregnancy has the best chance of a successful outcome, the birth of a healthy baby, if the blastocyst is implanted properly in the uterine wall. However, proper implantation does not always occur. Many offspring are lost before implantation occurs, often for unknown reasons.

As mentioned in the previous chapter, implantation outside the uterus results in an ectopic pregnancy. If the blastocyst implants in a region of endometriosis or normal peritoneal membrane, the pregnancy may be successful if there is room for the developing fetus to grow. Ectopic pregnancies that do succeed must be delivered by C-section rather than by normal vaginal birth. If an ectopic pregnancy occurs in a uterine tube, which cannot stretch to accommodate the developing offspring, the tube may rupture and cause life-threatening hemorrhaging. So-called *tubal pregnancies* are the most common type of ectopic pregnancy.

Occasionally, the blastocyst implants in the uterine wall near the cervix. This in itself may present no problem, but if the placenta grows too closely to the cervical opening a condition called **placenta previa** (PREE-vee-ah) results. The normal dilation and softening of the cervix that occurs in the third trimester often causes painless bleeding as the placenta near the cervix separates from the uterine wall. The massive blood loss that may result can be life threatening for both mother and offspring (Figure 23-10, *A*).

Separation of the placenta from the uterine wall can occur even when implantation occurs in the upper part of the uterus. When this occurs in a pregnancy of 20 weeks or more, the condition is called **abruptio placentae** (ab-RUP-chee-oh plah-SEN-tah). Complete separation of the placenta causes the immediate death of the fetus. The severe hemorrhaging that often results, sometimes hidden in the uterus, may cause circulatory shock and death of the mother within minutes. A cesarean section and perhaps also a hysterectomy must be performed immediately to prevent blood loss and death (Figure 23-10, *B*).

Preeclampsia

Preeclampsia (pree-ee-KLAMP-see-ah), also called *toxemia of pregnancy,* is a serious disorder that occurs in about 1 in every 20 pregnancies. This disorder is characterized by the onset of acute hypertension after the twenty-fourth week, accompanied by proteinuria and edema. The causes of preeclampsia are largely unknown, despite intense research efforts. Preeclampsia can result in complications such as abruptio placentae, stroke, hemorrhage, fetal malnutrition, and low birth weight. This condition can progress to *eclampsia,* a life-threatening form of toxemia that causes severe convulsions, coma, kidney failure, and perhaps death of the fetus and mother.

Fetal Death

A *miscarriage* is the loss of an embryo or fetus before the twentieth week (or a fetus weighing less than 500 g or 1.1 lb). Technically known as a **spontaneous abortion,** the most common cause of such a loss is a structural or functional defect in the developing offspring. Abnormalities of the mother, such as hypertension, uterine abnormalities, and hormonal imbalances, can also cause spontaneous abortions. After 20 weeks, delivery of a lifeless infant is termed a **stillbirth.**

Birth Defects

Developmental problems present at birth are often called **birth defects.** Such abnormalities may be structural or functional, perhaps even involving behavior and personality. Birth defects may be caused by genetic factors such as abnormal genes or inheritance of an abnormal number of chromosomes. Birth defects also may be caused by exposure to environmental factors called **teratogens** (TAYR-ah-toh-jenz).

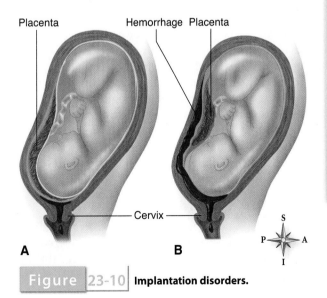

Figure 23-10 **Implantation disorders.**

A, Placenta previa. **B,** Abruptio placentae.

ANTENATAL DIAGNOSIS AND TREATMENT

Advances in **antenatal** (from the Latin *ante,* "before," *natus,* "birth") **medicine** now permit extensive diagnosis and treatment of disease in the fetus much like any other patient. This new dimension in medicine began with techniques by which Rh babies could be given transfusions before birth.

Current procedures using images provided by ultrasound equipment (see figures) allow physicians to prepare for and perform, before the birth of a baby, corrective surgical procedures such as bladder repair. These procedures also allow physicians to monitor the progress of other types of treatment on a developing fetus. Figure *A* shows placement of the ultrasound transducer on the abdominal wall. The resulting image is called an *ultrasonogram.* Figures *B* and *C* show two-dimensional and the newer three-dimensional types of ultrasonogram of a 20-week and 21-week fetus (respectively).

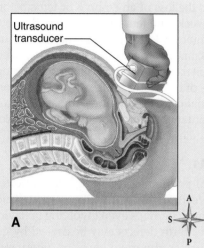

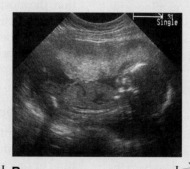

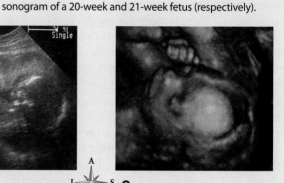

A **B** **C**

Teratogens include radiation (e.g., x-rays), chemicals (e.g., drugs, cigarettes, or alcohol), and infections in the mother (e.g., herpes or cytomegalovirus). Some teratogens are also mutagens because they do their damage by changing the genetic code in cells of the developing embryo. Nutritional deficiencies during pregnancy also can lead to birth defects.

As Figure 23-7 shows, the period during the first trimester when the tissues are beginning to differentiate and the organs are just starting to develop is the time that teratogens are most likely to cause damage. In fact, teratogens can cause spontaneous abortion (miscarriage) if significant damage occurs during the pre-embryonic stage.

Postpartum Disorders

Puerperal (pyu-ER-per-al) **fever,** or *childbed fever,* is a syndrome of postpartum mothers characterized by bacterial infection that progresses to septicemia (blood infection) and possibly death. Until the 1930s, puerperal fever was the leading cause of maternal death—claiming the lives of more than 20% of postpartum

women. Modern antiseptic techniques prevent most postpartum infections now. Puerperal infections that do occur are usually treated successfully by an immediate and intensive program of antibiotic therapy.

After a child is born, it needs the nourishment of mother's milk to survive. However, a number of disorders of lactation (milk production) may occur to prevent a mother from nursing her infant. For example, anemia, malnutrition, emotional stress, and structural abnormalities of the breast can all interfere with normal lactation. **Mastitis** (mas-TIE-tis), or breast inflammation, often caused by infection, can result in lactation problems or production of milk contaminated with pathogenic organisms. In many cultures, the availability of other nursing mothers or breast-milk substitutes allows proper nourishment of the infant when lactation problems develop. Most breast-milk substitutes are formulations of milk from another mammal, such as a cow. Infants who lack the enzyme *lactase* may not be able to digest the lactose present in human or animal milk, resulting in a condition called **lactose intolerance.** Infants with lactose intolerance are sometimes

FETAL ALCOHOL SYNDROME

Consumption of alcohol by the mother during pregnancy can have tragic effects on a developing fetus. Educational efforts to inform pregnant women about the dangers of alcohol are now receiving national attention. Even very limited consumption of alcohol during pregnancy poses significant hazards to the developing baby because alcohol can easily cross the placental barrier and enter the fetal bloodstream.

When alcohol enters the fetal blood, the potential result, called **fetal alcohol syndrome (FAS),** can cause tragic **congenital** abnormalities such as "small head," or **microcephaly** (my-kroh-SEF-ah-lee) (see figure), low birth weight, developmental disabilities such as mental retardation, and even fetal death.

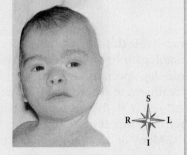

1. What is an *ectopic* pregnancy?
2. What disorders can result from improper implantation in the uterine wall?
3. What is a teratogen? Give some examples of teratogens.

sometimes given a lactose-free milk substitute made from soy or other plant products.

Postnatal Period

The **postnatal period** begins at birth and lasts until death. Although it is often divided into major periods for study, we need to understand and appreciate the fact that growth and development are continuous processes that occur throughout the life cycle.

Gradual changes in the physical appearance of the body as a whole and in the relative proportions of the head, trunk, and limbs are quite noticeable between birth and adolescence. Note in Figure 23-11 the obvious changes in the size of bones and in the proportionate sizes between different bones and body areas. The head, for example, becomes proportion-

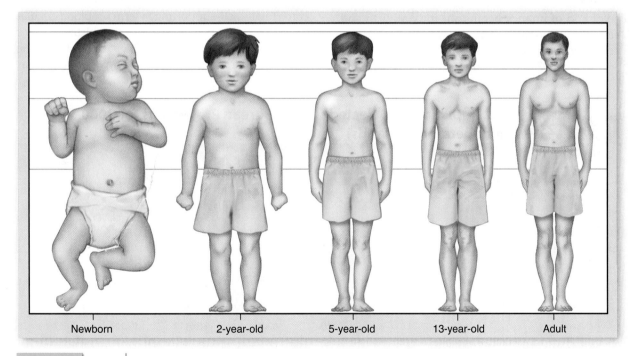

| Newborn | 2-year-old | 5-year-old | 13-year-old | Adult |

Figure 23-11 **Changes in the proportions of body parts from birth to maturity.**

Note the dramatic differences in head size.

ately smaller. Whereas the infant head is approximately one fourth the total height of the body, the adult head is only about one eighth the total height. The facial bones also show several changes between infancy and adulthood. In an infant the face is one eighth of the skull surface, but in an adult the face is half of the skull surface. Another change in proportion involves the trunk and lower extremities. The legs become proportionately longer and the trunk proportionately shorter. In addition, the thoracic and abdominal contours change, roughly speaking, from round to elliptical.

Such changes are good examples of the ever-changing and ongoing nature of growth and development. It is unfortunate that many of the changes that occur in the later years of life do not result in increased function. These degenerative changes are certainly important, however, and will be discussed later in this chapter. The following are the most common postnatal periods: (1) **infancy,** (2) **childhood,** (3) **adolescence,** (4) **adulthood,** and (5) **older adulthood.** Table 23-2 illustrates projected changes in U.S. population numbers in selected age-groups from 2000 through the year 2050.

Infancy

The period of infancy begins abruptly at birth and lasts about 18 months. The first 4 weeks of infancy are often referred to as the **neonatal** (nee-oh-NAY-tal) **period** (Figure 23-12). Dramatic changes occur at a

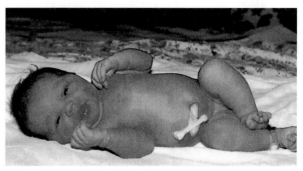

Figure 23-12 **The neonate infant.**

The umbilical cord has been cut.

rapid rate during this short but critical period. **Neonatology** (nee-oh-nay-TOL-oh-jee) is the medical and nursing specialty concerned with the diagnosis and treatment of disorders of the newborn or **neonate**. Advances in this area have resulted in dramatically reduced infant mortality.

Many of the changes that occur in the cardiovascular and respiratory systems at birth are necessary for survival. Whereas the fetus totally depends on the mother for life support, the newborn infant must become totally self-supporting in terms of blood circulation and respiration immediately after birth. A baby's first breath is deep and forceful. The stimulus to breathe results primarily from the increasing amounts of car-

Table 23-2	U.S. Population—Selected Census Bureau Projections for 2000-2050 (numbers in thousands)						
	2000	**2010**	**2020**	**2030**	**2040**	**2050**	**PERCENT CHANGE**
Total population	282,125	308,936	335,805	363,584	391,946	419,854	49%
INFANCY							
0-4 years	19,218	21,426	22,932	24,272	26,299	28,080	46%
CHILDHOOD/ADOLESCENCE							
5-19 years	61,331	61,810	65,955	70,832	75,326	81,067	32%
ADULTHOOD							
20-44 years	104,075	104,444	108,632	114,747	121,659	130,897	26%
45-64 years	62,440	81,012	83,653	82,280	88,611	93,104	49%
OLDER ADULTHOOD							
65-84 years	30,794	34,120	47,363	61,850	64,640	65,844	114%
85+ years	4,267	6,123	7,269	9,603	15,409	20,861	389%

bon dioxide (CO_2) that accumulate in the blood after the umbilical cord is cut following delivery.

Many developmental changes occur between the end of the neonatal period and 18 months of age. Birth weight doubles during the first 4 months and then triples by 1 year. The baby also increases in length by 50% by the twelfth month. The "baby fat" that accumulates under the skin during the first year begins to decrease, and the plump infant becomes leaner.

Early in infancy the baby has only one spinal curvature (Figure 23-13, *A*). The lumbar curvature appears between 12 and 18 months, and the once-helpless infant becomes a toddler who can stand (Figure 23-13, *B*). One of the most striking changes to occur during infancy is the rapid development of the nervous and muscular systems. This permits the infant to follow a moving object with the eyes (2 months); lift the head and raise the chest (3 months); sit when well supported (4 months); crawl (10 months); stand alone (12 months); and run, although a bit stiffly (18 months).

Childhood

Childhood extends from the end of infancy to sexual maturity or puberty—12 to 14 years in girls and 14 to 16 years in boys. Overall, growth during early childhood continues at a rather rapid pace, but month-to-month gains become less consistent. By the age of 6 years the child appears more like a preadolescent than an infant or toddler. The child becomes less chubby, the potbelly becomes flatter, and the face loses its babyish look. The nervous and muscular systems continue to develop rapidly during the middle years of childhood; by 10 years of age the child has developed numerous motor and coordination skills.

The *deciduous teeth*, which begin to appear at about 6 months of age, are lost during childhood, beginning at about 6 years of age. The *permanent teeth*, with the possible exception of the third molars, or wisdom teeth, all erupt by age 14.

Adolescence

The average age range of **adolescence** varies, but generally the teenage years (13 to 19) are referred to as adolescent years. The period is marked by rapid and intense physical growth, which ultimately results in sexual maturity. Many of the developmental changes that occur during this period are controlled by the secretion of sex hormones and are classified as **secondary sex characteristics.** Breast development is often the first sign of approaching

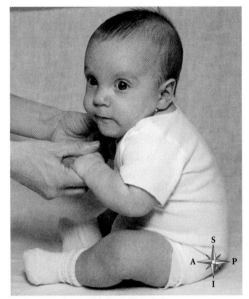

A

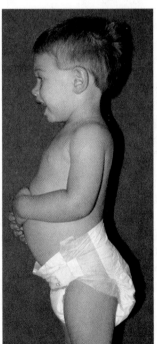

B

Figure 23-13

Spinal curvatures.

A, The infant spine. Photograph showing the normal rounded curvature of the vertebral column in an infant. **B**, Normal lumbar curvature of a toddler's spine.

puberty in girls, beginning about age 10. Most girls begin to menstruate at 12 to 13 years of age, which is about 3 years earlier than a century ago. In boys the first sign of puberty is often enlargement of the testicles, which begins between 10 and 13 years of age. Both sexes show a spurt in height during adolescence. In girls the spurt in height begins between the ages of 10 and 12 and is nearly complete by age 14 or 15. In boys the period of rapid growth begins between 12 and 13 and is generally complete by age 16.

Adulthood

Many developmental changes that begin early in childhood are not completed until the early or middle years of **adulthood.** Examples include the maturation of bone, resulting in the full closure of the growth plates, and changes in the size and placement of other body components such as the sinuses. Many body traits do not become apparent for years after birth. Normal balding patterns, for example, are determined at the time of fertilization by heredity but do not appear until maturity. As a general rule, adulthood is characterized by maintenance of existing body tissues. With the passage of years, the ongoing effort of maintenance and repair of body tissues becomes more and more difficult. As a result, degeneration begins. It is the process of aging, and it culminates in death.

Older Adulthood

Most body systems are in peak condition and function at a high level of efficiency during the early years of adulthood. As a person grows older, a gradual but certain decline takes place in the functioning of every major organ system in the body. The study of aging is called *gerontology*. Many of the biological changes associated with advancing age are shown in Figure 23-14. The illustration highlights the proportion of remaining function in a number of organs in older adulthood when compared with a 20-year-old person. Unfortunately, the mechanisms and causes of aging are not well understood.

Some gerontologists believe that an important aging mechanism is the limit on cell reproduction. Laboratory experiments have shown that many types of human cells cannot reproduce more than 50 times, thus limiting the maximum life span. Cells die continually, regardless of a person's age, but in older adulthood many dead cells are not replaced, causing degeneration of tissues. Perhaps the cells

are not replaced because the surrounding cells have reached their limit of reproduction. Perhaps differences in each individual's aging process result from differences in the reproductive capacity of cells. This mechanism seems to operate in individuals with **progeria** (proh-JAIR-ee-ah), a rare, inherited condition in which a person appears to age rapidly.

A variety of factors that affect the rates of cell death and cell reproduction have been cited as causes of aging. Some gerontologists believe that nutrition, injury, disease, and other environmental factors affect the aging process. A few have even proposed that aging results from cellular changes

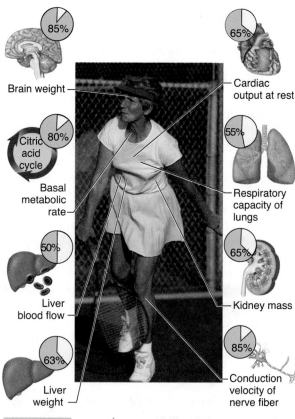

Figure 23-14 **Some biological changes associated with maturity and aging.**

Insets show proportion of remaining function in the organs of a person in late adulthood compared with that of a 20-year-old person. These data are for illustration only; individuals exhibit highly variable changes over the lifespan.

caused by slow-acting "aging" viruses found in all living cells. Other gerontologists have proposed that aging is caused by "aging" genes—genes in which aging is "preprogrammed." Yet another proposed cause of aging is autoimmunity. You may recall from Chapter 15 that autoimmunity occurs when the immune system attacks a person's own tissues.

One popular theory of aging states that oxygen *free radicals* play a major role in cellular aging (Figure 23-15). Free radicals are highly reactive forms of oxygen that normally result from cellular activities, but may damage the cell. As a person's cells produce more and more free radicals during the later years, more damage occurs to cellular structures and functions.

Although the causes and basic mechanisms of aging are yet to be understood, at least many of the signs of aging are obvious. The remainder of this chapter deals with a number of the more common degenerative changes that frequently characterize **senescence** (se-NES-ens), or older adulthood.

QUICK CHECK

1. Do the proportions of the human body change during postnatal development?

2. What is the neonatal period of development? Senescence?

3. During which phase of development do the deciduous teeth appear?

4. What biological changes happen during puberty?

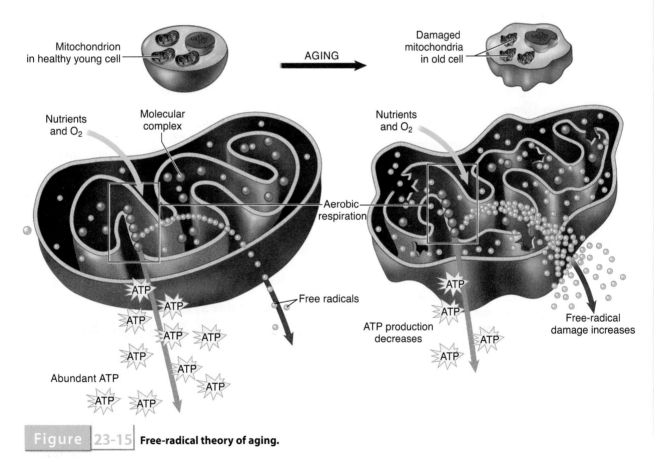

Figure 23-15   **Free-radical theory of aging.**

One of many possible mechanisms of the aging processes, free-radical production by cells may increase as a person gets older, increasing the amount of cellular damage. Free radicals are highly reactive forms of oxygen that are normal byproducts of cellular respiration in the mitochondria (shown) and other cell processes. As one ages, the number of free radicals increases as cellular efficiency decreases. Thus more cellular damage occurs, especially damage to cellular membranes, causing degeneration of the cell.

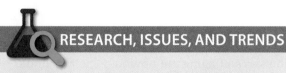

RESEARCH, ISSUES, AND TRENDS

PROGERIA

Progeria, also called Hutchinson-Gilford disease, is a rare, inherited condition in which a young child appears to age rapidly. In progeria (*pro-*, "before"; *-geras-*, "old age"; *-ia*, "condition of") the reproductive capacity of cells seems to be diminished. Thus the tissues of the body fail to maintain or repair themselves normally and many of the degenerative conditions more commonly seen in elderly individuals appear. Many of these conditions can be seen in this photograph of a young boy with progeria: thin, wrinkled skin; hair loss; loss of subcutaneous fat; and arthritis (causing stiff, partially flexed, and swollen joints). Most victims of progeria die of cardiovascular disease within the first or second decade of life.

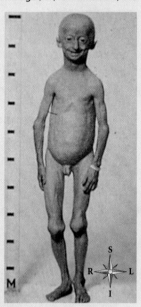

Effects of Aging

Skeletal System

In older adulthood, bones undergo changes in texture, degree of calcification, and shape. Instead of clean-cut margins, older bones develop indistinct and shaggy-appearing margins with spurs—a process called *lipping.* This type of degenerative change restricts movement because of the piling up of bone tissue around the joints. With advancing age, changes in calcification may result in reduction of bone size and in bones that are porous and subject to fracture. The lower cervical and thoracic vertebrae are the site of frequent fractures. The result is curvature of the spine and the shortened stature so typical of late adulthood. Degenerative joint diseases such as **osteoarthritis** (OS-tee-oh-ar-THRYE-tis) are also common in elderly adults.

Integumentary System (Skin)

With advancing age the skin becomes dry, thin, and inelastic. It "sags" on the body because of increased wrinkling and skinfolds. Pigmentation changes and the thinning or loss of hair are also common problems associated with the aging process.

Urinary System

The number of nephron units in the kidney decreases by almost 50% between the ages of 30 and 75. Also, because less blood flows through the kidneys as an individual ages, there is a reduction in overall function and excretory capacity or the ability to produce urine. In the bladder, significant age-related problems often occur because of diminished muscle tone. Muscle atrophy (wasting) in the bladder wall results in decreased capacity and inability to empty or void completely.

Respiratory System

In older adulthood the costal cartilages that connect the ribs to the sternum become hardened or calcified. This makes it difficult for the rib cage to expand and contract as it normally does during inspiration and expiration. In time the ribs gradually become "fixed" to the sternum, and chest movements become difficult. When this occurs, the rib cage remains in a more expanded position, respiratory efficiency decreases, and a condition called "barrel chest" results. With advancing years a generalized atrophy or wasting of muscle tissue takes place as the contractile muscle cells are replaced by connective tissue. This loss of muscle cells decreases the strength of the muscles associated with inspiration and expiration.

Cardiovascular System

Degenerative heart and blood vessel disease is one of the most common and serious effects of aging. Fatty deposits build up in blood vessel walls and narrow the passageway for the movement of blood, much as the buildup of scale in a water pipe decreases flow and pressure. The resulting condition, called **atherosclerosis** (ath-er-oh-skleh-ROH-sis), often leads to eventual blockage of the coronary arteries and a "heart attack" (myocardial infarction [MI]). If fatty accumulations or other substances in blood vessels calcify, actual hardening of the arteries, or **arteriosclerosis** (ar-teer-ee-oh-skleh-ROH-sis), occurs. Rupture of a hardened vessel in the brain (stroke), also called a cerebrovascular accident or CVA, is a frequent cause of serious disability or death in the older adult. **Hypertension,** or high blood pressure, is also more common in older adults.

Special Senses

The sense organs, as a group, all show a gradual decline in performance and capacity as a person ages. Most people are farsighted by age 65 because eye lenses become hardened and lose elasticity; the lenses cannot become curved to accommodate for near vision. This hardening of the lens is called **presbyopia** (pres-bee-OH-pee-ah), which means "old eye." Many individuals first notice the change at about 40 or 45 years of age, when it becomes difficult to do close-up work or read without holding printed material at arm's length. This explains the increased need, with advancing age, for bifocals, or glasses that incorporate two lenses, to automatically accommodate for near and distant vision. Loss of transparency of the lens or its covering capsule is another common age-related eye change. If the lens actually becomes cloudy and significantly impairs vision, it is called a **cataract** (KAT-ah-rakt) and must be removed surgically. The incidence of **glaucoma** (glaw-KOH-mah), the most serious age-related eye disorder, increases with age. Glaucoma causes an increase in the pressure within the eyeball and, unless treated, often results in blindness. The risk of retinal degeneration or detachment also increases with age.

In many elderly people a very significant loss of hair cells in the organ of Corti (spiral organ of the inner ear) causes a serious decline in the ability to hear certain frequencies. In addition, the eardrum and attached ossicles become more fixed and less able to transmit mechanical sound waves. Some degree of hearing impairment is universally present in the older adult.

The sense of smell and taste is also decreased. The resulting loss of appetite may be caused, at least in part, by the replacement of taste buds with connective tissue cells. Only about 40% of the taste buds present at age 30 remain in an individual at age 75

Reproductive Systems

Although most men and women remain sexually active throughout their later years, mechanisms of the

sexual response may change, and fertility declines. In men, erection may be more difficult to achieve and maintain, and urgency for sex may decline. In women, lubrication of the vagina may decrease. Although men can continue to produce gametes as they age, women experience a cessation of reproductive cycling between the ages of 45 and 60—**menopause.** Menopause results from a decrease in the cyclic production of gonadotropins from the pituitary, which in turn reduces estrogen secretion.

The process of menopause is not a disease condition and is considered a natural period of biological transition in a woman's life. However, in addition to the cessation of menstrual cycles, the decrease in blood estrogen levels during this period accounts for a number of common and often troubling symptoms which include hot flashes, sleep disturbances, and dryness and thinning of the vaginal wall in many women.

In the past, these menopause-related symptoms resulting from low estrogen levels were almost always treated with estrogen given as *hormone replacement therapy (HRT)* or more simply, *hormone therapy (HT)*. In recent years this practice has been used more carefully because of the increased risk of some forms of cancer, stroke, blood clotting disorders, and other serious side effects in some older women who had been using HRT for long periods or had begun HRT well after the onset of menopause. HRT continues to be used in many younger women when they first enter menopause. Fortunately, medications other than estrogen are also available to effectively treat or prevent most menopausal symptoms and other health problems, such as loss of bone mass, or osteoporosis (see Chapter 7), and heart disease, that increase in frequency in older women who have lower blood estrogen levels. As with any therapy, treatment for menopause-related symptoms requires careful, individualized risk-benefit analysis.

QUICK CHECK

1. What are some changes that occur in the skeleton as one ages?
2. How is kidney function affected during old age?
3. What changes in the cardiovascular system occur in older adults?
4. How does one's eyesight change during late adulthood?

RESEARCH, ISSUES, AND TRENDS

EXTENDING THE HUMAN LIFE SPAN

In the past few decades, the increased availability of better food, safer surroundings, and advanced medical care has extended quality living for many around the world. But even simple changes in lifestyle, regardless of modern medical wonders, can keep the effects of aging from creeping up too soon. Perhaps the three most important "low-tech" methods for improving the quality of life as you age are healthful diet, exercise, and stress management. A healthful diet is not available to some individuals, but it is available to most of us. We are learning more every day about what kind of diet is best, even to the point of being

able to manage specific diseases through diet. Exercise performed on a regular basis, even if light or moderate, can not only keep our skeletal and muscular systems more fit but can also decrease aging's effects on the nervous system, endocrine system, digestive system, immune system—the list seems endless. And last, even ancient and simple techniques of stress management such as meditation have been shown to help reduce the effects of aging and the diseases that often accompany aging such as heart disease and strokes.

In short, we can usually stay young longer if we *eat right*, *exercise*, and *relax*.

SCIENCE APPLICATIONS

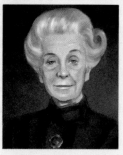

Rita Levi-Montalcini
(born 1909)

EMBRYOLOGY

Rita Levi-Montalcini had just finished a medical degree in her native Italy when in 1938 the Fascist government under Mussolini barred all "non-Aryans" from working in academic and professional careers. Being Jewish, Levi-Montalcini was forced to move to Belgium to work. But when Belgium was about to be invaded by the Nazis, she decided to return home to Italy and work in secret. Her home laboratory was very crude but in it she made some important discoveries about how the nervous system develops during embryonic growth. After World War II, she was invited to Washington University in St. Louis to work. There, she discovered the existence of *nerve growth*

factor (NGF), for which she later won the 1986 Nobel Prize. Her discovery of a chemical that regulates the growth of new nerves during early brain development has led to many different paths of investigation. For example, by learning more about growth regulators, we have gained knowledge about how the nervous system and also other tissues, organs, and systems of the body develop.

Today many professions make use of the discoveries of embryology—the study of early development. These discoveries are important not only for health professionals involved in obstetrics and prenatal health care but also for those studying and practicing adult medicine. Even the fields of gerontology (study of aging) and geriatrics (treatment of the aged) have benefited from embryological research. How? The insights gained on how tissue development is regulated in the embryo have given scientists a better understanding of how to possibly stimulate damaged tissues in older adults to repair or regenerate themselves.

Outline Summary

To download an MP3 version of the chapter summary for use with your iPod or portable media player, access the **Audio Chapter Summaries** on your CD.

Prenatal Period

A. Prenatal period begins at conception and continues until birth

B. Science of fetal growth and development is called *embryology*

C. Fertilization to implantation
    1. Fertilization normally occurs in outer third of oviduct (uterine or fallopian tube) (Figure 23-2)
    2. Fertilized ovum called a *zygote;* zygote is genetically complete—all that is needed for expression of hereditary traits is time and nourishment

3. After 3 days of cell division, the zygote has developed into a solid cell mass called a *morula*
4. Continued cell divisions of the morula produce a hollow ball of cells called a *blastocyst*
5. Blastocyst implants in the uterine wall about 10 days after fertilization
6. Blastocyst forms the amniotic cavity and chorion of the placenta (Figure 23-4)
7. Placenta provides for exchange of nutrients between the mother and fetus

D. Periods of development
1. Length of pregnancy or gestation period is about 39 weeks
2. Embryonic phase extends from third week after fertilization to the end of week 8 of gestation
3. Fetal phase extends from week 8 to week 39 of gestation

E. Formation of the primary germ layers—appear in the developing embryo after implantation of the blastocyst (Table 23-1):
1. Endoderm—inside layer
2. Ectoderm—outside layer
3. Mesoderm—middle layer
4. All organ systems are formed and functioning by month 4 of gestation (Figure 23-6)

F. Stem cells—unspecialized cells that reproduce to form specific lines of specialized cells

G. Histogenesis and organogenesis (Figure 23-7)
1. Formation of new organs (organogenesis) and tissues (histogenesis) occurs from specific development of the primary germ layers
2. Each primary germ layer gives rise to definite structures such as the skin and muscles
3. Growth processes include cell differentiation, multiplication, growth, and rearrangement
4. From 4 months of gestation until delivery, the development of the baby is mainly a matter of growth

Birth or Parturition

A. Process of birth called *parturition* (Figure 23-8)
1. At the end of week 39 of gestation, the uterus becomes "irritable"
2. Fetus takes head-down position against the cervix
3. Muscular contractions begin, and labor is initiated
4. Amniotic sac ("bag of waters") ruptures
5. Cervix dilates
6. Fetus moves through vagina to exterior

B. Stages of labor
1. Stage one—period from onset of uterine contractions until dilation of the cervix is complete
2. Stage two—period from the time of maximal cervical dilation until the baby exits through the vagina
3. Stage three—process of expulsion of the placenta through the vagina
4. Clinicians sometimes refer to the recovery period immediately following delivery of the placenta as the fourth stage of labor
5. Apgar score assesses general condition of a newborn infant
6. Cesarean section (C-section)—surgical delivery, usually through an incision in the abdomen and uterine wall

C. Multiple births—two or more infants from the same pregnancy
1. Identical siblings result from the splitting of tissue from the same zygote, making them genetically identical
2. Fraternal siblings develop from different ova that are fertilized separately

Disorders of Pregnancy

A. Implantation disorders
1. Ectopic pregnancy—implantation outside the uterus (e.g., tubal pregnancy)
2. Placenta previa—growth of the placenta at or near cervical opening, often resulting in separation of the placenta from the uterine wall
3. Abruptio placentae—separation of a normally placed placenta from the uterine wall

B. Preeclampsia (toxemia of pregnancy)—syndrome of pregnancy that includes hypertension, proteinuria, and edema; may progress to eclampsia, a severe toxemia that may result in death

C. Fetal death
1. Spontaneous abortion (miscarriage)—loss before week 20 (or 500 g)
2. Stillbirth—loss after 20 weeks

D. Birth defects
1. May be inherited (*congenital abnormalities*) or acquired
2. Acquired defects are caused by teratogens (agents that disrupt normal development)

E. Postpartum disorders
1. Puerperal fever is caused by bacterial infection that may progress to septicemia and death; occurs in mothers after delivery (postpartum)

2. Lactation and thus infant nutrition can be disrupted by anemia, malnutrition, and other factors
   a. Mastitis—inflammation or infection of the breast
   b. Milk can be supplied by another nursing mother or by breast-milk substitutes
   c. Lactose intolerance results from an infant's inability to digest lactose present in human or animal milk

Postnatal Period

A. Postnatal period begins at birth and lasts until death
B. Divisions of postnatal period into isolated time frames can be misleading; life is a continuous process; growth and development are continuous
C. Obvious changes in the physical appearance of the body—in whole and in proportion—occur between birth and maturity (Figure 23-11)
D. Divisions of postnatal period
   1. Infancy
   2. Childhood
   3. Adolescence and adulthood
   4. Older adulthood
E. Infancy
   1. First 4 weeks called *neonatal period* (Figure 23-12)
   2. Neonatology—medical and nursing specialty concerned with the diagnosis and treatment of disorders of the newborn
   3. Many cardiovascular changes occur at the time of birth; fetus is totally dependent on mother, whereas the newborn must immediately become totally self-supporting (respiration and circulation)
   4. Respiratory changes at birth include a deep and forceful first breath
   5. Developmental changes between the neonatal period and 18 months include:
      a. Doubling of birth weight by 4 months and tripling by 1 year
      b. 50% increase in body length by 12 months
      c. Development of normal spinal curvature by 15 months (Figure 23-13)
      d. Ability to raise head by 3 months
      e. Ability to crawl by 10 months
      f. Ability to stand alone by 12 months
      g. Ability to run by 18 months

F. Childhood
   1. Extends from end of infancy to puberty—13 years in girls and 15 in boys
   2. Overall rate of growth remains rapid but decelerates
   3. Continuing development of motor and coordination skills
   4. Loss of deciduous or baby teeth and eruption of permanent teeth
G. Adolescence
   1. Average age range of adolescence is from 13 to 19 years
   2. Period of rapid growth resulting in sexual maturity (adolescence)
   3. Appearance of secondary sex characteristics regulated by secretion of sex hormones
   4. Growth spurt typical of adolescence; begins in girls at about 10 and in boys at about 12
H. Adulthood
   1. Growth plates fully close in adult; other structures such as the sinuses acquire adult placement
   2. Adulthood characterized by maintenance of existing body tissues
   3. Degeneration of body tissue begins in adulthood
I. Older adulthood
   1. Degenerative changes characterize older adulthood, or senescence
   2. Every organ system of the body undergoes degenerative changes
      a. A variety of mechanisms of aging have been described
      b. The free-radical theory of aging states that the number of oxygen free radicals increases as one ages, thus increasing the rate of cellular damage
   3. Senescence culminates in death

Effects of Aging (Figure 23-14)

A. Skeletal system
   1. Aging causes changes in the texture, calcification, and shape of bones
   2. Bone spurs develop around joints
   3. Bones become porous and fracture easily
   4. Degenerative joint diseases such as osteoarthritis are common
B. Integumentary system (skin)

1. With age, skin "sags" and becomes thin, dry, and wrinkled (or inelastic)
2. Pigmentation problems are common
3. Frequent thinning or loss of hair occurs

C. Urinary system
   1. Nephron units decrease in number by 50% between ages 30 and 75
   2. Blood flow to kidney, and therefore ability to form urine, decreases
   3. Bladder problems such as inability to void completely are caused by muscle wasting in the bladder wall

D. Respiratory system
   1. Calcification of costal cartilages causes rib cage to remain in expanded position, resulting in barrel chest
   2. Wasting of respiratory muscles decreases respiratory efficiency
   3. Respiratory membrane thickens; movement of oxygen from alveoli to blood is slowed

E. Cardiovascular system
   1. Degenerative heart and blood vessel disease is among the most common and serious effects of aging
   2. Fat deposits in blood vessels (atherosclerosis) decrease blood flow to the heart and may cause complete blockage of the coronary arteries
   3. Hardening of arteries (arteriosclerosis) may result in rupture of blood vessels, especially in the brain (stroke)
   4. Hypertension or high blood pressure is common in older adulthood

F. Special senses
   1. All sense organs show a gradual decline in performance with age
   2. Eye lenses become hard and cannot accommodate for near vision; result is farsightedness in many people by age 45 (presbyopia)
   3. Loss of transparency of lens or cornea is common (cataract)
   4. Glaucoma (increase in pressure in eyeball) is often the cause of blindness in older adulthood
   5. Loss of hair cells in inner ear produces frequency deafness in many older people
   6. Decreased transmission of sound waves caused by loss of elasticity of eardrum and fixing of the bony ear ossicles is common in older adulthood
   7. Some degree of hearing impairment is universally present in the aged
   8. Only about 40% of the taste buds present at age 30 remain at age 75

G. Reproductive system
   1. Changes in the sexual response
      a. Men—erection is more difficult to achieve and maintain; urgency for sex may decline
      b. Women—lubrication during intercourse may decrease
   2. Changes in fertility
      a. Men—may continue to be fertile throughout later adult years
      b. Women—experience menopause (cessation of reproductive cycling) between the ages of 45 and 60

New Words

amniotic cavity	morula	
Apgar score	neonatal period	
blastocyst	neonate	
chorion	neonatology	
ectoderm	organogenesis	
embryology	parturition	
endoderm	postnatal period	
fertilization	prenatal period	
gestation period	primary germ layers	
histogenesis	senescence	
implantation	yolk sac	
mesoderm	zygote	

Diseases and Other Clinical Terms

abruptio placentae	lactose intolerance
antenatal medicine	laparoscope
birth defect	mastitis
cesarean section	microcephaly
congenital	placenta previa
fetal alcohol syndrome (FAS)	preeclampsia
fraternal (dizygotic) twins	progeria
identical (monozygotic) twins	puerperal fever
	spontaneous abortion
	stillbirth
	teratogen

Review Questions

1. Explain what occurs between the time of ovulation and the implantation of the fertilized egg into the uterus.
2. Explain the function of the chorion and placenta.
3. Name the three primary germ layers, and name three structures that develop from each layer.
4. Define histogenesis and organogenesis.
5. Describe and give the approximate length of each of the three stages of labor.
6. What is the difference between identical and fraternal twins?
7. What is an ectopic pregnancy? Where is it most likely to occur?
8. What is placenta previa? What is abruptio placentae?
9. What is preeclampsia?
10. What is a teratogen?
11. What is the stimulus for a baby's first breath?
12. Name three developmental changes that occur during infancy.
13. Briefly explain what biological developments occur during childhood.
14. Briefly explain what biological developments occur during adolescence.
15. Briefly explain what biological developments occur during adulthood.
16. What is progeria?
17. Explain the effects of aging on the skeletal system.
18. Explain the effects of aging on the respiratory system.
19. Explain the effects of aging on the cardiovascular system.
20. Explain the effects of aging on vision.

Critical Thinking

21. Where do the nutrients used by the zygote between the time of fertilization and implantation come from?
22. Explain the evolution of the function of the yolk sac.
23. What hormones are produced by the placenta? What is their function?

Chapter Test

1. The fertilized ovum is called a _____.
2. After about 3 days of mitosis, the fertilized ovum forms a solid mass of cells called the _____.
3. Mitosis continues, and by the time the developing egg reaches the uterus, it has become a solid ball of cells called the _____.
4. The _____ anchors the developing fetus to the uterus and provides a bridge for the exchange of substances between the mother and baby.
5. The _____ period lasts about 39 weeks and is divided into trimesters.
6. The three primary germ layers are the _____, the _____, and the _____.
7. The process by which the primary germ layers develop into tissues is called _____.
8. The process by which tissues develop into organs is called _____.
9. The process of birth is called _____.
10. Twins resulting from two different ova being fertilized by two different sperm are called _____ twins.
11. Twins resulting from the splitting of embryonic tissue from the same zygote are called _____ twins.
12. Agents that can disrupt normal histogenesis and organogenesis are called _____.
13. The first 4 weeks of infancy is referred to as the _____ period.
14. _____ is a degenerative joint disease that is common to older adults.
15. _____ is another name for "hardening of the arteries."
16. _____ means "old eye" and causes older adults to be farsighted.
17. If the lens of the eye becomes cloudy and impairs vision, the condition is called a _____.
18. _____s causes an increase in pressure within the eyeball.

Match each term in Column A with its corresponding description in Column B.

Column A
19. _____ infancy
20. _____ childhood
21. _____ adolescence
22. _____ adulthood
23. _____ older adulthood

Column B
a. period during which the deciduous teeth are lost
b. period during which closure of the bone growth plates occur
c. period that begins at birth
d. senescence
e. period during which the secondary sex characteristics usually begin to develop

Match each disorder in Column A with its corresponding description or cause in Column B.

Column A
24. _____ ectopic pregnancy
25. _____ abruptio placentae
26. _____ placenta previa
27. _____ preeclampsia
28. _____ puerperal fever
29. _____ mastitis
30. _____ progeria

Column B
a. a condition in which the blastocyst implants too close to the cervical opening of the uterus
b. inflammation of the breast
c. a postpartum disorder characterized by a bacterial infection that progresses to septicemia
d. an inherited condition in which the person seems to age very rapidly
e. separation of the placenta from the uterine wall in a pregnancy of 20 weeks or longer
f. a disorder characterized by acute hypertension after 24 weeks of pregnancy
g. the implantation of the blastocyst outside the uterus

Study Tips

continued from page 639

5. The stages of labor, the important events in the postnatal periods, and the effects of old age on various organ systems also can be put on flash cards to facilitate learning.
6. Make a chart of the disorders of pregnancy; organize it by mechanism or cause: implantation disorders, preeclampsia, birth defects, and postpartum disorders.

7. In your study group, go over the flash cards of the stages of development, making sure you know the proper sequence. Go over the flash cards for the primary germ layers and what organs come from each layer. Review the flash cards for the stages of labor, the postnatal periods, and the effects of aging, and review the chart of the disorders. Review the questions at the end of the chapter and discuss possible test questions.

Case Studies

1. Mary is pregnant with her first baby and is touring the maternity floor of a local hospital in preparation for the upcoming birth. She keeps asking about their precautions regarding aseptic technique in the "home-style" birthing rooms. She is concerned because her own grandmother died of an infection after delivering Mary's mother. Why should Mary be concerned? What might happen if aseptic techniques are not adhered to?
2. Two-year-old Abe has always been small for his age and is now diagnosed as having developmental disabilities. Abe's grandmother believes that these disabilities are associated with the moderate drinking done by Abe's mother during her pregnancy. Is Abe's grandmother simply trying to justify her meddling—or could his mother's drinking have caused his problems?
3. Lactose intolerance is sometimes treated by removing lactose from the diet. For example, infants with lactose intolerance may be given a lactose-free milk substitute to avoid the indigestion, diarrhea, abdominal discomfort, and other symptoms of this condition. Older children and adults with lactose intolerance may avoid dairy products and other foods high in lactose. Your friend Aileen, who has lactose intolerance, takes a tablet with her favorite ice cream (chocolate fudge) that helps her avoid any problems. What might this tablet contain?

Objectives

**After you have completed this chapter,
you should be able to:**

1. Explain how genes can cause disease.

2. Distinguish between dominant and
   recessive genetic traits.

3. Describe sex-linked inheritance.

4. List some important inherited diseases.

5. Describe how nondisjunction can
   result in trisomy or monosomy and list
   some disorders that result from it.

6. List some tools used in genetic
   counseling and explain how they are
   used to help clients.

7. Describe how genetic disorders can
   be treated.

24 Genetics and Genetic Diseases

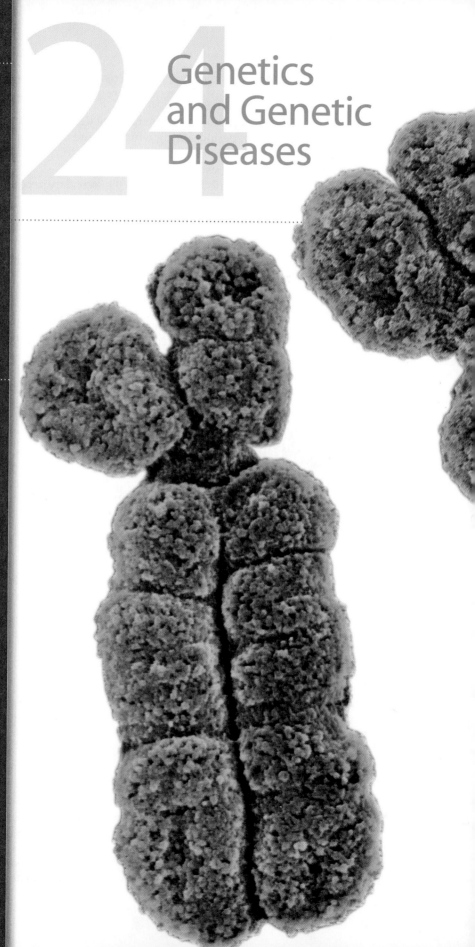

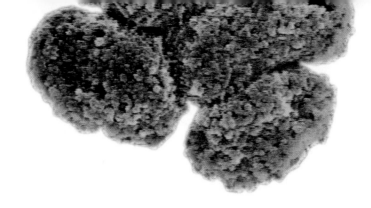

It seems that today we are hearing more and more about the relationship of **genetics,** the scientific study of inheritance, and human disease. Popular news magazines are running story after story on the revolution in treating fatal inherited disorders by using something called **gene therapy.** Health and science columns in newspapers keep us informed of the latest discoveries of genes involved with disease, human behavior, and even longevity. Television programs outline the progress of the largest coordinated biological quest that anyone can remember: mapping the entire human genetic code and listing all the proteins encoded there. Clearly, a person cannot be informed about the mechanisms of human disease today without some knowledge of basic genetics. In this chapter, we briefly review the essential concepts of genetics and explain how information in the genetic code can cause disease.

STUDY TIPS This chapter covers one of the most publicly discussed areas in biology. Stories on DNA fingerprinting, gene therapy, and genetically engineered medications and foods are often in the media. An understanding of the topics discussed in this chapter will allow you to better evaluate whether the stories you hear and read are based on good science.

1. The chapter requires an understanding of DNA; a review of the material in Chapter 3 may be helpful. It is important to understand how DNA controls the activity of the cell:

    DNA ⟶ mRNA ⟶ enzyme ⟶ biochemical reactions in the cell.

2. Make flash cards for the genetic terms. Be sure to understand how the genetic makeup of the parents determines the probability for traits in the offspring in both autosomal and sex-linked traits.

3. Understand the link between nondisjunction and both trisomy and monosomy. Mutations are changes in the DNA code; they can be harmful or beneficial.

4. Make a chart of the genetic disorders and organize them based on the mechanism or cause, single-gene or chromosomal.

continued on page 685

Genetics and Human Disease

History shows that humans have been aware of inheritance for thousands of years; however, it was not until the 1860s that the scientific study of inheritance—**genetics**—was born. At that time, a monk living in what is now part of the Czech Republic discovered the basic mechanism by which traits are transmitted from parents to offspring. That man, Gregor Mendel, demonstrated that independent units (which we now call *genes*) are responsible for the inheritance of biological traits.

The science of genetics developed from Mendel's quest to explain how normal biological characteristics are inherited. As time went by, and more genetic studies were done, it became clear that certain diseases have a genetic basis. As you may recall from Chapter 5, some diseases are inherited directly. For example, the blood-clotting disorder called *hemophilia* is inherited by children from a parent who has the genetic code for hemophilia. Other diseases are only partly determined by genetics; that is, they involve genetic risk factors (Chapter 5). For example, certain forms of skin cancer are thought to have a genetic basis. A person who inherits the genetic code associated with skin cancer will develop the disease only if the skin is also heavily exposed to the ultraviolet radiation in sunlight.

Chromosomes and Genes

Mechanisms of Gene Function

Mendel proposed that the genetic code is transmitted to offspring in discrete, independent units that we now call **genes** (jeans). Recall from Chapter 3 that each gene is a sequence of nucleotide bases in the deoxyribonucleic acid (DNA) molecule (also see Chapter 2). Each gene contains a genetic code that the cell transcribes to a messenger RNA (mRNA) molecule. Each mRNA molecule moves to a ribosome, where the code is translated to form a specific protein molecule. Many of the protein molecules thus formed are *enzymes*, functional proteins that permit specific biochemical reactions to occur (see Chapter 2). Because enzymes regulate the biochemistry of the body, they regulate the entire structure and function of the body. Thus genes determine the structure and function of the human body by producing a set of specific regulatory enzymes.

As described in Chapter 3, genes are simply segments of a DNA molecule. While the genetic codes of its genes are being actively transcribed, the DNA is in a threadlike form called *chromatin*. During cell division, each replicated strand of chromatin coils to form a compact mass called a *chromosome* (Figure 24-1). Thus each DNA molecule can be called either a *chromatin strand* or a *chromosome*. Genes may be actively transcribed in the chromatin form of DNA but not in the chromosome form. To make things easy, however, we will simply use the term *chromosome* for DNA and the term *gene* for each distinct encoding segment within a DNA molecule.

The Human Genome

The entire collection of genetic material in each typical cell of the human body is called the **genome** (JEEN-ome). The typical human genome includes 46 individual nuclear chromosomes and one mitochondrial chromosome. In 2003, the Human Genome Project—a publicly funded, worldwide collaboration to map all of the genes in the human genome—was completed. This landmark event coincided exactly with the 50th anniversary of the discovery of DNA. We now know that the human genome contains only about 20,000-25,000 or so genes. This is less than a quarter of the number originally estimated and only about one and a half times as many genes as in a fruit fly!

We also know that less than 2% of the DNA carries genes, the rest, called "junk DNA," either is not used or is edited out of mRNA before it is used to make proteins. Some of this noncoding DNA may actually be made up of broken bits of genes that are no longer functional—remnants of our evolutionary past. Termed **pseudogenes**, these bits of formerly functional genes are like genetic fossils that have begun to reveal an interesting history of our genetic past.

The current draft of the human genome shows us that most coding genes tend to lie in clusters, separated by long stretches of noncoding DNA. About 200 of the newly discovered genes in the human genome seem to be bacterial in origin, perhaps inserted there by bacteria in our distant ancestors.

Although we now have the essential picture of the details of the human genome, much work still lies ahead in the field of **genomics** (jen-OME-iks), the analysis of the genome's code. Besides filling in the remaining details of the rough draft, we have much work to do in discovering all the possible mutations that might exist (see the discussion later in this chapter) and all the proteins encoded by the genes that make up the human genome. In fact, this quest has generated another field called **proteomics** (proh-tee-OME-iks), the analysis of the proteins encoded by the genome. The entire group of proteins encoded by the human genome is called the human **proteome** (PROH-tee-ome). The ultimate goal of proteomics is to understand the role of each protein in the body. Understanding the roles of every single protein in the body will certainly go a long way toward improving our knowledge of the normal function of the body as well as the mechanisms for many diseases.

Information obtained about the human genome can be expressed in a variety of ways. As you can see in Figure 24-1, an **ideogram** (ID-ee-oh-gram), or simple cartoon of a chromosome, is often used in genomics to show the overall physical structure of a chromosome. The constriction in the ideogram shows the relative position of the chromosome's centromere. The shorter segment of the chromosome is called the **p-arm** and the longer segment is called the **q-arm**. The bands in an ideogram of a chromosome show staining landmarks and help identify the regions of the chromosome. Sometimes physical maps of genes will show exact positions of individual genes on the p-arm and q-arm of a chromosome. A more detailed representa-

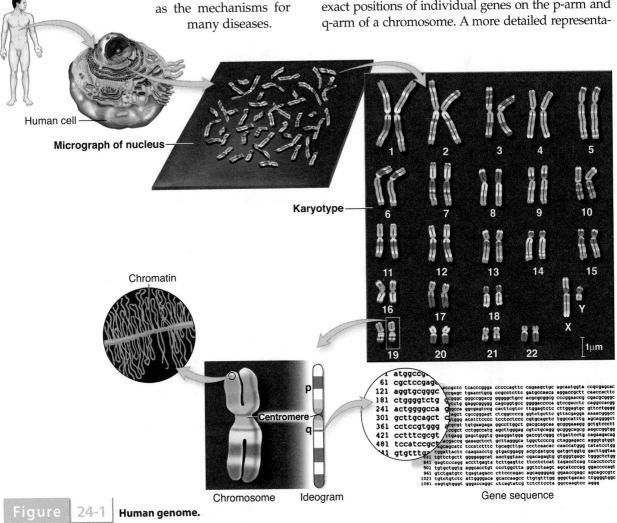

Figure 24-1 | **Human genome.**

A cell taken from the body is stained and photographed. A photograph of nuclear chromosomes is then cut and pasted, arranging each of the 46 chromosomes into numbered pairs of decreasing size to form a chart called the **karyotype.** Each chromosome is a coiled mass of chromatin (DNA). In this figure, differentially stained bands in each chromosome appear as different bright colors. Such bands are useful as reference points when identifying the locations of specific genes within a chromosome. The staining bands are also represented on an ideogram, or simple graph, of the chromosome as reference points to locate specific genes. The genes themselves are usually represented as the actual sequence of nucleotide bases, abbreviated as *a, c, g,* and *t*. In this figure, the sequence of one exon (segment) of a gene called *GPI* from chromosome 19 is shown. Each of these representations can be thought of as a type of "genetic map."

tion of a gene would show the actual sequence of nucleotide bases, abbreviated *a, c, g,* and *t* for *adenine, cytosine, guanine,* and *thymine,* as shown in Figure 24-1.

Distribution of Chromosomes to Offspring

Each cell of the human body contains 46 chromosomes. The only exceptions to this principle are the **gametes**—male *spermatozoa* and female *ova.* Recall from Chapter 22 that a special form of nuclear division called *meiosis* (Figure 24-2) produces gametes

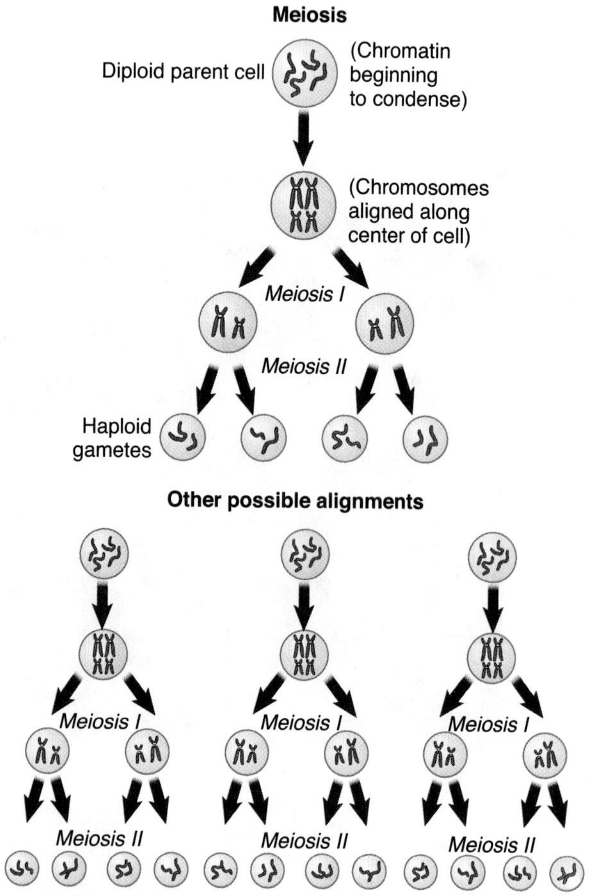

Figure 24-2 | **Meiosis.**

In meiosis, a series of two divisions results in the production of gametes with half the number of chromosomes of the original parent cell. In this figure, the original cell has four chromosomes and the gametes each have two chromosomes. During the first division of meiosis, pairs of similar chromosomes line up along the cell's equator for even distribution to daughter cells. Because different pairs assort independently of each other, any of four (2^2) different combinations of chromosomes may occur. Because human cells have 23 pairs of chromosomes, more than 8 million (2^{23}) different combinations are possible.

with only 23 chromosomes—exactly half the usual number. When a sperm (with its 23 chromosomes) unites with an ovum (with its 23 chromosomes) at conception, a *zygote* with 46 chromosomes is formed. Thus the zygote has the same number of chromosomes as each body cell in the parents.

As Figure 24-1 shows, the 46 human chromosomes can be arranged in 23 pairs according to size. One pair called the **sex chromosomes** may not match, but the remaining 22 pairs of **autosomes** (AW-toh-sohms) always appear to be nearly identical to each other.

Because half of an offspring's chromosomes are from the mother and half are from the father, a unique blend of inherited traits is formed. According to principles first discovered by Mendel, each chromosome asserts itself independently during meiosis (see Figure 24-2). This means that as sperm are formed, chromosome pairs separate and the maternal and paternal chromosomes get mixed up and redistribute themselves independently of the other chromosome pairs. Thus each sperm is likely to have a *different* set of 23 chromosomes. Because ova are formed in the same manner, each ovum is likely to be genetically different from the ovum that preceded it. Independent assortment of chromosomes ensures that each offspring from a single set of parents is very likely to be genetically unique—a phenomenon known as *genetic variation.*

The principle of independent assortment also applies to individual genes or groups of genes. During one phase of meiosis, pairs of matching chromosomes line up along the equator of the cell and exchange genes. This process is called *crossing-over* because genes from a particular location cross over to the same location on the matching gene (Figure 24-3). Sometimes a whole group stays together and crosses over as a single unit—a phenomenon called *gene linkage.* Crossing-over introduces additional possibilities for genetic variation among offspring of a set of parents.

QUICK CHECK

1. How do genes produce biological traits?
2. Who might be considered the founder of the scientific study of genetics?
3. What is the difference between an *autosome* and a *sex chromosome*?
4. List some mechanisms that increase genetic variation among human offspring.

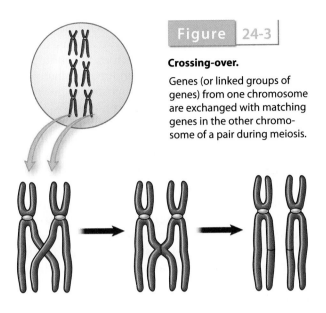

Figure 24-3

Crossing-over.

Genes (or linked groups of genes) from one chromosome are exchanged with matching genes in the other chromosome of a pair during meiosis.

Gene Expression

Hereditary Traits

Mendel discovered that the genetic units we now call *genes* may be expressed differently among individual offspring. After rigorous experimentation with pea plants, he discovered that each inherited trait is controlled by two sets of similar genes, one from each parent. We now know that each autosome in a pair matches its partner in the type of genes it contains. In other words, if one autosome has a gene for hair color, its partner will also have a gene for hair color—in the same location on the autosome. Although both genes specify hair color, they may not specify the *same* hair color. Mendel discovered that some genes are **dominant** and some are **recessive.** A dominant gene is one whose effects are seen and that is capable of masking the effects of a recessive gene for the same trait.

Consider the example of **albinism** (AL-bin-iz-em), a total lack of melanin pigment in the skin and eyes. Because they lack dark pigmentation, people with this condition have difficulty with seeing and protecting themselves from burns in direct sunlight. The genes that cause albinism are recessive; the genes that cause normal melanin production are dominant. By convention, dominant genes are represented by uppercase letters and recessive genes by lowercase letters. One can represent the gene for albinism as *a* and the gene for normal skin pigmentation as *A*. A person with the gene combination *AA* has two dominant genes—and so will exhibit a normal skin color. Someone with the gene combination *Aa* will also have normal skin color because the normal gene *A* is dominant over the recessive albinism gene *a*. Only a person with the gene combination *aa* will have albinism because there is no dominant gene to mask the effects of the two recessive genes.

In the example of albinism, a person with the gene combination of *Aa* is said to be a genetic **carrier** of albinism. This means that the person can transmit the albinism gene, *a*, to offspring. Thus two normal parents each having the gene combination *Aa* can produce both normal children and children that have albinism (Figure 24-4).

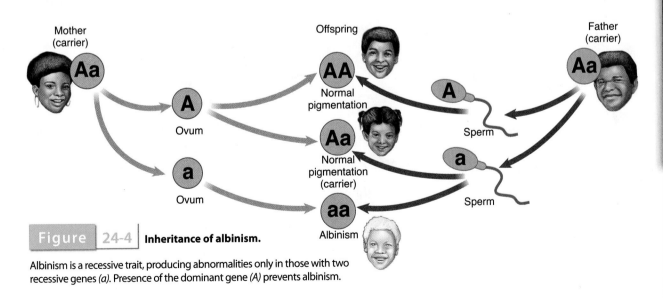

Figure 24-4 | **Inheritance of albinism.**

Albinism is a recessive trait, producing abnormalities only in those with two recessive genes *(a)*. Presence of the dominant gene *(A)* prevents albinism.

What happens if two different dominant genes occur together? Suppose there is a gene A^1 for light skin and a gene A^2 for dark skin. In a form of dominance called **codominance,** they will simply have equal effects and a person with the gene combination A^1A^2 will exhibit a skin color that is something between light and dark. Recall from Chapter 12 that the genes for sickle cell anemia behave this way. A person with two sickle cell genes will have *sickle cell anemia,* whereas a person with one normal gene and one sickle cell gene will have a milder condition called *sickle cell trait.*

Sex-Linked Traits

Recall from our earlier discussion that, in addition to the 22 pairs of autosomes, there is one pair of sex chromosomes. Notice in Figure 24-1 that the chromosomes of this pair do not have matching structures. The larger sex chromosome is called the *X chromosome,* and the smaller one is called the *Y chromosome.* The X chromosome is sometimes called the *female chromosome* because it has genes that determine female sexual characteristics. If a person has only X chromosomes, she is genetically a female. The Y chromosome is often called the *male chromosome* because anyone possessing a Y chromosome is genetically a male. Thus all normal females have the sex chromosome combination *XX* and all normal males have the combination *XY.* Because men produce both X-bearing and Y-bearing sperm, any two parents can produce male or female children (Figure 24-5).

These large X chromosomes contain many genes besides those needed for female sexual traits. Genes for producing certain clotting factors, the photopigments in the retina of the eye, and many other proteins are also found on the X chromosome. The tiny Y chromosome, on the other hand, contains few genes other than those that determine the male sexual characteristics. Thus males and females need at least one normal X chromosome; otherwise the genes for clotting factors and other essential proteins would be missing. Nonsexual traits thus carried on sex chromosomes are called sex-linked traits. Most **sex-linked traits** are called *X-linked traits* because they are determined by the genes in the large X chromosome.

Dominant X-linked traits appear in each person as one would expect for any dominant trait. In females, recessive X-linked genes are masked by dominant genes in the other X chromosome. Only females with two recessive X-linked genes can exhibit the recessive trait. Because males inherit only one X chromosome (from the mother), the presence of only one recessive X-linked gene is enough to produce the recessive trait. In short, in males, there are no matching genes in the Y chromosome to mask recessive genes in the X chromosome. For this reason, X-linked recessive traits appear much more often in males than in females.

An example of a recessive X-linked condition is *red-green color blindness,* which involves a deficiency of photopigments in the retina (see Chapter 10). In

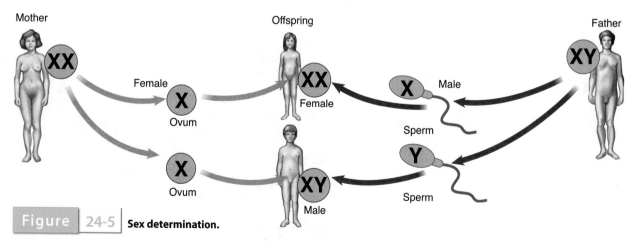

Mother

Offspring

Father

Female

Ovum

Male

Sperm

Female

Male

Ovum

Sperm

Figure 24-5 | **Sex determination.**

The presence of the Y chromosome specifies maleness. In the absence of a Y chromosome, an individual develops into a female.

this condition, male children of a parent who carries the recessive abnormal gene on an *X* chromosome may be color blind (Figure 24-6). A female can inherit this form of color blindness only if her father is color blind and her mother is color blind or is a color blindness carrier. The *X* chromosome has been studied in great detail by many researchers, and general locations for genes causing at least 59 distinct *X*-linked diseases have been identified.

 To learn more about sex-linked traits, go to **AnimationDirect** on your CD.

Genetic Mutations

The term *mutation* simply means "change." A *genetic mutation* is a change in the genetic code. Mutations may occur spontaneously, without the influence of factors outside the DNA itself. However, most genetic mutations are believed to be caused by **mutagens**—agents that cause mutations. Genetic mutagens include chemicals, some forms of radiation, and even viruses. Some mutations involve a change in the genetic code within a single gene, perhaps a slight rearrangement of the nucleotide sequence. Other mutations involve damage to a portion of a chromosome or a whole chromosome. For example, a portion of a chromosome may completely break away.

Beneficial mutations allow organisms to adapt to their environments. Because such mutant genes benefit survival, they tend to spread throughout a population over the course of several generations. Harmful mutations inhibit survival, so they are not likely to spread through the population. Most harmful mutations kill the organism in which they occur—or at least prevent successful reproduction—and so are never passed to offspring. If a harmful mutation is only mildly harmful, it may persist in a population over many generations.

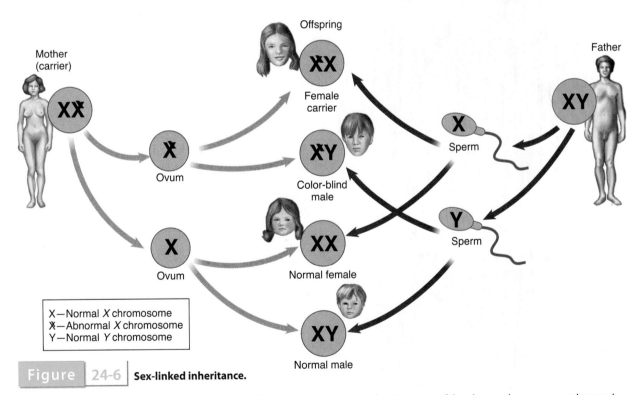

Figure 24-6 **Sex-linked inheritance.**

Some forms of color blindness involve recessive *X*-linked genes. In this case, a female carrier of the abnormal gene can produce male children who are color blind.

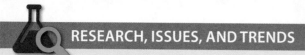
MITOCHONDRIAL INHERITANCE

Mitochondria are tiny, bacteria-like organelles present in every cell of the body (see Figure 3-2). Like a bacterium, each mitochondrion has its own circular DNA molecule, sometimes called *mitochondrial DNA* (mDNA or mtDNA). The figure shows an ideogram of the structure of a mitochondrial chromosome. Inheritance of mDNA occurs only through one's mother because the few mitochondria that a sperm may contribute to the ovum during fertilization do not survive. Because mDNA contains the only genetic code for several important enzymes, it has the potential for carrying mutations that produce disease. Mitochondrial inheritance is now known to transmit genes for several degenerative nerve and muscle disorders. One such disease is *Leber hereditary optic neuropathy*. In this disease, young adults begin losing their eyesight as the optic nerve degenerates—resulting in total blindness by age 30. Some medical researchers believe that at least some forms of several other diseases are associated with mDNA mutations. These diseases include *Parkinson disease, Alzheimer disease (AD), diabetes mellitis (DM)* with deafness, and maternally inherited forms of deafness, myopathy, and cardiomyopathy.

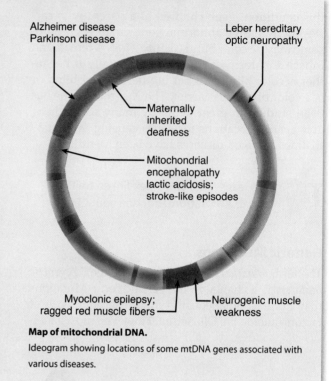

Map of mitochondrial DNA.

Ideogram showing locations of some mtDNA genes associated with various diseases.

QUICK CHECK

1. What is a *dominant* genetic trait? A *recessive* trait?
2. What is *codominance*?
3. How can a *mutant* gene benefit a human population?
4. What is *X-linked inheritance*?

Genetic Diseases

Mechanisms of Genetic Disease

As science writer Matt Ridley repeatedly and emphatically states in his best-selling book *Genome: The Autobiography of a Species in 23 Chapters*, "GENES ARE NOT THERE TO CAUSE DISEASE." Although we often hear of new "disease genes" being discovered and the pace is rapidly increasing—the function of these genes is not to cause disease any more than the function of an arm is to cause bone fractures. If you break an arm, a normal bone is broken and fails to serve its usual function. In genetic disorders, a normal gene or chromosome is broken (mutated) and fails to serve its usual function. Such a gene is sometimes called a "disease gene" because when it is broken, it is involved in the mechanism of a particular disease.

Keep this simple—but often overlooked—principle in mind as you read the following paragraphs.

As we just stated, genetic diseases are diseases produced by an abnormality in the genetic code. Many genetic diseases are caused by individual mutant genes that are passed from one generation to the next, making them *single-gene diseases*. The locations of some of the genes involved in selected single-gene diseases are shown in Figure 24-7. In single-gene diseases, the mutant gene may make an abnormal product that causes disease, or it may fail to make a product required for normal function. Some disease conditions result from the combined effects of inheritance and environmental factors. Because they are not solely caused by genetic mechanisms, such conditions are not genetic diseases in the usual sense of the word; they are instead said to involve a *genetic predisposition*.

Some genetic diseases do not result from an abnormality in a single gene. Instead, these diseases result from chromosome breakage or from the abnormal presence or absence of entire chromosomes. For example, a condition called **trisomy** (TRY-so-mee) may occur in which there is a triplet of autosomes rather than a pair. Trisomy results from a mistake in meiosis called *nondisjunction* when a pair of chromosomes fails to

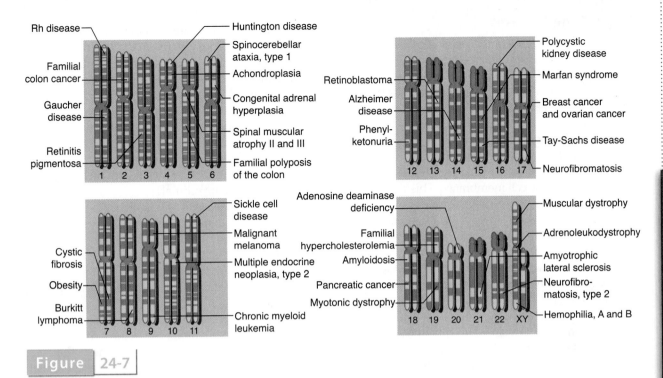

Figure 24-7

Location of genes involved in genetic diseases.

The ideogram of each chromosome is labeled with the location of just one or two examples of the many genes associated with genetic disease.

separate. This produces a gamete with two autosomes that are "stuck together" instead of the usual one. When this abnormal gamete joins with a normal gamete to form a zygote, the zygote has a triplet of autosomes (Figure 24-8). Usually trisomy of any autosome pair is fatal. However, if trisomy occurs in autosome pair 13, 15, 18, 21, or 22, a person may survive for a time but not without profound developmental defects. **Monosomy** (MAHN-oh-so-mee), the presence of only one autosome instead of a pair, also may result from conception involving a gamete produced by nondisjunction (see Figure 24-8). Like trisomy, monosomy

may produce life-threatening abnormalities. Because most trisomic and monosomic individuals die before they can reproduce, these conditions are not usually passed from generation to generation. Trisomy and monosomy are congenital conditions that are sometimes referred to as *chromosomal genetic diseases*.

> **QUICK CHECK**
>
> 1. How are *single-gene* diseases different from *chromosomal* conditions?
> 2. What is *nondisjunction*? How can it cause *trisomy*?

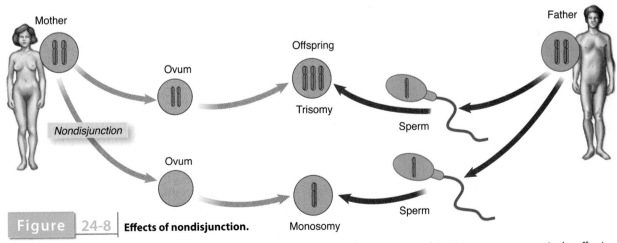

Figure 24-8 | **Effects of nondisjunction.**

Nondisjunction, failure of a chromosome pair to separate during gamete production, may result in trisomy or monosomy in the offspring.

Single-Gene Diseases

There are many single-gene diseases. Only a few are discussed here and summarized in Table 24-1.

Cystic fibrosis (SIS-tik fye-BROH-sis) **(CF)** is caused by a recessive gene in chromosome 7 that codes for *CFTR (CF transmembrane conductance regulator)*. CFTR normally regulates the transfer of sodium and chloride ions across cell membranes and serves as a chloride ion channel. When this gene is missing a single codon, the abnormal version of CFTR causes impairment of ion transport across cell membranes. This disruption causes exocrine cells to secrete thick mucus and sweat. The thickened mucus is especially troublesome in the gastrointestinal and respiratory tracts, where it can cause obstruction that leads to death.

Phenylketonuria (feen-il-kee-toh-NOO-ree-ah) **(PKU)** is caused by a recessive gene that fails to produce the enzyme *phenylalanine hydroxylase*. This is needed to convert the amino acid phenylalanine into another amino acid, tyrosine. Thus phenylalanine absorbed from ingested food accumulates, resulting in the abnormal presence of phenylketone in the urine (hence the name *phenylketonuria*). A high concentration of phenylalanine destroys brain tissue, so babies born with this condition are at risk of progressive mental retardation and perhaps death.

Many PKU victims are identified at birth by state-mandated tests. Once identified, PKU victims are put on diets low in phenylalanine, thus avoiding a toxic accumulation of it. You may be familiar with the printed warning for phenylketonurics commonly seen on products that contain aspartame (NutraSweet) or other substances made from phenylalanine. The mutant PKU gene may have originated among the Celts in western Europe, where it offered protection against the toxic effects of molds growing on grains stored in cold, damp climates.

Tay-Sachs disease (TSD) is a recessive condition involving failure to make a subunit of an essential lipid-processing enzyme, hexosaminidase. Abnormal lipids accumulate in the brain tissue of Tay-Sachs victims, causing severe retardation and death by 4 years of age. There is currently no specific therapy for this condition.

TSD is most prevalent among certain Jewish populations. Some epidemiologists believe that this ethnic distribution is related to the hypothesis that heterozygous carriers of the Tay-Sachs gene have a higher than normal resistance to tuberculosis (TB)—a potentially fatal disease that once killed millions in the crowded Jewish ghettos of many large cities. Residents of these TB-infested areas who carried the Tay-Sachs

Table 24-1 | Examples of Single-Gene Disorders

DISORDER	DOMINANCE	DESCRIPTION
Hemophilia (some forms)	Recessive (X-linked)	Group of blood-clotting disorders caused by a failure to form clotting factors VIII, IX, or XI
Albinism	Recessive	Lack of the dark-brown pigment melanin in the skin and eyes, resulting in vision problems and susceptibility to sunburn and skin cancer
Sickle cell anemia and sickle cell trait	Codominant	Blood disorder in which abnormal hemoglobin is produced, causing red blood cells to deform into a sickle shape
Red-green color blindness (X-linked)	Recessive	Inability to distinguish red and green light, resulting from a deficiency of photopigments in the cone cells of the retina
Cystic fibrosis (CF)	Recessive	Condition characterized by excessive secretion of thick mucus and concentrated sweat, often causing obstruction of the gastrointestinal (GI) or respiratory tracts
Phenylketonuria (PKU)	Recessive	Excess of phenylketone in the urine, which is caused by accumulation of phenylalanine in the tissues and may cause brain injury and death
Tay-Sachs disease	Recessive	Fatal condition in which abnormal lipids accumulate in the brain and cause damage that leads to death by age 4
Osteogenesis imperfecta	Dominant	Group of connective tissue disorders characterized by imperfect skeletal development that produces brittle bones
Multiple neurofibromatosis	Dominant	Disorder characterized by multiple, sometimes disfiguring, benign tumors of the Schwann cells (neuroglia) that surround nerve fibers
Duchenne muscular dystrophy (X-linked)	Recessive	Muscle disorder characterized by progressive atrophy of skeletal (DMD) muscle without nerve involvement
Hypercholesterolemia	Dominant	High blood cholesterol that may lead to atherosclerosis and other cardiovascular problems
Huntington disease (HD)	Dominant	Degenerative brain disorder characterized by chorea (purposeless movements), progressing to severe dementia and death by age 55
Severe combined immune deficiency (SCID)	Recessive	Failure of the lymphocytes to develop properly, in turn causing failure of the immune system's defense of the body; usually caused by adenosine deaminase (ADA) deficiency

gene apparently survived longer—and reproduced more frequently—than noncarriers.

Tay-Sachs is also found in higher than average frequencies in French Canadians in southeastern Quebec and Cajun French families in southern Louisiana—probably due to the gene's presence in several founders of these family groups, rather than natural selection by the threat of TB.

Chromosomal Diseases

Some genetic disorders are not inherited but result instead from nondisjunction during gamete formation. As Figure 24-8 shows, nondisjunction results in trisomy or monosomy.

The most well-known chromosomal disorder is *trisomy 21*, which produces a group of symptoms called **Down syndrome.** As Figure 24-9, *A*, shows, in this condition, there is a triplet of chromosome 21 rather than the usual pair. In the general population, trisomy 21 occurs in only 1 of every 600 or so live births. After age 35, however, a mother's chances of producing a trisomic child increase dramatically—to as high as 1 in 80 births by age 40. Down syndrome results from trisomy 21 and rarely from other genetic abnormalities (which can be inherited). This syndrome is characterized by mental retardation (ranging from mild to severe) and multiple defects that include distinctive facial appearance (Figure 24-9, *B*), enlarged tongue, short hands and feet with stubby digits, congenital heart disease, and susceptibility to acute leukemia. People with Down syndrome have a shorter-than-average life expectancy but can survive to old age.

Klinefelter syndrome is another genetic disorder resulting from nondisjunction of chromosomes (Figure 24-10, *B*). This disorder occurs in males with

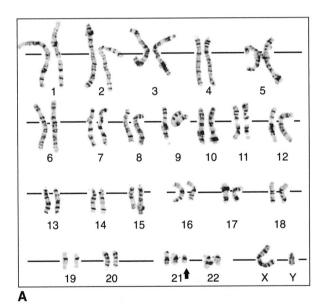

A

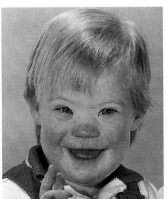

B

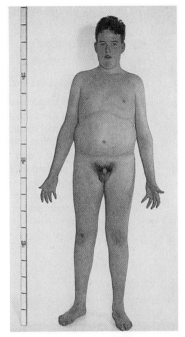

A

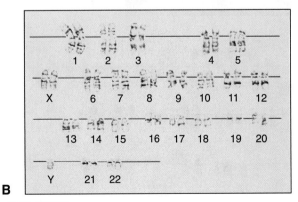

B

Figure 24-9

Down syndrome.

A, Down syndrome is usually associated with trisomy of chromosome 21, as you can see in this karyotype. **B,** A child with Down syndrome. Notice the distinctive anatomical features: folds around the eyes, flattened nose, round face, and small hands with short fingers.

Figure 24-10 Klinefelter syndrome.

A, This young man exhibits many of the characteristics of Klinefelter syndrome: small testes, some development of the breasts, sparse body hair, and long limbs. **B,** This syndrome results from the presence of two or more *X* chromosomes with a *Y* chromosome (genotypes XXY or XXXY, for example).

a *Y* chromosome and at least two *X* chromosomes, typically the *XXY* pattern. Characteristics of Klinefelter syndrome include long legs, enlarged breasts, low intelligence, small testes, sterility, and chronic pulmonary disease (Figure 24-10, *A*).

Turner syndrome, sometimes called *XO syndrome,* occurs in females with a single sex chromosome, *X*. Like the conditions described earlier, it results from nondisjunction during gamete formation (Figure 24-11, *B*). Turner syndrome is characterized by failure of the ovaries and other sex organs to mature (causing sterility), cardiovascular defects, dwarfism

or short stature, a webbed neck, and possible learning disorders (Figure 24-11, *A*). Symptoms of Turner syndrome can be reduced by hormone therapy using estrogens and growth hormone. Cardiovascular defects may be repaired surgically.

QUICK CHECK

1. How does avoidance of phenylalanine in the diet reduce the problems associated with *phenylketonuria (PKU)?*
2. What is trisomy 21?

Prevention and Treatment of Genetic Diseases

Genetic Counseling

The term *genetic counseling* refers to professional consultations with families regarding genetic diseases. Trained genetic counselors may help a family determine the risk of producing children with genetic diseases. Parents with a high risk of producing children with genetic disorders may decide to avoid having children. Genetic counselors may also help evaluate whether any offspring already born have a genetic disorder and offer advice on treatment or care. A growing list of tools is available to genetic counselors, some of which are described below.

Pedigree

A **pedigree** is a chart that illustrates genetic relationships in a family over several generations (Figure 24-12). Using medical records and family histories, the genetic counselors assemble the chart, beginning with the client and moving backward through as many generations as are known. Squares represent males; circles represent females. Fully shaded symbols represent affected individuals, whereas unshaded symbols represent normal individuals. Partially-shaded symbols represent **carriers** of a recessive trait. A horizontal line between symbols designates a sexual relationship that produced offspring.

The pedigree is useful in determining the possibility of producing offspring with certain genetic disorders. It also may tell a person whether he or she might have a genetic disorder that appears late in life, such as Huntington disease. In either case, a family can prepare emotionally, financially, and medically before a crisis occurs.

Figure 24-11

Turner syndrome.

A, This woman exhibits many of the characteristics of Turner syndrome, including short stature, webbed neck, and sexual immaturity. **B,** As this karyotype shows, Turner syndrome results from monosomy of sex chromosomes (genotype XO).

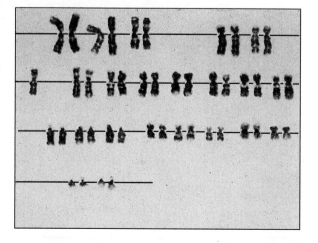

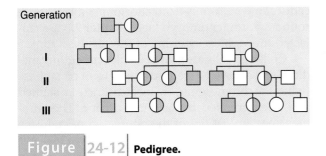

Generation

I

II

III

Figure 24-12 **Pedigree.**

Pedigrees chart the genetic history of family lines. Squares represent males, and circles represent females. Fully shaded symbols indicate affected individuals; partly shaded symbols indicate carriers, and unshaded symbols indicate unaffected noncarriers. Roman numerals indicate the order of generations. This pedigree reveals the presence of an *X*-linked recessive trait.

PUNNETT SQUARE

The **Punnett** (PUN-et) **square,** named after the English geneticist Reginald Punnett, is a grid used to determine the *probability* of inheriting genetic traits. As Figure 24-13, *A,* shows, genes in the mother's gametes are represented along one axis of the grid, and genes in the father's gametes are along the other axis. The ratio of different gene combinations in the offspring predicts their probability of occurrence in the next generation. Thus off-

spring produced by two carriers of PKU (a recessive disorder) have a one in four (25%) chance of inheriting this recessive condition (Figure 24-13, *A*). There is a two in four (50%) chance that an individual child produced will be a PKU carrier. Figure 24-13, *B,* shows that offspring between a carrier and a noncarrier cannot inherit PKU. What is the chance of an individual offspring being a PKU carrier in this case? Figure 24-13, *C,* shows the probability of producing an affected offspring when a PKU victim and a PKU carrier have children. Figure 24-13, *D,* shows the genetic probability when a PKU victim and a noncarrier produce children.

KARYOTYPE

Disorders that involve trisomy (extra chromosomes), monosomy (missing chromosomes), and broken chromosomes can be detected after a **karyotype** (KAIR-ee-o-type) is produced.

The first step in producing a karyotype is getting a sample of cells from the individual to be tested. This can be done by scraping cells from the lining of the cheek or from a blood sample containing white blood cells (WBCs). Fetal tissue can be collected by **amniocentesis** (am-nee-oh-sen-TEE-sis), a procedure in which fetal cells floating in the amniotic fluid are collected with a syringe

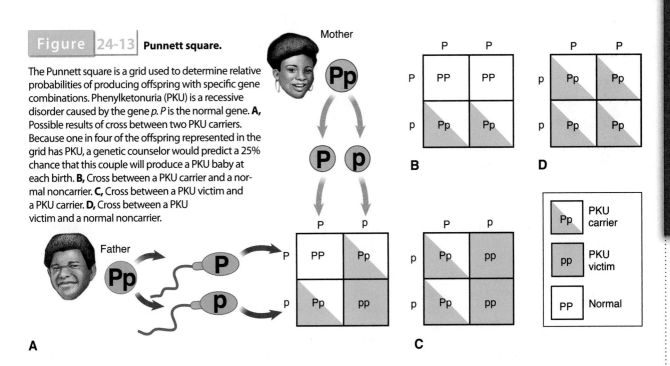

Figure 24-13 **Punnett square.**

The Punnett square is a grid used to determine relative probabilities of producing offspring with specific gene combinations. Phenylketonuria (PKU) is a recessive disorder caused by the gene *p. P* is the normal gene. **A,** Possible results of cross between two PKU carriers. Because one in four of the offspring represented in the grid has PKU, a genetic counselor would predict a 25% chance that this couple will produce a PKU baby at each birth. **B,** Cross between a PKU carrier and a normal noncarrier. **C,** Cross between a PKU victim and a PKU carrier. **D,** Cross between a PKU victim and a normal noncarrier.

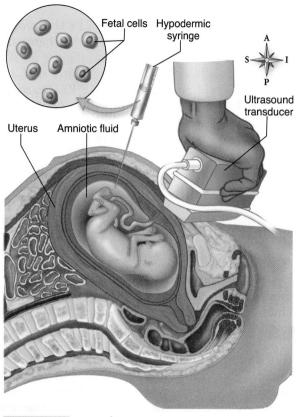

Fetal cells   Hypodermic syringe

Ultrasound transducer

Uterus   Amniotic fluid

Figure 24-14 **Amniocentesis.**

In amniocentesis, a syringe is used to collect amniotic fluid. Ultrasound imaging is used to guide the tip of the syringe needle to prevent damage to the placenta and fetus (see box on p. 650). Fetal cells in the collected amniotic fluid can then be chemically tested or used to produce a karyotype of the developing baby.

(Figure 24-14). **Chorionic villus sampling** is a procedure in which cells from chorionic villi that surround a younger embryo (see Chapter 23) are collected through the opening of the cervix.

Collected cells are grown in a special culture medium and allowed to reproduce. Cells in metaphase (when the chromosomes are most distinct) are stained and photographed using a microscope. The chromosomes are cut out of the photo and pasted on a chart in pairs according to size, as in Figures 24-1 and 24-9, *A*. Genetic counselors then examine the karyotype, looking for chromosome abnormalities. What chromosome abnormality is visible in Figure 24-9, *A*? Is this a male or female karyotype?

QUICK CHECK

1. What is genetic counseling?
2. How are pedigrees used by genetic counselors?
3. How is a Punnett square used to predict mathematical probabilities of inheriting specific genes?
4. How is a karyotype prepared? What is its purpose?

Treating Genetic Diseases

Until fairly recently, the only hope of treating any genetic disease was to treat the symptoms. In some diseases, such as PKU, this works well. If PKU victims simply avoid large amounts of phenylalanine in their diets, especially during critical stages of development, severe complications can be avoided. In Klinefelter and Turner syndromes, hormone therapy and surgery can alleviate some symptoms. However, there are no effective treatments for the vast majority of genetic disorders.

RESEARCH, ISSUES, AND TRENDS

GENETIC BASIS OF CANCER

Recall from Chapter 5 that some forms of cancer are thought to be caused, at least in part, by abnormal genes called *oncogenes*. One hypothesis states that most normal cells contain such cancer-causing genes. However, it is uncertain how these genes become activated and produce cancer. Perhaps oncogenes can transform a cell into a cancer cell only when certain environmental conditions occur.

Another hypothesis states that normal cells contain another class of genes, sometimes called *tumor suppressor genes*. According to this hypothesis, such genes regulate cell division so that it proceeds normally. When a tumor suppressor gene is nonfunctional because of a genetic mutation, it then allows cells to divide abnormally—possibly producing cancer.

Another possible genetic basis for cancer relates to the genes that govern the cell's ability to repair damaged DNA. As mentioned in Chapter 6, a rare genetic disorder called *xeroderma pigmentosum* is characterized by the inability of skin cells to repair genetic damage caused by ultraviolet radiation in sunlight. Individuals with this condition almost always develop skin cancer when exposed to direct sunlight. The genetic abnormality does not cause skin cancer directly but inhibits the cell's cancer-preventing mechanisms.

Researchers are working feverishly to determine the exact role various genes play in the development of cancer. The more we understand about the genetic basis of cancer, the more likely it is that we will find effective treatments—or even cures.

Fortunately, medical science now offers us some hope of treating genetic disorders through **gene therapy.**

In a therapy sometimes called *gene replacement,* genes that specify production of abnormal, disease-causing proteins are replaced by normal or "therapeutic" genes. To get the therapeutic genes to cells that need them, researchers are using genetically altered viruses as carriers. Recall from Chapter 5 that viruses are easily capable of inserting new genes into the human genome. If the therapeutic genes behave as expected, a cure may result. Thus the goal of gene replacement therapy is to genetically alter existing body cells in the hope of eliminating the cause of a genetic disease. Although called "gene replacement," this therapy does not actually replace the defective genes—it instead inserts normal genes so that normal proteins can "replace" abnormal or missing proteins in the body's metabolic pathways.

In a therapy called *gene augmentation,* normal genes are introduced with the hope that they will augment (add to) the production of the needed protein. In one form of gene augmentation, virus-altered cells are injected into the blood or implanted under the skin of a patient to produce adequate amounts of the missing protein. Another approach is to use bacterial DNA rings called **plasmids** that have been altered by recombinant DNA techniques to carry the therapeutic gene(s). A more recent approach used the *human engineered chromosome (HEC).* In the HEC approach, a set of therapeutic genes is incorporated into a separate strand of DNA that is inserted into a cell's nucleus, thus acting like an extra, or 47th, chromosome. Gene augmentation attempts to add genetically altered cells to the body, rather than to change existing body cells as in gene replacement therapy.

The use of genetic therapy began in 1990 with a group of young children having **adenosine deaminase (ADA) deficiency.** In this rare recessive disorder, the gene for producing the enzyme ADA is missing from both autosomes in pair 20. Deficiency of ADA results in *severe combined immune deficiency (SCID),* making its victims highly susceptible to infection (see Chapter 15). As Figure 24-15 shows, white blood cells from each pa-

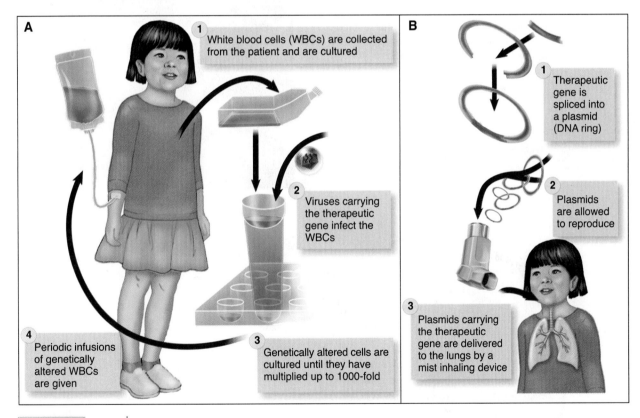

A

① White blood cells (WBCs) are collected from the patient and are cultured

② Viruses carrying the therapeutic gene infect the WBCs

③ Genetically altered cells are cultured until they have multiplied up to 1000-fold

④ Periodic infusions of genetically altered WBCs are given

B

① Therapeutic gene is spliced into a plasmid (DNA ring)

② Plasmids are allowed to reproduce

③ Plasmids carrying the therapeutic gene are delivered to the lungs by a mist inhaling device

Figure 24-15 **Gene therapy.**

A, This method of gene augmentation therapy was used to treat children stricken with a form of severe combined immune deficiency syndrome (SCID). White blood cells taken from the patient were infected with viruses carrying the therapeutic gene. The altered cells were reproduced and injected into the bloodstream, thereby reducing the immunity-inhibiting effects of SCID. **B,** Gene augmentation therapy in this example uses plasmids containing the therapeutic gene for cystic fibrosis (CF) and delivers them to the lung tissues by means of a common inhaler.

tient were collected and infected with viruses carrying therapeutic genes. After reproducing a thousand-fold, the genetically altered white blood cells were then injected into the patient. Because this treatment augments cells already present with genetically altered cells, it is a form of gene augmentation therapy. The first attempts at gene therapy in humans have met with some success, but many technical problems are yet to be overcome before it can be used widely.

Gene therapies for cystic fibrosis (CF) are also being tried. In one approach, researchers introduce therapeutic genes in cold viruses that are sprayed into the respiratory tract of CF victims. The viruses insert genes for normal chloride channels in the lung tissues, thus re-

---

CLINICAL APPLICATION

DNA ANALYSIS

As a result of the intense efforts under way to map the entire human genome, new techniques have been developed to analyze the genetic makeup of individuals. Automated machines can now chemically analyze chromosomes and "read" their sequence of nucleotides—the genetic code. One method by which this is done is called **electrophoresis** (eh-lek-troh-foh-REE-sis), which means "electric separation" *(A)*. In electrophoresis, DNA fragments are chemically processed, then placed in a thick fluid or *gel*. An electric field in the gel causes the DNA fragments to separate into groups according to their relative sizes. The pattern *(B)* that results represents the sequence of codons in the DNA fragment.

This process is also the basis for so-called *DNA fingerprinting*. Like a fingerprint pattern, each person's DNA sequence is unique. After the exact sequences for specific diseases have been discovered, genetic counselors will be able to provide more details about the genetic makeup of their clients. This technique is also used in forensic science to show that an individual was at the scene of the crime and left their DNA.

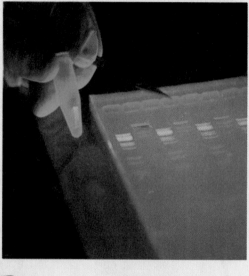
B

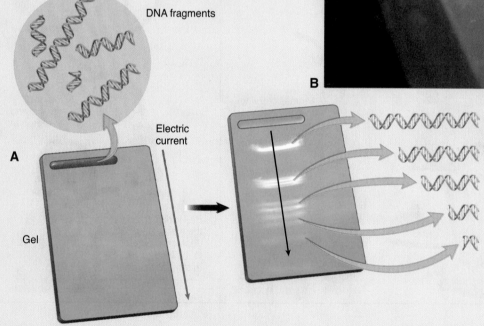

DNA fragments

Electric current

A

Gel

ducing the abnormally thick fluid secretions that characterize this disease. In another approach, shown in Figure 24-15, *B*, plasmids with the therapeutic gene are carried by a mist to lung tissues. There the plasmids enter the cells where they express the therapeutic gene. Early experiments proved that inhalation delivery is difficult, but research continues. These treatments are not expected to be one-time cures, but with ongoing use they should raise the average life expectancy of CF patients well beyond the current 27 years.

RNA interference (RNAi) may also become a weapon against genetic disorders in an approach called *RNAi therapy*. RNAi is a method of silencing particular genes. When harnessed in the laboratory, RNAi can turn off one gene at a time—greatly increasing the chances of figuring out which protein is encoded by that gene and what the function of that protein is. Currently hundreds of gene therapy trials for diverse genetic disorders, cancer, and even aging are proposed or ongoing. Thousands of laboratory experiments in anticipation of

human trials are also under way. Hurdles to overcome before we see widespread success of gene therapies include our lack of detailed knowledge of many of the "disease genes" and how multiple-gene diseases might be effectively treated—not to mention the high costs and risks involved. It is too early to say for sure, but there may soon come a time when many genetic diseases are treated—or even cured—with gene therapy.

 To learn more about vector-mediated gene therapy, go to **AnimationDirect** on your CD.

QUICK CHECK

1. How are most genetic disorders treated today?
2. How does *gene replacement* therapy work?

SCIENCE APPLICATIONS

GENETICS AND GENOMICS

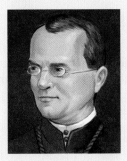

Gregor Mendel (1822–1884)

The Moravian-German Gregor Mendel was born to peasant farmers who taught him how plants and animals are bred for specific traits. Mendel's acceptance into a monastery allowed him to study the science that would later help him understand the mechanism of inheritance of biological traits.

Convinced that "particles" in the cells of the parents were responsible for inheritance of traits, Mendel carried out the now famous experiments with several generations of pea plants. In his report *Experiments with Plant Hybrids* Mendel outlined what has become the foundation of the science of genetics. Not only did he reveal the presence of genetic particles (which are now called *genes*) and the basic patterns of how they are transmitted to offspring, he also set in motion two important movements in modern biology.

First, Mendel was among the first to use mathematical analysis to support his theory about inheritance. Mendel's

work pioneered the systematic use of mathematics, quantified measurements, and applied statistics in biological research. Today, medical researchers often enlist the help of statisticians, mathematicians, computer programmers, and others in designing experiments, analyzing data, and interpreting results. In fact a whole field, sometimes called *biomathematics,* has now emerged to apply the principles of mathematics to biological study.

Second, Mendel was the first to discover how the biological mechanisms of inheritance worked in living organisms. This, of course, led to the science of genetics. Many disciplines have since grown from the study and application of genetics. For example, genetic counselors use principles of genetics to advise clients who wish to produce offspring but are worried about possible genetic disorders. Agricultural scientists use genetic principles in refining hybrid crop plants and livestock. Genetic engineers develop ways to manipulate the genetic code to produce a variety of therapies and enhanced biological characteristics of agricultural products. Genomics scientists analyze the genetic codes of organisms to help us better understand structure and function, which may lead to better treatments for genetic disorders.

Outline Summary

 To download an MP3 version of the chapter summary for use with your iPod or portable media player, access the **Audio Chapter Summaries** on your CD.

Genetics and Human Disease

A. Genetics, begun by Mendel more than 140 years ago, is the scientific study of inheritance
B. Inherited traits can produce disease (see Chapter 5)

Chromosomes and Genes

A. Mechanisms of gene function
   1. Gene—independent genetic units (DNA segments) that carry the genetic code
   2. Genes dictate the production of enzymes and other molecules, which in turn dictate the structure and function of a cell
   3. Genes are active in the chromatin (strand) form and inactive when DNA is in the chromosome (compact) form (Figure 24-1)
B. The human genome (Figure 24-1)
   1. Genome—entire set of human chromosomes (46 in nucleus of each cell, 1 mitochondrial chromosome)
      a. Rough draft of entire human genome (nearly all nucleotides in sequence) was published in 2001
      b. Contains about 30,000 genes and large amounts of non-coding DNA, termed pseudogenes
   2. Genomics—analysis of the sequence contained in the genome
   3. Proteomics—analysis of the entire group of proteins encoded by the genome, called the human *proteome*
   4. Genomic information can be expressed in various ways
      a. Ideogram—cartoon of a chromosome showing the centromere as a constriction and the short segment (p-arm) and long segment (q-arm)
      b. Genes are often represented as their actual sequence of nucleotide bases expressed by the letters *a, c, g,* and *t*

C. Distribution of chromosomes to offspring
   1. Meiotic cell division produces gametes with 23 chromosomes each (Figure 24-2)
   2. At conception, two gametes join and produce a zygote with 46 chromosomes—the complete human genome
   3. Twenty-two pairs of chromosomes are called *autosomes;* each member of a pair resembles its partner
   4. The remaining pair of chromosomes (pair 23) are called *sex chromosomes*
   5. Genetic variation among offspring is increased by:
      a. Independent assortment of chromosomes during gamete formation (Figure 24-2)
      b. Crossing-over of genes or linked groups of genes between chromosome partners during meiosis (Figure 24-3)

Gene Expression

A. Hereditary traits
   1. Dominant genes have effects that appear in the offspring (dominant forms of a gene are often represented by uppercase letters)
      a. A genetic carrier is a person who carries a recessive gene but does not show its effects because of masking effect of a dominant gene
      b. Codominant genes are two or more genes that are all dominant and when they appear together produce a combined effect in offspring
   2. Recessive genes have effects that do not appear in the offspring when they are masked by a dominant gene (recessive forms of a gene are represented by lowercase letters)
B. Sex-linked traits (Figures 24-5 and 24-6)
   1. The large X chromosome ("female chromosome") contains genes for female sexual characteristics and many other traits

2. The small *Y* chromosome ("male chromo-some") contains only genes for male sexual characteristics

3. Normal males have *XY* as pair 23; normal females have *XX* as pair 23

4. Nonsexual traits carried on sex chromo-somes are sex-linked traits; most are *X*-linked traits

C. Genetic mutations

  1. Can result in abnormalities in the genetic code that cause disease

  2. Most believed to be caused by mutagens

Genetic Diseases

A. Mechanisms of genetic disease

  1. Single-gene diseases result from individual mutant genes (or groups of genes) that are passed from generation to generation (Figure 24-7)

  2. Chromosomal diseases result from chromo-some breakage or from nondisjunction (failure of a chromosome pair to separate during gamete formation) (Figure 24-8)

    a. Trisomy—a chromosome triplet (instead of the usual pair)

    b. Monosomy—a single chromosome (instead of a pair)

B. Examples of single-gene diseases (Table 24-1)

  1. Cystic fibrosis—recessive autosomal condi-tion characterized by excessive secretion of mucus and sweat, often causing obstruction of the gastrointestinal or respiratory tracts

  2. Phenylketonuria (PKU)—recessive auto-somal condition characterized by excess phenylketone in urine, caused by accumu-lation of phenylalanine in tissues; may cause brain injury and death

  3. Tay-Sachs disease (TSD) is a recessive condi-tion involving failure to make a subunit of an essential lipid-processing enzyme

C. Examples of chromosomal diseases

  1. Down syndrome—usually caused by trisomy of chromosome 21; characterized by mental retardation and multiple struc-tural defects (Figure 24-9)

  2. Klinefelter syndrome—caused by the presence of two or more *X* chromosomes in a male (usually trisomy *XXY*); character-ized by long legs, enlarged breasts, low intelligence, small testes, sterility, chronic pulmonary disease (Figure 24-10)

  3. Turner syndrome—caused by monosomy of the *X* chromosome (*XO*); characterized by immaturity of sex organs (resulting in sterility), short stature, webbed neck, cardiovascular defects, and learning disorders (Figure 24-11)

Prevention and Treatment of Genetic Diseases

A. Genetic counseling—professional consultations with families regarding genetic diseases

  1. Pedigree—chart illustrating genetic relationships over several generations (Figure 24-12)

  2. Punnett square—grid used to determine the probability of inheriting genetic traits (Figure 24-13)

  3. Karyotype—arrangement of chromosome photographs used to detect abnormalities

    a. Amniocentesis—involves collection of fetal cells floating in the amniotic fluid (Figure 24-14)

    b. Chorionic villus sampling—involves collection of embryonic cells from outside of chorionic tissue

B. Treating genetic diseases

  1. Most current treatments for genetic diseases are based on relieving or avoiding symp-toms rather than attempting a cure

  2. Gene therapy—manipulates genes to cure genetic problems (Figure 24-15); most forms of gene therapy have not yet been proved effective in humans

    a. Gene replacement therapy—abnormal genes in existing body cells are replaced by therapeutic genes

    b. Gene augmentation therapy—cells carrying normal genes are introduced into the body to augment production of a needed protein

    c. RNAi therapy—RNA interference—silences individual genes that cause disease

New Words

autosome	pseudogene	albinism	mutagen
carrier	recessive gene	amniocentesis	p-arm
codominance	sex chromosome	chorionic villus sampling	pedigree
dominant gene	sex-linked trait	Down syndrome	phenylketonuria (PKU)
gamete		electrophoresis	plasmid
genetics	**Diseases and Other**	gene therapy	Punnett square
genome	**Clinical Terms**	ideogram	q-arm
genomics	adenosine deaminase	karyotype	Tay-Sachs disease
proteome	(ADA) deficiency	Klinefelter syndrome	trisomy
proteomics		monosomy	Turner syndrome

Review Questions

1. Explain how the DNA code is able to regulate the biochemistry of the cell.
2. As they are used in this chapter, define *chromosome* and *gene*.
3. What is meant by *independent assortment*?
4. Define or explain the terms *dominant, recessive,* and *codominant* in regard to genetics.
5. What is a sex-linked trait?
6. Define or explain the terms *nondisjunction, trisomy,* and *monosomy*.
7. What is a pedigree chart?
8. What is a Punnett square?
9. What is a karyotype? What are the two methods used to harvest cells for a karyotype?
10. Explain the difference between gene augmentation and gene replacement therapy.
11. Name and briefly describe the two single-gene diseases discussed in the chapter.
12. Name and briefly describe the three chromosomal diseases discussed in the chapter. Indicate whether the diseases are the result of trisomy or monosomy.

Critical Thinking

13. Explain why the particular sperm that fertilizes the egg determines the sex of the offspring.
14. What is crossing-over? How does this process add to genetic variation?
15. Explain why men have more sex-linked disorders than women.
16. Which type of genetic mutation has the greatest long-term impact on the population, harmful or beneficial? Explain your answer.
17. If parents are concerned that their child might be born with Down syndrome, what would be the best way to determine this: a pedigree, a Punnett square, or a karyotype? Explain your answer.

Chapter Test

1. _____ is the scientific study of inheritance.
2. The end product of protein synthesis is frequently an _____, which helps regulate the biochemistry of the body.
3. Most of the cells of the human body contain _____ chromosomes, but gametes contain _____ chromosomes.
4. A _____ gene is one whose effects are seen and is capable of masking a _____ gene for the same trait.

For questions 5, 6, and 7, let "A" stand for the dominant gene for normal skin pigment and let "a" stand for the recessive gene for albinism.

5. A father with *Aa* and a mother with *AA* have a _____% probability for having a child with albinism.
6. A father with *Aa* and a mother with *Aa* have a _____% probability for having a child with albinism.

7. A father with *Aa* and a mother with albinism have a _____% probability for having a child with albinism.
8. Nonsexual traits carried on the sex chromosome are called _____ traits.
9. Color blindness is carried on the *X* chromosome. If the father is color blind and the mother is not a carrier, the probability of having a color blind son would be _____%.
10. A change in the genetic code is called a _____.
11. A mistake in meiosis when a pair of chromosomes fails to separate is called _____.
12. _____ is a condition in which there is a triplet of autosomes rather than the normal pair.
13. _____ is a condition in which there is a single autosome rather than the normal pair.
14. A _____ is a chart that illustrates the genetic relationship in a family over several generations.
15. A _____ is a grid used to determine the probability of inheriting a genetic trait.
16. A _____ is a photograph of chromosomes arranged in pairs; amniocentesis can supply the cells for this.

Match each disorder in Column A with its corresponding cause or description in Column B.

Column A
17. _____ cystic fibrosis
18. _____ phenylketonuria
19. _____ Down syndrome
20. _____ Klinefelter syndrome
21. _____ Turner syndrome
22. _____ color blindness

Column B
a. a disorder caused by trisomy 21
b. a disorder caused by a recessive gene that fails to produce the enzyme phenylalanine hydroxylase
c. a disorder caused by the trisomy condition *XXY*
d. a condition caused by a recessive gene that causes an impairment in chloride ion transport across the cell membrane
e. a sex-linked trait that inhibits the production of certain photopigments
f. a disorder caused by the monosomy condition *XO*

Study Tips

continued from page 665

5. Pedigrees, Punnett squares, and karyotypes provide different types of genetic information; be sure you know what each of these can tell you.
6. Be able to differentiate between gene replacement and gene augmentation therapy.
7. In your study group, review the genetic terms using flash cards. Discuss the relationship between the DNA sequence and the biochemical activity of the cell. Quiz each other on the probability of various traits in the offspring based on the parental genes. Go over the disorders chart and the difference in the type of information gained by a pedigree, a Punnett square, and a karyotype. Go over the questions at the end of the chapter and discuss possible test questions.

Case Studies

1. Quentin's family physician suspects that Quentin may have Klinefelter syndrome. Quentin's long limbs, small testes, and enlarged breasts seem to support the diagnosis. What test might the physician order to confirm the syndrome? What test results would be expected? What causes the genetic abnormality that produces Klinefelter syndrome?

2. A young infant just born at Memorial Hospital has parents that both report a history of Tay-Sachs disease in their families. Assuming both parents have the Tay-Sachs gene, what is the probability that this infant will develop this deadly disease?

Examples of Pathological Conditions

Table 1 | Leading Health Problems

CONDITION	CHAPTER REFERENCE
Diseases of the heart and blood vessels	Chapters 13 and 14
Cancer	Chapter 5
Stroke	Chapter 9
Chronic lower respiratory diseases	Chapter 16
Accidents	Chapter 5
Diabetes mellitus	Chapter 11
Alzheimer disease (AD)	Chapter 9
Pneumonia and influenza	Chapters 5 and 16
Kidney disease	Chapter 19

Table 2 | Viral Conditions

DISEASE	VIRUS	DESCRIPTION
Acquired immunodeficiency syndrome (AIDS)	Human immunodeficiency virus (HIV)	Although not identified in the West until 1981, HIV may have existed in Africa for many years. It is transmitted by direct contact with body fluids, perhaps within white blood cells (WBCs) in blood or semen. AIDS is characterized by T-lymphocyte damage, resulting in immune dysfunction. Death results from secondary infections or tumors.
Acute T-cell lymphocytic leukemia (ATLL)	Human T-lymphotropic virus 1 (HTLV-1)	This form of cancer in adults can be caused by the *oncovirus* ("cancer virus") HTLV-1. This disease is one of many forms of leukemia and does not appear until at least 30 years after initial infection. HTLV-1 is transmitted in the same manner as HIV.
Chickenpox (varicella) and shingles (herpes zoster)	Varicella zoster virus (VZV)	Chickenpox is usually a childhood infection typically involving blisters and fever. Herpes zoster, commonly known as shingles, occurs later (in adulthood) in those who had the varicella infection at an earlier age. Shingles often involves a rash along a single dermatome on one side of the body and is accompanied by severe pain.
Common cold and upper respiratory infections (URIs)	Rhinoviruses	This mild, contagious infection is characterized by nasal inflammation, weakness, cough, and low-grade fever. Dozens of different rhinoviruses have been typed.
Fever blisters and herpes	Herpes simplex 1 and 2	This virus causes blisters on the hands or face (fever blisters) or genitals (genital herpes). The blisters may disappear temporarily but may reappear, especially as a result of stress.
Hantavirus pulmonary syndrome	Hantavirus	This serious viral disease is characterized by fever and flu-like symptoms that often progress to respiratory failure; it is spread by rodent excreta.

Table 2 | Viral Conditions (continued)

DISEASE	VIRUS	DESCRIPTION
Hepatitis (infectious)	Hepatitis A virus	The liver inflammation caused by this virus is characterized by slow onset and complete recovery. This virus is spread by direct contact or contaminated food or water.
Hepatitis (serum)	Hepatitis B virus	This acute-onset liver inflammation may develop into a severe chronic disease, perhaps ending in death.
Hepatitis (non A; non B)	Hepatitis C	This viral liver inflammation is transmitted by contaminated blood; initially mild cases may become chronic and over long periods progress to cirrhosis and liver failure.
Infectious mononucleosis	Epstein-Barr virus (EBV)	This acute infection is characterized by fever, sore throat, increased count and abnormal shape of lymphocytes, and liver, spleen, or lymph node swelling.
Influenza	Influenza A, B, C, etc.	This highly contagious respiratory infection is characterized by sore throat, fever, cough, muscle pain, and weakness. New strains of viruses A, B, and C appear at intervals—usually originating in Asia.
Measles	*Morbillivirus*	This acute, contagious respiratory infection is characterized by fever, headache, and the measles rash.
Mumps	*Paramyxovirus*	This acute infection is characterized by swollen parotid salivary glands, fever, and in adult males, swollen testes; mumps is most common in children but can occur at any age.
Poliomyelitis	Poliovirus 1, 2, and 3	This acute infection has several different forms (depending on extent of infection): asymptomatic, mild, nonparalyzing, and paralyzing. It is no longer common in the United States because of successful vaccination programs.
Rabies	Rabies virus	This fatal infection of the central nervous system is usually transmitted through the bites of infected animals.
Rubella (German measles)	Rubella virus	This contagious infection is characterized by upper respiratory inflammation, swollen lymph nodes, joint pain, and measles-like rash. In pregnant women, it can spread to the fetus and cause congenital defects.
Viral encephalitis	(Many different viruses)	*Viral encephalitis* is a general term for any brain inflammation caused by a virus. Brain damage may occur, perhaps causing death. Many different forms exist because many different viruses may infect the brain (e.g., St. Louis encephalitis, California encephalitis, and equine encephalitis). Most encephalitis viruses are transmitted by mosquitoes.
Warts, genital warts, and cervical cancer	Human papillomaviruses (HPV)	Warts are nipple-like neoplasms of the skin. Forty-six HPV types have been identified. HPV types 6 and 11 cause genital warts, a common sexually transmitted disease (STD).

Table 3 | Bacterial Conditions

DISEASE	ORGANISM	DESCRIPTION
Acute bacterial conjunctivitis	*Staphylococcus, Haemophilus, Proteus,* and other organisms	This acute inflammation of the conjunctiva covering the eye is characterized by a discharge of mucous pus; it is highly contagious (compare with trachoma).
Anthrax	*Bacillus anthracis*	Usually transmitted from farm animals, this infection is characterized by a reddish-brown skin lesion but can also infect the respiratory tract. It can be fatal.
Botulism	*Clostridium botulinum* (bacillus)	This is a possibly fatal food poisoning resulting from ingestion of food contaminated with toxins produced by *C. botulinum*.
Brucellosis	*Brucella* species (bacilli)	Also called *undulant fever,* this bacterial infection is transmitted from farm animals and is characterized by chills, fever, weight loss, and weakness. Serious complications can occur if it is not treated.

DISEASE	ORGANISM	DESCRIPTION
Cholera	*Vibrio cholerae* (curved)	This acute intestinal infection is characterized by diarrhea, vomiting, cramps, dehydration, and electrolyte imbalance caused by bacterial toxins. It can be fatal if untreated. It spreads through contaminated food or water.
Dental caries	*Streptococcus mutans* (coccus) and other organisms	Tooth demineralization is caused by acids formed when nutrients on the tooth's surface are metabolized by bacteria. It can progress to a bacterial invasion of the tooth's pulp cavity and beyond.
Diphtheria	*Corynebacterium diphtheriae* (bacillus)	Diphtheria is an acute, contagious disease characterized by systemic poisoning by bacterial toxins and development of a "false membrane" lining of the throat that may obstruct breathing. Untreated, it may be fatal.
Epiglottitis	*Haemophilus influenzae*	Acute inflammation of epiglottis is characterized by fever, sore throat, and swelling (emergency treatment to maintain airway may be necessary).
External otitis (swimmer's ear)	*Pseudomonas aeruginosa, Staphylococcus aureus, Streptococcus pyogenes,* etc.	Inflammation of the external ear canal is usually caused by bacteria but can also result from herpes infections, allergy, and other factors.
Gastroenteritis	(Many different bacteria)	*Gastroenteritis* is a general term for any inflammation of the gastrointestinal tract. Many different bacterial infections can cause this condition. (See Salmonellosis.)
Gonorrhea	*Neisseria gonorrhoeae* (coccus)	This common STD infects primarily the genital and urinary tracts but can affect the throat, conjunctiva, or lower intestines. It may progress to pelvic inflammatory disease (see later entry).
Legionnaires disease	*Legionella pneumophila* (bacillus)	This is a type of pneumonia characterized by influenza-like symptoms followed by high fever, muscle pain, and headache—possibly progressing to dry cough and pleurisy. It is spread by moist environmental sources (e.g., air conditioning cooling units and soil) rather than person-to-person contact.
Lyme disease	*Borrelia burgdorferi* (spirochete)	Although the first cases were known only near Lyme, Connecticut, this tick-borne disease is now endemic over much of the United States. It usually first presents as a "bull's-eye" rash but later may cause chronic nerve, heart, and joint problems.
Lymphogranuloma venereum (LGV)	*Chlamydia trachomatis* (small)	This chronic STD is characterized by genital ulcers, swollen lymph nodes, headache, fever, and muscle pain. *C. trachomatis* infection may cause a variety of other syndromes, including conjunctivitis, urogenital infections, and systemic infections. *C. trachomatis* infections constitute the most common STD in the United States.
Meningitis	*Streptococcus pneumoniae, Neisseria meningitidis, Haemophilus influenzae,* and other organisms	Meningitis is any inflammation of the meninges covering the brain and spinal cord. Several different bacteria can infect the meninges, as can several fungi; the condition can be mild, but if severe, it can cause death.
Parrot fever (psittacosis)	*Chlamydia psittaci* (small)	Also called *ornithosis*, this pneumonia-like infection is transmitted by parrots and other birds. It is characterized by cough, fever, loss of appetite, and severe headache.
Pelvic inflammatory disease (PID)	*Neisseria gonorrhoeae* (coccus), *Mycoplasma hominis* (small free-living), and other organisms	PID refers to any extensive inflammation of the female pelvic structures. Chronic inflammation associated with PID can cause tissue damage that leads to sterility.
Pertussis (whooping cough)	*Bordetella pertussis* (bacillus)	Pertussis is an acute, contagious infection of the respiratory tract characterized by coughs that end with "whooping" respirations.
Pneumonia	*Streptococcus pneumoniae* (coccus) and other organisms	An acute lung infection that commonly develops after the flu or some other condition that prevents clearance of the lungs. It is characterized by blockage of the pulmonary airways.

Table 3 | **Bacterial Conditions (continued)**

DISEASE	ORGANISM	DESCRIPTION
Q fever	*Coxiella burnetii* (small)	Q (for "query") fever usually involves respiratory infection and is characterized by fever, headache, and muscle pain. Acute and chronic forms may develop after exposure to infected animals or animal products; this is a rickettsial disease.
Rheumatic fever	Group A beta-hemolytic streptococci (cocci)	This inflammatory disease results from a delayed reaction to "strep" infection; it may affect heart, brain, joints, or skin.
Rocky Mountain spotted fever (RMSF)	*Rickettsia rickettsii* (small)	This sometimes fatal, tick-borne disease is characterized by fever, chills, headache, muscle pain, rash, constipation, and hemorrhagic lesions; it may progress to shock and renal failure.
Salmonellosis	*Salmonella* species (bacilli)	This type of bacterial gastroenteritis is caused by ingestion of contaminated food.
Shigellosis (Shigella dysentery and bacillary dysentery)	*Shigella* species (bacilli)	This common disease is characterized by bloody, mucous diarrhea, cramps, fever, and fatigue. It can cause dehydration, electrolyte imbalance, and acidosis if not treated. Antibiotic resistant strains of Shigella organisms make this condition a serious health threat—especially in areas with poor sanitation.
Staphylococcal infection	*Staphylococcus* species (cocci)	These bacterial infections are characterized by abscesses; one such infection is staphylococcal scalded skin syndrome (SSSS), a skin disorder of infants and young children.
Syphilis	*Treponema pallidum* (spirochete)	This sexually transmitted disease can affect any system. Primary syphilis is characterized by chancre sores on exposed areas of the skin. Untreated, secondary syphilis may appear 2 months after chancres disappear. The secondary stage occurs when the spirochete has spread throughout the body, presenting a variety of symptoms, and is still highly contagious—even through kissing. Tertiary syphilis may occur years later, possibly resulting in death.
Tetanus	*Clostridium tetani* (bacillus)	In this acute, sometimes fatal central nervous system infection, the bacteria usually enter a wound and then produce a toxin that causes headache, fever, and painful muscle spasms.
Toxic shock syndrome (TSS)	*Staphylococcus aureus* strains (cocci)	This acute, severe toxic infection is associated with the use of highly absorbent tampons but can occur under a variety of circumstances. It begins as a high fever, headache, sore throat, etc., and may progress to renal failure, liver failure, and possibly death.
Trachoma (chlamydial conjunctivitis)	*Chlamydia trachomatis* (small)	This chronic infection of the conjunctiva covering the eye is characterized by painful inflammation, photophobia (light sensitivity), and excessive production of tears; if untreated, it will progress to form granular lesions that eventually affect the cornea and cause blindness.
Tuberculosis	*Mycobacterium tuberculosis*	This chronic infection usually affects the lungs (pulmonary tuberculosis) and is characterized by fatigue, dyspnea, and chronic cough and is transmitted by inhalation or ingestion of bacteria.
Typhoid fever	*Salmonella typhi (bacillus)*	Also called *enteric fever,* this condition is characterized by fever, headache, cough, diarrhea, and rash; it is transmitted through contaminated food or water.

Table 4 | **Mycotic (Fungal) Conditions**

DISEASE	ORGANISM	DESCRIPTION
Aspergillosis	*Aspergillus* species (mold)	This uncommon, opportunistic mold infection by any of a number of different species has many different forms. It often affects the ear but can affect any organ, where it produces characteristic "fungus ball" lesions. If the infection becomes widespread, it can be fatal.

DISEASE	ORGANISM	DESCRIPTION
Blastomycosis	*Blastomyces dermatitidis* (mold*)	As with histoplasmosis, most cases of blastomycosis are asymptomatic. The most common symptomatic forms are skin ulcers and bone lesions, but the infection may spread to the lungs, kidneys, or nervous system.
Candidiasis	*Candida albicans* and other species (yeasts)	This opportunistic yeast infection is characterized by a white discharge, peeling, and bleeding; candidiasis has several forms, depending on the severity and where it occurs: thrush (skin), diaper rash (skin), vaginitis, endocarditis, etc. It can be transmitted sexually, making it a sexually transmitted disease (STD).
Coccidioidomycosis (San Joaquin fever)	*Coccidioides immitis* (mold*)	Also called *desert fever*, this condition is endemic to dry regions of the southwestern United States and Central and South America. It is characterized by cold- or influenza-like symptoms. A small number of cases develop into more serious infection.
Histoplasmosis	*Histoplasma capsulatum* (mold*)	Histoplasmosis is a fungal infection most common in the Midwestern United States, where it is spread through contaminated soil. In most cases, it is asymptomatic, but acute pneumonia may develop in a few cases.
Mycosis	(Many types)	*Mycosis* is a general term used to describe any disease caused by fungi. *Mycoses* is the plural form.
Tinea	*Epidermophyton, Microsporum,* and *Trichophyton* species (molds)	Examples of opportunistic cutaneous mycoses include tinea pedis (athlete's foot), tinea cruris (jock itch), tinea corporis (body ringworm), tinea capitis (scalp ringworm), and tinea unguium (nail fungus). All are characterized by inflammation accompanied by itching, scaling, and (occasionally) painful lesions.

*These molds are normally multicellular but transform to a unicellular phase when they infect humans.

| Table | 5 | **Conditions Caused by Protozoa** |

DISEASE	ORGANISM	DESCRIPTION
Amebiasis and amebic dysentery	*Entamoeba histolytica, Entamoeba polecki,* and other organisms (ameba)	Usually acquired through contaminated food and water, this condition is an amebic infection of the intestine or liver. Mild cases are asymptomatic. More severe forms are characterized by diarrhea, abdominal pain, jaundice, and weight loss.
Balantidiasis	*Balantidium coli* (ciliate)	*B. coli* can be carried asymptomatically in the gastrointestinal tract. The disease is characterized by abdominal pain, nausea, and diarrhea. It may progress to intestinal ulceration and subsequent secondary infections.
Giardiasis (traveler diarrhea)	*Giardia lamblia* (flagellate)	Intestinal infection is spread through contaminated food or water or through person-to-person contact. Symptoms range from mild diarrhea to malabsorption syndrome, with about half of all cases being asymptomatic.
Isosporiasis	*Isospora belli* (sporozoan)	Transmitted through contaminated food or oral-anal sexual contact, isosporiasis is an intestinal infection that may be asymptomatic. Symptomatic manifestations range from mild to severe, resembling giardiasis.
Malaria	*Plasmodium species* (sporozoa)	This serious disease is caused by blood-cell parasites that require two hosts: mosquitoes and humans (or other animals). Malaria is characterized by fever, anemia, swollen spleen, and possible relapse months or years later.
Toxoplasmosis	*Toxoplasma gondii* (sporozoan)	A common infection of blood and other tissue cells, this condition is often asymptomatic. It is transmitted through cat feces and undercooked meat. It is characterized by fever, lymphatic involvement, headache, fatigue, nervous disorders, and heart problems. If transmitted from mother to fetus, it can cause congenital defects that often lead to death.
Trichomoniasis	*Trichomonas vaginalis* (flagellate)	This urogenital infection is asymptomatic in most female patients and nearly all male patients. Vaginitis may occur, characterized by itching or burning and a foul-smelling discharge. It is usually spread through sexual contact.

| Table | 6 | Conditions Caused by Pathogenic Animals |

DISEASE	ORGANISM	DESCRIPTION
Ascariasis (roundworm infestation)	*Ascaris lumbricoides* (nematode)	This condition is transmitted through contaminated food or contact with contaminated surfaces (such as hands). Eggs hatch in the small intestine, and the larvae travel to the lungs, where they cause coughing and fever. Intestinal and liver involvement may also be serious.
Bites and stings	Arachnida and Insecta	Symptoms of bites and stings usually result from mechanical injury and the release of toxins at the injury site. Some individuals may be hypersensitive to certain toxins and thus exhibit an allergic reaction, perhaps even anaphylaxis and death. Bites and stings may also transmit pathogens when the culprit is a vector.
Enterobiasis (pinworm infestation)	*Enterobius vermicularis* (nematode)	This is a common parasite infestation in which eggs can be transmitted by contaminated hands (a common cause of reinfection) or on inhaled dust particles. The infestation is localized in the large intestine. The adult female lays eggs around the outside of the anus, causing itching and possibly insomnia.
Fish tapeworm infestation	*Diphyllobothrium latum* (platyhelminth)	Spread by eating undercooked, contaminated fish, this condition is usually asymptomatic but can cause pernicious anemia if too much vitamin B12 is absorbed from the host.
Liver fluke infestation	*Fasciola hepatica, Opisthorchis sinensis,* and other organisms (platyhelminths)	Transmitted through watercress contaminated by infected snails, especially in sheep-raising regions, this infestation causes inflammation and swelling of the liver. The symptoms may progress to include hepatitis, bile duct obstruction, and secondary infections.
Pork and beef tapeworm infestation	*Taenia solium* (pork tapeworm) and *Taenia saginata* (beef tapeworm) (platyhelminths)	This infestation is spread by eating undercooked, contaminated pork or beef. Adult tapeworms mature in the gastrointestinal tract, usually producing mild symptoms of diarrhea and weight loss. Larvae may spread to other tissue, sometimes causing serious infections.
Schistosomiasis (snail fever)	*Schistosoma mansoni, Schistosoma japonicum,* and *Schistosoma haematobium* (platyhelminths)	This is a parasitic condition transmitted in the form of skin-penetrating parasites released by freshwater snails in water contaminated by human feces. Characteristics of the disease depend on the organs involved and the species of fluke.
Trichinosis (threadworm infestation)	*Trichinella spiralis* (nematode)	This is an infestation characterized by diarrhea, nausea, and fever, possibly progressing to muscle pain and fatigue. In severe cases, the heart, lungs, and brain may become involved, sometimes resulting in death. The parasite is transmitted through undercooked pork, bear, and other meats.

| Table | 7 | Conditions Caused by Physical Agents |

CONDITION	PHYSICAL AGENTS	DESCRIPTION
Bone fracture	Mechanical injury (e.g., intense pressure, blow to the body, and abnormal turn while bearing weight)	Complete or incomplete break of hard bone tissue in one or more localized areas is often characterized by pain, swelling, and limited motion; compound fractures break the skin and may thus allow infection.
Burn	Chemical agents (e.g., acids and bases), intense heat, ionizing radiation (e.g., x-rays and gamma rays), non-ionizing radiation (e.g., ultraviolet), electricity	This is an injury to tissues caused by the factors listed in which the extent of the injury is proportional to exposure to the causative agent and percent of body area affected; it causes "burning" pain and resulting inflammation response. Untreated or severe burns may become infected and may cause severe fluid loss.
Cancer	Mechanical injury, ionizing radiation (e.g., x-rays and gamma rays), non-ionizing radiation (e.g., ultraviolet), chemical agents (e.g., irritants and carcinogens)	Malignant neoplasm (abnormal tissue growth) is characterized by invasion of surrounding tissue and metastasis (spread) to other parts of the body; it often progresses to death if not treated.

CONDITION	PHYSICAL AGENTS	DESCRIPTION
Chronic obstructive pulmonary disease (COPD)	Chemical pollutants (in air), airborne particulates	This group of disorders is characterized by progressive, irreversible obstruction of air flow in the lungs; it includes bronchitis, emphysema, asthma. The incidence in the U.S. population has increased with exposure to air pollutants, including cigarette smoke.
Contusion	Mechanical injury (e.g., blow to the body and intense pressure)	A contusion is a localized tissue lesion characterized by breakage of blood vessels and surrounding tissue cells without external bleeding; it is sometimes called a bruise.
Crush syndrome	Mechanical pressure (intense)	This severe, life-threatening condition is characterized by massive destruction of muscle and bone, hemorrhage, fluid loss, hypovolemic shock, hematuria (bloody urine), and kidney failure—often progressing to coma.
Diarrhea	Chemical agents (ingested), ionizing radiation (e.g., x-rays and gamma rays)	Frequent passing of loose, watery feces (stools) results from increased peristalsis (motility) of the colon, in this case resulting from irritation by physical agents; the resulting fluid and electrolyte imbalance may cause dehydration or another life-threatening condition.
Headache	Mechanical injury (e.g., blow to the head), chemical pollutants (e.g., inhaled organic compounds)	Pain in the head in this case results from injury by the agents listed.
Hearing impairment	High-volume (intensity) sound (e.g., noise pollution)	Chronic exposure to loud noise causes hearing loss proportional to exposure—resulting from damage to the organ of Corti.
Hypersensitivity reaction and physical allergy	Chemical substances in environment, light (as in photosensitivity), temperature (as in cold or heat sensitivity)	Inappropriate, intense immune reaction to otherwise harmless physical agents is characterized by urticaria (hives), edema, and other allergy symptoms; specific antigens are usually associated with the reaction.
Laceration	Mechanical injury (sharp-edged object)	This is a mechanical injury in which tissue is cut or torn, often characterized by bleeding; if untreated, it may become infected.
Nausea	Chemical agents (ingested), ionizing radiation (e.g., x-rays and gamma rays)	This is an unpleasant sensation of the gastrointestinal tract that commonly precedes the urge to vomit (that is, "upset stomach").
Pneumonia	Inhaled substances	This abnormal condition is characterized by acute inflammation of the lungs (in this case, triggered by irritation caused by inhaled substance) in which alveoli and bronchial passages become plugged with thick fluid (exudate).
Poisoning	Naturally occurring toxins, synthetic toxins, drugs (e.g., abuse, overdose, toxic interaction), environmental pollutants (e.g., air, water)	This condition results from exposure to a poison or toxin—a substance that impairs health or destroys life; effects may be local or systemic. Sometimes antidotes reverse toxicity, but sometimes the condition is irreversible. The toxin may be ingested, injected, inhaled, or absorbed through skin or may enter the body in some other way.
Radiation sickness	Ionizing radiation (e.g., x and gamma rays)	Depending on the length, intensity, and location of exposure to radiation, this condition may be mild (headache, nausea, vomiting, anorexia, and diarrhea) to severe (sterility, fetal injury, cancer, alopecia, and cataracts); excessive radiation exposure may cause death.
Visual impairment	Mechanical injury (e.g., blow to the head), intense light (e.g., direct sunlight and laser), ionizing radiation (e.g., x-rays and gamma rays), non-ionizing radiation (e.g., ultraviolet)	A blow to the head may cause detachment of the retina; intense light or other radiation may damage retinal tissue. Radiation may also cloud the lens or cornea, producing cataracts.
Windburn and abrasion burn	Abrasives (e.g., windblown particles and rough surfaces)	This injury is similar to a heat or chemical burn but is caused by mechanical abrasion of the skin or other tissues.

Table 8 | **Endocrine Conditions**

CONDITION	MECHANISM	DESCRIPTION
Acromegaly	Hypersecretion of growth hormone (GH) during adulthood	This is a chronic metabolic disorder characterized by gradual enlargement or elongation of facial bones and extremities.
Addison disease	Hyposecretion of adrenal cortical hormones *(adrenal cortical insufficiency)*	Caused by tuberculosis, autoimmunity, or other factors, this life-threatening condition is characterized by weakness, anorexia, weight loss, nausea, irritability, decreased cold tolerance, dehydration, increased skin pigmentation, and emotional disturbance; it may lead to an acute phase (adrenal crisis) characterized by circulatory shock.
Aldosteronism	Hypersecretion of aldosterone	Often caused by adrenal hyperplasia, this condition is characterized by sodium retention and potassium loss—producing Conn syndrome: severe muscle weakness, hypertension (high blood pressure), kidney dysfunction, and cardiac problems.
Cretinism	Hyposecretion of thyroid hormone during early development	This congenital condition is characterized by dwarfism, retarded mental development, facial puffiness, dry skin, umbilical hernia, and lack of muscle coordination.
Cushing disease	Hypersecretion of adrenocorticotropic hormone (ACTH)	Caused by secretory adenoma of the anterior pituitary; increased ACTH causes hypersecretion of adrenocortical hormones, producing Cushing syndrome.
Cushing syndrome	Hypersecretion (or injection) of glucocorticoids	This metabolic disorder is characterized by fat deposits on upper back, striated pad of fat on chest and abdomen, rounded "moon" face, muscular atrophy, edema, hypokalemia (low blood potassium), and possible abnormal skin pigmentation; it occurs in those with Cushing disease.
Diabetes insipidus	Hyposecretion of (or insensitivity to) antidiuretic hormone (ADH)	This metabolic disorder is characterized by extreme polyuria (excessive urination) and polydipsia (excessive thirst) caused by a decrease in the kidney's retention of water.
Gestational diabetes mellitus (GDM)	Temporary decrease in blood levels of insulin during pregnancy	This carbohydrate-metabolism disorder occurs in some pregnant women; it is characterized by polydipsia, polyuria, overeating, weight loss, fatigue, and irritability.
Gigantism	Hypersecretion of GH before age 25	This condition is characterized by extreme skeletal size caused by excess protein anabolism during skeletal development.
Graves disease (GD)	Hypersecretion of thyroid hormone	This inherited, possibly autoimmune disease is characterized by hyperthyroidism.
Hashimoto disease	Autoimmune damage to thyroid causing hyposecretion of thyroid hormone	Enlargement of thyroid (goiter) is sometimes accompanied by hypothyroidism, typically occurring between ages 30 and 50; it is 20 times more common in females than in males.

CONDITION	MECHANISM	DESCRIPTION
Hyperparathyroidism	Hypersecretion of parathyroid hormone (PTH)	This condition is characterized by increased reabsorption of calcium from bone tissue and kidneys and increased absorption by the gastrointestinal tract; it produces hypercalcemia, resulting in confusion, anorexia, abdominal pain, muscle pain, and fatigue, possibly progressing to circulatory shock, kidney failure, and death.
Hyperthyroidism (adult)	Hypersecretion of thyroid hormone	This condition, characterized by nervousness, exophthalmos (protruding eyes), tremor, weight loss, excessive hunger, fatigue, heat intolerance, heart arrhythmia, and diarrhea, is caused by a general acceleration of body function.
Hypothyroidism (adult)	Hyposecretion of thyroid hormone	This condition, characterized by sluggishness, weight gain, skin dryness, constipation, arthritis, and general slowing of body function, may lead to myxedema, coma, or death if untreated.
Insulin shock	Hypersecretion (or overdose injection) of insulin, decreased food intake, and excessive exercise	Hypoglycemic (low blood glucose) shock is characterized by nervousness, sweating and chills, irritability, hunger, and pallor—progressing to convulsion, coma, and death if untreated.
Myxedema	Extreme hyposecretion of thyroid hormone during adulthood	This is a severe form of adult hypothyroidism characterized by edema of the face and extremities, often progressing to coma and death.
Osteoporosis	Hyposecretion of estrogen in postmenopausal women	This bone disorder is characterized by loss of minerals and collagen from bone matrix, producing holes or porosities that weaken the skeleton.
Pituitary dwarfism	Hyposecretion of GH before age 25	This condition is characterized by reduced skeletal size caused by decreased protein anabolism during skeletal development.
Simple goiter	Lack of iodine in diet	Enlargement of thyroid tissue results from the inability of the thyroid to make thyroid hormone because of a lack of iodine; a positive-feedback situation develops in which low thyroid hormone levels trigger hypersecretion of thyroid-stimulating hormone (TSH) by the pituitary, which stimulates thyroid growth.
Sterility	Hyposecretion of sex hormones	This is a loss of reproductive function.
Type 1 diabetes mellitus (Type 1 DM)	Hyposecretion of insulin	This inherited condition with sudden childhood onset is characterized by polydipsia, polyuria, overeating, weight loss, fatigue, and irritability resulting from the inability of cells to secure and metabolize carbohydrates.
Type 2 diabetes mellitus (Type 2 DM)	Insensitivity of target cells to insulin	This carbohydrate-metabolism disorder with slow adult onset is thought to be caused by a combination of genetic and environmental factors and characterized by polydipsia, polyuria, overeating, weight loss, fatigue, and irritability.
Winter (seasonal affective disorder [SAD]) depression	Hypersecretion of (or hypersensitivity to) melatonin	This abnormal emotional state is characterized by sadness and melancholy resulting from exaggerated melatonin effects; melatonin levels are inhibited by sunlight so they increase when day length decreases during winter.

Table 9 | **Autoimmune Diseases**

DISEASE	POSSIBLE SELF-ANTIGEN	DESCRIPTION
Addison disease	Surface antigens on adrenal cells	Hyposecretion of adrenal hormones results in weakness, reduced blood sugar, nausea, loss of appetite, and weight loss.
Cardiomyopathy	Cardiac muscle	Disease of cardiac muscle (that is, the myocardium) results in a loss of pumping efficiency (heart failure).
Diabetes mellitus (type 1)	Pancreatic islet cells, insulin, and insulin receptors	Hyposecretion of insulin by the pancreas results in extremely elevated blood glucose levels (in turn causing a host of metabolic problems, even death if untreated).
Glomerulonephritis	Blood antigens that form immune complexes that are deposited in kidney	Disease of the filtration apparatus of the kidney (renal corpuscle) results in fluid and electrolyte imbalance and possibly total kidney failure and death.
Hemolytic anemia	Surface antigens on red blood cells (RBCs)	Condition of low RBC count in the blood results from excessive destruction of mature RBCs (hemolysis).
Graves disease (type of hyperthyroidism)	Thyroid-stimulating hormone (TSH) receptors on thyroid cells	Hypersecretion of thyroid hormone results in increase in metabolic rate.
Multiple sclerosis	Antigens in myelin sheaths of nervous tissue	Progressive degeneration of myelin sheaths results in widespread impairment of nerve function (especially muscle control).
Myasthenia gravis	Antigens at neuromuscular junction	Muscle disorder is characterized by progressive weakness and chronic fatigue.
Myxedema	Antigens in thyroid cells	Hyposecretion of thyroid hormone in adulthood causes decreased metabolic rate; it is characterized by reduced mental and physical vigor, weight gain, hair loss, and edema.
Pernicious anemia	Antigens on gastric parietal cells and intrinsic factor	Abnormally low RBC count results from the inability to absorb vitamin B12, a substance critical to RBC production.
Reproductive infertility	Antigens on sperm or tissue surrounding ovum (egg)	This is an inability to produce offspring (in this case, resulting from destruction of gametes).
Rheumatic fever	Cardiac cell membranes (cross-reaction with Group A streptococcal antigen)	This causes rheumatic heart disease and inflammatory cardiac damage (especially to the endocardium or valves).
Rheumatoid arthritis	Collagen	Inflammatory joint disease is characterized by synovial inflammation that spreads to other fibrous tissues.
Systemic lupus erythematosus	Numerous	Chronic inflammatory disease has widespread effects and is characterized by arthritis, a red rash on the face, and other signs.
Ulcerative colitis	Mucous cells of colon	Chronic inflammatory disease of the colon is characterized by watery diarrhea containing blood, mucus, and pus.

Table 10 | Deficiency Diseases*

CONDITION	DEFICIENT SUBSTANCE	DESCRIPTION
Avitaminosis K	Vitamin K	This occurs almost exclusively in children and is characterized by an impaired blood-clotting ability.
Beriberi	Vitamin B1 (thiamine)	Peripheral nerve condition is characterized by diarrhea, fatigue, anorexia, edema, heart failure, and limb paralysis leading to muscle atrophy.
Folate-deficiency anemia	Folic acid	Blood disorder is characterized by a decrease in red blood cell (RBC) count.
Iron-deficiency anemia	Iron (Fe)	Blood disorder is characterized by a decrease in size and pigmentation of RBCs that causes fatigue and pallor.
Kwashiorkor	Protein and calories	This form of protein-calorie malnutrition is characterized by wasting of muscle and subcutaneous tissue, dehydration, lethargy, edema and ascites, and retarded growth; it is caused by deficiency of proteins in the presence of adequate caloric intake (see marasmus).
Marasmus	Protein and calories	This form of protein-calorie malnutrition is characterized by progressive wasting of muscle and subcutaneous tissue accompanied by fluid and electrolyte imbalances; it is caused by deficiency of both protein and calories (see kwashiorkor).
Night blindness (nyctalopia)	Vitamin A	Relative inability to see in dim light results from failure to produce sufficient photopigment in the rods of the retina.
Osteomalacia	Vitamin D, calcium (Ca), and/or phosphorus (P)	Adult form of rickets is characterized by reduced mineralization of bone tissue accompanied by weakness, pain, anorexia, and weight loss.
Pellagra	Vitamin B3 (niacin) or tryptophan (an amino acid)	Disease is characterized by sun-sensitive scaly dermatitis, inflammation of mucosa, diarrhea, confusion, and depression.
Pernicious anemia	Vitamin B12	Blood disorder is characterized by a reduced number of RBCs, causing weakness, pallor, tingling of the extremities, and anorexia.
Protein-calorie malnutrition (PCM)	Protein and calories	Abnormal condition resulting from dietary deficiency of calories in general and protein in particular; its forms include kwashiorkor and marasmus.
Rickets	Vitamin D, calcium (Ca), and/or phosphorus (P)	Juvenile form of osteomalacia is characterized by weakness and abnormal skeletal formation resulting from reduced mineralization of bone tissue.
Scurvy	Vitamin C	Reduced manufacture and maintenance of collagen and other functions results in weakness, anemia, edema, weakness of gingiva and loosening of teeth, and hemorrhaging (especially in skin and mucous membranes).
Simple goiter	Iodine (I)	Enlargement of thyroid tissue results from inability of thyroid to make thyroid hormone because of lack of iodine; positive-feedback situation develops: low thyroid hormone levels trigger hypersecretion of thyroid-stimulating hormone (TSH) by pituitary, which stimulates thyroid growth.
Zinc deficiency	Zinc (Zn)	Condition is characterized by fatigue, decreased alertness, retarded growth, decreased smell and taste sensitivity, and impaired healing and immunity.

*Deficiency may be caused by dietary deficiency or an inability to absorb or chemically process the listed substances.

| Table | 11 | **Genetic Conditions** |

CHROMOSOME LOCATION	DISEASE	DESCRIPTION
SINGLE-GENE INHERITANCE (NUCLEAR DNA)		
Dominant		
7, 17	Osteogenesis imperfecta	Group of connective tissue disorders is characterized by imperfect skeletal development that produces brittle bones.
17	Multiple neurofibromatosis	Disorder is characterized by multiple, sometimes disfiguring benign tumors of the Schwann cells (neuroglia) that surround nerve fibers.
5	Hypercholesterolemia	High blood cholesterol may lead to atherosclerosis and other cardiovascular problems.
4	Huntington disease (HD)	Degenerative brain disorder is characterized by chorea (purposeless movements) progressing to severe dementia and death by age 55.
Co-dominant		
11	Sickle cell anemia Sickle cell trait	Blood disorder in which abnormal hemoglobin is produced, causing red blood cells (RBCs) to deform into a sickle shape; sickle cell anemia is the severe form, and sickle cell trait is the milder form.
11, 16	Thalassemia	Group of inherited hemoglobin disorders is characterized by production of hypochromic, abnormal RBCs.
Recessive (Autosomal)		
7	Cystic fibrosis (CF)	Condition is characterized by excessive secretion of thick mucus and concentrated sweat, often causing obstruction of the gastrointestinal or respiratory tracts.
15	Tay-Sachs disease	Fatal condition in which abnormal lipids accumulate in the brain and cause tissue damage; leads to death by age 4.
12	Phenylketonuria (PKU)	Excess of phenylketone in the urine is caused by accumulation of phenylalanine in the tissues; it may cause brain injury and death if phenylalanine (amino acid) intake is not managed properly.
11	Albinism (total)	Lack of the dark brown pigment melanin in the skin and eyes results in vision problems and susceptibility to sunburn and skin cancer.
20	Severe combined immune deficiency (SCID)	Failure of the lymphocytes to develop properly causes failure of the immune system's defense of the body; it is usually caused by adenosine deaminase (ADA) deficiency.

CHROMOSOME LOCATION	DISEASE	DESCRIPTION
Recessive (X-Linked)		
23 (X)	Hemophilia	Group of blood clotting disorders is caused by a failure to form clotting factors VIII, IX, or XI.
23 (X)	Duchenne muscular dystrophy (DMD)	Muscle disorder is characterized by progressive atrophy of skeletal muscle without nerve involvement.
23 (X)	Red-green color blindness	Inability to distinguish red and green light results from a deficiency of photopigments in the cone cells of the retina.
23 (X)	Fragile X syndrome	Mental retardation results from breakage of X chromosome in males.
23 (X)	Ocular albinism	Form of albinism in which the pigmented layers of the eyeball lack melanin; results in hypersensitivity to light and other problems.
23 (X)	Androgen insensitivity	Inherited insensitivity to androgens (steroid sex hormones associated with maleness) results in reduced effects of these hormones.
23 (X)	Cleft palate (X-linked form)	One form of a congenital deformity in which the skull fails to develop properly; it is characterized by a gap in the palate (plate separating mouth from nasal cavity).
23 (X)	Retinitis pigmentosa	Condition causes blindness, characterized by clumps of melanin in retina of eyes.
SINGLE-GENE INHERITANCE (MITOCHONDRIAL DNA)		
mDNA	Leber hereditary optic neuropathy	Optic nerve degeneration in young adults results in total blindness by age 30.
mDNA	Parkinson disease (?)	Nervous disorder is characterized by involuntary trembling and muscle rigidity.
CHROMOSOMAL ABNORMALITIES		
Trisomy		
21	Down syndrome	Condition is characterized by mental retardation and multiple structural defects.
23	Klinefelter syndrome	Condition is caused by the presence of two or more X chromosomes in a male (XXY); it is characterized by long legs, enlarged breasts, low intelligence, small testes, sterility, and chronic pulmonary disease.
Monosomy		
23	Turner syndrome	Condition is caused by monosomy of the X chromosome (XO); it is characterized by immaturity of sex organs (causing sterility), webbed neck, cardiovascular defects, and learning disorders.

Medical Terminology

Table 1 Word Parts Commonly Used as Prefixes
Table 2 Word Parts Commonly Used as Suffixes
Table 3 Word Parts Commnly Used as Roots

If you are unfamiliar with it, medical and scientific terminology can seem overwhelming. The length and apparent complexity of many medical terms seem completely foreign and mystifying to people who have not had any training or practice in scientific terminology. Although knowledge of some basic word parts and a few rules for using them are required, medical terminology is not as difficult as it seems. This appendix provides what you need to get you started on your way to understanding medical terminology. First, there are a handful of hints to help you learn and use medical terms. Second, there are several tables containing many of the most commonly used word parts and examples of how they are used. This appendix does not attempt to teach you the entire field of medical terminology, but with the information given here and a little practice, you will soon become comfortable with the basics.

Hints for Learning and Using Medical Terms

1. Many medical terms are derived from the Latin and Greek languages. This is because many of the anatomists, physiologists, and physicians around the world who discovered the basic principles of modern life science used these languages themselves so that they could communicate with each other without having to learn dozens of native languages. Thus Latin and Greek have become the "universal" language of scientific terminology. Not only many of the words but also some of the rules of usage are derived from these classical languages. The more useful of those rules are given later in this section.

2. One set of rules for using Latin and Greek is essential to understanding medical terminology. Both of these languages rely on the ability to combine word parts to make new words. Thus almost all medical terms are constructed by combining smaller word elements to make a meaningful term. Because of this combining

technique, many medical terms appear at first glance to be long and complex. However, if you read a new term as a series of word elements rather than a single word, you will find it less imposing. One of the easiest ways to learn medical terminology is to develop the ability to instantly analyze new terms to discover the word parts that compose them. Word parts differ in terms of exactly how they fit together with other word parts to form a complete term.

   a. A **prefix** is a word part that is added to the beginning of an existing word to alter its meaning. We use prefixes in English as well: the meaning of *sense* changes when we add the prefix *non-* to make the word *nonsense*.

   b. A **suffix** is a word part that is added to the end of an existing word to alter its meaning. Once again, suffixes are also sometimes used in English. For example, the meaning of *sense* changes when we add the suffix *-less* to make the word *senseless*. A complex term can have a series of suffixes, a series of prefixes, or both. For example, the word *senselessness* has two suffixes: *-less* and *-ness*.

   c. A **root** is a word part that serves as the starting point for forming a new term. In the previous examples in English, the word *sense* was the root to which was added a prefix or a suffix. Word parts commonly used as roots can also be used as suffixes or prefixes in forming a new term. Also, several roots are sometimes combined to form a larger root to which suffixes or prefixes can be added.

   d. **Combining vowels** are vowels (*a, e, i, o, u, y*) that are used to link word parts—often to make pronunciation of that new combination word easier. For example, to link the suffix *-tion* to the root *sense*, we must use the combining vowel *-a-* to form the new term *sensation*. Using the *-e* from the original root word would make the term difficult to pronounce. A root and a combining vowel together, such as *sensa-*, is often called the **combining form** of the word part.

3. Another set of rules for using Latin and Greek terms that you will find useful pertain to pluralization. To form a plural in English, we often

simply add -s or -es to a word. For example, the plural for *sense* is *senses*. Because we have adopted these medical terms and brought them into the English language, in many cases we simply use the pluralization rules of English and add the -s or -es when multiples are being discussed. Often, however, you will run across a term that has been pluralized according to Latin or Greek rules. This brief list will help you distinguish between many plural and singular forms:

4. Correct spelling of medical terms is essential to their meanings. This is especially true of terms that are very close in spelling but very different in meaning. For example, the *perineum* is the region of the trunk around the genitals and anus, whereas the *peritoneum* is a membrane that lines the abdominal cavity and covers abdominal organs. A mistake that involves just one letter can change the meaning of a word, as in the case of *ilium* (part of the bony pelvis) and *ileum* (part of the small intestine).

5. Communicating verbally is just as important as written communication, so correct pronunciation is as important as correct spelling. Medical terms can usually be pronounced phonetically—by sounding out each letter sound of each syllable. It is best to check the pronunciation keys given in each chapter and in the glossary if you are uncertain of how to pronounce any word presented in this text.

6. As you know, practice makes perfect. Practice using the medical terms in this or another book until you become comfortable with medical terminology. It won't take long—and you'll probably have fun doing it.

SINGULAR	PLURAL	EXAMPLE
-a	-ae	Ampulla, ampullae
-ax	-aces	Thorax, thoraces
-en	-ena	Lumen, lumena
-en	-ina	Foramen, foramina
-ex	-ices	Cortex, cortices
-is	-es	Neurosis, neuroses
-ix	-ices	Appendix, appendices
-on	-a	Mitochondrion, mitochondria
-um	-a	Datum, data
-ur	-ora	Femur, femora
-us	-I	Villus, villi
-yx	-yces	Calyx, calyces
-ma	-mata	Lymphoma, lymphomata

Table 1 | Word Parts Commonly Used as Prefixes

WORD PART	MEANING	EXAMPLE	MEANING OF EXAMPLE
a-	Without, not	Apnea	Cessation of breathing
af-	Toward	Afferent	Carrying toward
an-	Without, not	Anuria	Absence of urination
ante-	Before	Antenatal	Before birth
anti-	Against; resisting	Antibody	Unit that resists foreign substances
auto-	Self	Autoimmunity	Self-immunity
bi-	Two; double	Bicuspid	Two-pointed
circum-	Around	Circumcision	Cutting around
co-, con-	With; together	Congenital	Born with
contra-	Against	Contraceptive	Against conception
de-	Down from, undoing	Defibrillation	Stop fibrillation
dia-	Across; through	Diarrhea	Flow through (intestines)
dipl-	Twofold, double	Diploid	Two sets of chromosomes
dys-	Bad; disordered; difficult	Dysplasia	Disordered growth

WORD PART	MEANING	EXAMPLE	MEANING OF EXAMPLE
ectop-	Displaced	Ectopic pregnancy	Displaced pregnancy
ef-	Away from	Efferent	Carrying away from
em-, en-	In, into	Encyst	Enclose in a cyst
endo-	Within	Endocarditis	Inflammation of heart lining
epi-	Upon	Epimysium	Covering of a muscle
ex-, exo-	Out of, out from	Exophthalmos	Protruding eyes
extra-	Outside of	Extraperitoneal	Outside the peritoneum
eu-	Good	Eupnea	Good (normal) breathing
hapl-	Single	Haploid	Single set of chromosomes
hem-, hemat-	Blood	Hematuria	Bloody urine
hemi-	Half	Hemiplegia	Paralysis in half the body
hom(e)o-	Same; equal	Homeostasis	Staying the same
hyper-	Over; above	Hyperplasia	Excessive growth
hypo-	Under; below	Hypodermic	Below the skin
infra-	Below, beneath	Infraorbital	Below the (eye) orbit
inter-	Between	Intervertebral	Between vertebrae
intra-	Within	Intracranial	Within the skull
iso-	Same, equal	Isometric	Same length
macro-	Large	Macrophage	Large eater (phagocyte)
mega-	Large; million(th)	Megakaryocyte	Cell with large nucleus
mes-	Middle	Mesentery	Middle of intestine
meta-	Beyond, after	Metatarsal	Beyond the tarsals (ankle bones)
micro-	Small; millionth	Microcytic	Small-celled
milli-	Thousandth	Milliliter	Thousandth of a liter
mono-	One (single)	Monosomy	Single chromosome
neo-	New	Neoplasm	New matter
non-	Not	Nondisjunction	Not disjoined
oligo-	Few, scanty	Oliguria	Scanty urination
ortho-	Straight; correct, normal	Orthopnea	Normal breathing
para-	By the side of; near	Parathyroid	Near the thyroid
per-	Through	Permeable	Able to go through
peri-	Around; surrounding	Pericardium	Covering of the heart
poly-	Many	Polycythemia	Condition of having many blood cells
post-	After	Postmortem	After death
pre-	Before	Premenstrual	Before menstruation
pro-	First; promoting	Progesterone	Hormone that promotes pregnancy
quadr-	Four	Quadriplegia	Paralysis in four limbs
re-	Back again	Reflux	Backflow
retro-	Behind	Retroperitoneal	Behind the peritoneum
semi-	Half	Semilunar	Half-moon
sub-	Under	Subcutaneous	Under the skin
super-, supra-	Over, above, excessive	Superior	Above
trans-	Across; through	Transcutaneous	Through the skin
tri-	Three; triple	Triplegia	Paralysis of three limbs

Table 2 | Word Parts Commonly Used as Suffixes

WORD PART	MEANING	EXAMPLE	MEANING OF EXAMPLE
-al, -ac	Pertaining to	Intestinal	Pertaining to the intestines
-algia	Pain	Neuralgia	Nerve pain
-aps, -apt	Fit; fasten	Synapse	Fasten together
-arche	Beginning; origin	Menarche	First menstruation
-ase	Signifies an enzyme	Lipase	Enzyme that acts on lipids
-blast	Sprout; make	Osteoblast	Bone maker
-centesis	A piercing	Amniocentesis	Piercing the amniotic sac
-cide	To kill	Fungicide	Fungus killer
-clast	Break; destroy	Osteoclast	Bone breaker
-crine	Release; secrete	Endocrine	Secrete within
-ectomy	A cutting out	Appendectomy	Removal of the appendix
-emia	Refers to blood condition	Hypercholesterolemia	High blood cholesterol level
-emesis	Vomiting	Hematemesis	Vomiting blood
-flux	Flow	Reflux	Backflow
-gen	Creates; forms	Lactogen	Milk producer
-genesis	Creation, production	Oogenesis	Egg production
-gram*	Something written	Electroencephalogram	Record of brain's electrical activity
-graph(y)*	To write, draw	Electrocardiograph	Apparatus that records heart's electrical activity
-hydrate	Containing H_2O (water)	Dehydration	Loss of water
-ia, -sia	Condition; process	Arthralgia	Condition of joint pain
-iasis	Abnormal condition	Giardiasis	*Giardia* infestation
-ic, -ac	Pertaining to	Cardiac	Pertaining to the heart
-in	Signifies a protein	Renin	Kidney protein
-ism	Signifies "condition of"	Gigantism	Condition of gigantic size
-itis	Signifies "inflammation of"	Gastritis	Stomach inflammation
-lemma	Rind; peel	Neurilemma	Covering of a nerve fiber
-lepsy	Seizure	Epilepsy	Seizure upon seizure
-lith	Stone; rock	Lithotripsy	Stone-crushing
-logy	Study of	Cardiology	Study of the heart
-lunar	Moon; moonlike	Semilunar	Half-moon
-malacia	Softening	Osteomalacia	Bone softening
-megaly	Enlargement	Splenomegaly	Spleen enlargement
-metric, -metry	Measurement, length	Isometric	Same length
-oid	Like; in the shape of	Sigmoid	S-shaped
-oma	Tumor	Lipoma	Fatty tumor
-opia	Vision, vision condition	Myopia	Nearsightedness
-ose	Signifies a carbohydrate	Lactose	Milk sugar (especially sugar)
-osis	Condition, process	Dermatosis	Skin condition
-oscopy	Viewing	Laparoscopy	Viewing the abdominal cavity
-ostomy	Formation of an opening	Tracheostomy	Forming an opening in the trachea
-otomy	Cut	Lobotomy	Cut of a lobe
-philic	Loving	Hydrophilic	Water-loving
-penia	Lack	Leukopenia	Lack of white (cells)

*A term ending in *-graph* refers to an apparatus that results in a visual and/or recorded representation of biological phenomena, whereas a term ending in *-graphy* is the technique or process of using the apparatus. A term ending in *-gram* is the record itself. Example: In electrocardio*graphy*, an electrocardio*graph* is used in producing an electrocardio*gram*.

WORD PART	MEANING	EXAMPLE	MEANING OF EXAMPLE
-phobic	Fearing	Hydrophobic	Water-fearing
-phragm	Partition	Diaphragm	Partition separating thoracic and abdominal cavities
-plasia	Growth, formation	Hyperplasia	Excessive growth
-plasm	Substance, matter	Neoplasm	New matter
-plasty	Shape; make	Rhinoplasty	Reshaping the nose
-plegia	Paralysis	Triplegia	Paralysis in three limbs
-pnea	Breath, breathing	Apnea	Cessation of breathing
-(r)rhage, -(r)rhagia	Breaking out, discharge	Hemorrhage	Blood discharge
-(r)rhaphy	Sew, suture	Meningeorrhaphy	Suturing of meninges
-(r)rhea	Flow	Diarrhea	Flow through (intestines)
-some	Body	Chromosome	Stained body
-tensin, -tension	Pressure	Hypertension	High pressure
-tonic	Pressure, tension	Isotonic	Same pressure
-tripsy	Crushing	Lithotripsy	Stone-crushing
-ule	Small, little	Tubule	Small tube
-uria	Refers to urine condition	Proteinuria	Protein in the urine

Table	3	**Word Parts Commonly Used as Roots**

WORD PART	MEANING	EXAMPLE	MEANING OF EXAMPLE
acro	Extremity	Acromegaly	Enlargement of extremities
aden-	Gland	Adenoma	Tumor of glandular tissue
alveoli-	Small hollow; cavity	Alveolus	Small air sac in the lung
angi-	Vessel	Angioplasty	Reshaping a vessel
arthr-	Joint	Arthritis	Joint inflammation
asthen-	Weakness	Myasthenia	Condition of muscle weakness
bar-	Pressure	Baroreceptor	Pressure receptor
bili-	Bile	Bilirubin	Orange-yellow bile pigment
brachi-	Arm	Brachial	Pertaining to the arm
brady-	Slow	Bradycardia	Slow heart rate
bronch-	Air passage	Bronchitis	Inflammation of pulmonary passages (bronchi)
calc-	Calcium; limestone	Hypocalcemia	Low blood calcium level
capn-	Smoke	Hypercapnia	Elevated blood CO_2 level
carcin-	Cancer	Carcinogen	Cancer producer
card-	Heart	Cardiology	Study of the heart
cephal-	Head, brain	Encephalitis	Brain inflammation
cerv-	Neck	Cervicitis	Inflammation of (uterine) cervix
chem-	Chemical	Chemotherapy	Chemical treatment
chol-	Bile	Cholecystectomy	Removal of bile (gall) bladder
chondr-	Cartilage	Chondroma	Tumor of cartilage tissue
chrom-	Color	Chromosome	Stained body
corp-	Body	Corpus luteum	Yellow body
cortico-	Pertaining to cortex	Corticosteroid	Steroid secreted by (adrenal) cortex
crani-	Skull	Intracranial	Within the skull
crypt-	Hidden	Cryptorchidism	Undescended testis

Table 3	Word Parts Commonly Used as Roots (continued)		
WORD PART	**MEANING**	**EXAMPLE**	**MEANING OF EXAMPLE**
cusp-	Point	Tricuspid	Three-pointed
cut(an)-	Skin	Transcutaneous	Through the skin
cyan-	Blue	Cyanosis	Condition of blueness
cyst-	Bladder	Cystitis	Bladder inflammation
cyt-	Cell	Cytotoxin	Cell poison
dactyl-	Fingers, toes (digits)	Syndactyly	Joined digits
dendr-	Tree; branched	Oligodendrocyte	Branched nervous tissue cell
dent-	Tooth	Dentalgia	Toothache
derm-	Skin	Dermatitis	Skin inflammation
diastol-	Relax; stand apart	Diastole	Relaxation phase of heartbeat
dips-	Thirst	Polydipsia	Excessive thirst
ejacul-	To throw out	Ejaculation	Expulsion (of semen)
electr-	Electrical	Electrocardiogram	Record of electrical activity of heart
enter-	Intestine	Enteritis	Intestinal inflammation
eryth(r)	Red	Erythrocyte	Red (blood) cell
esthe-	Sensation	Anesthesia	Condition of no sensation
febr-	Fever	Febrile	Pertaining to fever
gastr-	Stomach	Gastritis	Stomach inflammation
gest-	To bear, carry	Gestation	Pregnancy
gingiv-	Gums	Gingivitis	Gum inflammation
glomer-	Wound into a ball	Glomerulus	Rounded tuft of vessels
gloss-	Tongue	Hypoglossal	Under the tongue
gluc-	Glucose, sugar	Glucosuria	Glucose in urine
glutin-	Glue	Agglutination	Sticking together (of particles)
glyc-	Sugar (carbohydrate); glucose	Glycolipid	Carbohydrate-lipid combination
hepat-	Liver	Hepatitis	Liver inflammation
hist-	Tissue	Histology	Study of tissues
hydro-	Water	Hydrocephalus	Water on the brain
hyster-	Uterus	Hysterectomy	Removal of the uterus
iatr-	Treatment	Podiatry	Foot treatment
kal-	Potassium	Hyperkalemia	Elevated blood potassium level
kary-	Nucleus	Karyotype	Array of chromosomes from nucleus
kerat-	Cornea	Keratotomy	Cutting of the cornea
kin-	To move; divide	Kinesthesia	Sensation of body movement
lact-	Milk; milk production	Lactose	Milk sugar
lapar-	Abdomen	Laparoscopy	Viewing the abdominal cavity
leuk-	White	Leukorrhea	White flow (discharge)
lig-	To tie, bind	Ligament	Tissue that binds bones
lip-	Lipid (fat)	Lipoma	Fatty tumor
lys-	Break apart	Hemolysis	Breaking of blood cells
mal-	Bad	Malabsorption	Improper absorption
melan-	Black	Melanin	Black protein
men-, mens-, (menstru-)	Month (monthly)	Amenorrhea	Absence of monthly flow
metr-	Uterus	Endometrium	Uterine lining
muta-	Change	Mutagen	Change-maker
my-, myo-	Muscle	Myopathy	Muscle disease

WORD PART	MEANING	EXAMPLE	MEANING OF EXAMPLE
myc-	Fungus	Mycosis	Fungal condition
myel-	Marrow	Myeloma	(Bone) marrow tumor
myx-	Mucus	Myxedema	Mucous edema
nat-	Birth	Neonatal	Pertaining to newborns (infants)
natr-	Sodium	Natriuresis	Elevated sodium in urine
nephr-	Nephron, kidney	Nephritis	Kidney inflammation
neur-	Nerve	Neuralgia	Nerve pain
noct-, nyct-	Night	Nocturia	Urination at night
ocul-	Eye	Binocular	Two-eyed
odont-	Tooth	Periodontitis	Inflammation (of tissue) around the teeth
onco-	Cancer	Oncogene	Cancer gene
ophthalm-	Eye	Ophthalmology	Study of the eye
orchid-	Testis	Orchiditis	Testis inflammation
osteo-	Bone	Osteoma	Bone tumor
oto-	Ear	Otosclerosis	Hardening of ear tissue
ov-, oo-	Egg	Oogenesis	Egg production
oxy-	Oxygen	Oxyhemoglobin	Oxygen-hemoglobin combination
path-	Disease	Neuropathy	Nerve disease
ped-	Children	Pediatric	Pertaining to treatment of children
phag-	Eat	Phagocytosis	Cell eating
pharm-	Drug	Pharmacology	Study of drugs
phleb-	Vein	Phlebitis	Vein inflammation
photo-	Light	Photopigment	Light-sensitive pigment
physio-	Nature (function) of	Physiology	Study of biological function
pino-	Drink	Pinocytosis	Cell drinking
plex-	Twisted; woven	Nerve plexus	Complex of interwoven nerve fibers
pneumo-	Air, breath	Pneumothorax	Air in the thorax
pneumon-	Lung	Pneumonia	Lung condition
pod-	Foot	Podocyte	Cell with feet
poie-	Make; produce	Hemopoiesis	Blood cell production
pol-	Axis, having poles	Bipolar	Having two ends
presby-	Old	Presbyopia	Old vision
proct-	Rectum	Proctoscope	Instrument for viewing the rectum
pseud-	False	Pseudopodia	False feet
psych-	Mind	Psychiatry	Treatment of the mind
pyel-	Pelvis	Pyelogram	Image of the renal pelvis
pyo-	Pus	Pyogenic	Pus-producing
pyro-	Heat; fever	Pyrogen	Fever producer
ren-	Kidney	Renocortical	Referring to the cortex of the kidney
rhino-	Nose	Rhinoplasty	Reshaping the nose
rigor-	Stiffness	Rigor mortis	Stiffness of death
sarco-	Flesh; muscle	Sarcolemma	Muscle fiber membrane
scler-	Hard	Scleroderma	Hard skin
semen-, semin-	Seed; sperm	Seminiferous tubule	Sperm-bearing tubule
sept-	Contamination	Septicemia	Contamination of the blood
sigm-	Greek Σ or Roman S	Sigmoid colon	S-shaped colon

Table 3	Word Parts Commonly Used as Roots (continued)		
WORD PART	**MEANING**	**EXAMPLE**	**MEANING OF EXAMPLE**
sin-	Cavity; recess	Paranasal sinus	Cavity near the nasal cavity
son-	Sound	Sonography	Imaging using sound
spiro-, -spire	Breathe	Spirometry	Measurement of breathing
stat-, stas-	A standing, stopping	Homeostasis	Staying the same
syn-	Together	Syndrome	Signs appearing together
systol-	Contract; stand together	Systole	Contraction phase of the heartbeat
tachy-	Fast	Tachycardia	Rapid heart rate
therm-	Heat	Thermoreceptor	Heat receptor
thromb-	Clot	Thrombosis	Condition of abnormal blood clotting
tom-	A cut; a slice	Tomography	Image of a slice or section
tox-	Poison	Cytotoxin	Cell poison
troph-	Grow; nourish	Hypertrophy	Excessive growth
tympan-	Drum	Tympanum	Eardrum
varic-	Enlarged vessel	Varicose vein	Enlarged vein
vas-	Vessel, duct	Vasoconstriction	Vessel narrowing
vesic-	Bladder; blister	Vesicle	Blister
vol-	Volume	Hypovolemic	Characterized by low volume

Chapter Test and Case Studies Answers

Chapter 1
Chapter Test
1. Anatomy
2. Physiology
3. Pathology
4. Chemical, cells, tissues, organs, systems
5. Supine, prone
6. transverse
7. frontal
8. sagittal
9. midsagittal
10. axial
11. appendicular
12. c
13. b
14. d
15. d
16. b
17. d
18. e
19. d
20. a
21. c
22. b

Case Studies
1. Mrs. Miller's mole is on the anterior (front) surface of her trunk, inferior to (below) the rib cage, and superior to (above) and left of the navel. With the choices given, it is best to ask Mrs. Miller to assume a supine (belly-up) position. Mrs. Miller's occipital mole is on the back of her head. This is best examined if she rolls to a prone (belly-down) position or sits up and tilts her head forward.
2. Mr. Sanchez's injury was at the end of his ring finger. A typical response to a sudden drop in blood pressure is to increase pumping of blood by the heart. Under normal circumstances, this response would bring the blood pressure back up to its average value. In this case, however, increased pumping by the heart will increase blood loss—causing a further drop in blood pressure and threatening Mr. Sanchez's homeostatic balance even more. If the blood loss is not stopped soon, Mr. Sanchez could lose a large volume of blood. Because this response amplifies the drop in blood pressure rather than returning it to its normal value, it is a case of positive feedback.

Chapter 2
Chapter Test
1. Matter
2. atoms
3. protons
4. energy
5. compounds
6. covalent
7. ion
8. electrolyte
9. organic
10. solvent
11. dehydration synthesis
12. Acids
13. buffers
14. d
15. f
16. g
17. e
18. a
19. c
20. b
21. c
22. a
23. d
24. b
25. c

Case Studies
1. A pH of 7.57 is significantly higher than the maximum (7.45) of the normal blood plasma pH range (7.35-7.45). Grania may be suffering from alkalosis, a condition in which the blood pH is higher than normal.
2. A "high-carb" diet is one in which a person eats a higher proportion of carbohydrates than usual. The primary dietary carbohydrates are those based on the saccharide group ($C_6H_{12}O_6$) and include monosaccharides, disaccharides, and polysaccharides. Monosaccharides in Baraka's diet may include glucose, fructose, or galactose. Disaccharides in his diet may include sucrose, maltose, and lactose. Polysaccharides in Baraka's food are known as glycogen and various starches. One of the main roles of carbohydrates in Baraka's body is to provide energy for cellular work. For example, the energy from carbohydrate molecules is transferred to ATP and then transferred to the fibers that power the contraction of muscles. Therefore, carbohydrates must be present in relatively large amounts for athletic use of muscles.
3. Although high overall cholesterol levels are associated with increased risks of health problems such as atherosclerosis and heart disease, there are different types of cholesterol with different roles in the body. HDLs (high-density lipoproteins) are a type of cholesterol that are associated with a lower risk of such health problems. Because Shane's HDL proportion has increased, he is now at a lower risk of health problems than before.

Chapter 3
Chapter Test
1. Phospholipid, cholesterol
2. Organelles
3. Active transport, passive transport
4. Pinocytosis
5. Cystic fibrosis
6. Translation
7. Transcription
8. Gene
9. Genome

10. Epithelial, connective, muscular, nervous
11. a
12. a
13. b
14. c
15. a
16. b
17. c
18. d
19. b
20. c
21. b
22. g
23. c
24. e
25. i
26. b
27. a
28. d
29. f
30. h

Case Studies

1. Glycogen-digesting enzymes are likely to be found within lysosomes. Recall that lysosomes are tiny sacs that contain enzymes used to digest food molecules within cells. The nonfunctional enzymes responsible for Pompe's disease were synthesized at ribosomes with information obtained from each cell's DNA—information that was incorrect. The incorrect genetic information in DNA originally came from the genetic code in the DNA passed from parent to offspring in the sperm and egg cells. A more detailed explanation of DNA inheritance is given in Chapter 24.

2. Drugs that interfere with formation of spindle fibers halt mitosis by preventing chromosomes from lining up during metaphase and from separating in an orderly fashion during anaphase. Mitosis cannot proceed without spindles to which chromosomes can attach. Drugs that prevent DNA synthesis affect cells before mitosis even begins—during interphase when DNA replication should be occurring. If DNA is not replicated, the cell will not enter prophase.

3. CF causes thickened secretions in many areas of the body. Thickened mucus secretions in the airways of the lungs often interfere with breathing and promote recurring infections. A traditional treatment for youngsters with CF is to put them over a pillow or other support, head down, and deliver a series of sharp slaps to the back of the thorax. This promotes drainage of the thick mucus out of the airways, making breathing easier and reducing the likelihood of pulmonary infection.

Chapter 4
Chapter Test

1. gastrointestinal tract *or* alimentary canal
2. Skeletal *or* Striated
3. Smooth *or* Visceral
4. nerve impulses
5. hair, nails, sense organs
6. thymus gland
7. urethra
8. testes; ovaries
9. cartilage, ligaments
10. Cochlear implant
11. Stem cells
12. f
13. k

14. a
15. i
16. b
17. g
18. c
19. j
20. d
21. e
22. h

Case Studies

1. The kidneys are part of the urinary system, so it is that system that is primarily involved in Tommy's condition. However, because the kidneys clear metabolic wastes from the blood and help maintain homeostasis of the entire internal environment, all systems will be affected if these functions are lost. Based on information given in this chapter, Tommy's physicians may recommend use of a dialysis machine or a similar procedure (see Chapter 19) for short-term use. Because the kidney failure is permanent, a kidney transplant may be recommended as a long-term solution.

2. The male urethra serves two functions: it conducts urine from the bladder to the outside of the body and it conducts sperm out of the body during the male sexual response. Thus both urinary and reproductive functions may be impaired by Mr. Davidson's condition.

Chapter 5
Chapter Test

1. Signs
2. Symptoms
3. idiopathic
4. pandemic
5. Vaccine
6. malignant
7. Metastasis
8. Sarcomas
9. Carcinomas
10. Mutagen
11. redness, heat, swelling, pain
12. d
13. d
14. a
15. b
16. a
17. c
18. e
19. b
20. d
21. g
22. a
23. d
24. c
25. g
26. b
27. f
28. b

Case Studies

1. An epidemiologist would probably label this outbreak of bacterial infection an epidemic. Bacterial pathogens can be transmitted by person-to-person contact (which can occur rapidly in crowded conditions or close-knit communities), by environmental contamination (such as unsanitary drinking water or improper waste disposal), by transmission by a vector (such as a mosquito), and by other means.

2. So-called "staph" infections are caused by *Staphylococcus* bacteria, round (coccus) bacteria that adhere to one another to form clusters of bacteria. Antibiotics are usually derived from living organisms such as fungi and bacteria and are thus classified as "natural" rather than synthetic. Chemists are able to produce synthetic copies or variants of natural compounds, so it is possible that the antibiotic was manufactured synthetically.

3. Fred's symptoms are classic symptoms of the inflammatory response. See Figures 5-13 and 5-14 for the details of how these symptoms are produced. In normal inflammatory responses, the body's defense mechanisms are called into play—thus taking care of the damage (including possible infection). If this normal response is inhibited, the body's defenses will be interrupted. This might increase the likelihood of a severe infection and will slow the healing process. Anti-inflammatory agents are normally used only when the inflammation response occurs at inappropriate times or is so great that it poses a threat of damage itself (as in allergic reactions or inflammatory disease).

Chapter 6
Chapter Test
1. Cutaneous, serous, mucous
2. basement membrane
3. parietal pleura
4. visceral peritoneum
5. synovial membrane
6. stratum corneum; stratum germinativum
7. keratin
8. dermal papillae
9. apocrine glands
10. eccrine glands
11. sebum
12. Protection, sensation, temperature regulation
13. burns
14. Decubitus ulcers
15. squamous cell
16. Acne
17. c
18. a
19. b
20. d
21. a
22. c
23. e
24. c
25. d
26. b
27. a
28. f

Case Studies
1. Dana can use the rule of nines. Each arm has about 9% of the total surface area of the body (4.5% in front, 4.5% in back). Both arms have about 18% of the total. If half of both arms are burned, and half of 18 is 9, then the patient has about 9% of the total skin surface affected by the burn.

2. Although one cannot be positive in this case, the characteristics and location of the lesion indicate that it is likely to be basal cell carcinoma. Aunt Gina might find some comfort in knowing that this form of cancer is less likely to spread (metastasize) than other types of skin cancer. She might also appreciate knowing that, because she is dark-skinned, she is in a lower risk group for developing this type of cancer.

3. The ringlike pattern, redness, and scaling of the skin lesion make it likely that the patient has ringworm, a type of fungal infection (mycosis) called *tinea*. Even after treatment with antifungal agents, some of the fungi responsible for the infection may remain—possibly causing a later opportunistic infection. Recurrence of tinea infections can be prevented by keeping the skin dry because dry conditions inhibit the growth of tinea-causing fungi.

Chapter 7
Chapter Test
1. articular cartilage
2. medullary cavity
3. trabeculae
4. Haversian system
5. lacunae
6. osteoclasts
7. osteoblasts
8. endochondral ossification
9. epiphyseal plate
10. axial; appendicular
11. synarthroses, amphiarthroses, diarthroses
12. ligaments
13. scoliosis
14. osteoporosis
15. osteomyelitis
16. compound *or* open
17. osteoarthritis
18. c
19. b
20. a
21. d
22. c
23. b
24. c
25. b
26. a
27. b
28. d
29. d
30. c
31. d
32. c
33. b
34. d
35. b
36. a
37. d
38. a
39. b
40. a
41. b
42. a

Case Studies
1. The term *greenstick fracture* refers to a type of incomplete fracture in which a bone bends and then breaks only along the outside curve of the bend. This type of fracture is so named because it imitates the incomplete break commonly seen when one tries to snap a green (fresh) wooden stick into two pieces. Greenstick fractures and other types of incomplete fractures heal more rapidly than other fractures because the broken edges of bone tissue remain close to one another after the injury—facilitating the repair process.

2. As Figure 7-16, *C* and *D*, shows, such an abnormality may result from scoliosis—abnormal lateral curvature of the vertebral column. Common among adolescent women, scoliosis can be treated in a variety of ways. The text mentions braces (e.g., the Milwaukee brace), transcutaneous muscle stimulation, and spinal fusion surgery as possible treatments. Other treatments you may know include prescribed exercises, traction (pulling on the vertebral column to straighten it), body casts, or other therapies.

3. Osteoporosis, literally "bone porosity," is characterized by the loss of bone volume as open spaces or pores develop in bone tissue. Such bone loss causes the skeleton to become brittle and thus easily broken. Sometimes the bone weakness is so profound that seemingly normal stresses cause fractures—often called *spontaneous fractures* because they seem to have no direct cause. Fractured bone, as with any broken or damaged tissue, may become infected—especially if proper medical treatment is delayed. Osteomyelitis is infection of bone tissue and may result from infection secondary to a fracture.

Chapter 8
Chapter Test
1. Muscle fiber
2. heart
3. insertion
4. origin
5. Actin
6. Myosin
7. sarcomere
8. movement, posture, heat production
9. ATP
10. Lactic acid
11. motor unit
12. Threshold stimulus
13. Isotonic
14. Isometric
15. Abduction
16. Extension
17. Supination
18. strain
19. fibromyositis
20. Poliomyelitis
21. Muscular dystrophy
22. Myasthenia gravis
23. b
24. a
25. a
26. b
27. d
28. a
29. d
30. b
31. c
32. d
33. a
34. c
35. d
36. b

Case Studies
1. Pseudohypertrophic muscular dystrophy, or Duchenne muscular dystrophy (DMD), is an *X-linked* inherited disorder, so the cause of Tom's condition is inheritance of a defective gene on the X chromosome. More information on X-linked traits is found in Chapter 24. It is unlikely that Geri will develop DMD because females rarely exhibit X-linked disorders. Your risk of developing DMD depends on several different factors. First, if you are female you are not likely to develop DMD. Second, Tom's defective X chromosome had to have been inherited from his mother (see Chapter 24)—so if you are related to Tom's mother you are more likely to have the defective gene than if you are not related to her. Third, because DMD typically strikes by age 3, you are unlikely to develop the disease now. The false (pseudo) enlargement (hypertrophy) of Tom's legs is the result of abnormal levels of a cytoskeletal protein in patients with DMD. The body replaces atrophied (reduced) muscle fibers with an overabundance of fat and fibrous tissue—a common occurrence in DMD.

2. Your friend has sustained a tear or overstretching of muscle fibers in a major lower leg muscle located in the "calf" region. Elena is likely suffering from myalgia (muscle pain) and myositis (muscle inflammation). The irritation of the injury and the resulting inflammation response may also cause muscle cramps. The gastrocnemius muscle plantar flexes the foot, causing the toes to point downward. Almost any movement of the lower leg is likely to disturb the injured tissue, so Elena should avoid leg movements as recommended by her physician. Walking or even standing are most likely to worsen Elena's injury.

3. Robert may have some increase, or hypertrophy, of his upper body muscles. However, because racquetball primarily involves endurance or "aerobic" exercise, the increase will not be great. Massive muscle hypertrophy, or "body building," results from strength training or "anaerobic" exercise such as weight-lifting. Robert seems out of breath because the aerobic exercise undertaken in a game of racquetball causes an oxygen debt that must be "repaid" after exercise by continued heavy breathing—perhaps making it difficult for Robert to speak to you.

Chapter 9
Chapter Test
1. Peripheral nervous system
2. Central nervous system
3. nerve
4. nervous; glia
5. reflex arc
6. nerve impulse
7. positive; negative
8. sodium
9. synapse
10. neurotransmitters
11. Dura mater, arachnoid layer, pia mater
12. 12; 31
13. Dermatomes
14. Parasympathetic nervous system
15. Sympathetic nervous system
16. acetylcholine; norepinephrine
17. acetylcholine; acetylcholine
18. cardiac muscle, smooth muscle, glandular epithelium
19. g
20. c
21. e
22. a
23. b
24. f
25. d
26. d
27. a
28. h

29. f
30. b
31. g
32. e
33. c
34. f
35. j
36. a
37. k
38. b
39. c
40. d
41. i
42. h
43. e
44. g

Case Studies

1. Many epileptics experience very mild seizures, which may appear to Tony's teachers as "daydreaming" or "not paying attention." Tony may indeed be simply daydreaming, but it is possible that he has epilepsy and his physician would be well advised to test him—perhaps by ordering an EEG (electroencephalogram). If Tony experiences an episode while the EEG machine is recording his brain waves, a sudden burst of increased, abnormal activity may be detected. Such a burst indicates a seizure.

2. Although the information given in this case study is limited, the description of Angela's condition fits that of multiple neurofibromatosis. This disease is characterized by tumors of the Schwann cells that wrap around the axons of cutaneous nerves—nerves near the surface of the skin—as well as other nerves. Thus a disorder of nerves in the skin can cause skin lesions. Similarly, the lesions of shingles are caused by viral (herpes) infection of cutaneous nerves, usually along a single dermatome.

3. A myelin disorder is caused by destruction of the myelin sheath that surrounds many neurons. Because the myelin sheath speeds up nerve conduction, damage to the myelin sheath decreases nerve conduction to below normal rates. Because coordination and precise timing is required for dancing, damage to the nerve conduction rates would cause some nerve pathways to carry information too slowly and therefore smooth body functions could not be facilitated. Multiple sclerosis (MS) is an example of a myelin disorder that could cause Baraka's symptoms. In MS, oligodendrocytes are destroyed and thus the myelin sheath in some areas is damaged. This causes lack of coordination in the body by slowing down some nerve pathways that would ordinarily be fast.

Chapter 10
Chapter Test

1. chemoreceptors; proprioceptors
2. organ of Corti
3. crista ampullaris
4. taste
5. sweet, sour, bitter, salty
6. papillae
7. olfactory receptors
8. e
9. i
10. j
11. b
12. a
13. g

14. c
15. f
16. h
17. d
18. k
19. f
20. g
21. a
22. b
23. e
24. c
25. d
26. d
27. j
28. b
29. f
30. i
31. a
32. c
33. h
34. e
35. g

Case Studies

1. Roger's condition, diabetic retinopathy, involves progressive degeneration of the retina. Early in this disease, small hemorrhages of retinal vessels disrupt the normal supply of blood to retinal cells. Later, the retina begins to form abnormal, thick vessels that block vision and may cause retinal detachment. The damage involved starts at the edges of the retina and progresses inward toward the optic nerve. Roger is legally blind, meaning that his vision is worse than 20-200. Roger may have seen the other pedestrian stumble in front him, if only as a very fuzzy image. Even without any vision, some blind individuals have learned to use their other senses—especially hearing—to detect changes in their environment.

2. Obviously, Mrs. Stark has a form of color blindness, or color deficiency. Because Mrs. Stark did not have difficulty in distinguishing colors until late adulthood, this could not have been one of the common, inherited forms of color blindness such as red-green color blindness. Being female, it is unlikely that she would have been born with such an X-linked condition anyway. Additionally, inherited forms of color blindness typically cause problems with specific ranges of color—not all colors. Considering her age and the suddenness of onset, it is likely that Mrs. Stark suffered a cerebrovascular accident (stroke) that damaged the color-perception centers of her brain. If damage was limited to that area only, she may not have any other symptoms besides color blindness. This condition has sometimes been called *acquired cortical color blindness*.

3. Otitis media is inflammation of the middle ear resulting from infection by bacterial or viral pathogens. A pathogen has entered the air-filled middle ear, possibly through the auditory (eustachian) tube, and infected the mucous lining. Inflammation and accumulation of exudate has likely occurred as a result. The swelling and fluid accumulation may affect your hearing—creating a conduction impairment. If left untreated, your body's immune system may be able to fight off the infection, and your ear tissues may repair themselves. On the other hand, the infection may become severe and spread to surrounding tissues. If the inner ear or vestibulocochlear nerve becomes involved, the infection may cause permanent hearing loss—a type of nerve impairment. In an extreme case, the infection may spread to yet other tissues, perhaps to the blood or to the brain, causing coma or death.

Chapter 11
Chapter Test
1. Exocrine
2. Endocrine; hormones
3. protein, steroid
4. target organ
5. cyclic AMP (cAMP)
6. cell membrane; nucleus
7. prostaglandins
8. posterior pituitary (neurohypophysis)
9. anterior pituitary (adenohypophysis)
10. posterior pituitary; hypothalamus
11. d
12. b
13. c
14. b
15. b
16. a
17. d
18. f
19. i
20. a
21. e
22. c
23. h
24. g
25. b
26. g
27. d
28. j
29. a
30. b
31. e
32. h
33. f
34. c
35. i

Case Studies
1. George's excessive level of activity and his abnormal heart rhythm (atrial fibrillation) are common characteristics of hyperthyroidism. Hypersecretion of thyroid hormone (T_3 and T_4) causes a general increase in the metabolism of all cells, and therefore increases activity in all organs. The heart is no exception, so many sufferers of hyperthyroidism experience heart problems such as atrial fibrillation. George's physicians will probably recommend surgical removal or destruction (via radiation) of some of the thyroid tissue in an attempt to reduce thyroid hormone secretion to normal levels.

2. George's surgeons will, as in any surgical procedure, be careful to avoid unnecessary injury to local blood vessels, nerves, and other tissues. Not only must George's surgeons be careful to avoid damaging George's trachea and larynx, they will probably be careful to avoid damaging or removing his parathyroid glands. As you know, these glands are necessary because they produce parathyroid hormone (PTH), which is essential to the vital calcium balance of the body.

3. Lynn's condition, type 1 diabetes mellitus, is caused by a reduction of insulin secretion by the pancreatic islets as described in the text. This fact suggests the most common form of treatment: insulin therapy. Usually, several small doses of insulin are injected into a person's body each day. There are a number of additional measures, such as diet control and exercise, that often supplement insulin therapy. Tissue grafts and other new methods of treatment are also

being explored. Type 1 DM results from hyposecretion of insulin, the hormone that allows glucose to enter cells. The hyperglycemia associated with diabetes results from accumulation of nutrients (glucose) that would otherwise have entered the cells for catabolism. Thus without sufficient insulin, the excess glucose really isn't available for cell use, and the body's cells literally "starve in the midst of plenty."

Chapter 12
Chapter Test
1. plasma
2. albumin, globulin, fibrinogen
3. serum
4. red blood cells, white blood cells, platelets
5. myeloid, lymphatic
6. hemoglobin
7. anemia
8. polycythemia
9. neutrophils
10. B-lymphocytes
11. calcium
12. fibrinogen; fibrin
13. K
14. thrombus
15. an embolus
16. Antigen
17. A and B; no
18. B, anti-A
19. O
20. AB
21. erythroblastosis fetalis
22. f
23. a
24. c
25. d
26. e
27. h
28. b
29. g

Case Studies
1. Angela's physician will probably order a test to determine which, if any, enzymes in Angela's blood plasma are abnormally elevated. In this chapter, you learned that transaminase is a plasma enzyme that increases after a heart attack.

2. Of course, the wisest course of action usually involves seeking and following professional medical advice rather than acting on one's own initiative. In this case, Yvonne's actions are not likely to help her because pernicious anemia is more often caused by a lack of intrinsic factor needed to absorb B_{12} into the blood. If this is true in Yvonne's case, no matter how many B_{12} tablets she takes, she will probably not absorb enough B_{12} to reverse her condition. Her physician would likely recommend an intramuscular injection of B_{12}—a method that bypasses the absorption problem.

3. The actual diagnosis can be made only by a qualified professional, but based on the results given and the data in Table 12-2, a good guess is a type of hemolytic anemia. Most types of hemolytic anemia, such as sickle-cell anemia and thalassemia, are inherited, so it is possible that you inherited the same defective gene or genes as your brother. Depending on the exact type, however, it is unlikely that you would have gotten this far in life without developing some symptoms already.

Chapter 13
Chapter Test
1. Ventricles
2. Atria
3. myocardium
4. interventricular septum
5. endocardium
6. epicardium
7. systole
8. diastole
9. tricuspid (right atrioventricular)
10. stroke volume
11. sinoatrial node
12. Purkinje fibers
13. QRS complex
14. P wave
15. a. 7
    b. 2
    c. 3
    d. 6
    e. 10
    f. 8
    g. 9
    h. 5
    i. 1
    j. 4
16. f
17. i
18. a
19. h
20. g
21. b
22. d
23. c
24. e

Case Studies
1. The large spikes (tall waves) on the ECG monitor are probably the QRS complexes, which represent depolarization of the ventricular myocardium—the point at which your friend's ventricles are about to pump blood out of the heart during each cardiac cycle. The observed change probably resulted from the electrical "noise" produced by a muscular movement made by the patient. If so, the ECG pattern will return to normal when she stops moving. However, the sudden change may be due to ventricular fibrillation, a judgment best made by a trained professional. As with any medical emergency, the first thing to do after determining that there is a problem is to summon help. First aid for such a problem may involve CPR (have you had your CPR refresher course this year?). A defibrillator or other treatments may be used to correct your friend's problem.
2. Vivian's mitral valve prolapse (MVP) is a condition in which the left atrioventricular (mitral) valve billows backward into the left atrium. Because of this defect, the edges of the mitral valve may not meet to form a tight seal. Thus blood may leak back into the left atrium during contraction of the left ventricle. The severity of Vivian's condition depends largely on the amount of blood leakage that occurs.
3. Your uncle's heart probably has blockage of some of the major coronary arteries. This blockage could be due to a number of factors, the most likely of which is atherosclerosis. In this condition, fatty deposits form in the wall of arteries—decreasing the diameter of the lumen and reducing blood flow. Without correction, your uncle may suffer a myocardial infarction resulting from oxygen deprivation of heart muscle supplied by the affected arteries. The triple-bypass surgery will graft new vessels into your uncle's coronary circulation to route blood around the blocked areas (Figure 13-7).

Chapter 14
Chapter Test
1. veins
2. arteries
3. capillaries
4. tunica intima
5. tunica adventitia
6. pulmonary
7. foramen ovale; ductus arteriosus
8. blood viscosity, heart rate
9. f
10. a
11. j
12. b
13. i
14. c
15. h
16. d
17. e
18. g

Case Studies
1. In Chapter 2, in the Blood Lipoproteins box, it states that exercise increases the ratio of "good" cholesterol, thus decreasing the ratio of the "bad" cholesterol that causes atherosclerosis. Atherosclerosis, which develops into hardening of the arteries (arteriosclerosis), may block vessels and cause myocardial infarction, ischemia or necrosis of other tissues, aneurysms, CVAs, and other serious problems.
2. Advanced atherosclerosis of a leg artery may reduce flow to skeletal muscles in the leg enough to make it difficult for them to get oxygen during walking. The muscles will use anaerobic respiration, which increases lactic acid levels and causes a burning pain often associated with muscle fatigue. Leo's physician has many choices of treatment. One choice would be to use vasodilator drugs, which will relax and expand the affected artery and thus improve blood flow. Another choice is angioplasty, in which the obstruction is mechanically altered to improve blood flow.
3. To reach the anterior tibial artery, the tip of the catheter must proceed through the femoral artery, then through the popliteal artery (see Figure 14-2). To reach the mitral (left AV) valve from the same point, the tip must pass superiorly through the femoral artery, through the external iliac artery, through the abdominal aorta, through the thoracic aorta, through the arch of the aorta, past the aortic valve, and through the left atrium (Figure 14-2).

Chapter 15
Chapter Test
1. Lymph
2. thoracic duct
3. right lymphatic duct
4. lymphedema
5. cisterna chyli
6. lymph node

7. afferent; efferent
8. T-lymphocytes (T-cells); thymosin
9. palatine, pharyngeal, lingual
10. spleen
11. inflammation
12. Complement fixation
13. monocytes
14. allergy
15. anaphylactic shock
16. autoimmunity
17. isoimmunity
18. tissue typing
19. SCID
20. HIV
21. c
22. b
23. d
24. a
25. B
26. B
27. T
28. B
29. T
30. T
31. B
32. T
33. B
34. T

Case Studies

1. One possible explanation is that the infection in the lymph nodes of the groin (area between the legs) produced scarring of the lymph nodes and/or the lymphatic vessels connected to the nodes. Scarring often occurs as a result of damage caused by infection. Such scarring may have blocked lymphatic drainage from the leg, causing tissue fluid to accumulate in the leg and produce swelling—a condition called *lymphedema*. If the scarring occurred on only one side, only one leg would be affected this way.

2. Although the spleen performs some im-portant functions, other organs can take over these functions well enough that Keith can survive without a spleen. This is fortunate because the usual treatment recommended for a ruptured spleen is immediate splenectomy, or surgical removal of the spleen. Without such treatment, Keith would lose a great deal of blood. He has probably already lost quite a bit of blood through hemorrhaging from the rupture because the spleen itself can hold more than a pint of blood.

3. Children with SCID are unable to defend themselves against infection by pathogens. Therefore such children are defenseless against the pathogenic bacteria found throughout the natural environment. Children without SCID have immune defenses that protect them from infection by these common pathogens. The "bubble" strategy was used to protect the boy from exposure to these pathogens. Recently, injections of antibodies have afforded partial, temporary immune protection to people with SCID. The boy in question died at age 12 after leaving the bubble to receive a bone marrow transplant. More recently, bone marrow transplants have been successful in treating some cases of SCID by replacing abnormal stem cells with normal donor cells.

Chapter 16
Chapter Test

1. air distribution, gas exchange
2. nose, pharynx, larynx

3. trachea, bronchial tree, lungs
4. respiratory membrane
5. respiratory mucosa
6. paranasal sinuses
7. lacrimal
8. conchae
9. pharynx
10. larynx
11. trachea
12. primary bronchi, secondary bronchi, bronchioles, alveolar ducts
13. surfactant
14. 3; 2
15. atelectasis
16. pneumothorax
17. hemothorax
18. Cheyne-Stokes
19. internal respiration
20. external respiration
21. diaphragm
22. oxyhemoglobin
23. bicarbonate; carbaminohemoglobin
24. medulla
25. Stretch receptors
26. Chemoreceptors
27. tidal
28. tidal, expiratory reserve, inspiratory reserve
29. residual
30. f
31. i
32. d
33. b
34. a
35. j
36. h
37. c
38. e
39. g

Case Studies

1. Because Curtis is obviously in *respiratory distress,* he is probably suffering from adult respiratory distress syndrome (ARDS). ARDS can be caused by impairment of the surfactant lining the alveoli of the lungs resulting from accidental inhalation of water in a swimming pool. The water has probably diluted the surfactant and thus increased the surface tension of the fluid lining the lungs. Many of Curtis's alveoli have probably collapsed as a result, restricting his breathing.

2. Aspergillosis is a mycotic or fungal condition in which a type of mold typically produces "fungus ball" lesions that can obstruct airways when they occur in the lung. Partial blockage of the bronchi, the principal airways leading into the lungs, constitutes an obstructive disorder. Obstructive disorders typically do not reduce lung volumes or capacities but rather obstruct normal inspiration and expiration. Thus a spirometry test should show an increased time for forced maximal inspiration or expiration.

3. Considering the circumstances (swallowing food) and the fact that your friend can't speak, indications are that the food has lodged in the larynx or upper trachea. The abdominal thrust maneuver (see the box) is the recommended first aid in this situation. Many people in such circumstances run to the rest room for privacy during their distress—often to their detriment because there may not be anyone to help them. Medical personnel may elect to perform an emergency tracheostomy if first aid procedures don't remove the obstruction. In a tracheostomy, an incision in the trachea (a tracheotomy) is made and a hollow tube is inserted into the airway, allowing the subject to breathe.

Chapter 17
Chapter Test

1. digestion, absorption
2. muscularis
3. submucosa
4. Mucosa
5. Serosa
6. uvula, soft palate
7. crown, neck, root
8. parotid, submandibular, sublingual
9. esophagus
10. fundus, body, pylorus
11. duodenum, jejunum, ileum
12. villi
13. lacteals
14. common hepatic duct; cystic duct
15. transverse colon
16. sigmoid colon
17. mesentery; greater omentum
18. absorption
19. e
20. i
21. j
22. k
23. b
24. l
25. f
26. g
27. d
28. c
29. a
30. h
31. g
32. d
33. a
34. j
35. i
36. b
37. c
38. f
39. h
40. e

Case Studies

1. Improper care of the teeth and gums may lead to gingivitis (gum inflammation). If untreated, the gingivitis may progress to periodontitis, which causes loosening of the teeth. Teeth may also be lost through a failure to treat caries (tooth decay), a condition that also results from poor dental hygiene.

2. Famotidine, like cimetidine, decreases secretion of stomach acid. Because hypersecretion of stomach acid is the usual cause of progressive ulceration of the gastrointestinal lining, this treatment should slow or stop the damage and allow healing of the ulcer. Because it is more potent than cimetidine, smaller, less frequent doses are required. Sucralfate helps in the treatment of ulcers by sticking to and protecting the areas of the gastrointestinal tract that have a damaged mucus coat—specifically the areas that already have damage (that is, the ulcer itself). The antipepsin effect prevents the stomach enzyme pepsin from digesting the proteins in exposed tissues lining the gastrointestinal tract and possibly perforating the gastrointestinal wall.

3. The barium swallow test, also called an *upper GI study*, stretches (fills) the stomach with barium contrast material and makes it easily visible in x-ray photography. In a hiatal hernia, the bottom of the esophagus may be abnormally stretched and the cardiac sphincter dilated. An x-ray photograph would

likely show the barium backing up into the lower esophagus. If stomach acid backed up in that way, it would produce the heartburn symptom experienced by Fred. Backflow, or reflux, would more likely occur when bending or reclining because gravity would pull the stomach contents toward the esophagus. When an individual is standing up, gravity pulls the stomach contents away from the esophagus.

Chapter 18
Chapter Test

1. assimilation
2. Catabolism
3. Anabolism
4. prothrombin, fibrinogen
5. A, D
6. water; fat
7. Total metabolic rate
8. Basal metabolic rate
9. total metabolic rate
10. convection
11. evaporation
12. Fat metabolism
13. protein
14. Nonessential amino acids
15. b
16. d
17. c
18. g
19. a
20. e
21. h
22. f
23. f
24. k
25. a
26. g
27. c
28. j
29. b
30. d
31. i
32. h
33. e

Case Studies

1. Your friend is probably suffering from heat exhaustion. Because of the loss of fluid and electrolytes while sweating, her body's internal environment has become imbalanced, producing the symptoms of nausea and muscle cramps (called heat cramps in this case). First aid for your friend should include rest in a cool environment—perhaps in an air-conditioned building or in the shade—and plenty of isotonic fluids (e.g., Gatorade).

2. Scurvy, an abnormal condition resulting from a deficiency of vitamin C, certainly can cause the loss of teeth, as well as other forms of degeneration or injury. Without sufficient vitamin C, the body cannot maintain the collagen fibers that hold together most of the body. The collagen forming the periodontal ligament (PDL) that holds each tooth in its socket can loosen enough to make tooth loss unavoidable (see Chapter 17). In the past, sailors were particularly vulnerable to scurvy because they often did not have sufficient fresh vitamin C–containing foods available to them on long voyages.

3. The body requires an assortment of 20 amino acids to synthesize proteins needed for normal body function. These proteins include functional proteins such as enzymes, neurotransmitters, and protein hormones, as well as structural

proteins such as collagen and keratin that hold the body together. Some of these 20 can be manufactured by the body from compounds already present, so they are considered nonessential in the diet. Some of them, however, cannot be made by the body so they are essential in the diet. Without sufficient essential amino acids in her diet, Andrea may suffer consequences such as an inability to produce one or more important proteins. She need not be overly concerned, however, because the proper combination of vegetables can easily supply all the essential amino acids Andrea needs.

Chapter 19
Chapter Test
1. 20
2. Bowman capsule; glomerulus
3. Henle loop *or* nephron loop; collecting tube
4. proximal convoluted tubule; distal convoluted tubule
5. reabsorption
6. filtration
7. secretion
8. ADH
9. atrial natriuretic hormone
10. aldosterone
11. urinalysis
12. casts
13. internal urethral sphincter
14. Suppression
15. Incontinence
16. Retention
17. g
18. a
19. k
20. b
21. d
22. f
23. j
24. h
25. c
26. e
27. i
28. d
29. b
30. a
31. e
32. g
33. f
34. c

Case Studies
1. The loss of the fatty pad that surrounds and supports the kidneys may cause them to drop from their normal positions, a condition called *nephroptosis*. In nephroptosis, the ureters may become kinked and cause urine to backflow into the kidneys and thereby produce hydronephrosis. Hydronephrosis, in turn, may prevent normal filtration of fluids into nephrons and thus cause kidney failure.
2. Thiazide diuretics lower blood pressure by inhibiting water reabsorption in the kidney, thus reducing the amount of water retained by the blood. As you may recall from Chapter 14, such a reduction in blood volume reduces the overall blood pressure. Because the water is prevented from re-entering the blood stream, it remains as urine, greatly increasing the volume of urine output. The term *diuretic* is applied to any agent that increases the volume of urine output.
3. The fluid used in CAPD is isotonic to normal body fluids, including blood plasma. If the fluid is significantly

hypertonic to plasma, it will draw water osmotically from the blood and cause dehydration of the body. If the fluid is significantly hypotonic to plasma, it will lose water osmotically to the blood, causing the blood cells to swell and burst. The dialyzing fluid is isotonic to plasma but contains a different mixture of solutes than plasma, a mixture devoid of metabolic wastes such as urea.

Chapter 20
Chapter Test
1. interstitial fluid, plasma
2. intracellular
3. fluid output
4. water from catabolism
5. kidneys, skin, lungs, intestines
6. aldosterone; atrial natriuretic hormone
7. ions
8. chloride
9. sodium
10. false
11. true
12. false
13. b
14. c
15. b
16. a

Case Studies
1. Tom's body can deal with an excessive input of sodium by excreting an increased amount of sodium in the urine. The specific mechanism involves decreased reabsorption of sodium ions in the kidney tubules (see Chapter 19).
2. If Jo has consumed a large amount of distilled water, especially without also consuming salts, she is likely to produce an excessive amount of urine. This occurs because the body attempts to maintain its homeostasis of fluid volume (so it gets rid of excess fluid) and its homeostasis of electrolyte and water concentration (so it gets rid of excess water to maintain the normal osmotic balance). A urinalysis might reveal a decreased specific gravity (density), perhaps one that is closer to the density of pure water (1.000). Because of the increased water content in Jo's urine, the remaining components (solutes) will be diluted. Thus the color may appear lighter than usual and the concentration of each solute will be less than normal.
3. Until and unless the body can reverse overhydration by increasing urinary output (see answer #2 above), the presence of excess water in the internal environment makes the blood volume greater than normal. Increased blood volume means increased blood pressure. If peripheral blood pressure increases, the heart must pump harder to exceed that pressure and thus maintain blood flow. (Recall from Chapter 14 that the heart must generate a pressure higher than peripheral vessels to maintain the pressure gradient that allows blood to flow through the circulatory system.)

Chapter 21
Chapter Test
1. carbonic anhydrase
2. Buffers
3. H_2CO_3
4. $NaHCO_3$
5. distal tubule
6. NaH_2PO_4
7. NH_4Cl
8. base

9. alkalosis
10. acidosis
11. 20
12. NaHCO$_3$
13. H$_2$CO$_3$
14. alkalosis
15. b
16. a
17. b
18. b
19. decreases
20. increases
21. increases
22. decreases
23. increases
24. decreases

Case Studies

1. Chronic obstruction of the airways, as in chronic bronchitis, may reduce the respiratory system's rate of CO$_2$ excretion. This elevates the concentration of carbonic acid (H$_2$CO$_3$) in the blood and thus decreases pH—respiratory acidosis. In such chronic disorders, the body compensates for this pH imbalance by increasing sodium bicarbonate (NaHCO$_3$–) levels to increase the pH to normal levels. One would expect to see blood pH within the normal range (because this is compensated acidosis), but an elevated level of H$_2$CO$_3$ and NaHCO$_3$.

2. There is indeed a connection; Larry's body is attempting to compensate for the reduced blood pH characteristic of metabolic acidosis. By hyperventilating, Larry is increasing the rate of CO$_2$ excretion by the lungs and thus reducing his blood CO$_2$ level. This in turn decreases his blood H$_2$CO$_3$ level. This sequence of events thus lowers the acid content of Larry's blood and increases blood pH toward the normal range.

3. If aldosterone increases secretion of H$^+$ into kidney tubules (i.e., into the urine) from the blood, then the urine is acidified (gaining H$^+$) and the blood becomes less acid (losing H$^+$). Thus the blood pH increases. In hypersecretion of aldosterone, the blood pH may rise dramatically. In hyposecretion, there is less aldosterone present and thus the blood will retain the H$^+$ it would have otherwise lost, decreasing the blood pH.

Chapter 22
Chapter Test

1. testes
2. scrotum
3. tunica albuginea
4. seminiferous tubule
5. interstitial cells
6. spermatogonium
7. meiosis (spermatogenesis)
8. acrosome
9. epididymis
10. ductus deferens (vas deferens)
11. prostate
12. seminal vesicles
13. corpora cavernosa
14. ovaries
15. graafian
16. oogenesis
17. polar bodies
18. uterine tubes (oviducts, fallopian tubes)
19. myometrium
20. cervix
21. endometrium
22. vagina

23. Bartholin
24. alveoli; lactiferous
25. h
26. c
27. a
28. b
29. d
30. e
31. i
32. g
33. f
34. g
35. k
36. a
37. i
38. h
39. b
40. e
41. c
42. l
43. d
44. f
45. j

Case Studies

1. Considering the anatomical position of the prostate under the urinary bladder (see Figure 22-1), the only way to palpate or "feel" the organ with the hands or fingers from the outside of the body is by a digital rectal examination. The prostate is just anterior to the rectum, so any swelling or other physical abnormality will probably be felt easily through the thin rectal wall. Benign prostatic hypertrophy, or any other disorder involving a physical change in the prostate, might be detected this way.

2. According to the definition, a couple that does not conceive after 1 year of normal sex without contraception is infertile; therefore Liz and Zeke could be said to be an infertile couple. Liz's PID could be a cause of infertility. PID can cause scarring or other damage that might impair ovulation, obstruct the uterine tubes, or prevent the uterine lining from sustaining a pregnancy. Only one partner needs to be infertile for the couple to be infertile. This couple's physician will likely recommend treatment of the PID.

3. Heather obviously did not follow recommended procedures for breast self-examination because her self-examinations were "brief" and infrequent. She should have asked her physician or another health professional for directions on how to examine her breasts properly. Perhaps Heather would still have missed the lumps, but proper self-examination often reveals lesions that improper examinations do not. Whether Heather has breast cancer cannot be deduced from the information given. The presence of lumps is a sign of possible breast cancer but is more likely to be a form of fibrocystic disease. *Fibrocystic disease* is a name for the extremely common, normal changes that sometimes occur in breast tissue. Although the lumps are probably benign, they should be studied thoroughly to rule out cancer—they could be cancerous, after all, and thus require prompt treatment.

Chapter 23
Chapter Test

1. zygote
2. morula
3. blastocyst
4. placenta
5. gestation

6. ectoderm, mesoderm, endoderm
7. histogenesis
8. organogenesis
9. parturition
10. fraternal (dizygotic)
11. identical (monozygotic)
12. teratogens
13. neonatal
14. Osteoarthritis
15. Arteriosclerosis
16. Presbyopia
17. cataract
18. Glaucoma
19. c
20. a
21. e
22. b
23. d
24. g
25. e
26. a
27. f
28. c
29. b
30. d

Case Studies

1. Until the 1930s, puerperal fever (childbed fever) was a leading cause of death associated with childbirth. Caused by infection during the birthing process, it can be avoided by using aseptic or clean technique in and around the delivery area. Mary is justified in her concern, given her family's sad experience and her knowledge of puerperal fever's cause. She was probably assured by the hospital staff that they do take precautions in safeguarding against infections before, during, and after the delivery procedure.

2. Although Abe's grandmother may indeed use this as an excuse for meddling in the affairs of her daughter, it is possible that even moderate drinking during pregnancy can cause congenital abnormalities. Alcohol is a teratogen that easily crosses the placental barrier between the mother's blood and that of the developing offspring. Fetal alcohol syndrome (FAS) is a pronounced collection of signs caused by maternal alcohol consumption. FAS may include microcephaly, low birth weight, and mental retardation or other developmental disabilities.

3. Lactose intolerance is also called *lactase deficiency,* a name that implies the mechanism of this condition. Deficiency of the lactose-digesting enzyme lactase causes congenital and adult-onset forms of this condition. Affecting a large segment of the human population (as high as 90% in some regions), this condition can be treated by avoiding lactose in the diet. Aileen has chosen to take a tablet that probably contains a powdered form of lactase to help her digest ice cream and thus avoid the unpleasant symptoms of her condition.

Chapter 24
Chapter Test
1. Genetics
2. enzyme
3. 46; 23
4. dominant; recessive
5. 0
6. 25
7. 50
8. sex-linked
9. 0
10. (genetic) mutation
11. nondisjunction
12. Trisomy
13. Monosomy
14. pedigree
15. Punnett square
16. karyotype
17. d
18. b
19. a
20. c
21. f
22. e

Case Studies

1. Quentin's physician might order a karyotype of Quentin. Blood or other tissue will be taken and cultured. Cells in metaphase will be stained and photographed, producing an image of Quentin's chromosomes. Because Klinefelter's syndrome occurs only when there is more than one X chromosome in a male, a result of XXY, XXXY, or a similar multiple-X result will confirm that the signs exhibited by Quentin do indeed constitute Klinefelter's syndrome. Such an abnormality usually results from nondisjunction during formation of gametes produced by Quentin's parents.

2. Tay-Sachs disease is a recessive disorder caused by an abnormal gene thought to be located on chromosome 15. Let T represent the normal, dominant gene and let t represent the recessive Tay-Sachs gene. Each parent must have the gene combination Tt, because each has the gene but does not have the disease. If either parent had the combination tt, they would have Tay-Sachs disease and would have died by age 4. Using a Punnett square, as in Figure 24-13, to determine probability, one would expect a 25% probability (1 in 4 chance) that the infant will exhibit Tay-Sachs disease.

Glossary

A

abdomen (AB-doh-men) body area between the diaphragm and pelvis

abdominal cavity (ab-DOM-i-nal KAV-i-tee) the cavity containing the abdominal organs

abdominal muscles (ab-DOM-i-nal MUSS-els) muscles supporting the anterior aspect of the abdomen

abdominal quadrants (ab-DOM-i-nal KWOD-rants) four topographic subdivisions of the abdomen determined by two imaginary lines dividing the body through the navel—one vertical, one horizontal; health professionals use these designations to help locate specific internal organs

abdominal regions (ab-DOM-i-nal REE-juns) nine topographic subdivisions of the abdomen determined by four imaginary lines configured in a tic-tac-toe pattern; anatomists use these named regions to identify the location of internal organs

abdominal thrusts (ab-DOM-i-nal thrusts) emergency procedure in which sudden pressure on the abdomen of a person who is choking may dislodge material from the airway; formerly called *Heimlich maneuver*

abdominopelvic cavity (ab-DOM-i-noh-PEL-vik KAV-i-tee) the single cavity containing the abdominal and pelvic organs

abduction (ab-DUK-shun) moving away from the midline of the body, opposite motion of **adduction**

ABO system human blood classification system based on RBC antigens (A, B, AB, and O) and their corresponding antibodies

abruptio placentae (ab-RUP-shee-oh plah-SEN-tay) separation of normally positioned placenta from the uterine wall; may result in hemorrhage and death of the fetus and/or mother

absorption (ab-ZORP-shun) passage of a substance through a membrane, such as skin or mucosa, into blood

accessory organ (ak-SES-oh-ree OR-gan) an organ that assists other organs in accomplishing their functions

acetabulum (ass-eh-TAB-yoo-lum) socket in the hip bone (ox coxae or innominate bone) into which the head of the femur fits

acetylcholine (ass-ee-til-KOH-lean) chemical neurotransmitter

acid (ASS-id) any substance that, when dissolved in water, contributes to an excess of H$^+$ ions (that is, a low pH)

acid-base balance (ASS-id bayse BAL-ans) maintaining the concentration of hydrogen ions in body fluids

acidosis (ass-i-DOH-sis) condition in which there is an excessive proportion of acid in the blood and thus an abnormally low blood pH; opposite of **alkalosis**

acne (AK-nee) a bacterial infection of the skin characterized by red pustules formed when hair follicles become infected

acne vulgaris (AK-nee vul-GAIR-iss) inflammatory skin condition affecting sebaceous gland ducts; *see* **comedones**

acquired immunodeficiency syndrome (AIDS) (ah-KWYERD IM-yoo-noh-deh-FISH-en-see SIN-drohm) disease in which the human immunodeficiency virus attacks T cells, thereby compromising the body's immune system

acquired immunity (ah-KWYERD i-MYOO-ni-tee) immunity that is obtained after birth through the use of injections or exposure to a harmful agent

acromegaly (ak-roh-MEG-ah-lee) condition caused by hypersecretion of growth hormone after puberty, resulting in enlargement of facial features (e.g., jaw, nose), fingers, and toes

acrosome (AK-ro-sohm) specialized structure covering the sperm head containing enzymes that break down the covering of the ovum to allow entry

actin (AK-tin) contractile protein found in the *thin* myofilaments of skeletal muscle

action potential (AK-shun poh-TEN-shal) nerve impulse

active transport (AK-tiv TRANS-port) movement of a substance into and out of a living cell requiring the use of cellular energy

acute (ah-KYOOT) intense; rapid onset, short in duration—as in acute disease

acute lymphocytic leukemia (ALL) (ah-KYOOT LIM-foh-sit-ik loo-KEE-mee-ah) type of acute (rapid onset and progression) blood cancer common in children 3 to 7 years of age; characterized by cancerous transformation and increased numbers of B lymphocytes

acute myeloid leukemia (AML) (ah-KYOOT MY-eh-loyd loo-KEE-me-ah) type of acute (rapid onset and progression) blood cancer most common in adults; characterized by cancerous transformation and increased numbers of myeloid precursor cells

Addison disease (AD-i-son dih-ZEEZ) disease of the adrenal gland resulting in low blood sugar, weight loss, weakness, increase in blood sodium and decrease in blood potassium

adduction (ad-DUK-shun) moving toward the midline of the body, opposite motion of **abduction**

adenine (ADD-en-een) one of several nitrogen-containing bases that make up nucleotides, which in turn make up nucleic acids such as DNA and RNA; in the cell, it can chemically bind to another nitrogenous base, thymine (T or t) or uracil (U or u), to form a more complex structure or in translating genetic codes; symbolized by the letter *A* or *a*; *see also* **guanine, cytosine, thymine, uracil**

adenocarcinoma (ad-eh-no-kar-sih-NO-mah) cancer of glandular epithelium

adenohypophysis (ad-eh-no-hye-POFF-i-sis) anterior pituitary gland, which has the structure of an endocrine gland

adenoid (AD-eh-noyd) literally, glandlike; adenoids, or *pharyngeal tonsils*, are paired lymphoid structures in the nasopharynx; *see also* **tonsils**

adenoma (ad-eh-NO-mah) benign tumor of glandular epithelium

adenosine deaminase (ADA) deficiency (ah-DEN-oh-seen dee-AM-i-nayse dee-FISH-en-see) rare, inherited condition in which production of the enzyme adenosine deaminase is deficient, resulting in severe combined immune deficiency (SCID); first human disorder treated by gene therapy

adenosine diphosphate (ADP) (ah-DEN-oh-seen dye-FAHS-fayt) molecule similar to adenosine triphosphate but containing only two phosphate groups

adenosine triphosphate (ATP) (ah-DEN-oh-seen try-FAHS-fayt) chemical compound that provides energy for use by body cells

adductor muscle (ad-DUK-tor MUSS-el) any of several muscles that adduct a joint, moving a body part in from the side (lateral) and thus toward the midline (median or midsagittal plane) of the body or of the body region; for example, the pectoralis major and latissimus dorsi muscles contract together to pull the upper arm toward the trunk, thus *adducting* the shoulder joint

adipose (AD-i-pohs) fat tissue; specialized tissue that stores lipids

adolescence (ad-oh-LESS-ens) period of life between puberty and adulthood

adrenal cortex (ah-DREE-nal KOR-teks) outer portion of adrenal gland that secretes hormones called *corticoids*

adrenal gland (ah-DREE-nal) glands that rest on the top of the kidneys, made up of the cortex and medulla

adrenal medulla (ah-DREE-nal meh-DULL-ah) inner portion of adrenal gland that secretes epinephrine and norepinephrine

adrenergic fibers (ad-ren-ER-jik FYE-bers) axons whose terminals release norepinephrine and epinephrine

adrenocorticotropic hormone (ACTH) (ah-dree-no-kor-teh-koh-TROH-pic HOR-mohn) hormone that stimulates the adrenal cortex to secrete larger amounts of hormones

adult polycystic kidney disease (ah-DULT pah-lee-siss-tic KID-nee dih-ZEEZ) hereditary condition characterized by development of multiple cystic spaces in one or both kidneys that often fill with clear fluid or blood

adult respiratory distress syndrome (ARDS) (ah-DULT RESS-per-ah-tohr-ee dis-TRESS sin-drohm) relative inability to inflate alveoli normally; caused by impairment or removal of surfactant following accidental inhalation of destructive substances

adulthood (ah-DULT-hood) period of life after adolescence

aerobic (air-OH-bik) requiring oxygen

aerobic respiration (air-OH-bik res-pih-RAY-shun) the stage of cellular respiration requiring oxygen

aerobic training (air-OH-bik TRAIN-ing) continuous vigorous exercise requiring the body to increase its consumption of oxygen and develop the muscles' ability to sustain activity over a long period

afferent (AF-fer-ent) carrying or conveying toward the center (e.g., an afferent neuron carries nerve impulses toward the central nervous system); opposite of **efferent**

agglutinate (ah-GLOO-tin-ayt) antibodies causing antigens to clump or stick together

aging process (AYJ-ing PRAH-sess) the gradual degenerative changes that occur after young adulthood as a person ages

AIDS-related complex (ARC) (AYDS ree-LAY-ted KOM-pleks) early manifestation of AIDS that produces fever, weight loss, and swollen lymph nodes in those whose immune systems are less deficient than those with full-blown AIDS

albinism (AL-bi-niz-em) recessive, inherited condition characterized by a lack of the dark brown pigment melanin in the skin and eyes, resulting in vision problems and susceptibility to sunburn and skin cancer; ocular albinism is a lack of pigment in the layers of the eyeball

albumin (AL-byoo-min) one of several types of proteins normally found in blood plasma; it helps thicken the blood

aldosterone (al-DOSS-ter-own) hormone that stimulates the kidney to retain sodium ions and water

alimentary canal (al-eh-MEN-tar-ee kah-NAL) principal tubelike structure of the digestive system extending from mouth to anus—sometimes called the **gastrointestinal (GI) tract**

alkaline (AL-kah-lin) base; any substance that, when dissolved in water, contributes to an excess of OH^- ions (thus creating a high pH value)

alkaline phosphatase (AL-kah-lin FOSS-fah-tays) enzyme present in blood plasma in high concentration during certain liver and malignant bone marrow disorders

alkalosis (al-kah-LOH-sis) condition in which there is an excessive proportion of alkali (base) in the blood; opposite of **acidosis**

allergen (AL-er-jen) harmless environmental antigen that stimulates an allergic reaction (hypersensitivity reaction) in a susceptible, sensitized person

allergy (AL-er-jee) hypersensitivity of the immune system to relatively harmless environmental antigens

all or none when stimulated, a muscle fiber will contract fully or not at all; whether a contraction occurs depends on whether the stimulus reaches the required threshold

alopecia (al-oh-PEE-shah) clinical term referring to hair loss

alpha cell (AL-fah sell) pancreatic cell that secretes glucagon

alveolar duct (al-VEE-oh-lar dukt) airway that branches from the smallest bronchioles; alveolar sacs arise from alveolar ducts

alveolar sac (al-VEE-oh-lar sak) sacs in the lungs that arise from the alveolar ducts and resemble a cluster of grapes

alveolus (al-VEE-oh-luss) (*pl.,* alveoli) literally, a small cavity; alveoli of lungs are microscopic saclike dilations of terminal bronchioles

Alzheimer disease (AHLZ-hye-mer dih-ZEEZ) brain disorder of the middle and late adult years characterized by loss of memory and dementia

amenorrhea (ah-men-oh-REE-ah) absence of normal menstruation

amino acid (ah-MEE-no ASS-id) structural units from which proteins are built

amniocentesis (AM-nee-oh-sen-TEE-sis) procedure in which a sample of amniotic fluid is removed with a syringe for use in genetic testing, perhaps to produce a karyotype of the fetus; compare with **chorionic villus sampling**

amniotic cavity (am-nee-OT-ik KAV-i-tee) cavity within the blastocyst that will become a fluid-filled sac in which the embryo will float during development

amoeba (ah-MEE-bah) protozoan of changing shape capable of causing infection

amphiarthrosis (am-fee-ar-THROH-sis) slightly movable joint such as the one joining the two pubic bones

amylase (AM-eh-lays) enzyme that digests carbohydrates; *also see* **salivary amylase**

anabolic steroid (an-ah-BAHL-ik STAIR-oyd) a lipid molecule of the steroid variety that acts as a hormone to stimulate anabolism (specifically protein synthesis) in body tissues such as muscle (e.g., testosterone)

anabolism (ah-NAB-oh-liz-em) process in which cells make complex molecules (e.g., hormones) from simpler compounds (e.g., amino acids), opposite of **catabolism**

anaerobic (an-air-OH-bik) requiring the absence of oxygen

anal canal (AY-nal kah-NAL) terminal portion of the rectum

anaphase (AN-ah-fayz) stage of mitosis; duplicate chromosomes move to poles of dividing cell

anaphylactic shock (an-ah-fih-LAK-tik shok) circulatory failure (shock) caused by a type of severe allergic reaction characterized by blood vessel dilation; may be fatal

anaplasia (an-ah-PLAY-zha) growth of abnormal (undifferentiated) cells, as in a tumor or neoplasm

anatomical position (an-ah-TOM-i-kal poh-ZISH-un) the standard neutral reference position for the body used to describe sites or motions of various body parts; gives meaning to directional terms

anatomy (ah-NAT-oh-mee) the study of the structure of an organism and the relationships of its parts

androgen (AN-droh-jen) male sex hormone

anemia (ah-NEE-mee-ah) deficient number of red blood cells or deficient hemoglobin

anesthesia (an-es-THEE-zhah) loss of sensation

aneurysm (AN-yoo-riz-em) abnormal widening of the arterial wall; aneurysms promote the formation of thrombi and also tend to burst

angina pectoris (an-JYE-nah PEK-tor-iss) severe chest pain resulting when the myocardium is deprived of sufficient oxygen

angioplasty (AN-jee-oh-plass-tee) medical procedure in which vessels occluded by arteriosclerosis are opened (that is, the channel for blood flow is widened)

Angstrom (ANG-strum) 0.1 mm (1/10,000,000,000 of a meter or about 1/250,000,000 of an inch)

anion (AN-eye-on) negatively charged particle

anorexia (an-oh-REK-see-ah) loss of appetite (a symptom, rather than a distinct disorder)

anorexia nervosa (an-oh-REK-see-ah ner-VOH-sah) behavioral eating disorder characterized by chronic refusal to eat, often related to an abnormal fear of becoming obese

antagonist muscle (an-TAG-oh-nist MUSS-el) those muscles having opposing actions; for example, muscles that flex the upper arm are antagonists to muscles that extend it

antebrachial (an-tee-BRAY-kee-al) refers to the forearm

antecubital (an-tee-KYOO-bi-tal) refers to the elbow

antenatal medicine (an-tee-NAY-tal MED-i-sin) prenatal medicine

anterior (an-TEER-ee-or) front or ventral; opposite of **posterior** or **dorsal**

anthrax (AN-thraks) bacterial infection caused by *Bacillus anthracis*, ordinarily affecting herbivores (sheep, cattle, goats, antelope) and often killing them; rarely it occurs in humans through accidental or intentional exposure to bacterial spores through inhalation or skin contact; inhalation anthrax is life-threatening but can be treated successfully with medication; cutaneous anthrax is less serious, characterized by a reddish-brown patch on the skin that ulcerates and then forms a dark, nearly black scab, followed by muscle pain, internal hemorrhage (bleeding), headache, fever, nausea, and vomiting

antibiotic (an-ti-by-OT-ik) compound usually produced by living organisms that destroys or inhibits microbes

antibody (AN-ti-bod-ee) substance produced by the body that destroys or inactivates a specific substance (antigen) that has entered the body

antibody-mediated immunity (AN-ti-bod-ee MEE-dee-ayt-ed i-MYOO-ni-tee) immunity that is produced when antibodies make antigens unable to harm the body; also referred to as *humoral immunity*

antidiuretic hormone (ADH) (an-tee-dye-yoo-RET-ik HOR-mohn) hormone produced in the posterior pituitary gland to regulate the balance of water in the body by accelerating the reabsorption of water

antigen (AN-ti-jen) substance that, when introduced into the body, causes formation of antibodies against it

antioxidant (an-tee-OK-seh-dent) substance such as vitamin E that can inhibit free radicals (oxidants), which are highly reactive, electron-seeking molecules occurring normally in cells but which may damage electron-dense molecules such as DNA or molecules in cell membranes

antrum (AN-trum) cavity

anuria (ah-NOO-ree-ah) absence of urine

anus (AY-nus) distal end or outlet of the rectum

aorta (ay-OR-tah) main and largest artery in the body

aortic body (ay-OR-tik BOD-ee) small cluster of chemosensitive cells that respond to carbon dioxide and oxygen levels

aortic semilunar valve (ay-OR-tik sem-ee-LOO-nar valv) valve between the aorta and left ventricle that prevents blood from flowing back into the ventricle

apex (AY-peks) pointed end of a conical structure

Apgar score (AP-gar) system of assessing general health of newborn infant, in which heart rate, respiration, muscle tone, skin color and response to stimuli are scored (a perfect total score is 10); named for the American physician Virginia Apgar

aplastic anemia (ay-PLAS-tik ah-NEE-mee-ah) blood disorder characterized by a low red blood cell count, caused by destruction of myeloid tissue in the bone marrow

apnea (APP-nee-ah) temporary cessation of breathing

apocrine (APP-oh-krin) sweat glands located in the axilla and genital regions; these glands enlarge and begin to function at puberty

apoptosis (app-op-TOH-sis) programmed cell death by means of several biochemical processes built into each cell; apoptosis clears space for newer cells, as in early embryonic development or in tissue repair

appendage (ah-PEN-dij) something that is attached; for example, an attached body part such as an arm

appendicitis (ah-pen-di-SYE-tiss) inflammation of the vermiform appendix

appendicular (ah-pen-DIK-yoo-lar) refers to the upper and lower extremities of the body

appendicular skeleton (ah-pen-DIK-yoo-lar SKEL-eh-ton) the bones of the upper and lower extremities of the body

appendix (ah-PEN-diks) see **vermiform appendix**

aqueous (AY-kwee-us) liquid mixture in which water is the solvent; for example, saltwater is an aqueous solution because water is the solvent

aqueous humor (AY-kwee-us HYOO-mohr) watery fluid that fills the anterior chamber of the eye, in front of the lens

aqueous solution (AY-kwee-us soh-LOO-shun) a mixture made up of molecules dissolved in water

arachnoid mater (ah-RAK-noyd MAH-ter) delicate, weblike middle membrane covering the brain, the meninges

archaea (ark-EE-ah) type of microbe resembling bacteria but with different chemical makeup (especially in the cell wall) and different metabolic pathways; often capable of thriving in very harsh environments (very hot, very acid, very salty, etc.); not known to infect humans

areola (ah-REE-oh-lah) (*pl.,* areolae) small space; the pigmented ring around the nipple

areolar connective tissue (ah-REE-oh-lar con-NEK-tiv TISH-yoo) a type of connective tissue consisting of fibers and a variety of cells embedded in a loose matrix of soft, sticky gel

arrector pili (ah-REK-tor PYE-lye) smooth muscles of the skin, which are attached to hair follicles; when contraction occurs, the hair stands up, resulting in "goose flesh" or "goose bumps"

arrhythmia (ah-RITH-mee-ah) see **dysrhythmia**

arteriole (ar-TEER-ee-ohl) small branch of an artery

arteriosclerosis (ar-teer-ee-oh-skleh-ROH-sis) hardening of arteries; materials such as lipids (as in atherosclerosis) accumulate in arterial walls, often becoming hardened via calcification

artery (AR-ter-ee) vessel carrying blood away from the heart

arthritis (ar-THRY-tis) inflammatory joint disease, characterized by inflammation of the synovial membrane and a variety of systemic signs or symptoms

arthropod (AR-throh-pod) type of animal capable of infesting or parasitizing humans

articular cartilage (ar-TIK-yoo-lar KAR-ti-lij) cartilage covering the joint ends of bones

articulation (ar-tik-yoo-LAY-shun) place of junction between two or more bones of the skeleton; also called a *joint*

artificial kidney (ar-ti-FISH-all KID-nee) mechanical device that removes wastes from the blood that would normally be removed by the kidney

artificial pacemaker (ar-ti-FISH-all PAYS-may-ker) an electrical device that is implanted into the heart to treat a heart block

ascites (ah-SYE-teez) abnormal accumulation of fluid in intraperitoneal space

aseptic technique (ay-SEP-tik tek-NEEK) approach to limiting the spread of infection by preventing or reducing contacts with contaminated surfaces

asexual (ay-SEKS-yoo-all) one-celled plants and bacteria that do not produce specialized sex cells

assimilation (ah-sim-i-LAY-shun) takes place when food molecules enter the cell and undergo chemical changes

association area (ah-so-see-AY-shun AIR-ee-ah) region of the cerebral cortex of the brain that functions to put together or "associate" information from many parts of the brain to help make sense of or analyze the information

asthma (AZ-mah) obstructive pulmonary disorder characterized by recurring spasms of muscles in bronchial walls accompanied by edema and mucus production, making breathing difficult

astigmatic keratotomy (AK) (AY-stig-mat-ic kair-ah-TOT-ah-mee) type of refractory eye surgery for treatment of astigmatism that involves placement of transverse cuts across the corneal surface to alter its shape

astigmatism (ah-STIG-mah-tiz-em) irregular curvature of the cornea or lens that impairs refraction of a well-focused image in the eye

astrocyte (ASS-troh-syte) a neuroglial cell

atelectasis (at-eh-LEK-tay-sis) total or partial collapse of the alveoli of the lung

atherosclerosis (ath-er-oh-skleh-ROH-sis) type of "hardening of the arteries" in which lipids and other substances build up on the inside wall of blood vessels

atom (AT-om) smallest particle of a pure substance (element) that still has the chemical properties of that substance; composed of protons, electrons, and neutrons (subatomic particles)

atomic mass (ah-TAH-mik MASS) combined total number of protons and neutrons in an atom

atomic number (ah-TAH-mik NUM-ber) total number of protons in an atom's nucleus; atoms of each element have a characteristic atomic number

atrial natriuretic hormone (ANH) (AY-tree-all nay-tree-yoo-RET-ik HOR-mohn) hormone secreted by the heart cells that regulates fluid and electrolyte homeostasis

atrioventricular node (ay-tree-oh-ven-TRIK-yoo-lar nohd) a small mass of special impulse-generating cardiac muscle tissue near the junction of the left atrium and ventricle; part of the conduction system of the heart

atrioventricular (AV) valves (ay-tree-oh-ven-TRIK-yoo-lar valvs) two valves that separate the atrial chambers from the ventricles

atrium (AY-tree-um) (*pl.*, atria) chamber or cavity; for example, atrium of each side of the heart

atrophy (AT-roh-fee) wasting away of tissue; decrease in size of a part; sometimes referred to as **disuse atrophy**

auditory tube (AW-di-toh-ree toob) tube extending from inside the middle ear to the throat to equalize air pressure; also called the **eustachian tube**

auricle (AW-ri-kul) part of the ear attached to the side of the head; earlike appendage of each atrium of the heart

autoimmunity (aw-toh-i-MYOO-ni-tee) process in which a person's immune system attacks the person's own body tissues—the underlying cause of several diseases

automated lamellar keratoplasty (ALK) (AW-toh-may-ted lah-MELL-ahr kair-AT-oh-plast-ee) type of refractory eye surgery that employs a microkeratome to cut off a cap of corneal tissue, which is replaced after the underlying tissue is reshaped

automatic external defibrillator (AED) (aw-toh-MAT-ik eks-TERN-all dee-FIB-rih-lay-tor) small, lightweight device that detects a person's heart rhythm using small electrode pads placed on the torso and, if ventricular fibrillation is detected, a nonmedical rescuer will be led through some simple steps to defibrillate the victim by applying brief electroshock to the heart

autonomic effector (aw-toh-NAHM-ik ef-FEK-tor) tissues to which autonomic neurons conduct impulses

autonomic nervous system (ANS) (aw-toh-NAHM-ik NER-vus SIS-tem) division of the human nervous system that regulates involuntary actions

autonomic neuron (aw-toh-NAHM-ik NOO-ron) motor neurons that make up the autonomic nervous system

autopsy (AW-top-see) systematic dissection and analysis of a dead body, often for the purpose of discovering the cause of death and/or the presence of health conditions; also called *necropsy*

autosome (AW-toh-sohm) one of the 44 (22 pairs) chromosomes in the human genome other than the two sex chromosomes; means "same body," referring to the fact that each member of a pair of autosomes match each other in size and other structural features

AV bundle (AV BUN-dul) fibers in the heart that relay a nerve impulse from the AV node to the ventricles; also known as the *bundle of His*

avitaminosis (ay-vye-tah-mi-NO-sis) general name for any condition resulting from a vitamin deficiency

avulsion fracture (ah-VUL-shun FRAK-chur) fracture occurring when a powerful muscle contraction pulling on a ligamentous or tendinous attachment to a bone forcibly pulls a fragment of bone free from underlying osseous tissue

axial (AK-see-all) refers to the head, neck, and torso or trunk of the body

axial skeleton (AK-see-all SKEL-eh-ton) the bones of the head, neck, and torso

axilla (AK-sil-ah) refers to the armpit

axillary (AK-si-lair-ee) pertaining to the area inside the shoulder joint or armpit

axon (AK-son) nerve cell process that transmits impulses away from the cell body

B

B cell (B sell) a lymphocyte; activated B cells develop into plasma cells, which secrete antibodies into the blood

bacillus (bah-SILL-us) (*pl.,* bacilli) rod-shaped bacterium

bacterium (bak-TEER-ee-um) microbe capable of causing disease; it is a primitive, single-celled organism without membranous organelles

Bard endoscopic suturing system (BARD en-doh-SKOP-ic SOO-chur-ing SISS-tem) use of an endoscope to place sutures in the lower esophageal sphincter to narrow the lumen

Barrett esophagus (BAHR-ett ee-SOFF-ah-guss) precancerous condition of esophageal lining

bartholinitis (bar-toh-lin-EYE-tis) inflammation of the Bartholin glands, accessory organs of the female reproductive tract

Bartholin glands (BAR-toh-lin) exocrine mucous glands located on either side of the vaginal outlet; also known as **greater vestibular glands**

basal cell carcinoma (BAY-sal sell car-sin-OH-mah) skin cancer, often occurring on upper face, with low potential for metastasizing

basal ganglia (BAY-sal GANG-glee-ah) islands of gray matter located in the cerebral cortex that are responsible for automatic movements and postures; also called **cerebral nuclei**

basal metabolic rate (BMR) (BAY-sal met-ah-BAHL-ik rayt) number of calories of heat that must be produced per hour by catabolism to keep the body alive, awake, and comfortably warm

base *1.* A chemical that, when dissolved in water, reduces the relative concentration of H^+ ions in the whole solution (sometimes by adding OH^- ions) *2.* In the context of nucleic acids (DNA and RNA), *base* or *nitrogen base* refers to one part of a nucleotide (sugar, phosphate, and base) that is the basic building block of nucleic acid molecules; possible bases include adenine, thymine, guanine, cytosine, and uracil

basement membrane (BAYSE-ment MEM-brayne) the connective tissue layer of the serous membrane that holds and supports the epithelial cells

basophil (BAY-so-fil) white blood cell that stains readily with basic dyes

BBB *see* **blood-brain barrier**

Bell palsy (bell PAWL-zee) temporary or permanent paralysis of facial features caused by damage to cranial nerve VII (facial nerve)

benign (be-NYNE) refers to a tumor or neoplasm that does not metastasize or spread to different tissues

benign prostatic hypertrophy (BPH) (be-NYNE pros-TAT-ik hye-PER-tro-fee) benign enlargement of the prostate, a condition common in older males

benign tumor (be-NYNE TOO-mer) a noncancerous and generally harmless neoplasm

beta cell (BAY-tah sell) pancreatic islet cell that secretes insulin

bicarbonate loading (bye-KAR-boh-net LOHD-ing) ingesting large amounts of sodium bicarbonate to counteract the effects of lactic acid buildup, thereby reducing fatigue; however, there are potentially dangerous side effects

biceps brachii (BYE-seps BRAY-kee-eye) the primary flexor of the forearm

biceps femoris (BYE-seps FEM-oh-ris) powerful flexor of the lower leg

bicuspid (bye-KUSS-pid) tooth with a large flat surface and two or three grinding cusps; also called **premolar**

bicuspid valve (bye-KUSS-pid valv) one of the two AV valves, it is located between the left atrium and ventricle and is sometimes called the **mitral valve**

bile (byle) substance that reduces large fat globules into smaller droplets of fat that are more easily broken down

bile duct (byle dukt) duct that drains bile into the small intestine and is formed by the union of the common hepatic and cystic ducts

biological filtration (bye-EH-lah-ji-kal fil-TRAY-shun) process in which cells alter the contents of the filtered fluid

biopsy (BYE-op-see) procedure in which living tissue is removed from a patient for laboratory examination, as in determining the presence of cancer cells

bioterrorism (bye-oh-TAIR-or-iz-em) unlawful release of biological agents (toxins or pathogens) for the purpose of intimidation

birth defect (DEE-fekt) any abnormality, whether caused by genetic or environmental factors, that exists at birth; *see* **teratogen**

blackhead description of sebum that accumulates, darkens, and enlarges some of the ducts of the sebaceous glands; also called a *comedo*

bladder (BLAD-der) a sac, usually referring to the urinary bladder

blastocyst (BLASS-toh-sist) postmorula stage of developing embryo; hollow ball of cells

blister (BLISS-ter) fluid-filled skin lesion; *see* **vesicle**

blood (blud) type of connective tissue characterized by a watery liquid matrix (blood plasma) and a variety of mobile cells that include red blood cells, white blood cells, and platelets

blood-brain barrier (BBB) (blud brayn BAYR-ee-er) structural and functional barrier formed by astrocytes and blood vessel walls in the brain; it prevents some substances from diffusing from the blood into brain tissue

blood doping (blud DOH-ping) a practice used to improve athletic performance by removing red blood cells weeks before an event and then reinfusing them just before competition to increase the oxygen-carrying capacity of the blood

blood pressure (blud PRESH-ur) pressure of blood in the blood vessels, expressed as systolic pressure over diastolic pressure (e.g., 120/80 mmHg)

blood pressure gradient (blud PRESH-ur GRAY-dee-ent) the difference between any two blood pressures in the body; for example, the pressure difference between the blood in the left ventricle of the heart and the blood in the aorta is a pressure gradient

blood types (blud) the different types of blood that are identified by certain antigens in red blood cells (A, B, AB, O, and Rh-negative or Rh-positive)

body (BOD-ee) unified and complex assembly of structurally and functionally interactive components

body composition (BOD-ee com-poh-ZISH-un) assessment that identifies the percentage of the body that is lean tissue and the percentage that is fat

boil (BOY-el) *see* **furuncle**

bolus (BOH-lus) a small, rounded mass of masticated food ready to be swallowed

bond a chemical bond or union between two or more atoms to form a molecule; *see* **ionic bond** and **covalent bond**

bone (bohn) highly specialized connective tissue whose matrix is hard and calcified

bone marrow (bohn MAIR-oh) soft material that fills cavities of the bones; red bone marrow is vital to blood cell formation; yellow bone marrow is inactive fatty tissue

bone marrow transplant (bohn MAIR-oh TRANZ-plant) treatment in which healthy blood-forming marrow tissue from a donor is intravenously introduced into a recipient

bony labyrinth (BOHN-ee LAB-eh-rinth) the fluid-filled complex maze of three spaces (the vestibule, semicircular canals, and cochlea) in the temporal bone

Bouchard nodes (boo-SHAR nohds) abnormal enlargements seen at the proximal interphalangeal joints in people with osteoarthritis

bovine spongiform encephalopathy (BSE) (BOH-vyne SPUNJ-i-form en-SEF-al-AH-path-ee [B-S-E]) also known as *mad cow disease*; a degenerative disease of the central nervous system caused by prions that convert normal proteins of the nervous system into abnormal proteins, causing loss of nervous system function; the abnormal form of the protein also may be inherited; *see also* **prion**

Bowman capsule (BOH-men KAP-sul) the cup-shaped beginning of a nephron that surrounds the glomerulus; also called *Bowman's capsule* or *glomerular capsule*

brachial (BRAY-kee-all) pertaining to the arm

bradycardia (bray-dee-KAR-dee-ah) slow heart rhythm (below 60 beats/minute)

brachytherapy placement of radioactive "seeds" in close or direct contact with cancerous tissue

breast (brest) anterior aspect of the chest; in females, also an accessory sex organ

bronchi (BRONG-kye) the branches of the trachea

bronchiole (BRONG-kee-ohl) small branch of a bronchus

bronchitis (brong-KYE-tiss) inflammation of the bronchi of the lungs, characterized by edema and excessive mucus production that causes coughing and difficulty in breathing (especially expiration); if the trachea is also inflamed, this condition may be referred to as *tracheobronchitis*

buccal (BUK-all) pertaining to the cheek

buffer (BUF-er) compound that combines with an acid or with a base to form a weaker acid or base, thereby lessening the change in hydrogen-ion concentration that would occur without the buffer

buffer pairs (BUFF-er) two kinds of chemical substances that prevent a sharp change in the pH of a fluid; for example, sodium bicarbonate ($NaHCO_3$) and carbonic acid (H_2CO_3)

buffy coat thin layer of white blood cells (WBCs) and platelets located between red blood cells (RBCs) and plasma in a centrifuged sample of blood

bulboid corpuscle (BUL-boyd KOHR-pus-ul) mucous membrane receptor that detects sensations of touch and vibration; also known as **Krause end bulb**

bulbourethral gland (BUL-boh-yoo-REE-thral) small glands located just below the prostate gland whose mucus-like secretions lubricate the terminal portion of the urethra and contribute less than 5% of the seminal fluid volume; also known as *Cowper gland*

bulimarexia (boo-lee-mah-REK-see-ah) condition in which people purposely induce the vomiting reflex to purge themselves of food they just ate; an eating disorder

bulimia (boo-LEE-mee-ah) behavioral eating disorder characterized by an alternating pattern of overeating followed by self-denial (and perhaps purging of GI contents)

bundle of His (BUN-dul of hiss) *see* **AV bundle**

burn (bern) an injury to tissues resulting from contact with heat, chemicals, electricity, friction, or radiant and electromagnetic energy; classified into three categories, depending on the number of tissue layers involved

bursa (BER-sah) (*pl.*, bursae) small, cushion-like sacs found between moving body parts, which make movement easier

bursitis (ber-SYE-tiss) inflammation of a bursa

C

cachexia (kah-KEK-see-ah) syndrome associated with cancer and other chronic diseases that involves loss of appetite, weight loss, and general weakness

calcaneus (kal-KAY-nee-us) heel bone; largest tarsal in the foot

calcitonin (CT) (kal-sih-TOH-nin) a hormone secreted by the thyroid gland that decreases calcium in the blood

calculi (KAL-kyoo-lie) hard, crystalline stones that form in the lumen of hollow organs such as the gallbladder or liver (biliary calculi) or renal passages (renal calculi)

callus (KAL-us) bony tissue that forms a sort of collar around the broken ends of fractured bone during the healing process

calorie (c) (KAL-ah-ree) heat unit; the amount of heat needed to raise the temperature of 1 g of water 1° C

Calorie (C) (KAL-ah-ree) heat unit; kilocalorie; the amount of heat needed to raise the temperature of 1 kilogram of water 1° C

calyx (KAY-liks) cup-shaped division of the renal pelvis

canaliculi (kan-ah-LIK-yoo-lye) an extremely narrow tubular passage or channel in compact bone

cancer (KAN-ser) tumor (neoplasm) capable of metastasizing (spreading) to other parts of the body

canine tooth (KAY-nyne) the tooth with the longest crown and the longest root, which is located lateral to the second incisor that serves to pierce or tear food being eaten; also called a **cuspid** tooth

capillary (KAP-i-lair-ee) tiny vessels that connect arterioles and venules

capillary blood pressure (KAP-i-lair-ee blud PRESH-ur) the blood pressure found in the capillary vessels

capsule (KAP-sul) hollowed out space found in diarthrotic joints, holds the bones of joints together while still allowing movement; made of fibrous connective tissue lined with a smooth, slippery synovial membrane

carbaminohemoglobin (karb-am-ee-no-hee-moh-GLOH-bin) compound formed by the union of carbon dioxide with hemoglobin

carbohydrate (kar-boh-HYE-drayt) organic compounds containing carbon, hydrogen, and oxygen in certain specific proportions (C, H, O in a 1:2:1 ratio); for example, sugars, starches, and cellulose

carbohydrate loading (kar-boh-HYE-drayt LOHD-ing) a method used by athletes to increase the stores of muscle glycogen, allowing more sustained aerobic exercise; also called *glycogen loading*

carbon (KAR-bun) one of the chemical elements found in great quantity in the human body and always found in organic compounds; symbolized by C, as in CO_2 (carbon dioxide)

carbon dioxide (KAR-bun dye-AHK-syde) molecule made up of one carbon atom and two oxygen atoms; symbolized by the formula CO_2; produced by processes of cellular respiration as a waste product that must be excreted from the body through the respiratory system

carbonic anhydrase (kar-BON-ik an-HYE-drays) the enzyme that converts carbon dioxide into carbonic acid

carbuncle (KAR-bung-kul) a mass of connected boils, pus-filled lesions associated with hair follicle infections; *see* **furuncle**

carcinogen (kar-SIN-oh-jen) substance that promotes the development of cancer

carcinoma (kar-sih-NO-mah) malignant tumor that arises from epithelial tissue

cardiac (KAR-dee-ak) refers to the heart

cardiac cycle (KAR-dee-ak SYE-kul) each complete heartbeat, including contraction and relaxation of the atria and ventricles

cardiac muscle (KAR-dee-ak MUSS-el) the involuntary type of muscle that makes up the heart wall

cardiac output (KAR-dee-ak OUT-put) volume of blood pumped by one ventricle per minute

cardiac sphincter (KAR-dee-ak SFINGK-ter) a ring of muscle between the stomach and esophagus that prevents food from reentering the esophagus when the stomach contracts

cardiac tamponade (KAR-dee-ak tam-pon-odd) compression of the heart caused by fluid buildup in the pericardial space, as in pericarditis or mechanical damage to the pericardium

cardiogenic shock (kar-dee-oh-JEN-ik shok) circulatory failure (shock) caused by heart failure; literally "heart-caused" shock

cardiologist (kar-dee-AH-lah-jist) physician or researcher who specializes in the structure and function of the heart and associated structures

cardiomyopathy (kar-dee-oh-my-OP-ah-thee) general term for disease of the myocardium (heart muscle)

cardiopulmonary resuscitation (CPR) (kar-dee-oh-PUL-moh-nair-ree ree-suss-i-TAY-shun) combined external cardiac (heart) massage and artificial respiration

cardiovascular (kar-dee-oh-VAS-kyoo-lar) pertaining to the heart and blood vessels

cardiovascular system (kar-dee-oh-VAS-kyoo-lar SIS-tem) the system that transports cells throughout the body by way of blood vessels; sometimes also called **circulatory system**

caries (KAIR-eez) decay of teeth or of bone; *see* **cavity**

carotid body (kah-ROT-id BOD-ee) chemoreceptor located in the carotid artery that detects changes in oxygen, carbon dioxide, and blood acid levels

carpal (KAR-pul) pertaining to the wrist

carpal tunnel syndrome (KAR-pul TUN-el SIN-drohm) muscle weakness, pain, and tingling in the radial side (thumb side) of the wrist, hand, and fingers—perhaps radiating to the forearm and shoulder; caused by compression of the median nerve within the carpal tunnel (a passage along the ventral concavity of the wrist)

carrier (KAIR-ee-er) in genetics, a person who possesses the gene for a recessive trait, but who does not actually exhibit the trait

cartilage (KAR-ti-lij) a specialized, fibrous connective tissue that has the consistency of a firm plastic or gristle-like gel

catabolism (kah-TAB-oh-liz-em) breakdown of food compounds or cytoplasm into simpler compounds; opposite of anabolism, the other phase of metabolism

catalyst (KAT-ah-list) chemical that speeds up reactions without being changed itself

cataract (KAT-ah-rakt) opacity of the lens of the eye

catecholamine (kat-eh-KOHL-ah-meen) category of signaling molecule tht includes norepinephrine and epinephrine

catheterization (kath-eh-ter-i-ZAY-shun) passage of a flexible tube (catheter) into the bladder through the urethra for the withdrawal of urine (urinary catheterization)

cation (KAT-eye-on) positively charged particle

cavity (KAV-i-tee) hollow place or space in a tooth resulting from decay; also referred to as *dental caries*

cecum (SEE-kum) blind pouch; the pouch at the proximal end of the large intestine

cell (sell) the basic biological and structural unit of the body consisting of a nucleus surrounded by cytoplasm and enclosed by a membrane

cell body (sell BOD-ee) the main part of a neuron from which the dendrites and axons extend

cell-mediated immunity (sell MEE-dee-ayt-ed i-MYOO-ni-tee) resistance to disease organisms resulting from the actions of cells; chiefly sensitized T cells

cellular respiration (SELL-yoo-lar res-pih-RAY-shun) enzymes in the mitochondrial wall and matrix using oxygen to break down glucose and other nutrients to release energy needed for cellular work

cementum (see-MEN-tum) bonelike dental tissue covering the neck and root areas of teeth

centimeter (SEN-ti-mee-ter) 1/100 of a meter; approximately 2.5 cm equal 1 inch

central canal (kah-NAL) longitudinal canal containing vascular elements and nervous tissue located in the center of an osteon, or Haversian system

central nervous system (CNS) (SEN-tral NER-vus SIS-tem) the brain and spinal cord

central venous pressure (SEN-tral VEE-nus PRESH-ur) venous blood pressure within the right atrium that influences the pressure in the large peripheral veins

centriole (SEN-tree-ohl) one of a pair of tiny cylinders in the centrosome of a cell; believed to be involved with the spindle fibers formed during mitosis

centromere (SEN-troh-meer) a beadlike structure that attaches one chromatid to another during the early stages of mitosis

cephalic (seh-FAL-ik) refers to the head

cerebellum (sair-eh-BELL-um) the second largest part of the human brain that plays an essential role in the production of normal movements

cerebral cortex (seh-REE-bral KOR-teks) a thin layer of gray matter made up of neuron dendrites and cell bodies that compose the surface of the cerebrum

cerebral nuclei (seh-REE-bral NOO-klee-eye) islands of gray matter located in the cerebral cortex that are responsible for autonomic movements and postures; also called **basal ganglia**

cerebral palsy (seh-REE-bral PAWL-zee) abnormal condition characterized by permanent, nonprogressive paralysis (usually spastic paralysis) of one or more extremities caused by damage to motor control areas of the brain before, during, or shortly after birth

cerebrospinal fluid (CSF) (SAIR-eh-broh-SPY-nal FLOO-id) fluid that fills the subarachnoid space in the brain and spinal cord and in the cerebral ventricles

cerebrovascular accident (CVA) (SAIR-eh-broh-VAS-kyoo-lar accident) a hemorrhage or cessation of blood flow through cerebral blood vessels resulting in destruction of neurons; commonly called a *stroke*

cerebrum (SAIR-eh-brum) the largest and uppermost part of the human brain that controls consciousness, memory, sensations, emotions, and voluntary movements

cerumen (seh-ROO-men) ear wax

ceruminous gland (seh-ROO-mih-nus) gland that produces a waxy substance called **cerumen** (ear wax)

cervical (SER-vih-kal) refers to the neck

cervicitis (ser-vih-SYE-tis) inflammation of the cervix of the uterus

cervix (SER-viks) neck; any necklike structure

cesarean section (seh-SAIR-ee-an SEK-shun) surgical removal of a fetus, often through an incision of the skin and uterine wall; also called *C-section*

chemical level (KEM-ih-kal LEV-el) the level of the body's organization that includes atoms and molecules; the chemical substances that make up the body's structure

chemoreceptors (kee-moh-ree-SEP-tors) receptors that respond to chemicals and are responsible for taste and smell

chemotaxis (kee-moh-TAK-sis) process in which white blood cells move toward the source of inflammation mediators

chemotherapy (kee-moh-THAYR-ah-pee) technique of using chemicals to treat disease (e.g., infections, cancer)

chest *see* **thorax**

Cheyne-Stokes respiration (CSR) (chain-stokes res-pih-RAY-shun) pattern of breathing associated with critical conditions such as brain injury or drug overdose and characterized by cycles of apnea and hyperventilation

childhood age period from infancy to puberty

chlamydia (klah-MID-ee-ah) small bacterium that infects human cells as an obligate parasite

cholangiography (kohl-an-jee-OG-rah-fee) specialized x-ray procedure used to visualize the gallbladder and the major bile and pancreatic ducts

cholecystectomy (kohl-eh-sis-TEK-toh-mee) surgical removal of the gallbladder

cholecystitis (koh-leh-sis-TYE-tis) inflammation of the gallbladder

cholecystokinin (CCK) (koh-leh-sis-toh-KYE-nin) hormone secreted from the intestinal mucosa of the duodenum that stimulates the contraction of the gallbladder, resulting in bile flowing into the duodenum

cholelithiasis (koh-leh-lih-THEE-ah-sis) condition of having gallstones (composed of cholesterol or bile salts), hard mineral deposits that may form and collect in the gallbladder

cholera (KAHL-er-ah) potentially fatal, infectious bacterial disease characterized by severe diarrhea, vomiting, cramps, dehydration; *see also* Appendix A, Table 3

cholesterol (koh-LESS-ter-ohl) steroid lipid found in many body tissues and in animal fat

cholinergic fiber (koh-leh-NER-jik FYE-ber) axon whose terminals release acetylcholine

chondrocyte (KON-droh-syte) cartilage cell

chondroma (kon-DROH-mah) benign tumor of cartilage

chondrosarcoma (kon-droh-sar-KOH-mah) cancer of cartilage tissue

chordae tendineae (KOR-dee ten-DIN-ee) stringlike structures that attach the AV valves to the wall of the heart

chorion (KOH-ree-on) structure that develops into an important fetal membrane in the placenta

chorionic gonadotropins (koh-ree-ON-ik goh-nah-doh-TROH-pins) hormones that are secreted as the uterus develops during pregnancy

chorionic villi (koh-ree-ON-ik VIL-eye) structures that connect the blood vessels of the chorion to the placenta

chorionic villus sampling (koh-ree-ON-ik VIL-lus SAM-pling) procedure in which a tube is inserted through the (uterine) cervical opening and a sample of the chorionic tissue surrounding a developing embryo is removed for genetic testing; compare with **amniocentesis**

choroid (KOH-royd) middle layer of the eyeball that contains a dark pigment to prevent the scattering of incoming light rays

choroid plexus (KOH-royd PLEK-sus) a network of brain capillaries that are involved with the production of cerebrospinal fluid

chromatids (KROH-mah-tids) a chromosome strand

chromatin granules (KROH-mah-tin GRAN-yoo-ulz) deep-staining substance in the nucleus of cells; divides into chromosomes during mitosis

chromosome (KROH-meh-sohm) DNA molecule that has coiled to form a compact mass during mitosis or meiosis; each chromosome is composed of regions called *genes,* each of which transmits hereditary information

chronic (KRON-ik) long-lasting, as in chronic disease

chronic lymphocytic leukemia (CLL) (KRON-ik LYM-foh-sit-ik loo-KEE-mee-ah) type of chronic (slow onset and progression) blood cancer most common in older adults; characterized by cancerous transformation and increased numbers of B lymphocytes

chronic myeloid leukemia (CML) (KRON-ik MY-loyd loo-KEE-mee-ah) type of chronic (slow onset and progression) blood cancer characterized by cancerous transformation and increased numbers of granulocytic white blood cells (WBCs)

chronic obstructive pulmonary disease (COPD) (KRON-ik ob-STRUK-tiv PUL-moh-nair-ee dih-ZEEZ) general term referring to a group of disorders characterized by progressive, irreversible obstruction of air flow in the lungs; *see* **bronchitis, emphysema**

chyme (kyme) partially digested food mixture leaving the stomach

cilia (SIL-ee-ah) hairlike projections of cells

ciliate (SIL-ee-at) type of protozoan having cilia

circulatory shock (SER-kyoo-lah-tor-ee) failure of the circulatory (cardiovascular) system to deliver adequate oxygen to the tissues of the body

circulatory system (SER-kyoo-lah-tor-ee SIS-tem) *see* **cardiovascular system**

circumcision (ser-kum-SIH-zhun) surgical removal of the foreskin or prepuce on the penis or clitoris

cirrhosis (sih-ROH-sis) degeneration of liver tissue characterized by the replacement of damaged liver tissue with fibrous or fatty connective tissue

cisterna chyli (sis-TER-nah KYE-lee) an enlarged pouch on the thoracic duct that serves as a storage area for lymph moving toward its point of entry into the venous system

citric acid cycle (SIT-rik ASS-id SYE-kul) the second series of chemical reactions in the process of glucose metabolism; it is an aerobic process; also referred to as the *Krebs cycle*

clavicle (KLAV-i-kul) collar bone, connects the upper extremity to the axial skeleton

cleavage furrow (KLEE-vij FUR-oh) appears at the end of anaphase and begins to divide the cell into two daughter cells

cleft lip (kleft) congenital defect resulting in one or more clefts in the upper lip

cleft palate (kleft PAL-ett) congenital defect resulting in a fissure of the palate in the roof of the mouth

clitoris (KLIT-oh-ris) erectile tissue located within the vestibule of the vagina

clone (klone) any of a family of many identical cells descended from a single "parent" cell

closed fracture (FRAK-chur) simple fracture; a bone fracture in which the skin is not pierced by bone fragments

coccus (KOK-us) spherical bacterial cell

cochlea (KOHK-lee-ah) snail shell or structure of similar shape; pertains to a structure within the inner ear

cochlear duct (KOHK-lee-ar dukt) membranous tube within the bony cochlea of the inner ear

cochlear implant (KOHK-lee-ar IM-plant) artificial hearing device that uses electronic circuits to perform the functions of the cochlea of the inner ear

codominance (koh-DOM-i-nance) in genetics, a form of dominance in which two dominant versions of a trait are both expressed in the same individual

coenzyme (koh-EN-zyme) molecule that assists an enzyme during metabolism, often by carrying a molecule (or molecule fragment) from one chemical pathway to another

colitis (koh-LIE-tis) any inflammatory condition of the colon and/or rectum

collagen (KAW-leh-jen) principal organic constituent of connective tissue

collecting duct (CD) (koh-LEK-ting dukt) a straight part of a renal tubule formed by distal tubules of several nephrons joining together

colloid (KOL-oyd) dissolved particles with diameters of 1 to 100 millimicrons (1 millimicron equals about 1/25,000,000 inch)

colon (KOH-lon) *see* **intestine**

color blindness (KUL-or BLIND-ness) X-linked inherited condition in which one or more photopigments in the cones of the retina are abnormal or missing

colorectal cancer (kohl-oh-REK-tal KAN-ser) common form of cancer, usually adenocarcinoma, associated with advanced age, low-fiber/high-fat diet, and genetic predisposition

colostomy (kah-LAH-stoh-mee) surgical procedure in which an artificial anus is created on the abdominal wall by cutting the colon and bringing the cut ends out to the surface to form an opening called a **stoma**

columnar (kah-LUM-nar) cell shape in which cells are higher than they are wide

combining sites (kom-BINE-ing) antigen-binding sites; antigen receptor regions on an antibody molecule; shape of each combining site is complementary to shape of a specific antigen

comedones (kom-eh-DOHNZ) (*sing.*, comedo) inflamed lesions associated with early stages of acne formed when sebaceous gland ducts become blocked

comminuted fracture (KOM-i-noo-ted FRAK-chur) bone fracture characterized by many bone fragments

communicable (koh-MYOO-nih-kah-ball) able to spread from one individual to another

compact bone (kom-PAKT) *see* **dense bone**

compensated metabolic acidosis (KOM-pen-say-ted met-ah-BOL-ik ass-i-DOH-sis) the body's successful adjustment of its body chemistry for the purpose of returning the blood pH value to near normal levels after metabolic acidosis has developed

complement (KOM-pleh-ment) any of several inactive protein enzymes normally present in blood, which when activated kill foreign cells by dissolving them

complement-binding sites (KOM-pleh-ment BIND-ing) locations on an antibody molecule that become available after exposure to an antigen and that bind to complement proteins in the blood plasma to trigger a complement cascade (immune system response) that harms the antigen-containing cell

complement cascade (KOM-pleh-ment kass-KAYD) rapid-fire series of chemical reactions involving proteins called *complements* (normally present in blood plasma) triggered by certain antibody-antigen reactions (and other stimuli) and resulting in the formation of tiny protein rings that create holes in a foreign cell and thus cause its destruction

complementary base pairing (kom-pleh-MEN-tah-ree bayse PAIR-ing) bonding purines and pyrimidines in DNA; adenine always binds with thymine, and cytosine always binds with guanine

complete fracture (kom-PLEET FRAK-chur) bone fracture characterized by complete separation of bone fragments

compound (KOM-pound) substance whose molecules have more than one kind of element in them

computed tomography (CT) (kom-PYOO-ted toh-MOG-rah-fee) radiographic imaging technique in which a patient is scanned with x-rays and a computer constructs an image that appears to be a cut section of the person's body

concave (KON-kave) a rounded, somewhat depressed surface

concentric lamella (kon-SEN-trik lah-MEL-ah) ring of calcified matrix surrounding the central (Haversian) canal

conchae (KONG-kee) shell-shaped structure; for example, bony projections into the nasal cavity

conduction (kon-DUK-shun) in regard to body temperature regulation, transfer of heat energy to the skin and then the external environment

cone receptor cell located in the retina that is stimulated by bright light

congenital (kon-JEN-i-tall) term that refers to a condition present at birth; congenital conditions may be inherited or may be acquired in the womb or during delivery

congestive heart failure (CHF) (kon-JES-tiv hart FAIL-yoor) left heart failure; inability of the left ventricle to pump effectively, resulting in congestion in the systemic and pulmonary circulations

conjunctiva (kon-junk-TIH-vah) mucous membrane that lines the eyelids and covers the sclera (white portion)

conjunctivitis (kon-junk-ti-VYE-tis) inflammation of the conjunctiva, usually caused by irritation, infection, or allergy

connective tissue (koh-NEK-tiv TISH-yoo) most abundant and widely distributed tissue in the body and has numerous functions

connective tissue membrane (koh-NEK-tiv TISH-yoo MEM-brane) one of the two major types of body membranes; composed exclusively of various types of connective tissue

constipation (kon-sti-PAY-shun) condition caused by decreased motility of the large intestine, resulting in the formation of small, hard feces and difficulty in defecation

contact dermatitis (KON-takt der-mah-TYE-tis) a local skin inflammation that lasts a few hours or days and is initiated by the skin being exposed to an antigen

continuous ambulatory peritoneal dialysis (CAPD) (kon-TIN-yoo-us AM-byoo-lah-tor-ee pair-i-toh-NEE-al dye-AL-i-sis) an alternative form of treatment for renal failure that may be used instead of the more complex and expensive **hemodialysis**

contractile unit (kon-TRAK-til YOO-nit) the sarcomere, the basic functional unit of skeletal muscle

contractility (kon-trak-TIL-i-tee) ability to contract a muscle

contraction (kon-TRAK-shun) ability of muscle cells to shorten or contract

control center (kon-TROHL SEN-ter) part of a homeostatic feedback loop that integrates (puts together) setpoint (pre-programmed) information with actual sensed information about a physiological variable and then possibly sends out a signal to an effector to change the variable

contusion (kon-TOO-zhun) local injury caused by mechanical trauma characterized by limited hemorrhaging under the skin, as in a muscle contusion or skin contusion caused by a blow to the body; a bruise

convection (kon-VEK-shun) transfer of heat energy to air that is flowing away from the skin

convex (KON-veks) a rounded, somewhat elevated surface

cor pulmonale (kohr pul-mah-NAL-ee) failure of the right atrium and ventricle to pump blood effectively, resulting from obstruction of pulmonary blood flow

coronal (koh-ROH-nal) literally "like a crown"; a coronal plane divides the body or an organ into anterior and posterior regions

coronary artery (KOHR-oh-nair-ee AR-ter-ee) the right and left coronary arteries are the first arteries to branch off the aorta; they supply blood to the myocardium (heart muscle)

coronary bypass surgery (KOHR-oh-nair-ee BYE-pass SER-jer-ee) surgery to relieve severely restricted coronary blood flow; veins are taken from other parts of the body and then reattached where needed to bypass the partial blockage

coronary circulation (KOHR-oh-nair-ee ser-kyoo-LAY-shun) delivery of oxygen and removal of waste product from the myocardium (heart muscle)

coronary embolism (KOHR-oh-nair-ee EM-boh-liz-em) blocking of a coronary blood vessel by a clot

coronary heart disease (KOHR-oh-nair-ee hart dih-ZEEZ) disease (blockage or other deformity) of the vessels that supply the myocardium (heart muscle); one of the leading causes of death among adults in the United States

coronary sinus (KOHR-oh-nair-ree SYE-nus) area that receives deoxygenated blood from the coronary veins and empties it into the right atrium

coronary thrombosis (KOHR-oh-nair-ee throm-BOH-sis) formation of a blood clot in a coronary blood vessel

coronary vein (KOHR-oh-nair-ee vane) any vein that carries blood from the myocardial capillary beds to the coronary sinus

coronavirus (koh-ROHN-ah-vye-rus) category of RNA-containing viruses that infect humans and other vertebrate animals, sometimes causing severe respiratory infections (and sometimes intestinal infections and neurological syndromes); for example, SARS **(severe acute respiratory syndrome)** is caused by a type of coronavirus, **SARS-associated coronavirus** (SARS-CoV)

corpora cavernosa (KOHR-pohr-ah kav-er-NO-sah) two columns of erectile tissue found in the shaft of the penis

corpus callosum (KOHR-pus kah-LOH-sum) brain structure at which the right and left cerebral hemispheres are joined

corpus luteum (KOHR-pus LOO-tee-um) a hormone-secreting glandular structure that is transformed after ovulation from a ruptured follicle; it secretes chiefly progesterone, with some estrogen secreted as well

corpus spongiosum (KOHR-pus spun-jee-OH-sum) a column of erectile tissue surrounding the urethra in the penis

cortex (KOHR-teks) outer part of an internal organ; for example, the outer part of the cerebrum and of the kidneys

cortical nephron (KOHR-tih-kahl NEFF-ron) microscopic unit of the kidney that makes up 85% of all nephron units in the kidney; is located almost entirely in the renal cortex

corticoids (KOHR-tih-koyds) hormones secreted by the three cell layers of the adrenal cortex

cortisol (KOHR-tih-sol) hormone secreted by the adrenal cortex to stimulate the availability of glucose in the blood; in large amounts, cortisol can depress immune functions, as when it is used as a drug treatment; *see* **hydrocortisone**

cotransport (koh-TRANZ-port) active transport process in which two substances are moved together across a cell membrane; for example, sodium and glucose may be transported together across a membrane

covalent bond (koh-VAYL-ent) chemical bond formed by two atoms sharing one or more pairs of electrons

Cowper gland *see* **bulbourethral gland**

coxal bone (kok-SAL) the pelvic bone or hipbone (also known as the *os coxae* or the *innominate bone*); formed by fusion of three distinct bones (ilium, ischium, and pubis) during skeletal development

cramps (kramps) painful muscle spasms (involuntary twitches) that result from irritating stimuli, as in mild inflammation, or from ion imbalances

cranial (KRAY-nee-all) toward the head

cranial cavity (KRAY-nee-all KAV-i-tee) space inside the skull that contains the brain

cranial nerve (KRAY-nee-all nerv) any of 12 pairs of nerves that attach to the undersurface of the brain and conduct impulses between the brain and structures in the head, neck, and thorax

craniosacral (kray-nee-oh-SAY-kral) pertaining to parasympathetic nerves

cranium (KRAY-nee-um) bony vault made up of eight bones that encases the brain

crenation (kreh-NAY-shun) abnormal notching in an erythrocyte caused by shrinkage after suspension in a hypertonic solution

cretinism (KREE-tin-iz-em) dwarfism caused by hyposecretion of the thyroid gland

crista ampullaris (KRIS-tah am-pyoo-LAIR-is) a specialized receptor located within the semicircular canals that detects head movements

Crohn disease (krohn dih-ZEEZ) chronic inflammatory bowel disease

croup (kroop) non–life-threatening type of laryngitis generally seen in children less than age 3; characterized by bark-like cough and caused by parainfluenza viruses

crown (krown) topmost part of an organ or other structure, such as a tooth

crural (KROOR-all) refers to the leg

crust (krust) scab; area of the skin covered by dried blood or exudate

cryptorchidism (krip-TOR-kih-diz-em) undescended testicles

cubital (KYOO-bi-tall) refers to the elbow

cuboid (KYOO-boyd) resembling a cube

cuboidal (kyoo-BOYD-al) cell shape resembling a cube

culture (KULT-chur) growth of microbes in a laboratory medium for the purpose of isolating and identifying pathogens from human body fluids

Cushing syndrome (KOOSH-ing SIN-drohm) condition caused by the hypersecretion of glucocorticoids from the adrenal cortex

cuspid (KUS-pid) having cusps or points; for example, the **canine tooth** located lateral to the second incisor that serves to pierce or tear food being eaten is also called a *cuspid tooth*

cutaneous (kyoo-TANE-ee-us) pertaining to the skin

cutaneous membrane (kyoo-TAYN-ee-us MEM-brane) primary organ of the integumentary system; the skin

cuticle (KYOO-ti-kul) skinfold covering the root of the nail

cyanosis (sye-ah-NO-sis) condition in which light-skinned individuals exhibit a bluish coloration resulting from relatively low oxygen content in the arterial blood; literally "blue condition"

cyclic AMP (SIK-lik A M P) (adenosine monophosphate) one of several second messengers that delivers information inside the cell and thus regulates the cell's activity

cystic duct (SIS-tik dukt) joins with the common hepatic duct to form the common bile duct

cystic fibrosis (SIS-tik fye-BROH-sis) inherited disease involving abnormal chloride ion (Cl⁻) transport; causes secretion of abnormally thick mucus and other problems

cystitis (sis-TYE-tis) inflammation or infection of the urinary bladder

cystoscope (SIS-toh-skohp) hollow instrument inserted through urethra into the bladder that permits passage of a light source and surgical instruments to be used for direct examination, biopsy, surgical removal, or treatment of bladder or other urinary tract lesions

cytoplasm (SYE-toh-plaz-em) the gel-like substance of a cell exclusive of the nucleus and other organelles

cytosine (SYE-toh-seen) one of several nitrogen-containing bases that make up nucleotides, which in turn make up nucleic acids such as DNA and RNA; in the cell, it can chemically bind to another nitrogenous base, guanine (*G* or *g*), to form a more complex structure or in translating genetic codes; symbolized by the letter *C* or *c*; *see also* **guanine, adenine, thymine, uracil**

D

deciduous (deh-SID-yoo-us) temporary; shedding of structures at a certain stage of growth; for example, deciduous teeth, which are commonly referred to as *baby teeth*, are shed to make way for the permanent adult teeth

decubitus ulcer (deh-KYOO-bi-tus UL-ser) pressure sore that often develops over a bony prominence, such as the heel, when lying in one position for prolonged periods

deep farther away (internally) from the body's surface

defibrillation (deh-fib-rih-LAY-shun) electrical stimulation of the heart in order to restore normal heart rhythm (used when the heart fibrillates, or gets out of rhythm); *see* **ventricular fibrillation** and **automatic external defibrillator**

degeneration (dee-jen-er-AY-shun) a biological process, still somewhat puzzling to scientists, in which tissues break down as a normal consequence of aging; degeneration of one or more tissues resulting from disease can occur at any time

deglutition (deg-loo-TISH-un) swallowing

dehydration (dee-hye-DRAY-shun) clinical term that refers to an abnormal loss of fluid from the body's internal environment

dehydration synthesis (dee-hye-DRAY-shun SIN-theh-sis) chemical reaction in which large molecules are formed by removing water from smaller molecules and joining them together

deltoid (DEL-toyd) having a triangular shape; for example, the deltoid muscle

dementia (deh-MEN-shah) syndrome of brain abnormalities that includes loss of memory, shortened attention span, personality changes, reduced intellectual capacity, and motor dysfunction

dendrite (DEN-dryte) branching or treelike; a nerve cell process that transmits impulses toward the body

dense bone bone that has a hard, dense outer layer; also called *compact bone*

dentin (DEN-tin) chief bonelike dental tissue covered by enamel in crown and by cementum in neck and root areas of tooth

deoxyribonucleic acid (DNA) (dee-ok-see-rye-boh-noo-klay-ik ASS-id) genetic material of the cell that carries the chemical "blueprint" of the body

depilatories (deh-PIL-ah-toh-rees) hair removers

depolarization (dee-poh-lar-i-ZAY-shun) the electrical activity that triggers a contraction of the heart muscle

dermal-epidermal junction (DER-mal-EP-i-der-mal JUNK-shun) junction between the thin epidermal layer of the skin and the dermal layer; provides support for the epidermis

dermal papilla (DER-mal pah-PIL-ah) (*pl.,* papillae [pah-PIL-ee]) upper region of the dermis that forms part of the dermal-epidermal junction and forms the ridges and grooves of fingerprints

dermatitis (der-mah-TYE-tis) general term referring to any inflammation of the skin

dermatome (DER-mah-tohm) skin surface area supplied by a single spinal nerve

dermatosis (der-mah-TOH-sis) general term meaning "skin condition"

dermis (DER-mis) the deeper of the two major layers of the skin, composed of dense fibrous connective tissue interspersed with glands, nerve endings, and blood vessels; sometimes called the "true skin"

developmental process (dee-vel-op-MEN-tal PROSS-es) changes and functions occurring during a human's early years as the body becomes more efficient and more effective

deviated septum (DEE-vee-ay-ted SEP-tum) abnormal condition in which the nasal septum (dividing wall between the two nasal air passages) is located far from its normal position, possibly obstructing normal nasal breathing

diabetes insipidus (dye-ah-BEE-teez in-SIP-i-dus) condition resulting from hyposecretion of ADH in which large volumes of urine are formed and, if left untreated, may cause serious health problems

diabetes mellitus (dye-ah-BEE-teez mell-EYE-tus) a condition resulting when the pancreatic islets secrete too little insulin, resulting in increased levels of blood glucose

diabetic ketoacidosis *see* **ketoacidosis**

diabetic retinopathy (dye-ah-BET-ik ret-in-AH-path-ee) growth or hemorrhage of blood vessels caused by diabetes mellitus

dialysis (dye-AL-i-sis) separation of smaller (diffusible) particles from larger (nondiffusable) particles through a semipermeable membrane

diaphragm (DYE-ah-fram) membrane or partition that separates one thing from another; the flat muscular sheet that separates the thorax and abdomen and is a major muscle of respiration

diaphysis (dye-AF-i-sis) (*pl.,* diaphyses) shaft of a long bone

diarrhea (dye-ah-REE-ah) defecation of liquid feces

diarthrosis (dye-ar-THROH-sis) (*pl.,* diarthroses) freely movable joint

diastole (dye-ASS-toh-lee) relaxation of the heart, interposed between its contractions; opposite of **systole**

diastolic pressure (dye-ah-STOL-ik PRESH-ur) blood pressure in arteries during diastole (relaxation) of the heart

diencephalons (dye-en-SEF-ah-lon) "between" brain; parts of the brain between the cerebral hemispheres and the mesencephalon, or midbrain

differential WBC count (dif-er-EN-shawl WBC count) special type of white blood cell (WBC) count in which proportions of each type of WBC are reported as percentages of the total count

differentiate (dif-er-EN-shee-ayt) a process by which daughter cells become different in structure and function (by using different genes from the genome, all cells of the body share), as when some of the original cells of early developmental stages differentiate to become muscle cells and other cells become nerve cells, and so on (*differentiation* is another form of this term)

diffusion (dih-FYOO-shun) spreading; for example, scattering of dissolved particles

digestion (dye-JES-chun) the breakdown of food materials either mechanically (that is, by chewing) or chemically (that is, by action of digestive enzymes)

digestive system (di-JES-tiv SIS-tem) organs that work together to ensure proper digestion and absorption of nutrients

digital (DIJ-i-tal) refers to fingers and toes

discharging chambers (dis-CHARJ-ing CHAYM-bers) the two lower chambers of the heart called *ventricles*

disease (dih-ZEEZ) any significant abnormality in the body's structure or function that disrupts a person's vital function or physical, mental, or social well-being

dislocation (dis-low-KAY-shun) abnormal movement of body parts, as in separation of bones of a joint; *see* **subluxation**

dissection (dye-SEK-shun) cutting technique used to separate body parts for study

dissociate (dih-SOH-see-ayt) action in which a compound breaks apart in solution

dissociation (dih-soh-see-AY-shun) separation of ions as they dissolve in water

distal (DIS-tall) toward the end of a structure; opposite of **proximal**

distal convoluted tubule (DCT) (DIS-tall KON-voh-loo-ted TOO-byoo-ul) the part of the tubule distal to the ascending limb of the Henle loop in the kidney

disuse atrophy (DIS-yoos AT-roh-fee) condition in which prolonged inactivity results in the muscles getting smaller in size; *see also* **atrophy**

diuretic (dye-yoo-RET-ik) a substance that promotes or stimulates the production of urine; diuretic drugs are among the most commonly used drugs in medicine

diverticulitis (dye-ver-tik-yoo-LYE-tis) inflammation of diverticula (abnormal outpouchings) of the large intestine, possibly causing constipation

dizygotic twins (dye-zye-GOT-il twinz) *see* **fraternal twins**

DNA (D N A) *see* **deoxyribonucleic acid**

DNA replication (D N A rep-lih-KAY-shun) the unique ability of DNA molecules to make copies of themselves

dominant (DOM-i-nant) in genetics, the term *dominant* refers to genes that have effects that appear in the offspring (dominant forms of a gene are often represented by upper case letters); compare with **recessive**

dopamine (DOH-pah-meen) chemical neurotransmitter

doping (DOH-ping) the addition of blood (or blood products), steroids, or other performance-enhancing substances to the bloodstream, a practice performed by some athletes that can have serious (even fatal) side effects and is outlawed worldwide

dorsal (DOR-sal) referring to the back; opposite of ventral; in humans, the posterior is dorsal

dorsal body cavity (DOR-sal BOD-ee KAV-i-tee) includes the cranial and spinal cavities

dorsal cavity *see* **dorsal body cavity**

dorsiflexion (dor-sih-FLEK-shun) movement in which the top of the foot is elevated (brought toward the front of the lower leg) with the toes pointing upward

double helix (HEE-lix) shape of DNA molecules; a double spiral

dowager hump (DOW-ah-jer) kyphosis (abnormal backward curvature of thoracic spine) caused by vertebral compression fractures in osteoporosis

Down syndrome (SIN-drohm) group of symptoms usually caused by trisomy of chromosome 21; characterized by mental retardation and multiple structural defects, including facial, skeletal, and cardiovascular abnormalities

Duchenne muscular dystrophy (DMD) (doo-SHEN MUSS-kyoo-lar DISS-troh-fee) form of muscular dystrophy (abnormal muscle development in which normal muscle is replaced with fat and fibrous tissue) inherited on the X chromosome and characterized by mild leg muscle weakness that progresses rapidly to include the shoulder muscles and eventually death from cardiac or respiratory muscle weakness; also called **pseudohypertrophy** ("false muscle growth")

ductless gland (DUKT-less) specialized gland that secretes hormones directly into the blood; endocrine gland

ductus arteriosus (DUK-tus ar-teer-ee-OH-sus) connects the aorta and the pulmonary artery, allowing most blood to bypass the fetus's developing lungs

ductus deferens (DUK-tus DEF-er-ens) a thick, smooth, muscular tube that allows sperm to exit from the epididymis and pass from the scrotal sac into the abdominal cavity; also known as the *vas deferens*

ductus venosus (DUK-tus veh-NO-sus) a continuation of the umbilical vein that shunts blood returning from the placenta past the fetus's developing liver directly into the inferior vena cava

duodenal papillae (doo-oh-DEE-nal pah-PIL-ee) ducts located in the middle third of the duodenum that empty pancreatic digestive juices and bile from the liver into the small intestine; there are two ducts, the major duodenal papilla and the minor papilla

duodenum (doo-oh-DEE-num) the first subdivision of the small intestine where most chemical digestion occurs

dura mater (DOO-rah MAH-ter) literally "strong or hard mother"; outermost layer of the meninges

dust cells macrophages that ingest particulate matter in the small air sacs of the lungs

dwarfism (DWARF-iz-em) condition of abnormally small stature, sometimes resulting from hyposecretion of growth hormone

dysentery (DISS-en-tayr-ee) inflammatory condition of colon characterized by frequent diarrhea that may contain blood or pus

dysfunctional uterine bleeding (DUB) (dis-FUNK-shun-all YOO-ter-in BLEED-ing) irregular or excessive bleeding from the uterus resulting from a hormonal imbalance

dysmenorrhea (dis-men-oh-REE-ah) painful menstruation

dyspnea (DISP-nee-ah) difficult or labored breathing

dysrhythmia (dis-RITH-mee-ah) any abnormality of cardiac rhythm

dysuria (diss-YOO-ree-ah) painful, burning urination

E

eardrum (EAR-drum) the tympanic membrane that separates the external ear and middle ear

eccrine (EK-rin) small sweat glands distributed over the total body surface

echocardiography (ek-oh-kar-dee-OG-rah-fee) heart imaging technique in which ultrasound waves echo back from heart tissues to form a continuous recording of heart structure movement during a series of cardiac cycles

ectoderm (EK-toh-derm) the innermost of the primary germ layers that develops early in the first trimester of pregnancy

ectopic pregnancy (ek-TOP-ik PREG-nan-see) a pregnancy in which the fertilized ovum implants someplace other than in the uterus

eczema (EK-zeh-mah) inflammatory skin condition associated with a variety of diseases and characterized by erythema, papules, vesicles, and crusts

edema (eh-DEE-mah) accumulation of fluid in a tissue, as in inflammation; swelling

effector (ef-FEK-tor) responding organ; for example, voluntary and involuntary muscle, the heart, and glands

effector cell (ef-FEK-tor) *see* **plasma cell**

efferent (EF-fer-ent) carrying from, as neurons that transmit impulses from the central nervous system to the periphery; opposite of **afferent**

ejaculation (ee-jak-yoo-LAY-shun) sudden discharging of semen from the body

ejaculatory duct (ee-JAK-yoo-lah-toh-ree dukt) duct formed by the joining of the ductus deferens and the duct from the seminal vesicle that allows sperm to enter the urethra

electrocardiogram (ECG) (eh-lek-troh-KAR-dee-oh-gram) graphic record of the heart's action potentials

electrocardiograph (e-lek-troh-KAR-dee-oh-graf) machine that produces electrocardiograms, graphic records of the heart's electrical activity (voltage fluctuations)

electroencephalogram (eh-lek-troh-en-SEF-ah-loh-gram) graphic representation of voltage changes in brain tissue used to evaluate nerve tissue function

electrolyte (eh-LEK-troh-lyte) substance that dissociates into ions in solution, rendering the solution capable of conducting an electric current

electrolyte balance (eh-LEK-troh-lyte BAL-ans) homeostasis of electrolytes

electron (ee-LEK-tron) small, negatively charged subatomic particle found in the outer regions of an atom

electron microscope (eh-LEK-tron MY-kroh-skope) a device that produces a greatly enlarged image of a tiny structure by using a beam of electrons focused by magnets (rather than a beam of light focused by glass lenses, as in a light microscope)

electron transport system (eh-LEK-tron TRANZ-port SIS-tem) cellular process within mitochondria that transfers energy from high-energy electrons from glycolysis and the citric acid cycle to ATP molecules so that the energy is available to do work in the cell

electrophoresis (eh-lek-troh-foh-REE-sis) laboratory procedure in which different types of molecules are separated according to molecular weight by passing a weak electric current through their liquid medium

element (EL-eh-ment) pure substance, composed of only one type of atom

elephantiasis (el-eh-fan-TYE-ah-sis) extreme lymphedema (swelling due to lymphatic blockage) in the limbs caused by a parasitic worm infestation, so called because the limbs swell to "elephant proportions"

embolism (EM-boh-liz-em) obstruction of a blood vessel by foreign matter carried in the bloodstream

embolus (EM-boh-lus) a blood clot or other substance (such as a bubble of air) that is moving in the blood and may block a blood vessel

embryo (EM-bree-oh) animal in early stages of intrauterine development; in humans, the first 3 months after conception

embryology (em-bree-OHL-oh-gee) study of the development of an individual from conception to birth

embryonic phase (em-bree-ON-ik fayz) the period extending from fertilization until the end of the eighth week of gestation; during this phase the term *embryo* is used

emesis (EM-eh-sis) vomiting

emphysema (em-fih-SEE-mah) abnormal condition characterized by trapping of air in alveoli of the lung that causes them to rupture and fuse to other alveoli

emptying reflex (EMP-tee-ing REE-fleks) the reflex that causes the contraction of the bladder wall and relaxation of the internal sphincter to allow urine to enter the urethra, which is followed by urination if the external sphincter is voluntarily relaxed

emulsify (eh-MULL-seh-fye) in digestion, when bile breaks up fats

endemic (en-DEM-ik) refers to a disease native to a local region of the world

endocarditis (en-doh-kar-DYE-tis) inflammation of the lining of the heart

endocardium (en-doh-KAR-dee-um) thin layer of very smooth tissue lining each chamber of the heart

endochondral ossification (en-doh-KON-drall os-i-fih-KAY-shun) the process in which most bones are formed from cartilage models

endocrine (EN-doh-krin) secreting into the blood or tissue fluid rather than into a duct; opposite of exocrine

endocrine glands (EN-doh-krin) ductless glands that are part of the endocrine system and secrete hormones into intercellular spaces

endocrine system (EN-doh-krin SIS-tem) the series of ductless glands that are found in the body

endocrinology (en-doh-krin-AHL-ah-jee) study of endocrine glands and their functions

endoderm (EN-doh-derm) the outermost layer of the primary germ layers that develops early in the first trimester of pregnancy

endometriosis (en-doh-mee-tree-OH-sis) presence of functioning endometrial tissue outside the uterus

endometrium (en-doh-MEE-tree-um) mucous membrane lining the uterus

endoneurium (en-doh-NOO-ree-um) the thin wrapping of fibrous connective tissue that surrounds each axon in a nerve

endoplasmic reticulum (ER) (en-doh-PLAZ-mik reh-TIK-yoo-lum) network tubules and vesicles in cytoplasm; two types: *rough* and *smooth*

endorphin (en-DOR-fin) chemical in the central nervous system that influences pain perception; a natural painkiller

endosteum (en-DOS-tee-um) a fibrous membrane that lines the medullary cavity

endothelium (en-doh-THEE-lee-um) squamous epithelial cells that line the inner surface of the entire circulatory system and the vessels of the lymphatic system

endotracheal intubation (en-doh-TRAY-kee-al in-too-BAY-shun) medical procedure in which a tube is placed through the mouth, pharynx, and larynx into the trachea to ensure an open airway

endurance training (en-DUR-ance TRAIN-ing) continuous vigorous exercise requiring the body to increase its consumption of oxygen and develop the muscles' ability to sustain activity over a prolonged period of time

energy level limited region surrounding the nucleus of an atom at a certain distance containing electrons; also called a *shell*

enkephalin (en-KEF-ah-lin) peptide chemical in the central nervous system that acts as a natural painkiller

enteritis (en-ter-EYE-tiss) inflammation of the small intestine

enuresis (en-yoo-REE-siss) involuntary urination

enzyme (EN-zyme) biochemical catalyst allowing chemical reactions to take place in a suitable timeframe

eosinophil (ee-oh-SIN-oh-fil) white blood cell that is readily stained by eosin

epicardium (ep-i-KAR-dee-um) the inner layer of the pericardium that covers the surface of the heart; it is also called the **visceral pericardium**

epidemic (ep-i-DEM-ik) refers to a disease that occurs in many individuals at the same time

epidemiology (EP-i-dee-mee-OHL-oh-jee) study of the occurrence, distribution, and transmission of diseases in human populations

epidermis (ep-i-DER-miss) "false" skin; outermost layer of the skin

epididymis (ep-i-DID-i-miss) one of two comma-shaped, long, tightly coiled tubes that carry sperm from testes to vas deferens

epididymitis (ep-i-did-i-MY-tis) inflammation of the epididymis

epiglottis (ep-i-GLOT-iss) lidlike cartilage overhanging the entrance to the larynx

epiglottitis (EPP-ih-glott-eye-tiss) life-threatening type of laryngitis generally seen in children 3 to 7 years of age; characterized by laryngeal edema and high fever and caused by *Haemophilus influenzae* virus

epilepsy (EP-i-lep-see) a seizure disorder characterized by recurring seizures

epinephrine (Epi) (ep-i-NEF-rin) adrenaline; hormone secreted by the adrenal medulla

epineurium (ep-i-NOO-ree-um) a tough fibrous sheath that covers the whole nerve

epiphyseal fracture (ep-i-FEEZ-ee-all FRAK-chur) when the epiphyseal plate is separated from the epiphysis or diaphysis; this type of fracture can disrupt the normal growth of the bone

epiphyseal line (ep-i-FEEZ-ee-all lyne) point of fusion seen in a mature bone that replaces the epiphyseal cartilage or growth plate that once separated the epiphysis and diaphysis of a growing bone

epiphyseal plate (ep-i-FEEZ-ee-all) the cartilage plate that is between the epiphysis and the diaphysis and allows growth to occur; sometimes referred to as a *growth plate*

epiphysis (eh-PIF-i-sis) (*pl.,* epiphyses) end of a long bone

episiotomy (eh-piz-ee-OT-oh-mee) a surgical procedure used during birth to prevent a laceration of the mother's perineum or the vagina

epispadias congenital defect in males characterized by opening of urethral meatus on dorsal (top) surface of glans or penile shaft

epistaxis (ep-i-STAK-sis) clinical term referring to a bloody nose

epithelial membrane (ep-i-THEE-lee-all MEM-brane) membrane composed of epithelial tissue with an underlying layer of specialized connective tissue

epithelial tissue (ep-i-THEE-lee-all TISH-yoo) covers the body and its parts; lines various parts of the body; forms continuous sheets that contain no blood vessels; classified according to shape and arrangement

erectile dysfunction (ED) *see* **impotence**

erythema (ayr-ith-EE-mah) redness or inflammation of the skin or mucous membranes

erythroblastosis fetalis (ee-rith-roh-blas-TOH-sis fee-TAL-iss) condition of a fetus or infant caused by the mother's Rh antibodies reacting with the baby's Rh-positive RBCs, characterized by massive agglutination of the blood and resulting in life-threatening circulatory problems

erythrocytes (eh-RITH-roh-sites) red blood cells

erythropoietin (eh-RITH-roh-POY-eh-tin) glycoprotein secreted to increase red blood cell production in response to oxygen deficiency (*erythro-* red, *-poiet-* make, *-in* substance)

esophagus (eh-SOF-ah-gus) the muscular, mucus-lined tube that connects the pharynx with the stomach; also known as the *foodpipe*

essential organs (ee-SEN-shal OR-gans) reproductive organs that must be present for reproduction to occur; known as **gonads**

estrogen (ES-troh-jen) sex hormone secreted by the ovary that causes the development and maintenance of the female secondary sex characteristics and stimulates growth of the epithelial cells lining the uterus

etiology (ee-tee-OHL-oh-jee) theory, or study, of the factors involved in causing a disease

eupnea (YOOP-nee-ah) normal respiration

eustachian tube (yoo-STAY-shun toob) *see* **auditory tube**

evaporation (ee-vap-oh-RAY-shun) heat being lost from the skin by sweat being vaporized

excimer laser surgery (EK-zim-er LAY-zer SIR-jer-ee) refractory eye surgery that uses an excimer or "cool" laser to vaporize corneal tissue in treating mild to moderate nearsightedness; also called **photorefractive keratectomy (PRK)**

excoriation (eks-koh-ree-AY-shun) skin lesion in which epidermis has been removed, as in a scratch wound

exhalation (eks-hah-LAY-shun) moving air out of the lungs; opposite of **inhalation,** or **inspiration;** also known as **expiration**

exocrine (EK-soh-krin) secreting into a duct; opposite of endocrine

exocrine gland (EK-soh-krin) glands that secrete their products into ducts that empty onto a surface or into a cavity; for example, sweat glands

experimental controls (eks-pair-i-MEN-tal kon-TROLZ) any procedure within a scientific experiment that ensures that the test situation itself is not affecting the outcome of the experiment

experimentation (eks-pair-i-men-TAY-shun) performing an experiment, which is usually a test of a tentative explanation of nature called a **hypothesis**

exophthalmos (ek-soff-THAL-mos) condition of abnormally protruding eyeballs, occurring in a form of hyperthyroidism called **Graves' disease;** also called *exophthalmia*

expiration (eks-pih-RAY-shun) moving air out of the lungs; opposite of **inhalation,** or **inspiration;** also known as **exhalation**

expiratory muscles (eks-PYE-rah-tor-ee MUSS-els) muscles that allow more forceful expiration to increase the rate and depth of ventilation; the internal intercostals and the abdominal muscles

expiratory reserve volume (ERV) (eks-PYE-rah-tor-ee ree-ZERV VOL-yoom) the amount of air that can be forcibly exhaled after expiring the tidal volume (TV)

extension (ek-STEN-shun) increasing the angle between two bones at a joint

external auditory canal (eks-TER-nal AW-dih-toh-ree kah-NAL) a curved tube (approximately 2.5 cm long) extending from the auricle into the temporal bone, ending at the tympanic membrane

external ear (eks-TER-nal) the outer part of the ear that is made up of the auricle and the external auditory canal

external genitalia (eks-TER-nal jen-i-TAIL-yah) external reproductive organs; also called *genitals* or simply *genitalia*

external intercostals (eks-TER-nal in-ter-KOS-talls) inspiratory muscles that enlarge the thorax, causing the lungs to expand and air to rush in

external nares (eks-TER-nal NAY-reez) nostrils

external oblique (eks-TER-nal oh-BLEEK) the outermost layer of the anterolateral abdominal wall

external otitis (eks-TER-nal oh-TYE-tis) a common infection of the external ear; also known as *swimmer ear*

external respiration (eks-TER-nal res-pih-RAY-shun) the exchange of gases between air in the lungs and in the blood

extracellular fluid (ECF) (eks-trah-SELL-yoo-lar FLOO-id) water found outside of cells located in two compartments between cells (interstitial fluid) and in the blood (plasma)

F

facial (FAY-shal) referring to the face

fallen arch condition in which the tendons and ligaments of the foot weaken, allowing the normally curved arch to flatten out

fallopian tubes (fal-LOH-pee-an toobs) *see* **uterine tubes**

false ribs the eighth, ninth, and tenth pairs of ribs, which are attached to the cartilage of the seventh ribs rather than the sternum

fascicle (FASS-i-kul) small bundle of fibers, as in a small bundle of nerve fibers or muscle fibers

fasciculus (fah-SIC-yoo-lus) little bundle

fat one of the three basic food types; primarily a source of energy

fatigue (fah-TEEG) loss of muscle power; weakness

fat tissue (TISH-yoo) *see* **adipose**

feces (FEE-seez) waste material discharged from the intestines

feedback control loop (FEED-bak kon-TROL loop) a highly complex and integrated communication control network, classified as negative or positive; negative feedback loops are the most important and numerous homeostatic control mechanisms

femoral (FEM-or-all) referring to the thigh

femur (FEE-mur) the thigh bone, which is the longest bone in the body

fertilization (FER-tih-lih-ZAY-shun) the action that takes place at the moment the female's ovum and the male's sperm cell unite

fetal alcohol syndrome (FAS) (FEE-tal AL-koh-hol SIN-drohm) a condition that may cause congenital abnormalities in a baby; it results from a woman consuming alcohol during pregnancy

fetal phase (FEE-tal fayz) period extending from the eighth to the thirty-ninth week of gestation; during this phase the term *fetus* is used

fetus (FEE-tus) unborn young, especially in the later stages; in human beings, from the third month of the intrauterine period until birth

fever (FEE-ver) elevated body temperature beyond the normal setpoint, usually triggered by the immune system in response to infection or injury

fibers (FYE-bers) threadlike structures; for example, nerve fibers

fibrillation (fih-brih-LAY-shun) condition in which individual muscle fibers, or small groups of fibers, contract asynchronously (out of time) with other muscle fibers in an organ, producing no effective movement

fibrin (FYE-brin) insoluble protein in clotted blood

fibrinogen (fye-BRIN-oh-jen) soluble blood protein that is converted to insoluble fibrin during clotting

fibroid (FYE-broyd) *see* **fibromyoma**

fibrous connective tissue (FYE-brus koh-NEK-tiv TISH-yoo) strong, nonstretchable, white collagen fibers that compose tendons

fibromyoma (fye-broh-my-OH-mah) benign tumor of smooth muscle and fibrous connective tissue commonly occurring in the uterine wall, where it is often called a *fibroid; see also* **myoma**

fibromyositis (fye-broh-my-oh-SYE-tis) inflammation of muscle tissue accompanied by inflammation of nearby tendon tissue

fibrosarcoma (fye-broh-sar-KOH-mah) cancer of fibrous connective tissue

fibula (FIB-yoo-lah) the slender non–weight-bearing bone located on the lateral aspect of the leg

fight-or-flight response (fyte or flyte) the changes produced by increased sympathetic impulses allowing the body to deal with any type of stress

filtration (fil-TRAY-shun) movement of water and solutes through a membrane by a higher hydrostatic pressure on one side

fimbriae (FIM-bree-ee) (*sing.,* fimbria) fringelike projection

first-degree burn minor burn with only minimal discomfort and no blistering; epidermis may peel but no dermal injury occurs; *also see* **partial-thickness burn**

flagellate (FLAJ-eh-lat) protozoan possessing flagella

flagellum (flah-JEL-um) (*pl.,* flagella) single projection extending from the cell surface; only example in human is the "tail" of the male sperm

flat bone one of the four types of bone; the frontal bone is an example of a flat bone

flat feet condition in which the tendons and ligaments of the foot are weak, allowing the normally curved arch to flatten out

flatulence (FLAT-yoo-lens) presence of air or other gases in the lumen of the gastrointestinal tract

flavivirus (FLAV-ih-vye-rus) category of RNA-containing viruses that typically require an insect vector to transmit them to humans; examples of flavivirus infections include yellow fever, dengue, St. Louis encephalitis, and West Nile virus (WNV)

flexion (FLEK-shun) act of bending; decreasing the angle between two bones at the joint

floating ribs (FLOW-ting) the eleventh and twelfth pairs of ribs, which are only attached to the thoracic vertebrae

fluid balance (FLOO-id BAL-ans) homeostasis of fluids; the volumes of interstitial fluid, intracellular fluid, and plasma and total volume of water remain relatively constant

fluid compartments (FLOO-id kom-PART-ments) the areas in the body where the fluid is located; for example, interstitial fluid

folate-deficiency anemia (FOH-layt–deh-FISH-en-see ah-NEE-mee-ah) blood disorder characterized by a decrease in the red blood cell count, caused by a deficiency of folic acid in the diet (as in malnourished individuals)

follicles (FOL-lih-kulz) specialized structures required for hair growth

follicle-stimulating hormone (FSH) (FOL-lih-kul STIM-yoo-lay-ting HOR-mohn) hormone present in males and females; in males, FSH stimulates the production of sperm; in females, FSH stimulates the ovarian follicles to mature and the follicle cells to secrete estrogen

fontanels (FON-tah-nelz) "soft spots" on an infant's head; unossified areas in the infant skull

foramen (foh-RAY-men) small opening; for example, the vertebral foramen, which allows the spinal cord to pass through the vertebral canal

foramen ovale (foh-RAY-men oh-VAL-ee) shunts blood from the right atrium directly into the left atrium allowing most blood to bypass the baby's developing lungs

foreskin (FORE-skin) a loose-fitting, retractable casing located over the glans of the penis; also known as the **prepuce**

formed elements cellular (RBC, WBC, and platelet) fraction of blood

fovea (FOH-vee-ah) small depression or pit in center of retinal macula lutea; site of acute image formation and color vision

fourth-degree burn complete destruction of epidermis, dermis, and subcutaneous tissue with additional damage below subcutaneous tissue to muscle and bone; see **full-thickness burn**

fractal geometry (FRAK-tul jee-OM-eh-tree) the study of surfaces with a seemingly infinite area, such as the lining of the small intestine

fraternal (dizygotic) twins (frah-TERN-al twinz) birth of two siblings at the same time that have developed from two separate zygotes (dizygotic); also called *dizygotic twins*; contrast with **identical (monozygotic) twins**

freckle (FREK-ull) small brown or red macules that are a common genetic variant of normal skin pigmentation

free nerve endings (nerv END-ings) specialized receptors in the skin that respond to pain

free radical (RAD-i-kal) highly reactive, electron-seeking molecules that occur normally in cells but may damage electron-dense molecules such as DNA or molecules in cell membranes; free radicals may be inhibited by antioxidants, such as vitamin E

frenulum (FREN-yoo-lum) the thin membrane that attaches the tongue to the floor of the mouth

frontal (FRUN-tall) lengthwise plane running from side to side, dividing the body into anterior and posterior portions

frontal muscle (FRUN-tall MUSS-el) one of the muscles of facial expression; it moves the eyebrows and furrows the skin of the forehead

frontal sinusitis (FRON-tall sye-nyoo-SYE-tis) inflammation in the frontal sinus

frostbite (FROST-byte) local tissue damage caused by extreme cold

full-thickness burn burn that (1) destroys epidermis, dermis, and subcutaneous tissue (*see* **third-degree burn**) and (2) extends below skin and subcutaneous tissue to reach muscle and bone (*see* **fourth-degree burn**)

functional protein (FUNK-shen-all PRO-teen) protein that has the role of regulating chemical reactions in the body, such as enzymes, some neurotransmitters, some hormones; compare to **structural protein**

fundus (of stomach) (FUN-duss) enlarged portion to the left of and above the opening of the esophagus into the stomach

fundus (of uterus) (FUN-duss of YOO-ter-us) bulging prominence above level where uterine tubes attach to the body of the uterus

fungus (FUNG-gus) (*pl.,* fungi [FUN-jye]) organism similar to plants but lacking chlorophyll and capable of producing mycotic (fungal) infections

furuncle (FUR-un-kul) boil; a pus-filled cavity formed by some hair follicle infections

G

G protein a protein molecule usually embedded in a cell's plasma membrane that plays an important role in getting a signal from a receptor (also in the plasma membrane) to the inside of the cell

gallstone (GAWL-stohn) solid concretions or stones, often composed of cholesterol or bile salts, found in the gallbladder; see also **cholelithiasis**

gametes (GAM-eets) either of the two sex cells, sperm (spermatozoa) and egg (ova), that have half the usual number of nuclear chromosomes (the haploid number)

ganglion (GANG-lee-un) (*pl.,* ganglia [GANG-lee-ah]) a region of unmyelinated nerve tissue (usually this term is used only for regions in the peripheral nervous system [PNS])

gangrene (GANG-green) tissue death (necrosis) that involves decay of tissue

gastric gland (GAS-trik) glands in stomach lining that secrete enzymes, mucus, or hydrochloric acid

gastritis (gas-TRY-tiss) inflammation of the lining of the stomach

gastrocnemius (GAS-trok-NEE-mee-us) superficial muscle of the calf of the leg, connected (along with the soleus muscle) to the calcaneus bone of the foot by way of the Achilles (calcaneal) tendon; its action is to dorsiflex the foot, bending the toes upward

gastroenteritis (gas-troh-en-ter-EYE-tis) inflammation of the stomach and intestines

gastroenterology (gas-troh-en-ter-AHL-oh-jee) study and treatment of diseases of the gastrointestinal (GI) tract

gastroesophageal reflux disease (gas-troh-eh-soff-eh-jee-all REE-fluks dih-SEEZ) a set of symptoms resulting from a hiatal hernia that allows stomach (gastric) contents to flow back (reflux) into the esophagus; symptoms include heartburn or chest pain and coughing or choking during or just after a meal; also known as *GERD*

gastroesophageal sphincter (gas-troh-eh-soff-eh-jee-all SFINK-ter) a ring of smooth muscle around the opening of the stomach at the lower end of the esophagus that acts as a valve to allow food to enter the stomach but prevents stomach contents from moving back into the esophagus

gastrointestinal (GI) tract (gas-troh-in-TESS-tih-nul trakt) principal tubelike structure of the digestive system extending from mouth to anus—sometimes called the **alimentary canal**

gene (jean) one of many segments of a chromosome (DNA molecule); each gene contains the genetic code for synthesizing a protein molecule such as an enzyme or hormone

gene therapy (jeen THER-ah-pee) manipulation of genes to cure genetic problems; most forms of gene therapy have not yet been proven effective in humans

genetics (jeh-NET-iks) scientific study of heredity and the genetic code

genital ducts (jen-i-tall dukts) tubelike structures in the embryo that develop into reproductive organs; also applies to adult reproductive ducts

genitals *see* **external genitalia**

genitalia (jen-i-TAIL-yah) reproductive organs; *see* **external genitalia**

genome (JEE-nome) entire set of chromosomes in a cell; the *human genome* refers to the entire set of human chromosomes

genomics (jeh-NOM-iks) field of endeavor involving the analysis of the genetic code contained in the human or other species' genome

gerontology (jair-on-TAHL-oh-jee) study of the aging process

gestation period (jes-TAY-shun) the length of pregnancy, approximately 9 months in humans

ghrelin (GRAY-lin) hormone secreted by epithelial cells lining the stomach; ghrelin boosts appetite, slows metabolism, and reduces fat burning; may be involved in the development of obesity

gigantism (jye-GAN-tiz-em) a condition produced by hypersecretion of growth hormone during the early years of life; results in a child who grows to gigantic size

gingivitis (jin-ji-VYE-tis) inflammation of the gum (gingiva), often as a result of poor oral hygiene

gland secreting structure

glandular epithelium (GLAN-dyoo-lar ep-i-THEE-lee-um) cells that are specialized for secreting activity

glans the distal end of the shaft of the penis or clitoris

glaucoma (glaw-KOH-mah) disorder characterized by elevated pressure in the eye

glia (GLEE-ah) supporting cells of nervous tissue; *see* **neuroglia**

glioma (glye-OH-mah) one of the most common types of brain tumors

globulin (GLOB-yoo-lin) a type of plasma protein that includes antibodies

glomerulonephritis (gloh-mer-yoo-loh-neh-FRY-tis) inflammatory disease of the glomerular-capsular membranes of the kidney

glomerulus (gloh-MAIR-yoo-lus) compact cluster; for example, capillaries in the kidneys

glottis (GLOT-iss) the space between the vocal cords

glucagon (GLOO-kah-gon) hormone secreted by alpha cells of the pancreatic islets

glucocorticoid (GC) (gloo-koh-KOR-tih-koyd) hormone that influences food metabolism; secreted by the adrenal cortex

gluconeogenesis (gloo-koh-nee-oh-JEN-eh-sis) formulation of glucose or glycogen from protein or fat compounds

glucose (GLOO-kohs) monosaccharide or simple sugar; the principal blood sugar

gluteal (GLOO-tee-al) of or near the buttocks

gluteus maximus (GLOO-tee-us MAX-i-mus) major extensor of the thigh and also supports the torso in an erect position

glycerol (GLIS-er-ohl) product of fat digestion

glycogen (GLYE-koh-jen) polysaccharide made up of a chain of glucose (monosaccharide) molecules; animal starch

glycogen loading (GLYE-koh-jen LOHD-ing) *see* **carbohydrate loading**

glycogenesis (glye-koh-JEN-eh-sis) formation of glycogen from glucose or from other monosaccharides, fructose, or galactose

glycogenolysis (glye-koh-jeh-NOL-i-sis) hydrolysis of glycogen to glucose-6-phosphate or to glucose

glycolysis (glye-KOHL-i-sis) the first series of chemical reactions in glucose metabolism; changes glucose to pyruvic acid in a series of anaerobic reactions

glycosuria (glye-koh-SOO-ree-ah) glucose in the urine; a sign of diabetes mellitus

goblet cells (GOB-let sells) specialized cells found in simple columnar epithelium that produce mucus

goiter (GOY-ter) enlargement of the thyroid gland

Golgi apparatus (GOL-jee ap-ah-RA-tus) small sacs stacked on one another near the nucleus that makes carbohydrate compounds, combines them with protein molecules, and packages the product in a globule

golgi tendon receptors (GOL-jee TEN-don ree-SEP-tors) sensors that are responsible for proprioception

gonads (GO-nads) essential organs of reproduction: **testes** in males; **ovaries** in females

gout (gowt) abnormal condition in which excess uric acid is deposited in joints and other tissues as sodium urate crystals—the crystals produce inflammation or *gout arthritis*

graafian follicle (GRAH-fee-en FOL-i-kul) a mature ovum in its sac

gradient (GRAY-dee-ent) a slope or difference between two levels; for example, blood pressure gradient: a difference between the blood pressure in two different vessels

gram the unit of measure in the metric system on which mass is based (approximately 454 grams equals 1 pound)

granulosa cell (gran-yoo-LOH-sah sell) cell layer surrounding the oocyte

Graves disease (gravz dih-ZEEZ) inherited, possibly immune endocrine disorder characterized by hyperthyroidism accompanied by exophthalmos (protruding eyes)

gray matter (MAT-er) tissue in the central nervous system made up of cell bodies and unmyelinated axons and dendrites

greater omentum (GRAYT-er oh-MEN-tum) a pouchlike extension of the visceral peritoneum

greater vestibular glands (ves-TIB-yoo-lar) exocrine mucous glands located on either side of the vaginal outlet; also known as **Bartholin glands**; *see also* **lesser vestibular glands**

growth hormone (GH) (HOR-mohn) hormone secreted by the anterior pituitary gland that controls the rate of skeletal and visceral growth

guanine (GWAH-neen) one of several nitrogen-containing bases that make up nucleotides, which in turn make up nucleic acids such as DNA and RNA; in the cell, it can chemically bind to another nitrogenous base, cytosine (*C* or *c*), to form more a complex structure or in translating genetic codes; symbolized by the letter *G* or *g; see also* **cytosine, adenine, thymine, uracil**

gustatory cell (GUS-tah-tor-ee sell) cells of taste

gyrus (JYE-rus) (*pl.,* gyri) convoluted ridge

H

hair follicle (FOHL-i-kul) a small tube where hair growth occurs

hair papilla (pah-PIL-ah) a small, cap-shaped cluster of cells located at the base of the follicle where hair growth begins

hamstring muscle (HAM-string MUSS-el) powerful flexor of the hip made up of the semimembranosus, semitendinosus, and biceps femoris muscles

Haversian canal (hah-VER-shun kah-NAL) the central canal in the osteon (Haversian system) that contains a blood vessel; named for English physician Clopton Havers

Haversian system (hah-VER-shun SIS-tem) structural unit of compact bone tissue made up of concentric layers (lamellae) of hard bone matrix and bone cells (osteocytes); named for English physician Clopton Havers; also called **osteon**

health (helth) physical, mental, and social well-being; the absence of disease

heart block (hart blok) a blockage of impulse conduction from atria to ventricles so that the heart beats at a slower rate than normal

heart disease (hart dih-ZEEZ) any of a group of cardiac disorders that together constitute the leading cause of death in the United States

heart failure (hart FAYL-yoor) inability of the heart to pump returned blood sufficiently

heart murmur (hart MUR-mur) abnormal heart sound that may indicate valvular insufficiency (leaking) or stenosing (narrowing; blockage) of the valve

heartburn (HART-bern) esophageal pain caused by backflow of stomach acid into esophagus

heat exhaustion (heet eg-ZAWS-chun) condition caused by fluid loss resulting from activity of thermoregulatory mechanisms in a warm external environment

heat stroke (heet) life-threatening condition characterized by high body temperature; failure of thermoregulatory mechanisms to maintain homeostasis in a very warm external environment

Heberden nodes (HEB-er-den nohds) abnormal enlargements seen at the distal interphalangeal joints in osteoarthritis

Heimlich maneuver *see* **abdominal thrusts**

Helicobacter pylori (HEEL-i-koh-BAK-ter pye-LOH-ree) spiral-shaped bacterium known to be a major cause of gastric and duodenal ulcers

hematocrit (hee-MAT-oh-krit) volume percent of blood cells in whole blood

hematopoiesis (hee-mah-toh-poy-EE-sis) blood cell formation

hematopoietic tissue (hee-mah-toh-poy-ET-ik TISH-yoo) specialized connective tissue that is responsible for the formation of blood cells and lymphatic system cells; found in red bone marrow, spleen, tonsils, and lymph nodes

hematuria (hem-ah-TOO-ree-ah) symptom of blood in the urine, often the result of a renal or urinary disorder

hemiplegia (hem-ee-PLEE-jee-ah) paralysis (lack of voluntary muscle control) of one entire side of the body

hemodialysis (hee-moh-dye-AL-i-sis) use of dialysis to separate waste products from the blood

hemoglobin (hee-moh-GLOH-bin) iron-containing protein in red blood cells

hemolytic anemia (hee-moh-LIT-ik ah-NEE-mee-ah) any of a group of blood disorders characterized by deficient or abnormal hemoglobin that causes deformation and fragility of red blood cells (e.g., sickle-cell anemia, thalassemia)

hemophilia (hee-moh-FIL-ee-ah) any of a group of X-linked inherited blood clotting disorders caused by a failure to form clotting factors VIII, IX, or XI

hemorrhagic anemias (HEM-oh-raj-ick ah-NEEM-ee-ahs) group of conditions characterized by low oxygen-carrying capacity of blood; caused by decreased red blood cell (RBC) life span and/or increased rate of RBC destruction

hemorrhoid (HEM-eh-royd) varicose vein in the rectum; hemorrhoids are also called *piles*

hemothorax (hee-moh-THOH-raks) abnormal condition in which blood is present in the pleural space surrounding the lung, possibly causing collapse of the lung

Henle loop (HEN-lee loop) extension of the proximal tubule of the kidney; also called *nephron loop*

heparin (HEP-ah-rin) naturally occurring substance that inhibits formation of a blood clot; has been used as a drug to inhibit clotting

hepatic colic flexure (heh-PAT-ik KOHL-ik FLEK-sher) the bend between the ascending colon and the transverse colon

hepatic ducts (heh-PAT-ik dukts) drain bile out of the liver

hepatic portal circulation (heh-PAT-ik POR-tall ser-kyoo-LAY-shun) the route of blood flow through the liver

hepatic portal vein (heh-PAT-ik POR-tall vane) delivers blood directly from the gastrointestinal tract to the liver

hepatitis (hep-ah-TYT-is) inflammation of the liver due to viral or bacterial infection; injury; damage from alcohol, drugs, or other toxins; or other factors

herniated ("slipped") disk (HER-nee-ayt-ed) rupture of a fibrocartilage intervertebral disk that permits the pulpy core of the disk to push against the spinal cord or spinal nerve roots, causing pain

herpes zoster (HER-peez ZOS-ter) viral infection that affects the skin of a single dermatome; commonly known as *shingles*

hiatal hernia (hye-AYT-al HER-nee-ah) a bulging out (hernia) of the stomach through the opening (hiatus) of the diaphragm through which the esophagus normally passes; this condition may prevent the valve between the esophagus and stomach from closing, thus allowing stomach contents to flow back into the esophagus; *see also* **gastroesophageal reflux disease**

hiccup (HIK-up) involuntary spasmodic contraction of the diaphragm

hip the joint connecting the legs to the trunk

histamine chemical released by basophils and mast cells in allergic and inflammatory reactions; results in blood vessel vasodilation and bronchoconstriction

histogenesis (hiss-toh-JEN-eh-sis) formation of tissues from primary germ layers of embryo

hives *see* **urticaria**

Hodgkin disease (HOJ-kin dih-ZEEZ) type of lymphoma (malignant lymph tumor) characterized by painless swelling of lymph nodes in the neck, progressing to other regions

homeostasis (hoh-mee-oh-STAY-sis) relative uniformity of the normal body's internal environment

homeostatic mechanism (hoh-mee-oh-STAT-ik MEK-ah-niz-em) a system that maintains a constant environment enabling body cells to function effectively

hormone (HOR-mohn) substance secreted by an endocrine gland

human immunodeficiency virus (HIV) (HYOO-man i-myoo-no-deh-FISH-en-see VYE-rus) the retrovirus that causes acquired immunodeficiency syndrome (AIDS)

human lymphocyte antigen (HLA) (HYOO-man LIM-foh-site AN-tih-jen) type of self-antigen that the immune system uses to distinguish one's own tissue from that of a foreign entity

humerus (HYOO-mer-us) the second longest bone in the body; the long bone of the arm

humoral immunity (HYOO-mor-al i-MYOO-nih-tee) *see* **antibody-mediated immunity**

Huntington disease (HD) (HUNT-ing-tun dih-ZEEZ) degenerative, inherited brain disorder characterized by chorea (purposeless movements) progressing to severe dementia and death by age 55

hybridoma (hye-brid-OH-mah) fused or hybrid cells that continue to produce the same antibody as the original lymphocyte

hydrocele (HYE-droh-seel) abnormal accumulation of watery fluid, as can occur in the scrotum

hydrocephalus (hye-droh-SEF-ah-lus) abnormal accumulation of cerebrospinal fluid; "water on the brain"

hydrocortisone (hye-droh-KOR-tih-zohn) a hormone ordinarily secreted by the adrenal cortex as cortisol, but as hydrocortisol it is used as a drug to reduce inflammation or other immune functions; *see* **cortisol**

hydrogen (HYE-droh-jen) one of the chemical elements found in great quantity in the human body; symbolized by H, as in H_2O (water); may form ions such as H^+ (hydrogen ion) or OH^- (hydroxide ion)

hydrogen ion (HYE-droh-jen eye-on) found in water and water solutions; produces an acidic solution; H^+

hydrolysis (hye-DROHL-i-sis) chemical reaction in which water is added to a large molecule, causing it to break apart into smaller molecules

hydronephrosis (HYE-droh-neff-ROH-siss) pathological swelling or enlargement of renal pelvis or calyces caused by blockage of urine outflow

hydrostatic pressure (hye-droh-STAT-ik PRESH-ur) the force of a fluid pushing against some surface

hydroxide ion (hye-DROK-side eye-on) found in water and water solutions; produces an alkaline solution; OH^+

hydroxyurea (hye-DROK-see-yoo-REE-ah) an antineoplastic (antitumor) drug

hymen (HYE-men) Greek for "membrane"; mucous membrane that may partially or entirely occlude the vaginal outlet

hyperacidity (hye-per-ah-SID-i-tee) excessive secretion of acid; an important factor in the formation of ulcers

hypercalcemia (hye-per-kal-SEE-mee-ah) a condition in which harmful excesses of calcium are present in the blood

hypercholesterolemia (hye-per-koh-les-ter-ohl-EE-mee-ah) condition of high blood cholesterol content

hyperglycemia (hye-per-glye-SEE-mee-ah) higher than normal blood glucose concentration

hyperkalemia (hy-per-kal-EE-mee-ah) abnormally high blood potassium level

hypernatremia (hy-per-nah-TREE-mee-ah) abnormally high blood sodium level

hyperopia (hye-per-OH-pee-ah) refractive disorder of the eye caused by a shorter than normal eyeball; farsightedness

hyperplasia (hye-per-PLAY-zha) growth of an abnormally large number of cells at a local site, as in a neoplasm or tumor

hypersecretion (hye-per-seh-KREE-shun) too much of a substance is being secreted

hypersensitivity (hye-per-SEN-sih-tiv-i-tee) inappropriate or excessive response of the immune system

hypertension (hye-per-TEN-shun) abnormally high blood pressure

hyperthyroidism (hye-per-THYE-royd-iz-em) oversecretion of thyroid hormones, which increases metabolic rate resulting in loss of weight, increased appetite, and nervous irritability

hypertonic (hye-per-TON-ik) a solution containing a higher level of salt (NaCl) than is found in a living red blood cell (above 0.9% NaCl)

hypertrophy (hye-PER-troh-fee) increased size of a part caused by an increase in the size of its cells

hyperventilation (hye-per-ven-tih-LAY-shun) very rapid, deep respirations

hypervitaminosis (hye-per-vye-tah-mih-NO-sis) general name for any condition resulting from an abnormally high intake of vitamins

hypoalbuminemia (hye-poh-al-byoo-min-EE-mee-ah) condition of low albumin (protein) in the blood plasma; it often results from renal disorders or malnutrition; loss of plasma protein usually causes edema of the tissue spaces

hypocalcemia (hye-poh-kal-SEE-mee-ah) abnormally low blood calcium level

hypochondriac regions (hye-poh-KON-dree-ak REE-junz) the left and right upper regions of the abdominopelvic cavity, just under the lower part of the rib cartilage and on either side of the epigastric region; used when the abdominopelvic cavity is visualized as being subdivided into nine regions as in a tic-tac-toe grid

hypodermis (hye-poh-DER-mis) the loose ordinary (areolar) tissue just under the layers of skin and superficial to the muscles; made of loose connective tissue and fat: also called *subcutaneous tissue* or *superficial fascia*

hypogastric region (hye-poh-GAST-rik REE-jun) the central lower region of the abdominopelvic cavity, below the stomach and umbilicus (navel) and between the left and right iliac regions; used when the abdominopelvic cavity is visualized as being subdivided into nine regions as in a tic-tac-toe grid

hypoglycemia (hye-poh-glye-SEE-mee-ah) lower-than-normal blood glucose concentration

hypokalemia (hye-poh-kal-EE-mee-ah) abnormally low blood potassium level

hyponatremia (hye-poh-nah-TREE-mee-ah) abnormally low blood sodium level

hyposecretion (hye-poh-seh-KREE-shun) too little secretion of a substance

hypospadias (hye-poh-SPAY-dee-us) congenital defect in males characterized by opening of urethral meatus on underside of the glans or penile shaft

hypothalamus (hye-poh-THAL-ah-muss) portion of the floor and lateral wall of the third ventricle of the brain

hypothermia (hye-poh-THER-mee-ah) failure of thermoregulatory mechanisms to maintain homeostasis in a very cold external environment

hypothesis (hye-POTH-eh-sis) (*pl.*, hypotheses) a proposed explanation of an observed phenomenon

hypothyroidism (hye-poh-THYE-royd-iz-em) undersecretion of thyroid hormones; early in life results in cretinism; later in life results in myxedema

hypotonic (hye-poh-TON-ik) a solution containing a lower level of salt (NaCl) than is found in a living red blood cell (below 0.9% NaCl)

hypoventilation (hye-poh-ven-tih-LAY-shun) slow and shallow respirations

hypovitaminosis (hye-poh-VYTE-ah-min-oh-sis) condition of having too few vitamin molecules in the body for normal function

hypovolemic shock (hye-poh-voh-LEE-mik) circulatory failure (shock) caused by a drop in blood volume that causes blood pressure (and blood flow) to drop; literally "low volume" shock

hypoxia (hye-POCK-see-ah) abnormally low concentration of oxygen in the blood or tissue fluids

hysterectomy (hiss-teh-REK-toh-mee) surgical removal of the uterus

I

identical (monozygotic) twins birth of two siblings at the same time that have developed from a single zygote that splits into two offspring early during development; also called *monozygotic twins;* contrast with **fraternal (dizygotic) twins**

ideogram (ID-ee-oh-gram) a simple cartoon of a chromosome used in genomics to show the overall structure of the chromosome, including staining landmarks and the relative position of the centromere

idiopathic (id-ee-oh-PATH-ik) refers to a disease of undetermined cause

ileocecal valve (il-ee-oh-SEE-kal valv) the sphincter-like structure between the end of the small intestine and the beginning of the large intestine

ileum (IL-ee-um) the distal portion of the small intestine

iliac crest (IL-ee-ak krest) the superior edge of the ilium

iliac regions (ILL-ee-ak REE-junz) the left and right lower regions of the abdominopelvic cavity, near the iliac region of the pelvis and on either side of the hypogastric region; terminology used to describe the abdominopelvic cavity when it is visualized as being subdivided into nine regions as in a tic-tac-toe grid; also called *left and right inguinal regions*

iliopsoas (il-ee-oh-SO-ass) a flexor of the thigh and an important stabilizing muscle for posture

ilium (IL-ee-um) one of the three separate bones that fuse to form the os coxae or hip bone

immune deficiency (i-MYOON deh-FISH-en-see) general term for complete or relative failure of the immune system to defend the internal environment of the body

immune system (i-MYOON SIS-tem) the body's defense system against disease

immunization (i-myoo-nih-ZAY-shun) deliberate artificial exposure to disease to produce acquired immunity in the body

immunosuppressive drugs (i-myoo-no-soo-PRES-iv) compounds that suppress, or reduce, the capacity of the immune system; such drugs are sometimes used to prevent rejection of transplanted tissues

immunotherapy (im-yoo-no-THAYR-ah-pee) therapeutic technique that bolsters a person's immune system in an attempt to control a disease

impacted fracture (im-PAK-ted FRAK-chur) fracture in which bone fragments are driven into each other

impetigo (im-peh-TYE-go) a highly contagious bacterial skin infection that occurs most often in children

implantation (im-plan-TAY-shun) occurs when a fertilized ovum implants in the uterus

impotence (IM-poh-tense) failure to achieve erection of the penis, results in an inability to reproduce; also called *erectile dysfunction (ED)*

inborn immunity (IN-born i-MYOO-nih-tee) immunity to disease that is inherited

incisor (in-SYE-zor) refers to the front teeth, which are adapted for cutting

incompetent (cardiac) valves (in-KOM-peh-tent [KAR-dee-ak] valvs) cardiac valves that "leak," allowing some blood to flow back into the chamber from which it came

incomplete fracture (in-kom-PLEET FRAK-chur) bone fracture in which the bone fragments remain partially joined

incontinence (in-KON-tih-nens) condition in which an individual voids urine involuntarily

incubation (in-kyoo-BAY-shun) early, latent stage of an infection, during which an infection has begun but signs or symptoms have not yet developed

incus (IN-kus) the anvil, the middle ear bone that is shaped like an anvil

induced abortion (in-DOOST ah-BOR-shun) purposeful termination of a pregnancy before the fetus is able to survive outside the womb

infancy (IN-fan-see) refers to age range from birth to about 18 months of age

infant respiratory distress syndrome (IRDS) (IN-fant RES-pih-rah-toh-ree dih-STRESS SIN-drohm) leading cause of death in premature babies, caused by a lack of surfactant in the alveolar air sacs

infectious arthritis (in-FEK-shuss ahr-TRHYE-tiss) inflammation of joint tissues caused by a variety of pathogens (e.g., Lyme arthritis)

infectious mononucleosis (in-FEK-shuss MAHN-oh-NOO-klee-OH-sus) a viral (noncancerous) white blood cell (WBC) disorder common in young adults; characterized by leukocytosis of atypical lymphocytes and severe fatigue

inferior (in-FEER-ee-or) lower; opposite of **superior**

inferior vena cava (in-FEER-ee-or VEE-nah KAY-vah) one of two large veins carrying blood into the right atrium

infertility (in-fer-TIL-i-tee) lower-than-normal ability to reproduce

inflammation (in-flah-MAY-shun) group of responses to a tissue irritant marked by signs of redness, heat, swelling, and pain

inflammation mediators (in-flah-MAY-shun MEE-dee-ay-tors) chemicals (e.g., prostaglandins, histamine, kinins) released by irritated tissues that promote the events of the inflammation response

inflammatory exudate (in-FLAM-ah-toh-ree EKS-oo-dayt) fluid that accumulates in inflamed tissues as a result of increased permeability of blood vessels

inflammatory response (in-FLAM-ah-toh-ree ree-SPONS) nonspecific immune process produced in response to injury and resulting in redness, pain, heat, and swelling and promoting movement of white blood cells to the affected area

inguinal (ING-gwih-nal) of the groin

inguinal hernia (ING-gwih-nal HER-nee-ah) protrusion of abdominopelvic organs through the inguinal canal and into the scrotum

inhalation (in-hah-LAY-shun) breathing in; opposite of **exhalation,** or **expiration;** also called **inspiration**

inherited immunity (in-HAIR-i-ted i-MYOO-nih-tee) *see* **inborn immunity**

inhibiting hormone (in-HIB-i-ting HOR-mohn) hormone produced by the hypothalamus that slows the release of anterior pituitary hormones

inorganic compound (in-or-GAN-ik KOM-pownd) compound whose molecules do not contain carbon-carbon or carbon-hydrogen bonds

INR acronym for international normalized ratio

insertion (in-SER-shun) attachment of a muscle to the bone that it moves when contraction occurs (as distinguished from its origin)

inspiration (in-spih-RAY-shun) moving air into the lungs; opposite of **exhalation** or **expiration;** also referred to as **inhalation**

inspiratory muscle (in-SPY-rah-tor-ee MUSS-el) the muscles that increase the size of the thorax, including the diaphragm and external intercostals, and allow air to rush into the lungs

inspiratory reserve volume (IRV) (in-SPY-rah-tor-ee ree-SERV VOL-yoom) the amount of air that can be forcibly inspired over and above a normal respiration

insulin (IN-suh-lin) hormone secreted by the pancreatic islets

integument (in-TEG-yoo-ment) refers to the skin

integumentary system (in-teg-yoo-MEN-tar-ee SIS-tem) the skin; the largest and most important organ in the body

intercalated disks (in-TER-kah-lay-ted) connections that form unique dark bands between cardiac muscle fibers

intercostal muscle (in-ter-KOS-tal MUSS-el) the respiratory muscles located between the ribs

interferon (in-ter-FEER-on) small proteins produced by the immune system that inhibit virus multiplication

internal oblique (in-TER-nal oh-BLEEK) the middle layer of the anterolateral abdominal walls

internal respiration (in-TER-nal reh-spih-RAY-shun) the exchange of gases that occurs between the blood and cells of the body

international normalized ratio (INR) (in-ter-NASH-en-ul NOR-mah-lyzed RAY-shee-oh) method of expressing the **prothrombin time** (time it takes for a blood sample to clot after tissue thromboplastin [prothrombin activator] is added) based on international standards

interneuron (in-ter-NOO-ron) nerve that conducts impulses from a sensory neuron to a motor neuron

interphase (IN-ter-fayz) the phase immediately before the visible stages of cell division when the DNA of each chromosome replicates itself

interstitial cell (in-ter-STISH-al sell) small specialized cells in the testes that secrete the male sex hormone, testosterone

interstitial cell-stimulating hormone (ICSH) (in-ter-STISH-al sell STIM-yoo-lay-ting HOR-mohn) the previous name for luteinizing hormone in males; causes testes to develop and secrete testosterone

interstitial fluid (IF) (in-ter-STISH-al FLOO-id) fluid located in the microscopic spaces between the cells

intestine (in-TES-tin) the part of the digestive tract through which food remains pass after leaving the stomach; separated into two segments, the small and the large

intestinal gland (in-TES-tih-nal) thousands of glands found in the mucous membrane of the mucosa of the small intestines; secrete intestinal digestive juices

intracellular fluid (ICF) (in-trah-SELL-yoo-lar FLOO-id) fluid located within the cells; largest fluid compartment

in vitro (in VEE-troh) occuring in a test tube, dish, or other laboratory apparatus

involuntary muscle (in-VOL-un-tair-ee MUSS-el) smooth muscle that is not under conscious control and is found in organs such as the stomach and small intestine; cardiac muscle is also an involuntary type of muscle; *see* **smooth muscle** and **cardiac muscle**

involution (in-voh-LOO-shun) return of an organ to its normal size after an enlargement; also after retrograde or degenerative change

ion (EYE-on) electrically charged atom or group of atoms

ionic bond (eye-ON-ik) chemical bond formed by the positive-negative attraction between two ions

iris (EYE-riss) circular, pigmented ring of muscle tissue behind the cornea; the center of the iris is perforated by the pupil

iron-deficiency anemia (EYE-ern deh-FISH-en-see ah-NEE-mee-ah) condition in which there are inadequate levels of iron in the diet causing less hemoglobin to be produced; results in extreme fatigue

ischemia (is-KEE-mee-ah) reduced flow of blood to tissue resulting in impairment of cell function

ischium (IS-kee-um) one of three separate bones that forms the os coxae

islets of Langerhans *see* **pancreatic islets**

isoimmunity (eye-soh-i-MYOO-nih-tee) immune response to antigens of another human, as in transplanted (grafted) tissues; in some cases it is called *rejection syndrome*

isometric contraction (eye-soh-MET-rik) type of muscle contraction in which muscle does not shorten

isotonic contraction (eye-soh-TON-ik) type of muscle contraction that maintains uniform tension or pressure

isotope (EYE-soh-tope) atom with the same atomic number as another atom but with a different atomic weight (that is, with a different number of neutrons in the nucleus of the atom)

J

jaundice (JAWN-dis) abnormal yellowing of skin, mucous membranes, and white of eyes

jejunum (jeh-JOO-num) the middle third of the small intestine

joint capsule (joynt CAP-sool) fibrous connective tissue sleeve, lined with synovial membrane, that holds together opposing ends of articulating bones in a synovial joint

joint (joynt) *see* **articulation**

juvenile rheumatoid arthritis (JRA) (JOO-veh-neye-al ROO-mah-toyd arth-REYE-tis) form of rheumatoid arthritis affecting people under 16 years of age; it may affect bone development

juxtaglomerular (JG) apparatus (JUX-tah-gloh-mair-yoo-lar app-ah-RAT-us) complex of cells in nephron near the glomerulus and adjacent to distal tubule and afferent arteriole; secretes enzyme (renin) important in regulation of blood pressure

juxtamedullary nephron (JUX-tah-MED-oo-lair-ee NEFF-ron) nephron units with renal corpuscles located near junction between cortex and medullary layers of kidney; *see also* **nephron**

K

Kaposi sarcoma (KS) (KAH-poh-see sar-KOH-mah) a malignant neoplasm (cancer) of the skin characterized by purplish spots

karyotype (KAIR-ee-oh-type) ordered arrangement of photographs of chromosomes from a single cell used in genetic counseling to identify chromosomal disorders such as trisomy or monosomy

keloid (KEE-loyd) an unusually thick, irregularly shaped, progressively enlarging fibrous scar on the skin

keratin (KAIR-ah-tin) protein substance found in hair, nails, outer skin cells, and horny tissues

ketoacidosis (kee-toh-ass-i-DOH-sis) a condition of abnormally low blood pH (acidity) caused by the presence of an abnormally large number of ketone bodies or "keto acids" that are produced when fats are converted to forms of glucose to be used for cellular respiration; often occurs in those with diabetes mellitus, when it is more specifically called *diabetic ketoacidosis*; *see also* **acidosis**

ketone bodies (KEE-tohn) acidic products of lipid metabolism that may accumulate in blood of individuals with uncontrolled type 1 diabetes

kidney (KID-nee) organ that cleanses the blood of waste products produced continually by metabolism

kilocalorie (Kcal) (KIL-oh-kal-oh-ree) 1000 calories

kinesthesia (kin-es-THEE-zee-ah) "muscle sense"; that is, sense of position and movement of body parts

Klinefelter syndrome (KLINE-fel-ter SIN-drohm) genetic disorder caused by the presence of two or more X chromosomes in a male (typically trisomy XXY); characterized by long legs, enlarged breasts, low intelligence, small testes, sterility, chronic pulmonary disease

Krause end bulb (krows) mucous membrane receptor that detects sensations of touch and vibration; also known as **bulboid corpuscle**

Krebs cycle *see* **citric acid cycle**

Kupffer cell (KOOP-fer sell) phagocytic cell found in spaces between liver cells

kyphosis (kye-FOH-sis) abnormally exaggerated thoracic curvature of the vertebral column

L

labia majora (LAY-bee-ah mah-JO-rah) "large lips" of the vulva

labia minora (LAY-bee-ah mih-NO-rah) "small lips" of the vulva

labor (LAY-bor) the process that results in the birth of the baby

lacrimal gland (LAK-rih-mall) gland that produces tears; one gland located in the upper lateral portion of each eye orbit

lacteal (LAK-tee-al) a lymphatic vessel located in each villus of the intestine; serves to absorb fat materials from the chyme passing through the small intestine

lactiferous duct (lak-TIF-er-us dukt) the duct that drains the grapelike cluster of milk-secreting glands in the breast

lactogenic hormone (lak-toh-JEN-ik HOR-mohn) *see* prolactin

lactose intolerance (LAK-tose in-TOL-er-ans) lack of the enzyme lactase, resulting in an inability to digest lactose (a disaccharide present in milk and dairy products)

lacuna (lah-KOO-nah) (*pl.,* lacunae) space or cavity; for example, lacunae in bone contain bone cells

lambdoidal suture (LAM-doyd-al SOO-chur) the immovable joint formed by the parietal and occipital bones

lamella (lah-MEL-ah) (*pl.,* lamellae) thin layer, as of bone

lanugo (lah-NOO-go) the extremely fine and soft hair found on a newborn infant

laparoscope (LAP-ah-roh-skope) specialized optical viewing tube

large intestine (in-TESS-tin) part of GI tract that includes cecum, ascending, transverse, descending and sigmoid colons, rectum, and anal canal

laryngitis (lar-in-JYE-tis) inflammation of the mucous tissues of the larynx (voice box)

laryngopharynx (lah-ring-go-FAIR-inks) the lowest part of the pharynx

larynx (LAIR-inks) the voice box located just below the pharynx; the largest piece of cartilage making up the larynx is the thyroid cartilage, commonly known as the *Adam's apple*

laser-assisted in situ keratomileusis (LASIK) (LAY-zer ah-SIS-ted in SYE-too kair-at-oh-mill-YOO-sis) refractory eye surgery using a microkeratome to cut a corneal cap, which is replaced after an excimer laser is used to vaporize and reshape underlying corneal tissue

laser therapy (LAY-zer THAYR-ah-pee) use of laser (intense beams of light) to destroy a tumor, abnormal tissue, damaged tissue, or scars

laser thermal keratoplasty (LTK) (LAY-zer THER-mull kair-AT-oh-plast-ee) refractory eye surgery employing ultrashort bursts (3 seconds) of laser energy to reshape the cornea

lateral (LAT-er-all) of or toward the side; opposite of medial

lateral longitudinal arch (LAT-er-all lawnj-i-TOOD-in-all) outer lengthwise (anteroposterior) support structure of the foot

latissimus dorsi (lah-TIS-i-muss DOR-sye) an extensor of the upper arm

law a scientific law is a theory, or explanation, of a scientific principle that is based on experimentation results and supported by scientists who have an extraordinarily high degree of confidence in its validity

lens (lenz) the refracting mechanism of the eye that is located directly behind the pupil

leptin (LEHP-tin) hormone, secreted by fat-storing cells, that regulates how hungry or full we feel and how fat is metabolized by the body

lesion (LEE-zhun) any objective abnormality in a body structure

lesser vestibular glands (ves-TIB-yoo-lar) exocrine mucus glands located on either side of the urinary outlet in women; *see also* **greater vestibular glands**

leukemia (loo-KEE-mee-ah) blood cancer characterized by an increase in white blood cells

leukocyte (LOO-koh-syte) white blood cells

leukocytosis (loo-koh-sye-TOH-sis) abnormally high white blood cell numbers in the blood

leukopenia (loo-koh-PEE-nee-ah) abnormally low white blood cell numbers in the blood

leukoplakia (loo-koh-PLAY-kee-ah) white patches in the mouth, commonly seen in chronic cigarette smokers; may lead to mouth cancer

leukorrhea (loo-koh-REE-ah) whitish discharge from the urogenital tract

levodopa (LEV-oh-doh-pah) chemical manufactured by the brain cells and then converted into the neurotransmitter dopamine; has been used to treat disorders involving dopamine deficiencies such as Parkinson disease; also called *L-dopa* (el DOH-pah)

ligament (LIG-ah-ment) bond or band connecting two objects; in anatomy, a band of white fibrous tissue connecting bones

limbic system (LIM-bik) a collection of various small regions of the brain that act together to produce emotion and emotional response; sometimes called "the emotional brain"

linear fracture (LIN-ee-ar FRAK-chur) bone fracture characterized by a fracture line that is parallel to the bone's long axis

lingual tonsil *see* **tonsils**

lipase (LYE-payse) fat-digesting enzymes

lipid (LIP-id) organic molecule usually composed of glycerol and fatty acid units; types include triglycerides, phospholipids, and cholesterol; a fat, wax, or oil

lipoma (lip-OH-mah) benign tumor of adipose (fat) tissue

lithotriptor (LITH-oh-trip-tor) a specialized ultrasound generator that is used to pulverize kidney stones

liver glycogenolysis (LIV-er glye-koh-jeh-NOL-i-sis) chemical process by which liver glycogen is converted to glucose

lobectomy (loh-BEK-toh-mee) surgical removal of a single lobe of an organ, as in the removal of one lobe of a lung

lock-and-key model (lok and kee MAHD-el) concept that explains how molecules react when they fit together in a complementary way in the same manner that a key fits into a lock to cause the lock to open or close; the analogy is often used to explain the action of hormones, enzymes, and other biological molecules

longitudinal arch (lon-jih-TOO-dih-nal) two arches, the medial and lateral, that extend lengthwise in the foot

loop of Henle (loop of HEN-lee) *see* **Henle loop**

lordosis (lor-DOH-sis) abnormally exaggerated lumbar curvature of the vertebral column

lower esophageal sphincter (ee-SOFF-ah-JEE-ull SFINK-ter) ring of muscular tissue (sphincter) located between terminal esophagus and stomach

lumbar (LUM-bar) lower back, between the ribs and pelvis

lumbar puncture (LUM-bar PUNK-chur) when some cerebrospinal fluid is withdrawn from the subarachnoid space in the lumbar region of the spinal cord

lumbar regions (LUM-bar REE-junz) the left and right middle regions of the abdominopelvic cavity, near the lumbar area of the vertebral column and on either side of the umbilical region; terminology used when the abdominopelvic cavity is visualized as being subdivided into nine regions as in a tic-tac-toe grid

lumen (LOO-men) the hollow space within a tube

lung organ of respiration; the right lung has three lobes and the left lung has two lobes

lunula (LOO-nyoo-lah) crescent-shaped white area under the proximal nail bed

luteinization (loo-tee-in-i-ZAY-shun) the process of development of a corpus luteum (golden body) in the ovary after an ovum is released from the follicle; stimulated by the action of luteinizing hormone (LH) from the anterior pituitary

luteinizing hormone (LH) (loo-tee-in-EYE-zing HOR-mohn) anterior pituitary hormone that stimulates the development of a corpus luteum (literally "yellow body") that secretes hormones at the surface of the ovary after a follicle has released its ovum; a tropic hormone also known as *LH*

lymph (limf) specialized fluid formed in the tissue spaces that returns excess fluid and protein molecules to the blood via lymphatic vessels

lymph node (limf) performs biological filtration of lymph on its way to the circulatory system

lymph nodule (limf NOD-yool) is a mass of lymphoid tissue (developing white blood cells) within a lymph node or making up a patch of lymph nodules (as in the tonsils)

lymphadenitis (lim-FAD-in-eye-tiss) inflammation of a lymph node, usually caused by a bacterial infection or occasionally a neoplasm (benign or cancerous), and characterized by swelling and tenderness

lymphangiogram (lim-FAN-jee-oh-gram) radiograph (x-ray) of a part of the lymphatic network, which is produced by injecting a special dye that is opaque to x-rays into the soft tissues drained by the lymphatic network

lymphangitis (lim-fan-JYE-tis) inflammation of lymph vessels, usually caused by infection, characterized by fine red streaks extending from the site of infection; may progress to septicemia (blood infection)

lymphatic capillaries (lim-FAT-ik CAP-i-lair-ees) tiny, blind-ended tubes distributed in the tissue spaces

lymphatic duct (lim-FAT-ik dukt) terminal vessel into which lymphatic vessels empty lymph; the duct then empties the lymph into the circulatory system

lymphatic system (lim-FAT-ik SIS-tem) a system that plays a critical role in the functioning of the immune system, moves fluids and large molecules from the tissue spaces and fat-related nutrients from the digestive system to the blood

lymphatic tissue (lim-FAT-ik TISH-yoo) tissue that is responsible for manufacturing lymphocytes and monocytes; found mostly in the lymph nodes, thymus, and spleen

lymphatic vessels (lim-FAT-ik VES-els) vessels that carry lymph to its eventual return to the circulatory system

lymphedema (lim-feh-DEE-mah) swelling (edema) of tissues caused by partial or total blockage of the lymph vessels that drain the affected tissue

lymphocyte (LIM-foh-sytes) one type of white blood cell

lymphoid neoplasm (LIM-foyd NEE-oh-plaz-em) abnormal proliferation of lymphoid tissue or lymphoid precursor cells often associated with cancerous transformation

lymphoma (lim-FOH-mah) cancer of lymphatic tissue

lyse (lize) disintegration of a cell

lysosome (LYE-so-sohm) membranous organelles containing various enzymes that can dissolve most cellular compounds; thus called *digestive bags* or *suicide bags* of cells

M

macrophage (MAK-roh-fayje) phagocytic cells in the immune system

macula lutea (MAK-yoo-lah LOO-tee-ah) yellowish area near center of retina filled with cones permitting acute image formation and color vision

macular degeneration (MAK-yoo-lahr dee-jen-er-AY-shun) progressive deterioration of macula lutea of retina causing loss of central visual field

macule (MAK-yool) a flat skin lesion distinguished from the surrounding tissue by a difference in coloration

mad cow disease *see* **bovine spongiform encephalopathy**

magnetic resonance imaging (MRI) (mag-NET-ik REZ-oh-nans IM-ah-jing) scanning technique that uses a magnetic field to induce tissues to emit radio waves that can be used by computer to construct a sectional view of a patient's body

malabsorption syndrome (mal-ab-SORP-shun SIN-drohm) group of symptoms associated with the failure to absorb food properly: anorexia, ascites, cramps, anemia, fatigue

male erectile dysfunction (ED) (ee-REK-tyl dis-FUNK-shun) disorder in which the penis fails to become erect during the male sexual response, usually due to a lack of relaxation in smooth muscles in the wall of blood vessels in the penis; the drug Viagra (sildenafil) treats ED by promoting the same response in the penis as NO (nitric acid), which relaxes smooth muscles in the vessel walls

malignant (mah-LIG-nant) refers to a tumor or neoplasm that is capable of metastasizing or spreading to new tissues (i.e., cancer)

malignant hyperthermia (MH) (mah-LIG-nant hye-per-THERM-ee-ah) inherited condition characterized by an abnormally increased body temperature (hyperthermia) and muscle rigidity when a person is exposed to certain anesthetics (e.g., succinylcholine)

malleus (MAL-ee-us) hammer; the tiny middle ear bone that is shaped like a hammer

malnutrition (mal-noo-TRISH-un) insufficient or imbalanced intake of nutrients, often causing any of a variety of diseases

malocclusion (MAL-oh-clew-zhun) abnormal contact between the teeth of the upper and lower jaw

mammary gland (MAM-ar-ee) breasts; classified as external accessory sex organs in females

masseter (mass-EET-er) large muscle of the cheek, used to lift the lower jaw (mandible) and thus provide chewing movement

mast cells immune system cells (related to basophils) that secrete histamine and other inflammatory chemicals

mastication (mass-tih-KAY-shun) chewing

mastitis (mass-TYE-tis) inflammation or infection of the breast

mastoiditis (mass-toyd-EYE-tis) inflammation of the air cells within the mastoid portion of the temporal bone; usually caused by infection

matrix (MAY-triks) the intracellular substance of a tissue; for example, the matrix of bone is calcified, whereas that of blood is liquid

matter any substance that occupies space and has mass

mature follicle (mah-CHUR FOL-li-kul) *see* **graafian follicle**

maximum oxygen consumption (VO$_{2max}$) (MAX-i-mum OKS-i-jen kon-SUMP-shun) the maximum amount of oxygen taken up by the lungs, transported to the tissues, and used to do work

mechanoreceptor (mek-an-oh-ree-SEP-tor) receptors that are mechanical in nature; for example, equilibrium and balance sensors in the ears

medial (MEE-dee-al) of or toward the middle; opposite of lateral

medial longitudinal arch (MEE-dee-all lawnj-i-TOOD-in-all) inner lengthwise (anteroposterior) support structure of the foot

mediastinum (mee-dee-ass-TIH-num) a subdivision in the midportion of the thoracic cavity

medulla (meh-DUL-ah) Latin for "marrow"; the inner portion of an organ in contrast to the outer portion or cortex

mvedulla oblongata (meh-DUL-ah ob-long-GAH-tah) the lowest part of the brainstem; an enlarged extension of the spinal cord; the vital centers are located within this area

medullary cavity (med-OO-lair-ee KAV-i-tee) hollow area inside the diaphysis of the bone that contains yellow bone marrow

meiosis (my-OH-sis) nuclear division in which the number of chromosomes are reduced to half their original number; produces gametes

Meissner corpuscle (MEYES-ner KOR-pus-ul) a sensory receptor located in the skin close to the surface that detects light touch; also known as **tactile corpuscle**

melanin (MEL-ah-nin) brown skin pigment

melanocyte (MEL-ah-no-syte) specialized cells in the pigment layer that produce melanin

melanocyte-stimulating hormone (MSH) (MEL-ah-no-syte STIM-yoo-lay-ting HOR-mohn) responsible for a rapid increase in the synthesis and dispersion of melanin granules in specialized skin cells

melanoma (mel-ah-NO-mah) a malignant neoplasm (cancer) of the pigment-producing cells of the skin (melanocytes); also called *malignant melanoma*

melatonin (mel-ah-TOH-nin) important hormone produced by the pineal gland; believed to regulate the onset of puberty and the menstrual cycle; also referred to as the *third eye* because it responds to levels of light and is thought to be involved with the body's internal clock

membrane (MEM-brane) thin layer or sheet

membranous labyrinth (MEM-brah-nus LAB-i-rinth) a membranous sac that follows the shape of the bony labyrinth and is filled with endolymph

memory cell (MEM-oh-ree sell) cell that remains in reserve in the lymph nodes until its ability to secrete antibodies is needed

menarche (meh-NAR-kee) beginnings of the menstrual function

Ménière disease (men-ee-AIR dih ZEEZ) chronic inner ear disorder characterized by tinnitus, progressive nerve deafness, and vertigo

meninges (meh-NIN-jeez) fluid-containing membranes surrounding the brain and spinal cord

meningitis (men-in-JYE-tis) inflammation of the meninges caused by a variety of factors including bacterial infection, mycosis, viral infection, and tumors

menopause (MEN-oh-pawz) termination of menstrual cycles

menses (MEN-seez) menstrual flow

menstrual cycle (MEN-stroo-all SYE-kul) the cyclical changes in the uterine lining

mesentery (MEZ-en-tair-ee) a large double fold of peritoneal tissue that anchors the loops of the digestive tract to the posterior wall of the abdominal cavity

mesoderm (MEZ-oh-derm) the middle layer of the primary germ layers

messenger RNA (mRNA) (MES-en-jer R N A) a duplicate copy of a gene sequence on the DNA that passes from the nucleus to the cytoplasm

metabolic acidosis (met-ah-BOL-ik ass-i-DOH-sis) a disturbance affecting the bicarbonate element of the bicarbonate-carbonic acid buffer pair; bicarbonate deficit

metabolic alkalosis (met-ah-BOL-ik al-kah-LOH-sis) disturbance affecting the bicarbonate element of the bicarbonate-carbonic acid buffer pair; bicarbonate excess

metabolism (meh-TAB-oh-liz-em) complex process by which food is used by a living organism

metacarpal (met-ah-KAR-pal) the part of the hand between the wrist and fingers

metaphase (MET-ah-fayz) second stage of mitosis, during which the nuclear membrane and nucleolus disappear

metastasis (meh-TASS-tah-sis) process by which malignant tumor cells fall off a primary tumor, then migrate to a new tissue to colonize a secondary tumor

metatarsal arch (met-ah-TAR-sal) the arch that extends across the ball of the foot; also called the *transverse arch*

metatarsals (met-ah-TAR-salz) the five bones that form the foot; articulate with tarsal bones proximally and the first row of toe phalanges distally

meter (MEE-ter) a measure of length in the metric system; equal to about 39.5 inches

microbe (MY-krobe) refers to any microscopic organism

microcephaly (my-kroh-SEF-ah-lee) a congenital abnormality in which an infant is born with a small head

microglia (my-KROG-lee-ah) one type of connective tissue found in the brain and spinal cord

micron (MY-kron) measurement that equals 1/1000 millimeter; 1/25,000 inch

microvilli (my-kroh-VIL-ee) brushlike border made up of epithelial cells found on each villus in the small intestine and other areas of the body; increases the surface area (as for absorption of nutrients)

micturition (mik-too-RISH-un) urination, voiding

midbrain (MID-brain) one of the three parts of the brainstem

middle ear (MID-ul eer) a tiny and very thin epithelium-lined cavity in the temporal bone that houses the ossicles; in the middle ear, sound waves are amplified

midsagittal plane (mid-SAJ-i-tal) a cut or plane that divides the body or any of its parts into two equal halves

minerals (MIN-er-als) inorganic elements or salts found naturally in the earth that are vital to the proper functioning of the body

mineralocorticoid (MC) (min-er-al-oh-KOR-tih-koyd) hormone that influences mineral salt metabolism; secreted by adrenal cortex; aldosterone is the chief mineralocorticoid

mitochondria (my-toh-KON-dree-ah) threadlike structures

mitochondrial DNA (my-toh-KON-dree-al D N A) DNA located in the mitochondria of each cell, constituting a single chromosome; also called *mtDNA* or *mDNA*

mitosis (my-TOH-sis) indirect cell division involving complex changes in the nucleus

mitral valve (MY-tral valv) heart valve located between the left atrium and ventricle: also known as the **bicuspid valve**

mitral valve prolapse (MVP) (MY-tral valv PROH-laps) condition in which the bicuspid (mitral) valve extends into the left atrium, causing incompetence (leaking) of the valve

molar *see* **tricuspid**

mold large fungus (compared to a yeast, which is a small fungus)

molecule (MOL-eh-kyool) particle of matter composed of one or more smaller units called **atoms**

monoclonal antibody (mon-oh-KLONE-al AN-tih-bod-ee) specific antibody produced from a population of identical cells

monocyte (MON-oh-syte) largest type of white blood cell; a type of agranular leukocyte; often involved in phagocytosis of abnormal cells or particles

mononucleosis (MAHN-oh-NOO-klee-OH-sis) condition characterized by an increase in the number of mononuclear leukocytes; can be caused by the Epstein-Barr virus (EBV); also commonly called *"mono"*

monosaccharide (mon-oh-SAK-ah-ryde) a "simple sugar" composed of only a single saccharide group ($C_6H_{12}O_6$); examples include glucose, fructose, galactose

monosomy (MON-oh-so-mee) abnormal genetic condition in which cells have only one chromosome where there should be a pair; usually caused by nondisjunction (failure of chromosome pairs to separate) during gamete production

monozygotic twins (mon-oh-zye-GOT-ik twinz) twins that develop from a single zygote that has split during early development into two separate, but genetically identical, offspring; *see also* **identical twins**

mons pubis (monz PYOO-bis) skin-covered pad of fat over the symphysis pubis in the female

morbidity (mor-BID-i-tee) illness or disease; the rate of incidence of a specific illness or disease in a specific population

mortality (mor-TAL-i-tee) death; the rate of deaths caused by a specific disease within a specific population

morula (MOR-yoo-lah) a solid mass of cells formed by the divisions of a fertilized egg

motor neuron (MOH-tor NOO-ron) neuron that transmits nerve impulses from the brain and spinal cord to muscles and glandular epithelial tissues

motor unit (MOH-tor YOO-nit) a single motor neuron along with the muscle cells it innervates

mucocutaneous junction (myoo-koh-kyoo-TAY-nee-us JUNK-shun) the transitional area where the skin and mucous membrane meet

mucosa (myoo-KOH-sah) mucous membrane

mucous membrane (MYOO-kus MEM-brane) epithelial membranes that line body surfaces opening directly to the exterior and secrete a thick, slippery material called **mucus**

mucus (MYOO-kus) thick, slippery material that is secreted by the mucous membrane and keeps the membrane moist

multiple myeloma (MUL-tih-pul my-LOH-mah) cancer of plasma cells

multiple neurofibromatosis (MUL-tih-pul noo-roh-fye-broh-mah-TOH-sis) disorder characterized by multiple, sometimes disfiguring, benign tumors of the Schwann cells (neuroglia) that surround nerve fibers

multiple sclerosis (MS) (MUL-tih-pul skleh-ROH-sis) the most common primary disease of the central nervous system; a myelin disorder

muscle fiber (MUSS-el FYE-ber) the specialized contractile cells of muscle tissue that are grouped together and arranged in a highly organized way

muscle strain (MUSS-el strayne) muscle injury resulting from overexertion or trauma and involving overstretching or tearing of muscle fibers

muscular dystrophy (MUSS-kyoo-lar DIS-troh-fee) a group of muscle disorders characterized by atrophy of skeletal muscle without nerve involvement; Duchenne muscular dystrophy (DMD) is the most common type

muscular system (MUSS-kyoo-lar SIS-tem) the muscles of the body

muscularis (muss-kyoo-LAIR-is) two layers of muscle surrounding the digestive tube that produce wavelike, rhythmic contractions called **peristalsis**, which move food material

mutagen (MYOO-tah-jen) agent capable of causing mutation (alteration) of DNA

myalgia (my-AL-jee-ah) general term referring to the symptom of pain in muscle tissue

myasthenia gravis (my-ass-THEE-nee-ah GRAH-vis) autoimmune muscle disorder characterized by progressive weakness and chronic fatigue

mycotic infection (my-KOT-ik in-FEK-shun) fungal infection

myelin (MY-eh-lin) lipoid substance found in the myelin sheath around some nerve fibers

myelinated fiber (MY-eh-lih-nay-ted FYE-ber) axons outside the central nervous system that are surrounded by a segmented wrapping of myelin

myeloid (MY-eh-loyd) pertaining to bone marrow

myeloid neoplasm (MY-eh-loyd NEE-oh-plaz-em) abnormal proliferation of myeloid tissue or myeloid precursor cells often associated with cancerous transformation

myeloma (my-eh-LOH-mah) malignant tumor of bone marrow

myocardial infarction (my-oh-KAR-dee-al in-FARK-shun) death of cardiac muscle cells resulting from inadequate blood supply, as in coronary thrombosis

myocardium (my-oh-KAR-dee-um) muscle of the heart

myofilaments (my-oh-FIL-ah-ments) ultramicroscopic, threadlike structures found in myofibrils; two types: *thick* and *thin*

myoglobin (MY-oh-GLO-bin) a red, oxygen-storing protein pigment similar to hemoglobin found in muscle fibers

myoma (my-OH-mah) benign tumor of smooth muscle commonly occurring in the uterine wall; *see also* **fibromyoma**

myometrium (my-oh-MEE-tree-um) muscle layer in the uterus

myopathy (my-OP-ah-thee) general term referring to any muscle disease

myopia (my-OH-pee-ah) refractive disorder of the eye caused by an elongated eyeball; nearsightedness

myosin (MY-oh-syn) contractile protein found in the thick myofilaments of skeletal muscle

myositis (my-oh-SYE-tis) general term referring to muscle inflammation, as in infection or injury

myxedema (mik-seh-DEE-mah) condition caused by deficiency of thyroid hormone in adults

N

nail body (BOD-ee) the visible part of the nail

nail root the part of the nail hidden by the cuticle

nanometer (NAN-oh-mee-ter) a measure of length in the metric system; one billionth of a meter

nares (NAY-reez) nostrils

nasal cavity (NAY-zal KAV-i-tee) the moist, warm cavities lined by mucosa located just beyond the nostrils; olfactory receptors are located in the mucosa

nasal polyp (NAY-zal PAH-lip) painless, non-cancerous tissue growths that project from nasal mucosa

nasal septum (NAY-zal SEP-tum) a partition that separates the right and left nasal cavities

nasopharynx (nay-zoh-FAIR-inks) the uppermost portion of the tube just behind the nasal cavities

nausea (NAW-zee-ah) unpleasant sensation of the gastrointestinal tract that commonly precedes the urge to vomit; upset stomach

necrosis (neh-KROH-sis) death of cells in a tissue, often resulting from ischemia (reduced blood flow)

negative feedback (NEG-ah-tiv FEED-bak) homeostatic control system in which information feeding back to the control center causes the level of a variable to be changed in the direction opposite to that of the initial stimulus

nematode (NEM-ah-tohd) roundworms—large parasites capable of infesting humans

neonatal period (nee-oh-NAY-tal PEER-ee-od) stage of early human development that corresponds to approximately the first 4 weeks after birth

neonate (NEE-oh-nayt) another name for an infant during the first 4 weeks after birth; *see* **neonatal period**

neonatology (nee-oh-nay-TOL-oh-jee) diagnosis and treatment of disorders of the newborn infant

neoplasm (NEE-oh-plaz-em) an abnormal mass of proliferating cells that may be either benign or malignant

nephritis (neh-FRY-tis) general term referring to inflammatory or infectious conditions of renal (kidney) tissue

nephron (NEF-ron) anatomical and functional unit of the kidney, consisting of the renal corpuscle and the renal tubule

nephropathy (neh-FROP-ah-thee) kidney disease

nephrotic syndrome (neh-FROT-ik SIN-drohm) group of symptoms and signs that often accompany glomerular disorders of the kidney: proteinuria, hypoalbuminemia, and edema

nerve (nerv) collection of nerve fibers

nerve impulse (nerv IM-puls) signals that carry information along the nerves

nervous tissue (NER-vus TISH-yoo) consists of neurons and neuroglia and provides rapid communication and control of body function

neuralgia (noo-RAL-jee-ah) general term referring to nerve pain

neurilemma (noo-rih-LEM-mah) nerve sheath

neuritis (noo-RYE-tis) general term referring to nerve inflammation

neuroblastoma (noo-roh-blas-TOH-mah) malignant tumor of sympathetic nervous tissue, found mainly in young children

neurogenic bladder (noo-roh-JEN-ik BLAD-der) condition in which the nervous control of the urinary bladder is impaired, causing abnormal or obstructed flow of urine from the body

neurogenic shock (noo-roh-JEN-ik shock) circulatory failure (shock) caused by a nerve condition that relaxes (dilates) blood vessels and thus reduces blood flow; literally "nerve-caused" shock

neuroglia (noo-ROG-lee-ah) supporting cells of nervous tissue; also called simply *glia*

neurohypophysis (noo-roh-hye-POFF-i-sis) posterior pituitary gland

neuroma (noo-ROH-mah) general term for nervous tissue tumors

neuromuscular junction (noo-roh-MUSS-kyoo-lar JUNK-shun) the point of contact between the nerve endings and muscle fibers

neuron (NOO-ron) nerve cell, including its processes (axons and dendrites)

neurotransmitter (noo-roh-trans-MIT-ter) chemicals by which neurons communicate

neutron (NOO-tron) electrically neutral particle within the nucleus of an atom

neutrophil (NOO-troh-fil) white blood cell that stains readily with neutral dyes

nevus (NEE-vus) small, pigmented benign tumor of the skin (e.g., a mole)

nitric oxide (NO) (NYE-trik AWK-side) small-molecule neurotransmitter

nitrogen (NYE-troh-jen) one of the chemical elements found in great quantity in the human body, especially in nucleic acids (DNA, RNA), proteins and amino acids; symbolized by N, as in NH_3 (ammonia)

Nobel prize (no-BELL) international award created by the late Alfred Nobel and awarded each year to up to three recipients in each of several categories such as chemistry, physics, and medicine or physiology (each Nobel laureate [prizewinner] receives a diploma, a medal, and a cash prize at a ceremony in Stockholm, Sweden)

nodes of Ranvier (rahn-vee-AY) indentations found between adjacent Schwann cells

nodule (NOD-yool) *see* **lymph nodule**

nonelectrolyte (non-ee-LEK-troh-lyte) compound that does not dissociate into ions in solution; for example, glucose

non-Hodgkin lymphoma (non-HOJ-kin lim-FOH-mah) type of lymphoma (malignant lymph tumor) characterized by swelling of lymph nodes and progressing to other areas

nonsteroid hormone (nahn-STAYR-oyd HOR-mohn) general type of hormone that does not have the lipid steroid structure (derived from cholesterol) but is instead a protein or protein derivative; also sometimes called **protein hormone**

norepinephrine (NR) (nor-ep-i-NEF-rin) hormone secreted by adrenal medulla; released by sympathetic nervous system; also known as *noradrenaline*

normal saline (SAY-leen) sodium chloride solution isotonic with body fluids

nose respiratory organ

nosocomial infection (no-zoh-KOAM-ee-al in-FEK-shun) infection that begins in the hospital or clinic

NSAID (EN-sayd) acronym for nonsteroidal antiinflammatory drug, the term is applied to aspirin, ibuprofen, acetaminophen, and many other antiinflammatory agents that do not contain steroid hormones or their derivatives

nuclear envelope (NOO-klee-ar AHN-vel-ohp) the boundary of a cell's nucleus, made up of a double layer of cellular membrane

nuclear membrane (NOO-klee-ar MEM-brane) membrane that surrounds the cell nucleus

nucleic acids (noo-KLAY-ik ASS-ids) the two nucleic acids are ribonucleic acid (RNA), found in the cytoplasm, and deoxyribonucleic acid (DNA), found in the nucleus and mitochondrion; made up of units called **nucleotides** that each include a phosphate, a five-carbon sugar, and a nitrogen base

nucleolus (noo-KLEE-oh-lus) intercellular structure critical to protein formation because it "programs" the formation of ribosomes in the nucleus

nucleoplasm (NOO-klee-oh-plaz-em) a special type of cytoplasm found in the nucleus

nucleotide (NOO-klee-oh-tyde) molecule that connects to other nucleotides to form a nucleic acid such as DNA or RNA; each nucleotide has three parts: a phosphate group, a sugar (ribose or deoxyribose) and a nitrogenous base (adenine, thymine [or uracil], guanine, or cytosine)

nucleus (NOO-klee-us) spherical structure within a cell; a group of neuron cell bodies in the brain or spinal cord; central core of the atom, made up of protons and (sometimes) neutrons

nutrition (noo-TRIH-shun) food, vitamins, and minerals that are ingested and assimilated into the body

nyctalopia (nik-tah-LOH-pee-ah) condition caused by retinal degeneration or avitaminosis A and characterized by the relative inability to see in dim light; night blindness

O

obesity (oh-BEES-i-tee) condition characterized by abnormally high proportion of body fat

oblique fracture (oh-BLEEK FRAK-chur) bone fracture characterized by a fracture line that is diagonal to the long axis of the broken bone

occipital (ok-SIP-it-al) pertaining to the area at the back of the lower skull

old age *see* **senescence**

olecranal (oh-LEK-reh-nal) pertaining to olecranon (back of elbow)

olecranon fossa (oh-LEK-rah-nohn FOSS-ah) a large depression on the posterior surface of the humerus

olecranon process (oh-LEK-rah-nohn PROSS-es) the large bony process of the ulna; commonly referred to as the tip of the elbow

olfaction (ohl-FAK-shun) sense of smell

olfactory receptor (ohl-FAK-tor-ee ree-SEP-tor) chemical receptors responsible for the sense of smell; located in the epithelial tissue in the upper part of the nasal cavity

oligodendrocyte (ohl-i-go-DEN-droh-syte) a cell that holds nerve fibers together and produces the myelin sheath around axons in the CNS

oligospermia (ohl-i-go-SPER-mee-ah) low sperm production

oliguria (ohl-i-GOO-ree-ah) scanty amounts of urine

oncogene (ON-koh-jeen) gene (DNA segment) thought to be responsible for the development of a cancer

onycholysis (ahn-ik-oh-LYE-sis) separation of nail from the nail bed that begins at the distal or free edge of the affected nail

oocyte (OH-oh-site) immature stage of the female sex cell

oogenesis (oh-oh-JEN-eh-sis) production of female gametes

oophorectomy (oh-off-eh-REK-toh-mee) surgical procedure to remove the ovaries

oophoritis (oh-off-eh-RYE-tis) inflammation of the ovaries

open fracture (OH-pen FRAK-chur) compound fracture; bone fracture in which bone fragments pierce the skin

ophthalmic (off-THAL-mik) pertaining to the eye

ophthalmoscope (off-THAL-mah-skohp) lighted instrument fitted with optical devices to permit examination of the retina and internal eye structures

opposition (op-oh-ZISH-un) moving the thumb to touch the tips of the fingers; the movement used to hold a pencil to write

optic disc (OP-tik disk) the area in the retina where the optic nerve fibers exit and there are no rods or cones; also known as a *blind spot*

oral candidiasis *see* **thrush**

oral cavity (OR-al KAV-i-tee) mouth

orbicularis oculi (or-bik-yoo-LAIR-is OK-yoo-lye) facial muscle that causes a squint

orbicularis oris (or-bik-yoo-LAIR-is OH-ris) facial muscle that puckers the lips

orbital (OR-bi-tal) pertaining to orbit of the eye

orchitis (or-KYE-tis) inflammation of the testes, often caused by infection

organ (OR-gan) group of several tissue types that performs a special function

organelle (or-gah-NELL) intercell organ; for example, the ribosome

organic compound (or-GAN-ik KOM pownd) compound whose large molecules contain carbon and that include C-C bonds and/or C-H bonds

organism (OR-gah-niz-em) an individual living thing

organization (or-gan-i-ZAY-shun) the characteristic of the body of being organized, that is, structured in different levels of complexity and coordinated in function; the human body is often said to be organized into different levels of organization: chemical, cell, tissue, organ, system, and body

organ of Corti (OR-gan of KOR-tee) the organ of hearing located in the cochlea and filled with endolymph; also called *spiral organ*

organogenesis (or-gah-no-JEN-eh-sis) formation of organs from the primary germ layers of the embryo

origin (OR-i-jin) the attachment of a muscle to the bone, which does not move when contraction occurs, as distinguished from insertion

oropharynx (oh-roh-FAIR-inks) the portion of the pharynx that is located behind the mouth

orthodontics (or-thoh-DON-tics) dental specialty dealing with diagnosis and treatment of malocclusion of the teeth

orthopnea (or-THOP-nee-ah) dyspnea (difficulty in breathing) that is relieved after moving into an upright or sitting position

os coxae (os KOK-see) hip bones; *see also* **coxal bone**

osmosis (os-MOH-sis) movement of a fluid through a semipermeable membrane

ossicles (OS-si-kuls) little bones (malleus, incus, stapes); found in the ears

osteoarthritis (os-tee-oh-ar-THRY-tis) degenerative joint disease; a noninflammatory disorder of a joint characterized by degeneration of articular cartilage

osteoblast (OS-tee-oh-blast) bone-forming cell

osteoclast (OS-tee-oh-klast) bone-absorbing cell

osteocyte (OS-tee-oh-syte) bone cell

osteogenesis imperfecta (os-tee-oh-JEN-eh-sis im-per-FEK-tah) dominant, inherited disorder of connective tissue characterized by imperfect skeletal development, resulting in brittle bones

osteoma (os-tee-OH-mah) benign bone tumor

osteomalacia (os-tee-oh-mah-LAY-shee-ah) bone disorder usually caused by vitamin D deficiency and characterized by loss of mineral in the bone matrix; the adult form of rickets

osteomyelitis (os-tee-oh-my-eh-LYE-tis) bacterial (usually staphylococcus) infection of bone tissue

osteon (AHS-tee-on) structural unit of compact bone tissue made up of concentric layers (lamellae) of hard bone matrix and bone cells (osteocytes); also called **Haversian system**

osteoporosis (os-tee-oh-poh-ROH-sis) bone disorder characterized by loss of minerals and collagen from bone matrix, reducing the volume and strength of skeletal bone

osteosarcoma (os-tee-oh-sar-KOH-mah) bone cancer

otitis (oh-TYE-tis) general term referring to inflammation or infection of the ear; otitis media involves the middle ear

otitis media (oh-TYE-tis MEE-dee-ah) a middle ear infection

otosclerosis (oh-toh-skleh-ROH-sis) inherited bone disorder involving structural irregularities of the stapes in the middle ear and characterized by tinnitus progressing to deafness

otoscope (OH-toh-skohp) lighted device used to examine external ear canal and eardrum

ova (OH-vah) (*sing.,* ovum) female sex cells

oval window (OH-val WIN-doh) a small, membrane-covered opening that separates the middle and inner ear

ovarian cyst (oh-VAIR-ee-an CIST) smooth fluid-filled sac that forms in ovarian tissue

ovarian follicle (oh-VAIR-ee-an FOL-i-kuls) each contains an oocyte

ovaries (OH-var-ees) female gonads that produce ova (sex cells)

overactive bladder (OH-ver-ak-tiv BLADD-er) refers to frequent urination characterized by sensation of urgency and pain

overhydration (oh-ver-hye-DRAY-shun) too much fluid input in the body, which can put a burden on the heart

oviducts (OH-vih-dukts) also called *uterine* or *fallopian tubes; see* **uterine tubes** for definition

oxygen (AHK-sih-jen) one of the chemical elements found in great quantity in the human body; symbolized by O, as in H_2O (water) or O_2 (oxygen gas)

oxygen concentrator (AHK-sih-jen KON-sen-tray-tor) a device used in health care that increases the proportion of oxygen gas in the air of the room in which it is placed; sometimes used in treatment of persons in respiratory distress and in other such conditions that produce hypoxia (low oxygen concentration in the blood)

oxygen debt (AHK-si-jen det) continued increased metabolism that occurs in a cell to remove excess lactic acid that resulted from exercise

oxygen therapy (AHK-sih-jen) administration of oxygen gas to individuals suffering from low oxygen concentration in the blood (hypoxia)

oxyhemoglobin (ahk-see-HEE-moh-GLO-bin) hemoglobin combined with oxygen

oxytocin (OT) (ahk-see-TOH-sin) hormone secreted by the posterior pituitary gland in a woman before and after she has delivered a baby; thought to initiate and maintain labor and also causes the release of breast milk into the mammary ducts to provide nourishment for the baby

P

p-arm (PEE-arm) the short segment of a chromosome that is divided into two segments by a centromere

pacemaker (PASE-may-ker) *see* **sinoatrial node**

Pacinian corpuscle (pah-SIN-ee-an KOHR-pus-ul) a receptor found deep in the dermis that detects pressure on the skin surface

Paget disease (PAJ-et dih-ZEEZ) osteitis deformans; a common, often mild bone disorder characterized by replacement of normal spongy bone with disorganized bone matrix

palate (PAL-let) the roof of the mouth; made up of the hard (anterior portion of the mouth) and soft (posterior portion of the mouth) palates

palatine tonsil *see* **tonsils**

palmar (PAHL-mar) palm of the hand

palpable (PAL-pah-bul) can be felt or touched

pancreas (PAN-kree-ass) endocrine gland located in the abdominal cavity; contains pancreatic islets that secrete glucagon and insulin

pancreatic islets (pan-kree-AT-ik eye-lets) endocrine portion of the pancreas; made up of alpha and beta cells, among others; also called *islets of Langerhans*

pancreatitis (pan-cree-ah-TYE-tiss) inflammation of the pancreas

pandemic (pan-DEM-ik) refers to a disease that affects many people worldwide

Papanicolaou test (pah-pah-NIH-kah-lah-oo) cancer-screening test in which cells swabbed from the uterine cervix are smeared on a glass slide and examined for abnormalities; also called *Pap smear* or *Pap test*

papillae (pah-PIL-ee) (*sing.*, papilla) small, nipple-shaped elevations

papilloma (pap-i-LOH-mah) benign skin tumor characterized by finger-like projections (e.g., a wart)

papule (PAP-yool) raised, firm skin lesion less than 1 cm in diameter

paralysis (pah-RAL-i-sis) loss of the power of motion, especially voluntary motion

paranasal sinus (pair-ah-NAY-sal SYE-nus) four pairs of sinuses that have openings into the nose

paraplegia (pair-ah-PLEE-jee-ah) paralysis (loss of voluntary muscle control) of both legs

parasite (PAIR-ah-syte) any organism that lives in or on another organism (a host) to obtain its nutrients; parasites may be harmless to the host, or they may disrupt normal body functions of the host and thus cause disease

parasympathetic nervous system (PNS) (pair-ah-sim-pah-THET-ik NER-vus SIS-tem) part of the autonomic nervous system; ganglia are connected to the brainstem and the sacral segments of the spinal cord; controls many visceral effectors under normal conditions

parathyroid glands (pair-ah-THYE-royd) endocrine glands located in the neck on the posterior aspect of the thyroid gland; secrete parathyroid hormone

parathyroid hormone (PTH) (pair-ah-THYE-royd HOR-mohn) hormone released by the parathyryoid gland that increases the concentration of calcium in the blood

parietal (pah-RYE-i-tal) of the walls of an organ or cavity

parietal pericardium (pah-RYE-i-tal pair-i-KAR-dee-um) pericardium surrounding the heart like a loose-fitting sack to allow the heart enough room to beat

parietal peritonium (pah-RYE-i tal payr-i-TOHN-ee-um) serous membrane that lines and is adherent to the wall of the abdominal cavity

parietal pleura (pah-RYE-i tal PLOO-rah) serous membrane that lines and is adherent to the wall of the thoracic cavities

parietal portion (pah-RYE-i-tal POR-shun) serous membrane that lines the walls of a body cavity

Parkinson disease (PARK-in-son dih-ZEEZ) a chronic disease of the nervous system characterized by a set of signs called *parkinsonism* that results from a deficiency of the neurotransmitter dopamine in certain regions of the brain that normally inhibit overstimulation of skeletal muscles; parkinsonism is characterized by muscle rigidity and trembling of the head and extremities, forward tilt of the body, and shuffling manner of walking

parotid ducts (per-AH-tid dukts) the ducts of the parotid salivary glands; also known as **Stensen ducts**

parotid glands (per-AH-tid) paired salivary glands that lie just below and in front of each ear at the angle of the jaw

partial-thickness burn term used to describe both minor burn injury (see **first-degree burn**) and more severe burns that injure both epidermis and dermis (see **second-degree burn**)

parturition (pahr-too-RI-shun) act of giving birth

patella (pah-TEL-ah) small, shallow pan; the kneecap

pathogenesis (path-oh-JEN-eh-sis) pattern of a disease's development

pathology (pah-THOL-oh-jee) the scientific study of disease

pathophysiology (path-oh-fiz-ee-OL-oh-jee) study of the underlying physiological aspects of disease

pectoral girdle (PEK-teh-rel GIR-dul) shoulder girdle; the scapula and clavicle

pectoralis major (pek-teh-RAH-liss MAY-jor) major flexor of the upper arm

pedal (PEED-al) foot

pedigree (PED-i-gree) chart used in genetic counseling to illustrate genetic relationships over several generations

pelvic (PEL-vik) pertaining to the pelvis or hip bones

pelvic cavity (PEL-vik KAV-i-tee) the lower portion of the ventral cavity; the distal portion of the abdominopelvic cavity

pelvic girdle (PEL-vik GIR-dul) connects the legs to the trunk

pelvic inflammatory disease (PID) (PEL-vik in-FLAM-ah-tor-ee dih-ZEEZ) acute inflammatory condition of the uterus, fallopian tubes, and/or ovaries—usually the result of a sexually transmitted infection (STI)

pelvis (PEL-vis) basin- or funnel-shaped structure

penis (PEE-nis) structure that forms part of the male genitalia; when sexually aroused, becomes stiff to enable it to enter and deposit sperm in the vagina

pepsinogen (pep-SIN-oh-jen) component of gastric juice that is converted into pepsin by hydrochloric acid

peptide bond (PEP-tyde) covalent bond linking amino acids within a protein molecule

pericarditis (pairr-i-kar-DYE-tis) condition in which the pericardium becomes inflamed

pericardium (pair-i-KAR-dee-um) membrane that surrounds the heart

perilymph (PAIR-i-limf) a watery fluid that fills the bony labyrinth of the ear

perinatal infection (pair-ih-NAY-tal in-FEK-shun) infection passed from a mother to an infant during the time of the birth process

perineal (pair-i-NEE-al) area between the anus and genitals; the **perineum**

perineum (pair-i-NEE-um) *see* **perineal**

periodontitis (pair-ee-oh-don-TYE-tis) inflammation of the periodontal membrane (periodontal ligament) that anchors teeth to jaw bone; common cause of tooth loss among adults

periosteum (pair-ee-OS-tee-um) tough, connective tissue covering the bone

perineurium (pair-i-NOO-ree-um) connective tissue that encircles a bundle (fascicle) of nerve fibers within a nerve

periodontal membrane (pair-ee-oh-DON-tull MEM-brayne) fibrous tissue that lines each tooth socket and serves to attach the tooth to underlying bone

peripheral (peh-RIF-er-all) pertaining to an outside surface

peripheral nervous system (PNS) (peh-RIF-er-all NER-vus SIS-tem) the nerves connecting the brain and spinal cord to other parts of the body

peripheral resistance (peh-RIF-er-all) resistance (blocked effort) to blood flow encountered in the peripheral arteries (arteries that branch off the aorta and pulmonary arteries)

peristalsis (pair-i-STAWL-sis) wavelike, rhythmic contractions of the stomach and intestines that move food material along the digestive tract

peritoneal space (pair-i-toh-NEE-all) small, fluid-filled space between the visceral and parietal layers that allows the layers to slide over each other freely in the abdominopelvic cavity

peritoneum (pair-i-toh-NEE-um) large, moist, slippery sheet of serous membrane that lines the abdominopelvic cavity (parietal layer) and its organs (visceral layer)

peritonitis (pair-i-toh-NYE-tis) inflammation of the serous membranes in the abdominopelvic cavity; sometimes a serious complication of an infected appendix

permeable membrane (PER-mee-ah-bul MEM-brayne) a membrane that allows passage of substances

permease system (PER-mee-ayz SIS-tem) a specialized cellular component that allows a number of active transport mechanisms to occur

pernicious anemia (per-NISH-us ah-NEE-mee-ah) deficiency of red blood cells caused by a lack of vitamin B_{12}

peroneal muscles (per-oh-NEE-al MUSS-els) plantar flexors and evertors of the foot; the peroneus longus forms a support arch for the foot

peroneous group (per-on-EE-uss groop) group of lateral muscles of the lower leg that act to pronate the foot, rotating it toward the midline, and plantar flex the foot, pulling it toes-downward

perspiration (per-spih-RAY-shun) transparent, watery liquid released by glands in the skin that eliminates ammonia and uric acid and helps maintain body temperature; also commonly known as **sweat**

pH (p H) mathematical expression of relative H^+ concentration (acidity); pH value higher than 7 is basic, pH value less than 7 is acidic, pH value equal to 7 is neutral

phagocyte (FAG-oh-syte) white blood cell that engulfs microbes and digests them

phagocytosis (fag-oh-sye-TOH-sis) ingestion and digestion of particles by a cell

phalanges (fah-LAN-jeez) the bones that make up the fingers and toes

pharmacology (farm-ah-KAHL-ah-jee) study of drugs and their actions in the body

pharyngeal tonsil *see* adenoid

pharyngitis (fair-in-JYE-tis) sore throat; inflammation or infection of the pharynx

pharynx (FAIR-inks) organ of the digestive and respiratory systems; commonly called the *throat*

phenylketonuria (PKU) (feen-il-kee-toh-NOO-ree-ah) recessive, inherited condition characterized by excess of phenylketone in the urine, caused by accumulation of phenylalanine (an amino acid) in the tissues; may cause brain injury and death if phenylalanine intake is not managed properly

phimosis (fih-MOH-sis) abnormal condition in which the prepuce (foreskin) fits tightly over the glans of the penis

phlebitis (fleh-BYE-tis) inflammation of a vein

phospholipid (fos-foh-LIP-id) phosphate-containing fat molecule

photodynamic therapy (foh-toh-dye-NAM-ic) use of laser energy to trigger photosensitizing drugs in specialized treatment of superficial cancers and "wet" age-related macular degeneration

photopigments (foh-toh-PIG-ments) chemicals in retinal cells that are sensitive to light

photoreceptor (FOH-toh-ree-sep-tor) specialized nerve cell stimulated by light

photorefractive keratectomy (PRK) (FOH-toh-ree-frak-tiv kair-ah-TEK-toh-mee) refractory eye surgery that uses an excimer or "cool" laser to vaporize corneal tissue in treating mild to moderate nearsightedness; also called **excimer laser surgery**

phrenic nerve (FREN-ik nerv) the nerve that stimulates the diaphragm to contract

physiology (fiz-ee-OL-oh-jee) the study of body function

pia mater (PEE-ah MAH-ter) the vascular innermost covering (meninx) of the brain and spinal cord

pigment layer (PIG-ment LAY-er) the layer of the epidermis that contains the melanocytes that produce melanin to give skin its color

pineal gland (PIN-ee-al gland) endocrine gland located in the third ventricle of the brain; produces melatonin

pinocytosis (pin-oh-sye-TOH-sis) active transport mechanism used to transfer fluids or dissolved substances into cells

pitting edema (pitt-ing eh-DEE-mah) depressions in swollen subcutaneous tissue that do not rapidly refill after exerted pressure is removed

pituitary gland (pih-TOO-i-tair-ee) endocrine gland located in the skull; made up of the adenohypophysis and the neurohypophysis

placenta (plah-SEN-tah) anchors the developing fetus to the uterus and provides a "bridge" for the exchange of nutrients and waste products between the mother and developing baby

placenta previa (plah-SEN-tah PREE-vee-ah) abnormal condition in which a blastocyst implants in the lower uterus, developing a placenta that approaches or covers the cervical opening; placenta previa involves the risk of placental separation and hemorrhage

planes (of body) (playnz) any completely flat cut through the body or any of its parts; a body plane can be oriented in any of several directions (e.g., sagittal, midsagittal, frontal [coronal], transverse [horizontal]) and is used to visualize the body from different perspectives; *see also* **sections (of body)**

plantar (PLAN-tar) pertaining to the sole of the foot

plantar flexion (PLAN-tar FLEK-shun) movement in which the bottom of the foot is directed downward; this motion allows a person to stand on tiptoe

plaque (plak) raised skin lesion greater than 1 cm in diameter

plasma (PLAZ-mah) the liquid part of the blood

plasma cell (PLAZ-mah sell) cell that secretes copious amounts of antibody into the blood; also called *effector cell*

plasma membrane (PLAZ-mah MEM-brayne) membrane that separates the contents of a cell from the tissue fluid; encloses the cytoplasm and forms the outer boundary of the cell

plasma protein (PLAZ-mah PRO-teen) any of several proteins normally found in the plasma; includes albumins, globulins, and fibrinogen

plasmid (PLAS-mid) small circular ring of bacterial DNA

platelet plug (PLAYT-let) a temporary accumulation of platelets (thrombocytes) at the site of an injury; it precedes the formation of a blood clot

platyhelminth (plat-ih-HEL-minth) flatworm or fluke—animal parasite capable of infesting humans

pleura (PLOOR-ah) the serous membrane in the thoracic cavity

pleural cavity (PLOOR-al KAV-i-tee) a subdivision of the thorax

pleural space (PLOOR-al) the space between the visceral and parietal pleurae filled with just enough fluid to allow them to glide effortlessly with each breath

pleurisy (PLOOR-i-see) inflammation of the pleura

plexus (PLEK-sus) complex network formed by converging and diverging nerves, blood vessels, or lymphatic vessels

plica (PLYE-kah) (*pl.*, plicae) multiple circular folds

pneumocystosis (noo-moh-sis-TOH-sis) a protozoan infection, most likely to invade the body when the immune system has been compromised

pneumonectomy (noo-moh-NEK-toh-mee) surgical procedure in which an entire lung is removed

pneumonia (noo-MOH-nee-ah) abnormal condition characterized by acute inflammation of the lungs in which alveoli and bronchial passages become plugged with thick fluid (exudate)

pneumothorax (noo-moh-THOH-raks) abnormal condition in which air is present in the pleural space surrounding the lung, possibly causing collapse of the lung

polar body (POH-lar BOD-ee) small, nonfunctional cell produced during meiotic divisions in the formation of female sex cells (gametes); incapable of being fertilized

poliomyelitis (poh-lee-oh-my-eh-LYE-tis) viral disease that damages motor nerves, often progressing to paralysis of skeletal muscles

polycystic ovary syndrome (PCOS) (pahl-ee-SIS-tik OH-var-ee) condition that is characterized by ovaries usually twice the normal size and that are studded with fluid-filled cysts

polycythemia (pol-ee-sye-THEE-mee-ah) an excessive number of red blood cells

polyuria (pol-ee-YOO-ree-ah) unusually large amounts of urine

pons (ponz) the part of the brainstem between the medulla oblongata and the midbrain

popliteal (pop-lih-TEE-al) behind the knee

pore (por) pinpoint-size openings on the skin that are outlets of small ducts from the eccrine sweat glands

port-wine stain pigmented, benign tumor of the skin present at birth and ranging in color from pale red to a deep reddish purple; also called *nevus flammeus* (*see* **nevus**)

positive feedback (POZ-it-iv FEED-bak) homeostatic control system in which information feeding back to the control center causes the level of a variable to be pushed farther in the direction of the original deviation, causing an amplification of the original stimulus; ordinarily this mechanism is used by the body to amplify a process and quickly finish it, as in labor contractions and blood clotting

posterior (pohs-TEER-ee-or) located behind; opposite of **anterior**

posterior pituitary gland (pohs-TEER-ee-or pih-TOO-i-tair-ee) neurohypophysis; produces hormones ADH and oxytocin

posterior root ganglion (pohs-TEER-ee-or GANG-lee-on) ganglion located near the spinal cord; where the neuron cell body of the dendrites of the sensory neuron is located

postganglionic neurons (post-gang-glee-ON-ik NOO-rons) autonomic neurons that conduct nerve impulses from a ganglion to cardiac or smooth muscle or glandular epithelial tissue

postherpetic neuralgia (post-her-PET-ik noo-RAL-jee-ah) pain (often severe) along nerve pathways previously affected by an outbreak of shingles (herpes zoster)

postnatal period (POST-nay-tal PEER-ee-odd) the period beginning after birth and ending at death

postsynaptic neuron (post-sih-NAP-tik NOO-ron) a neuron situated distal to a synapse

posture (POS-chur) position of the body

precapillary sphincter (pree-CAP-pih-lair-ee SFINGK-ter) smooth muscle cells that guard the entrance to the capillary

preeclampsia (pree-eh-KLAMP-see-ah) syndrome of abnormal conditions in pregnancy of uncertain cause; syndrome includes hypertension, proteinuria, and edema; also called *toxemia of pregnancy*, it may progress to eclampsia—severe toxemia that may cause death

preganglionic neurons (pree-gang-glee-ON-ik NOO-rons) autonomic neurons that conduct nerve impulses between the spinal cord and a ganglion

premature (cardiac) contractions (pree-mah-TUR [KAR-dee-ak] kon-TRAK-shuns) contractions of the heart wall that occur before expected; extrasystoles

premenstrual syndrome (PMS) (pree-MEN-stroo-all SIN-drohm) syndrome of psychological changes (such as irritability) and physical changes (localized edema) that occur before menstruation in many women

premolar *see* **bicuspid**

prenatal period (PREE-nay-tall PEER-ee-odd) the period after conception until birth

prepuce *see* **foreskin**

presbycusis (pres-bih-KYOO-sis) progressive hearing loss associated with advanced age

presbyopia (pres-bee-OH-pee-ah) farsightedness associated with advancing age

presynaptic neuron (pree-sih-NAP-tik NOO-ron) a neuron situated proximal to a synapse

primary bronchi (PRI-mayr-ee BRAHN-kye) first branches of the trachea (right and left primary bronchi)

primary follicles (PRYE-mayr-ee FOL-i-kuls) the ovarian follicles present at puberty; covered with granulosa cells

primary germ layers (PRYE-mayr-ee jerm LAY-ers) three layers of specialized cells that give rise to definite structures as the embryo develops

primary protein (PRYE-mayr-ee PRO-teen) the preliminary structure of a protein: the sequence of amino acids held together with peptide bonds (this structure will then fold to become the secondary protein structure)

primary spermatocyte (SPER-mah-toh-syte) specialized cell that undergoes meiosis to ultimately form sperm

prime mover the muscle responsible for producing a particular movement

prion (PREE-ahn) shortened form of the term "PROteinaceous INfectious particle"; pathogenic protein molecule that converts normal proteins of the body into abnormal proteins, causing abnormalities of function (the abnormal form of the protein also may be inherited by offspring of an affected person); *see also* **bovine spongiform encephalopathy**

product any substance formed as a result of a chemical reaction

progesterone (pro-JES-ter-ohn) hormone produced by the corpus luteum; stimulates secretion of the uterine lining; with estrogen, helps to initiate the menstrual cycle in girls entering puberty

progeria (pro-JEE-ree-ah) rare, inherited condition in which a person appears to age rapidly as a result of abnormal, widespread degeneration of tissues; adult and childhood forms exist, with the childhood form resulting in death by age 20 or so

prognosis (prog-NO-sis) in medicine, the probable outcome of a disease

prolactin (pro-LAK-tin) hormone secreted by the anterior pituitary gland during pregnancy to stimulate the breast development needed for lactation; also called *lactogenic hormone*

proliferative phase (PROH-lif-eh-rah-tiv faze) phase of menstrual cycle that begins after the menstrual flow ends and lasts until ovulation

pronate (PROH-nayt) to make a rotational movement of the forearm (turning the palm medially to face backward) or of the leg and ankle (turning the foot so toes point outward and the medial edge of the sole hits the ground); opposite of **supinate**

pronation (PROH-nay-shun) action in which the forearm or leg and ankle **pronates;** opposite of **supination**

prone used to describe the body lying in a horizontal position facing downward

prophase (PRO-fayz) first stage of mitosis during which chromosomes become visible

proprioceptors (proh-pree-oh-SEP-tors) receptors located in the muscles, tendons, and joints; allow the body to recognize its position

prostaglandins (PG) (pross-tah-GLAN-dins) a group of naturally occurring fatty acids that affect many body functions

prostatectomy (pross-tah-TEK-toh-mee) surgical removal of part or all of the prostate gland

prostate gland (PROSS-tayt) lies just below the bladder; secretes a fluid that constitutes about 30% of the seminal fluid volume; helps activate sperm and helps them maintain motility

prostate-specific antigen (PSA) (PROSS-tayt-speh-CIF-ik AN-tih-jen) a protein (antigen) produced by prostate tissue that may be elevated in the blood of men with prostate cancer

prosthesis (pros-THEE-sis) an artificial body part or device that assists the functioning of a body part

protease (PRO-tee-ayz) protein-digesting enzyme

protein (PRO-teen) one of the basic nutrients needed by the body; a nitrogen-containing organic compound composed of a folded strand of amino acids

protein-calorie malnutrition (PCM) (PRO-teen-KAL-or-ee mal-noo-TRISH-un) abnormal condition resulting from a deficiency of calories in general and protein in particular; likely to result from reduced intake of food but may also be caused by increased nutrient loss or increased use of nutrients by the body

protein hormone (PRO-teen HOR-mohn) a nonsteroid; *see* **nonsteroid hormone**

proteinuria (pro-teen-YOO-ree-ah) presence of abnormally high amounts of plasma protein in the urine; usually an indicator of kidney disease

proteome (PRO-tee-ohm) the entire group of proteins encoded by the genome; *see* **genome**

proteomics (pro-tee-OH-miks) the endeavor that involves the analysis of the proteins encoded by the genome, with the ultimate goal of understanding the role of each protein in the body

prothrombin (pro-THROM-bin) a protein present in normal blood that is required for blood clotting

prothrombin activator (pro-THROM-bin AK-tih-vay-tor) combination of clotting factors and circulating plasma proteins that initiates conversion of prothrombin to thrombin in the clotting mechanism

prothrombin time (pro-THROM-bin tyme) time it takes for a blood sample to clot after tissue thromboplastin (prothrombin activator) is added—a way to assess efficiency of a person's extrinsic clotting mechanism; see also **international normalized ratio (INR)**

proton (PRO-ton) positively charged particle within the nucleus of an atom

protozoa (proh-toh-ZOH-ah) single-celled organisms with nuclei and other membranous organelles that can infect humans

proximal (PROK-sih-mal) next or nearest; located nearest the center of the body or the point of attachment of a structure; opposite of **distal**

proximal convoluted tubule (PCT) (PROK-sih-mal kon-voh-LOO-ted TOOB-yool) the first segment of a renal tubule

pseudo (SOO-doh) false

pseudohypertrophy (soo-doh-hye-PER-troh-fee) literally, "false muscle growth"; another name for **Duchenne muscular dystrophy (DMD)**

pseudostratified epithelium (SOOD-oh-STRAT-i-fyde ep-i-THEE-lee-um) type of tissue similar to simple columnar epithelium that forms a membrane made up of a single layer of cells that are tall and narrow but that are squeezed together in a way that pushes the nuclei into two layers and thus gives an initial impression that it is stratified (having more than one layer of cells); compare to **simple columnar epithelium**

psoriasis (so-RYE-ah-sis) chronic, inflammatory skin disorder characterized by cutaneous inflammation and scaly plaques

psychogenic (sye-koh-JEN-ik) pertaining to anything caused by psychological mechanisms; for example, psychogenic disorders are often caused by stress or other psychological trauma

pubis (PYOO-biss) joint in the midline between the two pubic bones

puerperal fever (pyoo-ER-per-al FEE-ver) condition caused by bacterial infection in a woman after delivery of an infant, possibly progressing to septicemia and death; also called *childbed fever*

pulmonary artery (PUL-moh-nair-ee AR-ter-ee) artery that carries deoxygenated blood from the right ventricle to the lungs

pulmonary circulation (PUL-moh-nair-ee ser-kyoo-LAY-shun) venous blood flow from the right atrium to the lung and then to the left atrium

pulmonary embolism (PUL-moh-nair-ee EM-boh-liz-em) blockage of the pulmonary circulation by a thrombus or other matter; may lead to death if blockage of pulmonary blood flow is significant

pulmonary semilunar valve (PUL-moh-nair-ee sem-i-LOO-nar valv) valve located at the beginning of the pulmonary artery

pulmonary vein (PUL-moh-nair-ee vayne) any vein that carries oxygenated blood from the lungs to the left atrium

pulmonary ventilation (PUL-moh-nair-ee ven-tih-LAY-shun) breathing; process that moves air in and out of the lungs

Punnett square (PUN-it skwair) grid used in genetic counseling to determine the probability of inheriting genetic traits

pupil (PYOO-pill) the opening in the center of the iris that regulates the amount of light entering the eye

Purkinje fibers (pur-KIN-jee FYE-bers) specialized cells located in the walls of the ventricles; relay nerve impulses from the AV node to the ventricles, causing them to contract

pus accumulation of white blood cells, dead bacterial cells, and damaged tissue cells at the site of an infection

pustule (PUS-tyool) small, raised skin lesion filled with pus

P wave deflection on an ECG that occurs with depolarization of the atria

pyelonephritis (pye-eh-loh-neh-FRY-tis) infectious condition characterized by inflammation of the renal pelvis and connective tissues of the kidney

pyloric sphincter (pye-LOR-ik SFINGK-ter) sphincter that prevents food from leaving the stomach and entering the duodenum

pyloric stenosis (pye-LOR-ik steh-NO-sis) anatomical abnormality in which the opening through the pylorus or pyloric sphincter is unusually narrow

pylorospasm (pye-LOHR-oh-spaz-um) spasm of pyloric sphincter of stomach

pylorus (pye-LOR-us) the small narrow section of the stomach that joins the first part of the small intestine

pyramids (PEER-ah-mids) triangular-shaped divisions of the medulla of the kidney; *see* **renal pyramid**

Q

q-arm (KYU-arm) the long segment of a chromosome that is divided into two segments by a centromere

QRS complex (Q R S KOM-pleks) deflection on an ECG that occurs as a result of depolarization of the ventricles

quadrant (KWOD-runt) *see* **abdominal quadrants**

quadriceps femoris (KWOD-reh-seps feh-MOR-iss) extensor of the lower leg

quadriplegia (kwod-rih-PLEE-jee-ah) paralysis (loss of voluntary muscle control) in all four limbs

quaternary protein (KWAT-er-nair-ee PRO-teen) the fourth level of structure in a protein formed when two or more tertiary (third-level) proteins unite to form a larger protein molecule

quickening (KWIK-en-ing) when a pregnant woman first feels recognizable movements of the fetus

R

radiation (ray-dee-AY-shun) flow of heat waves away from the blood

radiation therapy (ray-dee-AY-shun THAYR-ah-pee) treatment often used for cancer in which high-intensity radiation is used to destroy cancer cells; also called *radiotherapy*

radical mastectomy (RAD-i-kal mas-TEK-toh-mee) surgical procedure in which a cancerous breast is removed along with nearby muscle tissue and lymph nodes

radioactive isotope (ray-dee-oh-AK-tiv EYE-soh-tohp) form of an element in which atoms have a unique atomic number (*see also* **isotope**) and also release particles or waves of radiation

radiography (ray-dee-OG-rah-fee) imaging technique using x-rays that pass through some tissues more easily than others, allowing an image of tissues to form on a photographic plate or other sensitive surface; invented by Wilhelm Röntgen in 1895

radius (RAY-dee-us) one of the two bones in the forearm; located on the thumb side of the forearm

reabsorption (ree-ab-SORP-shun) process of absorbing again that occurs in the kidneys

reactant (ree-AK-tant) any substance entering (and being changed by) a chemical reaction

receiving chambers (ree-SEE-ving CHAYM-bers) atria of the heart; receive blood from the superior and inferior venae cavae

receptor (ree-SEP-tor) peripheral beginning of a sensory neuron's dendrite

recessive (ree-SES-iv) in genetics, the term *recessive* refers to genes that have effects that do not appear in the offspring when they are masked by a dominant gene (recessive forms of a gene are represented by lowercase letters); compare with **dominant**

rectum (REK-tum) distal portion of the large intestine

rectus abdominis (REK-tus ab-DOM-i-nis) muscle that runs down the middle of the abdomen; protects the abdominal viscera and flexes the spinal column

reflex (REE-fleks) involuntary action

reflex arc (REE-fleks ark) allows an impulse to travel in only one direction

reflux (REE-fluhks) backflow, as in flow of stomach contents back into esophagus

refraction (ree-FRAK-shun) bending of a ray of light as it passes from a medium of one density to one of a different density

regeneration (ree-jen-er-AY-shun) the process of replacing missing tissue with new tissue by means of cell division

rejection reaction (ree-JEK-shun re-AK-shun) immune responses to a donated or grafted tissue or organ; *see also* **isoimmunity**

releasing hormones (ree-LEE-sing HOR-mohns) hormone produced by the hypothalamus gland that causes the anterior pituitary gland to release its hormones

remission (ree-MISH-un) stage of a disease during which a temporary recovery from symptoms occurs

renal calculi (REE-nal KAL-kyoo-lye) kidney stones

renal colic (REE-nal KOL-ik) pain caused by the passage of a kidney stone

renal columns (REE-nall coll-ums) extensions of cortical tissue that dip down into the medulla of the kidney between the renal pyramids

renal corpuscle (REE-nal KOR-pus-ul) the part of the nephron located in the cortex of the kidney

renal cortex (REE-nal KOR-teks) outer portion of the kidney; *pl.*, cortices

renal failure (REE-nal FAIL-yoor) acute or chronic loss of kidney function; acute kidney failure is often reversible, but chronic kidney failure slowly progresses to total loss of renal function (and death if kidney function is not restored through a kidney transplant or use of an artificial kidney)

renal medulla (REE-nal meh-DUL-ah) inner portion of the kidney; *pl.*, medullae or medullas

renal papilla (REE-nal pah-PIL-uh) (*pl.*, papillae) nipple-like point of a renal pyramid, from which urine drips out of the kidney tubules

renal pelvis (REE-nal PEL-vis) basin-like upper end of the ureter that is located inside the kidney

renal ptosis (REE-nal TOH-sis) condition in which one or both kidneys descend, often because of loss of the fat pad that surrounds each kidney

renal pyramid (PEER-ah-mid) triangular-shaped division of the medulla of the kidney

renal tubule (REE-nal TOOB-yool) one of the two principal parts of the nephron

renin (REE-nin) enzyme produced by the kidney that catalyzes the formation of angiotensin, a substance that increases blood pressure

renin-angiotensin-aldosterone system (RAAS) (REE-nin-an-jee-oh-TEN-sin-al-DAH-stair-ohn) causes changes in blood plasma volume and blood pressure mainly by controlling aldosterone secretion

repolarization (ree-poh-lah-rih-ZAY-shun) begins just before the relaxation phase of cardiac muscle activity

reproductive system (ree-proh-DUK-tiv SIS-tem) produces hormones that permit the development of sexual characteristics and the propagation of the species

residual volume (RV) (reh-ZID-yoo-al VOL-yoom) the air that remains in the lungs after the most forceful expiration

respiration (res-per-AY-shun) breathing or pulmonary ventilation

respiratory acidosis (RES-pih-rah-tor-ee ass-i-DOH-sis) a respiratory disturbance that results in a carbonic acid excess

respiratory alkalosis (RES-pih-rah-tor-ee al-kah-LOH-sis) a respiratory disturbance that results in a carbonic acid deficit

respiratory arrest (RES-pih-rah-tor-ee ah-REST) cessation of breathing without resumption

respiratory control centers (RES-pih-rah-tor-ee kon-TROL SEN-ters) centers located in the medulla and pons that stimulate the muscles of respiration

respiratory distress syndrome (RES-pih-rah-tor-ee dih-STRESS SIN-drohm) difficulty in breathing caused by absence or failure of the surfactant in fluid lining the alveoli of the lung; IRDS is infant respiratory distress syndrome; ARDS is adult respiratory distress syndrome

respiratory membrane (RES-pih-rah-tor-ee MEM-brayne) the single layer of cells that makes up the wall of the alveoli

respiratory mucosa (RES-pih-rah-tor-ee myoo-KOH-sah) mucus-covered membrane that lines the tubes of the respiratory tree

respiratory muscles (RES-pih-rah-tor-ee MUSS-els) muscles responsible for the changing shape of the thoracic cavity that allows air to move in and out of the lungs

respiratory system (RES-pih-rah-tor-ee SIS-tem) the organs that allow the exchange of oxygen from the air with the carbon dioxide from the blood

respiratory therapist (RES-pih-rah-tor-ee THAYR-ah-pist) health professional who helps patients increase respiratory function and/or overcome or cope with the effects of respiratory conditions

respiratory tract (RES-pih-rah-tor-ee trakt) the two divisions of the respiratory system are the upper and lower respiratory tracts

reticular formation (reh-TIK-yoo-lar for-MAY-shun) located in the medulla where bits of gray and white matter mix intricately

retina (RET-i-nah) innermost layer of the eyeball; contains rods and cones and continues posteriorly with the optic nerve

retroperitoneal (reh-troh-pair-i-toh-NEE-al) area outside of the peritoneum

rheumatic heart disease (roo-MAT-ik hart dih-ZEEZ) cardiac damage (especially to the endocardium, including the valves) resulting from a delayed inflammatory response to streptococcal infection

rheumatoid arthritis (ROO-mah-toyd ar-THRY-tis) an autoimmune inflammatory joint disease characterized by synovial inflammation that spreads to other tissue

rhinitis (rye-NYE-tis) inflammation of the nasal mucosa often caused by nasal infections

Rh-negative (R H NEG-ah-tiv) red blood cells that do not contain the antigen called *Rh factor*

RhoGAM (ROH-gam) an injection of a special protein given to an Rh-negative woman who is pregnant to prevent her body from forming anti-Rh antibodies, which may harm an Rh-positive baby

Rh-positive (R H POZ-i-tiv) red blood cells that contain an antigen called *Rh factor*

Rh system classification of blood based on the presence (Rh^+) or absence (Rh^-) of a unique antigen on the surface of RBCs

ribonucleic acid (RNA) (rye-boh-noo-KLAY-ik ASS-id) a nucleic acid found in the cytoplasm that is crucial to protein synthesis

ribosomal RNA (rye-boh-SOHM-al R-N-A) also called *rRNA*, it is a form of RNA that makes up most of the structures (subunits) of the ribosome organelle of the cell

ribosome (RYE-boh-sohm) organelle in the cytoplasm of cells that synthesizes proteins; also known as a *protein factory*

rickets (RIK-ets) childhood form of osteomalacia, a bone-softening condition caused by vitamin D deficiency

rickettsia (rih-KET-see-ah) small bacterium that infects human cells as an obligate parasite

rigor mortis (RIG-or MOR-tis) literally "stiffness of death," the permanent contraction of muscle tissue after death caused by the depletion of ATP during the actin-myosin reaction—preventing myosin from releasing actin to allow relaxation of the muscle

risk factor (FAK-tor) predisposing condition; factor that puts one at a higher than usual risk for developing a particular disease

RNA (R N A) *see* **ribonucleic acid**

rods receptors located in the retina that are responsible for night vision

rotation (roh-TAY-shun) movement around a longitudinal axis; for example, shaking your head "no"

rugae (ROO-gee) (*sing.*, ruga [ROO-gah]) wrinkles or folds

rule of nines a frequently used method to determine the extent of a burn injury; the body is divided into 11 areas of 9% each to help estimate the amount of skin surface burned in an adult

S

sagittal (SAJ-i-tal) longitudinal; like an arrow

salivary amylase (SAL-i-vair-ee AM-i-layz) digestive enzyme found in the saliva that begins the chemical digestion of carbohydrates (begins conversion of starch to smaller carbohydrate molecules)

salpingitis (sal-pin-JYE-tis) inflammation of the uterine (fallopian) tubes

salt compound formed when an acid and a base combine; sometimes specifically refers to the common salt, sodium chloride (NaCl)

saltatory conduction (SAL-tah-tor-ee kon-DUK-shun) when a nerve impulse encounters myelin and "jumps" from one node of Ranvier to the next

sarcoma (sar-koh-mah) tumor of muscle tissue

sarcomere (SAR-koh-meer) contractile unit of muscle; length of a myofibril between two Z bands

SARS-associated coronavirus (SARS-CoV) (SARZ ass-OH-see-ayt-ed koh-ROH-nah-vye-rus [SARZ koh-VEE]) a type of coronavirus shown to be the cause of severe acute respiratory syndrome (SARS); *see also* **severe combined acute respiratory syndrome (SARS)** and **coronavirus**

scabies (SKAY-bees) contagious skin condition caused by the itch mite (*Sarcoptes scabei*)

scapula (SKAP-yoo-lah) shoulder blade

scar (skahr) thickened mass of tissue, usually fibrous connective tissue, that remains after a damaged tissue has been repaired

Schwann cells (shwon sells) large nucleated cells that form myelin

sciatica (sye-AT-i-kah) neuralgia (pain) of the sciatic nerve

scientific method (sye-en-TIF-ik METH-odd) any logical and systematic approach to discovering principles of nature, often involving testing of tentative explanations called **hypotheses**

sclera (SKLEER-ah) white outer coat of the eyeball

scleroderma (skleer-oh-DER-mah) rare disorder affecting the vessels and connective tissue of skin and other tissues, characterized by tissue hardening

scoliosis (skoh-lee-OH-sis) abnormal lateral (side-to-side) curvature of the vertebral column

scotoma (skoh-TOH-mah) loss of the central visual field caused by nerve degeneration, it sometimes occurs with neuritis associated with multiple sclerosis

scrotum (SKROH-tum) pouchlike sac that contains the testes

scurvy (SKER-vee) condition caused by avitaminosis C (lack of vitamin C), which impairs the normal maintenance of collagen-containing connective tissues, causing bleeding and ulceration of the skin, gums, and other tissues

sebaceous gland (seh-BAY-shus) oil-producing glands found in the skin

sebum (SEE-bum) secretion of sebaceous glands

second-degree burn burn injury that is more severe than a first-degree burn and often involves damage to the dermis; *see also* **partial-thickness burn**

second messenger (SEK-und MESS-en-jer) molecule that provides communication within the target cell of a chemical signal such as a hormone; for example, cyclic AMP

second messenger mechanism (SEK-und MESS-en-jer MEK-an-is-em) a system of cellular communication (signal transduction) in which a molecule provides a communication link within the target cell of a chemical signal such as a hormone; for example, cyclic AMP links the external signal (arrival of the hormone or neurotransmitter) to the internal cellular processes that produce changes in the target cell

secondary infection (SEK-on-dair-ee in-FEK-shun) infection that occurs as a consequence of the weakened state of the body or damage caused by a previously existing disease

secondary protein (SEK-on-dair-ee PRO-teen) second level of protein structure formed by the folding of the primary protein (string of amino acids) into helices (spirals) and pleated folds

secondary sexual characteristics (SEK-on-dair-ee SEK-shoo-al kair-ak-ter-ISS-tiks) external physical characteristics of sexual maturity resulting from the action of the sex hormones; they include growth of male and female patterns of body hair and fat distribution, as well as development of the external genitals

secondary bronchi (SEK-un-dayr-ee BRAHN-kye) smaller bronchial branches that result from division of the primary bronchi

secretion (seh-KREE-shun) in kidney function refers to active movement of substances such as electrolytes, waste products, or drugs through kidney tubule cells into the urine

secretory phase phase of menstrual cycle that begins at ovulation and lasts until the next menses begins

sections (of body) a cut, ordinarily flat, through the body or any body part; *see also* **planes (of body)**

seizure (SEE-zhur) sudden onset of abnormal body function, as in a brain seizure when a sudden disruption in the normal firing of neurons in the brain causes mild to severe neurological symptoms such as involuntary muscle spasms, changes in consciousness, or abnormal sensations

sella turcica (SEL-lah TER-si-kah) small depression of the sphenoid bone that contains the pituitary gland

semen (SEE-men) male reproductive fluid or **seminal fluid**

semicircular canals (sem-i-SIR-kyoo-lar kah-nals) located in the inner ear; contain a specialized receptor called *crista ampullaris* that generates a nerve impulse on movement of the head

semilunar (SL) valves (sem-i-LOO-nar valvs) valves located between the two ventricular chambers and the large arteries that carry blood away from the heart; valves found in the veins

seminal fluid (SEM-i-nal FLOO-id) *see* **semen**

seminal vesicle (SEM-i-nal VES-i-kul) paired, pouchlike glands that contribute about 60% of the seminal fluid volume; rich in fructose, which is a source of energy for sperm

seminiferous tubule (seh-mih-NIF-er-us TOOB-yool) long, coiled structure that forms the bulk of the testicular mass

senescence (seh-NES-enz) older adulthood; aging

sensor (SEN-sor) part of a homeostatic feedback loop that detects (senses) changes in the physiological variable that is regulated by the feedback loop

sensory neurons (SEN-sor-ee NOO-rons) neurons that transmit impulses to the spinal cord and brain from all parts of the body

sensory receptors (SEN-soh-ree ree-sep-tohrs) sense organs in skin, internal organs, and muscles that allow body to respond to various stimuli

septic shock (SEP-tik shock) circulatory failure (shock) resulting from complications of septicemia (toxins in blood resulting from infection)

serosa (seh-ROH-sah) outermost covering of the digestive tract; composed of the parietal pleura in the abdominal cavity

serotonin (sair-oh-TOH-nin) a neurotransmitter that belongs to a group of compounds called **catecholamines**

serous membrane (SEER-us MEM-brayne) a two-layer epithelial membrane that lines body cavities and covers the surfaces of organs

serum (SEER-um) blood plasma minus its clotting factors, still contains antibodies

severe acute respiratory syndrome (SARS) (seh-VEER ah-KYOOT res-pir-ah-TOR-ee SIN-drohm [sarz]) viral infection characterized by pneumonia and symptoms of fever, dry cough, dyspnea (shortness of breath), headache, hypoxia (low oxygen concentration in the blood), and sometimes progressing to death due to respiratory failure caused by damage to alveoli of the lungs

severe combined immune deficiency (SCID) (seh-VEER kom-BYNED i-MYOON deh-FISH-en-see) nearly complete failure of the lymphocytes to develop properly, in turn causing failure of the immune system's defense of the body; very rare congenital immune disorder

sex chromosomes (seks KRO-moh-sohms) pair of chromosomes in the human genome that determine gender; normal males have one X chromosome and one Y chromosome (XY), whereas normal females have two X chromosomes (XX)

sex hormone (seks HOR-mohn) any hormone that has a direct effect on sexual structure or function, such as testosterone (male) and estrogens (female)

sex-linked trait (seks-linked trayt) nonsexual, inherited trait governed by genes located in a sex chromosome (X or Y); most known sex-linked traits are X-linked

sexually transmitted disease (STD) (SEKS-yoo-al-ee trans-MIH-ted dih-ZEEZ) any communicable disease that is commonly transmitted through sexual contact; compare to **sexually-transmitted infection (STI)**

sexually transmitted infection (STI) (SEKS-yoo-al-ee trans-MIH-ted in-FEK-shun) any infection that is commonly transmitted through sexual contact and which may or may not produce symptoms; a sexually transmitted infection that produces symptoms (makes a person sick) may also be called a **sexually transmitted disease (STD)**

shingles (SHING-guls) *see* **herpes zoster**

sickle cell anemia (SIK-ul sell ah-NEE-mee-ah) severe, possibly fatal, hereditary disease caused by an abnormal type of hemoglobin

sickle cell trait (SIK-ul sell trayt) condition in which only one defective gene is inherited and only a small amount of hemoglobin that is less soluble than usual is produced

sigmoid colon (SIG-moyd KOH-lon) S-shaped segment of the large intestine that terminates in the rectum

sign (syne) objective deviation from normal (perceived by an examiner) that marks the presence of a disease

signal transduction (tranz-DUK-shen) term that refers to the whole process of getting a chemical signal (such as a hormone or neurotransmitter) to the inside of a cell; in a way, signal transduction is really "signal translation" by the cell

simple columnar epithelium (SIM-pul KAHL-um-nar ep-i-THEE-lee-um) type of tissue that forms a membrane made up of a single layer of cells that are taller than they are wide

simple cuboidal epithelium (SIM-pul KYOO-boyd-ul ep-i-THEE-lee-um) type of tissue that forms a membrane made up of a single layer of cube-like cells

simple squamous epithelium (SIM-pul SKWAY-muss ep-i-THEE-lee-um) type of tissue that forms a membrane made up of a single layer of flattened cells

sinoatrial (SA) node (sye-no-AY-tree-al) the heart's pacemaker; where the impulse conduction of the heart normally starts; located in the wall of the right atrium near the opening of the superior vena cava

sinus (SYE-nus) a space or cavity inside some structures of the body, as inside the cranial bones (paranasal sinuses) and inside a lymph node; some large veins are also called *sinuses*

sinus dysrrhythmia (SYE-nus dis-RITH-mee-ah) variation in the rhythm of heart rate during the breathing cycle (inspiration and expiration)

sinusitis (sye-nyoo-SYE-tis) sinus infection

skeletal muscle (SKEL-eh-tal MUSS-el) muscles under willed or voluntary control; also known as *voluntary muscle*

skeletal system (SKEL-eh-tal SIS-tem) the bones, cartilage, and ligaments that provide the body with a rigid framework for support and protection

skin *see* **cutaneous membrane**

skull bony structure of the head

sliding filament model (SLY-ding FILL-ah-ment MAH-del) concept in muscle physiology describing the contraction of a muscle fiber in terms of the sliding of microscopic protein filaments past each other within the myofibrils in a manner that shortens the myofibrils and thus the entire muscle

small intestine (in-TEST-in) part of GI tract that includes duodenum, jejunum, and ileum

smooth muscle (MUSS-el) muscle that is not under conscious control; also known as *involuntary* or *visceral muscle*; forms the walls of blood vessels and hollow organs such as the stomach and small intestine

snuff dipper pouch precancerous leukoplakia (white patches) in fold between cheek and gum caused by use of smokeless tobacco

sodium-potassium pump (SO-dee-um poh-TAS-ee-um) a system of coupled ion pumps that actively transports sodium ions out of a cell and potassium ions into the cell at the same time—found in all living cells

solute (SOL-oot) substance that dissolves into another substance; for example, in saltwater the salt is the solute dissolved in water

solvent (SOL-vent) substance in which other substances are dissolved; for example, in saltwater the water is the solvent for salt

somatic nervous system (so-MAH-tik NER-vus SIS-tem) the motor neurons that control the voluntary actions of skeletal muscles

spastic paralysis (SPAS-tik pah-RAL-i-sis) loss of voluntary muscle control characterized by involuntary contractions of affected muscles

specific immunity (spih-SIH-fik i-MYOON-i-tee) the protective mechanisms that provide specific protection against certain types of bacteria or toxins

sperm the male spermatozoon; sex cell

spermatids (SPER-mah-tids) the resulting daughter cells from the primary spermatocyte undergoing meiosis; these cells have only half the genetic material and half the chromosomes of other body cells

spermatogenesis (sper-mah-toh-JEN-eh-sis) production of sperm cells

spermatogonia (sper-mah-toh-GO-nee-ah) sperm precursor cells

spermatozoa (sper-mah-tah-ZOH-ah) (*sing.,* spermatozoon) sperm cells or male sex cells

sphincter (SFINGK-ter) ring-shaped muscle

sphygmomanometer (sfig-moh-mah-NOM-eh-ter) device for measuring blood pressure in the arteries of a limb

spinal cavity (SPY-nal KAV-i-tee) the space inside the spinal column through which the spinal cord passes

spinal nerves (SPY-nal nervs) nerves that connect the spinal cord to peripheral structures such as the skin and skeletal muscles

spinal tracts (SPY-nal trakts) the white columns of the spinal cord that provide two-way conduction paths to and from the brain; ascending tract carries information to the brain, whereas descending tracts conduct impulses from the brain

spindle fiber (SPIN-dul FYE-ber) a network of tubules formed in the cytoplasm between the centrioles as they are moving away from each other

spirometer (spih-ROM-eh-ter) an instrument used to measure the amount of air exchanged in breathing

spleen largest lymphoid organ; filters blood, destroys worn-out red blood cells, salvages iron from hemoglobin, and serves as a blood reservoir

splenectomy (spleh-NEK-toh-mee) surgical removal of the spleen

splenic colic flexure (SPLEN-ik KOHL-ik FLEK-shur) point at which the descending colon turns downward on the left side of the abdomen

splenomegaly (spleh-no-MEG-ah-lee) condition of enlargement of the spleen

spongy bone (SPUN-jee) porous bone in the end of the long bone, which may be filled with marrow

spontaneous abortion (spon-TAY-nee-us ah-BOR-shun) miscarriage; loss of an embryo or fetus before the twentieth week of gestation (or fetus under a weight of 500 g)

spore (spor) nonreproducing form of a bacterium that resists adverse environmental conditions; spores revert to the active multiplying form when conditions improve

sporozoa (spor-oh-ZOH-ah) coccidia; parasitic protozoan that enters a host cell during one phase of a two-part life cycle

sprain (sprayn) an acute injury to soft tissues surrounding a joint, including muscle, tendon, and/or ligament

squamous (SKWAY-muss) scalelike

squamous cell carcinoma (SKWAY-muss sell car-sih-NO-mah) malignant tumor of the epidermis; slow-growing cancer that is capable of metastasizing; the most common type of skin cancer

squamous suture (SKWAY-muss SOO-chur) the immovable joint between the temporal bone and the sphenoid bone

stapes (STAY-peez) tiny, stirrup-shaped bone in the middle ear

staph (staf) a short word form for *Staphylococcus*, a category of bacteria that can infect the skin and other organs, sometimes seriously

stem cells cells capable of dividing to produce new cell types

stenosed (cardiac) valves (steh-NOST KAR-dee-ak valvs) valves that are narrower than normal, slowing blood flow from a heart chamber

Stensen ducts (STEN-sen dukts) the ducts of the parotid salivary glands; also known as **parotid ducts**

sternoclavicular joint (ster-no-klah-VIK-yoo-lar joynt) the direct point of attachment between the bones of the upper extremity and the axial skeleton

sterility (steh-RIL-i-tee) as applied to humans, the inability to reproduce

sternocleidomastoid (stern-oh-klye-doh-MAS-toyd) the "strap" muscle located on the anterior aspect of the neck

steroid hormones (STER-oyd HOR-mohns) lipid-soluble hormones that pass intact through the cell membrane of the target cell and influence cell activity by acting on specific genes

stillbirth (STILL-berth) delivery of a dead fetus (after twentieth week of gestation; before 20 weeks it is termed a **spontaneous abortion**)

stimulus (STIM-yoo-lus) (*pl.,* stimuli) agent that causes a change in the activity of a structure

stoma (STO-mah) an opening, such as the opening created in a colostomy procedure

stomach (STUM-ak) an expansion of the digestive tract between the esophagus and small intestine

strabismus (strah-BIS-muss) abnormal condition in which lack of coordination of, or weakness in, the muscles that control one or both eyes cause improper focusing of images on the retina, thus making depth perception difficult

strain (strayn) injury involving any component of the "musculotendinous unit"; although muscle is usually involved, the tendon, the junction between the two, as well as their attachments to bone, also may be involved

stratified squamous epithelium (STRAT-i-fyde SKWAY-muss ep-i-THEE-lee-um) type of tissue that forms a membrane made up of several layers of cells, with flattened cells in the surface layer(s)

stratified transitional epithelium (STRAT-i-fyde tran-ZISH-en-al ep-i-THEE-lee-um) type of tissue that forms a membrane made up of several layers of cells that can stretch out and flatten without breaking

stratum corneum (STRAH-tum KOR-nee-um) the tough outer layer of the epidermis; cells are filled with keratin

stratum germinativum (STRAH-tum JER-mih-nah-tiv-um) the innermost layer of the tightly packed epithelial cells of the epidermis; cells in this layer are able to reproduce themselves

strawberry hemangioma (hem-an-jee-OH-mah) common pigmented and generally transient birthmark caused by a collection of dilated blood vessels

strength training (STREN-th TRAIN-ing) contracting muscles against resistance to enhance muscle hypertrophy

Stretta procedure (STRETT-ah proh-see-jur) procedure using an endoscope to deliver radiofrequency energy to burn, tighten, and reduce the size of the lumen of the lower esophageal sphincter in a person with gastroesophageal reflux disease (GERD)

striae (STRYE-ay) (*sing.,* stria) "stretch marks" caused by stretching of the skin beyond its ability to rebound

striated muscle (STRYE-ay-ted MUSS-el) *see* **skeletal muscle**

stroke volume (VOL-yoom) the amount of blood that is ejected from the ventricles of the heart with each beat

structural protein (STRUK-shur-al PRO-teen) protein that has the role of building structures in the body, such as collagen fibers or keratin fibers; compare to **functional protein**

subcutaneous injection (sub-kyoo-TAY-nee-us in-JEK-shun) injection of liquid or pelleted material into the spongy and porous subcutaneous layer beneath the skin

subcutaneous tissue (sub-kyoo-TAY-nee-us TISH-yoo) *see* **hypodermis**

sublingual glands (sub-LING-gwall) salivary glands that drain saliva into the floor of the mouth

subluxation (sub-luks-AY-shun) abnormal, partial separation of the bones in a joint; also called *incomplete dislocation*

submandibular glands (sub-man-DIB-yoo-lar) salivary glands that drain saliva into the mouth on either side of the lingual frenulum

submucosa (sub-myoo-KOH-sah) connective tissue layer containing blood vessels and nerves in the wall of the digestive tract

sudden infant death syndrome (SIDS) unexpected death of unknown origin in apparently normal infants; sometimes called "crib death"

sudoriferous gland (soo-doh-RIF-er-us) glands that secrete sweat; also referred to as *sweat glands*

sulcus (SUL-kus) (*pl.,* sulci) furrow or groove

superficial (soo-per-FISH-all) near the body surface

superior (soo-PEER-ee-or) higher, opposite of **inferior**

superior vena cava (soo-PEER-ee-or VEE-nah KAY-vah) one of two large veins returning deoxygenated blood to the right atrium

supinate (SOO-pih-nayt) to make a rotational movement of the forearm (turning the palm laterally to face forward) or of the leg and ankle (turning the foot so toes point inward and the lateral edge of the sole hits the ground); opposite of **pronate**

supination (soo-pih-NAY-shun) action in which the forearm or leg and ankle supinates; opposite of **pronation**

supine (SOO-pyne) description of the body lying in a horizontal position facing upward

supraclavicular (soo-prah-klah-VIK-yoo-lar) area above the clavicle

surfactant (sur-FAK-tant) a substance covering the surface of the respiratory membrane inside the alveolus; it reduces surface tension and prevents the alveoli from collapsing

suture (SOO-chur) immovable joint

sweat (swet) see **perspiration**

sweat gland (swet) see **sudoriferous gland**

sympathetic nervous system (sim-pah-THET-ik NER-vus SIS-tem) part of the autonomic nervous system; ganglia are connected to the thoracic and lumbar regions of the spinal cord; functions as an emergency system

sympathetic postganglionic neurons (sim-pah-THET-ik post-gang-glee-ON-ik NOO-rons) dendrites and cell bodies are in sympathetic ganglia and axons travel to a variety of visceral effectors

sympathetic preganglionic neurons (sim-pah-THET-ik pree-gang-glee-ON-ik NOO-rons) dendrites and cell bodies are located in the gray matter of the thoracic and lumbar segments of the spinal cord; leaves the cord through an anterior root of a spinal nerve and terminates in a collateral ganglion

symptom (SIMP-tum) subjective deviation from normal that marks the presence of a disease (perceived by a patient)

synapse (SIN-aps) junction between adjacent neurons

synaptic cleft (si-NAP-tik kleft) the space between a synaptic knob and the plasma membrane of a postsynaptic neuron

synaptic knob (sih-NAP-tik nob) a tiny bulge at the end of a terminal branch of a presynaptic neuron's axon that contains vesicles with neurotransmitters

synarthrosis (sin-ar-THROH-sis) a joint in which fibrous connective tissue joins bones and holds them together tightly; commonly called **sutures**

syndrome (SIN-drohm) collection of signs or symptoms, usually with a common cause that defines or gives a clear picture of a pathological condition

synergist (SIN-er-jist) muscle that assists a prime mover

synovial fluid (sih-NO-vee-all FLOO-id) the thick, colorless lubricating fluid secreted by the synovial membrane

synovial membrane (sih-NO-vee-all MEM-brayne) connective tissue membrane lining the spaces between bones and joints that secretes synovial fluid

system (SIS-tem) group of organs arranged so that the group can perform a more complex function than any one organ can perform alone

systemic circulation (sis-TEM-ik ser-kyoo-LAY-shun) blood flow from the left ventricle to all parts of the body and back to the right atrium

systemic lupus erythematosus (SLE) (sis-TEM-ik LOO-pus er-i-them-ah-TOH-sus) chronic inflammatory disease caused by widespread attack of self-antigens by the immune system (autoimmunity); characterized by a red rash on the face and other signs

systole (SIS-toh-lee) contraction of the heart muscle

T

tachycardia (tak-i-KAR-dee-ah) rapid heart rhythm (greater than 100 beats/minute)

tactile corpuscle (TAK-tyle KOR-pus-ul) a sensory receptor located in the skin close to the surface that detects light touch; also known as **Meissner corpuscle**

target organ cell (TAR-get OR-gan sell) organ or cell that is acted on by a particular hormone and then responds to it

tarsals (TAR-sals) seven bones of the heel and back part of the foot; the calcaneus is the largest

taste buds chemical receptors that generate nerve impulses, resulting in the sense of taste

Tay-Sachs disease (TAY-saks dih-ZEEZ) recessive, inherited condition in which abnormal lipids accumulate in the brain and cause tissue damage that leads to death by age 4

telemetry (tel-EM-eh-tree) technology by which data, such as heart activity monitored by an electrocardiograph, can be sent to a remote location through telephone wires, radio waves, or other communication pathway

telophase (TEL-oh-fayz) last stage of mitosis in which the cell divides

temporal (TEM-poh-ral) muscle that assists the masseter in closing the jaw

tendons (TEN-dons) bands or cords of fibrous connective tissue that attach a muscle to a bone or other structure

tendon sheath (TEN-don sheeth) tube-shaped structure lined with synovial membrane that encloses certain tendons

tenosynovitis (ten-oh-sin-oh-VYE-tis) inflammation of a tendon sheath

teratogen (TER-ah-toh-jen) any environmental factor that causes a birth defect (abnormality present at birth); common teratogens include radiation (e.g., x-rays), chemicals (e.g., drugs, cigarettes, or alcohol), and infections in the mother (e.g., herpes or rubella)

tertiary protein (TER-shee-air-ee PRO-teen) third level of protein structure formed by further folding of the secondary protein structure

testes (TES-teez) male gonad responsible for production of sex cells or gametes (sperm) and testosterone

testosterone (tes-TOS-teh-rohn) male sex hormone produced by the interstitial cells in the testes; the "masculinizing hormone"

tetanic contraction (teh-TAN-ik kon-TRAK-shun) sustained contraction

tetanus (TET-ah-nus) sustained muscular contraction

thalamus (THAL-ah-muss) located just above the hypothalamus; its functions are to help produce sensations, associate sensations with emotions, and play a part in the arousal mechanism

thalassemia (thal-ah-SEE-mee-ah) any of a group of inherited hemoglobin disorders characterized by production of hypochromic, abnormal red blood cells

theory (THEE-ah-ree) an explanation of a scientific principle that has been tested experimentally and found to be true; compare to hypothesis and law

thermoregulation (ther-moh-reg-yoo-LAY-shun) maintaining homeostasis of body temperature

third-degree burn involves complete destruction of both epidermis and dermis with injury extending into subcutaneous tissue; see **full-thickness burn**

thoracic (tho-RASS-ik) pertaining to the chest area of the body (upper trunk)

thoracic cavity (tho-RASS-ik KAV-it-ee) organ-containing space inside the rib cage or chest of the body that includes the mediastinum and left and right pleural cavities

thoracic duct (tho-RASS-ik dukt) largest lymphatic vessel in the body

thorax (THOR-aks) bony cage of the upper torso formed by 12 pairs of ribs, the sternum, and thoracic vertebrae; also called the *chest*

threshold stimulus (THRESH-hold STIM-yoo-lus) minimal level of stimulation required to cause a muscle fiber to contract

thrombin (THROM-bin) protein important in blood clotting

thrombocytes (THROM-boh-sytes) blood cells that play a role in blood clotting; also called *platelets*

thrombocytopenia (throm-boh-sye-toh-PEE-nee-ah) general term referring to an abnormally low blood platelet count

thrombophlebitis (throm-boh-fleh-BYE-tis) vein inflammation (phlebitis) accompanied by clot formation

thrombosis (throm-BOH-sis) formation of a clot in a blood vessel

thrombus (THROM-bus) stationary blood clot

thrush candidiasis of mouth (mouth infection) characterized by white, creamy patches of exudate on inflamed oral mucosa and tongue; caused by yeastlike fungal organism

thymine (THYE-meen) one of several nitrogen-containing bases that make up nucleotides, which in turn make up nucleic acids such as DNA (but not RNA); in the cell, it can chemically bind to another nitrogenous base, adenine (*A* or *a*), to form a more complex structure or in translating genetic codes; symbolized by the letter *T* or *t*; *see also* **guanine, adenine, cytosine, uracil**

thymosin (THY-moh-sin) hormone produced by the thymus that is vital to the development and functioning of the body's immune system

thymus gland (THY-muss) endocrine gland located in the mediastinum; vital part of the body's immune system

thyroid gland (THY-royd) endocrine gland located in the neck that stores its hormones until needed; thyroid hormones regulate cellular metabolism

thyroid-stimulating hormone (TSH) (THY-royd STIM-yoo-lay-ting HOR-mohn) a tropic hormone secreted by the anterior pituitary gland that stimulates the thyroid gland to increase its secretion of thyroid hormone

thyroxine (T₄) (thy-ROK-sin) thyroid hormone that stimulates cellular metabolism

tibia (TIB-ee-ah) shinbone

tibialis anterior (tib-ee-AL-is an-TEER-ee-or) dorsiflexor of the foot

tic douloureux (doo-loh-ROO) *see* **trigeminal neuralgia**

tidal volume (TV) (TYE-dal VOL-yoom) amount of air breathed in and out with each breath

tinea pedis (TIN-ee-ah PED-is) athlete's foot, a fungal infection of the skin characterized by redness and itching

tinnitus (tih-NYE-tus) abnormal sensation of ringing or buzzing in the ear

tissue (TISH-yoo) group of similar cells that perform a common function

tissue fluid (TISH-yoo FLOO-id) a dilute saltwater solution that bathes every cell in the body

tissue hormone (TISH-yoo HOR-mohn) prostaglandins; produced in a tissue and diffused only a short distance to act on cells within the tissue

tissue plasminogen activator (TPA or tPA) (TISH-yoo plaz-MIN-oh-jen AK-ti-vay-tor) naturally occurring substance that activates plasminogen and converts it to the active enzyme plasmin, which in turn dissolves fibrin blood clots

tissue typing (TISH-yoo TYE-ping) a procedure used to identify tissue compatibility before an organ transplant

T lymphocytes (T LIM-foh-sytes) cells that are critical to the function of the immune system; produce cell-mediated immunity

tonic contraction (TAHN-ik kon-TRAK-shun) special type of skeletal muscle contraction used to maintain posture

tonsillectomy (tahn-sih-LEK-toh-mee) surgical procedure used to remove the tonsils

tonsillitis (tahn-sih-LIE-tis) inflammation of the tonsils, usually caused by infection

tonsils (TAHN-sils) masses of lymphoid tissue; protect against bacteria; three types: palatine tonsils, located on each side of the throat; pharyngeal tonsils (adenoids), near the posterior opening of the nasal cavity; and lingual tonsils, near the base of the tongue

tophi (TOH-fee) calculus-like growths or deposits in tissues or around joints; may contain urate crystals in patients with gout

total metabolic rate (TMR) (TOH-tal met-ah-BOL-ik rayt) total amount of energy used by the body per day

trabeculae (trah-BEK-yoo-lee) needle-like threads of spongy bone that surround a network of spaces

trachea (TRAY-kee-ah) the windpipe; the tube extending from the larynx to the bronchi

tracheostomy (tray-kee-OS-toh-mee) medical procedure involving the cutting of an opening into the trachea

trachoma (trah-KOH-mah) chronic infection of the conjunctiva covering the eye caused by the bacterium *Chlamydia trachomatis*; also called *chlamydial conjunctivitis*

tract (trakt) a single nerve pathway made up of several bundles of axons and extending through the central nervous system; compare to **nerve**

transaminase (trans-AM-i-nayz) enzyme released from damaged tissues; high blood concentration may indicate a heart attack or other pathological event

transcription (trans-KRIP-shun) action that occurs when the double-stranded DNA molecule unwinds and forms mRNA

transfer RNA (TRANS-fer R N A) type of ribonucleic acid (RNA) that temporarily binds to specific amino acids and transfers them to specific sequences (codons) on a messenger RNA (mRNA) molecule; also known as *tRNA*

transitional epithelium (tranz-I-shen-al ep-i-THEE-lee-um) type of epithelial tissue that forms membranes capable of stretching without breaking, as in the urinary bladder; cells in this type of tissue can stretch from a roughly columnar shape out to a flattened (squamous) shape and back again without sustaining damage

translation (trans-LAY-shun) the synthesis of a protein by ribosomes

transplant (trans-PLANT) tissue or organ graft; procedure in which a tissue (e.g., skin, bone marrow) or an organ (such as kidney, liver) from a donor is surgically implanted into a recipient

transverse arch (TRANS-vers) *see* **metatarsal arch**

transverse fracture (TRANS-vers FRAK-chur) bone fracture characterized by a fracture line that is at a right angle to the long axis of the bone

transverse plane (tranz-VERS playn) a flat cut through the body (or a body part) that is horizontal or crosswise and thus divides the body (or body part) into upper and lower portions; see also **sections (of body)**

transversus abdominis (trans-VER-sus ab-DOM-i-nis) the innermost layer of the anterolateral abdominal wall

trapezium (trah-PEE-zee-um) the carpal bone of the wrist that forms the saddle joint that allows the opposition of the thumb

trapezius (trah-PEE-zee-us) triangular muscle in the back that elevates the shoulder and extends the head backward

triceps brachii (TRY-seps BRAY-kee-eye) extensor of the elbow

tricuspid (try-KUS-pid) tooth with rather large flat surface with two or three grinding "cusps"; also called *molar*

tricuspid valve (try-KUS-pid valv) the valve located between the right atrium and ventricle

trigeminal neuralgia (try-JEM-i-nal noo-RAL-jee-ah) pain in one or more (of three) branches of the fifth cranial nerve (trigeminal nerve) that runs along the face; also called *tic douloureux*

triglyceride (try-GLISS-er-yde) lipid that is synthesized from fatty acids and glycerol or from excess glucose or amino acids; stored mainly in adipose tissue cells

trigone (TRY-gon) triangular area on the wall of the urinary bladder

triiodothyronine (T₃) (try-eye-oh-doh-THY-roh-neen) thyroid hormone that stimulates cellular metabolism

triple therapy (TRIP-pul THAYR-ah-pee) treatment of ulcers using a combination of bismuth subsalicylate (Pepto-Bismol) and two antibiotics

triplegia (try-PLEE-jee-ah) paralysis (loss of voluntary muscle control) in three limbs, often two legs and one arm

trisomy (TRY-so-mee) abnormal genetic condition in which cells have three chromosomes (a triplet) where there should be a pair; usually caused by nondisjunction (failure of chromosome pairs to separate) during gamete production

tropic hormone (TROH-pik HOR-mohn) hormone that stimulates another endocrine gland to grow and secrete its hormones

true ribs the first seven pairs of ribs, which are attached to the sternum

tubal pregnancy (TOO-bal PREG-nan-see) ectopic pregnancy that occurs in a uterine (fallopian) tube

tuberculosis (TB) (too-ber-kyoo-LOH-sis) chronic bacterial (bacillus) infection of the lungs or other tissues caused by *Mycobacterium tuberculosis* organisms

tumor (TOO-mer) growth of tissues in which cell proliferation is uncontrolled and progressive

tunica albuginea (TOO-nih-kah al-byoo-JIN-ee-ah) a tough, whitish membrane that surrounds each testis and enters the gland to divide it into lobules

tunica externa (TOO-nih-kah eks-TER-nah) the outermost layer found in blood vessels

tunica intima (TOO-nih-kah IN-tih-mah) endothelium that lines blood vessels; also called *tunica interna*

tunica media (TOO-nih-kah MEE-dee-ah) the muscular middle layer found in blood vessels; the tunica media of arteries is more muscular than that of veins

Turner syndrome (TUR-ner SIN-drohm) genetic disorder caused by monosomy of the X chromosome (XO) in females; characterized by immaturity of sex organs (causing sterility), webbed neck, cardiovascular defects, and learning disorders

T wave deflection on an electrocardiogram that occurs with repolarization of the ventricles

twitch a quick, jerky response to a single stimulus

tympanic (tim-PAN-ik) drumlike

tympanic membrane (tim-PAN-ik MEM-brayn) eardrum; membrane that separates external ear canal from middle ear

type 1 diabetes mellitus (dye-ah-BEE-teez mell-EYE-tus) a condition in which the pancreatic islets secrete too little insulin, resulting in increased levels of blood glucose; formerly known as *juvenile-onset diabetes* or *insulin-dependent diabetes mellitus*

type 2 diabetes mellitus (dye-ah-BEE-teez mell-EYE-tus) a condition in which cells of the body become less sensitive to the hormone insulin and perhaps the pancreatic islets secrete too little insulin, resulting in increased levels of blood glucose; formerly known as *maturity-onset diabetes* or *non–insulin-dependent diabetes mellitus*

U

ulcer (UL-ser) a necrotic open sore or lesion

ulna (UL-nah) one of the two forearm bones; located on the little finger side

ultrasonogram (ul-trah-SOHN-oh-gram) a record obtained by using sound to produce images

ultrasonography (ul-trah-son-OG-rah-fee) an imaging technique in which high-frequency sound waves are reflected off tissue to form an image

umami (oo-MOM-ee) "meaty" taste proposed as a "primary taste sensation" comparable to sweet, sour, bitter, and salty

umbilical (um-BIL-i-kul) pertaining to the navel or umbilicus, a structure made up of blood vessels connecting the developing fetus to the placenta

umbilical artery (um-BIL-i-kul AR-ter-ee) two small arteries that carry oxygen-poor blood from the developing fetus to the placenta

umbilical cord (um-BIL-i-kul) flexible structure connecting the fetus to the placenta, which allows the umbilical arteries and vein to pass

umbilical region (um-BIL-ik-al REE-jun) the very center region of the abdominopelvic cavity, near the umbilicus (navel) and between the left and right lumbar regions; terminology used when the abdominopelvic cavity is visualized as being subdivided into nine regions as in a tic-tac-toe grid

umbilical vein (um-BIL-i-kul vayn) a large vein carrying oxygen-rich blood from the placenta to the developing fetus

universal donor blood blood type O

universal recipient blood blood type AB

upper esophageal sphincter (ee-soff-ah-JEE-al SFINK-ter) ring of muscular tissue (sphincter) located between laryngopharynx and proximal end of esophagus

uracil (YOOR-ah-sill) one of several nitrogen-containing bases that make up nucleotides, which in turn make up nucleic acids such as RNA (but not DNA); in the cell, it can chemically bind to another nitrogenous base, adenine (*A* or *a*), to form a more complex structure or in translating genetic codes; symbolized by the letter *U* or *u*; *see also* **guanine, adenine, thymine, cytosine**

urea (yoo-REE-ah) nitrogen-containing waste product

uremia (yoo-REE-mee-ah) condition in which blood urea concentration is abnormally elevated, expressed as a high BUN (blood urea nitrogen) value; uremia is often caused by renal failure; also called *uremic poisoning*

uremic poisoning (yoo-REE-mik POY-zon-ing) *see* **uremia**

ureter (YOO-ree-ter) muscular tube that conducts urine from the kidney to the urinary bladder

urethra (yoo-REE-thrah) passageway for elimination of urine; in males, also acts as a genital duct that carries sperm to the exterior

urethritis (yoo-reh-THRY-tis) inflammation or infection of the urethra

urinary meatus (YOOR-i-nair-ee mee-AY-tus) external opening of the urethra

urinary retention (YOOR-in-ayr-ee ree-TEN-shun) condition in which no urine is voided

urinary suppression (YOOR-in-ayr-ee supp-PRESH-un) condition in which kidneys do not produce urine

urinary system (YOOR-i-nair-ee SIS-tem) system responsible for excreting liquid waste from the body

urination (yoor-i-NAY-shun) passage of urine from the body; emptying of the bladder

urine (YOOR-in) fluid waste excreted by the kidneys

urticaria (er-tih-KAIR-ee-ah) an allergic or hypersensitivity response characterized by raised red lesions; also referred to as *hives*

uterine tubes (YOO-ter-in toobs) the pair of tubes that conduct the ovum from the ovary to the uterus; also called *fallopian tubes* or *oviducts*

uterus (YOO-ter-us) hollow, muscular organ where a fertilized egg implants and grows

uvula (YOO-vyoo-lah) cone-shaped process hanging down from the soft palate that helps prevent food and liquid from entering the nasal cavities

V

vaccine (VAK-seen) application of killed or attenuated (weakened) pathogens (or portions of pathogens) to a patient to stimulate immunity against that pathogen

vagina (vah-JYE-nah) internal tube from uterus to vulva

vaginitis (vaj-i-NYE-tis) inflammation of the vagina

variant Creutzfeldt-Jakob disease (vCJD) (VAYRE-ee-ant KROYTS-felt YAH-kohb dih-ZEEZ [V-C-J-D]) a degenerative disease of the central nervous system caused by prions (proteinaceous infectious particles) that convert normal proteins of the nervous system into abnormal proteins, causing loss of function; *see* **prion**

varicose vein (VAIR-i-kohs vayn) enlarged vein in which blood pools; also called *varix*

varix (VAIR-iks) (*pl.,* varices) *see* **varicose vein**

vas deferens (vas DEF-er-enz) *see* **ductus deferens**

vasomotor mechanism (vay-so-MOH-tor MEK-ah-niz-em) factors that control changes in the diameter of arterioles by changing the tension of smooth muscles in the vessel walls

vastus (VAS-tus) wide; of great size

vector (VEK-tor) arthropod that carries an infectious pathogen from one organism to another

vein (vayn) vessel carrying blood toward the heart

ventral (VEN-tral) of or near the belly; in humans, front or **anterior;** opposite of **dorsal** or **posterior**

ventral body cavity (VEN-trul BOD-ee KAV-it-ee) organ-containing space in the anterior trunk of the body that includes the thoracic and abdominopelvic cavities; compare with **dorsal body cavity**

ventral cavity (VEN-trul KAV-it-ee) *see* **ventral body cavity**

ventricles (VEN-tri-kuls) small cavities

ventricular fibrillation (VF or V-fib) (ven-TRIK-yoo-lar fib-ril-LAY-shun) life-threatening condition in which the lack of ventricular pumping suddenly stops the flow of blood to vital tissues; unless ventricular fibrillation is corrected immediately by defibrillation or some other method, death may occur within minutes; *see also* **automatic external defibrillator**

venule (VEN-yool) small blood vessels that collect blood from the capillaries and join to form veins

vermiform appendix (VERM-i-form ah-PEN-diks) a tubular structure attached to the cecum and composed of lymphatic tissue

vertebrae (VER-teh-bray) bones that make up the spinal column

vertebral column (ver-TEE-bral KOL-um) the spinal column, made up of a series of separate vertebrae that form a flexible, curved rod

vertigo (VER-tih-go) abnormal sensation of spinning; dizziness

vesicle (VES-i-kul) a clinical term referring to blisters, fluid-filled skin lesions

vestibular nerve (ves-TIB-yoo-lar nerv) a division of the vestibulocochlear nerve (the eighth cranial nerve)

vestibule (VES-tih-byool) located in the inner ear; the portion adjacent to the oval window between the semicircular canals and the cochlea

vestibule (of the vulva) the area between the labia minora; the clitoris and the orifice of the urethra are located in the vestibule

villi (VIL-eye) (*sing.,* villus) fingerlike folds covering the plicae of the small intestines

Vincent infection (VIN-sent in-FEK-shun) bacterial (spirochete) infection of the gum, producing gingivitis; also called *Vincent angina* and *trench mouth*

virilizing tumor (VEER-il-eye-zing TOOM-er) neoplasm of the adrenal cortex that stimulates overproduction of testosterone and therefore an increase in masculinization, even of women

virus (VYE-rus) microscopic, parasitic entity consisting of a nucleic acid bound by a protein coat and sometimes a lipoprotein envelope

visceral (VISS-er-al) pertaining to the viscera or internal organs

visceral effector (VISS-er-al ee-FEK-tor) any muscle or gland (effector) found within the cavities of the body and controlled by the autonomic nervous system; examples include cardiac muscle tissue, smooth muscle tissue, and internal glands

visceral muscle (VISS-er-al MUSS-el) *see* **smooth muscle** and **involuntary muscle**

visceral pericardium (VISS-er-al payr-i-KAR-dee-um) the pericardium that covers the heart; also called **epicardium**

visceral peritoneum (VISS-er-al payr-i-TOHN-ee um) serous membrane that covers and is adherent to the abdominal viscera

visceral pleura (VISS-er-al PLOO-rah) serous membrane that covers and is adherent to the surface of the lungs

visceral portion (VISS-er-al POR-shun) serous membrane that covers the surface of organs found in the body cavity

vital capacity (VC) (VYE-tal kah-PASS-i-tee) largest amount of air that can be moved in and out of the lungs in one inspiration and expiration

vitamins (VYE-tah-mins) organic molecules needed in small quantities to help enzymes operate effectively or to otherwise regulate metabolism in the body

vitiligo (vit-i-LYE-go) patchy areas of light skin caused by acquired loss of epidermal melanocytes

vitreous humor (VIT-ree-us HYOO-mor) the jelly-like fluid found in the eye, posterior to the lens

vocal cords (VOH-kull kords) bands of tissue in larynx responsible for production of sound (speech)

voiding (VOYD-ing) emptying of the bladder

volar (VOH-lar) palm or sole

voluntary muscle (VOL-un-tair-ee MUSS-el) *see* **skeletal muscle**

vulva (VUL-vah) external genitals of the female

vulvitis (vul-VYE-tis) inflammation of the vulva (the external female genitals)

W

wart raised bump that is a benign neoplasm (tumor) of the skin caused by viruses

water intoxication (WAH-ter in-TOK-sih-kay-shen) possibly life-threatening neurological impairment caused by severe overhydration and accompanying electrolyte imbalance

West Nile virus (WNV) (nyle VY-rus [W-N-V]) sometimes fatal viral infection caused by a type of flavivirus transmitted to humans by an insect vector such as a mosquito, sand fly, or tick; characterized by sudden onset of fever and often accompanied by malaise, anorexia, nausea/vomiting, eye pain, headache, myalgia (muscle pain), rash, swollen lymph nodes, and sometimes progressing to severe neurological disease

wheal (weel) raised red skin lesion often associated with severe itching, as in hives

white matter (MAT-ter) tissue made up of nerve tracts covered with white myelin

withdrawal reflex (with-DRAW-al REE-fleks) a reflex that moves a body part away from an irritating stimulus

Y

yeast (yeest) single-celled fungus (compared to mold, which is a multicellular fungus)

yolk sac (yohk sak) in humans, involved with the production of blood cells in the developing embryo

Z

Z disk *see* **Z line**

Z line dark band often seen in micrographs of the myofibrils of skeletal muscle fibers, separating one structural unit (sarcomere) of the myofibril from the next unit of the myofibril; also called Z *disk*

zona fasciculata (ZOH-nah fas-sic-yoo-LAY-tah) middle zone of the adrenal cortex that secretes **glucocorticoids**

zona glomerulosa (ZOH-nah gloh-mair-yoo-LOH-sah) outer zone of the adrenal cortex that secretes mineralocorticoids

zona reticularis (ZOH-nah reh-tik-yoo-LAIR-is) inner zone of the adrenal cortex that secretes small amounts of sex hormones

zygomaticus (zye-goh-MAT-ik-us) muscle that elevates the corners of the mouth and lips; also known as the *smiling muscle*

zygote (ZYE-goht) a fertilized ovum

Chapter 1

1-1, 1-3, 1-5, 1-6: Barbara Cousins. **1-2:** Copyright Kevin Patton, Lion Den Inc, Weldon Spring, MO. **1-4:** Rolin Graphics. **Modern Anatomy box:** (Portrait): Joe Kulka. (Photo): National Library of Medicine (National Institute of Health).

Chapter 2

Biochemistry box: Joe Kulka.

Chapter 3

3-3, *A:* Courtesy Charles Flickinger, University of Virginia. **3-3,** *B:* Lennart Nilsson, Albert Bonniers Forlag AB, Stockholm Sweden. **3-7:** Courtesy Ingalls AJ, Salerno MC: *Maternal and child health nursing,* ed 6, St Louis, 1987, Mosby. **3-12, 3-13,** *B,* **3-14,** *B,* **3-15,** *B,* **3-16,** *B:* Barbara Cousins. **3-13,** *A,* **3-14,** *A,* **3-15,** *A,* **3-16,** *A,* **3-22:** From Gartner LP, Hiatt JL: *Color textbook of histology,* ed 3, Philadelphia, 2007, Saunders. **3-17:** From Erlandsen SL, Magney J: *Color atlas of histology,* St Louis, 1992, Mosby. **3-18, 3-19, 3-20, 3-21, 3-23, 3-25, 3-26:** Dennis Strete. **3-24:** Ed Reschke. **3-27:** From Callen J, Greer K, Hood A et al: *Color atlas of dermatology,* Philadelphia, 1993, Saunders. **Tables 3-2, 3-3:** Network Graphics. **Microscopy box:** Joe Kulka.

Chapter 4

4-2, 4-6: Barbara Cousins. **Radiography box:** (Portrait): Joe Kulka. (Photo): Photo Researchers.

Chapter 5

5-1, 5-3: Centers for Disease Control and Prevention, Atlanta, Georgia. **5-4:** Barbara Cousins. **5-5:** Travis J: Drugs counter mad cow agent in cells, *Science News* 160(7):100, 2001, © Fred Cohen. **5-6, 5-7 (Micrographs), 5-9:** David M. Phillips/Visuals Unlimited. **5-8:** From Schuster FL, Visvesvara GS: Free-living amoebae as opportunistic and non-opportunistic pathogens of humans and animals, *Int J Parasitol* 34(9): 1001-1027, 2004. **5-10, 5-11:** Rolin Graphics. **5-12,** *A:* From LeTreut AL: *Mammography,* St Louis, 1991, Mosby. **5-12,** *B:* Courtesy Williams AL, Haughton VM: *Cranial computed tomography,* St Louis, 1985, Mosby. **5-12,** *C:* Courtesy Runge VM: *Enhanced magnetic resonance imaging,* St Louis, 1989, Mosby. **Laboratory Identification of Pathogens box:** Courtesy Stratford BC: *An Atlas of medical microbiology: common human pathogens,* Edinburgh, 1977, Blackwell Scientific Publications. **Disease as a Weapon box:** From Beeching NJ, Nye FD: *Diagnostic picture tests in clinical infectious diseases,* St Louis, 1996, Mosby. **Medical Imaging of the Body box,** *A, B, C* **(Photos):** Photo Researchers. **Medical Imaging of the Body box,** *D* **(Photo):** From Ballinger PW, Frank ED: *Merrill's atlas of radiographic positions and radiologic procedures,* ed 10, St Louis, 2003, Mosby.

Chapter 6

6-3: Ed Reschke. **6-4:** Courtesy James A. Ischen, MD, Baylor College of Medicine. **6-5:** Copyright Kevin Patton, Lion Den Inc, Weldon Spring, MO. **6-6, 6-10,** *B:* From Habif TP: *Clinical dermatology,* ed 4, St Louis, 2004, Mosby. **6-7:** Copyright © by David Scharf, 1986, 1993. **6-8:** From Goldstein B, editor: *Practical dermatology,* ed 2, St Louis, 1997, Mosby. **6-10,** *A,* **6-11,** *B,* **6-20,** *B, C,* **Table 6-1 (Plaque, vesicle, wheal photos):** From Habif TP: *Clinical dermatology: a color guide to diagnosis and therapy,* ed 3, St Louis, 1996, Mosby. **6-11,** *A:* From Habif TP: *Clinical dermatology,* ed 2, St Louis, 1990, Mosby. **6-12:** From Callen JP et al: *Color atlas of dermatology,* ed 2, Philadelphia, 2000, Saunders. **6-13:** From McCance K, Huether S: *Pathophysiology,* ed 5, St Louis, 2006, Mosby. **6-14:** From Wong DL: *Whaley & Wong's nursing care of infants and children,* ed 5, St Louis, 1995, Mosby. **6-17:** From Copstead-Kirkhorn L, Banasik J: *Pathophysiology,* ed 2, St Louis, 1999, Saunders. **6-18:** Barbara Cousins. **6-19,** *A:* From Emond RTD, Welsby PD, Rowland HAK: *Colour atlas of infectious diseases,* ed 3, London, 1995, Mosby. **6-19,** *D:* Courtesy Jaime A. Tschen, MD, Department of Dermatology, Baylor College of Medicine, Houston, TX. **6-20,** *A:* From Potter P, Perry A: *Fundamentals of nursing,* ed 7, St Louis, 2009, Mosby. **6-20,** *D,* **Table 6-1 (Papule photo):** From Kumar V, Abbas A, Fausto N: *Robbins and Cotran pathologic basis of disease,* ed 7, Philadelphia, 2005, Saunders. **6-21,** *A:* From Goldman L, Ausiello D: *Cecil textbook of medicine,* ed 23, Philadelphia, 2008, Saunders. **6-21,** *B:* From Noble J: *Textbook of primary care medicine,* ed 3, Philadelphia, 2001, Mosby. **6-21,** *C:* From Townsend C, Beauchamp RD, Evers BM, Mattox K: *Sabiston textbook of surgery,* ed 18, Philadelphia, 2008, Saunders. **6-21,** *D:* From Rakel R: *Textbook of family medicine,* ed 7, Philadelphia, 2007, Saunders. **Table 6-1 (Pustule, crust, patch, excoriation, atrophy, ulcer, fissure photos):** From Seidel HM, Ball JW, Dains JE, Benedict GW: *Mosby's guide to physical examination,* ed 5, St Louis, 2003, Mosby. **Table 6-1 (Macule photo):** From Lemmi FO, Lemmi CAE: *Physical assessment findings multi-user CD-ROM,* St Louis, 2001, Saunders. **Secrets of the Skin box:** Joe Kulka.

Chapter 7

7-3, C: From Gartner LP, Hiatt JL: *Color textbook of histology,* ed 3, Philadelphia, 2007, Saunders. **7-4:** Adapted from McCance K, Huether S: *Pathophysiology,* ed 4, St Louis, 2002, Mosby. **7-5:** Dennis Strete. **7-7:** Network Graphics. **7-8, 7-19, 7-20, C:** From Lumley J: *Surface anatomy,* ed 3, Edinburgh, 2002, Churchill Livingstone. **7-10, 7-14, 7-18 (Drawing), 7-21 (Drawing), 7-27:** Barbara Cousins. **7-12:** Courtesy Dr. N. Blevins, New England Medical Center, Boston. **7-15:** From Hockenberry MJ, Wilson D: *Wong's essentials of pediatric nursing,* ed 8, St Louis, 2009, Mosby. **7-16, D:** From Barkauskas V, Baumann L, Stoltenberg-Allen K, Darling-Fisher C: *Health and physical assessment,* ed 2, St Louis, 1998, Mosby. **7-16, E:** Courtesy Nancy Lynch. **7-18, C, F, 7-20, B, 7-21, B, D:** Courtesy Vidic B, Suarez FR: *Photographic atlas of the human body,* St Louis, 1984, Mosby. **7-23, C:** From Seidel HM, Ball JW, Dains JE, Benedict GW: *Mosby's guide to physical examination,* ed 5, St Louis, 2003, Mosby. **7-29:** From Damjanov I, Linder J: *Anderson's pathology,* ed 10, St Louis, 1996, Mosby. **7-30, 7-31, 7-34:** From Kumar V, Abbas A, Fausto N: *Robbins and Cotran pathologic basis of disease,* ed 7, Philadelphia, 2005, Saunders. **7-32:** From Browner B, Jupiter J, Trafton P: *Skeletal trauma: basic science, management, and reconstruction,* ed 3, Philadelphia, 2003, Saunders. **7-33, Total Hip Replacement box:** From Canale ST: *Campbell's operative orthopaedics,* ed 9, St Louis, 1998, Mosby. **7-37, 7-38, A:** From Swartz MH: *Textbook of physical diagnosis,* ed 4, Philadelphia, 2002, Saunders. **7-38, B:** From Habif TP: *Clinical dermatology,* ed 4, St Louis, 2004, Mosby. **Epiphyseal and Avulsion Fractures box:** Courtesy JM Booher, GA Thibodeau. **Palpable Bony Landmarks box:** Terry Cockerham/Synapse Media Production. **The Knee Joint box (Photo):** From Cummings N, Stanley-Green S, Higgs P: *Perspectives in athletic training,* St Louis, 2009, Mosby. **Arthroscopy box:** From Johnson LL: *Diagnostic and surgical arthroscopy,* ed 2, St Louis, 1981, Mosby. **Bones and Joints box:** Joe Kulka.

Chapter 8

8-3, B: Courtesy Dr. H.E. Huxley. **8-5:** Courtesy Dr. Paul C. Letourneau, Department of Anatomy, Medical School, University of Minnesota, Minneapolis. **8-7, 8-8, 8-9, Intramuscular Injections box:** John V Hagen. **8-10, A, C, 8-11, A, C:** Rolin Graphics. **8-13 (Photo):** Courtesy Rob Williams, from Booher JM, Thibodeau GA: *Athletic injury assessment,* ed 2, St Louis, 1989, Mosby. **Muscle Function box:** Joe Kulka.

Chapter 9

9-2, C: Dennis Strete. **9-5:** From Feldman M, Friedman L, Brandt L: *Sleisenger & Fordtran's gastro-intestinal and liver disease,* ed 8, Philadelphia, 2006, Saunders. **9-6 (Micrograph):** Courtesy Dr. Richard Kessel, Professor of Biological Sciences, University of Iowa, Iowa City. **9-10:** Rolin Graphics. **9-12, B, 9-13 (Photo), 9-17:** Courtesy Vidic B, Suarez FR: *Photographic atlas of the human body,* St Louis, 1984, Mosby. **9-13, B:** William Ober. **9-14:** From Zitelli BJ, Davis HW: *Atlas of pediatric physical diagnosis,* ed 5, Philadelphia, 2007, Mosby. **9-15:** James King-Holmes and Science Photo Library. **9-25:** From Habif TP: *Clinical dermatology,* ed 2, St Louis, 1990, Mosby. **Antidepressants box:** From Harkreader H, Hogan MA, Thobaben M: *Fundamentals of nursing: caring & clinical judgement,* ed 3, St Louis, 2008, Saunders. **Brain Studies box:** Courtesy John Nolte, PhD, University of Arizona College of Medicine. **Lumbar Puncture box (Photos):** From Forbes CD, Jackson WD: *Color atlas and text of clinical medicine,* ed 3, London, 2003, Mosby. **Neuroscience box:** Joe Kulka.

Chapter 10

10-2: Copyright Kevin Patton, Lion Den Inc, Weldon Spring, MO. **10-4:** From Palay DA, Krachmer JH: *Ophthalmology for the primary care physician,* St Louis, 1997, Mosby. **10-5, 10-14, A:** From Swartz MH: *Textbook of physical diagnosis,* ed 5, Philadelphia, 2006, Saunders. **10-6, 10-11:** From Newell FW: *Ophthalmology: principles and concepts,* ed 7, St Louis, 1992, Mosby. **10-7:** From Zitelli BJ, Davis HW: *Atlas of pediatric physical diagnosis,* ed 5, Philadelphia, 2007, Mosby. Courtesy Stephen Ludwig, MD, Children's Hospital of Philadelphia. **10-12:** From Seidel HM, Ball JW, Dains JE, Benedict GW: *Mosby's guide to physical examination,* ed 3, St Louis, 2003, Mosby. **10-13:** From *Ishihara's tests for colour deficiency,* Tokyo, Japan, 1973, Kanehara Trading Co, Copyright Isshinkai Foundation. **10-14, B:** From Wilson SF, Giddens JF: *Health assessment for nursing practice,* ed 3, St Louis, 2008, Mosby. **10-14, C:** Courtesy Richard A. Buckingham, Clinical Professor, Otolaryngology, Abraham Lincoln School of Medicine, University of Illinois, Chicago. **10-15:** From Kliegman RM, Behrman RE, Jenson HB, Stanton BF: *Nelson textbook of pediatrics,* ed 18, Philadelphia, 2007, Saunders. **Swimmer's Ear box:** From Zitelli BJ, Davis HW: *Atlas of pediatric physical diagnosis,* ed 5, Philadelphia, 2007, Mosby. Courtesy Michael Hawke, MD. **The Senses box:** Joe Kulka.

Chapter 11

11-9: From Stein HA, Slatt BJ, Stein RM: *The ophthalmic assistant: fundamentals and clinical practice,* ed 7, Philadelphia, 2000, Mosby. **11-10:** From Seidel HM, Ball JW, Dains JE, Benedict GW: *Mosby's guide to physical examination,* ed 3, St Louis, 2003, Mosby. **11-15:** Courtesy Gower Medical

Publishers. **Synthetic Human Insulin box:** Perry A, Potter P: *Clinical nursing skills and techniques,* ed 6, St Louis, 2006, Mosby. **Endocrinology box:** Joe Kulka.

Chapter 12

12-1, 12-2: Barbara Cousins. **12-2 (Photos):** From Belcher AE: *Blood disorders,* St Louis, 1993, Mosby. **12-3, 12-7:** Courtesy Bevelander G, Ramalay JA: *Essentials of histology,* ed 8, St Louis, 1979, Mosby. **12-4:** From Carr J, Rodak B: *Clinical hematology atlas,* St Louis, 1999, Elsevier. **12-6:** Christine Oleksyk. **12-9:** Dennis Strete. **12-10:** Courtesy A Arlan Hinchee. **12-11, 12-15:** From Kumar V, Abbas A, Fausto N: *Robbins and Cotran pathologic basis of disease,* ed 7, Philadelphia, 2005, Saunders. **12-12:** Courtesy Dr. JV Melo. **12-13:** From Copstead-Kirkhorn L, Banasik J: *Pathophysiology,* ed 2, St Louis, 2005, Saunders. **12-14:** From Skarin A: *Atlas of diagnostic oncology,* ed 2, Philadelphia, 1996, Mosby. **12-16, *B:*** Copyright Dennis Kunkel Microscopy, Inc. **12-17:** From Cotran R, Kumar V, Collins T: *Robbins pathologic basis of disease,* ed 6, Philadelphia, 1999, Saunders. **Cardiac Blood Tests box:** From Warekois R, Robinson R: *Phlebotomy,* ed 2, St Louis, 2007, Saunders. **Hematology box:** Joe Kulka.

Chapter 13

13-2, 13-10: Barbara Cousins. **13-4, 13-13:** From Cotran R, Kumar V, Collins T: *Robbins pathologic basis of disease,* ed 6, Philadelphia, 1999, Saunders. **13-5 (Photo):** From Cotran R, Kumar V, Collins T: *Robbins pathologic basis of disease,* ed 6, Philadelphia, 1999, Saunders. Courtesy William D. Edwards, MD, Mayo Clinic, Rochester, MN. **13-11:** From Aehlert B: *ACLS Quick Review Study Cards,* ed 2, St Louis, 2004, Mosby. **13-12:** From Libby P, Bonow RO, Mann DL, Zipes DP: *Braunwald's heart disease: a textbook of cardiovascular medicine,* ed 8, Philadelphia, 2008, Saunders. **13-14:** Courtesy Patricia Kane, Indiana University Medical School. **Cardiology box:** Joe Kulka.

Chapter 14

Reynaud Phenomenon box: From Barkauskas VH, Baumann LC, Darling-Fisher CS: *Health and physical assessment,* ed 3, St Louis, 2002, Mosby. **Blood Pressure Readings box:** Barbara Cousins. **Circulation of the Blood box:** Joe Kulka.

Chapter 15

15-4: Courtesy Walter Tunnesen, MD, The American Board of Pediatrics, Chapel Hill, NC. **15-5:** From Zitelli BJ, Davis HW: *Atlas of pediatric physical diagnosis,* ed 4, Philadelphia, 2002, Mosby. **15-6:** From Goldstein B, editor: *Practical dermatology,* ed 2, St Louis, 1997, Mosby. **15-8:** Courtesy Ballinger P, Frank E: *Merrill's atlas of radiographic positions and radiologic procedures,* vol 1,

ed 10, St Louis, 2003, Mosby. **15-10:** From Stevens A, Lowe JS, Young B: *Wheater's basic histopathology,* ed 4, Edinburgh, 2002, Churchill Livingstone. **15-15:** Courtesy Emma Shelton. **15-18:** Courtesy James T Barrett. **15-20:** Courtesy Cerio R, Jackson WF: *Colour atlas of allergic skin disorders,* London, 1992, Mosby-Wolfe. **15-21:** From Habif TP: *Clinical dermatology: a color guide to diagnosis and therapy,* ed 3, St Louis, 1996, Mosby. **Monoclonal Antibodies box:** David Scharf/Peter Arnold, Inc. **Interferon box:** National Cancer Institute. **Vaccines box:** Joe Kulka.

Chapter 16

16-1, 16-18, Heimlich Maneuver box: Barbara Cousins. **16-6:** From Zitelli BJ, Davis HW: *Atlas of pediatric physical diagnosis,* ed 4, Philadelphia, 2002, Mosby. **16-7, *C:*** Custom Medical Stock Photo, Chicago, IL. **16-9:** Network Graphics. **16-17:** From Cotran R, Kumar V, Collins T: *Robbins pathologic basis of disease,* ed 6, Philadelphia, 1999, Saunders. **Lung Volume Reduction Surgery box:** Courtesy Andrew P Evan, Indiana University School of Medicine. **Respiratory Medicine box:** Joe Kulka.

Chapter 17

17-2, *C:* From Zitelli BJ, Davis HW: *Atlas of pediatric physical diagnosis,* ed 5, Philadelphia, 2007, Mosby. **17-2, *D:*** Dennis Strete. **17-3:** Barbara Cousins. **17-5, *A:*** From Regezi JA, Sciubba JJ, Pogrel MA: *Atlas of oral and maxillofacial pathology,* Philadelphia, 2000, Saunders. **17-5, *B,* 17-24 (Photo):** From Swartz MH: *Textbook of physical diagnosis,* ed 4, Philadelphia, 2002, Saunders. **17-5, *C:*** From Grundy JR, Jones JG: *A color atlas of clinical operative dentistry: crowns and bridges,* ed 2, London, 1993, Mosby-Wolfe. **17-6:** From Christensen GJ: *A consumer's guide to dentistry,* ed 2, St Louis, 2002, Mosby. **17-7, 17-9, *B:*** From Emond R, Welsby P, Rowland H: *Colour atlas of infectious diseases,* ed 4, Edinburgh, 2003, Mosby. **17-8, *A:*** From Wilson SF, Giddens JF: *Health assessment for nursing practice,* ed 2, St Louis, 2001, Mosby. **17-8, *B:*** From Greig JD, Garden OJ: *Color atlas of surgical diagnosis,* London, 1996, Times Mirror International Publishers. **17-9, *A:*** Rolin Graphics. **17-9, *C:*** From Zitelli BJ, Davis HW: *Atlas of pediatric physical diagnosis,* ed 5, Philadelphia, 2007, Mosby. Courtesy GDW McKendrick, MD. **17-13, 17-20, *A:*** Copyright Kevin Patton, Lion Den Inc, Weldon Spring, MO. **17-16, *B:*** From Cotran R, Kumar V, Collins T: *Robbins pathologic basis of disease,* ed 6, Philadelphia, 1999, Saunders. **17-17, *B:*** From Weir J, Abrahams PH: *Imaging atlas of human anatomy,* ed 3, St Louis, 2004, Mosby. **17-17, *C,* 17-18 (X-ray):** From Abrahams P, Marks S, Hutchings R: *McMinn's color atlas of human anatomy,* ed 5, Philadelphia, 2003, Mosby. **17-19, 17-22, *B:*** Courtesy Thompson JM, Wilson

SF: *Health assessment for nursing practice,* St Louis 1996, Mosby. **17-21:** Courtesy Vidic B, Suarez RF: *Photographic atlas of the human body,* St Louis, 1984, Mosby. **17-22, *C:*** From Chabner DE: *The language of medicine,* ed 8, St Louis, 2008, Mosby. **17-22, *D:*** From Zitelli BJ, Davis HW: *Atlas of pediatric physical diagnosis,* ed 3, Philadelphia, 1997, Mosby. **Upper Gastrointestinal X-ray Study box:** Photo Researchers, Inc. **Gastroenterology box:** Joe Kulka.

Chapter 18

18-4: From Morgan S, Weinsier R: *Fundamentals of clinical nutrition,* St Louis, 1993, Mosby. **18-6, *A, B:*** From Zitelli BJ, Davis HW: *Atlas of pediatric physical diagnosis,* ed 5, Philadelphia, 2007, Mosby. **18-8:** Barbara Cousins. **Food Science box:** Joe Kulka.

Chapter 19

19-1, *B,* 19-2, *B:* From Abrahams P, Marks S, Hutchings R: *McMinn's color atlas of human anatomy,* ed 5, Philadelphia, 2003, Mosby. **19-3, *C:*** Courtesy Andrew P Evan, Indiana University School of Medicine. **19-7:** From Kerr J: *Atlas of functional histology,* London, 1999, Mosby. **19-9, *A,* 19-11, *A, B:*** From Kumar V, Abbas A, Fausto N: *Robbins and Cotran pathologic basis of disease,* ed 7, Philadelphia, 2005, Saunders. **19-9, *B:*** From Cotran R, Kumar V, Collins T: *Robbins pathologic basis of disease,* ed 6, Philadelphia, 1999, Saunders. **19-10, *A:*** Barbara Cousins. **19-10, *B:*** From Skarin A: *Atlas of diagnostic oncology,* ed 3, Philadelphia, 2003, Mosby. **Fighting Infection box:** Joe Kulka.

Chapter 20

20-4 (Photo): Copyright Kevin Patton, Lion Den Inc, Weldon Spring, MO. **20-6:** From Bloom A, Ireland J: *Color atlas of diabetes,* ed 2, St Louis, 1992, Mosby. **20-9:** From Barkauskas V, Baumann L, Stoltenberg-Allen K, Darling-Fisher C: *Health and physical assessment,* ed 2, St Louis, 1998, Mosby. **The Constancy of the Body box:** Joe Kulka.

Chapter 21

The Body in Balance box: Joe Kulka.

Chapter 22

22-2, *A:* Lennart Nilsson, Albert Bonniers Forlag AB, Stockholm Sweden. **22-4, *A:*** From Kerr J: *Atlas of functional histology,* London, 1999, Mosby. **22-5, *A:*** Carolyn Coulam and John A McIntyre. **22-6:** From Abrahams P, Marks S, Hutchings R: *McMinn's color atlas of human anatomy,* ed 5, Philadelphia, 2003, Mosby. **22-7, *B:*** Courtesy Vidic B, Suarez FR: *Photographic atlas of the human body,* St Louis, 1984, Mosby. **22-8 (Photo):** From Zitelli BJ, Davis HW: *Atlas of pediatric physical diagnosis,* ed 5, Philadelphia, 2007, Mosby. **22-16:** From Kumar V, Abbas A, Fausto N: *Robbins and Cotran pathologic basis of disease,* ed 7, Philadelphia, 2005, Saunders. **22-17, *B, C:*** From Cotran R, Kumar V, Collins T: *Robbins pathologic basis of disease,* ed 6, Philadelphia, 1999, Saunders. **Reproductive Sciences box:** Joe Kulka.

Chapter 23

23-1 (Micrograph): Lennart Nilsson, Albert Bonniers Forlag AB, Stockholm Sweden. **23-3:** Courtesy Lucinda L. Veeck, Jones Institute for Reproductive Medicine, Norfolk, VA. **23-5, *B:*** From Cotran R, Kumar V, Collins T: *Robbins pathologic basis of disease,* ed 6, Philadelphia, 1999, Saunders. **23-6:** Lennart Nilsson, Albert Bonniers Forlag AB, Stockholm Sweden. **23-11:** Barbara Cousins. **23-12:** Courtesy Marjorie M Pyle for Lifecircle, Costa Mesa, California. **23-13, *A:*** From Hockenberry MJ, Wilson D: *Wong's essentials of pediatric nursing,* ed 8, St Louis, 2009, Mosby. **23-13, *B,* Antenatal Diagnosis and Treatment box, *B, C:*** Copyright Kevin Patton, Lion Den Inc, Weldon Spring, MO. **Freezing Umbilical Cord Blood box:** Courtesy Craig Borck, St Paul Pioneer Press. **Fetal Alcohol Syndrome box:** Courtesy Claus Simon/Michael Janner. **Embryology box:** Joe Kulka.

Chapter 24

24-9, *A:* Courtesy Lois McGavran, Denver Children's Hospital. **24-9, *B:*** From Zitelli BJ, Davis HW: *Atlas of pediatric physical diagnosis,* ed 5, Philadelphia, 2007, Mosby. **24-10, 24-11:** Courtesy Nancy S. Wexler, PhD, Columbia University. **Genetics and Genomics box:** Joe Kulka.

Index

Page numbers followed by *f* indicate
figures; *t* indicates tables.